S0-AIX-962

The American Psychiatric Publishing

Textbook of GERIATRIC PSYCHIATRY

FOURTH EDITION

The American Psychiatric Publishing

Textbook of GERIATRIC PSYCHIATRY

FOURTH EDITION

Edited by

Dan G. Blazer, M.D., Ph.D.

David C. Steffens, M.D., M.H.S.

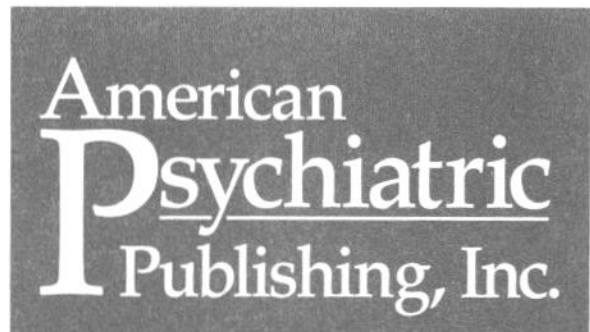

Washington, DC

London, England

Note: The authors have worked to ensure that all information in this book is accurate at the time of publication and consistent with general psychiatric and medical standards, and that information concerning drug dosages, schedules, and routes of administration is accurate at the time of publication and consistent with standards set by the U.S. Food and Drug Administration and the general medical community. As medical research and practice continue to advance, however, therapeutic standards may change. Moreover, specific situations may require a specific therapeutic response not included in this book. For these reasons and because human and mechanical errors sometimes occur, we recommend that readers follow the advice of physicians directly involved in their care or the care of a member of their family.

Books published by American Psychiatric Publishing, Inc., represent the views and opinions of the individual authors and do not necessarily represent the policies and opinions of APPI or the American Psychiatric Association.

If you would like to buy between 25 and 99 copies of this or any other APPI title, you are eligible for a 20% discount; please contact APPI Customer Service at appi@psych.org or 800-368-5777. If you wish to buy 100 or more copies of the same title, please e-mail us at bulksales@psych.org for a price quote.

Manufactured in the United States of America on acid-free paper
13 12 11 10 09 5 4 3 2 1
Fourth Edition

Typeset in Adobe's Bembo and Futura Condensed.

American Psychiatric Publishing, Inc.
1000 Wilson Boulevard
Arlington, VA 22209-3901
www.appi.org

Library of Congress Cataloging-in-Publication Data
The American Psychiatric Publishing textbook of geriatric psychiatry / edited by Dan G. Blazer, David C. Steffens. -- 4th ed.
p. ; cm.
Includes bibliographical references and index.
ISBN 978-1-58562-277-1 (alk. paper)
1. Geriatric psychiatry. I. Blazer, Dan G. (Dan German), 1944- II. Steffens, David C., 1962- III. Title: Textbook of geriatric psychiatry.
[DNLM: 1. Mental Disorders. 2. Aged. 3. Aging--physiology. 4. Geriatric Psychiatry--methods. WT 150 A5126 2009]
RC451.4.A5A518 2009
618.97'689--dc22

2008035653

British Library Cataloguing in Publication Data
A CIP record is available from the British Library.

Contents

Part I
The Basic Science of Geriatric Psychiatry

Part II
The Diagnostic Interview in Late Life

Part III
Psychiatric Disorders in Late Life

Part IV
Treatment of Psychiatric Disorders in Late Life

Part V
Special Topics

Contributors

Marc E. Agronin, M.D.
Director of Mental Health Services, Miami Jewish Home & Hospital for the Aged; Associate Professor of Psychiatry, University of Miami Miller School of Medicine, Miami, Florida

Deborah K. Attix, Ph.D.
Associate Professor of Medical Psychology, Department of Psychiatry and Behavioral Sciences, and Director, Clinical Neuropsychology Service, Division of Neurology, Duke University Medical Center, Durham, North Carolina

Connie Watkins Bales, Ph.D., R.D.
Associate Director, Geriatrics Research, Education, and Clinical Center, Durham VA Medical Center; Associate Professor, Department of Medicine, Duke University Medical Center, Durham, North Carolina

John L. Beyer, M.D.
Assistant Professor of Psychiatry, Duke University Medical Center, Durham, North Carolina

Dan G. Blazer, M.D., Ph.D.
J.P. Gibbons Professor of Psychiatry and Behavioral Sciences and Professor of Community and Family Medicine, Duke University Medical Center, Durham, North Carolina

Elise J. Bolda, M.S.P.H., Ph.D.
Associate Research Professor and Director, NPO Institute for Health Policy, University of Southern Maine, Portland, Maine

Patrick S. Calhoun, Ph.D.
Clinical Assistant Professor, Department of Psychiatry and Behavioral Sciences, Duke University Medical Center; Staff Psychologist, Durham VA Medical Center; Health Services Research Core Director, VA Mid-Atlantic Mental Illness Research, Education, and Clinical Center, Durham, North Carolina

Steven S. Chin, M.D., Ph.D.
Associate Professor of Pathology and Neurology and Director of Neuropathology, Department of Pathology, University of Utah Health Sciences Center, Salt Lake City, Utah

Peggye Dilworth-Anderson, Ph.D.
Professor, Health Policy and Administration/School of Public Health, and Associate Director, UNC Institute on Aging, University of North Carolina, Chapel Hill

P. Murali Doraiswamy, M.D.
Associate Professor of Psychiatry and Chief, Division of Biological Psychiatry, Duke University Medical Center, Durham, North Carolina

Jack D. Edinger, Ph.D.
Senior Psychologist, Durham VA Medical Center; Clinical Professor, Department of Psychiatry and Behavioral Sciences, Duke University Medical Center, Durham, North Carolina

Michael A. Fearing, Ph.D.
Postdoctoral Research Fellow, Aging Brain Center, Institute for Aging Research, Hebrew SeniorLife; Fellow in Medicine, Department of Medicine, Beth Israel Deaconess Medical Center, Harvard Medical School, Boston, Massachusetts

Linda K. George, Ph.D.
Professor of Sociology and Associate Director, Center for the Study of Aging and Human Development, Duke University, Durham, North Carolina

Harold W. Goforth, M.D.
Assistant Professor of Psychiatry, Department of Psychiatry and Behavioral Sciences, Duke University Medical Center, Durham, North Carolina

Lisa P. Gwyther, M.S.W.
Associate Clinical Professor, Department of Psychiatry and Behavioral Sciences, Duke University Medical Center, Durham, North Carolina

Judith C. Hays, R.N., Ph.D.
Associate Professor, Duke University School of Nursing, Center for the Study of Aging and Human Development, Durham, North Carolina

Celia F. Hybels, Ph.D.
Assistant Professor, Department of Psychiatry and Behavioral Sciences, Center for the Study of Aging and Human Development, Duke University Medical Center, Durham, North Carolina

Sharon K. Inouye, M.D., M.P.H.
Director and Milton and Shirley F. Levy Family Chair, Aging Brain Center, Institute for Aging Research, Hebrew SeniorLife; Professor of Medicine, Department of Medicine, Beth Israel Deaconess Medical Center, Harvard Medical School, Boston, Massachusetts

Dilip V. Jeste, M.D.
Estelle and Edgar Levi Chair in Aging; Director, Sam and Rose Stein Institute for Research on Aging; and Distinguished Professor of Psychiatry and Neurosciences, University of California, San Diego; Chief, Division of Geriatric Psychiatry, VA San Diego Healthcare System, San Diego, California

Robert M. Kaiser, M.D., M.H.Sc.
Associate Professor of Clinical Medicine, Division of Gerontology and Geriatric Medicine; University of Miami Miller School of Medicine; Geriatric Research, Education and Clinical Center Investigator, Miami VA GRECC, Miami, Florida

Jason H.T. Karlawish, M.D.
Associate Professor, Departments of Internal Medicine and Medical Ethics, University of Pennsylvania, Philadelphia, Pennsylvania

Ira R. Katz, M.D., Ph.D.
Professor of Psychiatry, Department of Psychiatry, University of Pennsylvania, Philadelphia, Pennsylvania

Jason D. Kilts, Ph.D.
Senior Research Associate, Department of Psychiatry and Behavioral Sciences, Duke University Medical Center; Durham VA Medical Center, Durham, North Carolina

Harold G. Koenig, M.D., M.H.Sc.
Professor of Psychiatry and Behavioral Sciences and Associate Professor of Medicine, Duke University, Durham, North Carolina

Andrew D. Krystal, M.D., M.S.
Director, Sleep Research Laboratory, and Associate Professor, Department of Psychiatry and Behavioral Sciences, Duke University Medical Center, Durham, North Carolina

Nicole M. Lanouette, M.D.
Postdoctoral Research Fellow, Department of Psychiatry, University of California, San Diego, VA San Diego Healthcare System, San Diego, California

Eric J. Lenze, M.D.
Associate Professor of Psychiatry, Washington University School of Medicine, St. Louis, Missouri

J. Pierre Loebel, M.D.
Clinical Professor Emeritus of Psychiatry, Department of Psychiatry, University of Washington, Seattle, Washington

Constantine G. Lyketsos, M.D., M.H.S.
The Elizabeth Plank Althouse Professor and Chair of Psychiatry for Johns Hopkins Bayview, Department of Psychiatry and Behavioral Sciences, Johns Hopkins University School of Medicine, Baltimore, Maryland

Thomas R. Lynch, Ph.D.
Professor of Clinical Psychology, Mood Disorders Centre, School of Psychology, University of Exeter, and Academic Lead, Human Sciences, Peninsula College of Medicine and Dentistry, Exeter, United Kingdom

David J. Madden, Ph.D.
Professor of Medical Psychology, Department of Psychiatry and Behavioral Sciences, Duke University Medical Center, Durham, North Carolina

George L. Maddox, Ph.D.
Professor Emeritus, Department of Sociology, and Program Director, Long Term Care Resources Program, Duke University Medical Center, Durham, North Carolina

Peter Martin, Ph.D.
Professor, Human Development and Family Studies, and Director, Gerontology Program, Iowa State University, Ames, Iowa

Christine E. Marx, M.D., M.A.
Associate Professor, Department of Psychiatry and Behavioral Sciences, Duke University Medical Center; Staff Psychiatrist, Durham VA Medical Center; Clinical Interventions Core Director, VA Mid-Atlantic Mental Illness Research, Education, and Clinical Center, Durham, North Carolina

Shahrzad Mavandadi, Ph.D.
Investigator, Philadelphia VA Medical Center VISN 4 Mental Illness Research, Education, and Clinical Center, Philadelphia, Pennsylvania

Diane E. Meglin, M.S.W.
Medical Instructor, Clinical Social Workers, Duke University Medical Center, Durham, North Carolina

Scott D. Moore, M.D., Ph.D.
Associate Professor of Biological Psychiatry, Duke University Medical Center, Durham, North Carolina

Benoit H. Mulsant, M.D.
Clinical Director, Geriatric Mental Health Program, and Physician in Chief, Centre for Addiction and Mental Health, Toronto, Ontario, Canada; Professor and Vice-Chair, Department of Psychiatry, University of Toronto, Toronto, Ontario, Canada

Jennifer C. Naylor, Ph.D.
Research Associate, Department of Psychiatry and Behavioral Sciences, Duke University Medical Center; Durham VA Medical Center; Mid-Atlantic Mental Illness Research, Education, and Clinical Center, Durham, North Carolina

David W. Oslin, M.D.
Associate Professor, University of Pennsylvania and Philadelphia VA Medical Center VISN 4 Mental Illness Research, Education, and Clinical Center, Philadelphia, Pennsylvania

Thomas E. Oxman, M.D.
Professor Emeritus of Psychiatry, Dartmouth Medical School, Lebanon, New Hampshire

Martha Elizabeth Payne, Ph.D., R.D., M.P.H.
Assistant Professor, Department of Psychiatry and Behavioral Sciences, Duke University, Durham, North Carolina

Victoria M. Payne, M.D.
Psychiatry Research Fellow, Durham VA Medical Center; VA Mid-Atlantic Mental Illness Research, Education, and Clinical Center, Durham, North Carolina

Bruce G. Pollock, M.D., Ph.D.
Vice President, Research, Centre for Addiction and Mental Health, Toronto, Ontario, Canada; Sandra A. Rotman Chair in Neuropsychiatry, Rotman Research Institute, Toronto, Ontario, Canada; Professor and Head, Division of Geriatric Psychiatry, Faculty of Medicine, University of Toronto, Toronto, Ontario, Canada

Leonard W. Poon, Ph.D.
Professor of Public Health and Psychology and Director, Institute of Gerontology and the Georgia Geriatric Education Center, College of Public Health, The University of Georgia, Athens, Georgia

William E. Reichman, M.D.
Professor of Psychiatry, Baycrest Centre for Geriatric Care and Department of Psychiatry, University of Toronto, Ontario, Canada

K. Warner Schaie, Ph.D., Sc.D. (hon.), Dr.Phil.H.C.
Evan Pugh Professor of Human Development and Psychology, Pennsylvania State University, University Park; Affiliate Professor of Psychiatry and Behavioral Science, University of Washington, Seattle

Burton Scott, Ph.D., M.D.
Associate Clinical Professor, Division of Neurology, Department of Medicine; Duke University Movement Disorders Clinic, Duke University Medical Center, Durham, North Carolina

Ilene C. Siegler, Ph.D., M.P.H.
Professor of Medical Psychology, Department of Psychiatry and Behavioral Sciences, Duke University Medical Center, and Professor of Psychology and Neuroscience, Duke University, Durham, North Carolina; Adjunct Professor of Epidemiology, School of Public Health, University of North Carolina at Chapel Hill, North Carolina

Moria J. Smoski, Ph.D.
Clinical Associate, Department of Psychiatry and Behavioral Sciences, Duke University Medical Center, Durham, North Carolina

David C. Steffens, M.D., M.H.S.
Professor of Psychiatry and Medicine and Head, Division of Geriatric Psychiatry, Duke University Medical Center, Durham, North Carolina

Jennifer L. Strauss, Ph.D.
Assistant Professor, Department of Psychiatry and Behavioral Sciences, Duke University Medical Center; Durham VA Medical Center; VA Mid-Atlantic Mental Illness Research, Education, and Clinical Center, Durham, North Carolina

Joel E. Streim, M.D.
Professor of Psychiatry, Department of Psychiatry, University of Pennsylvania; VISN 4 Mental Illness Research, Education, and Clinical Center, Philadelphia VA Medical Center, Philadelphia, Pennsylvania

Robert A. Sweet, M.D.
Professor of Psychiatry and Neurology, University of Pittsburgh; Co-Associate Director for Research, Mental Illness Research, Education, and Clinical Center, VA Pittsburgh Healthcare System, Pittsburgh, Pennsylvania

Warren D. Taylor, M.D.
Associate Professor of Psychiatry and Behavioral Sciences, Duke University Medical Center, Durham, North Carolina

Mugdha Thakur, M.D.
Assistant Professor of Psychiatry, Duke University Medical Center, Durham, North Carolina

Larry W. Thompson, Ph.D.
Professor of Medicine (Research), Emeritus, Stanford University School of Medicine, Stanford, California

Ipsit V. Vahia, M.D.
Stein Institute for Research on Aging, Department of Psychiatry, University of California, San Diego; VA San Diego Healthcare System, San Diego, California

Richard D. Weiner, M.D., Ph.D.
Professor, Department of Psychiatry and Behavioral Sciences, Duke University Medical School; Chief, Mental Health Service Line, Durham VA Medical Center, Durham, North Carolina

Kathleen A. Welsh-Bohmer, Ph.D.
Professor of Medical Psychology, Department of Psychiatry, and Director, Joseph and Kathleen Bryan Alzheimer's Disease Research Center, Division of Neurology, Department of Medicine, Duke University Medical Center, Durham, North Carolina

Julie Loebach Wetherell, Ph.D.
Associate Professor of Psychiatry, University of California, San Diego; Staff Psychologist, VA San Diego Healthcare System, San Diego, California

Patricia A. Wilkosz, M.D., Ph.D.
Postdoctoral Research Scholar, University of Pittsburgh School of Medicine, Pittsburgh, Pennsylvania

Sherry L. Willis, Ph.D.
Professor of Human Development, The Pennsylvania State University, University Park; Affiliate Research Professor, Department of Psychiatry, University of Washington, Seattle

William K. Wohlgemuth, Ph.D.
Research Associate Professor, Departments of Psychology and Neurology, University of Miami, Miami, Florida

Disclosure of Interests

The following contributors to this book have indicated a financial interest in or other affiliation with a commercial supporter, a manufacturer of a commercial product, a provider of a commercial service, a nongovernmental organization, and/or a government agency, as listed below:

Marc E. Agronin, M.D. *Research support:* Elan, Forest, Novo Nordisk, Ono, Ortho Biotech, Solvay, Takeda. *Speaker's bureau:* Abbott, AstraZeneca, Forest, Janssen, Ortho-McNeil Neurologics.

John L. Beyer, M.D. *Advisory committee:* Eli Lilly. *Research support:* Bristol-Myers Squibb, Eisai, Elan, Eli Lilly, GlaxoSmithKline, Myriad Genetics, National Institute of Mental Health, Novartis, Pfizer, Sanofi-Aventis. *Speaker's bureau:* Bristol-Myers Squibb, Eli Lilly, Pfizer.

P. Murali Doraiswamy, M.D. *Honoraria:* Alzheimer Foundation of America, American Psychiatric Association, AVID, Eli Lilly, Forest, Myriad Genetics, Otsuka/Bristol Myers-Squibb, National Institutes of Health, Neuroptix, Wyeth. *Research support:* AVID, Boehringer-Ingelheim, Eisai, Elan, GlaxoSmithKline, Myriad Genetics, National Institutes of Health, Novartis, Pfizer, Sanofi, University of California. *Equities:* Fidelity (403), Sonexa.

Jack D. Edinger, Ph.D. *Consulting:* Philips Respironics. *Honorarium:* Takeda. *Research support:* Helicor, Philips Respironics. *Speaker's bureau:* Sleep Medicine Education Institute.

Harold W. Goforth, M.D. *Consulting:* Bristol-Myers Squibb. *Research support:* Forest, Sepracor.

Dilip V. Jeste, M.D. *Consulting:* Bristol-Myers Squibb, Otsuka, Solvay, Wyeth. *Donations:* AstraZeneca, Bristol-Myers Squibb, and Eli Lilly donate antipsychotic medications for the NIMH-funded R01 grant "Metabolic Effects of Newer Antipsychotics in Older Patients." *Research support:* Department of Veterans Affairs, National Institute of Mental Health (grant MH66248).

Eric J. Lenze, M.D. *Research support:* Forest Research Institute, Ortho-McNeil Neurologics, Pfizer.

Constantine G. Lyketsos, M.D., M.H.S. *Continuing medical education support, honoraria, research support, and travel support:* Bristol-Myers Squibb, Forest, GlaxoSmithKline, Janssen, Johnson & Johnson, Novartis, Ortho, Pfizer.

Christine E. Marx, M.D., M.A. *Donations:* Bristol-Myers Squibb, study drug and matching placebo for a randomized, controlled trial of aripiprazole in posttraumatic stress disorder. *Patent application (provisional):* "Neurosteroid Compositions and Methods of Use Therefor."

Benoit H. Mulsant, M.D. [1999–2006 interests] *Consulting:* AstraZeneca, Bristol-Myers Squibb, Eli Lilly, Forest, Fox Learning System, GlaxoSmithKline, Janssen, Lundbeck Research, Pfizer. *Honoraria:* AstraZeneca, Eisai, Forest, Janssen, Lundbeck Research, GlaxoSmithKline, Pfizer. *Research support:* AstraZeneca, Corcept, Eisai, Eli Lilly, Forest, GlaxoSmithKline, Janssen, National Institutes of Health (current), Pfizer (current). *Equities* (as of April 2008): AkzoNobel, Alkermes, AstraZeneca, Biogen Idec, Celsion, Elan, Eli Lilly, Forest, General Electric, Orchestra Therapeutics. *Other material or financial support:* Forest, Janssen.

Bruce G. Pollock, M.D., Ph.D. *Advisory board:* Forest Laboratories, Takeda. *Research support:* Janssen, National Institutes of Health.

Burton Scott, Ph.D., M.D. *Research support:* Boehringer-Ingelheim, Cephalon, GlaxoSmithKline, Merz, Schwarz, Teva. *Speaker's bureau:* Boehringer-Ingelheim, GlaxoSmithKline, UCB.

Warren D. Taylor, M.D. *Research support:* National Institutes of Health.

Julie Loebach Wetherell, Ph.D. *Research support:* Forest Laboratories.

The following authors have no competing interests to report:

Deborah K. Attix, Ph.D.
Connie Watkins Bales, Ph.D., R.D.
Dan G. Blazer, M.D., Ph.D.
Elise J. Bolda, M.S.P.H., Ph.D.
Patrick S. Calhoun, Ph.D.
Steven S. Chin, M.D., Ph.D.
Peggye Dilworth-Anderson, Ph.D.
Michael A. Fearing, Ph.D.
Linda K. George, Ph.D.
Lisa P. Gwyther, M.S.W.
Judith C. Hays, R.N., Ph.D.
Celia F. Hybels, Ph.D.
Sharon K. Inouye, M.D., M.P.H.
Robert M. Kaiser, M.D., M.H.Sc.
Jason H.T. Karlawish, M.D.
Ira R. Katz, M.D., Ph.D.
Jason D. Kilts, Ph.D.
Harold G. Koenig, M.D., M.H.Sc.
Andrew D. Krystal, M.D., M.S.
Nicole M. Lanouette, M.D.
J. Pierre Loebel, M.D.
Thomas R. Lynch, Ph.D.
David J. Madden, Ph.D.
George L. Maddox, Ph.D.
Peter Martin, Ph.D.
Shahrzad Mavandadi, Ph.D.
Diane E. Meglin, M.S.W.
Scott D. Moore, M.D., Ph.D.
Jennifer C. Naylor, Ph.D.
David W. Oslin, M.D.
Thomas E. Oxman, M.D.
Martha Elizabeth Payne, Ph.D., R.D., M.P.H.
Victoria M. Payne, M.D.
Leonard W. Poon, Ph.D.
William E. Reichman, M.D.
K. Warner Schaie, Ph.D., Sc.D. (hon.), Dr.Phil.H.C.
Ilene C. Siegler, Ph.D., M.P.H.
Moria J. Smoski, Ph.D.
David C. Steffens, M.D., M.H.Sc.
Jennifer L. Strauss, Ph.D.
Joel E. Streim, M.D.
Robert A. Sweet, M.D.
Mugdha Thakur, M.D.
Larry W. Thompson, Ph.D.
Ipsit V. Vahia, M.D.
Richard D. Weiner, M.D., Ph.D.
Kathleen A. Welsh-Bohmer, Ph.D.
Patricia A. Wilkosz, M.D., Ph.D.
Sherry L. Willis, Ph.D.
William K. Wohlgemuth, Ph.D.

PREFACE

The current edition of the *American Psychiatric Publishing Textbook of Geriatric Psychiatry* is the first that has not involved Dr. Ewald W. Busse, the senior editor for the first two editions. Dr. Busse died very soon after the publication of the last edition. We were thankful that he was able to see the product of his work, and he had a copy by his bedside at his death. Drs. Blazer and Steffens hope to continue the eclectic, interdisciplinary, and developmental perspective, which was so important to Dr. Busse, in subsequent editions including this one. We therefore dedicate this edition to the memory of Dr. Busse.

Many new findings now inform our field, and this edition reflects those changes. The reader will find more new material and alterations of existing materials. The first edition of this textbook, entitled *Geriatric Psychiatry,* was published in 1989; the second edition was published with the title *The American Psychiatric Press Textbook of Geriatric Psychiatry* in 1996; and a third edition with the same title appeared in 2004. The decision to publish a fourth edition rested on an appreciation of the enormous expansion of scientific knowledge about aging and the diseases of late life, as well as on advances in biological psychiatry and neuropsychiatry that have greatly altered the practice of geriatric psychiatry. *The American Psychiatric Publishing Textbook of Geriatric Psychiatry,* Fourth Edition, is designed to provide both the scholar and the clinician with the current state of scientific understanding as well as the practical skills and knowledge base required for dealing with mental disorders in late life. Consequently, this volume covers not only the wide range of important mental diseases of late life but also the so-called normal age changes that result in biological, social, and behavioral changes in older adults.

As in previous editions, the chapters are presented in a sequential and integrated fashion, which we have found enhances the accessibility and usefulness of the information presented. The contributors include both basic and clinical scholars who have a clear ability to make complex material understandable to our readers. We maintained an eclectic orientation regarding theory and practice in geriatric psychiatry. Although most contributors are psychiatrists, we also called on colleagues from relevant biomedical and behavioral disciplines—especially for chapters covering the basic sciences—because of their expertise and ability to incorporate such knowledge into a comprehensive approach to patient care.

We targeted this text to psychiatrists and other health professionals who have an interest in and a commitment to older adults. This book is of particular value to candidates seeking certification in geriatrics from the American Board of Psychiatry and Neurology, the American Board of Internal Medicine, and the American Board of Family Practice. All of these bodies' examinations place considerable emphasis on geriatric psychiatry and the behavioral aspects of aging.

Dan Blazer and David Steffens
Durham, North Carolina

PART I

The Basic Science of Geriatric Psychiatry

CHAPTER 1

THE MYTH, HISTORY, AND SCIENCE OF AGING

DAN G. BLAZER, M.D., PH.D.

Scholars, physicians, theologians, philosophers, and others have written on the subjects of life, aging, and death for many years. Some of their observations and conclusions are casual, many are frivolous or reek of quackery, and some are based on careful study and considered judgment. These older explorations are interesting because they provide information about social values, the influence of political and economic factors, the level of scientific knowledge, and, in particular, the interpretation of the significance and application of existing knowledge. In addition, the geriatric psychiatrist constantly works against the background of normal aging, despite the immediate presence of physical and psychiatric disorders that demand her or his attention.

The Prolongation of Youth in Retrospect

Attempts to prolong youth or to restore sexual vigor and physical vitality have been made for many centuries and still occur today. Many such attempts at rejuvenation carry a distinct risk (be careful what you pray for because your prayers may be answered). The goddess Aurora (also called Eos) with great effort persuaded Zeus to grant her husband Tithonus immortality. Regrettably, she neglected to mention that she also wanted him to remain eternally young. As the years passed, Tithonus became more and more disabled, praying frequently for death. Eternal life did not equate with eternal youth.

The belief that in remote parts of the world there are people who enjoy remarkably long lives appears in the mythology of many cultures. In Greek legend, the Hyperboreans, a group of people who lived beyond the north wind in a region of perpetual sunshine, were free from all natural ills. Writing in the first century, Pliny (23–79 A.D.) noted that the Hyperboreans were extremely happy and "aloof from toil and conflict" and that they lived to an extreme old age until "sated with life and luxury, they leaped into the sea" (Gruman 1966, p. 22). This idea of people living in remote parts of the world who enjoy a long life persists in the mythology of the centenarians that recurs periodically in news media and scientific literature (see section "The Centenarians" later in this chapter).

The Fountain of Youth

In America, the myth of the fountain of youth was instrumental in Ponce de Leon's discovery of what is now the state of Florida. The fountain of youth legend is traced by scholars to several possible origins. In ancient

Note: Much of the material in this chapter was compiled by Ewald W. Busse, M.D., and Dan G. Blazer, M.D., Ph.D., for previous editions of this textbook. Dr. Busse, since deceased, did not have the opportunity to review this current revision of the chapter, and it was his wish that he not be included as an author.

Greek and Roman writings, there are two interesting references to fountains with properties that conferred a prolonged life span. Hera, the wife of Zeus, bathed each year in a spring that renewed her maidenhood. In another classical reference, Herodotus (ca. 484–425 B.C.) recounted a search for a spring and pool whose constant use made people live longer.

Roger Bacon (ca. 1214–ca. 1292) promoted his belief that the life span of his day, which usually was not more than 45–50 years, could be tripled. His reasoning was in part based on the long life spans of Methuselah and Noah: if life spans had once been that long and then had shortened, some reversal must be possible. Bacon became a Franciscan monk in order to pursue a moral and physically clean life. He did recommend the rejuvenating breath of a young virgin, but as a monk he cautioned against any accompanying licentiousness. Bacon reasoned that if disease were contagious, why not vitality (Gruman 1966)?

The Myth of Cell Immortality

Alexis Carrel (1873–1944), a surgeon, devoted much work to wound healing. This interest in wound healing led him to an interest in growing tissues outside the body. For his surgical contributions, he won the 1912 Nobel Prize for physiology and medicine. He subsequently developed his studies in tissue culture, and on the basis of some of his own apparent successes, he became convinced that some human cells grown in culture were immortal. This claim of possible cell immortality was reported by Carrel and Ebeling beginning in 1912. Despite numerous objections to his work, Carrel was very persuasive, and his belief was widely accepted. In January 1912, Carrel established a series of chick heart fibroblast cultures, one of which was destined to become the "immortal" cell strain.

Subsequently, it was shown that Carrel and Ebeling had made an error in their methodology that resulted in improper conclusions. The Carrel-Ebeling cell culture was fed an extract taken from chick embryos. This extract actually contained a small but significant number of new viable cells; hence, the introduction of new cells permitted the culture to survive. If the extract was carefully prepared, removing all new cells, the cell colony would die. Although other experiments have suggested that animal and human cells have the capacity to be immortal, all such immortal cell colonies are abnormal in one way or another. At present, it appears that the only human cells that may be immortal are transformed or abnormal mixoploid cells such as the HeLa cells, which were originally taken from cancerous cervical tissue and grown in culture by Gey (1955).

Hayflick and Moorhead (1961) first described the finite replicative capacity of cultured normal human fibroblasts and interpreted this phenomenon as aging at the cellular level. They reported that even when normal human embryonic cells were grown under the most favorable conditions, death was inevitable after about 50 population doublings. Thus, the death of the cell line was an inherent property of the cells themselves.

In 1965, Hayflick reported that culture fibroblasts derived from older human donors divided fewer times than did those derived from embryos. Since then, several investigators have replicated the work of Hayflick, finding that the number of population doublings of cultured human cells is inversely proportional to donor age. It was subsequently shown that freezing viable normal human cells at subzero temperatures does not alter the memory in the cells for the number of doublings that had previously occurred. These cells had been held for more than 24 years in a frozen state and, when thawed, replicated only the same number of times that they would have done had they never been frozen.

Zhores Medvedev, a Russian scientist, made many contributions to the study of biological aging, including the redundant theory of aging (i.e., that the amount of DNA reserve within the genome that can be called on to maintain vital function plays an important role in determining life span [Busse 1983]). Of particular interest to the geriatric psychiatrist is Medvedev's account of a technique of rejuvenation advocated by a woman named O.B. Lepeshinskaya. Around 1949, Lepeshinskaya began to advocate the use of soda baths to prolong life and restore vigor. This approach quickly moved to the drinking of soda water and finally to the introduction of soda into the body by enema. Apparently the latter two techniques were used as alternatives for those who were unable to take frequent soda baths. Lepeshinskaya also claimed that she could make living matter from nonliving material—a vivid example of how vulnerable geriatrics is to the practice of pseudoscience.

The Centenarians

Reports of life spans exceeding 100 years have involved three pockets of people in wide-ranging locales. One group, the Viejos ("Old Ones"), live in Vilcabamba, a small mountain village in Ecuador. The other two pockets are in widely separated regions of Asia—the Hunzukuts of the Karakoram region in Kashmir and the Abkhazians of the Republic of Georgia in the former Soviet Union. Over the past decades, a number of individuals have visited the two groups in Ecuador and Georgia. In February 1978, the National Institute on Aging brought together several scientists who had visited Vilcabamba. After three visits to Vilcabamba, the scientists concluded that the oldest person in the community was 96 years old. Similar visits to the Soviet Caucasus and reevaluations found that the reports of longevity there had been grossly exaggerated (Palmore 1984).

In recent years, however, centenarians are becoming more prevalent, not because the life span is extended but rather because more people are pushing the limits of the life span. In addition, centenarians are found to be more heterogeneous. In 1990, approximately 37,000 centenarians lived in the United States (U.S. Census Bureau 1999). By 2050, the number could reach 1 million! Centenarians were more likely to be women, to have lower educational levels than younger cohorts, and to be widowed; one-half were living in nursing homes. There will be increasing diversity from a racial and ethnic perspective, and biological diversity is apparent now as well (Hazzard 2001). For example, the ε2 allele of apolipoprotein E (APOE), either homozygous or heterozygous, is found more frequently but not exclusively in centenarians compared with younger persons. The ε2 allele appears to be associated with lower cholesterol levels in persons at these advanced ages.

In a more recent effort involving the U.S. state of Georgia, the National Institute on Aging is supporting a project, "The Georgia Centenarian Study." Led by Leonard Poon, Ph.D., at the University of Georgia, this study will establish longitudinal cohorts of centenarians, octogenarians, and sexagenarians (Dai et al. 2006). In this multisite collaboration, the investigators seek to identify and isolate longevity genes, neuropathology, and functional capacity of a population-based sample of centenarians in 31 counties in northern Georgia.

Attitudes Toward Aging

Marcus Tullius Cicero, the Roman orator and statesman of the first century (106–43 B.C.), incorporated into his elegant speeches and writings the philosophical views and social values of his time (Gruman 1966). Cicero, at age 62, produced an essay on senescence ("de Senectute"; 44 B.C.) in which he suggested that old age was not welcomed equally by different human races. The status the elderly held within a society apparently made a difference. The Spartans capitalized on the experience of older men, and the gerotes, a council of 28 men past 60 years old, controlled the city-state (Thewlis 1924). Cicero argued that successful aging was attainable if one developed an appropriate attitude and dealt effectively with the four major complaints associated with aging. It is interesting that these same four complaints exist today.

The first complaint was that society excluded older adults from important work of the world. Cicero replied by saying that courageous elders can find a way to make themselves useful in various advisory, intellectual, and administrative functions. The second complaint was that aging undermines physical strength and reduces the individual's value. Cicero answered that bodily decline counts for little compared with the cultivation of mind and character. The third complaint was that aging prevents or reduces the enjoyment of sensual pleasures, particularly sexual enjoyment. Cicero replied that such a loss has some merit because it allows the elderly person to concentrate on the promotion of reason and virtue. The fourth, and final, complaint was that old age brings with it increasing anxiety about death. In response to this charge, Cicero followed Plato by saying that death could be considered a blessing, freeing individuals and their immortal souls from their bodily prison on this very imperfect earth. Cicero concluded by saying that the wise individual is one who submits to the dictates of nature and passes through the vicissitudes of life with a tranquil mind. He implied that the prolongation of life seemed undesirable, particularly if, in old age, one had to go back to being "a crying child in the cradle."

Gerontocomia, perhaps the first practical manual on the problems of old age, was published in Latin by Gabriele Zerbi in 1482. Zeman (1967) reported finding this fascinating volume and noted that Zerbi's work had not previously been quoted by any medical or lay writer since its original publication. Zerbi dealt with the care of the elderly in a rest home that had been especially selected with regard to climate, exposure, equipment, and staff. He described all of his ideas regarding longevity and maintenance of health, advocating exercise, bathing, massage, rest, and diet. He referred to medications that are useful to old people and discussed their ingredients and dosages. One of Zerbi's most fascinating recommendations was the continuing use of human milk for the elderly. Recognizing that death and old age are inevitable, Zerbi stated, "It is impossible therefore to prevent the wasting away of old age, but it is possible to combat and resist it considerably" (Lind 1988, p. 26).

Sir William Osler, an astute observer, teacher, and scholar (Belkin and Neelon 1992), delivered his farewell address to the Johns Hopkins faculty in 1905 at age 56 (Berk 1989). In that address, he expressed the belief that with advancing age, professors often lose their usefulness. Osler held the position that productivity in life occurs before age 40. This farewell speech resulted in negative reaction both from his colleagues and the public press. An effort was made to explain it away by characterizing it as an attempt in humor. However, in answer to this storm, Osler said the following:

> The criticisms have not shaken my convictions that the telling work of the world has been done and is done by men under forty years of age. The exceptions which have been given only illustrate the rule. It would also be to the general good if men at sixty were retired from active work. We should miss the energies of some young-old men, but on the whole be of greater service to the sexagenarii themselves. (Belkin and Neelon 1992, p. 863)

Osler died in 1919 at age 70. In contrast to his observations, until approximately a year before his death he is said to have remained an active teacher, researcher, and statesman.

Freud (1905/1957) was quite pessimistic about the value of psychotherapy with older adults (i.e., older than 55), believing them to be unanalyzable despite the fact that he continued to self-analyze until his death. Freud's negative views led to a lack of attention to psychotherapy with older adults until a number of empirical studies were launched during the 1980s, especially studies of psychotherapy for depression.

Palmore (1979), in contrast, documented what he believed to be some major advantages of aging. These include the fact that the elderly are the most law-abiding of all age groups, except for young children. Older adults are much better citizens and are interested and active in public issues and political affairs. They make an enormous contribution to society by maintaining voluntary participation in community organizations, churches, and recreational groups. Although many are not gainfully employed, they are quite capable of participating in performance tasks. Older workers are stable and dependable and have less absenteeism. Although older persons are equally exposed to crimes of certain types, they are much less likely to be the victims of crime in general than are people in other age groups.

Although some of the apparent advantages of aging are under constant pressure, it is obvious that Social Security and other pension systems have improved the economic status of older individuals, as have lower taxes and other economic benefits such as reduced rates in many hotels, motels, and recreational facilities. Medicare, in spite of its limitations, provides health insurance for many older people who otherwise would not be covered. Undoubtedly there are other advantages. The disadvantages appear repeatedly throughout this book, as is true in all medical publications.

A Definition of Aging

Aging, in living organisms, usually refers to a series of time-dependent anatomical and physiological changes that reduce physiological reserve and functional capacity, although occasionally the term refers to the positive processes of maturating or acquiring a desirable quality (Ahmed and Tollefsbol 2001). Biological aging is not necessarily confined to the later years of life; some declines begin with conception. In general, the term does designate those physical changes that develop in adulthood, result in a decline in efficiency of function, reduce homeostasis, and terminate in death.

The multiple processes of decline that are associated with growing old can be separated into primary and secondary aging (Busse 1987). *Primary aging* is held to be intrinsic to the organism, and the decremental factors are determined by inherent or hereditary influences. The rate of aging as a functional decline varies widely between individuals. Furthermore, there are extreme aging variations in systems, organs, and cells. *Secondary aging* refers to the appearance of defects and disabilities that are caused by hostile factors in the environment, including trauma and acquired disease.

This operational separation of primary and secondary aging processes has limitations because both inherent (hereditary) and acquired decremental age changes often have multiple etiologies. Inherent defects that make the organism vulnerable may not appear unless and until the organism is exposed to hostile precipitating events. Definitions of aging that have been offered, including those for primary and secondary aging, are not consistently accepted and applied. The aging of living organisms is a universal phenomenon, but the rate of aging can vary between individuals and groups. In humans, aging differences are in part genetically determined but also are substantially influenced by nutrition, lifestyle, and environment (Busse 1987). Some scientists define primary aging as the first cause and secondary aging as the pathological processes that ensue from the first cause.

Many age-related changes are relatively benign and allow a person to continue to function, meet personal needs, and maintain a place in society. Age-related changes are recognized as a decline in efficiency or performance but in the extreme are often labeled a disease. Examples of age changes that can become sufficiently severe to be a disease include a decline in kidney function (creatinine clearance), reduced respiratory performance (forced expiratory volume), an increase in systolic blood pressure (isolated systolic hypertension), and an impaired response to oral glucose tolerance tests (type 2 diabetes mellitus; Tobin 1984).

The chronological age of a person is often estimated by changes in appearance and the person's ability to perform tasks associated with activities of daily living and working. As humans age, the skin often becomes wrinkled, dry, and seborrheic, and actinic keratosis appears. Hair becomes gray and thinner; baldness increases. Teeth decay and are lost. In addition, height tends to decrease, as does weight. Chest depth and abdominal depth both increase. The ears lengthen and the nose broadens. Fat cells invade muscle, and muscle strength decreases. Posture and height are affected by musculoskeletal changes. Bone densities, influenced by gender and race, decrease with age; in women especially, the trabecular bones of the hip, wrist, and vertebrae are particularly affected.

The metabolic dimensions that are affected by age include drug absorption, distribution, destruction, and excretion; the kinetics of drug binding; and alterations in biological rhythms. Drugs are therefore metabolized differently in elderly people than in younger adults.

Another important age change is the loss of irreplaceable cells, most noticeably in the skeletal muscle tissue, heart, and brain (although recent studies suggest that cells originally thought not to have the capability to reproduce, such as neurons, may under certain circumstances reproduce). Striated musculature diminishes by about one-half by approximately age 80 years. As these muscle cells disappear, they are replaced by fat cells and fibrous connective tissue. Hence, the body achieves increased storage capacities for certain drugs that are stored in fat cells. The loss of brain cells alters important aspects of body metabolism and affects circadian rhythms. The decrease in heart cells results in alterations in certain cardiac functions. Cellular and supportive tissue changes cause pulmonary changes.

In the brain, neurons shrink and are lost, and alterations occur in neuronal synapses and networks. The loss of nerve cells, particularly those in vulnerable areas of the hypothalamus, may contribute to placing the elderly at risk for certain physiological changes and associated mental and emotional aberrations. Aging results in a decline of neurotransmitters such as dopamine, norepinephrine, serotonin, tyrosine hydroxylase, and cholinesterase. The activity of monoamine oxidase increases with age.

Biological Theories of Aging

There are many theories and processes of aging, but a satisfactory, unified theory of aging does not exist. In part, this is due to variability in the "aging" of various organs and tissues. Similar age changes have been identified in one or two of the body components, but rarely are the same changes seen in all simultaneously. Some theories of aging lack adequate scientific proof. For example, at present, there is substantial—although not conclusively definitive—evidence that intrinsic cellular or molecular aging changes underlie many of the neuronal or endocrine changes associated with the brain.

In 1993, the National Institute on Aging published a booklet, "In Search of the Secrets of Aging" (National Institute on Aging 1993a, 1993b), which divides the major theories of aging into two categories: program theories and error theories. *Program theories* hold that aging is the result of sequential switching on and off of certain genes. Defects develop during this switching on and off, and these defects are manifested by senescence. Those who subscribe to *error theories* maintain that aging is the result of wear-and-tear processes; these theorists hold that in many mechanisms, important parts wear out and cannot be replaced or repaired. Included among the error theories is the somatic mutation theory, whose proponents maintain that genetic mutations occur and accumulate with increasing age, causing cells to deteriorate and malfunction.

In a review of biological theories of aging, Hart and Turturro (1985) categorized theories into cellular, organ, and population-based theories; integrative approaches; and meta-aging theories.

The cellular-based theories are those that emphasize the importance of the inherent limited potential proliferation of cells. These theories are consistent with the fact that animals have decreased cellularity in several organs as aging advances. Consequently, aging stem cells have a progressively limited ability to repopulate differentiated daughter cells. The capacity for limited proliferation is linked to some experiments that have shown that the limited proliferation of cells is the result of stochastic changes. Other experiments have been concerned with the somatic mutation theory of aging and the closely associated error theory. Finally, cellular aging may be attributed to accumulated effects of damage from the expression of "cell death genes" important to development. The theory of cell death genes is linked to the observation that during embryogenesis the number of cells retained for further development is reduced by some genetic mechanism. Because cell numbers are reduced in late life, it would be important to understand the underlying mechanism that is needed by the organism early in life but that may be detrimental late in life. In a similar manner, Hart and Turturro's (1985) review identified those theories of aging that are related to mechanisms of cell death.

The final category of aging theories mentioned by Hart and Turturro is meta-aging. This encompasses what the authors referred to as "the theory of the theory of aging." The complexity of such a discussion is obvious, and the development of a unified theory of aging will be extremely difficult because such a theory of biosenescence would have to take into consideration all of the processes an individual undergoes as well as the sequence of environmental interactions that occurs within the individual over a lifetime.

The Watch-Spring Theory

One early biological explanation of aging rested on the assumption that a living organism contains a fixed store of energy not unlike that contained within a coiled watch spring. When the spring of the watch is unwound, life ends. This is a type of exhaustion theory. Another simple theory relates to the accumulation of deleterious material. This particular theory is given some support by the observation that pigments such as lipofuscin accumulate in some cells throughout life. Although these two simple theories may make some contribution to the aging process, there is little evidence that they have any substantial role.

The "Master Clock"

The hypothalamus is said to be the location of the "master clock." Age changes within the hypothalamus play a particularly important role in losses of homeostatic mechanisms in the body. Cell loss, an event that is common in late life, occurs within clusters of cells in the hypothalamus. The disappearance of a few critical cells in the hypothalamus may have far-reaching consequences. The remaining aging cells may become less efficient. These changes in the hypothalamus undoubtedly cause important changes within the pituitary that affect other glands and organs within the body. As a consequence, the aging body undergoes many endocrine changes. Alterations within the hypothalamus also affect numerous connections within the brain and play a major role in age changes associated with chemical messengers of the brain. Nevertheless, there is debate as to where this timing mechanism might lie or how it might control aging from molecule to organ (Miller 1999).

Stochastic Theories

Processes of aging that are associated with random changes such as cell loss or mutation are often termed *stochastic* processes. Stochastic implies "a process or a series of events for which the estimate of the probability of certain outcomes approaches the true possibility as the number of events increases" (Busse 1977, p. 16). The atomic scientist Leo Szilard advanced a stochastic theory based on what he termed a "hit." A hit is not solely the result of radiation but rather can be considered any event that alters a chromosome. In addition, Szilard believed that every animal carries a load of what he termed "faults." A fault is a congenital absence or impairment of one of the genes essential to cell function. A cell is capable of operating as long as one of the pair of genes continues to function; however, when both members of a pair of essential genes are incapable of functioning, the cell declines and dies. Therefore, a cell will cease to function effectively if one of the pair carries the fault and the other is the victim of a hit or if both of the pair are the victims of hits.

Deliberate Biological Programming

The theory of deliberate biological programming has received considerable attention. This theory holds that within a normal cell are stored the memory and the capability of determining the life of a cell. This theory is consistent with the research and conclusions of Hayflick (1965). The memory and capacity to terminate life are found in all normal human diploid cells. In mixoploid or cancer cells, this memory or capacity apparently is destroyed, and the cells can duplicate indefinitely.

Cristafalo (1972) reported that the number of doublings is the same for both male and female cells. (Female cells are easily identified by the presence of a Barr body, the second sex chromosome.) This observation suggests that the difference in life expectancy between human males and females cannot be attributed to intracellular differences (Weiss 1974).

The Telomere Theory

A variant of the deliberate biological programming theory and also of the genetic theories is the telomere theory. DNA damage is the centerpiece of many theories of aging. Telomere shortening has been described to be associated with DNA damage (Ahmed and Tollefsbol 2001). Located at the ends of eukaryotic chromosomes, telomeres are specialized DNA sequences that maintain the length of chromosomes. When they are lost, DNA damage results. Telomere shortening and cellular senescence have been well established in the laboratory. In addition, many human cancer cells (which replicate without control) show high telomerase activity (telomerase being the enzyme that stimulates telomere activity). In other words, telomerase activity is essential for cellular immortalization, and its absence may constitute a fundamental basis for cellular aging.

The Free Radical Theory

A free radical is a chemical molecule or compound that has an odd number of electrons (an unpaired electron) and is highly reactive, in contrast to most chemical compounds, which have an even number of electrons and are stable. Often considered molecular fragments, free radicals are highly reactive and destructive, but they are produced by normal metabolic processes and are ubiquitous in living substances. They can also be produced by ionizing radiation, ozone, and chemical toxins such as insecticides. The oxygen free radical, superoxide, is an important agent of oxygen toxicity and the aging process. Scavengers of oxygen free radicals exist within cells. Enzymatic defenses involve superoxide dismutase, catalases, and perioxidases. Oxygen free radicals have been linked to DNA damage, the cross-linkage of collagen, and the accumulation of age pigments and cancers (Busse 1983). Nutrient antioxidants include vitamins C and E and beta-carotene (National Institute on Aging 1993a).

The Immune System Theory

The immune system performs both surveillance and protective tasks. It is a complex, widespread bodily function that is essential for the preservation of life (Suskind 1980). The destruction of the immune system is well known to people because it is identified with acquired immunodeficiency syndrome (AIDS) (Laurence 1985). Traditionally the immune system has been considered to have two major components. One is the humoral immune response, characterized by the production of antibody molecules that specifically bind the introduced foreign substance. The second is the cellular immune response, by which cells are mobilized that can specifically react with and destroy the invader. There has been considerable evidence that a decrease in the immune competence and alterations in the regulation of the immune system are associated with aging. With increasing age, surveillance is impaired, and the efficiency of the protective mechanism declines. Furthermore, there is a loss of control in which immune functions become so distorted that they are self-destructive. The impairment of the immune system results in an increased incidence of certain diseases in the aging population. Certain tumors in older adults appear to be related to the failure of the body to recognize and eliminate abnormal cells. Autoantibodies increase with the passage of time, and the presence of autoantibodies identifies subpopulations at risk for early death. The older body has an increased susceptibility to infection, and, in general, effective immunization cannot be induced in late life (Finkelstein 1984).

The Eversion (Cross-Linkage) Theory

The eversion, or cross-linkage, theory of aging is based on the observation that changes in collagen structure are associated with aging. Collagen is probably the most important protein in the human body. The two types of collagen are interstitial and basement membrane. With the passage of time, the ester bonds from within the collagen molecule switch to binding together individual collagen molecules. This aging chain alters the characteristics of connective tissue. Modification of proteins may, in addition, be caused by glycosylation. Glycated forms of human collagen do accumulate with age in tendon and skin (Miller 1999).

Genetics of Human Aging

Brown and Wisniewski (1983) stated that the genetic nature of the aging process is reflected by the wide range of maximal life spans that animal species may attain. Among mammals, the life span range is from 1 year in the smoky shrew to more than 114 years in humans. This wide variation in life spans emphasizes that the aging process is likely to have an underlying basis that is in part encoded in our genes. The genetic basis may involve two types of inherited species-specific differences. The first type relates to development of the organism. This mechanism governs program timings in developmental stages as well as rates of maturation. The second genetic determinant relates to self-maintenance. This mechanism influences the efficiency of enzymatic systems as well as protection and repair of internal and external insults to the machinery.

If the DNA process is damaged or declines in efficiency, the functioning capacity of the organism will be severely impaired. The numerous biological changes that take place over the life span are complicated, and it is likely that many interacting genes are involved. However, specific genetic defects have been identified that are particularly relevant to certain life-shortening conditions. It is possible that there are other genes that contribute to longer life; however, at this stage of our knowledge, only rarely have specific "longevity" genes been identified that are consistently associated with increased life expectancy. Examples are genes that overproduce superoxide dismutase and catalase; such genes are antioxidants and appear to increase life expectancy (National Institute on Aging 1993b).

Martin (1978) reviewed a long list of human genetic conditions to select out those in which physical and physiological changes usually were associated with senescence. He identified the 10 genetic disorders that had the highest number of senescent features and thus that were considered to be associated with the aging process: Down syndrome, Werner's syndrome, Cockayne's syndrome, progeria, ataxia-telangiectasia, Lawrence-Seip syndrome, cervical lipodysplasia, Klinefelter's syndrome, Turner's syndrome, and myotonic dystrophy.

The progerias are syndromes that are linked with premature aging. The presence of these disorders does, to a limited extent, provide an opportunity to study accelerated bodily changes that resemble those attributable to aging. Although all of these syndromes are quite rare, two have received particular attention: Hutchinson-Gilford syndrome (Hastings 1904; Hutchinson 1886) and Werner's syndrome.

The early-onset Hutchinson-Gilford syndrome is characterized by dwarfism, physical immaturity, and pseudosenility. Individuals with this syndrome have a peculiar form of hypermetabolism, and they generally die during their mid-teens of coronary heart disease. Hutchinson-Gilford syndrome affects both sexes and has been described in white, black, and Asian races. The affected individuals look like very old, wizened, small humans with distorted features. This is because their heads are large in comparison with the face, and their ears and nose are small. They have no scalp hair, eyebrows, or eyelashes. Some of the features that are commonly associated with aging, including tumors, cataracts, and osteoporosis, are not increased in Hutchinson-Gilford syndrome. A biochemical defect found in patients with Hutchinson-Gilford syndrome or Werner's syndrome is decreased excretion of urinary hyaluronic acid.

The search for the mode of inheritance of Hutchinson-Gilford syndrome continues. The syndrome has been considered to be a rare autosomal recessive condition, but it has been argued that it is more likely a sporadic autosomal dominant mutation because of several observations, including 1) a lower frequency of consanguinity than might be expected, 2) the low frequency of recurrence in families, and 3) a possible parental age effect. The vast majority of cases occur with no siblings affected. For this reason, all of the progerias, and particularly Hutchinson-Gilford syndrome, may be sporadic dominant-type mutations.

Although the life span of fibroblasts of progeria is affected, reports on the life spans of individuals with these disorders have varied, making it unclear whether the reduction in life span is modest or severe. Furthermore, the suspicion that a basic defect in protein synthesis fidelity is a basic defect in progeria lacks confirmation (Goldstein et al. 1985). Similarly, there is confusion regarding the existence or nonexistence of definitive immune abnormalities. As to DNA repair capability, although such a defect is not uncommon, it is not a consistent marker for progeria. One must conclude that the basic metabolic defect is, at this time, unknown.

Werner's syndrome is a later-onset type of progeria. In his doctoral dissertation entitled "Cataract in Connection With Scleroderma," Werner (1904) described an unusual disorder. He reported the condition in siblings, two brothers and two sisters, between ages 36 and 40 years, whose parents, grandparents, and one sister were healthy. Because Werner's syndrome differs from normal aging in several respects, Martin (1985) classified this condition as a "segmental progeroid syndrome." The appearance of an individual affected by Werner's syndrome is indeed striking because the initial impression is that the person is very old. As the disease develops, affected individuals look 20–30 years older than their actual years, and their life span is shortened. Because the disease usually appears before growth is completed, patients with this syndrome frequently have thin limbs and typically are of smaller stature and are less developed than would be expected. Their face develops a tightly drawn, pinched expression. Pseudoexophthalmos (bulging eyes), a beak nose, protuberant teeth, and a recessive chin are characteristic features. Cataracts develop early, and, in addition to hypogonadism, individuals are likely to have diabetes. Not infrequently, they develop cancer, which contributes to their shortened life expectancy. The connective tissue cells and fibroblasts of these patients have been studied. For instance, Hayflick (1977) mentioned that fibroblast cells that are derived from individuals with Werner's syndrome and cultured in vitro undergo significantly fewer doublings than do cell samples from age-matched control subjects. The *WRN* locus on chromosome 8 produces a base that encodes a special protein, a helicase. Loss of function of this protein via mutation, which appears in Werner's syndrome, can result in genomic instability and subsequently a hastening of the aging process (Turner and Martin 1999).

Finch (1990) suggested that approximately 35% of the factors that influence life span are inherited. The remainder are chance events that occur during biological development and random environmental changes during the life span. Species and even populations can vary tremendously with regard to the duration of the developmental phase and the adult life span as well as phenotypic variations. Finch concluded that there is little evidence indicating that the life span is generally set by molecular or cellular mechanisms that are intrinsically time dependent.

Studies of the genetic components of aging have considered the gene regulation of simple organisms, such as the soil roundworm *Caenorphabditis elegans* (*C. elegans*; Kenyon 2001), the first multicellular organism to have its genome completely sequenced. Some years ago, it was reported that a mutant strain of *C. elegans* lived twice as long as normal, the largest proportional life span extension of any animal known at the time. This long-lived mutant strain arose from a defect in a hormone-triggered cascade of molecular signals that resembles one in humans that is prompted by the hormone insulin. It turns out that quite a large number of genes control this hormone cascade, yet two genes had major effects: *daf-2* and *daf-16*. The *daf-16* gene promotes longevity, but the *daf-2* gene suppresses this genetic activity. Some have therefore been quite interested in how the *daf-16* gene might promote longevity.

Sex Differences in Longevity

In humans and in many other animal species, females outlive males. It is easy to assume that the differences between the two sexes are genetically determined by the presence or absence of the Y chromosome. It has been suggested that the greater constitutional weakness of males may be the result of their having only one X chromosome.

In countries where data are available, there seemed to be slightly more older men than older women before 1900. After the turn of the twentieth century, this situation gradually changed, and by 1940 the situation had reversed itself. Thereafter, the preponderance of older women increased rapidly. In 2003 in the population older than 65 years, the sex ratio was 58% women to 42% men.

Contrary to the reasonable expectation of the equal balance in males and females at birth, there are in the United States approximately 106–110 white males born for every 100 white females and approximately 104 black males born for every 100 black females. It has been reported, but not confirmed, that in black populations of several islands in the West Indies, there are fewer males than females at birth (American Association of Retired Persons 1987).

The female in the more developed nations has a life expectancy of 8 or more years beyond that of the male. In 1978, France had the most extreme female/male differences for life expectancy at birth: 8.21 years. In Japan this female/male difference is increasing: in 2007 the life expectancy in Japan was 86 years for females and 79 years for males.

Waldron (1986) reviewed the literature as to causes of sex differences in mortality. She noted that in contemporary industrial societies, the single most important cause of higher mortality for males has been a greater incidence of cigarette smoking among men. Other sex differences in mortality are related to behaviors that contribute to the males' higher mortality. Such behaviors include heavier alcohol consumption and employment in hazardous occupations. In many nonindustrial societies, where in many instances the sex differences in mortality are not as great as in the industrial societies, these factors play a less important role.

In nonindustrial societies, women are more vulnerable to infectious diseases. This greater susceptibility may be related to less adequate nutrition and health care for women. Waldron (1987) described a wide variety of factors that influence sex differences in mortality. In contrast to men in undeveloped nations, men in the United States tend to have a higher death rate from infectious and parasitic diseases than do women; American men were more vulnerable in 1930 than in 1978. However, one must be cautious in interpreting this information because, as Waldron pointed out, sex differences do vary somewhat for different types of infections and parasitic diseases.

Death rates by accidents and other violent causes are much higher for men than for women. Motor vehicle accidents account for a significant percentage of these differences. The difference caused by motorcycle accidents involving young men is a significant and perhaps growing factor. Men have a much higher death rate than do women from accidental drownings and fatal gun accidents as well. Suicide is also more prevalent among men, and the incidence increases with age. As noted above, the higher death rate among men may be related to behavioral factors such as heavier alcohol consumption and other types of risk-taking behavior; these behaviors may or may not have a biological component, and cultural influences also may have an effect.

Ischemic heart disease has been consistently higher for men than for women in almost all available international and historical data. However, the magnitude of sex differences for ischemic heart disease has varied considerably in different regions, historical periods, and ethnic groups. The relation between cigarette smoking and heart disease cannot be ignored. Interestingly, women who smoke do not have the same risk as men. This difference is attributable to different smoking habits. Men not only smoke more cigarettes per day but also inhale more deeply. Coronary-prone behavior also plays a significant role. There is a greater prevalence of type A coronary-prone behavior among men than among women. Type A behavior is marked by impatience, competitive drive, and hostility (Busse and Walker 1986).

As to the influence of menopause, there is contradictory evidence regarding the risk for women before or after menopause. There continues to be a debate regarding early onset of menopause. Early onset of natural menopause has been reported to be higher among women who smoke, and this may account in part for the increased risk of myocardial infarction among women with early natural menopause (Waldron 1986).

Mortality due to malignancies is more frequent among males than among females over most of the life span. Because of the large variety of cancers, the patterns and causes of sex differences vary for the many different types of malignant neoplasms. Furthermore, occupational exposures contribute to the higher cancer rate among men (Centers for Disease Control and Prevention National Center for Health Statistics 2005).

Behavioral factors cannot be ignored for either sex. It is clear that the complex interaction of cultural, anatomical, physiological, and behavioral characteristics must be taken into consideration when sex differences in aging, longevity, and mortality are discussed.

A Note on Stem Cells and Aging

Stem cell research will have a significant effect on the biology of aging and perhaps on the prevention and treatment of the diseases common in late life. Various types of stem cells are associated with stages of embryonic development, including totipotential cells (which develop into a genetically identical organism), pluripotential cells (which can produce many but not all types of cells necessary for fetal development), and multipotential cells (which can produce limited types of cells that have a specific function, such as blood stem cells that can supplement existing blood cells). Of special interest are the cells capable of producing specialized cells that can potentially supplement cells that have been destroyed or that deteriorate with aging.

For example, conditionally immortal neuroepithelial stem cell grafts appear to reverse age-associated memory impairments in rats (Hodges et al. 2000), which have been linked to degeneration of cholinergic neurons. The rats were divided into two groups, impaired and unimpaired, on the basis of prior performance in a water maze. One-half of the impaired rats were grafted with a hippocampal stem cell line. In a subsequent water maze test, the engrafted rats were substantially superior to the control rats in this task (improving function to the level of unimpaired, aged control rats). The results suggest that the cognitive decline was not simply retarded but actually reversed. The findings demonstrate the capacity of a migratory stem cell line to repair diffuse damage in the aged brain.

Psychological Theories of Aging

Birren and Renner (1977) expressed the opinion that there was no pressure on the field of psychology to formulate a unified theory of aging or to explain how behavior is organized over time. They did offer a definition of aging for the behavioral sciences that recognizes that there can be incremental functions as well as decremental changes that occur over the adult life span. "Aging refers to the regular changes that occur in mature, genetically representative organisms living under representative environmental conditions" (Birren and Renner 1977, p. 4). Later, Birren and Cunningham (1985) stated, "The psychology of aging is concerned with differences in behavior, changes in behavior with age, and patterns of behavior shown by persons of different ages in different periods of time" (p. 18). They also noted that "much of contemporary psychology of aging is a collection of segments of knowledge" (p. 19). This statement implies that most theories of the psychology of aging are actually microtheories because they do not embrace large amounts of data derived from various domains of behavior.

Baltes and Willis (1977) reached a somewhat similar conclusion: "All existing theories of psychologic aging and development are of the prototheoretical kind and are incomplete" (p. 148). The psychological theories that have appeared are often the extension of personality and developmental theories into middle and late life. Personality theories usually consider the innate human needs and forces that motivate thought and behavior and a modification of these biologically based energies by the experience of living in a physical and social environment.

Baltes (1993) later extended and clarified his concept of the process of the aging mind. He emphasized that it is important to know the full range of human mental performance and potential. Baltes begins with two major aggregations of mental processes: fluid and crystallized intelligence (Hebb 1949). *Fluid intelligence* is described as the cognitive mechanics and *crystallized intelligence* as the cognitive pragmatics. The fluid mechanisms are considered the basic information processes and are referred to as the hardware. In contrast, the crystallized pragmatics are culturally based and acquired; this cognitive function is the software of the mind. Baltes is also interested in reaching a better understanding of wisdom, because it is often believed to be a characteristic of many elderly persons. According to Baltes, wisdom is the ability to deal with important and difficult matters that are associated with how people conduct their lives and the meaning of life. Wisdom reflects a superior knowledge and includes judgment and sound advice; it is one of the few attributes of late life that is frequently recognized by a large segment of the population. One characteristic of wisdom that leads directly to better adaptation to aging is selective optimization and compensation. The wise elder selects carefully where her or his effort should be placed, optimizes the chances of success, and compensates when success is not attainable according to previous expectations.

Schaie (1977–1978) advanced what he called a "stage theory of adult cognitive development" (p. 129). His tentative scheme involved four possible cognitive stages: 1) acquisitive (childhood, adolescence); 2) achieving (young adulthood); 3) responsible and executive (middle age); and 4) reintegrative (old age). Schaie postulated two overlapping cognitive patterns during middle life—a "responsible" component and "executive" abilities—neither of which can be judged by common psychometric testing. He suggested that during the life span, a transition occurs from "what should I know" through "how should I use what I know" to a "why should I know" phase of life. Schaie stated that numerous new strategies and techniques will have to be developed to fully test a stage theory and that alterations in the theory will emerge.

Yet another theory is the socioemotional selectivity theory proposed by Carstensen, which holds that older people tend to focus on positive emotion; this theory is discussed in more detail in Chapter 15 of this volume ("Mood Disorders"). There are obvious limitations in the psychological theories of aging; these are quite realistic, however, in view of the complexity of the research. Furthermore, recognizing the complexity of psychological experimentation and theory is essential to an awareness of the considerable psychological investigations that have contributed to a better understanding of human aging.

Social Theories of Aging

Palmore (1981) proposed five categories of social theories of aging: 1) disengagement, activity, and continuity theories; 2) age stratification; 3) minority group theory; 4) life events and stress theory; and 5) homogeneity versus heterogeneity. To this can be added attachment theory. *Disengagement theory* states that aging invariably causes physical, psychological, and social disengagement (Cumming and Henry 1961). Physical disengagement is attributable to a decline in physical energy, a decline in strength, and the slowing of responses. Psychological disengagement refers to the withdrawal of concern from a rather diffuse interest in many people to a focus on those who are directly related to the individual. Some describe this as a shift of attention from the outer world to the inner world of one's own feelings and thoughts. Social disengagement means the reduction of all types of social interaction, including activities related to family, friends, community actions, church participation, and so forth. This theory of disengagement originally held that it was actually good—both for the older person and for society—for the older person to disengage. It was proposed that disengaged older persons tend to be happier and healthier than those who remain active.

Shortly after the appearance of the disengagement theory, the *activity theory* was proposed (Havighurst 1963). This theory holds that activity positively affects health, happiness, and longevity and that remaining active is good for both the aging individual and society.

The *continuity approach* is something of a compromise position between the disengagement and activity theories (Neugarten 1964). Proponents of the continuity approach maintain that older people tend to behave according to a pattern that has been established before late life. At times the person may disengage and at other times remain active. It is also apparent that some elderly people will drop one type of activity only to replace it with something that is more suitable to their health status and environment.

Age stratification is really a model of life span development but obviously includes late life as a part of the conceptualization. According to Palmore (1981), age stratification conceptualizes society as being composed of different age groups with different roles and different expectations. Each age group must move up through time while responding to changes in environment. Age stratification focuses on distinguishing between age, period, and cohort effects.

The *minority group theory* relates to differences such as those attributed to race and ethnic groups. According to this theory, the elderly are a minority group and frequently experience the same kind of discrimination that society inflicts on other minority groups (Busse 1970). The *life events and stress theory* holds that those major events usually associated with advancing age are particularly important to health and well-being in late life. A study using this approach must distinguish events that may be welcomed or resisted from those that do not affect all people in a similar manner. Some people resist retirement, whereas others welcome it. Some are unhappy in retirement, whereas others see it as an opportunity to attain life satisfactions.

Some social theories are related to the age distribution of the population and economic influences. One of these theories holds that the status of the elderly is high in static societies and tends to decline with the acceleration of social change (Ogburn and Nimkoff 1940). Another theory is that the status of older adults is inversely related to their proportion in the population. For the most part, the elderly are highly valued in societies in which they are scarce, and their value and status decrease as they become more numerous. The modernization theory of Cowgill and Holmes (1972) suggests that elderly persons are more highly respected in agricultural societies than they are in urbanized societies and that the status of the older adults is inversely proportional to the rate of social change. Another study suggests that in some societies in the process of modernization, the status of the elderly population goes through phases. During a developmental phase toward modernization, family control of resources increases, but as modernization continues, the status of elderly people is likely to decline (Gilleard and Gurkan 1987).

Homogeneity and heterogeneity are concerned with the issue of whether individuals become more like one another or increasingly different from one another as they age (Maddox and Douglass 1974). One interesting consideration is the possibility that those who survive into late life (i.e., those who are 85 years and older) have identifiable characteristics that are very similar, whereas these individuals may have been quite different from others in the same age group 10 to 5 years earlier. Another consideration concerns the differences between men and women. Do men and women become increasingly different or increasingly similar as they age?

Kalish and Knudtson (1976) recommended the extension of *attachment theory*, common in infant and child psychology, to a lifetime conceptual scheme for understanding the relationships and involvements of older people. They further stated that the concept of disengagement is not functional and that it should be eliminated. Attachment is a relationship established and maintained by social bonds and is distinguished from social contact. Elderly people lose significant early objects of attachment, such as parents, siblings, and spouses. New attachments are often much weaker, frequently are not mutual, and therefore are vulnerable. Kalish and Knudtson argued that an appreciation and understanding of attachments will provide a better approach to explaining the psychological changes in elderly people. Relevant to the attachment concept is the finding by Lowenthal and Haven (1968) that, more than any other single factor, having a confidant appeared to discriminate between elderly persons who were institutionalized and those who could remain in the community.

Key Points

- Many theories have been proposed through the years to explain aging, and these theories have been characterized as much by pseudoscience as by true science.
- To date, no factor has been discovered that significantly extends the life span of humans.
- Centenarians are of interest to gerontologists in part because they may possess biological, psychological, and social characteristics that facilitate longevity.
- Genetic factors will undoubtedly be found to contribute to longevity, yet the genes associated with longevity are likely to be many and to have complex interrelationships.
- Among the psychological theories of aging, wisdom and varying approaches to time appear to facilitate successful aging.
- On balance, older adults are more healthy and happy if they remain active in their later years rather than disengage from the social environment.

References

Ahmed A, Tollefsbol T: Telomeres and telomerase: basic science implications for aging. J Am Geriatr Soc 49:1105–1109, 2001

American Association of Retired Persons: A Profile of Older Americans, 1986. Washington, DC, American Association of Retired Persons, 1987

Baltes PB: The aging mind: potential and limits. Gerontologist 33:580–594, 1993

Baltes PB, Willis SL: Toward psychological theories of aging and development, in Handbook of the Psychology of Aging. Edited by Birren JE, Schaie KW. New York, Van Nostrand Reinhold, 1977, pp 128–154

Belkin BM, Neelon FA: The art of observation: William Osler and the method of Zadig. Ann Intern Med 116:863–866, 1992

Berk SL: Sir William Osler, ageism, and "the fixed period": a secret revealed. J Am Geriatr Soc 37:263–266, 1989

Birren JE, Cunningham WR: Research on the psychology of aging: principles, concepts, and theory, in Handbook of the Psychology of Aging, 2nd Edition. Edited by Birren JE, Schaie KW. New York, Van Nostrand Reinhold, 1985, pp 5–45

Birren JE, Renner VJ: Research on the psychology of aging, in Handbook of the Psychology of Aging. Edited by Birren JE, Schaie KW. New York, Van Nostrand Reinhold, 1977, pp 3–34

Brown TW, Wisniewski HM: Genetics of human aging. Review of Biological Research in Aging 1:81–99, 1983

Busse EW: The aged: a deprived minority. N C J Ment Health 4:3–7, 1970

Busse EW: Theories of aging, in Behavior and Adaptation in Late Life, 2nd Edition. Edited by Busse EW, Pfeiffer E. Boston, MA, Little, Brown, 1977, pp 11–32

Busse EW: Biologic and psychosocial bases of behavioral changes in aging, in Psychiatry Update: The American Psychiatric Association Annual Review, Vol 2. Edited by Grinspoon L. Washington, DC, American Psychiatric Press, 1983, pp 96–106

Busse EW: Primary and secondary aging, in The Encyclopedia of Aging. Edited by Maddox GL, Roth G, Atchley R, et al. New York, Springer, 1987, pp 5–34

Busse EW, Walker JI: Heart and neuropsychiatric disorders, in The International Text of Cardiology. Edited by Cheng TO. New York, Pergamon, 1986, pp 976–987

Carrel A: On the permanent life of tissues outside of the organism. J Exp Med 15:516–528, 1912

Centers for Disease Control and Prevention National Center for Health Statistics: Fast Stats A to Z: Death and Mortality. 2005. Available at http://www.cdc.gov/nchs/fastats/deaths.htm. Accessed July 2008.

Cowgill D, Holmes L (eds): Aging and Modernization. New York, Appleton-Century-Crofts, 1972

Cristafalo VS: Animal cell cultures as a model for the study of aging, in Advances in Gerontological Research. Edited by Strehler BL. New York, Academic Press, 1972, pp 68–72

Cumming E, Henry W: Growing Old. New York, Basic Books, 1961

Dai J, Davey A, Siegler IC, et al. GCSDB: an integrated database system for the Georgia Centenarian Study. Bioinformation 1:214–219, 2006

Finch CE: Longevity, Senescence and the Genome. Chicago, IL, University of Chicago Press, 1990

Finkelstein MS: Defenses against infection in the elderly: the compromises of aging. Triangle 23:57–64, 1984

Freud S: On psycho-therapy (1905), in The Standard Edition of the Complete Psychological Works of Sigmund Freud, Vol 7. Translated and edited by Strachey J. London, Hogarth Press, 1957, pp 257–268

Gey GO: Some aspects of the constitution and behavior of normal and malignant cells maintained in continuous culture. Harvey Lectures 50:154–229, 1955

Gilleard CJ, Gurkan AA: Socioeconomic development and the status of elderly men in Turkey: a test of modernization theory. J Gerontol 42:353–357, 1987

Goldstein S, Wojtyk RI, Harley CB, et al: Protein synthetic fidelity in aging human fibroblasts, in Werner's Syndrome and Human Aging (Advances in Experimental Medicine and Biology, Vol 190). Edited by Salk D, Fujiwara Y, Martin GM. New York, Plenum, 1985, pp 495–508

Gruman GJ: A History of Ideas About the Prolongation of Life: The Evolution of Prolongevity Hypotheses to 1880. Philadelphia, PA, American Philosophical Society, 1966

Hart RW, Turturro A: Review of recent biological research theories of aging. Review of Biological Research in Aging 2:3–12, 1985

Hastings G: Progeria: a form of senilism. Practitioner 73:188–217, 1904

Havighurst R: Successful aging, in Processes of Aging. Edited by Williams R, Tibbitts C, Donahue W. New York, Atherton Press, 1963, pp 81–90

Hayflick L: The limited in vitro lifetime of human diploid cell strains. Exp Cell Res 37:614–616, 1965

Hayflick L: Cellular basis for biological aging, in Handbook of Biology of Aging. Edited by Finch CE, Hayflick L. New York, Van Nostrand Reinhold, 1977, pp 73–86

Hayflick L, Moorhead PS: The serial cultivation of human diploid cell strains. Exp Cell Res 25:585–621, 1961

Hazzard WR: What heterogeneity among centenarians can teach us about genetics, aging, and longevity. J Am Geriatr Soc 49:1568–1569, 2001

Hebb DO: The Organization of Behavior. New York, Wiley, 1949

Hodges H, Veizovic T, Bray N, et al: Conditionally immortal neuroepithelial stem cell grafts reverse age-associated memory impairments in rats. Neuroscience 101:945–955, 2000

Hutchinson J: Case of congenital absence of hair and mammary glands with atrophic condition of the skin and its appendages. Lancet 1:473–477, 1886

Kalish RA, Knudtson FW: Attachment versus disengagement: a life-span conceptualization. Hum Dev 19:171–181, 1976

Kenyon C: A conserved regulatory system for aging. Cell 105:165–168, 2001

Laurence J: The immune system in AIDS. Sci Am 252:84–93, 1985

Lind LR (trans): Gabriele Zerbi, Gerontocomia: On the Care of the Aged and Maximianus, Elegies on Old Age and Love. Philadelphia, PA, American Philosophical Society, 1988

Lowenthal MF, Haven C: Interaction and adaptation: intimacy as a critical variable, in Middle Age and Aging. Edited by Neugarten BL. Chicago, IL, University of Chicago Press, 1968, pp 390–400

Maddox GL, Douglass EB: Aging and individual differences. J Gerontol 29:555–563, 1974

Martin GM: Genetic syndromes in man with potential relevance to the pathobiology of aging: genetics of aging. Birth Defects Orig Artic Ser 14:5–39, 1978

Martin GM: Genetics and aging: the Werner syndrome as a segmental progeroid syndrome, in Werner's Syndrome and Human Aging (Advances in Experimental Medicine and Biology, Vol 190). Edited by Salk D, Fujiwara Y, Martin GM. New York, Plenum, 1985, pp 161–170

Miller RA: The biology of aging and longevity, in Principles of Geriatric Medicine and Gerontology, 4th Edition. Edited by Hazzard WR, Blass JP, Ettinger WH, et al. New York, McGraw-Hill, 1999, pp 1–19

National Institute on Aging: Biochemistry and aging, in In Search of the Secrets of Aging (NIH Publ No 93-2756). Washington, DC, National Institute on Aging, May 1993a. Also available at http://www.healthandage.net/html/min/nih/content/booklets/in_search_of_the_secrets/in_search_of_the_secrets.htm. Accessed October 20, 2003.

National Institute on Aging: The genetic connection, in In Search of the Secrets of Aging (NIH Publ No 93-2756). Washington, DC, National Institute on Aging, September 1993b. Also available at http://www.healthandage.net/html/min/nih/content/booklets/in_search_of_the_secrets/in_search_of_the_secrets.htm. Accessed October 20, 2003.

Neugarten B: Personality in Middle and Later Life. New York, Atherton Press, 1964

Ogburn WF, Nimkoff MF: Sociology. Boston, MA, Houghton Mifflin, 1940

Palmore E: Advantages of aging. Gerontologist 19:220–223, 1979

Palmore E: Social Patterns in Normal Aging: Findings From the Duke Longitudinal Study. Durham, NC, Duke University Press, 1981

Palmore EB: Longevity in Abkhasia: a reevaluation. Gerontologist 24:95–96, 1984

Schaie KW: Toward a stage theory of adult cognitive development. Int J Aging Hum Dev 8:129–138, 1977–1978

Suskind GW: Immunological aspects of aging: an overview. Paper presented at the National Institute on Aging Conference on Biological Mechanisms of Aging, Washington, DC, 1980

Thewlis MW: The history of geriatrics, in The Care of the Aged. Edited by Thewlis MW. St. Louis, MO, CV Mosby, 1924

Tobin JD: Physiological indices of aging, in The Baltimore Longitudinal Study of Aging (NIH Publ No 84-2450). Edited by Shock NW. Rockville, MD, National Institutes of Health, 1984, pp 387–395

Turner MS, Martin GM: Genetics of human disease, longevity, and aging, in Principles of Geriatric Medicine and Gerontology, 4th Edition. Edited by Hazzard WR, Blass JP, Ettinger WH, et al. New York, McGraw-Hill, 1999, pp 21–44

U.S. Census Bureau: Centenarians in the United States. Washington, DC, U.S. Department of Health and Human Services, 1999

Waldron I: What do we know about causes of sex differences in mortality: a review of the literature. Population Bulletin of the United Nations 18:59–76, 1986

Waldron I: Causes of the sex differential in longevity. J Am Geriatr Soc 35:365–366, 1987

Weiss AK: Biomedical gerontology: the Hayflick hypothesis. Gerontologist 14:491–493, 1974

Werner O: [Cataract in connection with scleroderma] (in German). Doctoral dissertation, Ophthalmological Clinic, Kiel, Germany, 1904

Zeman FD: Some little-known classics of old-age medicine. JAMA 200:150–152, 1967

Suggested Readings

Austad SN, Masoro EJ (eds): Handbook of the Biology of Aging. New York, Academic Press, 2005

Binstock RH, George LK (eds): Handbook of Aging and the Social Sciences. New York, Academic Press, 2005

Birren JE, Schaie KW (eds): Handbook of the Psychology of Aging. New York, Academic Press, 2005

Finch CE: Longevity, Senescence and the Genome. Chicago, IL, University of Chicago Press, 1990

Hayflick L: Cellular basis for biological aging, in Handbook of Biology of Aging. Edited by Finch CE, Hayflick L. New York, Van Nostrand Reinhold, 1977, pp 73–86

U.S. Census Bureau: Centenarians in the United States. Washington, DC, U.S. Department of Health and Human Services, 1999

CHAPTER 2

Demography and Epidemiology of Psychiatric Disorders in Late Life

Celia F. Hybels, Ph.D.
Dan G. Blazer, M.D., Ph.D.
Judith C. Hays, R.N., Ph.D.

Epidemiology is traditionally defined as the distribution or pattern of disease within a specified population and determinants or factors that affect these disease patterns (MacMahon and Pugh 1970). The epidemiology of psychiatric disorders in late life, therefore, is the study of the distribution of psychiatric disorders and psychiatric symptoms among older adults and the variables that affect the distribution. In this chapter, the findings of demographers and epidemiologists are reviewed as they relate to the care of the psychiatrically impaired older adult.

Demography

In 2000, approximately 35 million persons ages 65 years and older lived in the United States, accounting for more than 12% of the population. Over the last century, the number of persons in this age group steadily increased, from 3.1 million in 1900 and 12.3 million in 1950 to the current estimate. As shown in Figure 2–1, the size of the elderly population is projected to continue to increase over the next several decades and to reach 71.5 million by the year 2030, and then 86.7 million by 2050. Even more astounding, in 2000, the number of "oldest old," or persons ages 85 years and older, was 4.2 million and was projected to reach 20.9 million by 2050 (Federal Interagency Forum on Aging-Related Statistics 2006). The oldest old are more likely to experience poverty, to have less education, and to receive far more federal transfer payments (Blazer 2000). Although nursing home residence has declined in recent years, the rate among those age 65 years or older in 1999 was 43.3 per 1,000, and the rate for those age 85 or older was 182.5 per 1,000 (Federal Interagency Forum on Aging-Related Statistics 2006). Many of these residents are placed in nursing homes because of psychiatric disorders, especially the behavior problems that result from Alzheimer's disease.

The current older population of the United States is predominantly female and white. In 2003, women accounted for 58% of the population ages 65 and older and 69% of those ages 85 and older (Federal Interagency Forum on Aging-Related Statistics 2004). The racial and ethnic composition of the older population is projected to change over the next several decades. In 2004, 81.9% of those age 65 or older were non-Hispanic white, 8.4% black, 6.0% Hispanic, 2.9% Asian, and 1.2% other race/ethnic group. By 2050, the proportion of blacks is projected to be 12.0%, Asians 7.8%, and Hispanics of any race 17.5%, while the proportion of non-Hispanic whites is expected to decrease to 61.3% (Federal Interagency Forum on Aging-Related Statistics 2006).

In 1900, life expectancy in the United States was 48.3 years for females and 46.3 years for males, whereas in 2004, the life expectancy at birth was 80.4 years for

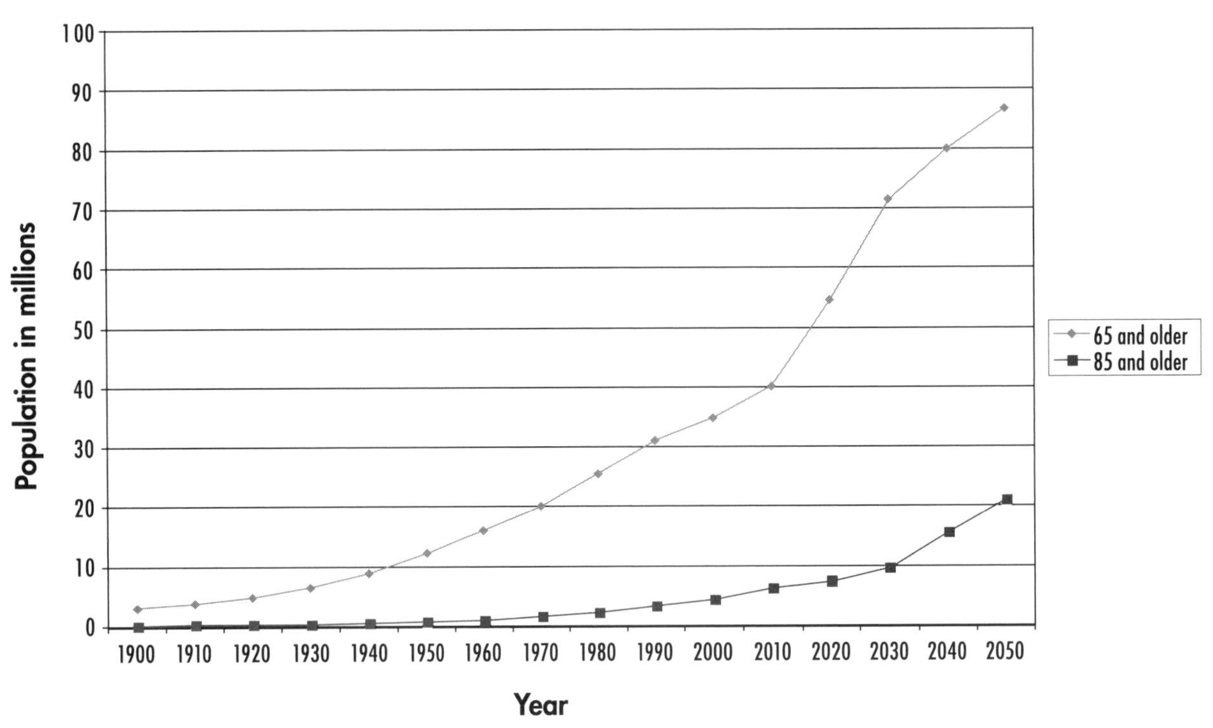

FIGURE 2–1. Population of older adults in the United States (in millions) from 1900 to 2004 and projected to 2050.

Source. Data from Federal Interagency Forum on Aging-Related Statistics 2006.

females and 75.2 years for males. In 2004, a 65-year-old could expect to live an average of 18.7 more years, and a 75-year-old could expect to live 11.9 additional years (National Center for Health Statistics 2006). The higher percentage of elderly who are women and the increased life expectancy of women compared with men have been the subject of much discussion. Contributions to this difference in longevity may derive from both environmental and genetic factors. Cigarette smoking, more prevalent among men, has contributed to this difference. The more stressful and physically demanding occupations in which men engaged through much of the twentieth century may partially explain the difference as well. These potential mortality risks are dynamic across the sexes because more women are entering the workplace at all levels and more women are smoking. Women, however, may have a genetic advantage in life expectancy.

The percentage of older adults in the labor force—those who are either working or looking for work—has changed over the last four decades. The percentage of men ages 65–69 years in the labor force declined from 1963 (40.9%) to 1983 (26.1%) and then increased to 32.8% by 2003. The percentage of men ages 70 years and older in the labor force declined from 20.8% in 1963 to 12.3% in 2003. The percentage of women ages 65–69 years in the labor force increased from 16.5% in 1963 to 22.7% in 2003 (Federal Interagency Forum on Aging-Related Statistics 2004). Even if adults continue to retire at a later age, the effect of an aging population on the economy of the United States—not to mention the need for health care—will be dramatic. This can be seen in the profound increase in the age-to-dependency ratio—that is, the ratio of persons in the workforce compared with children or retired people. Flexibility in retirement and other social and economic changes will help modify the effect of the "squaring" of the population pyramid. Nevertheless, this demographic revolution will affect every individual and every institution in U.S. society (Pifer and Bronte 1986).

If an older person develops a psychiatric disorder, the disorder may become chronic and the person may live many years with a decreased quality of life because of psychiatric morbidity. In addition, the great majority of older persons with psychiatric disorders experience a comorbid physical illness (Blazer 2000). Currently, the proportion of younger and middle-aged adults with a psychiatric disorder is higher than the proportion of older adults, suggesting that as the younger adults age, the proportion of older adults with a psychiatric disorder may also increase and create a potential crisis in geriatric mental health (Jeste et al. 1999).

What can psychiatric epidemiologic studies contribute to mental health services for older adults? Morris (1975) suggested the following uses of epidemiology:

- Identify cases (e.g., determine whether the symptom pattern of depression in elderly persons can be readily identified in community-dwelling and clinical [e.g., hospitalized] populations of older adults)
- Reveal the distribution of psychiatric disorders in the population (e.g., determine the prevalence and/or incidence of dementia)
- Trace historical trends of mental illness among elderly persons (e.g., find out whether the incidence of suicide has increased among this population over the past 10 years)
- Determine the etiology of psychiatric disorders in late life (e.g., determine whether social factors contribute more to the etiology of late-life psychiatric disorders than to such disorders in midlife, given lower potential for genetic contributions)
- Examine the use of psychiatric and other mental health services by elderly persons (e.g., establish whether psychiatrically impaired older adults in the community underutilize psychiatric services)

Each of these functions of epidemiology is reviewed in this chapter.

Case Identification

Clinicians constantly face the task of distinguishing abnormality from normality. Although most epidemiologists and clinicians agree on the core symptoms of psychiatric disorders throughout the life cycle, the absolute distinction between cases and noncases—that is, persons requiring psychiatric attention versus those who do not require such care—is not easily established. Many of the symptoms and signs of a psychiatric disorder in late life may be ubiquitous with the aging process, thus blurring the distinction between cases and noncases. Epidemiologists can assist the clinician in identifying meaningful clusters of symptoms and significant degrees of symptom severity. Case identification is also the foundation of descriptive epidemiology: "cases" are the numerator of the equation from which *prevalence* (the proportion of disease that is present in the population during a specified time period) and *incidence* (the proportion of new cases that develop in a population at risk over a specified time period) estimates are derived in community and clinical samples (the denominator).

What is a case? Copeland (1981) suggested that this question be turned by epidemiologists, with advantage, to "A case for what?" The choice of a construct for a case depends on the particular scientific or clinical inquiry of the investigator. If, to determine a value of a new short-acting sedative-hypnotic agent, the clinician wishes to identify a group of older adults with initial insomnia, the prevalence and severity of a target symptom (initial insomnia) define the case. The sleep difficulty may result from several different underlying disorders, but diagnosis would be irrelevant to the purpose of the study. For most clinicians, however, the goal of case identification is to identify subjects experiencing uniform underlying psychopathology, as is implicit in DSM-IV and DSM-IV-TR (American Psychiatric Association 1994, 2000)

Diagnostic categories that approximate true disease processes have several characteristics, including the following (Weissman and Klerman 1978):

1. A category should be distinguished on the basis of patterns of symptomatology (e.g., the clustering of symptoms in vascular depression [Alexopoulas et al. 1997]).
2. A category should predict the outcome of a disorder (e.g., Alzheimer's disease should predict a steady decline in cognitive functioning [Shoghi-Jadid et al. 2002]).
3. A category should reflect underlying biological reality, confirmed by family and genetic studies (e.g., Alzheimer's disease [Roses 1994]).
4. Laboratory studies should eventually validate a diagnostic category (e.g., the use of specific imaging studies to diagnose Alzheimer's disease [Roses 1997]).
5. The classification scheme should identify persons who may respond to a specific therapeutic intervention, such as a particular form of psychotherapy or a specific group of medications (e.g., the use of combined pharmacotherapy and interpersonal psychotherapy to treat late-life depression [Reynolds et al. 1999]).

The goal of DSM-IV-TR is to provide categories that eventually will meet each of these characteristics.

At present, however, these categories are defined by operational criteria (e.g., the symptom criteria for the diagnosis of major depression). One method of case identification is the use of diagnostic instruments. These instruments (usually standardized interviews) have been developed and used in community- and clinic-based epidemiologic studies to identify persons with symptoms that meet these criteria. The Composite International Diagnostic Interview (CIDI; World Health Organization 1990), the Structured Clinical Interview for DSM-IV (First et al. 1997), and the Diagnostic Interview Schedule (DIS; Robins et al. 1981) are examples of frequently used interview schedules.

For example, the World Mental Health Survey version of the CIDI was used in the National Comorbidity Survey Replication (NCS-R), which reported that the lifetime prevalence of major depressive disorder was 10.6% among those ages 60 years and older compared to 15.4% among those ages 18–29, 19.8% among those ages 30–44, and 18.8% among those ages 45–59 (Kessler et al. 2005). The DIS was used in the landmark Epidemiologic Catchment Area (ECA) study conducted over two decades ago, from which a 1-month national estimate of the prevalence of affective disorders in persons ages 65 years and older was 2.5% (compared with 6.4% for persons ages 25–44 years) (Regier et al. 1988).

A second approach to case identification is the use of self-administered symptom scales and personality inventories. Frequently used scales in epidemiologic surveys include the Center for Epidemiologic Studies—Depression Scale (Radloff 1977) and the Geriatric Depression Scale (Yesavage et al. 1983), which screen for depressive symptoms, and the Short Portable Mental Status Questionnaire (Pfeiffer 1975) and the Mini-Mental State Examination (Folstein et al. 1975), which screen for cognitive impairment. The advantage of these scales is that, unlike diagnostic interviews, they do not subjectively assign patients to a particular diagnostic category; a disadvantage is the lack of diagnostic specificity that can be achieved with their use. For example, the severity of depressive symptoms after the loss of a loved one may be similar to that associated with a major depressive episode with melancholia; however, a symptom checklist cannot be used to distinguish one from the other, although the diagnosis of, and intervention for, these two disorders would be very different. For example, Blazer et al. (1991a) estimated the prevalence of clinically significant depression symptoms among community-dwelling elders in North Carolina to be 9%, although most of these individuals would not receive diagnoses of major depression.

Other authors define a case on the basis of severity of physical, psychological, and social impairment secondary to the symptoms. This approach to case identification is less popular among clinicians, who are more inclined to "treat a disease" than to "improve function." Improved function, in theory, should derive from remission of the disease. Nevertheless, function has special relevance in the care of older adults, especially the oldest old (Blazer 2000). When managing chronic psychiatric disorders, such as primary degenerative dementia of the Alzheimer's type, the improvement or maintenance of physical, psychological, and social functioning is a clinician's primary goal (Hazzard 1994). Family members are often more concerned with improved functioning than with alleviation of symptoms. Improved sleep and appetite and a decline in suicidal ideation in a depressed older adult may not translate into a perceived recovery from a depressive episode by the family. Rather, the family may focus on the quality of interpersonal interactions and social functioning.

Whichever approach is used to identify cases, most clinicians and clinical investigators want to achieve perfection in the separation of cases from noncases (e.g., case identification is critical for entry into a clinical trial). The epidemiologic method depends, for the most part, on a clear distinction between cases and noncases (Kleinbaum et al. 1982), yet most older adults do not ideally fit the psychiatric diagnosis they receive (Strauss et al. 1979).

Regardless of the diagnostic system, unusual or borderline cases exist that cannot be clearly placed in a single category. This has led some investigators to consider the possibility of "fuzzy sets" as a means by which cases can be more realistically distinguished (Blazer et al. 1989). Not infrequently, older adults manifest more than one disease simultaneously (e.g., major depression and primary degenerative dementia). In addition, the prescribed categories of DSM-IV-TR do not always match the symptoms that individuals in this population may be experiencing; generalized anxiety, for instance, is not always disentangled from a major depressive episode in an agitated older adult. Krishnan (2007) suggested that it may be advantageous to separate etiology from clinical manifestation in future classification of disease.

Most natural clustering of older adults into categories is perceptually "fuzzy" (Rosch 1978), for natural processes rarely show necessary and sufficient criteria for sharp distinctions. Boundaries between closely related categories are ill defined. Some of the methods of case identification, such as the symptom checklist and standardized interview approaches that archive symptoms, are adaptive to the development of clusters of both symptoms and subjects with fuzzy boundaries. For example, depressed elderly persons are more likely to express cognitive dysfunction than are depressed middle-aged persons, yet cognitive dysfunction is part of the depressed syndrome across the life cycle (Blazer et al. 1988). Therefore, psychiatric syndromes—rather than discrete disorders—are more realistic as diagnostic entities in geriatric psychiatry. The most common of these syndromes are memory loss, confusion, depression, anxiety, suspiciousness and agitation, sleep disturbance, and hypochondriasis (Blazer 2000).

Recent research has focused on latent subtypes of psychiatric disorders, which offer new directions in case definition, suggesting that cases may differ in their symptom presentation or risk factors within a disorder. For example, Lyketsos et al. (2001) identified three latent classes of neuropsychiatric disturbance in a sample of older adults with Alzheimer's disease.

A diagnosis must be reliable and valid for it to be a useful means of communicating clinical information. To pass the test of reliability, a diagnosis must be consistent and repeatable. Standardized or operational methods for identifying psychiatric symptoms and the availability of specific criteria for psychiatric diagnoses have greatly improved the reliability of case identification by psychiatrists and by lay interviewers in psychiatric epidemiologic surveys. Reliability, however, does not ensure validity—that is, the test of whether a case identified by a particular method reflects underlying reality (Blazer and Kaplan 2000).

Distribution of Psychiatric Disorders

Epidemiologic studies of psychiatric impairment in older adults have generally concentrated on either overall mental health functioning or the distribution of specific psychiatric disorders in the population. Reports from these studies usually begin as general observations of the association of impairment or specific disorders to characteristics such as age, gender, race/ethnicity, and socioeconomic status. These trends provide the template for more in-depth studies of the hereditary, biological, and psychosocial contributors to the etiology of disorders and the effect of the distribution of the disorders on mental health care utilization. Frequencies of disorders within the population are usually presented in terms of prevalence. Almost all epidemiologic studies provide estimates based on community samples of larger populations. Smaller studies of the prevalence of impairment or specific disorders in institutional or clinical settings provide important data about service use. Longitudinal epidemiologic studies of older adults can also provide data on the incidence of impairment or psychiatric disorders. Longitudinal studies provide data on outcomes associated with impairment or specific psychiatric disorders.

One of the landmark studies of the prevalence of psychiatric disorders in the United States was the ECA survey conducted over two decades ago. The National Institute of Mental Health established the ECA program to determine the prevalence of specific psychiatric disorders in both community and institutional populations (Regier et al. 1984). Data were collected in five communities, and the DIS was used to identify persons who met criteria for specific disorders. DIS diagnoses were based on DSM-III criteria (American Psychiatric Association 1980), the nomenclature in effect at the time the data were collected. More than 18,000 persons were interviewed in the ECA study, including 5,702 persons who were ages 65 and older. All disorders, with the exception of cognitive impairment, were more prevalent in younger or middle-aged adults than in older adults. Of those ages 65 and older, 12.3% (13.6% of the women and 10.5% of the men) met criteria for one or more psychiatric disorders in the month prior to the interview. The two most prevalent disorders in this age group were any anxiety disorder (5.5%) and severe cognitive impairment (4.9%) (Regier et al. 1988). The National Comorbidity Survey was conducted in the United States from 1990 to 1992 using a nationally representative sample, enabling national estimates of the prevalence of psychiatric disorders using DSM-III-R criteria (American Psychiatric Association 1987); however, the sample only included people ages 15–54 years.

Two large-scale epidemiologic surveys provide more recent estimates of lifetime and current prevalence of psychiatric disorders. The National Epidemiologic Survey on Alcohol and Related Conditions (NESARC) was sponsored by the National Institute on Alcohol Abuse and Alcoholism. From 2001 to 2002, in-person interviews were conducted with 43,093 participants ages 18 years and older, and the data were weighted to represent the U.S. population at the time of the 2000 census, enabling national estimates of the prevalence of psychiatric disorders using DSM-IV criteria (Grant et al. 2005b). The diagnostic interview used was the Alcohol Use Disorder and Associated Disabilities Interview Schedule—DSM-IV Version (Grant et al. 2001).

The World Health Organization (WHO) World Mental Health (WMH) surveys were conducted from 2001 to 2003 in 14 countries, and a total of 60,463 adults were interviewed. DSM-IV psychiatric diagnoses were assessed using the WMH version of the WHO Composite International Diagnostic Interview (Kessler and Ustun 2004; WHO World Mental Health Survey Consortium 2004). In the United States, the WMH survey was called the National Comorbidity Survey Replication (NCS-R) and included data from 9,282 adults ages 18 years and older (Kessler et al. 2005). These large-scale studies have added to the rich data provided earlier by the ECA surveys and by numerous smaller studies conducted in various geographic locations.

Specific disorders are addressed in detail in subsequent chapters, but Tables 2–1 through 2–5 provide summaries of the prevalence of both psychiatric symptoms and disorders in both community and clinical populations based on selected studies conducted in the United States and other countries over the last several decades.

The prevalence of cognitive impairment in selected community and institutional populations of older adults is presented in Table 2–1. The prevalence of cognitive impairment reported from the ECA two decades ago was 4.9% (Regier et al. 1988), within the range found in three of the community sites of the Established Populations for Epidemiologic Studies of the Elderly (EPESE) conducted by the National Institute on Aging (Cornoni-Huntley et al. 1986, 1990). As shown in Table 2–1, the prevalence of cognitive impairment may range from 1% to over 18%, depending on the age of the sample. The Canadian Study of Health and Aging (Graham et al. 1997) reported a prevalence of 16.8% for a diagnosis they identified as "cognitive impairment, no dementia" in their sample of both community-dwelling and institutionalized older adults. Since the late 1990s much attention has focused on mild cognitive impairment, and studies listed in Table 2–1 report prevalence estimates ranging from 2% to 29% depending on the age group assessed and the research setting (community vs. institutional). These examples show that the prevalence of cognitive impairment is higher in samples that include patients from primary care or long-term care facilities. Also, as shown in Table 2–1, studies conducted since 2003 have begun to focus on the prevalence of different subtypes of mild cognitive impairment.

It is important to note that the studies in Table 2–1 reporting the prevalence of cognitive impairment measured cognitive function using standardized screening tests such as the Short Portable Mental Status Questionnaire (Pfeiffer 1975) and the Mini-Mental State Examination (Folstein et al. 1975). Therefore, these studies do not report the prevalence of dementia or Alzheimer's disease or actual cerebral impairment, although some of the more recent studies have augmented their test results with imaging data (Lopez et al. 2003). The prevalence of cognitive impairment as assessed through these screening tests can be affected by the educational level of the population being studied, as well as by other sociocultural factors that may affect performance on cognitive tasks.

The prevalence of dementia and Alzheimer's disease in both community and institutional samples is shown in Table 2–2. Overall, the prevalence of dementia is lower than that of cognitive impairment or mild cognitive impairment and is estimated to be 0%–23% in the community. The prevalence of dementia in primary care samples is higher than that observed in community samples (Olafsdottir et al. 2001) and lower than that observed in long-term care samples, which often have a higher mean age (Bland et al. 1988; Rovner et al. 1986).

In the East Boston EPESE, the prevalence of probable Alzheimer's disease increased with age. Specifically, the prevalence was 3.0% in those ages 65–74 years, 18.7% in those ages 75–84 years, and 47.2% in those ages 85 years and older. In recent years research has focused more on earlier stages of cognitive decline, such as mild cognitive impairment, than the prevalence of subtypes of dementia (Panza et al. 2005) assessed using techniques such as imaging data (Feldman and Jacova 2005), resulting in fewer recent studies of the prevalence of Alzheimer's disease.

The prevalence of psychiatric symptoms in community samples of older adults is presented in Table 2–3. The most frequently reported symptoms are generally problems with sleep and feelings of anxiety. Psychotic symptoms are less prevalent in community samples than anxiety symptoms, but may be as high as 10% in the oldest old. The prevalence of alcohol use in older adults is low, but the proportion of drinkers who drink in excess is greater than 19% (P.A. Saunders et al. 1989).

TABLE 2–1. Prevalence of cognitive impairment in community and institutional populations of older adults

Authors	Sample	*N*	Age (years)	Prevalence
Trollor et al. 2007	Community, Australia	1,792	65+	7.4%
Di Carlo et al. 2007	Community and institutional, Italy	2,830	65–84	9.5% CIND
				16.1% MCI
Rait et al. 2005	Community-based controlled trial, United Kingdom	15,051	75+	18.3%
Manley et al. 2005	Community, New York	1,315	65+	5.0% amnestic MCI
				2.1%–6.2% other MCI
Ganguli et al. 2004	Community, MoVIES	1,248	Mean age = 74.6	2.9%–4.0% amnestic MCI over 10 years
Lopez et al. 2003	Cardiovascular Health Study—Cognition Study[a]	2,470	65+	19% MCI <75 years
				29% MCI 85+ years
Busse et al. 2003	Community, Germany	1,045	75+	3.1% MCI
				8.8% age-associated cognitive decline
Hanninen et al. 2002	Population-based sample, eastern Finland	806	60–76	5.3% MCI
Graham et al. 1997	Community and institution, Canadian Study of Health and Aging	2,914	65+	16.8% CIND
Callahan et al. 1995	Primary care patients, Indiana	3,594	60+	15.7%
Regier et al. 1988	Five U.S. communities, ECA	5,702	65+	4.9% (2.9% ages 65–74; 6.8% ages 75–84; 15.8% ages 85+)
Cornoni-Huntley et al. 1986	Iowa EPESE	3,673	65+	1.3%
Cornoni-Huntley et al. 1986	New Haven, Connecticut, EPESE	2,811	65+	5.3%
Cornoni-Huntley et al. 1986	East Boston, Massachusetts, EPESE	3,812	65+	6.0%

Note. CIND = cognitive impairment, no dementia; ECA = Epidemiologic Catchment Area; EPESE = Established Populations for Epidemiologic Studies of the Elderly; MCI = mild cognitive impairment; MoVIES = Monongahela Valley Independent Elders Survey.

[a]Participants in the Cardiovascular Health Study were age 65 or older and were selected from Medicare eligibility lists in four U.S. communities (Fried et al. 1991).

TABLE 2–2. Prevalence of dementia and Alzheimer's disease in community and institutional populations

Authors	Sample	*N*	Age (years)	Prevalence
Li et al. 2007	Community, Beijing, China	1,593	60+	2.5% dementia
Stevens et al. 2002	Community, Islington, England	1,085	65+	9.9% dementia *Among those with dementia:* 31.3% Alzheimer's disease 21.9% vascular dementia 10.9% dementia with Lewy bodies 7.8% frontal lobe dementia
Olafsdottir et al. 2001	Primary care center, Sweden	350	70+	16.0% dementia
Riedel-Heller et al. 2001	Community, Leipzig, Germany (Leipzig Longitudinal Study of the Aged)	1,692	75+	17.4% DSM-III-R dementia 12.4% ICD-10 dementia
Canadian Study of Health and Aging Working Group 1994	Canada	10,263	65+	8.0% dementia 5.1% Alzheimer's disease
Copeland et al. 1992	Community, Liverpool, England	1,070	65+	3.3% Alzheimer's disease
Heeren et al. 1991	Community, The Netherlands	1,259	85+	23% dementia (moderate or severe dementia 11%)
Evans et al. 1989	Community, East Boston EPESE	467	65+	10.3% probable Alzheimer's disease
Bland et al. 1988	Community and institution, Edmonton, AB, Canada	358 community 199 institutional	65+	*Severe cognitive impairment:* Community: 0.0% Institutional: 42% female; 36.1% male
Copeland et al. 1987	Community, Liverpool, England	1,070	65+	5.2% probable dementia
Rovner et al. 1986	Institution, Maryland	50	Mean age=83	56% primary degenerative dementia 18% multi-infarct dementia 4% Parkinson's dementia

Note. EPESE=Established Populations for Epidemiologic Studies of the Elderly; ICD-10= *International Statistical Classification of Diseases and Related Health Problems*, 10th Revision (World Health Organization 1992).

TABLE 2–3. Prevalence of psychiatric symptoms in community populations of older adults

Authors	Sample	*N*	Age (years)	Symptoms/syndrome	Prevalence
Anstey et al. 2007	Australia	1,116	65+	Depressive symptoms	14.4% comm; 32% inst
Stek et al. 2004	Leiden, The Netherlands	500	85+	Depressive symptoms	15.4%
Copeland et al. 1999	EURODEP	13,808	65+	Cases/subcases of depression	12.3%: 8.6% male; 14.1% female
Black et al. 1998	Hispanic EPESE	2,823	65+	Depressive symptoms	25.6%: 17.3% male; 31.9% female
Beekman et al. 1995	LASA	3,056	55–85	Minor depression	12.9%
Cornoni-Huntley et al. 1986	New Haven, Connecticut, EPESE	2,811	65+	Depressive symptoms	15.1%
Ostling and Skoog 2002	Sweden	347	85+	Psychotic symptoms	10.1% (5.5% delusions; 6.9% hallucinations; 6.9% paranoid ideation)
Livingston et al. 2001	Islington, England	720	65+	Persecutory symptoms and perceptual disturbance	3.9%
Henderson et al. 1998	Australia	1,377	70+	Psychotic symptoms	5.7%
Christenson and Blazer 1984	North Carolina	997	65+	Persecutory ideation	4%
Blazer and Houpt 1979	North Carolina	997	65+	Hypochondriasis	14%
Cornoni-Huntley et al. 1986	Iowa EPESE	3,673	65+	Trouble falling asleep	14.1%
				Awakening during night	33.7%
				Daytime sleepiness	30.7%
Thomas and Rockwood 2001	Canadian Study of Health and Aging	2,873	65+	Alcohol abuse	8.9%
				Questionable alcohol abuse	3.7%
P.A. Saunders et al. 1989	Liverpool, England	1,070	65+	Drinkers exceeding sensible limits	19.6% females; 19.5% males
Forsell and Winblad 1998	Stockholm, Sweden	966	78+	Feelings of anxiety	24.4%

Note. Comm=community; inst=institutional; EPESE=Established Populations for Epidemiologic Studies of the Elderly; EURODEP=European Concerted Action on Depression of Older People; LASA=Longitudinal Aging Studies Amsterdam.

Numerous studies have reported a high prevalence of depressive symptoms among older adults. As shown in Table 2–3, the prevalence of depressive symptoms may be as high as 25% in community samples. The prevalence is even higher in residential care settings (Anstey et al. 2007) and is generally higher in females than males (Copeland et al. 1999).

Across the entire life cycle, many psychiatric symptoms, especially hypochondriasis and sleep disorders, have their highest frequencies among elderly adults. A relatively high frequency of certain symptoms in elderly populations, however, does not necessarily signify an increased frequency of specific psychiatric disorders. The paradox of relatively high reports of depressive symptoms and relatively low reports of the prevalence of major depressive episodes illustrates this point (Blazer 1982). Diagnostic categories, such as those found in DSM-IV-TR, are clusters of symptoms and signs that derive their validity not from the overall weight of symptomatology but rather from regularities in the clustering of history, the persistence of symptoms over time, a predictable outcome, a common pathophysiology, and possible biochemical disturbances. As biological markers of psychiatric disorders are identified, laboratory diagnostic techniques will provide information that is complementary to the symptoms reported. As knowledge progresses in the area of nomenclature, new categories of symptoms may be lumped together to define a particular syndrome. As Morris (1975) noted, each succeeding generation will split and lump groups of symptoms and signs to suit its own purposes, given the current biomedical and clinical understanding of disease entities.

Symptoms, the most objective clinical indicators of psychopathology, may reflect more than one diagnostic entity. On the other hand, symptoms may not be associated with any disorder of interest to the clinician. For example, decreased appetite can result from several sources. At a given time, grief reactions, more frequent in late life than at other stages of the life cycle, may be virtually indistinguishable from major depressive episodes if appetite alone is considered. Loss of appetite also accompanies major life adjustments such as a forced change of residence or a decline in economic resources. Most commonly, loss of appetite in late life is a result of poor physical health.

The prevalence of selected psychiatric disorders in community populations, shown in Table 2–4, is lower than the prevalence of related psychiatric symptoms (Table 2–3). The disorder with the highest 12-month prevalence among participants ages 65 and older reported from the NESARC was specific phobia (7.5%) (Stinson et al. 2007), whereas the disorder with the highest lifetime prevalence was any alcohol use disorder (16.1%) (Hasin et al. 2007). In the NCS-R, the disorder with the highest lifetime prevalence among participants age 60 years or older was major depression (10.6%) (Kessler et al. 2005). The presentation of studies in Table 2–4 provides an opportunity to note several important points to consider when comparing prevalence estimates across studies. Lifetime prevalence is generally higher than but can be equal to point prevalence. Similarly, prevalence is dependent on both the incidence and duration of the disorder within the period of risk, so 12-month prevalence is generally higher than 1-month prevalence. Prevalence estimates also can vary depending on the diagnostic instruments used (which may explain in part the differences between the lifetime prevalence estimates reported in the NCS-R and the NESARC).

As shown in Table 2–4, the current prevalence of major depression reported from these studies ranges from 0.7% reported from the ECA (Regier et al. 1988) to 3% reported from a survey in France (Ritchie et al. 2004), and somewhat higher in the Cache County (Utah) survey (Steffens et al. 2000). Overall, the findings are fairly consistent, with prevalence estimates from the rest of the studies presented falling within that range of 1%–3%. The prevalence is higher in older females than males (Regier et al. 1988; Steffens et al. 2000). The current prevalence of anxiety disorders is higher than that of major depression, and the estimates depend in part on whether specific phobia is included. As shown in Table 2–4, the prevalence of individual disorders is highest for phobic disorders (3%–10%) and lowest for panic disorder (<1%). The prevalence of generalized anxiety disorder is approximately 1%–2.2%. The prevalence of any anxiety disorder among adults age 65 or older in the ECA studies was 5.5%, with a higher prevalence in females (6.8%) than in males (3.6%) (Regier et al. 1988). The current prevalence of alcohol abuse/dependence is low (0.1% to 1.5%) (Regier et al. 1988; Trollor et al. 2007), with higher lifetime prevalence. Similarly, the 1-month prevalence of schizophrenia among persons age 65 or older in the ECA was 0.1% (Regier et al. 1988).

Overall, psychiatric disorders are found at a lower prevalence among elderly people than in people at other stages of the life cycle. In the ECA, the 1-month prevalence of any Diagnostic Interview Schedule disorder (including cognitive impairment) was 16.9% in those ages 18–24 years, 17.3% in those ages 25–44 years, 13.3% in those ages 45–64 years, and 12.3% in those ages 65 years and older (Regier et al. 1988). The virtual absence of alcohol abuse or dependence and of schizophrenia in those ages 65 and older may reflect selective mortality. It may also reflect changes in drinking patterns (the lifetime prevalence in the NESARC was 16.1% compared to a 12-month prevalence of 1.5%) (Hasin et al. 2007). On the other hand, it may also reflect the case findings techniques used. For example, the investigators in the ECA, the NCS-R, and the NESARC did not attempt to assess the homeless population. The community data do not include persons in institutions, and many persons in late life with chronic schizophrenia may be institutionalized. In addition, early-onset schizophrenia may be associated with a "burned-out" symptom picture; this pattern, coupled with poor reporting, may mean that an individual's clinical presentation does not meet the criteria for a diagnosis of schizophrenia.

Another question derives from these data: Do unique late-life symptom presentations render the DSM-IV-TR inadequate as a system of nomenclature? DSM-IV-TR provides age-specific categories for children but not for elderly persons. Clinicians who work with older adults, however, have often commented that depression may be masked in late life by symptoms of poor physical health or pseudodementia. Yet there is no compelling evidence for developing a new classification specific to older adults. Although DSM-IV-TR may not identify all persons with significant psychiatric symptoms, those older persons who do qualify for a DSM-IV-TR diagnosis are not unlike persons at other stages of the life cycle (Blazer 1980a; Blazer et al. 1987b). The deficiency inherent in DSM-IV-TR is that it poorly differentiates psychiatric symptoms from symptoms that signify the presence of physical illness and impaired cognition—a situation that may also occur in younger individuals, although it is far more common as a diagnostic problem in late life than in middle life.

The prevalence of psychiatric symptoms and disorders, especially major depression, in treatment settings is presented in Table 2–5. Burns et al. (1988) found among nursing home patients with mental disorders, excluding organic brain syndrome, an average of 1.3 mental disorder diagnoses per person. As is evident in Table 2–5, the prevalence of both symptoms and disorders is much higher than found in community populations. The prevalence of major depression in nursing homes or long-term care facilities is estimated to be 6.0%–14.4%, and the prevalence of minor depression to be as high as 30.5%. As shown in Table 2–5, the prevalence of major depression in both acute care hospitals and primary care is higher than that found in the community. Many older adults may be selectively admitted to medical inpatient units or long-term care facilities (because older adults are less likely to use specialty psychiatric care). The lower prevalence in the community, therefore, should not lull clinicians into believing that psychiatric problems are of little consequence to older adults.

Fewer data regarding the incidence of psychiatric disorders in late life are available because most disorders begin early in adulthood. In a study of 875 nondepressed older adults with a mean age of 85 years, the 3-year incidence of depression was 4.1% (Forsell and Winblad 1999). Henderson et al. (1997) reported that the 3- to 6-year incidence of depression in a sample of community-dwelling elders age 70 or older was 2.5%. The 2-year incidence of depression defined by the Geriatric Depression Scale (not necessarily first-onset) was 8.4% in adults ages 65 and older in a community sample in London (Harris et al. 2006). Incidence of depression appears to rise with age and differ by gender. In a Swedish population of adults followed from age 70 to age 85, the incidence of first-onset depression was 12 per 1,000 person-years for men and 30 per 1,000 person-years for women (Palsson et al. 2001). The incidence of schizophrenia among older adults is estimated to be 3 per 100,000 persons per year for new cases (Copeland et al. 1998). The incidence of dementia also increases with age. Bachman et al. (1993) reported from the Framingham data that the 5-year incidence of dementia was 7 per 1,000 in those ages 65–69 and 118 per 1,000 at ages 85–89. A similar increase with age in the 1-year incidence of Alzheimer's disease was reported from the East Boston EPESE: 0.6% in those age 65–69 years and 8.4% in those age 85 or older (Hebert et al. 1995). The 1-year incidence (per 100 person-years) reported from the ECA among those age 65 years or older was 1.25 for major depression, 0.04 for panic disorder, 4.29 for phobic disorder, and 0.63 for alcohol abuse/dependence (Eaton et al. 1989).

TABLE 2–4. Prevalence of selected psychiatric disorders in community populations of older adults

Authors	Sample	*N*	Age	Disorder	Period	Prevalence
Hasin et al. 2007	National Epidemiologic Survey on Alcoholism and Related Conditions	8,205 65+ (from total U.S. representative sample of 43,093)	65+	Alcohol use disorder	12 months	1.5%
					Lifetime	16.1%
Hasin et al. 2005	"	"	"	Major depression	12 months	2.7%
					Lifetime	8.2%
Grant et al. 2006	"	"	"	Panic disorder	12 months	0.8%
					Lifetime	2.8%
Grant et al. 2005a	"	"	"	Social anxiety disorder	12 months	1.6%
					Lifetime	3.0%
Grant et al. 2005b	"	"	"	Generalized anxiety	12 months	1.0%
					Lifetime	2.6%
Stinson et al. 2007	"	"	"	Specific phobia	12 months	7.5%
Trollor et al. 2007	Australian National Mental Health and Well-Being Survey	1,792	65+	Major depression	1 month	1.2%
				Dysthymia		0.2%
				Panic disorder/agoraphobia		0.3%
				Social phobia		0.1%
				Generalized anxiety disorder		0.8%
				Posttraumatic stress disorder		0.2%
				Alcohol abuse/dependence		0.3%
Kessler et al. 2005	National Comorbidity Survey Replication	1,837 60+ (from total U.S. representative sample of 9,282)	60+	Major depression	Lifetime	10.6%
				Dysthymia		1.3%
				Panic disorder		2.0%
				Agoraphobia without panic		1.0%
				Specific phobia		7.5%
				Social phobia		6.6%
				Generalized anxiety disorder		3.6%
				Posttraumatic stress disorder		2.5%
				Obsessive-compulsive disorder		0.7%
				Alcohol abuse		6.2%
				Alcohol dependence		2.2%
Ritchie et al. 2004	Montpelier district of France	1,873	65+	Anxiety disorders	Current	14.2%
				Phobia		10.7%
				Major depression		3.0%
				Psychosis		1.7%

TABLE 2–4. Prevalence of selected psychiatric disorders in community populations of older adults *(continued)*

Authors	Sample	*N*	Age	Disorder	Period	Prevalence
ESEMeD/MHEDEA 2000 Investigators 2004	European Study of the Epidemiology of Mental Disorders (ESEMeD)	4,401 age 65+ (from total sample of 21,425)	65+	Any mood disorder	12 months	3.2%
				Any anxiety disorder		3.6%
				Any alcohol disorder		0.1%
Steffens et al. 2000	Cache County (UT) study	4,559	65+	Major depression	Current	4.4% female 2.7% male
Beekman et al. 1995	LASA	3,056	55–85	Major depression	Current	2.0%
Blazer et al. 1991b	Durham, North Carolina, ECA	784	65+	Generalized anxiety disorder		2.2%
Lindesay et al. 1989	Guy's/Age Concern Survey	890	65+	Phobic disorder	Current	10.0%
Bland et al. 1988	Edmonton, AB, Canada	358	65+	Major depression	Current	1.2%
				Phobic disorder		3.0%
				Panic disorder		0.3%
Regier et al. 1988	ECA in five U.S. communities	5,702 age 65+ (from total sample of 18,571)	65+	Major depression	1 month	0.7%
				Dysthymia		1.8%
				Any anxiety disorder		5.5%
				Phobic disorder		4.8%
				Schizophrenia		0.1%
				Alcohol abuse/dependence		0.9%
Copeland et al. 1987	Liverpool, England	1,070	65+	Depressive neurosis	Current	8.3%
				Depressive psychosis		2.9%

Note. ECA=Epidemiologic Catchment Area; LASA=Longitudinal Aging Studies Amsterdam.

TABLE 2–5. Prevalence of selected psychiatric symptoms and disorders among older adults in selected treatment settings

Authors	Sample	*N*	Age (years)	Disorder	Prevalence
McCusker et al. 2005	Two acute care hospitals	380	65+	Major depression Minor depression	14.2%–44.5% 7.9%–9.4%
Smalbrugge et al. 2005	AGED study nursing home patients on somatic wards	333	55+	Any anxiety disorder Subthreshold anxiety disorder Anxiety symptoms	5.7% 4.2% 29.7%
Jongenelis et al. 2004	AGED study nursing home patients on somatic wards	333	55+	Major depression Minor depression Subclinical depression	8.1% 14.1% 24%
Sheehan et al. 2003	Primary care	140	65+	Hypochondriacal neurosis	5.0%
Bruce et al. 2002	Elderly home health care patients	539	65+	Major depression	13.5%
Kvaal et al. 2001	Geriatric inpatients	98	70+	Anxiety symptoms	47% male 41% female
Teresi et al. 2001	Nursing homes	319	Mean=84.5	Major depression	14.4%
Lyness et al. 1999	Primary care	224	60+	Major depression Minor depression	6.5% 5.2%
Parmelee et al. 1989	Nursing homes and congregate housing	708	Mean=84	Major depression Minor depression	12.4% 30.5%
Koenig et al. 1988	Acute care facility	171	70+	Major depression Other depressive syndromes	11.5% 23.0%
Rovner et al. 1986	Intermediate care facility	50	Mean=83	Major depression	6.0%

Note. AGED=Amsterdam Groningen Elderly Depression.

Historical Studies

Historical studies in psychiatric epidemiology yield an important perspective on the causal web of mental illness over time. With the caveat that case identification methods change over time and place, rendering the detection of historical trends subject to misclassification error, historical studies have contributed importantly to estimating the separate effects of age, historical events, and cohort behavior on the incidence of mental illness. For example, the benefits of historical studies can be seen in recent research on suicide mortality among older adults.

Suicide mortality is positively correlated with age. Suicide mortality worldwide in 2000 was more than twice as high for older men (50.0 per 100,000 men ages 75 years and older) as for young men (22.0 per 100,000 men ages 15–24 years), according to pooled data from the WHO (2000). Among women, although the incidence of suicide mortality has long been lower than among men, the age differential in suicide mortality is greater. Older women were 3.22 times more likely to die from suicide than young women (4.9 per 100,000 women ages 15–24 years vs. 15.8 per 100,000 women ages 75 years and older) in 2000 (World Health Organization 2000).

Pooled data obscure significant differences among older persons across nations and in gender, racial, and rural-urban subgroups. For example, the marked age disadvantage of older women worldwide is weaker among U.S. women, where women ages 75–84 years were only 30% more likely to commit suicide than women ages 15–24 years in 2000 (National Center for Health Statistics 2006). In the United States, the age disadvantage is largely explained by the elevated rates of suicide among white men older than 75 years (see Figure 2–2). Yet minority elders are not uniformly advantaged. African American men are at highest risk of suicide mortality both at ages 20–30 years and at ages 70 years and older (a bimodal distribution); older African

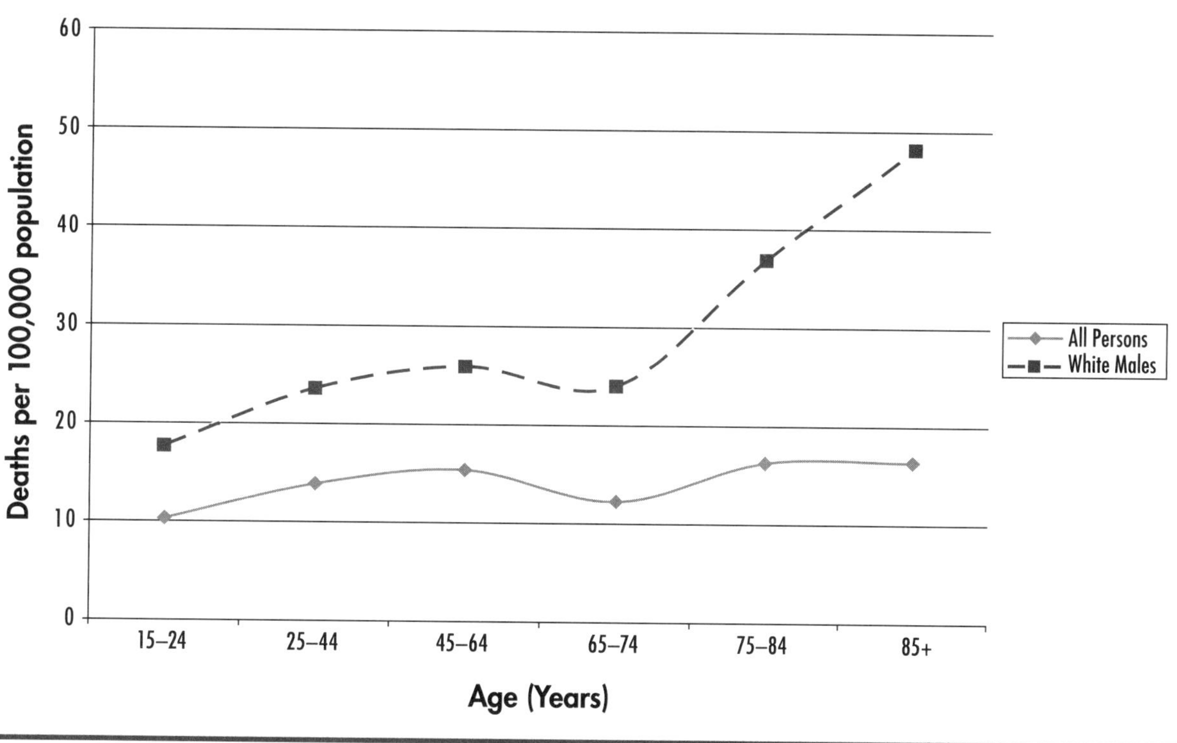

FIGURE 2–2. Suicide deaths per 100,000 in the United States by age in 2004.
Source. Data from National Center for Health Statistics 2006.

American women are at lower risk than women ages 30–34 years (Joe 2006). Rural dwelling also has had differential effects on suicide mortality by age and gender. Rural dwelling has increasingly protected older U.S. women (compared to younger women) against suicide mortality over time but has elevated the risk for all U.S. men, regardless of age (Singh and Siahpush 2002).

Age-related increases in suicide rates have flattened over the past century. Although suicide has continued to increase with age generally, later-born cohorts demonstrate lower suicide rates as they age across time than earlier cohorts. For example, Haas and Hendin (1983) showed that persons born in the United States in 1923 had lower suicide mortality rates at every age until 1970 than did persons born in the United States in 1908. Joe (2006) also showed a declining trend in late-life suicide mortality across successive birth cohorts among U.S. African Americans.

Suicide trends vary not only by age and cohort but also by historical period. Cross-national studies have provided intriguing comparisons of change in suicide mortality rates over time, as well as hypotheses about the period effects of historical events and policies on rate changes during the last half century (see Table 2–6). For example, the sharply declining trends in suicide mortality since 1950 among persons ages 60 years and older in England and Wales were briefly but significantly interrupted in the late 1970s and early 1980s—a period coinciding with economic recession in the British Isles (Gunnell et al. 2003). WHO mortality data collected between 1979 and 1999 from 10 Western countries with populations greater than 16 million showed that suicide mortality among persons ages 65 and older declined in 7 of these, and most dramatically in England and Wales, where psychogeriatric and community services were expanded coincidentally (Pritchard and Hansen 2005). Likewise, falling rates in northern Finland are hypothesized to have resulted from targeted prevention measures during the 1990s (Koponen et al. 2007). However, even where rates of suicide mortality fell overall between 1990 and 2000, rates among the oldest-old men (ages 85+ years) were stubbornly resistant to change; in Austria, for example, rates remained seven times higher than the average total Austrian suicide rate (Etzerdorfer et al. 2005). These researchers noted the absence of an Austrian national suicide prevention plan and the need for a strategy targeted at restricting access to firearms, which, with jumping from heights, have replaced poisoning and hangings as the most prevalent suicide methods in Austria.

TABLE 2–6. Change in risk of suicide mortality over historical time period by race[a], gender[a], and age[b] subgroups of the older populations in specific countries

			Relative risk/trend[c]						
			Men			*Women*			
Locale	Historical time period	Race	Young-old	Mid-old	Old-old	Young-old	Mid-old	Old-old	Reference
Australia	1979–1999		0.91	1.05		0.58	0.84		Pritchard and Hansen 2005
Australia	1986–2000		0.80	0.79	0.85	0.69	0.70	0.59	Hall et al. 2003
Austria	1990–2000		–	1.15	1.25	–	Decrease		Etzerdorfer et al. 2005
Brazil	1980–2000		1.23	1.14		0.80	0.70		Mello-Santos et al. 2005
Canada	1979–1999		0.76	0.95		0.56	0.78		Pritchard and Hansen 2005
England/Wales	1979–1999		0.56	0.78		0.31	0.42		Pritchard and Hansen 2005
England/Wales	1950–1998			0.29			0.29		Gunnell et al. 2003
Finland	1989–2003				0.48				Koponen et al. 2007
France	1979–1999		0.77	0.93		0.65	0.81		Pritchard and Hansen 2005
Germany	1979–1999		0.65	0.99		0.47	0.73		Pritchard and Hansen 2005
India	1995–1997			1.21			1.20		Mayer and Ziaian 2002
Italy	1979–1999		0.87	1.17		0.71	0.96		Pritchard and Hansen 2005
Japan	1979–1999		0.96	0.78		0.62	0.59		Pritchard and Hansen 2005
Japan	1970–2002		1.00		0.56	0.56		0.39	Yamamura et al. 2006
Netherlands	1979–1999		0.70	0.77		0.58	0.77		Pritchard and Hansen 2005
Quebec, Canada	1950–1999			6.3			3.7		Preville et al. 2005
Russia	1984–1986			Decrease			Decrease		Nemtsov 2003
Russia	1991–1994		Increase	Stable	Increase	Increase	Stable	Increase	Nemtsov 2003
South Africa	1968–1990	Asian	Decrease+inconsistent increase			Inconsistent			Flisher et al. 2004
		White	Marked consistent increase			Consistent increase			
		Colored/Black	Stable			Stable			
South Korea	1985–2000		Stable	Increasing		Stable	Increasing		Chiu et al. 2003
Spain	1979–1999		1.48	1.54		1.49	1.59		Pritchard and Hansen 2005
United States	1979–1999		0.88	1.0		0.72	0.94		Pritchard and Hansen 2005
	1981–2002	African American	Inconsistent			–	–	–	Joe 2006

[a]Where specified.
[b]Age group cutoffs vary by study, generally 60–74 years (young-old), 75–84 years (mid-old), 85+ years (old-old); risk estimates/trends that overlie gender and/or age group columns indicate that only pooled data were reported.
[c]Relative risk <1.00 indicates declining risk over the historical time period indicated.

Interpretations of the findings from historical studies are often prey to the ecologic fallacy, which assumes that putative exposures and effects measured in aggregates and not for individuals are causal. That suicide prevention measures coincide with a drop in suicide mortality rates—or conversely that economic recession coincides with a rise in rates—does not indicate causality. Such conclusions require well-designed etiological studies.

Etiological Studies

One of the basic contributions of epidemiology is to identify determinants of disease or to identify causal factors that can offer the possibility of disease prevention (MacMahon and Pugh 1970). Within geriatric psychiatry, it is important to identify factors that can either predispose individuals to developing psychiatric disorders or precipitate such disorders. These disorders may have their initial onset in late life, or the disorders may have an early onset and recur later in life. Other factors can be identified that are associated with the prevalence of a disorder, but the antecedent-consequent relationship has not been established. For practical purposes in this discussion, we identify all of these as risk factors. These factors generally fall into several categories, including genetic or biological factors, environmental or chemical factors, and social factors. Examples of each are provided in the following sections. In addition, the presence of a comorbid physical or mental condition or disorder often leads to the development of psychiatric symptoms or another disorder, and these are described in chapters related to specific disorders throughout this textbook.

Genetic Factors

Heston et al. (1981) studied the relatives of 125 probands who had dementia of the Alzheimer's type (as identified at autopsy). The risk of dementia in first-degree relatives varied with the age of the person at the onset of dementia. Those persons who were first-degree relatives of someone with Alzheimer's disease were more likely to develop the disease earlier in life, suggesting that the inherited form of Alzheimer's disease is associated with an accelerated onset. Barclay et al. (1986) reported that a family history for dementia was positive in 35.9% of the patients with Alzheimer's disease, compared with 5.6% of the individuals who were cognitively intact.

Genetic research in Alzheimer's disease and dementia has focused on the ε4 allele of the apolipoprotein E (*APOE*) gene (Evans et al. 1997; A.M. Saunders et al. 1993). That is, the ε4 allele is a susceptibility gene in that some (but not all) persons with the allele develop dementia. Some studies have also found a relationship between the *APOE*E3* and *APOE*E4* alleles and the onset of late-life depression (Krishnan et al. 1996), whereas other studies did not find a link between genotype and change in the number of depressive symptoms (Mauricio et al. 2000).

Investigators have proposed an association between early-onset Alzheimer's disease and Down syndrome, suggesting a common biological or genetic mechanism. Heyman et al. (1983) studied 68 patients with Alzheimer's disease who had experienced clinical onset before age 70 years. Secondary cases of dementia were found in 17 (25%) of the families, affecting 22 of the probands' siblings and parents. An increased frequency of Down syndrome was observed among relatives of the probands, at a rate of 3.6 per 1,000 compared with the expected rate of 1.3 per 1,000.

Current research that focuses on the interaction between genetic and environmental factors and the occurrence of disease (Hernandez and Blazer 2006) can potentially offer new information on the etiology of psychiatric disorders. One example of a possible gene-environment interaction is evident in Hendrie et al.'s (2004) work in Indianapolis, Indiana, and Ibadan, Nigeria. Hendrie et al. reported a significant association between *APOE*E4* and Alzheimer's disease in African Americans in Indianapolis, but the alleles were not associated with an increased risk for Alzheimer's disease among Yoruba living in Ibadan, suggesting that an interaction between gene and environment may play a role in the etiology of the disease. Gatz et al. (1992) studied genetic and environmental contributions to self-reported depressive symptoms in older adults in a sample of twin pairs. Genetic influence accounted for 16% of the variance in depression score and for 19% of the variance in psychomotor and somatic complaints, but heritability was minimal for depressed mood and well-being. Although shared experiences contributed to the variance, the most important correlate of late-life depressive symptoms was nonshared experiences.

Physical Agents in the Environment

Physical agents in the environment may lead to cognitive problems and other psychiatric symptoms. One such relationship is the effect of diet on psychiatric disorder. Susser and Lin (1992) examined the risk of schizophrenia onset in birth cohorts exposed to prenatal food deprivation during the Dutch Hunger Winter of 1944–1945. They reported an increased risk of schizophrenia for women in the area of the country exposed to severe famine. Researchers examined the effect of this Dutch famine on brain morphology and found that nutritional deficiency during the first trimester of gestation was associated with brain abnormalities, particularly white matter hyperintensities, and aberrant early brain development in patients with schizophrenia, suggesting that stunted brain development during the first trimester may be a risk factor for developing schizophrenia (Hulshoff Pol et al. 2000).

Environmental agents such as bodily injuries can also be factors. Studies of the association between prior head trauma and the development of Alzheimer's disease have been inconclusive. Mortimer et al. (1991) pooled data from 11 retrospective studies and concluded that head trauma increased the risk of Alzheimer's disease (relative risk=1.82). In a prospective study of 6,645 patients ages 55 years and older, however, mild head trauma was not a risk factor for dementia or Alzheimer's disease (Mehta et al. 1999). Epidemiologic studies have also suggested that elevated levels of aluminum and other metals such as copper, zinc, and iron in the brain may be a risk factor for the development or progression of Alzheimer's disease (Shcherbatykh and Carpenter 2007). Other chemical agents such as medication have the potential to affect the brain. Estrogen has been shown in some studies to have a protective effect against dementia (Kawas et al. 1997), yet other studies have found that estrogen was not protective against cognitive decline (Fillenbaum et al. 2001). Yaffe et al. (2005) reported that older women taking 120 mg/day of raloxifene had a 33% lower 3-year risk of mild cognitive impairment and somewhat lower risk of Alzheimer's disease and any cognitive impairment. Some research has found a protective effect of nonsteroidal anti-inflammatory drug use in Alzheimer's disease (Anthony et al. 2000). The use of statins and similar lipid-lowering agents was associated with a lower risk of dementia and Alzheimer's disease among those younger than age 80 years (but not those ages 80 years and older) in the Canadian Study of Health and Aging (Rockwood et al. 2002).

Social Factors

By far the most frequently investigated environmental factors associated with psychiatric disorders are social factors. Many investigators believe that the changing roles and circumstances of older adults can cause stress and thereby contribute to the onset of psychiatric disorders and cognitive difficulties. In a study of 986 community-dwelling older adults, Blazer (1980b) found the crude estimate of relative risk for mental health impairment to be 2.14, given a life event score of 150 or greater on the Schedule of Recent Events (Holmes and Rahe 1967). A relative risk of 1.73 ($P<0.01$) was estimated when a binary regression procedure was used, controlling for physical health, economic status, social support, and age. In a study of individuals ages 55 years and older, Murrell et al. (1983) found that social factors, including widowhood, divorce, separation, and decreased income, were related to depressive symptomatology in the community. In the Hispanic EPESE, economic stressors and conditions such as chronic financial strain were associated with depressive symptoms in Mexican American elders (Black et al. 1998).

In the Longitudinal Aging Study Amsterdam (LASA), major depression was associated with unmarried status, functional limitation, perceived loneliness, internal locus of control, poorer self-perceived health, and lack of instrumental social support (Beekman et al. 1995). In the Duke ECA study, the recent experience of negative life events and poor social support were associated with major depression (Blazer et al. 1987a). Perceived health and loneliness were also some of the correlates of depressive symptoms in the Leiden 85-plus study (Stek et al. 2004). Depression has also been linked with variables suggesting increased dependency (Anstey et al. 2007). Impairment or dissatisfaction with one's social network has been reported to be associated with anxiety symptoms in late life (Forsell and Winblad 1998). Nevertheless, the study of social factors in relation to psychiatric disorders must not be viewed simplistically. The mitigating effect of social support, the perception of a stressful life event (as well as the actual occurrence of the event), the expectancy of an event, and the perceived importance of an event all may contribute to the effect of environmental stress on the older adult.

Epidemiologic research has also focused on the impact of contextual factors such as the poverty level or residential stability of the neighborhood and the prevalence of psychiatric disorders. More than 60 years ago, Faris and Dunham (1939) looked at the addresses of psychiatric patients and found that patients with schizophrenia and substance use disorders tended to have addresses in areas within Chicago that were more deteriorated and disorganized than the neighborhoods of those patients with affective disorders. But these and similar findings were subject to "ecologic fallacy" or drawing conclusions about individuals from group data. Improved statistical software has made the process of separating individual and contextual effects easier, and more recent studies have explored the association between neighborhood characteristics and psychiatric symptoms in older adults. For example, using data from the New Haven EPESE, Kubzansky et al. (2005) reported that living in a poor neighborhood increased the risk of depressive symptoms beyond that attributed to individual vulnerabilities, and that the presence of more older adults in the neighborhood was protective.

From these examples, it is clear that both psychiatric disorders and symptoms in late life can have multiple causes and that these factors may interact with one another to produce adverse outcomes. Skoog (2004) suggested that the science of epidemiology has much to contribute to increased knowledge of the etiology of mental disorders in older adults and that to maximize that contribution, future population studies should be longitudinal and should include assessments of psychosocial risk factors as well as biological markers such as brain imaging, neurochemical analyses, and genetic information.

Health Service Utilization

Community-based epidemiologic studies provide an opportunity not only to estimate the prevalence of psychiatric disorders, but also to examine service use among those with psychiatric symptoms or disorders. More than two decades ago, in a study of three of the ECA communities (New Haven, Connecticut; Baltimore, Maryland; and St. Louis, Missouri), Shapiro et al. (1984) found that 6%–7% of older adults had made a visit to a health care provider for mental health reasons during the previous 6 months. Those in the group age 65 years or older infrequently received care from mental health specialists, even if they were identified in the community as having a DSM-III psychiatric disorder or severe cognitive impairment. German et al. (1985) analyzed the ECA data from Baltimore in greater detail. Of those persons younger than age 65 years, 8.7% had made a visit to a specialty or primary care provider for mental health care during the 6 months prior to the interview. For those ages 64–74 years, the rate was 4.2%; of those ages 75 and older, only 1.4% received such care. In the age 75 and older group, not one person among the 292 individuals interviewed saw a specialty mental health care provider. The investigators concluded that the likeliest source of care for older individuals with emotional or psychiatric problems was their primary care provider, within the context of a visit for physical medical problems.

Since the ECA was conducted, the United States has seen changes in the service sectors used for mental health care, with the general medical sector experiencing the largest proportional increase (Wang et al. 2006). In the NCS-R, participants ages 60 years and older were less likely than those in younger age groups to receive any mental health treatment in the last 12 months. Among those who received treatment, those age 60 years and older were less likely to receive treatment in the health care setting, and among those who did receive treatment in the health care setting, less likely to receive treatment in a mental health specialty (Wang et al. 2005b). Being in an older cohort was also associated with failure to make initial contact for mental health treatment after initial onset of the disorder, and with delay among those who eventually made treatment contact (Wang et al. 2005a). One study reported that older adults who met criteria for a psychiatric disorder were less likely than younger adults to perceive a need for mental health care, to receive specialty mental health care or counseling, and to receive referrals from primary care to mental health specialty care (Klap et al. 2003). Older patients seen in primary care who receive a diagnosis of depression are more likely to have increased total ambulatory costs, tests, and consultations than older primary care patients without this diagnosis (Luber et al. 2001).

In contrast to less treatment use by older adults than younger adults, the use of psychotropic drugs is high among older adults. Hanlon et al. (1992) found that 12.5% of community-dwelling persons older than 65 years during 1986 were taking central nervous system drugs, and psychotropic medications were the second most frequently used therapeutic class of medication. Blazer and colleagues noted an increase in the use of antianxiety, sedative, and hypnotic medication in community-dwelling older adults from 1986 to 1996 (Blazer et al. 2000b), as well as a simultaneous increase in the use of antidepressants in this population (Blazer et al. 2000a), and, more recently, reported that factors that predict antidepressant use changed during this period (Blazer et al. 2005).

Even though a high proportion of older adults use psychotropic medications, their disorders, such as depression, remain untreated. Unutzer et al. (2000) found in a study of health maintenance organization enrollees that 4%–7% of the older adults received treatment for depression but that most individuals with probable depression did not receive treatment. Similarly, Steffens et al. (2000) found in the Cache County study that only 35.7% of the older adults with major depression were taking antidepressants and 27.4% of those with major depression were taking sedative-hypnotic medications.

The value of community surveys does not end, however, with a description of patterns of health services use. Such investigations are especially useful for determining the need for service for noninstitutionalized and institutionalized elderly persons. By sampling elderly community-dwelling populations, researchers can collect data on the proportion of older adults with impairment, those with a need or a perceived need for services, and the current use of services. This information can be used by government and private agencies to chart effective assessment, treatment, and prevention patterns. This development is especially relevant to the care of older adults because they tend to be isolated, their psychiatric impairment may be masked, and they are less active advocates for their mental health needs than are younger persons. In summary, community studies of older adults have shown that the prevalence rates of psychiatric disorders and psychiatric symptoms in older adults are significant, and this has implications for all types of health service utilization.

Key Points

- The proportion of older adults in the United States is expected to dramatically increase over the next 50 years and to be accompanied by an increase in the number of older adults with psychiatric disorders.
- The prevalence of clinically significant psychiatric symptoms is generally higher than the prevalence of psychiatric disorders, and the prevalence of both symptoms and disorders is higher in clinical samples than in community samples. Psychiatric syndromes, rather than disorders, are the more realistic diagnostic entities in geriatric psychiatry.
- Alzheimer's disease is the most prevalent form of dementia, and its prevalence increases with age.
- Sleep problems, anxiety symptoms, and depressive symptoms are the most prevalent psychiatric symptoms among older adults.
- Besides dementia, anxiety disorders (particularly phobic disorders) are the most prevalent psychiatric disorders in older adults in community samples.
- Genetic, environmental, and social factors, as well as their interaction, can predispose individuals to psychiatric disorders in late life or be risk factors for the recurrence of psychiatric symptoms.
- The high suicide rate among older adults is due primarily to the high rate in older white males.
- Older adults are less likely than younger adults to seek treatment for mental health problems, and if treatment is sought, it is likely to be within the primary care setting.
- Even though a high proportion of older adults use psychotropic medications, psychiatric disorders, particularly depression, are generally untreated in older persons.

References

Alexopoulas G, Meyers B, Young R, et al: "Vascular depression" hypothesis. Arch Gen Psychiatry 54:915–922, 1997

American Psychiatric Association: Diagnostic and Statistical Manual of Mental Disorders, 3rd Edition. Washington, DC, American Psychiatric Association, 1980

American Psychiatric Association: Diagnostic and Statistical Manual of Mental Disorders, 3rd Edition, Revised. Washington, DC, American Psychiatric Association, 1987

American Psychiatric Association: Diagnostic and Statistical Manual of Mental Disorders, 4th Edition. Washington, DC, American Psychiatric Association, 1994

American Psychiatric Association: Diagnostic and Statistical Manual of Mental Disorders, 4th Edition, Text Revision. Washington, DC, American Psychiatric Association, 2000

Anstey KJ, von Sanden C, Sargent-Cox K, et al: Prevalence and risk factors for depression in a longitudinal, population-based study including individuals in the community and residential care. Am J Geriatr Psychiatry 15:497–505, 2007

Anthony JC, Breitner JC, Zandi PP, et al: Reduced prevalence of AD in users of NSAIDs and H_2 receptor antagonists: the Cache County study. Neurology 54:2066–2071, 2000

Bachman DL, Wolf PA, Linn RT, et al: Incidence of dementia and probable Alzheimer's disease in a general population: the Framingham study. Neurology 43:515–519, 1993

Barclay LL, Kheyfets S, Zemcov A, et al: Risk factors in Alzheimer's disease, in Alzheimer's Disease and Parkinson's Disease: Strategies for Research and Development. Edited by Fisher A, Hanin I, Lachman C. New York, Plenum, 1986, pp 141–146

Beekman ATF, Deeg DJH, van Tilberg T, et al: Major and minor depression in later life: a study of prevalence and risk factors. J Affect Disord 36:65–75, 1995

Black SA, Markides KS, Miller TQ: Correlates of depressive symptomatology among older community-dwelling Mexican Americans: the Hispanic EPESE. J Gerontol B Psychol Sci Soc Sci 53B:S198–S208, 1998

Bland RC, Newman SC, Orn H: Prevalence of psychiatric disorders in the elderly in Edmonton. Acta Psychiatr Scand 77 (suppl 338):57–63, 1988

Blazer DG: The diagnosis of depression in the elderly. J Am Geriatr Soc 28:52–58, 1980a

Blazer DG: Life events, mental health functioning and the use of health care services by the elderly. Am J Public Health 70:1174–1179, 1980b

Blazer DG: The epidemiology of late life depression. J Am Geriatr Soc 30:587–592, 1982

Blazer DG: Psychiatry and the oldest old. Am J Psychiatry 157:1915–1924, 2000

Blazer DG, Houpt JL: Perception of poor health in the healthy older adult. J Am Geriatr Soc 27:330–334, 1979

Blazer D, Kaplan B: Controversies in community-based psychiatric epidemiology. Arch Gen Psychiatry 57:227–228, 2000

Blazer DG, Bachar JR, Hughes DC: Major depression with melancholia: a comparison of middle-aged and elderly adults. J Am Geriatr Soc 35:927–932, 1987a

Blazer D, Hughes DC, George LK: The epidemiology of depression in an elderly community population. Gerontologist 27:281–287, 1987b

Blazer D, Swartz M, Woodbury M, et al: Depressive symptoms and depressive diagnoses in a community population. Arch Gen Psychiatry 45:1078–1084, 1988

Blazer D, Woodbury M, Hughes D, et al: A statistical analysis of the classification of depression in a mixed community and clinical sample. J Affect Disord 16:11–20, 1989

Blazer D, Burchett B, Service C, et al: The association of age and depression among the elderly: an epidemiologic exploration. J Gerontol A Biol Sci Med Sci 46:M210–M215, 1991a

Blazer D, Hughes D, George L: Generalized anxiety disorder, in Psychiatric Disorders in America: The Epidemiologic Catchment Area Study. Edited by Robins L, Regier D. New York, Free Press, 1991b, pp 180–203

Blazer DG, Hybels CF, Simonsick E, et al: Marked differences in antidepressant use by race in an elderly community sample: 1986–1996. Am J Psychiatry 157:1089–1094, 2000a

Blazer DG, Hybels CF, Simonsick E, et al: Sedative, hypnotic and anti-anxiety medication use in an aging cohort over ten years: a racial comparison. J Am Geriatr Soc 48:1073–1079, 2000b

Blazer DG, Hybels CF, Fillenbaum GG, et al: Predictors of antidepressant use among older adults: have they changed over time? Am J Psychiatry 162:705–710, 2005

Bruce ML, McAvay GJ, Raue PJ, et al: Major depression in elderly home health care patients. Am J Psychiatry 159:1367–1374, 2002

Burns BJ, Larson DB, Goldstrom ID, et al: Mental disorder among nursing home patients: preliminary findings from the National Nursing Home Survey Pretest. Int J Geriatr Psychiatry 3:27–35, 1988

Busse A, Bischkopf J, Riedel-Heller SG, et al: Mild cognitive impairment: prevalence and incidence according to different diagnostic criteria: results of the Leipzig Longitudinal Study of the Aged (LEILA 75+). Br J Psychiatry 182:449–454, 2003

Callahan CM, Hendrie HC, Tierney WM: Documentation and evaluation of cognitive impairment in elderly primary care patients. Ann Intern Med 122:422–429, 1995

Canadian Study of Health and Aging Working Group: Canadian Study of Health and Aging: study methods and prevalence of dementia. CMAJ 150:899–913, 1994

Chiu H, Takahashi Y, Suh G: Elderly suicide prevention in East Asia. Int J Geriatr Psychiatry 18:973–976, 2003

Christenson R, Blazer D: Epidemiology of persecutory ideation in an elderly population in the community. Am J Psychiatry 141:1088–1091, 1984

Copeland J: What is a "case"? A case for what? In What Is a Case: The Problem of Definition in Psychiatric Community Surveys. Edited by Wing J, Bebbington P, Robins L. London, Grant McIntyre, 1981, pp 9–11

Copeland JRM, Dewey ME, Wood N, et al: Range of mental illness among the elderly in the community: prevalence in Liverpool using the GMS-AGECAT package. Br J Psychiatry 150:815–823, 1987

Copeland JRM, Davidson IA, Dewey ME, et al: Alzheimer's disease, other dementias, depression, and pseudodementia: prevalence, incidence, and three-year outcome in Liverpool. Br J Psychiatry 161:230–239, 1992

Copeland JRM, Dewey ME, Scott A, et al: Schizophrenia and delusional disorder in older age: community prevalence, incidence, comorbidity, and outcome. Schizophr Bull 24:153–161, 1998

Copeland JRM, Beekman ATF, Dewey ME, et al: Depression in Europe: geographic distribution among older people. Br J Psychiatry 174:312–321, 1999

Cornoni-Huntley J, Brock D, Ostfeld A, et al: Established Populations for Epidemiologic Studies of the Elderly: Resource Data Book (NIH Publ No 86-2443). Bethesda, MD, National Institutes of Health, 1986

Cornoni-Huntley J, Blazer DG, Lafferty ME, et al: Established Populations for Epidemiologic Studies of the Elderly: Resource Data Book, Vol. II (NIH Publ No 90-495). Washington, DC, National Institutes of Health, 1990

Di Carlo A, Lamassa M, Baldereschi M, et al: CIND and MCI in the Italian elderly: frequency, vascular risk factors, progression to dementia. Neurology 68:1909–1916, 2007

Eaton WW, Kramer M, Anthony JC, et al: The incidence of specific DIS/DSM-III mental disorders: data from the NIMH Epidemiologic Catchment Area program. Acta Psychiatr Scand 79:163–178, 1989

ESEMeD/MHEDEA 2000 Investigators: Prevalence of mental disorders in Europe: results from the European Study of the Epidemiology of Mental Disorders (ESEMeD) project. Acta Psychiatr Scand 109 (suppl 420):21–27, 2004

Etzerdorfer E, Voracek M, Kapusta N, et al: Epidemiology of suicide in Austria 1990–2000: general decrease, but increased suicide risk for old men. Wien Klin Wochenschr 117:31–35, 2005

Evans DA, Funkenstein HH, Albert MS, et al: Prevalence of Alzheimer's disease in a community population of older persons: higher than previously reported. JAMA 262:2551–2556, 1989

Evans DA, Beckett LA, Field T, et al: Apolipoprotein E ε4 and incidence of Alzheimer's disease in a community population of older persons. JAMA 277:822–824, 1997

Faris RE, Dunham HW: Mental Disorders in Urban Areas: An Ecological Study of Schizophrenia and Other Psychoses. Chicago, IL, University of Chicago Press, 1939

Federal Interagency Forum on Aging-Related Statistics: Older Americans 2004: Key Indicators of Well-Being. Washington, DC, U.S. Government Printing Office, 2004

Federal Interagency Forum on Aging-Related Statistics: Older Americans Update 2006: Key Indicators of Well-Being. Washington, DC, U.S. Government Printing Office, 2006

Feldman HH, Jacova C: Mild cognitive impairment. Am J Geriatr Psychiatry 13:645–655, 2005

Fillenbaum GG, Hanlon JT, Landerman LR, et al: Impact of estrogen use on decline in cognitive function in a representative sample of older community-resident women. Am J Epidemiol 153:137–144, 2001

First MB, Spitzer RL, Gibbon M, et al: Structured Clinical Interview for DSM-IV Axis I Disorders, Research Version. Washington, DC, American Psychiatric Association, 1997

Flisher AJ, Liang H, Laubscher R, et al: Suicide trends in South Africa, 1968–90. Scand J Public Health 32:411–418, 2004

Folstein MF, Folstein SE, McHugh P: "Mini-mental state": a practical method for grading the cognitive state of patients for clinicians. J Psychiatr Res 12:189–198, 1975

Forsell Y, Winblad B: Feelings of anxiety and associated variables in a very elderly population. Int J Geriatr Psychiatry 13:454–458, 1998

Forsell Y, Winblad B: Incidence of major depression in a very elderly population. Int J Geriatr Psychiatry 14:368–372, 1999

Fried LP, Borhani NO, Enright P, et al: The Cardiovascular Health Study: design and rationale. Ann Epidemiol 1:263–276, 1991

Ganguli M, Dodge HH, Shen C, et al: Mild cognitive impairment, amnestic type: an epidemiologic study. Neurology 63:115–121, 2004

Gatz M, Pedersen N, Plomin R, et al: Importance of shared genes and shared environments for symptoms of depression in older adults. J Abnorm Psychol 101:701–708, 1992

German PS, Shapiro S, Skinner EA: Mental health of the elderly: use of health and mental health services. J Am Geriatr Soc 33:246–252, 1985

Graham JE, Rockwood K, Beattie BL, et al: Prevalence and severity of cognitive impairment with and without dementia in an elderly population. Lancet 349:1793–1796, 1997

Grant BF, Dawson DA, Hasin DS: The Alcohol Use Disorder and Associated Disabilities Interview Schedule DSM-IV. Bethesda, MD, National Institute on Alcohol Abuse and Alcoholism, 2001

Grant BF, Hasin DS, Blanco C, et al: The epidemiology of social anxiety disorder in the United States: results from the National Epidemiologic Survey on Alcohol and Related Conditions. J Clin Psychiatry 66:1351–1361, 2005a

Grant BF, Hasin DS, Stinson FS, et al: Prevalence, correlates, comorbidity, and comparative disability of DSM-IV generalized anxiety disorder in the USA: results from the National Epidemiologic Survey on Alcohol and Related Conditions. Psychol Med 35:1747–1759, 2005b

Grant BF, Hasin DS, Stinson FS, et al: The epidemiology of DSM-IV panic disorder and agoraphobia in the United States: results from the National Epidemiologic Survey on Alcohol and Related Conditions. J Clin Psychiatry 67:363–374, 2006

Gunnell D, Middleton N, Whitley E, et al: Why are suicide rates rising in young men but falling in the elderly? A time-series analysis of trends in England and Wales 1950–1998. Soc Sci Med 57:595–611, 2003

Haas AP, Hendin H: Suicide among older people: projections for the future. Suicide Life Threat Behav 13:147–154, 1983

Hall WD, Mant A, Mitchell PB, et al: Association between antidepressant prescribing and suicide in Australia 1991–2000: trend analysis. BMJ 326:1008–1011, 2003

Hanlon JT, Fillenbaum GG, Burchett B, et al: Drug-use patterns among black and nonblack community-dwelling elderly. Ann Pharmacother 26:679–685, 1992

Hanninen T, Hallikainen M, Tuomainen S, et al: Prevalence of mild cognitive impairment: a population-based study in elderly subjects. Acta Neurol Scand 106:148–154, 2002

Harris T, Cook DG, Victor C, et al: Onset and persistence of depression in older people: results from a 2-year community follow-up study. Age Ageing 35:25–32, 2006

Hasin DS, Goodwin RD, Stinson FS, et al: Epidemiology of major depressive disorder: results from the National Epidemiologic Survey on Alcohol and Related Conditions. Arch Gen Psychiatry 62:1097–1106, 2005

Hasin DS, Stinson FS, Ogburn E, et al: Prevalence, correlates, disability, and comorbidity of DSM-IV alcohol abuse and dependence in the United States: results from the National Epidemiologic Survey on Alcohol and Related Conditions. Arch Gen Psychiatry 64:830–842, 2007

Hazzard W: Introduction: the practice of geriatric medicine, in Principles of Geriatric Medicine and Gerontology. Edited by Hazzard W, Bierman E, Blass J, et al. New York, McGraw-Hill, 1994, pp xxiii–xxiv

Hebert LE, Scherr PA, Beckett LA, et al: Age-specific incidence of Alzheimer's disease in a community population. JAMA 273:1354–1359, 1995

Heeren TJ, Lagaay AM, Hijmans W, et al: Prevalence of dementia in the "oldest old" of a Dutch community. J Am Geriatr Soc 39:755–759, 1991

Henderson AS, Korten AE, Jacomb PA, et al: The course of depression in the elderly: a longitudinal community-based study in Australia. Psychol Med 27:119–129, 1997

Henderson AS, Korten AE, Levings C, et al: Psychotic symptoms in the elderly: a prospective study in a population sample. Int J Geriatr Psychiatry 13:484–492, 1998

Hendrie HC, Hall KS, Ogunniyi A, et al: Alzheimer's disease, genes, and environment: the value of international studies. Can J Psychiatry 49:92–99, 2004

Hernandez LM, Blazer DG: Beyond the Nature/Nurture Debate: Connecting Genes, Behavior, and the Social Environment. Washington, DC, National Academies Press, 2006

Heston LL, Mastri AR, Anderson VE, et al: Dementia of the Alzheimer type: clinical genetics, natural history, and associated conditions. Arch Gen Psychiatry 38:1085–1090, 1981

Heyman A, Wilkinson WE, Hurwitz BJ, et al: Alzheimer's disease: genetic aspects and associated clinical disorders. Ann Neurol 14:507–515, 1983

Holmes TH, Rahe RH: The Social Readjustment Rating Scale. J Psychosom Res 11:213–218, 1967

Hulshoff Pol HE, Hoek HW, Susser E, et al: Prenatal exposure to famine and brain morphology in schizophrenia. Am J Psychiatry 157:1170–1172, 2000

Jeste DV, Alexopoulos GS, Bartels SJ, et al: Consensus statement on the upcoming crisis in geriatric mental health. Arch Gen Psychiatry 56:848–853, 1999

Joe S: Explaining changes in the patterns of black suicide in the United States from 1981 to 2002: an age, cohort, and period analysis. J Black Psychol 32:262–284, 2006

Jongenelis K, Pot AM, Eisses AMH, et al: Prevalence and risk indicators of depression in elderly nursing home patients: the AGED study. J Affect Disord 83:135–142, 2004

Kawas C, Resnick S, Morrison A, et al: A prospective study of estrogen replacement therapy and the risk of developing Alzheimer's disease: the Baltimore Longitudinal Study of Aging. Neurology 48:1517–1521, 1997

Kessler RC, Ustun TB: The World Mental Health (WMH) Survey Initiative Version of the World Health Organization (WHO) Composite International Diagnostic Interview (CIDI). Int J Methods Psychiatr Res 13:93–121, 2004

Kessler RC, Berglund P, Demler O, et al: Lifetime prevalence and age-of-onset distributions of DSM-IV disorders in the National Comorbidity Survey Replication. Arch Gen Psychiatry 62:593–602, 2005

Klap R, Unroe KT, Unutzer J: Caring for mental illness in the United States: a focus on older adults. Am J Geriatr Psychiatry 11:517–524, 2003

Kleinbaum DG, Kupper LL, Morgenstern H: Epidemiologic Research. New York, Van Nostrand Reinhold, 1982, pp 320–376

Koenig HG, Meador KG, Cohen HJ, et al: Depression in elderly hospitalized patients with medical illness. Arch Intern Med 148:1929–1936, 1988

Koponen HJ, Viilo K, Hakko H, et al: Rates and previous disease history in old age suicide. Int J Geriatr Psychiatry 22:38–46, 2007

Krishnan KRR: Concept of disease in geriatric psychiatry. Am J Geriatr Psychiatry 15:1–11, 2007

Krishnan KRR, Tupler LA, Ritchie JC, et al: Apolipoprotein E ε4 frequency in geriatric depression. Biol Psychiatry 40:69–71, 1996

Kubzansky LD, Subramanian SV, Kawachi I, et al: Neighborhood contextual influences on depressive symptoms in the elderly. Am J Epidemiol 162:253–260, 2005

Kvaal K, Macijauskiene J, Engedal K, et al: High prevalence of anxiety symptoms in hospitalized geriatric patients. Int J Geriatr Psychiatry 16:690–693, 2001

Li S, Yan F, Chen C, et al: Is the dementia rate increasing in Beijing? Prevalence and incidence of dementia 10 years later in an urban elderly population. Acta Psychiatr Scand 115:73–79, 2007

Lindesay J, Briggs K, Murphy E: The Guy's/Age Concern Survey: prevalence rates of cognitive impairment, depression and anxiety in an urban elderly community. Br J Psychiatry 155:317–329, 1989

Livingston G, Kitchen G, Manela M, et al: Persecutory symptoms and perceptual disturbance in a community sample of older people: the Islington study. Int J Geriatr Psychiatry 16:462–468, 2001

Lopez OL, Jagust WJ, DeKosky ST, et al: Prevalence and classification of mild cognitive impairment in the Cardiovascular Health Study Cognition Study. Arch Neurol 60:1385–1389, 2003

Luber MP, Meyers BS, Williams-Russo PG, et al: Depression and service utilization in elderly primary care patients. Am J Geriatr Psychiatry 9:169–176, 2001

Lyketsos CG, Sheppard JE, Steinberg M, et al: Neuropsychiatric disturbance in Alzheimer's disease clusters into three groups: the Cache County study. Int J Geriatr Psychiatry 16:1043–1053, 2001

Lyness JM, King DA, Cox C, et al: The importance of subsyndromal depression in older primary care patients: prevalence and associated functional disability. J Am Geriatr Soc 47:647–652, 1999

MacMahon B, Pugh TF: Epidemiology: Principles and Methods. Boston, MA, Little, Brown, 1970

Manley JJ, Bell-McGinty S, Tang M-X, et al: Implementing diagnostic criteria and estimating frequency of mild cognitive impairment in an urban community. Arch Neurol 62:1739–1746, 2005

Mauricio M, O'Hara R, Yesavage JA, et al: A longitudinal study of apolipoprotein-E genotype and depressive symptoms in community-dwelling older adults. Am J Geriatr Psychiatry 8:196–200, 2000

Mayer P, Ziaian T: Suicide, gender, and age variations in India: are women in Indian society protected from suicide? Crisis: The Journal of Crisis Intervention and Suicide Prevention 23:98–103, 2002

McCusker J, Cole M, Dufouil C, et al: The prevalence and correlates of major and minor depression in older medical inpatients. J Am Geriatr Soc 53:1344–1353, 2005

Mehta KM, Ott A, Kalmijn S, et al: Head trauma and risk of dementia and Alzheimer's disease: the Rotterdam Study. Neurology 53:1959–1962, 1999

Mello-Santos CD, Bertolote JM, Wang Y-P: Epidemiology of suicide in Brazil (1980–2000): characterization of age and gender rates of suicide. Revista Brasileira de Psiquiatria 27:131–134, 2005

Morris JN: Uses of Epidemiology, 3rd Edition. London, Churchill Livingstone, 1975

Mortimer JA, van Duijn CM, Chandra V, et al: Head trauma as a risk factor for Alzheimer's disease: a collaborative re-analysis of case-control studies: EURODEM Risk Factors Research Group. Int J Epidemiol 20 (suppl 2):S28–S35, 1991

Murrell SA, Himmelfarb S, Wright K: Prevalence of depression and its correlates in older adults. Am J Epidemiol 117:173–185, 1983

National Center for Health Statistics: Health, United States 2006 With Chartbook on Trends in the Health of Americans. Hyattsville, MD, National Center for Health Statistics, 2006

Nemtsov A: Suicides and alcohol consumption in Russia, 1965–1999. Drug Alcohol Depend 71:161–168, 2003

Olafsdottir M, Marcusson J, Skoog I: Mental disorders among elderly people in primary care: the Linkoping study. Acta Psychiatr Scand 104:12–18, 2001

Ostling S, Skoog I: Psychotic symptoms and paranoid ideation in a nondemented population-based sample of the very old. Arch Gen Psychiatry 59:53–59, 2002

Palsson SP, Ostling S, Skoog I: The incidence of first-onset depression in a population followed from the age of 70 to 85. Psychol Med 31:1159–1168, 2001

Panza F, D'Introno A, Colacicco AM, et al: Current epidemiology of mild cognitive impairment and other predementia syndromes. Am J Geriatr Psychiatry 13:633–644, 2005

Parmelee PA, Katz IR, Lawton MP: Depression among institutionalized aged: assessment and prevalence estimation. J Gerontol A Biol Sci Med Sci 44:M22–M29, 1989

Pfeiffer E: A short portable mental status questionnaire for the assessment of organic brain deficit in elderly patients. J Am Geriatr Soc 23:433–441, 1975

Pifer A, Bronte D: Introduction: squaring the pyramid. Daedalus 115:1–12, 1986

Preville M, Boyer R, Hebert R, et al: Correlates of suicide in the older adult population in Quebec. Suicide Life Threat Behav 35:91–105, 2005

Pritchard C, Hansen L: Comparison of suicide in people aged 65–74 and 75+ by gender in England and Wales and the major Western countries 1979–1999. Int J Geriatr Psychiatry 20:17–25, 2005

Radloff LS: The CES-D scale: a self-report depression scale for research in the general population. Applied Psychological Measurement 1:385–401, 1977

Rait G, Fletcher A, Smeeth L, et al: Prevalence of cognitive impairment: results from the MRC trial of assessment and management of older people in the community. Age Ageing 34:242–248, 2005

Regier DA, Myers JK, Kramer M, et al: The NIMH Epidemiologic Catchment Area Program: historical context, major objectives and study population characteristics. Arch Gen Psychiatry 41:934–941, 1984

Regier DA, Boyd JH, Burke JD, et al: One-month prevalence of mental disorders in the United States. Arch Gen Psychiatry 45:977–986, 1988

Reynolds C, Frank E, Perel J, et al: Nortriptyline and interpersonal psychotherapy as maintenance therapies for recurrent major depression: a randomized controlled trial in patients older than 59 years. JAMA 281:39–45, 1999

Riedel-Heller SG, Busse A, Aurich C, et al: Prevalence of dementia according to DSM-III-R and ICD-10. Br J Psychiatry 179:250–254, 2001

Ritchie K, Artero S, Beluche I, et al: Prevalence of DSM-IV psychiatric disorder in the French elderly population. Br J Psychiatry 184:147–152, 2004

Robins LN, Helzer JE, Croughan J, et al: National Institute of Mental Health Diagnostic Interview Schedule: its history, characteristics, and validity. Arch Gen Psychiatry 38:381–389, 1981

Rockwood K, Kirkland S, Hogan DB, et al: Use of lipid lowering agents, indication bias, and the risk of dementia in community-dwelling elderly people. Arch Neurol 59:223–227, 2002

Rosch E: Principles of categorization, in Cognition and Categorization. Edited by Rosch E, Lloyd B. Hillsdale, NJ, Erlbaum, 1978, pp 3–27

Roses A: Apolipoprotein E affects the rate of Alzheimer disease expression: β-amyloid burden is a secondary consequence dependent on *APOE* genotype and duration of disease. J Neuropathol Exp Neurol 53:429–437, 1994

Roses A: Genetic testing for Alzheimer disease: practical and ethical issues. Arch Neurol 54:1226–1229, 1997

Rovner BW, Kafonek S, Filipp L, et al: Prevalence of mental illness in a community nursing home. Am J Psychiatry 143:1446–1449, 1986

Saunders AM, Schmader K, Breitner J, et al: Apolipoprotein E ε4 allele distributions in late-onset Alzheimer's disease and in other amyloid-forming diseases. Lancet 342:710–711, 1993

Saunders PA, Copeland JRM, Dewey ME, et al: Alcohol use and abuse in the elderly: findings from the Liverpool Longitudinal Study of Continuing Health in the Community. Int J Geriatr Psychiatry 4:103–108, 1989

Shapiro S, Skinner EA, Kessler LG, et al: Utilization of health and mental health services: three Epidemiologic Catchment Area sites. Arch Gen Psychiatry 41:971–978, 1984

Shcherbatykh I, Carpenter DO: The role of metals in the etiology of Alzheimer's disease. J Alzheimer's Dis 11:191–205, 2007

Sheehan B, Bass C, Briggs R, et al: Somatization among older primary care attenders. Psychol Med 33:867–877, 2003

Shoghi-Jadid K, Small G, Agdeppa E, et al: Localization of neurofibrillary tangles and β-amyloid plaques in the brains of living patients with Alzheimer disease. Am J Geriatr Psychiatry 10:24–35, 2002

Singh GK, Siahpush M: Increasing rural-urban gradients in U.S. suicide mortality 1970–1997. Am J Public Health 92:1161–1167, 2002

Skoog I: Psychiatric epidemiology of old age: the H70 study—the NAPE Lecture 2003. Acta Psychiatr Scand 109:4–18, 2004

Smalbrugge M, Pot AM, Jongenelis K, et al: Prevalence and correlates of anxiety among nursing home patients. J Affect Disord 88:145–153, 2005

Steffens DC, Skoog I, Norton M, et al: Prevalence of depression and its treatment in an elderly population: the Cache County study. Arch Gen Psychiatry 57:601–607, 2000

Stek ML, Gussekloo J, Beekman ATF, et al: Prevalence, correlates and recognition of depression in the oldest old: the Leiden 85-plus study. J Affect Disord 78:193–200, 2004

Stevens T, Livingston G, Kitchen G, et al: Islington study of dementia subtypes in the community. Br J Psychiatry 180:270–276, 2002

Stinson FS, Dawson DA, Chou SP, et al: The epidemiology of DSM-IV specific phobia in the USA: results from the National Epidemiologic Survey on Alcohol and Related Conditions. Psychol Med 37:1047–1059, 2007

Strauss J, Gabriel K, Kokes R, et al: Do psychiatric patients fit their diagnoses? Patterns of symptomatology as described with the biplot. J Nerv Ment Dis 167:105–113, 1979

Susser ES, Lin SP: Schizophrenia after prenatal exposure to the Dutch Hunger Winter of 1944–45. Arch Gen Psychiatry 49:983–988, 1992

Teresi J, Abrams R, Holmes D, et al: Prevalence of depression and depression recognition in nursing homes. Soc Psychiatry Psychiatr Epidemiol 36:613–620, 2001

Thomas VS, Rockwood KJ: Alcohol abuse, cognitive impairment, and mortality among older people. J Am Geriatr Soc 49:415–420, 2001

Trollor JN, Anderson TM, Sachdev PS, et al: Prevalence of mental disorders in the elderly: the Australian National Mental Health and Well-Being Survey. Am J Geriatr Psychiatry 15:455–466, 2007

Unutzer J, Simon G, Belin T, et al: Care for depression in HMO patients aged 65 or older. J Am Geriatr Soc 48:871–878, 2000

Wang PS, Berglund P, Olfson M, et al: Failure and delay in initial treatment contact after first onset of mental disorders in the National Comorbidity Survey Replication. Arch Gen Psychiatry 62:603–613, 2005a

Wang PS, Lane M, Olfson M, et al: Twelve-month use of mental health services in the United States. Arch Gen Psychiatry 62:629–640, 2005b

Wang PS, Demler O, Olfson M, et al: Changing profiles of service sectors used for mental health care in the United States. Am J Psychiatry 163:1187–1198, 2006

Weissman M, Klerman G: Epidemiology of mental disorders: emerging trends in the United States. Arch Gen Psychiatry 25:705–715, 1978

WHO World Mental Health Survey Consortium: Prevalence, severity, and unmet need for treatment of mental disorders in the World Health Organization World Mental Health Surveys. JAMA 291:2581–2590, 2004

World Health Organization: Composite International Diagnostic Interview, Version 1.0. Geneva, World Health Organization, 1990

World Health Organization: International Statistical Classification of Diseases and Related Health Problems, 10th Revision. Geneva, World Health Organization, 1992

World Health Organization: Distribution of suicide rates (per 100,000) by gender and age, 2000. Available at http://www.who.int/mental_health/prevention/suicide/suicide_rates_chart/en/index.html. Accessed September 4, 2007.

Yaffe K, Krueger K, Cummings S, et al: Effect of raloxifene on prevention of dementia and cognitive impairment in older women: the Multiple Outcomes of Raloxifene Evaluation (MORE) randomized trial. Am J Psychiatry 162:683–690, 2005

Yamamura T, Kinoshita H, Nishiguchi M, et al: A perspective in epidemiology of suicide in Japan. Vojnosanit Pregl 63:575–583, 2006

Yesavage JA, Brink TL, Rose TL, et al: Development and validation of a geriatric depression screening scale. J Psychiatr Res 17:37–49, 1983

Suggested Readings

Beekman ATF, Deeg DJH, van Tilberg T, et al: Major and minor depression in later life: a study of prevalence and risk factors. J Affect Disord 36:65–75, 1995

Blazer DG: Psychiatry and the oldest old. Am J Psychiatry 157:1915–1924, 2000

Jeste DV, Alexopoulos GS, Bartels SJ, et al: Consensus statement on the upcoming crisis in geriatric mental health. Arch Gen Psychiatry 56:848–853, 1999

Kessler RC, Berglund P, Demler O, et al: Lifetime prevalence and age-of-onset distributions of DSM-IV disorders in the National Comorbidity Survey Replication. Arch Gen Psychiatry 62:593–602, 2005

Krishnan KRR: Concept of disease in geriatric psychiatry. Am J Geriatr Psychiatry 15:1–11, 2007

Wang PS, Lane M, Olfson M, et al: Twelve-month use of mental health services in the United States. Arch Gen Psychiatry 62:629–640, 2005b

CHAPTER 3

Physiological and Clinical Considerations of Geriatric Patient Care

Robert M. Kaiser, M.D., M.H.Sc.

> Grow old along with me!
> The best is yet to be…
> —*Robert Browning*

> Will you still need me,
> Will you still feed me
> When I'm sixty-four?
> —*John Lennon and Paul McCartney*

The burgeoning of the geriatric population is an unquestioned demographic fact in the early twenty-first century. The retirement of the generation born after World War II, the baby boomers, is imminent, and policymakers must soon make crucial decisions (Peterson 2004). People older than 65 years constitute one of the fastest-growing segments of the U.S. population (Fried 2000; Hobbs 2001). The conquest of childhood infectious disease, improvements in sanitation, and better nutrition all have contributed to increased survival (McKeown 1979), and medical innovation also has had a beneficial effect on morbidity and mortality (Hunick et al. 1997). People are living longer, and the numbers of elderly grow with each passing year. The average life span has lengthened significantly (Fried 2000; Hall 1997; Vaillant and Mukamal 2001). Reaching the age of 100 years is no longer the anomaly it once was, and centenarians are now the focus of rigorous scientific investigation (Perls 2005). Careful and sophisticated longitudinal studies of elderly populations in the United States, such as the Established Populations for the Epidemiological Studies of the Elderly (Cornoni-Huntley et al. 1986) and the Baltimore Longitudinal Study of Aging (Shock 1984), have addressed how and why people are living to the eighth decade and beyond. Basic science has yielded fundamental anatomical, physiological, and genetic information about the aging process. A more complete picture of what aging entails has emerged.

The hallmarks of physiological change in elderly people are twofold: impaired homeostasis (also called *homeostenosis*) and increased vulnerability because of decreased reserve capacity (Armbrecht 2001; Taffet 1999). Homeostasis—that is, the ability of the organism to maintain a steady state—lessens with time. Consider two straightforward, representative examples: First, in elderly people, the baroreceptor reflex, which triggers vasoconstriction in order to maintain normal blood pressure, is less robust, and elderly people are less able to respond quickly to intravascular volume depletion. Second, when faced with repelling an invading microorganism, an older patient is less able to mount a strong immune response, therefore making it more difficult to fight infection effectively. Both of these situations clearly show that altered physiology leads the elderly patient to be more susceptible to harm. In the first example above, an older person might become lightheaded and possibly fall to the floor; in the second situation, the inability to repel a virulent streptococcus might lead to a severe upper respiratory infection or perhaps even a life-threatening pneumonia.

"Grow old along with me! The best is yet to be," proclaims Robert Browning optimistically in his famous poem. One might endorse Browning's belief that human relationships become deeper and richer with time, but the inevitability of physiological decline is also a reality that all humans must face as they age. Lennon and McCartney's rather endearing song, which has a young man wondering what life will be like in the seventh decade, underscores that widespread apprehension about approaching infirmity. As time passes, none of us can expect—like an aspiring Olympic athlete—to run faster, throw farther, and leap higher. Age brings with it expected decrements in function. This chapter details the various physiological changes that occur with "normal" aging—in other words, those progressive changes that take place over time but not as a result of disease. The following topics are covered:

- Physiological changes in the major organ systems
- Special implications for prescribing medications in elderly patients because of age-related physiological changes
- Chronic diseases
- Geriatric syndromes
- Fundamental principles of geriatric assessment that follow from those expected physiological changes

Physiological Changes in Major Organ Systems

Sensory Systems: Vision and Hearing

Older adults develop significant age-related changes in the eye, which have important effects on vision. The weakening of the ciliary muscle, combined with decreased curvature of the lens, results in a loss of accommodation; therefore, it becomes difficult for an individual to focus on near objects, and bifocals may be needed. It is also difficult for elderly people to adapt to light because of rigidity of the pupil and increasing size and opacity of the lens. As the lens changes with age, the increased scattering of light produces glare, which may be bothersome to elderly people. The pupil becomes smaller in diameter (more miotic) with age, due to atrophy of the dilator muscle fibers and increased rigidity of the blood vessels of the iris. This anatomical alteration in the pupil, combined with the increased thickness of the lens, contributes to the impairment of the visual performance of older persons at twilight. The growth in lens thickness causes a change in the absorption of light, with a decreased sensitivity at the violet end of the spectrum and a decreased ability to distinguish between blues and greens. Elderly people also show a decline in their ability to view objects at rest (static acuity) and in motion (dynamic acuity). Reportedly, 93.5% of individuals ages 40–44 years have a corrected visual acuity of 20/20 or better compared with 41.9% of those ages 70–74 years (Weymouth 1960). With age, the lens opacifies (i.e., becomes less transparent as a result of protein aggregations), and a cataract can form. Elderly patients are also at risk for age-related macular degeneration, which causes loss of central vision when drusen (yellowish-white deposits) accumulate in the retina. Age-related macular degeneration is the most common cause of blindness in elderly people (Haegerstrom-Portnoy and Morgan 2007; Harvey 2003).

In addition to changes in vision, older adults can expect alterations in the ear, which may lead to hearing loss in both high and low frequencies. In the middle ear, thickening of the tympanic membrane and degenerative changes in the ossicles occur, but these changes have an insignificant effect on function. In the inner ear, cochlear neurons are lost, and there are changes in the organ of Corti, basilar membrane, stria vascularis, and spiral ligament that also affect hearing. The degeneration of the organ of Corti is associated with high-frequency sensorineural hearing loss, whereas atrophy of the stria vascularis may cause hearing loss across all frequencies. The stiffening of the basilar membrane and atrophy of the spiral ligament both can result in loss of speech discrimination (Mills et al. 2003; Taffet 1999).

Cardiovascular System

The heart and blood vessels of aging people undergo significant anatomical alterations. These structural changes lead to changes in function. In addition, age-associated changes occur in the autonomic nervous system and in the response of the cardiovascular system to it, and these changes have important physiological effects. The ability of the heart to beat faster and pump efficiently and the ease with which blood vessels dilate or constrict are markedly affected. Both cardiac output and cardiac reserve decrease (O'Rourke and Hashimoto 2006; Seals and Esler 2000).

With age, human blood vessels stiffen. Anatomically, the intima and media both thicken with age, but according to autopsy studies, this thickening occurs disproportionately in the intima, with intimal hyperplasia observed. The vessels are thicker and less distensible. The ability of arterial vessels to transmit blood is not appreciably affected, but the cushioning effect of the arterial system is adversely altered. The physiological results are a greater pulse wave velocity, early reflected pulse waves, and higher systolic blood pressures and aortic pulse pressures in older individuals. Higher pressures can increase the load on the heart and lead to left ventricular enlargement as well as increased left ventricular oxygen requirements, thereby increasing the risk of congestive heart failure. There is an increased need for coronary blood flow oxygen, but there is a decreased ability to provide such flow due to decreased aortic pressure during diastole as well as a reduced period of diastole. This situation may cause cardiac ischemia by worsening ventricular function and cardiac perfusion during diastole. Increased pressures can also result in damage to the endothelium and media in the microcirculation of the brain and kidneys and may be connected with organ dysfunction (O'Rourke and Hashimoto 2006).

The function of the heart during exercise, including the force and rate of contraction, is mediated by the sympathetic nervous system. Age-related changes in that system affect the adaptability of the heart and blood vessels to stress. In general, sympathetic nervous activity rises in elderly patients, as evidenced by higher circulating levels of norepinephrine. Norepinephrine fills cardiac and vascular surface cell receptors, making them less sensitive. The β-adrenergic response of the heart during exercise is attenuated; a lower maximum heart rate and decreased force of contraction are the result. Similarly, large arteries do not respond as well to β-adrenergic stimulation, and their ability to dilate is reduced (Lakatta 1999; Seals and Esler 2000).

The older heart dilates during exercise to increase end-diastolic volume and maintain stroke volume, but cardiac output nonetheless declines with age. Because the heart stiffens, it empties less completely. This is the result of several factors, including increased afterload, decreased contractility of the heart, and the reduced inotropic effect of β-adrenergic stimulation to the heart. The decline in cardiac output also adversely affects oxygen use in older adults. The decline in cardiac function with age may explain 50% of the reduction in maximum oxygen consumption that occurs (Lakatta 1999).

Respiratory System

As individuals age, the chest wall becomes stiffer and less compliant. From age 24 to age 75 years, compliance declines by 31%. A number of factors contribute to stiffening of the chest wall, including degenerative joint disease and the calcification of the costal cartilages and chondrosternal junction. In older persons, osteoporosis may cause partial or wedge fractures of the vertebrae, with resulting kyphosis and an increase in the anteroposterior diameter of the thorax; these physical alterations can in turn adversely affect chest wall mechanics. When an older adult generates a breath, the relative contribution of the diaphragm and abdominal muscles is increased compared with the thoracic muscles, as a result of decreased chest wall compliance. Respiratory muscle function also declines because of changes in the rib cage, decreased chest wall compliance, and decreased elastic recoil of the lung. Respiratory muscles weaken with age, as a result of nutritional deficiencies, anatomical changes in skeletal muscle, and physiological decline (Janssens 2005).

Changes in the lung itself and in the control of breathing negatively affect the respiratory system. A loss of elastic tissue in the lung occurs, with a loss of elastic recoil, and the alveolar ducts and respiratory bronchioles enlarge. This enlargement leads to a loss of alveolar surface area; less tissue is available for gas exchange, and partial pressure of oxygen (PO_2) decreases with age but the decline is not uniform. The diffusing capacity of the lung also declines. Higher closing volumes make full expansion of the airways more difficult, especially in the dependent areas of the lung. The loss of surface area combined with decreased expansion results in ventilation-perfusion mismatch and decreased oxygenation. The control of breathing is also altered in elderly patients. Low oxygen tension and high carbon dioxide levels fail to provide the same physiological stimulus to breathe, but the decreased response to hypercapnia is not consistent in all studies.

In older people, the lung is less able to guard itself against infection (Taffet 1999). The mucociliary tree lining the respiratory tract is slower in ridding the lung of invading particles and microorganisms. With age, the person's ability to generate a sufficiently strong cough declines. The development of higher closing volumes further complicates defense against infection by making it harder to expel secretions from the lower areas of the lungs.

Some studies suggest that exercise training can slow the respiratory decline that occurs with aging. The age-related decrease in maximum oxygen consumption, as well as the decreased responsiveness to low oxygen tension or high carbon dioxide levels, can improve with exercise. Although exercise is helpful, it cannot prevent the ultimate decline in pulmonary function (Schwartz and Kohrt 2003).

Gastrointestinal System

As people age, numerous anatomical changes take place throughout the gastrointestinal tract, some of which are functionally significant (Firth and Prather 2002; Hall and Wiley 2003; Majumdar et al. 1997; Taffet 1999). For the most part, the production of saliva is adequately maintained. Receding gums make the teeth more susceptible to dental caries and subsequent tooth loss. The mastication of food may be incomplete. There are fewer myenteric ganglion cells, which affects the coordination of swallowing and may predispose some elderly patients to aspiration. The strength of esophageal contractions is diminished, but food nonetheless traverses the length of the esophagus uneventfully. The production of acid and pepsin by the stomach is mostly preserved. Both the stomach and the small intestine do not dilate as easily as a bolus of food enters, and transit through the large bowel may be slower. The small bowel is less effective at absorbing vitamins and minerals (such as vitamin D, calcium, and iron) and sugars (such as xylose and lactose). The motor function of the colon is not significantly affected by aging.

The liver, gallbladder, and pancreas continue to function well in elderly patients (Hall and Wiley 2003; Majumdar et al. 1997; Oskvig 1999; Taffet 1999). The liver loses hepatocytes and becomes smaller; those cells remaining are less able to regenerate. In general, the liver's ability to manufacture binding proteins and metabolize drugs is stable, although considerable variability can be found between individuals. The liver makes fewer vitamin K–dependent factors. Liver transaminases and alkaline phosphatase remain unchanged. Few significant anatomical changes occur in the gallbladder, and its function remains intact. In the aging pancreas, there is parenchymal fibrosis, acinar atrophy, and fatty infiltration but no resulting impairment in the synthesis of pancreatic enzymes and bicarbonate. The role of the pancreas in digestive function is therefore unaffected.

Endocrine System

Prolactin

Levels of prolactin in aging women have been reported to increase, decrease, or remain the same, whereas those in aging men are slightly increased. None of these changes is believed to have an effect on normal function (Gruenewald and Matsumoto 2003).

Antidiuretic Hormone

Aging causes significant changes in antidiuretic hormone (ADH) and the body's response to it, which alter the older patient's ability to excrete free water—resulting in hyponatremia—or to prevent volume losses—resulting in dehydration. Basal ADH levels are normal to increased in older adults; because renal free water clearance decreases with age, hyponatremia can more easily occur. However, when volume loss takes place, with subsequent hypotension, less ADH is released in older persons. In this particular clinical situation, other age-related changes are also at work to produce dehydration: 1) the kidney is less responsive to ADH, which impairs its effort to make more concentrated urine, and 2) aldosterone activity decreases and natriuretic hormone activity increases, both of which inhibit renal conservation of sodium and restoration of normal volume. The impaired thirst mechanism in elderly people further exacerbates this scenario by preventing them from drinking adequate amounts of fluid to correct free water losses, thereby contributing further to dehydration (Gruenewald and Matsumoto 2003; Oskvig 1999; Perry 1999).

Corticotropin and Cortisol

Basal corticotropin levels are normal in elderly people. Neither the corticotropin pulse frequency nor its circadian rhythm of secretion is altered. Stimulation of the hypothalamic-pituitary-adrenal (HPA) axis by exogenous corticotropin produces the expected cortisol response, but the cortisol secretion rate actually declines. Cortisol levels remain the same because of a decrease in the cortisol metabolic clearance rate. When subjected to stress, the HPA axis produces higher peak cortisol levels, which then dissipate more slowly; this occurs because the negative feedback of cortisol on the HPA axis is less effective (Gruenewald and Matsumoto 2003).

Adrenal Androgens

Both dehydroepiandrosterone (DHEA) and dehydroepiandrosterone sulfate (DHEA-S) decrease significantly in older adults. DHEA production peaks at age 20 and then declines (Fried and Walston 2003; Gruenewald and Matsumoto 2003).

Adrenal Medulla and Sympathetic Nervous System

In older people, secretion of norepinephrine increases and clearance decreases; plasma levels therefore increase. Epinephrine secretion and clearance both increase with age, so the level of epinephrine does not change. The level of sympathetic nervous system activity is increased in older persons, but both α-adrenergic and β-adrenergic receptors are less sensitive to stimulation (Gruenewald and Matsumoto 2003; Oskvig 1999; Seals and Esler 2000).

Renin, Angiotensin, and Aldosterone

An age-related decrease in plasma renin activity leads to reduced aldosterone secretion; aldosterone levels are thus reduced significantly. The rise in natriuretic hormone secretion in older adults also serves to decrease aldosterone levels; higher levels of natriuretic hormone suppress renin secretion, plasma renin activity, and angiotensin II, further lowering aldosterone secretion. In addition, natriuretic hormone itself can inhibit aldosterone secretion. The ability of corticotropin to stimulate aldosterone secretion is unchanged in the aging adult. The overall decrease in aldosterone adversely affects sodium retention in the kidney and predisposes elderly people to dehydration, as discussed earlier in this chapter. Another consequence of lower aldosterone levels is an increased likelihood of hyperkalemia (Gruenewald and Matsumoto 2003).

Growth Hormone

Growth hormone levels peak at puberty and then decrease by 14% per decade. Both a decrease in growth hormone–releasing hormone secretion and an increase in somatostatin are responsible for the decline in growth hormone. Insulin-like growth factor (IGF-1), which is produced by the liver and mediates the actions of growth hormone in the body, also diminishes gradually, at a rate of 7%–13% per decade. The decline in growth hormone with age may result in a decrease in both lean body mass and bone mass (Gruenewald and Matsumoto 2003; Perry 1999).

Parathyroid Hormone, Vitamin D, and Calcium Regulation

Older adults generally consume insufficient calcium in their diet; in addition, calcium is less efficiently absorbed in the small intestine. Vitamin D is essential to that absorption, and levels of vitamin D, 25-hydroxy (25,D) and vitamin D, 1,25-dihydroxy (1,25D) both decrease as a result of several factors, including 1) decreased sunlight exposure and less efficient photoconversion in the skin of 2-dehydrocholesterol to vitamin D_3; 2) insufficient dietary intake of vitamin D; 3) intestinal malabsorption of, or resistance to, vitamin D; 4) decreased 1-α-hydroxylase activity in the kidney; and 5) the use of medications that cause the liver to break down vitamin D.

The decline in both serum calcium and 1,25D levels triggers a compensatory increase in parathyroid hormone (PTH). PTH then 1) stimulates osteoclasts to resorb bone and 2) acts on the renal distal tubule to promote calcium reabsorption, thereby increasing serum calcium levels. PTH levels are higher in elderly individuals because of increased secretion and decreased renal clearance. This is thought to represent a form of secondary, rather than primary, hyperparathyroidism and can have a deleterious effect on bone mass in older patients (Perry 1999; Prestwood and Duque 2003).

Testosterone

As men age, the number of Leydig cells in the testis declines and testosterone secretion gradually decreases. Two other factors influence the age-related decline in testosterone: 1) a loss of the circadian variation in testosterone levels and 2) an increase in sex hormone–binding globulin levels, which limits the amount of free testosterone available. The action of the hypothalamus and pituitary on the testis also may be affected by aging. The pituitary in some older men may be less responsive to gonadotropin-releasing hormone, with lower follicle-stimulating hormone and luteinizing hormone levels as a result. The overall decline in testosterone causes a decrease in both the number of Sertoli's cells and daily sperm production; the sperm produced may have defects in motility as well as chromosomal abnormalities. The volume of the seminiferous tubules and the testis itself also decreases. Both libido and fertility may decline. Declining testosterone levels are thought to have less effect on sexual function than chronic medical or psychiatric illness, vascular disease, neuropathy, or medications. Declining testosterone may indeed adversely affect bone mass as well as muscle mass and strength in older men. The changes in testosterone secretion are common but not universal, and some men have normal serum testosterone levels as they age (Gruenewald and Matsumoto 2003; Perry 1999). Testing for testosterone deficiency is generally recommended only for those patients with clinical symptoms of hypogonadism, including both specific symptoms—decreased libido, erectile dysfunction, loss of body hair, small testes, loss of height, and reduced muscle size and strength—and nonspecific symptoms—decreased energy, depression, anemia, and decline in physical performance (Bhasin et al. 2006; Sadovsky et al. 2007). Screening all patients with erectile dysfunction for testosterone deficiency is not universally endorsed by experts; in fact, only 2% of men with erectile dysfunction have an endocrine disorder (Sadovsky et al. 2007). The Endocrine Society has established clinical practice guidelines for testosterone replacement (Bhasin et al. 2006). Replacement has a number of potential benefits, including improved libido, sexual functioning, and sense of well-being, as well as increased muscle mass and strength and better physical functioning (Matsumoto 2002).

Estrogen

Estrogen declines precipitously with menopause. Both fibrosis and involution of the ovary, as well as atrophy of the uterus and vagina, take place. The number of ovarian follicles declines, and a corresponding decrease in the secretion of both estrogen and androgens occurs; after menopause, the ratio of estrogens to androgens decreases. Menopause is also marked by an alteration in gonadotropin-releasing hormone secretion and high follicle-stimulating hormone levels, although luteinizing hormone levels remain the same. The loss of estrogen affects bone mass and places women at risk for osteoporosis. Women also lose the beneficial effects of estrogen on lipids, with rising low-density lipoprotein levels, and are at higher risk for cardiovascular disease. The lack of estrogen causes atrophy of the vaginal endothelium; the endothelium thins, less lubrication occurs with intercourse, and dyspareunia can result (Gruenewald and Matsumoto 2003; Perry 1999; Taffet 1999). The results of a widely cited randomized clinical trial, the Women's Health Initiative, demonstrated that estrogen replacement in postmenopausal women did not produce the expected reductions in cardiovascular events, stroke, fractures, and dementia that had been anticipated based on previous observational studies (Grimes and Lobo 2002; Nelson et al. 2002). Some obstetricians and gynecologists have nonetheless suggested that estrogen can be safely prescribed, at lower doses than those given in the Women's Health Initiative trial, for the relief of common postmenopausal symptoms such as hot flashes (Grimes and Lobo 2002).

Thyroid

Although there are age-related changes in the thyroid gland, these changes have no corresponding effect on thyroid function. The aging thyroid is more fibrotic and nodular in composition; there have been conflicting reports about whether its size increases, decreases, or remains unchanged. The renal and thyroidal iodide clearance rate declines in older persons. Thyrotropin has been reported to be higher, lower, or normal in elderly patients. A study of older men documented decreased responsiveness to thyrotropin-releasing hormone stimulation, with decreased thyrotropin production, but other studies have reported no change or an increase in response to thyrotropin-releasing hormone. Although the thyroid continues to make sufficient amounts of thyroxine (T_4), it fails to metabolize T_4 as well. The synthesis of T_4 actually declines, but its level is unchanged. Peripheral deiodination of T_4 to triiodothyronine (T_3) also decreases, and the level of T_3 declines by 10%–20% in elderly people. Reverse T_3 levels do not change. Thyroxine-binding globulin levels remain normal with age (Hassani and Hershman 2003; Perry 1999).

Insulin

Elderly patients have a tendency toward hyperglycemia. Circulating insulin levels may rise but are less efficiently utilized. Although insulin secretion by the pancreatic β cells is preserved with age, insulin clearance declines and insulin levels increase. Peripheral uptake of insulin is affected by insulin resistance in peripheral tissues; some of these tissues, particularly adipocytes, have fewer receptors, thereby decreasing their sensitivity to insulin.

The presence in the bloodstream of free fatty acids and inflammatory adipocytokines may also contribute to pancreatic β cell dysfunction. Elderly patients have decreased muscle mass and a higher percentage of fat and therefore an increased number of adipocytes. These notable changes in insulin secretion and tissue sensitivity in the periphery may lead to observed increases in fasting glucose in older adults. Another factor that leads to higher glucose levels is that IGF-1, which acts at insulin receptors to promote glucose uptake, is less abundant in older adults (Halter 2003; Perry 1999; Rizvi 2007; Taffet 1999). A number of other factors contribute to the increased prevalence of glucose intolerance and type II diabetes mellitus in elderly people, including changes in body composition, a reduction in physical activity, and increased comorbid illness and medication use. According to estimates of the Centers for Disease Control and Prevention, 10.3 million (20.9%) people ages 60 years and older in the United States have diabetes (Rizvi 2007).

Musculoskeletal System

In general, elderly people are weaker and less muscular. Sarcopenia, a decline in skeletal muscle mass, occurs. In the fourth decade, both muscle mass and strength begin to decrease. There are smaller numbers of type II fast-twitch fibers and fewer motor units and synapses; slow muscle fibers predominate. The motor units may enlarge. There are fewer and smaller ventral spinal motor neurons in the cervical and lumbar regions. Age, however, does not affect conduction velocity. Biochemical changes also occur, with decreased activity of glycolytic enzymes, including triosephosphate dehydrogenase, lactate dehydrogenase, glycerolphosphate dehydrogenase, and citrate synthase. Exercise may modify age-associated changes in muscle mass and strength. Sarcopenia places older people at risk for significant physical disability and a decline in their ability to perform activities of daily living and may ultimately undermine their ability to live independently (Loeser and Delbono 2003; Taffet 1999).

Elderly people also develop demonstrable changes in cartilage, tendons, and ligaments. Cartilage becomes less cellular with age. Alterations in the structure of proteoglycans affect the ability of these molecules to bind water and maintain the hydration of cartilage. Cartilage weakens as the number of proteoglycan monomers decreases and the protein links between the monomers are broken. An increase in collagen cross-linking and in the diameter of collagen fibrils occurs, which makes collagen stiffer; this stiffness results in the compression of proteoglycans, which further interferes with water retention. The overall effect of age-related changes in cartilage is to decrease both its tensile strength and its stiffness, adversely affecting its response to mechanical stress (Loeser and Delbono 2003; Taffet 1999).

Older tendons and ligaments may be stiffer because of an increase in cross-linking of type I collagen, and their water content is also decreased. These alterations may make them less able to withstand mechanical stress and more susceptible to fatigue. Biomechanical studies confirm the weakening of tendons and ligaments with age. These changes may decrease the range of motion of joints in older adults and make them more prone to tendonitis, ligament tears, and ligament ruptures (Loeser and Delbono 2003; Taffet 1999).

Age-related changes in the structure of both cortical and trabecular bone occur. Cortical bone becomes thinner and more porous; trabecular bone also thins, and whole trabeculae are lost. Bones are therefore weaker. As a person ages, the number of osteoblasts and osteocytes may decrease. Osteoclasts continue to function normally. Mechanical strain, an important stimulus to bone formation, has less of an effect in older people, and less bone is made. Older individuals are at increased risk for bone loss. Without estrogen replacement, women can lose significant bone mass after menopause. Elderly men with testosterone deficiency also may develop osteoporosis. Other factors that contribute to bone loss in both men and women include low peak bone density, poor calcium intake, secondary hyperparathyroidism (as discussed earlier), and insufficient exercise (Prestwood and Duque 2003).

Hematological and Immune Systems

Despite a decrease in bone marrow mass, the aging adult does not lose the ability to produce normal numbers of red blood cells, white blood cells, and platelets; however, when challenged to produce more red blood cells by the occurrence of blood loss or by the presence of hypoxic conditions, the bone marrow is less able to respond quickly. Red blood cells and white blood cells retain normal function. The red blood cell's capacity to carry oxygen is essentially unchanged. The white blood cell continues to engulf and kill bacteria, but the respiratory burst activity of polymorphonuclear neutrophils decreases with age. Platelets, however, may be more sensitive to substances that trigger them to form blood clots. Although the prothrombin time and partial thromboplastin time are unchanged, fibrinogen increases, and factor VII, factor VIII, and D-dimer are all elevated (Chatta and Lipschitz 2003; Taffet 1999).

When confronted with a new infection, older people are less able to mount an adequate cell-mediated response. With age, the thymus decreases in size, the number of T lymphocytes is diminished, and the individual's capacity to respond is adversely affected. Although the number of memory T lymphocytes increases with age, these are less easily activated. Natural killer cells do not function as well with age, with decreased cytotoxicity and reduced production of cytokines and chemokines. The humoral, or antibody, response in elderly people is also impaired. Older adults respond less vigorously to the first presentation of an antigen as well as to the reintroduction of antigen. There is decreased production of immunoglobulin-producing B lymphocytes and a loss of immunoglobulin diversity and affinity. These decreased primary and secondary responses may explain why older adults respond less well to vaccination (Aw et al. 2007; Miller 1999; Taffet 1999).

The body's primary defenses against infection are also affected by age. The thinner skin of elderly people is more vulnerable to injury; when the integrity of this barrier is compromised, surface bacteria may enter, resulting in cellulitis or a potentially serious bacteremia. The mucous membranes of the genitourinary and respiratory tracts of elderly people may become more easily colonized with gram-negative organisms, thereby serving as a potential source of infection. In urine, the amount, concentration, and acidity of urea are decreased, depriving the urine of an intrinsic defense against possible bacterial infection. Microorganisms also may find their way into the body by other means; those elderly patients with swallowing dysfunction may subsequently aspirate bacteria from the oral cavity, or those unable to produce an adequate cough will leave infectious material in the airways (Taffet 1999).

Renal System

As a person ages, a progressive decrease occurs in the size of the kidney due to fatty infiltration, fibrosis, and the dropout of cortical nephrons. The rate of decline of nephrons is 0.5%–1.0% per year; by age 60, 30%–50% of functioning glomeruli have been eliminated. Cortical nephrons become diffusely sclerotic. Glomeruli outside the cortex have fewer capillary loops and epithelial cells, but more mesangial cells. Other areas of the kidney may also be affected; interstitial fibrosis may adversely affect the renal pyramids. These losses do not automatically lead to a failure of the kidney to keep fluids and electrolytes in balance, but decreased reserve capacity does predispose the kidney to possible dysfunction or failure. Creatinine clearance, a widely accepted measure of kidney function, declines 7.5%–10.0% per decade (Oskvig 1999; Taffet 1999).

These anatomical changes have important physiological consequences, including the decreased ability of the kidney to acidify urine or to excrete an acid or a water load. The response of the renin-angiotensin-aldosterone system is less supple, renin activity declines, and less renin is produced in the face of decreased intravascular volume or a depletion of salt. The kidney is able to maintain its output of erythropoietin, but the hydroxylation of vitamin D declines. Levels of atrial natriuretic peptide rise. The kidney less reliably metabolizes hormones such as glucagon, calcitonin, and parathyroid hormone; drug metabolism is also significantly affected (Oskvig 1999; Taffet 1999), as discussed below in "Effects of Aging on Pharmacokinetics and Pharmacodynamics."

Considerations in Geriatric Prescribing

Effects of Aging on Pharmacokinetics and Pharmacodynamics

The effect of aging on pharmacokinetics (absorption, volume of distribution, clearance rate, and elimination half-life) and pharmacodynamics (the effect of a drug at a given dose) is crucial to understanding how drugs should be prescribed in the elderly patient (Schwartz 1999; Semla and Rochon 2006).

Pharmacokinetics

Absorption. Age has no significant effect on absorption. Although acid secretion, gastrointestinal perfusion, and membrane transport all may decrease and thereby *lower* absorption, gastrointestinal transit time is prolonged and *increases* absorption, and thus no net change occurs.

Volume of distribution. The volume of distribution is significantly affected by the changes in body mass and total body water that occur with aging. Older patients, with decreased lean body mass and total body water, have a smaller volume of distribution. This is particularly relevant when choosing proper doses for drugs, such as antibiotics or lithium, that are primarily distributed in water. Protein binding also can affect the volume of distribution; it is generally unaffected by age. In frail elderly patients, there may be significant decreases in albumin levels, which affect the binding of potentially harmful drugs such as warfarin, which must be vigilantly titrated.

Clearance rate. With age, renal mass and renal blood flow are decreased, resulting in a decline in glomerular filtration rate and creatinine clearance. This decrease in clearance can alter the rate at which drugs are excreted, and dosages must be appropriately adjusted. Certain drugs, such as nonsteroidal anti-inflammatory drugs and angiotensin-converting enzyme inhibitors, also may alter renal blood flow and thereby depress kidney function. Hepatic drug clearance is decreased by an age-related decline in hepatic blood flow; oxidative metabolism in the cytochrome P450 system is slower, thereby affecting elimination, but conjugation is not. Underlying hepatic disease and drug interactions also may significantly affect the metabolism of drugs by the liver.

Elimination half-life. The elimination half-life—the time required for the drug concentration to decrease by half—of certain drugs increases in older adults. This may require adjustment of the drug dosing interval. For example, aspirin, certain antibiotics (e.g., vancomycin), digoxin, and the calcium channel blockers (diltiazem, felodipine, and nifedipine) all have higher elimination half-lives, and the dosages must be adjusted downward.

Pharmacodynamics

The pharmacodynamic effects of drugs in elderly patients must also be considered. Frequently, older adults are more sensitive to medications, and drugs often must be given in lower doses. For example, because their response to anticholinergic drugs is increased, elderly patients develop side effects, including constipation, urinary retention, and delirium, more frequently than younger patients. Other notable examples of drugs with enhanced pharmacodynamic effects in elderly people include diazepam, morphine, and theophylline.

Chronic Disease in Older Adults

Some chronic diseases are more prevalent in older people, and these predominantly occur as a result of "usual aging." The cumulative effect of environment and heredity on the individual over time makes these diseases more common, and they account for significant morbidity and mortality. Among the most formidable and omnipresent are cardiovascular disease, cerebrovascular disease, and cancer. Hypercholesterolemia and hypertension are frequently diagnosed. As people age, weight and the incidence of obesity increase; patients are at higher risk for the development of type 2 diabetes mellitus. Aging also leads to an increased occurrence of joint problems, particularly osteoarthritis, which can result in chronic pain and the need for joint replacement. Elderly people can develop cataracts and macular degeneration and therefore impaired vision; hearing loss in the elderly, caused by either previous noise exposure or age-related anatomical changes in the ear, is also prevalent. Postmenopausal women and some hypogonadal elderly men are prone to develop osteoporosis. Benign prostatic hypertrophy, often with resultant urinary frequency and nocturia, becomes more of a clinical problem as men age. Polymyalgia rheumatica and temporal arteritis are collagen vascular diseases that occur often in elderly patients. The increasing prevalence of multisystem disease in the older patient can impose a substantial burden on the individual; in the face of already diminished physiological reserves, such an individual is considerably more vulnerable to declining health (Fried 2000).

Geriatric Syndromes

In addition, several common syndromes—known generally as *geriatric syndromes*—are found more frequently in older patients. Geriatric syndromes include falls, a multifactorial phenomenon that increases with age. Both elderly men and elderly women often develop chronic difficulty with control of urination, or urinary incontinence. Elderly people can be predisposed to delirium, a waxing and waning disorder of inattention; many elderly patients develop dementia, which doubles in the population every 5 years after age 65. The tendency of the elderly to use multiple drugs—or polypharmacy—is also a well-known geriatric syndrome. Frailty is a complex geriatric syndrome in which the health of the elderly individual declines after cumulative loss of physiological reserve, with sarcopenia, osteopenia, weight loss, and progressive functional deterioration. Four of the most characteristic geriatric syndromes—dementia, falls, urinary incontinence, and polypharmacy—are discussed in the following subsections; frailty is discussed later in conjunction with geriatric assessment.

Memory Loss and Dementia

Various studies have documented a decline in cognitive function with age. Such decline may occur in several areas, including intelligence, ability to maintain attention, language, memory, learning, visuospatial function, and psychomotor function. These deficits do not occur uniformly across all areas and do not occur in every person. Although the capacity to recognize words does not change in older age, elderly adults are less able to name items. Short-term, or working, memory is unaffected, but there may be problems in accessing data from long-term memory. The time needed to learn new information is increased for older adults. Visuospatial tasks are more difficult, and both motor speed and response times decline with aging. Some evidence suggests that executive function, or the ability to conceive, organize, and carry out a plan or activity, may remain intact in the elderly (Craft et al. 2003).

Dementia is a prevalent condition in elderly people but not a result of normal aging (Morris 1999). Dementia is defined as the development of significant deficits in two or more areas of cognition—an impairment of memory and at least one other area, such as abstract thinking, judgment, language, or visuospatial ability—that are severe enough to affect the individual's day-to-day functioning (Nyenhuis and Gorelick 1998). With the inevitable decline in intellectual functioning and in the ability to perform activities of daily living that occurs, dementia poses particular challenges for the clinician and special burdens for caregivers.

Two-thirds of all dementia is caused by Alzheimer's disease. Alzheimer's disease is present in about 5% of the population over age 65, and beyond that age, the prevalence of the disease doubles every 5 years (Klafki et al. 2006). Vascular dementia accounts for 15%–25% of dementia (Gomez-Tortosa et al. 1998), and Lewy body dementia constitutes 10%. The natural history and symptomatology of dementia vary according to its etiology (Marin et al. 2002).

The accurate diagnosis of dementia requires a comprehensive assessment by the clinician, including a detailed history; thorough physical, neurological, and mental status examinations; and a depression screen. Because the patient may have significant deficits, the history needs to be gathered from the patient along with someone who is extremely familiar with the history of the patient's illness, medications, and social history. The evaluating clinician should order laboratory studies to rule out vitamin B_{12} deficiency, syphilis, and hypothyroidism and should examine the patient for evidence of anemia, electrolyte abnormalities, renal failure, and liver dysfunction. This laboratory evaluation enables the clinician to detect reversible causes of dementia and uncover evidence of metabolic abnormalities that might point to a diagnosis of delirium rather than dementia (Marin et al. 2002).

Above all, the treatment of dementia involves the building of a proper support system for the patient. Pharmacological treatment of Alzheimer's disease may be appropriate in some cases. Acetylcholinesterase inhibitors, including donepezil, galantamine, and rivastigmine, have shown some effectiveness in clinical trials of patients with mild to moderate disease, with documented improvements in the Alzheimer's Disease Assessment Scale Cognitive Subscale score (Clark and Karlawish 2003; Frisoni 2001; Klafki et al. 2006; Sramek et al. 2001). Patients with moderate to severe Alzheimer's disease who took memantine, an *N*-methyl-D-aspartate (NMDA) receptor inhibitor, in randomized clinical trials demonstrated a benefit in measures of cognition and function (Klafki et al. 2006; McShane et al. 2006; Tariot et al. 2004). New drugs that target amyloid production and tau phosphorylation are being investigated but are not yet approved for clinical use (Klafki et al. 2006). Patients with Alzheimer's disease are at risk for the development of depressive symptoms as well as major depression, for which clinicians can provide effective medical treatment. Because agitation is also a prevalent symptom, particularly in patients with late disease, this symptom also may require treatment; atypical antipsychotic agents such as risperidone may be helpful in this context (Defilippi and Crismon 2000; Tune 2001).

Falls

Falls are a common phenomenon in older patients; every year, one-half of all nursing home residents and one-third of all community-dwelling elderly have a fall. These falls produce notable morbidity: 2% cause hip fractures, 5% cause other fractures, and 10% cause head injuries or other significant injuries. Half of the persons who fall experience minor injuries. In the aftermath of falls, disability may result. Those people who fall frequently are at risk for a decline in their instrumental activities of daily living and their activities of daily living (assessment of such functions is discussed later in this chapter in "Fundamentals of Geriatric Assessment"). A decline in these functions can ultimately undermine independence and also might result in hospitalization (Fried 2000; King and Tinetti 1995; Rubenstein and Josephson 2006; Rubenstein et al. 1994).

Falls are generally multifactorial and are caused by 1) intrinsic factors, 2) situational factors, 3) extrinsic factors, and 4) medications (Alexander 1999; King and Tinetti 1995). *Intrinsic factors* are disease-specific deficits in an individual patient that might contribute to falling;

these factors include neurological problems (central, neuromuscular, vestibular, visual, and proprioceptive) as well as systemic illness. *Situational factors* relate to the particular activity that is taking place. *Extrinsic factors* relate to the demands and hazards of a particular environment. *Medications* may adversely affect mental status, cognition, balance, circulation, and neuromuscular function and therefore predispose patients to falls.

The proper evaluation of a fall requires 1) taking a detailed history and review of systems and 2) performing a thorough physical examination and neurological examination (Rubenstein and Josephson 2006). The fall may indeed be a nonspecific presentation of a serious medical illness such as cardiac ischemia, infection, intravascular volume depletion, or hypothyroidism, and these should be initially considered. The clinician should ask about any symptoms and situational or extrinsic factors that might have led to the fall and determine exactly how the fall occurred. A medication list should be compiled. The physical examination should rule out any cardiac abnormalities; the neurological examination must carefully assess the patient for any deficits in vision, strength, sensation, joint mobility, balance, cerebellar function, gait, or proprioception.

The prevention of falls focuses on altering both intrinsic and extrinsic factors (Gillespie et al. 2003; King and Tinetti 1995; Rubenstein and Josephson 2006). With regard to intrinsic factors, one can 1) prescribe medication appropriately, 2) optimally treat disease, 3) improve balance and gait through physical therapy, and 4) improve conditioning and strength through exercise. With regard to extrinsic factors, one can 1) improve the environment by reducing or eliminating hazards, 2) monitor patients more carefully by increasing staff supervision and using motion detection, 3) eliminate restraints and the risk of injury they pose, 4) encourage patients to wear hip protectors, and 5) install protective flooring. Preventing falls ultimately requires multiple steps to produce successful results.

A meta-analysis of five randomized clinical trials suggested that vitamin D supplementation may reduce the risk of falls in ambulatory or institutionalized older individuals by more than 20% (Bischoff-Ferrari et al. 2004).

Urinary Incontinence

Urinary incontinence is a prevalent condition in older adults that causes significant morbidity and affects quality of life (DuBeau 2006; Tannenbaum et al. 2001). One-half of all nursing home residents and up to one-third of persons older than age 65 years who reside in the community carry the diagnosis. It is a condition with multiple causes, including age-related changes, genitourinary tract abnormalities, and coexisting illnesses.

Urinary incontinence can be classified into two main categories: 1) transient incontinence and 2) established incontinence. Transient incontinence is reversible and can be easily treated. For example, transient incontinence could be a consequence of an acute urinary tract infection, inadequately controlled diabetes mellitus, or a recent prescription of a diuretic and will resolve with the correction of those conditions. Established incontinence is further subdivided into the following three subcategories:

1. *Urge incontinence.* This is the most prevalent form of incontinence in older patients. Urge incontinence results from detrusor overactivity, sometimes with simultaneous impaired contractility. Detrusor overactivity is more common with aging but can also occur for other reasons, including neurological dysfunction (e.g., stroke) or irritation of the bladder (secondary to cancer, urolithiasis, or infection); it can also occur in elderly patients without other illnesses. Patients usually complain of a sudden urge to urinate. They also classically have urinary frequency and nocturia. They experience varying amounts of leakage.
2. *Stress incontinence.* Stress incontinence occurs when increased abdominal pressure, triggered by cough or sneezing, results in urinary leakage. It happens commonly in women with weak pelvic muscles, although it also may occur as a consequence of failed anti-incontinence surgery or vaginal mucosal atrophy in women or prostatectomy in men. It is a frequent form of incontinence among elderly women, ranking second.
3. *Overflow incontinence.* Detrusor underactivity and bladder outlet obstruction can both produce overflow incontinence. Detrusor underactivity can be caused by fibrosis of the detrusor muscle, peripheral neuropathy, disc herniation, or spinal stenosis. Detrusor underactivity is an infrequent cause of urinary incontinence in older adults. Urethral strictures, benign prostatic hypertrophy, and prostate cancer can cause bladder outlet obstruction in elderly men; this form of incontinence is the second

most prevalent in this population. Bladder outlet obstruction in women occurs much less frequently; the etiology is either the presence of a large cystocele or a history of anti-incontinence surgery.

In general, the treatment of incontinence in elderly people begins with behavioral interventions, which are followed by medical treatment. Surgery is considered the last option and is appropriate only for stress incontinence or outlet obstruction. Because urinary incontinence in the elderly is invariably the result of more than one cause, clinicians must appreciate that a single intervention may not be effective. Medications must be reviewed to determine whether they are contributing to incontinence. Patients must be cautioned against intake of fluids such as alcohol, coffee, tea, and soft drinks, which stimulate urination. Fluid restriction at bedtime may be appropriate to decrease nocturia.

Several specific interventions can be undertaken to treat the three forms of established incontinence:

1. Urge incontinence is best treated by frequent voluntary voiding and bladder retraining. Patients are placed on a voiding schedule that corresponds to their usual minimal interval of urination. They are taught how to voluntarily inhibit the urge to void. The goal of therapy is to increase gradually the interval between urination. For patients with cognitive impairment, bladder retraining is not appropriate; instead, timed voiding, scheduled voiding, or prompted voiding is instituted to decrease episodes of incontinence. For those who fail behavioral methods, medications such as oxybutynin, tolterodine, or imipramine may be helpful, but patients should be monitored carefully for anticholinergic side effects.
2. Stress incontinence is also amenable to nonmedical therapy. The mainstay of this approach is strengthening the pelvic muscles that support the urethra by performing repeated isometric exercises, thereby preventing urinary leakage. The patient should be referred to a physical therapist to initiate an exercise program. In some cases, medical treatment also may be helpful. In women, oral or topical estrogen sometimes has been beneficial. Propanolamine also can be a useful adjunct, although this is not an option in patients with hypertension. For women who fail physical therapy and medical treatment, surgery remains another option.
3. Overflow incontinence in men is most often the result of outlet obstruction due to benign prostatic hypertrophy, which can be treated by both medical and surgical modalities. In clinical trials, α-adrenergic blocking agents have been proven most effective for benign prostatic hypertrophy, although finasteride may be used as a second-line treatment. Transurethral resection of the prostate and prostatectomy are available options for those who fail medical therapy. In women, previous vaginal or urethral surgery may be the cause of overflow incontinence; this is surgically correctable by lysis of adhesions or unilateral suture removal. For cases of overflow incontinence caused by detrusor underactivity, appropriate interventions include avoidance of constipation as well as careful management of medications to exclude those that adversely affect detrusor function. Intermittent catheterization is most often recommended for treatment of detrusor underactivity.

Incontinence can ultimately have harmful medical consequences, including pressure ulcers, cellulitis, falls, and fractures. It can interfere with sleep. It can also result in sexual dysfunction and depression. The proper treatment of incontinence is therefore important and can yield significant benefits.

Polypharmacy

Defined as the simultaneous use of multiple medications or the prescribing of more medications than is clinically appropriate, polypharmacy is a common problem in older adults (Hanlon et al. 2001; Stewart 2001). The high use of drugs by elderly people is attributable to several factors. Older patients more commonly have chronic illness and experience more symptoms. They are also more frequent consumers of medical care. Drug use is also influenced by individual physician prescribing practices and by drug advertising. According to studies conducted in outpatients, elderly patients typically use 3.1–7.9 prescription and nonprescription drugs simultaneously. Polypharmacy carries with it certain consequences, including adverse drug reactions, drug interactions, and patient noncompliance; polypharmacy also increases the incidence of geriatric syndromes such as urinary incontinence, falls, cognitive impairment, and delirium.

Clinicians should take several steps to ensure that medicines are prescribed appropriately. They should take a careful, comprehensive medication history, including allergies and adverse drug reactions. Current use of alcohol, tobacco, and recreational drugs should be documented. Medicines should be prescribed only if they have a known benefit, and they should be given at the lowest effective dose. Instructions about medication use should be communicated clearly to patients. Patients taking medication should be carefully monitored for therapeutic effectiveness and for side effects (Semla and Rochon 2006). A systematic review of 14 clinical trials on optimizing prescribing in older patients reported that certain clinical interventions, including geriatric medicine services, the participation of a pharmacist in clinical care, and computerized decision support, had beneficial effects on prescribing (Spinewine et al. 2007).

Geriatric Assessment

The presentation of acute illness in older adults may not be typical of that in younger adults, and diagnosis in the geriatric patient therefore poses special challenges. For example, the geriatric patient may experience a change in mental status that suggests an acute neurological event but is instead due to pneumonia, urinary tract infection, myocardial infarction, or an adverse reaction to medication. The symptoms of the older patient are very often nonspecific. The astute clinician must consider this carefully when constructing a differential diagnosis. Something as straightforward as functional decline might signal a more serious medical problem. The physiological changes that occur in the elderly also may alter markedly how patients present. Older persons may not always develop fever and leukocytosis in response to infection, and the clinician must recognize other clues. The decline in functional reserve in many organ systems may predispose elderly people to harm even when a precipitating event seems minor. An elderly person with an impaired thirst mechanism may not replenish water losses quickly enough on a hot summer day, and dehydration could then happen very suddenly. The challenges of deciphering symptoms and preventing harm are heightened by the difficulty of gathering information from elderly patient. Those who are capable of giving a good history may be reluctant to report that anything is wrong; they may be depressed, fearful of a new diagnosis, convinced that their problem is nothing but "old age," or skeptical that any doctor or medical system can help them. In some cases, medical illness can exacerbate psychiatric illness—making the depressed patient more disengaged or the schizophrenic patient more agitated—and clinicians must be willing to consider diagnoses beyond mere worsening of an ongoing psychiatric condition and other possibilities.

Frailty

The sum effect of physiological decline in the older patient, combined with the cumulative and simultaneous burden of chronic disease, may result in the geriatric syndrome known as frailty (Cohen 2000; Hamerman 1999; Morley et al. 2006). *Frailty* has been defined by Fried and Walston (2003) as "a state of age-related physiologic vulnerability resulting from impaired homeostatic mechanisms and a reduced capacity of the organism to withstand stress" (p. 1489). Older patients have less pulmonary, cardiac, and renal reserve. They are less able to mount an effective immune response. They also have higher sympathetic nervous tone, which may increase cortisol production and further impair the immune system. In older patients, cortisol also may have catabolic effects on bone and muscle and result in insulin resistance. These patients also may have higher levels of circulating cytokines—such as interleukin-6, interleukin-1B, and tumor necrosis factor-α—which also may have deleterious catabolic effects on muscle. Changes in neuroendocrine function—the decline in sex steroids, growth hormone, and DHEA—can have corresponding negative effects on the size and strength of muscle and, in the case of estrogen and testosterone, on bone mass. The frail older individual is characteristically weak as a result of declining muscle and bone mass; a tendency toward a sedentary state may lead to deconditioning, further weakness, and fatigue. Poor oral intake may lead to weight loss and nutritional compromise, adding even more to the tendency to tire easily. Progressive weakness may adversely affect balance and the ability to ambulate. Ultimately, the frail older patient loses the capacity to function independently and may require skilled assistance in a facility outside the home. Frailty also carries with it a higher risk of medical illness and mortality (Fried and Walston 2003).

Fundamentals of Geriatric Assessment

The effective evaluation and treatment of the geriatric patient—from the fully functioning community-dwelling older adult to the frail older adult in decline—require a global approach, which includes, but reaches beyond, a consideration of the patient's medical problems. Reuben (2003) defined *geriatric assessment* as a comprehensive patient evaluation, conducted by an individual clinician or an interdisciplinary team, which considers the effect of key medical, social, psychological, and environmental factors on health and pays careful attention to function. During the medical assessment, the clinician performs a complete history and physical examination. He or she reviews the medication list for appropriateness and evidence of polypharmacy; checks for deficits in vision, hearing, ambulation, and balance; and screens for common geriatric problems such as falling, incontinence, and malnutrition. Vision is tested with Snellen's eye chart. Hearing is screened with the "whispering voice test" or a handheld audiometer. The patient's weight and height are measured, and the body mass index is calculated. In addition to the standard neurological examination, the patient's mobility and balance can be determined by a "get up and go" test; the patient is asked to stand, walk 10 feet, turn around, return, and be seated. The task is timed; a time greater than 20 seconds suggests that more extensive evaluation is needed.

Cognitive assessment is performed with the Mini-Mental State Examination (Folstein et al. 1975). The Geriatric Depression Scale (Yesavage and Brink 1983) is used to screen for depression. Fundamental day-to-day functioning is determined by documenting activities of daily living—bathing, dressing, toileting, feeding, and transferring—and instrumental activities of daily living—driving, shopping, cooking, housekeeping, using the telephone, and managing finances. The clinician also must gather other important information about function: 1) the extent, strength, and reliability of the patient's social support system (most often the patient's family); 2) the patient's economic resources; and 3) the safety of the patient's home and its proximity to medical care and other essential services. The patient's spiritual preferences and needs are also assessed. After the assessment is completed, recommendations are developed and a care plan is implemented.

Although the results across clinical trials have not been consistent, the effectiveness of comprehensive geriatric assessment and management has been validated in several studies. Increased diagnostic accuracy has been noted. Patients have shown significant improvements in functional status. Affect and cognition have improved. The use of health care services, as measured by nursing home days, hospital services, and medical costs, has been reduced. The use of medications has improved, with fewer drugs being prescribed (Hanlon et al. 2001; Reuben 2003; Spinewine et al. 2007; Stuck et al. 1993). In-home geriatric assessment of older patients may postpone the onset of disability, as well as reduce the number of patients requiring permanent placement in nursing homes (Stuck et al. 1995). A multi-institutional randomized, controlled trial of geriatric evaluation and management units in the Veterans Affairs Health Care System showed a positive effect on functional status and quality of life for inpatients and on mental health and quality of life for outpatients, with overall costs equivalent to those for usual care, but no effect on morbidity or mortality (Cohen et al. 2002). As suggested by the evidence, comprehensive geriatric assessment and management may serve as a useful tool for the diagnosis and the care of older patients, and the geriatrician has a valuable and essential role in the evaluation and treatment of this population.

Key Points

- People older than age 65 years constitute one of the fastest-growing segments of the U.S. population, and the average life span has lengthened significantly.
- The hallmarks of physiological change in older adults are twofold: impaired homeostasis (also called homeostenosis) and increased vulnerability because of decreased reserve capacity.
- The time needed for older adults to learn new information increases, and they may have more difficulty accessing data from long-term memory.
- Older persons develop significant age-related changes in vision—including decreases in accommodation, ability to adapt to light, color discrimination, and visual acuity—and in hearing, with loss of hearing ability in both high and low frequencies.
- Aging results in arterial stiffening and subsequent increased systolic blood pressure and aortic pulse pressure, with resultant susceptibility to left ventricular hypertrophy, cardiac ischemia, left ventricular failure, cerebrovascular ischemia, and renal dysfunction.
- The immune response of the older individual is less vigorous, with decreased cell-mediated response, impaired humoral response, and increased susceptibility to infection.
- The decline in renal clearance and the increase in the elimination half-life in elderly people may require adjustment of the dosing interval of medications; because older adults are more sensitive to medications, drugs must often be given in lower doses.
- Some chronic diseases are more prevalent in older adults, predominantly occurring as a result of "usual

aging"; these include obesity, hypertension, hypercholesterolemia, type 2 diabetes mellitus, osteoarthritis, cerebrovascular disease, cardiovascular disease, and cancer.

- Several common syndromes—known generally as geriatric syndromes—are found more frequently in older patients, including dementia, falls, urinary incontinence, polypharmacy, and frailty.
- The effectiveness of comprehensive geriatric assessment and management has been validated in several large randomized studies, and the geriatrician has a valuable and essential role in the evaluation and treatment of this population.

References

Alexander NB: Falls and gait disturbances, in Geriatrics Review Syllabus: A Core Curriculum in Geriatric Medicine. Edited by Cobbs E, Duthie EH, Murphy JB. Dubuque, IA, Kendall/Hunt, 1999, pp 145–149

Armbrecht HJ: The biology of aging. J Lab Clin Med 138:220–225, 2001

Aw D, Silva AB, Palmer DB: Immunosenescence: emerging challenges for an ageing population. Immunology 120:435–446, 2007

Bhasin S, Cunningham GR, Hayes FJ, et al: Testosterone deficiency in men with androgen deficiency syndromes: an Endocrine Society clinical practice guideline. J Clin Endocrinol Metab 91:1995–2010, 2006

Bischoff-Ferrari HA, Dawson-Hughes B, Willett WC, et al: Effect of vitamin D on falls: a meta-analysis. JAMA 291:1999–2006, 2004

Chatta GS, Lipschitz DA: Aging of the hematopoietic system, in Principles of Geriatric Medicine and Gerontology, 5th Edition. Edited by Hazzard WR, Blass JP, Halter JB, et al. New York, McGraw-Hill, 2003, pp 763–770

Clark CM, Karlawish JH: Alzheimer disease: current concepts and emerging diagnostic and therapeutic strategies. Ann Intern Med 138:400–410, 2003

Cohen HJ: In search of underlying mechanisms of frailty. J Gerontol A Biol Sci Med Sci 55:M706–M708, 2000

Cohen HJ, Feussner JR, Weinberger M, et al: A controlled trial of inpatient and outpatient geriatric evaluation and management. N Engl J Med 346:905–912, 2002

Cornoni-Huntley J, Brock DB, Ostfield A, et al (eds): Established Populations for the Epidemiologic Study of the Elderly: Resource Data Book. Bethesda, MD, National Institutes of Health, 1986

Craft S, Cholerton B, Reger M: Aging and cognition: what is normal? In Principles of Geriatric Medicine and Gerontology, 5th Edition. Edited by Hazzard WR, Blass JP, Halter JB, et al. New York, McGraw-Hill, 2003, pp 1355–1372

Defilippi JL, Crismon ML: Antipsychotic agents in patients with dementia. Pharmacotherapy 20:23–33, 2000

DuBeau CW: Urinary incontinence, in Geriatrics Review Syllabus: A Core Curriculum in Geriatric Medicine, 6th Edition. Edited by Pompei P, Murphy JB. New York, American Geriatrics Society, 2006, pp 184–195

Firth M, Prather CM: Gastrointestinal motility problems in the elderly patient. Gastroenterology 122:1688–1700, 2002

Folstein MF, Folstein SE, McHugh PR: "Mini-mental state": a practical method for grading the cognitive state of patients for the clinician. J Psychiatr Res 12:189–198, 1975

Fried LP: Epidemiology of aging. Epidemiol Rev 22:95–106, 2000

Fried LP, Walston J: Frailty and failure to thrive, in Principles of Geriatric Medicine and Gerontology, 5th Edition. Edited by Hazzard WR, Blass JP, Halter JB, et al. New York, McGraw-Hill, 2003, pp 1487–1502

Frisoni GB: Treatment of Alzheimer's disease with acetylcholinesterase inhibitors: bridging the gap between evidence and practice. J Neurol 248:551–557, 2001

Gillespie LD, Gillespie WJ, Robertson MC, et al: Interventions for preventing falls in elderly people. Cochrane Database Syst Rev Issue 4. Art. No.: CD000340. DOI: 10.1002/14651858.CD000340, 2003

Gomez-Tortosa E, Ingraham AO, Irizarry MC, et al: Dementia with Lewy bodies. J Am Geriatr Soc 46:1449–1458, 1998

Grimes DA, Lobo RA: Perspectives on the Women's Health Initiative trial of hormone replacement therapy. Obstet Gynecol 100:1344–1353, 2002

Gruenewald DA, Matsumoto AM: Aging of the endocrine system, in Principles of Geriatric Medicine and Gerontology, 5th Edition. Edited by Hazzard WR, Blass JP, Halter JB, et al. New York, McGraw-Hill, 2003, pp 819–836

Haegerstrom-Portnoy G, Morgan MW: Normal age-related vision changes, in Rosenbloom and Morgan's Vision and Aging. Edited by Rosenbloom AA Jr. St. Louis, MO, Elsevier, 2007, pp 31–48

Hall KE, Wiley JW: Age-associated changes in gastrointestinal function, in Principles of Geriatric Medicine and Gerontology, 5th Edition. Edited by Hazzard WR, Blass JP, Halter JB, et al. New York, McGraw-Hill, 2003, pp 593–600

Hall WJ: Update in geriatrics. Ann Intern Med 127:557–564, 1997

Halter JB: Diabetes mellitus, in Principles of Geriatric Medicine and Gerontology, 5th Edition. Edited by Hazzard WR, Blass JP, Halter JB, et al. New York, McGraw-Hill, 2003, pp 855–874

Hamerman D: Toward an understanding of frailty. Ann Intern Med 130:945–950, 1999

Hanlon JT, Schmader KE, Ruby CM, et al: Suboptimal prescribing in older inpatients and outpatients. J Am Geriatr Soc 49:200–209, 2001

Harvey PT: Common eye diseases of elderly people: identifying and treating causes of vision loss. Gerontology 48:1–11, 2003

Hassani S, Hershman JM: Thyroid diseases, in Principles of Geriatric Medicine and Gerontology, 5th Edition. Edited by Hazzard WR, Blass JP, Halter JB, et al. New York, McGraw-Hill, 2003, pp 837–854

Hobbs FB: The elderly population. U.S. Census Bureau, Population Division and Housing and Household Economic Statistics Division, 2001. Available at http://www.census.gov/population/www/pop-profile/elderpop.html. Accessed February 2, 2008.

Hunick MG, Goldman L, Tosteson AN, et al: The recent decline in mortality from coronary heart disease. JAMA 277:535–542, 1997

Janssens JP: Aging of the respiratory system: impact on pulmonary function tests and adaptation to exertion. Clin Chest Med 26:469–484, 2005

King MB, Tinetti ME: Falls in community-dwelling older persons. J Am Geriatr Soc 43:1146–1154, 1995

Klafki HW, Staufenbiel S, Kornhuber J, et al: Therapeutic approaches to Alzheimer's disease. Brain 129:2840–2855, 2006

Lakatta EG: Cardiovascular aging research: the next horizons. J Am Geriatr Soc 47:613–625, 1999

Loeser RF, Delbono O: Aging and the musculoskeletal system, in Principles of Geriatric Medicine and Gerontology, 5th Edition. Edited by Hazzard WR, Blass JP, Halter JB, et al. New York, McGraw-Hill, 2003, pp 905–918

Majumdar AP, Jaszewski R, Dubick MA: Effect of aging on gastrointestinal tract and the pancreas. Proc Soc Exp Biol Med 215:134–144, 1997

Marin DB, Sewell MC, Schlecter A: Alzheimer's disease: accurate and early diagnosis in the primary care setting. Geriatrics 57:36–40, 2002

Matsumoto AM: Andropause: clinical implications of the decline in serum testosterone levels with aging in men. J Gerontol A Biol Sci Med Sci 57:M76–M99, 2002

McKeown T: The role of medicine: dream, mirage, or nemesis. Princeton, NJ, Princeton University Press, 1979

McShane R, Areosa Sastre A, Minakaran N: Memantine for dementia. Cochrane Database Syst Rev, Issue 2. Art. No.: CD003154. DOI: 10.1002/14651858.CD003154.pub5, 2006

Miller RA: The biology of aging and longevity, in Principles of Geriatric Medicine and Gerontology. Edited by Hazzard WR, Blass JP, Ettinger WH, et al. New York, McGraw-Hill, 1999, pp 3–19

Mills JH: Age-related changes in the auditory system, in Principles of Geriatric Medicine and Gerontology, 5th Edition. Edited by Hazzard WR, Blass JP, Halter JB, et al. New York, McGraw-Hill, 2003, pp 1239–1251

Morley JE, Haren MT, Rolland YR, et al: Frailty. Med Clin North Am 90:837–847, 2006

Morris JC: Is Alzheimer's disease inevitable with age? Lessons from clinicopathologic studies of healthy aging and very mild Alzheimer's disease. J Clin Invest 104:1171–1173, 1999

Nelson, HD, Humphrey LL, Nygren P, et al: Postmenopausal hormone replacement therapy: scientific review. JAMA 288:872–881, 2002

Nyenhuis DL, Gorelick PB: Vascular dementia: a contemporary review of epidemiology, diagnosis, prevention and treatment. J Am Geriatr Soc 46:1437–1448, 1998

O'Rourke MF, Hashimoto J: Mechanical factors in arterial aging: a clinical perspective. J Am Coll Cardiol 50:1–13, 2006

Oskvig RM: Special problems in the elderly. Chest 155 (suppl): 158S–164S, 1999

Perls T: The different paths to age one hundred. Ann NY Acad Sci 1055:13–25, 2005

Perry HM: The endocrinology of aging. Clin Chem 45:1369–1376, 1999

Peterson PG: Running on Empty: How the Democratic and Republican Parties Are Bankrupting Our Future and What Americans Can Do About It. New York, Farrar, Straus, and Giroux, 2004

Prestwood K, Duque G: Osteoporosis, in Principles of Geriatric Medicine and Gerontology, 5th Edition. Edited by Hazzard WR, Blass JP, Halter JB, et al. New York, McGraw-Hill, 2003, pp 973–985

Reuben DB: Principles of geriatric assessment, in Principles of Geriatric Medicine and Gerontology, 5th Edition. Edited by Hazzard WR, Blass JP, Halter JB, et al. New York, McGraw-Hill, 2003, pp 99–110

Rizvi AA: Management of diabetes in older adults. Am J Med Sci 333:35–47, 2007

Rubenstein LZ, Josephson KR: Falls and their prevention in elderly people: what does the evidence show? Med Clin North Am 90:807–824, 2006

Rubenstein LZ, Josephson KR, Robbins AS: Falls in the nursing home. Ann Intern Med 121:442–451, 1994

Sadovsky R, Dhindsa S, Margo K: Testosterone deficiency: which patients should you screen and treat? J Fam Pract 56 (5 Suppl Testosterone):S1–S20, 2007

Schwartz JB: Clinical pharmacology, in Principles of Geriatric Medicine and Gerontology, 4th Edition. Edited by Hazzard WR, Blass JP, Ettinger WH, et al. New York, McGraw-Hill, 1999, pp 303–332

Schwartz RS, Kohrt WM: Exercise in elderly people: physiological and functional effects, in Principles of Geriatric Medicine and Gerontology, 5th Edition. Edited by Hazzard WR, Blass JP, Halter JB, et al. New York, McGraw-Hill, 2003, pp 931–946

Seals DR, Esler MD: Human ageing and the sympathoadrenal system. J Physiol 528:407–417, 2000

Semla TP, Rochon PA: Pharmacotherapy, in Geriatrics Review Syllabus: A Core Curriculum in Geriatric Medicine, 6th Edition. Edited by Pompei P, Murphy JB. New York, American Geriatrics Society, 2006, pp 72–80

Shock NW: Normal Human Aging: The Baltimore Longitudinal Study of Aging. Washington, DC, National Institute on Aging, U.S. Government Printing Office, 1984

Spinewine A, Schmader KE, Barber N, et al: Appropriate prescribing in elderly people: how well can it be measured and optimised? Lancet 370:173–184, 2007

Sramek JJ, Alexander BD, Cutler NR: Acetylcholinesterase inhibitors for the treatment of Alzheimer's disease. Annals of Long Term Care 9(10):15–22, 2001

Stewart RB: Drug use in the elderly, in Therapeutics in the Elderly, 3rd Edition. Edited by Delafuente JC, Stewart RB. Cincinnati, OH, Harvey Whitney, 2001, pp 235–256

Stuck AE, Siu AL, Wieland GD, et al: Comprehensive geriatric assessment: a meta-analysis of controlled trials. Lancet 342:1032–1036, 1993

Stuck AE, Aronow HU, Steiner A, et al: A trial of annual in-home comprehensive geriatric assessments for elderly people living in the community. N Engl J Med 333:1184–1189, 1995

Taffet GE: Age-related physiologic changes, in Geriatrics Review Syllabus: A Core Curriculum in Geriatric Medicine, 5th Edition. Edited by Cobbs E, Duthie EH, Murphy JB. Dubuque, IA, Kendall/Hunt, 1999, pp 10–23

Tariot PN, Farlow MR, Grossberg GT, et al: Memantine treatment in patients with moderate to severe Alzheimer's disease already receiving donepezil: a randomized controlled trial. JAMA 291:317–324, 2004

Tannenbaum C, Perrin L, DuBeau CE, et al: Diagnosis and management of urinary incontinence in the older patient. Arch Phys Med Rehabil 82:134–138, 2001

Tune LE: Risperidone for the treatment of behavioral and psychological symptoms of dementia. J Clin Psychiatry 62 (suppl 21):29–32, 2001

Vaillant GE, Mukamal K: Successful aging. Am J Psychiatry 158:839–847, 2001

Weymouth F: Effect of age on visual acuity, in Vision of the Aging Patient. Edited by Hirsh MJ, Wick RE. Philadelphia, PA, Chilton, 1960, pp 37–62

Yesavage JA, Brink TL: Development and validation of a geriatric depression screening scale: a preliminary report. J Psychiatr Res 17:37–49, 1983

Suggested Readings

Aw D, Silva AB, Palmer DB: Immunosenescence: emerging challenges for an ageing population. Immunology 120:435–446, 2007

Bischoff-Ferrari HA, Dawson-Hughes B, Willett WC, et al: Effect of vitamin D on falls: a meta-analysis. JAMA 291:1999–2006, 2004

Cohen HJ, Feussner JR, Weinberger M, et al: A controlled trial of inpatient and outpatient geriatric evaluation and management. N Engl J Med 346:905–912, 2002

Fried LP: Epidemiology of aging. Epidemiol Rev 22:95–106, 2000

Klafki HW, Staufenbiel S, Kornhuber J, et al: Therapeutic approaches to Alzheimer's disease. Brain 129:2840–2855, 2006

O'Rourke MF, Hashimoto J: Mechanical factors in arterial aging: a clinical perspective. J Am Coll Cardiol 50:1–13, 2006

Perls T: The different paths to age one hundred. Ann NY Acad Sci 1055:13–25, 2005

Rubenstein LZ, Josephson KR: Falls and their prevention in elderly people: what does the evidence show? Med Clin North Am 90:807–824, 2006

Spinewine A, Schmader KE, Barber N, et al: Appropriate prescribing in elderly people: how well can it be measured and optimised? Lancet 370:173–84, 2007

Vaillant GE, Mukamal K: Successful aging. Am J Psychiatry 158:839–847, 2001

CHAPTER 4

Neuroanatomy, Neurophysiology, and Neuropathology of Aging

Warren D. Taylor, M.D.
Scott D. Moore, M.D., Ph.D.
Steven S. Chin, M.D., Ph.D.

Neuroanatomy and the Aging Brain

Much has been revealed about the human brain in the past few decades. In vivo visualization of the human brain is more accessible to psychiatrists and other clinicians with the emergence of high-resolution magnetic resonance imaging (MRI). Functional neuroimaging research has rapidly expanded, first with positron emission tomography (PET) and single-photon emission computed tomography (SPECT), and more recently with functional MRI (fMRI), a technique that offers improved resolution and wider access.

As neuroimaging has become more readily available to the clinician, a working knowledge of neuroanatomy has become very useful. Unfortunately, neuroanatomy tends to be overwhelming, indigestible, and frustrating. Given that the understanding of the brain is still quite limited, especially regarding the qualities and functionality unique to the human brain, many clinicians lack a clear understanding of the basic framework of brain anatomy and function. Few clinicians have the time to read neuroanatomy textbooks cover to cover. As a result, most clinicians have a working knowledge of neuroanatomy that tends to be patchy and vague.

This discussion is intended to be a brief and concise review of neuroanatomy—almost a contradiction in terms. To enhance the basic understanding of how the brain may work, it is helpful to step back and look at a simplified, more essential picture. This review will err on the side of being too simple, perhaps glossing over controversy, but also will avoid misrepresenting speculation as fact. The intent is to allow the reader to obtain a picture of the whole brain, a simple functional framework, which will allow the clinician and other readers to have a better idea of where to dig more deeply for more comprehensive information.

Several concepts can facilitate gaining a basic but sophisticated understanding of brain function. First, for those of us raised on cellular physiology, is the obvious but important fact that *the brain is not the liver.* In the brain, precise anatomical connections are virtually everything. That drugs can act on a particular cell type belies the fact that neuronal systems in the brain mediate experience and behavior. Neurons with a particular type of receptor may respond to a drug, but it is the anatomical connections of that neuron that determine what parts of the brain have their activity altered. The targets of the given neuron may be distant in the brain, may be myriad, and may respond in a variety of ways to the given neuronal impulse. A certain type of drug may influence several (or more) neuronal types simultaneously and may interact with a given cell type to

The authors wish to acknowledge Dr. Christine Hulette, Division of Neuropathology, Duke University Medical Center, for contributions made to the previous edition of this chapter, some of which were retained in the current edition.

produce quite different changes in neuronal activity in different target areas in the brain. For this reason, pharmacological treatments are determined empirically. The basic concept is this: in the brain, anatomy and function are inseparable; therefore, any discussion of any part of the brain will be in terms of its known or suspected function.

Second, probably the most important concept in neuroanatomy today is that of *distributed systems*. It has become abundantly clear that cortical and subcortical structures are so extensively interconnected that it is not possible to assign a behavior or an emotional or cognitive experience to a discrete area of the brain. Individual neurons in the human brain can receive thousands of afferent connections, and each neuron may in turn directly influence many other neurons simultaneously, some nearby and some in relatively remote areas of the central nervous system (CNS). Some functional systems in the brain are relatively well defined, other systems are becoming clearer, and others lie undiscovered. As research progresses, behaviors and experiences are now being seen to arise from one or more distributed systems in the brain, with components that may lie in far-flung parts of the brain, including the brain stem. This is not to say that every locus in the distributed system performs some homogeneous or interchangeable function. A particular part of the system may contribute some unique or relatively unique aspect to the overall brain function. Moreover, a given brain structure may participate in several or more systems, perhaps contributing its unique processing to a multitude of behaviors and experiences. An example of a distributed system is the limbic system (Parent 1996).

Terminology

To understand anatomy, one must understand the terminology used by radiologists and neuroanatomists to describe brain orientation. Literature describing the animal CNS includes terms such as *dorsal* and *ventral*, which do not really fit when applied to the human neuraxis. The dorsal and ventral horns of the spinal cord are not dorsal and ventral in the human spinal cord, but rather anterior and posterior. However, especially in the spinal cord, the animal nomenclature is retained.

This nomenclature persists to some degree for the human brain stem, though a preference is seen for the more precise terms *rostral* (or *cranial*) and *caudal*—meaning toward the forebrain and toward the spinal cord, respectively. In the human cerebrum, these terms are less useful. The preferred terms are *anterior* and *posterior*, referring to the front and back of the brain (i.e., toward the frontal pole and the occipital pole, respectively). The terms *superior* and *inferior* mean toward the top of the brain (the vertex) and toward the bottom of the brain (i.e., toward the base of the skull). The term *neuraxis* refers to the entire CNS, excluding cranial nerves and spinal nerves, and *extra-axial* refers to anything outside the CNS, including the skull and vertebral column and the dural and vascular spaces, as well as the nerves traversing the spaces.

Brain Stem

Although the initial impression may be that the brain stem has little to do with issues of mood or cognition that are relevant to geriatric psychiatry, this is definitely not the case. The brain stem is of central importance in neurological dysfunction because of its control of vegetative functions and because it either mediates or gives passage to the great majority of sensory and motor impulses. The brain stem can be a locus of important and serious drug side effects, and these frequently need to be differentiated from acute neurological events. In addition, the neurons associated with the monoamine systems are in the brain stem, and these systems can affect virtually any part of the brain and can affect the brain in a global way. Thus, a brief description of the brain stem from a functional standpoint is important and will make a neuroanatomical survey more complete.

The brain stem, or *rhombencephalon*, is composed of several subdivisions (from caudal to rostral): the medulla, the pons, and the midbrain, plus the cerebellum, which has large and direct connections with all three. From an anatomical and functional (and even embryological) perspective, the brain stem is the cranial extension of the spinal cord and shares the basic anatomical organization. The brain stem contains elements of both motor and sensory systems, including systems intrinsic to the brain stem (the cranial nerves) as well as prominent ascending and descending *fibers of passage*, which pass through the brain stem to or from the spinal cord without synapsing in the brain stem.

Although from a gross anatomical perspective the pons is most notable for the corticocerebellar connections making up the middle cerebellar peduncle, it otherwise is fairly similar to the medulla, and for our purposes, we consider them as a unit. The medulla and pons contain the subcortical aspects of the sensory systems for all the cranial nerves (CNs) except CNs I (olfaction) and II (vision). The massive somatosensory system of the head and neck is mediated by the sensory division of the trigeminal nerve (CN V). The cochlear (and some secondary auditory structures) and the vestibular nuclei of CN VIII, now known as the vestibulocochlear nerve, mediate the sense of hearing and the special sense related to the vestibular system. The sense of taste (gustation) is mediated by the solitary nucleus in the medulla, with input from CNs VII, IX, and X. Sensory input from the viscera is considered a special sense and is mediated by the sensory division of the vagus nerve (CN X). The somatosensory, auditory, and gustatory senses send fiber bundles ascending toward the thalamus, joining the sensory pathways ascending from the spinal cord. The auditory system has special characteristics, projecting first to the tectum of the midbrain and then to the thalamus.

The medulla and pons contain the motor nuclei and related pathways mediating control of skeletal muscle of the head and neck. They are also involved in the parasympathetic control of visceral organs, pupillary responses, and exocrine function. The facial motor nucleus (CN VII) controls all the muscles of facial expression. The motor division of the trigeminal nerve (CN V) controls the muscles of mastication. The nucleus of the spinal accessory nerve (CN XI) controls the large muscles responsible for rotating and tilting the head. This nucleus has important connections with the tectum of the midbrain, constituting special systems mediating head and neck reflexes such as orienting and tracking in response to auditory or visual stimuli.

The tongue is controlled by the hypoglossal nerve (CN XII). The muscles of the larynx and pharynx are controlled by the nucleus ambiguus, with its motor fibers split between the glossopharyngeal (CN IX) and vagus (CN X) nerves. Other motor fibers of the vagus nerve, part of the parasympathetic arm of the autonomic nervous system (ANS), originate in the dorsal motor nucleus of the vagus nerve and modulate the intrinsic activity of the cardiac muscle and the smooth muscle of the viscera.

The extraocular muscles of the eyes are controlled by the nuclei of CNs III and IV (midbrain) and VI (pontomedullary), which are tightly interconnected with one another and with the vestibular nuclei. Another small nucleus in the midbrain, the Edinger-Westphal nucleus, contributes to parasympathetic control of the iris and pupillary reflexes.

The cerebellum is best known for controlling balance, posture, coordination, and gait. The system is extensive and includes precerebellar nuclei (including the inferior olivary nucleus and several reticular formation nuclei) and their connection to the cerebellum through the inferior cerebellar peduncle. The corticocerebellar pathway includes the massive corticopontine tract, the pontine gray nuclei, and their connection to the cerebellum through the middle cerebellar peduncle. The output of cerebellar cortical activity is mediated by the deep cerebellar nuclei, which project via the superior cerebellar peduncle mainly to the motor nuclei of the thalamus. The vestibular part of the cerebellum also projects to the spinal cord via the red nucleus and the rubrospinal tract, directly facilitating balance and posture.

Prominent fiber bundles course through all three subdivisions of the brain stem, including the large *corticospinal tract*, composed mainly of descending cortical motor neuron axons. At the level of the medulla, the corticospinal tract is relatively superficial, forming bulges on the anterior surface known as the pyramids, giving the more common name *pyramidal tract*. Rostrally, at the level of the pons, the corticospinal tract is broken up into many fascicles by the pontine gray nuclei. At the most rostral level of the brain stem—the midbrain—the corticospinal tract is again united into single bundles bilaterally, now completely superficial and known as the *cerebral peduncles*. Among the many descending motor neuron axons of the corticospinal tract, some terminate in the brain stem (*corticobulbar* fibers) to influence the cranial nerve motor nuclei. A large proportion of the descending corticospinal axons are *corticopontine* fibers, which synapse in the pontine gray nuclei (thus, *corticospinal tract* is a misnomer), giving rise to axons that innervate the cerebellum through the middle cerebellar peduncle. The remaining fibers course through the brain stem to the spinal cord. Similarly, ascending sensory neuron axons from the spinal cord and cranial nerve sensory nuclei form several large bundles as they pass through the brain stem toward the thalamus.

The sensory and motor nuclei of the cranial nerves and the ascending and descending fiber bundles are embedded in a loose matrix of many short neurons, collectively called the *reticular formation*. The reticular formation extends throughout the brain stem from the medulla into the diencephalon. In addition to other roles, these neurons constitute the *reticular activating system*, which plays a critical role in regulating the sleep-wake cycle and level of arousal or vigilance. The reticular formation has several other roles, including that of a slower sensory pathway from the spinal cord and brain stem to the thalamus. The sensory information transmitted along this pathway serves less to provide specific information about stimulus features, instead functioning to change the level of arousal in relation to stimuli. The reticular formation also contains centers for control of the primary functions, including respiration and cardiac and vascular control of blood pressure. This is mediated through the ANS, via direct connections from reticular formation cells to sympathetic preganglionic cells in the spinal cord and through the parasympathetic influence of the vagus nerve (CN X).

The midbrain differs somewhat from the medulla-pons, although the reticular formation (called the *tegmentum* in the midbrain) continues to be prominent. The ascending fiber tracts remain embedded in the reticular formation, but the corticospinal/pontine/bulbar tract is superficial to the tegmentum as the cerebral peduncles. The posterior aspect of the midbrain (covered by the cerebellum at lower levels) forms four bumps known as the *superior* and *inferior colliculi* and collectively known as the *tectum*. The superior and inferior colliculi receive direct visual and auditory input, respectively, and mediate head and neck reflexes (via the tectospinal tract) and other functions not involving the cerebral sensory cortex. The core of the midbrain is composed of a dense area of neurons surrounding the cerebral aqueduct and is known as the *periaqueductal gray*, an area significantly involved in pain control.

Finally, the brain stem gives rise to the monoamine systems. All three subdivisions of the brain stem contain neuronal cell bodies of the monoamine systems—small groups of cells that together innervate virtually the entire CNS. The monoamines include *norepinephrine* (a catecholamine), which arises from several groups, the largest and most compact of which is the *locus coeruleus*. The locus coeruleus innervates virtually the entire forebrain, giving it the potential to profoundly influence the cerebrum and is considered critical in mood disorders, anxiety, and certain types of drug withdrawal. A second catecholamine, *dopamine*, arises from the midbrain in a large, compact group known as the *substantia nigra* and from a smaller, diffuse group lying in the anterior tegmental area known as the *ventral tegmental area*. Dopamine deficiencies and excesses figure prominently in certain neurological and psychiatric diseases.

Another monoamine, *serotonin*, is an indoleamine rather than a catecholamine. Some small groups of serotonergic neurons lie throughout the brain stem along the midline anterior to the ventricular system. These collectively are known as the *raphe nuclei*, and individually these groups each innervate certain areas of the CNS from spinal cord to cerebellum to forebrain. The largest and most rostral of the raphe nuclei is called the *dorsal raphe nucleus*, and like the locus coeruleus, it innervates virtually the entire cerebrum, giving the dorsal raphe nucleus the capacity to influence the brain in a global way.

Prosencephalon

The prosencephalon, or forebrain, contains all the parts of the "higher brain" that makes us human but more importantly contains all of the higher control of the critical physiological machinery that keeps us alive. The forebrain, which is synonymous with cerebrum, has two main parts: the diencephalon and the telencephalon.

Diencephalon

The diencephalon forms the core of the forebrain, both anatomically and functionally. Some neuroanatomists include the diencephalon as part of the brain stem, an idea that is based mainly on the continuity of the reticular formation from the midbrain tegmentum into the hypothalamus and thalamus. No discrete border exists between the posterior hypothalamus and the reticular formation of the midbrain. This reticular formation also continues rostrally from the midbrain into the thalamus, forming the intralaminar nuclei. This is a less obvious continuation than is seen in the hypothalamus but in fact is a very clear continuity from a functional standpoint. The intralaminar nuclei, especially the centromedian nuclei, form a critical part of the reticular activating system, essentially governing the level of activation of the forebrain, from deep sleep to waking to a state of hypervigilance.

Conversely, the hypothalamus and thalamus are integral parts of the cerebral systems and participate fully in cortical functioning on multiple levels. In contrast to the anatomical landmarks, from a functional standpoint the boundary between the diencephalon and telencephalon is arbitrary. Thus, the term *cerebrum* is synonymous with *prosencephalon*, which represents the diencephalon and telencephalon as an anatomical and functional unit.

The diencephalon is mainly composed of the hypothalamus and thalamus but generally is considered to include several smaller structures as well. These include the subthalamus, functionally part of the basal ganglia, and the epithalamus, which lumps together the habenula (part of the limbic system) and the pineal body or gland, which secretes the hormone melatonin into the cerebrospinal fluid in relation to circadian rhythms. Finally, the pituitary gland hangs off the bottom of the hypothalamus, forming the endocrine interface between the hypothalamus and the body.

Hypothalamus. The hypothalamus is a relatively small, heterogeneous structure at the base of the cerebrum. It is roughly divisible into medial and lateral halves, which are extensively interconnected. The medial portion is characterized by discrete nuclei embedded in a loose matrix of small neurons, whereas the lateral half of the hypothalamus more closely resembles the reticular formation of the brain stem. The lateral hypothalamus is dominated by a large fiber bundle known as the *median forebrain bundle*, which runs longitudinally from brain stem to basal forebrain. This bundle contains many short axons interconnecting nuclei in the midbrain, hypothalamus, and basal forebrain. However, it also contains many important fibers of passage—most notably, the monoamine projections from noradrenergic and serotonergic cell groups in the brain stem that innervate virtually the entire forebrain. The *fornix*, another prominent fiber bundle that serves to delineate lateral from medial hypothalamus, interconnects the hippocampus with the mamillary nuclei of the hypothalamus and several other structures important in the formation, storage, and retrieval of memories.

The hypothalamus plays multiple roles, reflecting its diverse anatomical makeup. Most notably, the hypothalamus serves to coordinate endocrine, autonomic, and somatic motor responses to a broad array of physiological and psychological information to maintain physiological homeostasis. Among the factors regulated by the hypothalamus are body temperature, heart rate, blood pressure, blood osmolarity, metabolism, digestion, and water and food intake. The hypothalamus regulates sexual and reproductive functioning and growth. The hypothalamus also plays roles in the body's responses to stress, including control of adrenal cortical secretion of cortisol, which is part of the body's mechanism for coping with stress. These functions are mediated by a distributed system of interconnected hypothalamic nuclei.

The hypothalamus controls the endocrine system through the pituitary gland. This gland hangs by a stalk (the infundibulum) from the medial hypothalamus, and the two are linked by a system of small (portal) capillaries (anterior pituitary or adenohypophysis) and by a direct neuronal connection (posterior pituitary or neurohypophysis). Nuclei of the medial half of the hypothalamus produce many peptide hormones and hormone-releasing factors. The hypothalamus also has receptors for the hormones it controls, as well as thermoreceptors and osmoreceptors. Control of the ANS occurs through projections from the lateral hypothalamus to the preganglionic sympathetic and parasympathetic neurons in the brain stem and spinal cord. Some functional division can be appreciated, with the anterior hypothalamus manifesting mainly parasympathetic aspects of the ANS and the posterior hypothalamus manifesting mainly the sympathetic autonomic responses.

The hypothalamus has widespread and often reciprocal connections with the brain stem, limbic structures, and prefrontal cortex. In addition to its well-defined role in maintaining physiological homeostasis, the hypothalamus participates in emotional expression and motivation through its broad interconnections with limbic structures, especially the amygdala. The hypothalamus integrates cortical and subcortical aspects of emotional states and coordinates concomitant physiological manifestations.

Thalamus. The thalamus is located superior to the hypothalamus, enclosing the upper part of the third ventricle. It is bounded laterally by the white matter of the internal capsule. The thalamus is divided into lateral, medial, and anterior groups by white matter laminae.

The thalamus plays a critical role in the functioning of the cerebral cortex. No information enters the cortical mantle without going through the thalamus, with the notable exception of the olfactory system, the most primitive of the sensory systems.

The thalamus contains two different types of subnuclei. The first is called the *specific* (or *relay*) type. Each nucleus of the specific type receives a specific type of input that is projected to a discrete area of cerebral cortex. These nuclei do not function as simple relays between afferent input and efferent projection to its area of neocortex. Each of these nuclei receives reciprocal afferent input from the area of cortex it is projecting to, allowing the thalamic nucleus to modulate its own output. A considerable amount of processing takes place at the level of the thalamus.

Each *lateral thalamic nucleus* receives either unimodal (only one sensory type) sensory input or specially processed information related to control of movement, and each projects to and receives input from a specific region of sensory, motor, or association cortex. The lateral group also receives information related to movement from the cerebellum and basal ganglia, and relays information to the primary motor cortex. The *ventral tier* of the lateral nuclear group of the thalamus contains nuclei for each of the senses except olfaction. Each of these thalamic nuclei then sends its sensory-specific information to the appropriate primary sensory cortex for that modality.

The *dorsal tier* of the lateral thalamic nuclear group contains the pulvinar, the largest of the thalamic nuclei. The pulvinar processes sensory information, but the information is polymodal (i.e., representing the integration of two or more sensory modalities). The pulvinar receives input from the superior colliculus, parietal-temporal-occipital association cortex, and primary visual cortex and, in turn, projects back to the parietal-temporal-occipital association cortex. Its diverse connections suggest that the pulvinar is performing a high-level integration of sensory information (see discussion of multimodal association cortex in the "Association Cortex" section later in this chapter).

Other specific-type nuclei in the thalamus receive input from limbic structures and project to limbic association cortex. The anterior nuclear group receives input from the hippocampus by way of the mamillary nuclei and the mamillothalamic tract and projects to the limbic association cortex of the cingulate gyrus. Similarly, the dorsomedial nucleus of the medial thalamic group receives afferent input from the amygdaloid complex and temporal neocortex, projecting in turn to the limbic association cortex of the prefrontal lobe.

In contrast to the specific nuclei, the other type of thalamic nuclei is known as the *diffuse projection* type. These include the intralaminar nuclei, which have precisely organized connections with the striatum and also project diffusely to several cortical areas in the frontal lobe, influencing the sensitivity of cortical neurons. The reticular thalamic nucleus, a second type of diffuse projection nucleus, forms a shell around the lateral aspect of the thalamus on each side so that corticothalamic and thalamocortical fibers are contacted as they pass through it. The reticular nucleus does not project to the cerebral cortex and instead has an inhibitory influence on the activity of the specific-type nuclei. The activity of the reticular nucleus is closely correlated with electroencephalographic activity during sleep and wakefulness and is associated with the control of attention to sensory stimuli.

Telencephalon

The telencephalon, which is about 40% white matter by volume, consists of huge bundles of glial cells and myelinated axons that provide vital connectivity within the cerebral hemispheres and that connect the cerebral cortex with subcortical structures and the rest of the CNS. In addition to the thin layer of gray matter of the cerebral cortex, the forebrain contains several subcortical gray matter structures. The basal ganglia lie deep in the cerebrum, forming a sort of outer core surrounding the diencephalon. A loose group of nuclei and diffuse cell groups collectively called the *basal forebrain* lies anterior to the diencephalon. Unlike the basal ganglia, this gray matter is superficial and does not form anything resembling a layered cortical structure. The amygdalohippocampal complex forms the ventromedial surface of the temporal lobes, overlapping with the olfactory brain (rhinencephalon) that comprises the anterior region of the temporal lobes. The phylogenetically old hippocampal formation and the olfactory structures are cortical structures but differ from the rest of the cerebral cortex in their cytoarchitecture and are designated as the *allocortex* (discussed later in the "Classification and Parcellation of the Cerebral Cortex" section). The amygdaloid complex is a heterogeneous collection of subnuclei that has been called *corticoid* (i.e., showing only a suggestion of the neuronal layering characteristic of cortex).

At the level of the midbrain, ascending and descending tracts of myelinated axons coalesce to form the large white matter fiber bundles called the *cerebral peduncles* (discussed earlier in this chapter in the "Brain Stem" section). Rostral to the midbrain, at the most inferior levels of the cerebrum, the cerebral peduncles spread to form a capsule around the diencephalon and are given the name *internal capsule*. At this level, a large amount of two-way traffic leading into and out of the thalamus mixes with the fibers of the corticospinal tract, forming a thick sheet of white matter, which separates the gray matter of the thalamus from the gray matter of the globus pallidus and also splits the caudate nucleus from the putamen. Superior to the level of the basal ganglia, the internal capsule splays out anteriorly, laterally, and posteriorly to form the *corona radiata*. These fibers are joined by the medial and laterally oriented fibers of the corpus callosum to form a dense core of white matter in the superior part of the cerebrum known as the *centrum semiovale*. This collection of myelinated axons includes corticothalamic and thalamocortical fibers, commissural fibers from the corpus callosum (interhemispheric association fibers), descending projections from motor cortex to multiple levels of the CNS, and long intrahemispheric association fibers interconnecting areas of cortex. Finally, just below the thin layer of gray matter making up the cerebral cortex are short association fibers interconnecting neurons in one gyrus with those in the next gyrus.

Basal ganglia. Deep in the cerebrum are several nuclei constituting the basal ganglia, although a sometimes confusing multitude of names are given to these structures in various combinations. The superior portion of the basal ganglia is known as the *dorsal striatum*, which includes the caudate nucleus and the putamen; these are very similar in structure and essentially split into the two nuclei by fibers of the internal capsule. The striped appearance of the small white matter bundles of the internal capsule and the gray matter bridges still joining the two nuclei in places gave rise to their original, collective name of *striatum* (or rarely *neostriatum*). Ventromedial to the putamen are the inner and outer segments of the globus pallidus, making up the third major element of the dorsal striatum. This structure is sometimes just called the *pallidum* (or rarely the *paleostriatum*), so named because the greater content of whitish myelinated axons gives this structure a pale appearance in fresh sections. The putamen and globus pallidus are nestled snugly together, giving the appearance of a lens shape with the convex surface oriented laterally and narrowing to somewhat of a point ventromedially, pointing toward the base of the diencephalon. The term *lenticular nucleus* is given to the putamen–globus pallidus combination; this term has usefulness as a gross anatomical term but little usefulness from a functional standpoint.

The inferior division of the basal ganglia, known as the *ventral striatum*, has a structure that parallels that of the dorsal striatum but differs significantly in connectivity and function. The ventral striatum is usually considered to include the nucleus accumbens and the olfactory tubercle; the nucleus accumbens represents the fused inferior extent of the caudate and putamen. Similarly, the ventral pallidum is the inferior extent of the globus pallidus, so no clear separation exists between dorsal and ventral striatopallidum from a gross anatomical standpoint, although the differences in connectivity clearly justify the nomenclature.

The basal ganglia consist of input nuclei and output nuclei. The input nuclei, comprising the caudate, putamen, and ventral striatum, receive afferent input from virtually all areas of cortex. Cortical input to the striatum has a distinctly regional pattern. The putamen is innervated by sensorimotor cortex, whereas the caudate nucleus preferentially receives input from association areas of frontal, temporal, parietal, and cingulate cortex. Furthermore, afferent input from limbic and paralimbic cortex, hippocampus, and amygdala primarily terminates in the ventral striatum. Based on this corticostriatal innervation pattern, the striatum is divided into sensorimotor, associative, and limbic territories. This regional organization is maintained throughout the basal ganglia as parallel, segregated pathways from input to output. In addition to the massive cortical innervation, the striatum receives prominent afferent input from the thalamus, originating primarily in the intralaminar nuclei. Both striatal divisions are innervated by dopaminergic cell groups in the midbrain; the dorsal striatum receives input from the substantia nigra (considered part of the basal ganglia), and the ventral division receives input from the more diffuse *ventral tegmental area*. In addition, like most of the forebrain, both divisions receive serotonergic input from the dorsal raphe nucleus and noradrenergic input from the locus coeruleus.

The striatal nuclei project exclusively to the globus pallidus, which is the main output nucleus of the basal ganglia, and to the substantia nigra. The effects exerted by the dorsal striatopallidum on other parts of the nervous system are mediated primarily by efferent fibers from the internal segments of the globus pallidus and from the substantia nigra to the thalamus (the ventral tier and centromedian nuclei). The ventral striatopallidum similarly projects to the thalamus, to the limbic-related dorsomedial nucleus. However, in contrast to the globus pallidus, which has connections exclusively to other elements of the basal ganglia and the thalamus, the ventral pallidum also has direct reciprocal connections with limbic structures, especially the amygdala.

The basal ganglia are thus intercalated in a loop of neuronal connections from the cerebral cortex and back to the cerebral cortex via the thalamus (corticostriatal-thalamocortical loops). Although the basal ganglia receive afferent input from almost all parts of the cortex, a high degree of topographic organization is maintained throughout the basal ganglia, from input to output. It is now believed that the basal ganglia process different kinds of information in parallel rather than being primarily concerned with integration of information from large parts of the cortex. Thus, every cortical area has a separate functional pathway through the striatum that lies adjacent to and interdigitates with that of functionally related cortical areas. In other words, the striatum is processing information of different kinds simultaneously, although it remains segregated.

There are thought to be five or more lines or circuits through the basal ganglia in which the flow of information remains segregated. Presumably, the basal ganglia are performing some particular type of processing common to all the pathways. Because of the parallel processing and the segregation, the output of each functional pathway will be dissimilar, reflecting the unique and varying type of input to each pathway. Within each pathway, convergence on a local scale is evident, reflecting the considerable processing that is occurring during the transit through the basal ganglia system.

The nature of the processing that occurs in the basal ganglia system is unclear; thus, the function of the basal ganglia system, within each pathway and as a whole, remains speculative. It is believed, at least for the systems involving sensorimotor cortex, that the basal ganglia system is involved in the planning and production of movement. In contrast to the putamen, which mainly receives input from sensorimotor cortex and projects back to sensorimotor cortex via the thalamus, the caudate nucleus receives highly processed information from association areas and acts primarily on prefrontal cortex. Several corticostriatal-thalamocortical loops involving the caudate nucleus and prefrontal cortex have been proposed, which may involve primarily cognitive tasks. A similar corticostriatal-thalamocortical loop exists between limbic cortex of orbitofrontal and temporal lobes and the cingulate gyrus through the ventral striatopallidum to the dorsomedial thalamus and back to the same cortex. The connections of the ventral striatopallidum with limbic structures suggest involvement in motivation and emotion. The specific role played by the various loops of the basal ganglia system may act to suppress or select potentially competing cognitive or limbic mechanisms.

As a final note, diseases affecting the basal ganglia have long been known to affect motor functioning, resulting in disturbances of movement and of resting muscle tone. Before modern tract-tracing technologies, it was believed there was a second, *extrapyramidal* pathway from motor cortex to the brain stem and spinal cord. This has been proven incorrect, so the term *extrapyramidal* is inappropriate and misleading. However, the term *extrapyramidal* is fairly entrenched in psychiatric literature in relation to medication side effects and may continue to persist as an occasionally confusing relic.

Basal forebrain. The basal forebrain is one of several subcortical gray matter areas in the telencephalon. Unlike the basal ganglia or the amygdalohippocampal complex, the basal forebrain does not have a real structure. Rather, it is largely a collection of diffuse cholinergic cell groups and several nuclei of apparently unrelated function. The basal forebrain region lies anterior to the diencephalon and inferomedial to the basal ganglia. The basal forebrain has three functional entities:

1. The ventral striatopallidum or ventral striatum, which was discussed with the basal ganglia.
2. The *extended amygdala*, which primarily comprises the bed nucleus of the stria terminalis. The stria terminalis is one of two main efferent pathways from the amygdala, and the extended amygdala thus represents a rostral extension of the medial amygdala, with which it shares neurotransmitter properties.
3. A system of large cholinergic neurons in a thin disk close to the basal surface of each hemisphere, which is the most diffuse component of the basal forebrain. The most lateral collection of these magnocellular cholinergic neurons is known as the *basal nucleus* (or the basal nucleus of Meynert). The basal nucleus, which receives an extensive and diverse afferent input, provides cholinergic innervation to virtually the entire neocortex, in a manner analogous to the monoamine systems originating in the locus coeruleus and raphe system. The loss of acetylcholine in the cerebral cortex associated with degenerative dementias has been traced to degeneration of this small group of neurons. The other magnocellular cholinergic neurons are found in the septal nuclei, the most medial and least diffuse grouping of these neurons. The septal nuclei are part of the limbic system and, with some adjacent neurons, provide cholinergic innervation of the hippocampal formation.

Classification and Parcellation of the Cerebral Cortex

In the adult human brain, the cerebral cortex has about 1,500–2,200 cm^2 of surface area, with a thickness that

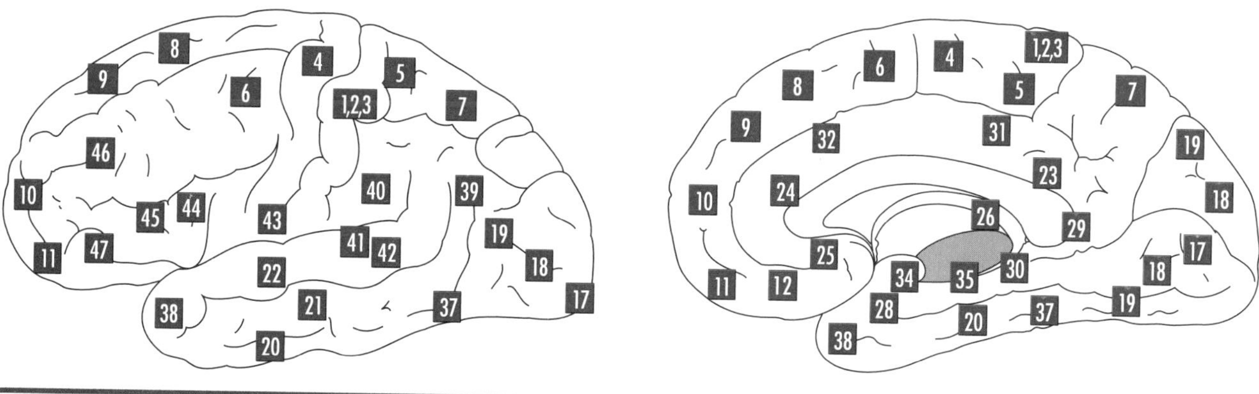

FIGURE 4–1. Illustration of cortical (*left*) and sagittal (*right*) views of the brain, marked with selected Brodmann areas.

TABLE 4–1. Brodmann areas of selected brain regions

Brain region	Brodmann area(s)
Auditory cortex, primary	41, 42
Cingulate cortex	
Dorsal anterior	32
Dorsal posterior	31
Subgenual	25
Ventral anterior	24
Ventral posterior	23
Dorsolateral prefrontal cortex	9, 46
Motor cortex, primary	4
Motor cortex, secondary (premotor, supplementary motor)	6
Orbitofrontal area (orbital gyrus and gyrus rectus)	11
Somatosensory cortex, primary	1, 2, 3
Temporal gyrus	
Inferior	20
Middle	21
Superior	22
Visual cortex, primary	17

varies from 1.5 to 4.5 mm. Only about one-fourth of the cortex is visible, with the rest buried in sulci and fissures.

The cerebral cortex can be classified in several different ways: 1) by the pattern of layering of cortical neurons; 2) by the sizes and shapes and arrangements of neuronal perikarya, or *cytoarchitectonics*; or 3) by connectivity. One fundamental classification of the cerebral cortex looks at the layering of small and large neurons and neuronal axons in different areas of cortex. Most (≥95%) of the cerebral cortex consists of six layers and is known as *neocortex*, *isocortex*, or *homotypic cortex*. Phylogenetically older parts of the cerebral cortex contain fewer layers and are known as *allocortex* or *heterotypic cortex*. The allocortex contains only three layers and includes areas related to olfaction and the hippocampal formation. Notably, whereas the neocortex develops in parallel with the thalamus and receives most of its subcortical afferents from the thalamus, the allocortex receives afferents from other subcortical nuclei.

A second classification scheme was developed by Brodmann based on cytoarchitectonics. Brodmann identified 47 different areas of neocortex, which can be approximately classified into three functional categories. One category is termed *agranular cortex* and is characteristic of motor cortex (Brodmann areas [BAs] 4 and 6). This type of cortex is characterized by a poorly developed inner granular layer and prominent pyramidal cell layers. The large pyramidal cells provide long axons to project long distances to the brain stem or spinal cord. A second cytoarchitectonic category is termed the *granular cortex* or *koniocortex*, characterized by a prominent inner granular layer and a paucity of large projection neurons. The inner granular layer, so named for the many small neurons concentrated there, is specialized to receive afferent axons and is best developed in sensory cortex. The large remaining areas of cortex are designated *association cortex*, with variable cytoarchitectonics reflecting both input and output functions. Brodmann area designations are shown in Figure 4–1 and are related to key regions in Table 4–1.

The third classification scheme is based on connectivity. All areas of cortex receive thalamic input, which in a real sense determines the identity of each cortical area. Cerebral cortex can thus be divided into sensory, motor, and association areas. Some areas of association cortex are identified as limbic cortex, based on their connections with subcortical limbic structures.

Afferent and Efferent Connections of the Cerebral Cortex

Afferent input to the cerebral cortex is of several types: thalamocortical, corticocortical, and the diffuse modulatory neurotransmitter systems. As described earlier, two types of thalamic input reach the cerebral cortex. The first arises from specific thalamic nuclei, which contribute topographically organized projections to all parts of the neocortex. These are generally reciprocated and are not simple relays (i.e., some degree of processing takes place at the level of the thalamus). The second arises from the diffuse projection thalamic nuclei, which contribute diffusely organized connections and represent primarily the projections of the intralaminar thalamic nuclei. These nuclei exert general effects on the excitability of cortical neurons. Corticocortical connections include association fibers and commissural fibers. Association fibers interconnect areas of cortex within the hemispheres, are generally reciprocal, and are a vital part of the distributed neuronal systems mediating many brain activities. Commissural fibers generally interconnect corresponding areas in the two hemispheres, virtually all crossing in the corpus callosum.

In addition to the diffuse thalamic innervation, most of the forebrain, including the entire cerebral cortex, is diffusely innervated by two monoamine neurotransmitter systems that originate in the brain stem: the locus coeruleus provides noradrenergic innervation, and the dorsal raphe nucleus provides serotonergic innervation. In both cases, a relatively small number of neurons innervate vast areas of cortex, as well as subcortical structures, by widely ramifying axonal collaterals. Thus, the modulatory actions mediated by these systems act in a global way, perhaps affecting the whole of distributed systems simultaneously. A third monoamine system in the ventral tegmental area of the midbrain that uses dopamine affects more restricted areas of cortex, primarily frontal and temporal neocortex. A fourth neurotransmitter system that uses acetylcholine arises in the basal nucleus in the basal forebrain and diffusely innervates the cerebral neocortex. By virtue of their extremely widespread distribution, these systems can affect the brain in comprehensive ways. Each of these systems is now known to have profound implications for geriatric psychiatry.

Efferent connections of cerebral cortex include the corticocortical connections described above, in addition to the subcortical targets of cortical projection neurons. These targets include the thalamus, in part reciprocating corticothalamic projections, and the striatum, which receives projections from all areas of cortex except primary auditory and visual cortex. The remaining subcortical projections of cerebral cortical neurons are corticopontine (innervating the cerebellum via the pontine gray nuclei and the middle cerebellar peduncle), corticobulbar (innervating various brain stem nuclei), and corticospinal (projecting primarily to spinal motor neurons).

Organization of Sensorimotor Systems

The sensory cortex is organized such that thalamic projections for each sensory modality innervate a single area of neocortex, designated the *primary sensory cortex*. The *olfactory cortex* is exceptional because it is allocortical and because the thalamus is bypassed, but the organization is similar. Adjacent to the primary sensory cortex for each modality are one or two areas of secondary sensory cortex, which receive sensory input from the primary sensory cortex after initial processing. In the case of *visual cortex*, the area surrounding the calcarine sulcus near the posterior (occipital) pole of the brain (BA 17), known as *striate cortex* or *calcarine cortex*, receives direct thalamic input from the lateral geniculate nucleus (ventral tier of the lateral thalamus). The striate cortex sends its output to secondary and then to tertiary visual cortex (BAs 18 and 19), which lie adjacent to primary visual cortex. There are extensive, reciprocal connections between these three areas of visual cortex. Different aspects of visual processing take place in different areas, with the development of progressively more complex analysis. For example, recognition of stimuli in the visual system goes from simple spots of light or color in primary visual cortex to detection of shapes, direction, and speed of movement in secondary and tertiary visual cortex. Thus, the overall movement of information from primary to secondary to tertiary visual cortex shows a progressively higher level of processing at each step, but the information being analyzed remains unimodal and still lacks meaningful context.

The *somatosensory (somesthetic) cortex* has some unique features because of its relationship with the motor cortex. These cortices can be seen as a unitary system, not only because of their proximity but also because they are extensively interconnected. Activation of muscles can occur with electrical stimulation of somesthetic cortex, albeit at higher stimulus intensities than direct stimulation of motor cortex. The primary somesthetic cortex (S-1) is located in the postcentral gyrus and its medial extension (BAs 1–3). Thalamic input comes from the lateral and medial ventral posterior thalamic nuclei (VPL and VPM). An additional unique feature is that the secondary somesthetic area (S-2) also receives direct input from VPL and VPM and from S-1 bilaterally. Both S-1 and S-2 project to multimodal sensory association cortex in the posterior parietal lobe (BAs 5 and 7). However, both somesthetic areas also project directly to primary motor cortex, and, moreover, both make a significant contribution to the corticospinal tract, allowing direct control of sensory signal transmission from caudal levels of the CNS.

The primary *motor cortex* (M-1), located in the precentral gyrus (BA 4), is the locus of voluntary movement control and is the main source of corticospinal tract axons. M-1 receives afferent input from primary and secondary somesthetic areas. Thalamic input to M-1 comes from the ventral anterior and ventral lateral thalamic nuclei, which provide critical input from the two subcortical adjunctive motor control systems: the basal ganglia and the cerebellum, respectively. BA 6 contains "supramotor" areas: the premotor area and the supplementary motor area. Both of these adjunctive motor areas receive afferent input from prefrontal cortex and project primarily to M-1 and are important for precise movements of the hands (especially rhythmic movements). The supplementary motor area is important for organizing and planning fairly complex movements and for mediating an appropriate motor response to sensory stimuli. The premotor area is important for control of visually guided movements. Just anterior to the premotor area is the frontal eye field, the center for voluntary eye movements.

The primary *auditory cortex* (A-1) is located in a part of the superior temporal gyrus of the posterior temporal lobe known as *Heschl's gyrus* (BAs 41 and 42) and receives thalamic input from the medial geniculate body (ventral tier of lateral thalamus). The rest of the superior temporal gyrus represents secondary auditory cortex (A-2), necessary for the interpretation of auditory information. Damage to A-2 can result in *acoustic agnosia*, the inability to recognize tones in particular patterns, such as laughter or the sounds of various animals, in the absence of impaired hearing.

The *gustatory cortex* is found in BA 43, part of insular cortex buried in the lateral sulcus (also known as the *sylvian fissure*). This primary sensory cortex is less well defined than other sensory cortices.

The oldest part of the human cerebral cortex is the *rhinencephalon*, or *olfactory brain*. This includes the olfactory structures, the anterior olfactory nucleus, the corticomedial and anterior parts of the amygdaloid complex, and the piriform lobe in the anteromedial temporal lobe. Part of the piriform lobe is *allocortex* and represents the primary sensory cortex of the olfactory system. The other subdivision of the piriform lobe is the *entorhinal cortex*, which is *neocortex* (BA 28) and represents secondary olfactory cortex. This area, located on the parahippocampal gyrus, forms the *uncus*, a gross anatomical landmark that can have critical clinical significance in cases of traumatic brain injury. Notably, olfactory cortex receives input directly from olfactory structures, making the olfactory system unique among the sensory systems in that the thalamus does not intervene between sensory neurons and sensory cortex.

Sensory Association Cortex

The sensorimotor cortex occupies a relatively small proportion of cerebral cortex, leaving a large amount of neocortex designated *association cortex*. The association cortex is found in parietal, temporal, and frontal lobes. Sensory and association cortices form a functional hierarchy, with primary sensory cortex forming the most basic level (Table 4–2). What has been traditionally described as secondary and tertiary sensory cortex for each sensory modality is *unimodal sensory association cortex*. This level of association cortex is responsible for integrating the most basic elements of sensory information that have been identified by the primary sensory cortex. For example, the visual association cortex could integrate information such as the shape and color of an object and the direction and velocity of its movement.

Within each primary sensory cortex and unimodal sensory association cortex, sensory information is processed sequentially, operating in parallel. Subsequently, sensory information from the unimodal sensory association cortices converges in *multimodal sensory association cortex*. This level of association cortex takes highly processed unimodal sensory information from several

TABLE 4–2. Hierarchical distribution and location of major cortical types

Cortical type	Specific type	Lobe	Location in lobe
Primary sensorimotor cortex	Motor	Frontal	Precentral gyrus
	Somesthetic	Parietal	Postcentral gyrus
	Visual	Occipital	Calcarine fissure
	Auditory	Temporal	Heschl's gyrus
	Olfactory	Temporal	Piriform cortex (anteromedial temporal lobe)
	Gustatory	Parietal	Insular cortex
Unimodal sensory association cortex	Somesthetic	Parietal	Anterior inferior parietal lobe at the lateral sulcus (sylvian fissure)
	Visual	Occipital	Gyri surrounding calcarine fissure
	Auditory	Temporal	Superior temporal gyrus
	Olfactory	Temporal	Entorhinal cortex (parahippocampal gyrus)
Multimodal sensory association cortex	Somesthetic-visual	Parietal, occipital	Parietal-occipital junction
	Auditory-visual	Temporal	Middle and inferior temporal gyri
Nonsensory association cortex	Premotor	Frontal	Anterior to precentral gyrus
	Limbic	Temporal, parietal, frontal	Cingulate gyrus, parahippocampal gyrus, temporal pole, orbitofrontal cortex
Integrative association cortex	Posterior: final sensory integration	Parietal, temporal, occipital	Junction of parietal, temporal, occipital lobes
	Anterior: higher cortical functions	Frontal	Dorsolateral prefrontal cortex

sensory modalities and begins the process of weaving a comprehensive sensory experience. Multimodal sensory association cortex is found at the junction of parietal, temporal, and occipital lobes, near the visual, auditory, and somesthetic cortices.

The multimodal sensory association cortex in the posterior parietal area is responsible for the integration of visual and somesthetic information, which is essential for defining spatial relationships. This area is important for movement and motor control, specifically for execution of more complex movements. Lesions of parietal association areas can result in a variety of neurological deficits, including apraxias (inability to perform certain learned complex movements in the absence of paralysis, sensory loss, or ataxia). Other deficits include agnosias (impairment of the ability to recognize or comprehend the meaning of various sensory stimuli), neglect (the inability to recognize or interact with part of one's personal or extrapersonal space), and problems with visually guided movements.

The multimodal sensory association cortex in the temporal area (the middle and inferior temporal gyri) is responsible for the integration of visual and auditory information, essential for language. This area is important for object identification, with discrete lesions resulting in area-specific agnosias, such as the inability to recognize faces (prosopagnosia). The inferior temporal gyrus is dominated by input of processed visual information from extrastriate visual areas and is of importance for the interpretation and categorization of complex visual stimuli. As noted earlier in this chapter, the superior temporal gyrus comprises primary and unimodal auditory association cortex.

The motor and premotor cortices act on the progressive integration of sensory, emotional, motivational, and physiological information from other association areas. The premotor areas are in themselves integrative, receiving stimuli from integrative association cortices as well as directly from the unimodal somesthetic cortex. The influence of bias introduced by noradrenergic, serotonergic, cholinergic, and possibly dopaminergic innervation is integrated with excitatory input from the thalamus, which represents the influence of the cerebellum and basal ganglia.

Nonsensory Association Cortex: Limbic System

A "limbic system" was originally proposed as the neuroanatomical substrate of emotion. It was conceived as a discrete, closed system of cortical and subcortical structures and addressed the mechanism by which the cerebral cortex influences the hypothalamus and vice versa. As sophisticated tract-tracing techniques have clarified the extensive interconnections between limbic and nonlimbic structures and the existence of distributed systems throughout the CNS, the limbic system is now accepted as an open system thoroughly integrated with structures at all levels of the CNS (Parent 1996).

The subcortical limbic structures include the amygdaloid complex, ventral striatum, mamillary nuclei, hypothalamus, and several thalamic nuclei. Cortical regions considered limbic include the parahippocampal gyrus, cingulate gyrus, orbitofrontal cortex, piriform cortex, and hippocampus. Several limbic structures, including the amygdaloid complex, hippocampal formation, and cingulate gyrus, have extensive interconnections with broad areas of neocortex, including virtually all areas of multimodal sensory association cortex and integrative association cortex (discussed in the following section).

The limbic system may form the gateway for neocortical cognitive influences on hypothalamic mechanisms associated with motivation and emotion, and vice versa. The limbic system directly influences neuroendocrine, autonomic, and behavioral mechanisms associated with the diencephalon. Functions such as the fight-or-flight response, homeostasis, self-maintenance, feeding, and sexuality are thought to be linked to limbic structures. The limbic system is also involved in more complex behaviors, including production of an emotional response, learning, and memory. For example, the amygdala is the CNS locus that attaches emotional significance to extensively processed sensory stimuli. Additionally, the hippocampal formation–mamillary body–fornix system is crucial in the formation of new memories.

Integrative Association Cortex

After sensory modalities are integrated in the multimodal sensory association cortices, information next progresses to the *integrative association cortex*. The two areas of integrative association cortex are extensively interconnected, so they should be considered as two aspects of a distributed system. The smaller of the two areas—the *posterior integrative association cortical area*—is found where the parietal, occipital, and temporal lobes converge. This area can be considered the locus of final multimodal sensory integration. Along with adjacent multimodal sensory association areas, it is in this area that object identification and other meaningful features of sensory experiences are appreciated. This suggests an area where a completely integrated perceptual world might be accessed and an area where dysfunction, as in degenerative dementias, could leave a person essentially lost in the world.

The *anterior integrative association cortical area* is found in the broad convexity of the frontal lobes, usually designated *dorsolateral prefrontal cortex*. This area manifests extensive connections with occipital, parietal, and temporal lobes, especially the posterior integrative association cortical area, and the cingulate gyrus. Afferent input from the dorsomedial thalamic nucleus provides input from the amygdala and other limbic structures. It also has reciprocal connections with premotor and supplementary motor areas, the caudate nucleus, and the hypothalamus.

The frontal association cortex thus receives information from all sensory modalities, from all other cortical association areas, from subcortical structures such as the basal ganglia and limbic system, and from the hypothalamus, the master of the body's physiology and autonomic nervous system. Limbic input, both cortical and subcortical, introduces the influence of emotion, attention, and motivation to the integrated and interpreted sensory information. The frontal association cortex is considered the locus of executive functioning, insight, judgment, planning, abstract thought, and the ability to anticipate consequences of actions. This area uniquely does not fully mature until early adulthood, so some of these are capabilities of adult humans. Other abilities conferred by the frontal association cortex include the ability to form and retain inner conceptions of objects, with dysfunction resulting in increased distractibility. Lesions restricted to the frontal lobes can produce disturbances of mood, including depression or mania, as well as marked personality changes and impairment of judgment.

Hemispheric Lateralization of Function

Lateralization of speech is the most extreme example of lateralization of function (or *hemispheric dominance*). Speech centers are located in the dominant hemisphere, which is the left hemisphere in at least 90% of people. The anterior speech area (Broca's area) is located in prefrontal association cortex, just anterior to the most inferior part of the motor strip, corresponding approximately to BA 44. This region is an essential component of the motor mechanisms governing articulated speech, and lesions of Broca's area result in nonfluent or *expressive aphasia*. Despite preservation of control of motor systems and preservation of language comprehension in individuals with this aphasia, the ability to produce more than a few words is markedly impaired. The impairment of speech production is often accompanied by *agraphia*, the inability to generate written communication. Thus, the inability to express oneself through language characterizes this form of aphasia.

The posterior speech area (Wernicke's area) is located in the superior part of the temporal lobe, corresponding approximately to BA 22. Lesions of Wernicke's area result in fluent or *receptive aphasia*. Receptive aphasia is characterized by impairment of the appreciation of the meaning of both spoken and written words. Speech can appear normal in terms of flow, but the content of the communication is notable for a paucity of meaning and the use of incorrect words. Other forms of aphasia are seen when lesions interrupt the fiber bundle interconnecting the anterior and posterior speech areas.

Although we have just stated that speech centers are located in the dominant hemisphere in most people, this is an oversimplification. In fact, the verbal aspect of speech occupies the dominant hemisphere in most people. The nondominant hemisphere has corresponding speech centers that govern *nonverbal* aspects of speech, or *prosody*. Lesions can result in impairment of the ability to imbue speech with the intonation and melody that lend emotional meaning to speech (anterior area) or in impairment of the ability to appreciate or understand the prosody of other people's speech (posterior area).

Electrophysiological Studies in the Psychiatric Evaluation of the Elderly Patient

Electroencephalography

Electroencephalography is the oldest functional imaging technique in continued use by psychiatry and neurology. Although lacking the spatial resolution of newer imaging techniques, it retains an exceptionally high degree of temporal resolution, as electroencephalographic (EEG) recordings reflect brain activity essentially on the same time scale as the activity of cortical neurons. Electroencephalography has traditionally been used to assist diagnosis of epilepsy, delirium, and gross neuropathology. Although no qualitatively specific EEG markers exist for psychopathology, the electroencephalogram is highly sensitive to a variety of neuropathological conditions. In addition, the introduction of quantitative EEG analysis has greatly expanded the usefulness of the technique in the evaluation of dementia and delirium. Quantitative electroencephalography has been an important research tool, showing promise for enhancing our understanding of the neurophysiology and neuropathology underlying these conditions (Cook and Leuchter 1996; Holschneider and Leuchter 1999; Knott et al. 2001). The APA Task Force on Quantitative Electrophysiological Assessment (1991) suggested that the technique has particular clinical utility for detection of slow-wave abnormalities.

The surface and scalp electroencephalograph measures the integrated electrical activity of neuronal processes in the superficial layers of the cortex. The specific neuronal events constituting the EEG signal likely result from summated postsynaptic potentials rather than the relatively short-duration action potentials (Creutzfeldt et al. 1966). Although activity in only the most superficial layers of cortex is thought to produce the EEG signal, the influence of deeper brain structures on the activity of these cortical neurons is reflected in the frequency spectra and synchrony of the electroencephalogram (Holschneider and Leuchter 1999). In particular, synchronous pacemaker activity is thought to be generated by thalamocortical networks, whereas desynchronization (which reflects increased arousal) may be mediated by monoaminergic inputs from the brain stem and basal forebrain. Normally, the resistive and capacitative characteristics of the scalp and skull significantly attenuate the electrical signal. Thus, pathologies that may reduce electrical resistance (skull fractures) or increase resistance (subdural hematomas) may result in localized alterations in the amplitude of the electroencephalogram (Pfurtscheller and Cooper 1975). On occasion, the electroencephalogram may provide the initial clue to the presence of these conditions.

The electroencephalogram is typically recorded with the patient awake and at rest in a comfortable position. Specific studies also may use sleep deprivation or hyperventilation to increase sensitivity for detection of abnormal electrical activity. Electrodes are placed on the scalp in an array, or *montage*, of 10–20 leads, although special studies may warrant the addition of nasopharyngeal or ethmoid electrodes. Visual inspection by a qualified electroencephalographer remains the best method for distinguishing paroxysmal activity, epileptiform activity, and asymmetries from artifacts. Subsequently, portions of the signal may be digitized and the various frequency spectra of background activity quantified with a computer. The spectra of EEG frequencies are conventionally divided into bands defined as delta (<4 Hz), theta (4–8 Hz), alpha (8–13 Hz), and beta (>13 Hz). These frequency bands can be characterized on the basis of *absolute power* (the magnitude of the signal amplitude of a specific frequency band, measured in microvolts squared) and *relative power* (the percent contribution of a specific frequency band to the total power), in addition to measures of ratios of particular frequencies (called *spectral ratios*). Alterations in the frequency spectrum associated with neuropathology may be global (often seen in metabolic, toxic, or anoxic encephalopathy) or localized (seen in focal lesions such as tumors or strokes). Other useful quantitative EEG measures are *coherence*, which indicates the functional coupling of distinct brain regions based on common time-locked frequency elements, and *cordance*, which normalizes power across electrode sites and combines absolute and relative power into a single measure (Holschneider and Leuchter 1999). Cordance, in particular, appears to best correlate with measures of cerebral perfusion (Leuchter et al. 1999).

EEG Changes With Normal Aging

The electroencephalogram of a healthy awake adult is dominated by frequencies in the alpha range. This pattern shows little change with normal aging (Duffy et al. 1984). A small decline in the mean alpha frequency may be seen beginning in the fifth decade, but a significant drop suggests underlying neuropathology. When comparing healthy subjects across the entire span of the adult years, a small increase in beta frequency activity often correlates with age (Holschneider and Leuchter 1995). Small increases in theta activity are frequently seen in healthy older adults but also may be associated with the subclinical onset of cerebrovascular disease; however, normal aging is generally not associated with significant increases in delta activity (Holschneider and Leuchter 1999).

EEG Changes With Dementia

The most characteristic EEG findings associated with dementia are an increase in low-frequency (delta and theta) activity, along with a decrease in high-frequency beta activity and slowing of the dominant alpha frequencies. These separate findings are not necessarily statistically associated within populations of subjects with dementia, suggesting that they may reflect independent underlying processes (Claus et al. 2000; Leuchter et al. 1993a). Abnormal findings with conventional electroencephalography are most evident in the later stages of dementia but may be common even in the early stages (Leuchter et al. 1993b). The probability of early detection of these abnormalities is increased by combining several complementary quantitative EEG measures (Leuchter et al. 1993a). Thus, the change in the low-frequency band is best able to distinguish subjects with dementia from control subjects, although inclusion of additional parameters has cumulative diagnostic significance. Several studies have also shown decreased coherence in dementia, which may reflect the loss of long corticocortical connections (Knott et al. 2000; Leuchter et al. 1992). This "disconnection" hypothesis is supported by a study reporting that dementia patients exhibit decreased global EEG synchronization in alpha, beta, and gamma bands (but increased delta bands) (Koenig et al. 2005). By combining measures of spectral ratios and coherence variables, quantitative EEG testing has accurately discriminated between subjects with Alzheimer's dementia, subjects with vascular dementia, and control subjects without dementia (Leuchter et al. 1987). A recent report has suggested that quantitative EEG measures may be used to accurately predict subsequent cognitive decline and dementia in persons initially presenting with only subjective memory complaints (Prichep et al. 2006).

The cognitive dysfunction seen in Alzheimer's dementia is associated with loss of central cholinergic systems. Following treatment of dementia with the acetylcholinesterase inhibitor physostigmine (Gustafson 1993), tetrahydroaminoacridine (Minthon et al. 1993; Perryman and Fitten 1991), or rivastigmine (Adler and Brassen 2001), the quantitative electroencephalogram shows a decrease in slow-frequency power and an increase in high-frequency power. Thus, the quantitative electroencephalogram may parallel response to agents that enhance cognitive function in subjects with dementia (although this effect may not necessarily be specific to cholinergic agents).

EEG Changes With Delirium

Delirium refers to an acute confusional state, characterized by clouding of consciousness and impaired attentional capacity. The causes of delirium are numerous, with the most common being drug toxicity and metabolic imbalances. Electroencephalography is a standard tool in the evaluation of delirium because EEG slowing is an almost universal finding in delirium. The quantitative electroencephalogram may be more sensitive than the conventional electroencephalogram to changes in slow-wave power during the course of delirium (Leuchter and Jacobson 1991). The quantitative EEG signal correlates with the severity and duration of the delirium (Koponen et al. 1989), whereas the normalization of the signal parallels and occasionally precedes the course of recovery (Leuchter and Jacobson 1991). The degree of slowing reflects the severity of the delirium even in the context of preexisting dementia and therefore may be of particular use in detecting delirium as a complication of dementia (Jacobson et al. 1993).

EEG Changes With Depression

The standard awake electroencephalogram is expected to have normal findings in otherwise healthy depressed subjects (Heyman et al. 1991). Thus, in the context of cognitive dysfunction suggestive of dementia, a normal EEG result may be useful in identifying depression-related pseudodementia (Brenner et al. 1989). However, several studies of subjects with pseudodementia or depression still documented more EEG abnormalities than in nondepressed control subjects (Brenner et al. 1986, 1989; Visser et al. 1985). In depressed elderly subjects, abnormal EEG findings are associated with an increased risk for subsequent cognitive dysfunction and may be indicative of underlying cerebrovascular disease. The electroencephalogram recorded during sleep (polysomnographic recording) often shows depression-related phenomena such as reduced slow-wave sleep and decreased rapid eye movement latency (see Chapter 22, "Sleep and Circadian Rhythm Disorders," in this volume).

Epilepsy in the Elderly

The incidence of seizures in the elderly is quite high and may account for up to one-quarter of new epilepsy cases (Sander et al. 1990). Approximately half of these seizures are related to either strokes or tumors, whereas up to one-quarter have unknown causes; as many as 80% become recurrent (Luhdorf et al. 1986b). Alzheimer's dementia is also a risk factor for refractory seizures in the elderly (Mendez et al. 1994). The electroencephalogram is commonly used to confirm epileptiform activity and to assist in classification of the seizure disorder. However, a high percentage of persons with seizures may have normal EEG findings, depending on the type of seizure and the interval between the seizure activity and the recording (Luhdorf et al. 1986a). In addition, the presence of interictal epileptiform activity (spike-and-wave complexes) alone does not establish a diagnosis of epilepsy. Various other clinical conditions can predispose a person to paroxysmal electrical activity unrelated to seizures. For example, elderly patients with syncopal episodes show an almost 50% incidence of epileptiform events (Hughes and Zialcita 2000). Increased diagnostic reliability may be facilitated by simultaneous electroencephalography and videotape monitoring to assess motor and behavioral disturbance with concomitant EEG activity (Bridgers and Ebersole 1985). Ultimately, the diagnosis of epilepsy and the decision to treat with anticonvulsant medication should rely primarily on the clinical presentation.

Evoked Potentials

Evoked potentials refer to EEG signals recorded in response to a specific sensory stimulus. However, the amplitude of background EEG activity is typically 10–100 times that of single evoked responses. Averaging the stimulus-locked signal over multiple trials causes the background activity to average out to zero, allowing accurate measure of the amplitude and latency of the evoked response. Evoked potentials are frequently used to assess neuroanatomical pathways underlying the response to visual, auditory, or somatosensory stimuli. Most studies focus on particular components of the evoked potential waveform, designated according to the eliciting conditions or the electrophysiological signature (e.g., the P300, or P3, wave, seen as a positive-going wave 300 milliseconds after the trigger stimulus). The P3 wave is elicited in response to infrequent target stimuli to which the subject must attend; these stimuli are typically intermixed with multiple irrelevant stimuli. As such, the P3 wave is thought to reflect neural processes underlying attention and immediate memory (Polich and Kok 1995). The P3 wave has been shown to increase in latency with age in neurologically normal subjects (Goodin et al. 1978a), with little age-related change occurring in other components of the evoked waveform (Polich 1997). The P3 latency is increased further in most patients with dementia (Goodin et al. 1978b; Polich 1991). The P3 latency is related to the severity of the dementia, although less so with mild dementia (Polich et al. 1986), whereas variability in P3 wave amplitude is highly correlated with decrements in cognitive performance (Hogan et al. 2006). Although studies of the P3 latency have not been able to distinguish between subtypes of cortical dementias (Polich et al. 1986), other studies have suggested that evoked potentials may distinguish between cortical dementias (e.g., Alzheimer's) and subcortical dementias (Parkinson's or Huntington's disease) (Goodin and Aminoff 1986, 1987).

The use of evoked potentials in the evaluation of dementias remains primarily a research tool, although studies to date suggest that, like quantitative electroencephalograms, evoked potentials may serve to elucidate aspects of the underlying neuropathologies of dementias (Polich 1991).

Magnetoencephalography

Magnetoencephalography involves recording magnetic fields generated by neural activity, which, according to the "right-hand rule," occur at right angles to the direction of current flow across the neuronal membranes. Thus, the magnetoencephalographic (MEG) signal is related to the electroencephalogram but has the advantage of more accurately detecting current sources from deep brain structures (Reeve et al. 1989). For example, MEG recordings have localized the neural generators of the P3 wave in the frontal and posterior parietal cortices and have shown age-related decreases in the magnetic signal from these areas that parallel the P3 signal (Anderer et al. 1998). MEG studies have reported delayed preconscious auditory processing in patients with mild to moderate Alzheimer's dementia (Pekkonen et al. 1999). Recent studies indicate that magnetoencephalography may be used to discriminate between normal aging, mild cognitive impairment, and Alzheimer's dementia (Fernández et al. 2006). In addition, source modeling with MEG studies has suggested that the decrease in EEG frequency observed in dementia patients may not be due so much to slowing of activity of existing oscillatory sources, but rather due to a shift to enhanced signal strength from brain regions (e.g., temporal) with slower intrinsic oscillation (Osipova et al. 2005). However, magnetoencephalography remains primarily a research tool largely because of cost and technical constraints of the recording.

Neuroanatomical and Neuropathological Processes of Aging

The faculty of cognition is that function of the human brain that sets humans apart from other animals. Unfortunately, this unique ability is subject to degeneration as a consequence of aging. Much more extensive degeneration with significant loss of cognitive function occurs during the evolution of Alzheimer's disease and other neurodegenerative disorders that uniquely afflict the aging population.

We focus on the neuroanatomical and neuropathological processes that occur during normal aging. Subsequently, we address abnormal aging, discussing each of the major neurodegenerative disorders that affect the human brain and cause dementia.

Neuroanatomy

The average adult male human brain weighs 1,400 g (Sunderman and Boerner 1949). The organ is composed of neurons and supporting cells and structures. The supporting elements include astrocytes, oligodendroglia, and ependyma, collectively known as *glia, blood vessels*, and *myelin*. Myelin is a complex lipoprotein that serves to protect axonal processes and to facilitate neurotransmission.

It has been estimated that the adult human brain contains some 20 billion neurons. Each neuron is an individual unit that can be thought of as a microprocessor. Individual neurons are functionally integrated into networks of allied nerve cells. Networks of neurons are assembled within subcortical structures that are known as *nuclei* (Vogel 1996). Networks of neurons in the neocortex, the outer layer of the cerebrum, are also organized into functional units so that some parts of the neocortex are devoted to cognitive function, whereas other parts command motor skills and the major senses, including vision, hearing, and smell.

The neuron develops during embryonic intrauterine life. Both neurons and glia originate from the germinal zone in the subpial and subependymal regions. During intrauterine development, neurons undergo mitotic division and then migrate to the cerebral cortex.

They are assisted in their migration by glial filaments that stretch from the subependymal germinal zone to the cortex (Marín-Padilla 1995). Once the neurons have reached their permanent location, they differentiate and develop synaptic connections. Development of synaptic connections continues to progress rapidly after birth (Vogel 1996). The neuron is no longer capable of division after birth, but synaptic connections are continuously remodeled. This is the neuroanatomical basis of memory and learning. Loss of some of these synaptic connections is the neuroanatomical cause of normal age-related memory impairment. Pathological loss of these synaptic connections is the basis of dementia.

Each neuron is surrounded by a three-layer plasma membrane that is regionally specialized to form axons, dendrites, and synapses. As with all cells in the body, the plasma membrane of neurons controls the movement of metabolites between the neuron and its environment. Selected areas serve as synaptic sites. Synaptic transmission transfers messages from one neuron to other neurons and to end organs (Vogel 1996).

The neuronal nucleus is located in the cell body. It varies in size from 5 to 100 μm. The area around the nucleus, or perikaryon, contains ribosomes that synthesize the proteins that are necessary to maintain metabolism and synaptic transmission. Ribosomes may reside free within the cytoplasm, or they may be attached to the endoplasmic reticulum. The endoplasmic reticulum, being largely composed of proteins, is acidic in nature, and it appears as a blue granular Nissl substance on histological preparations (Vogel 1996).

Neurons are metabolically very active cells and thus require numerous mitochondria. Most of the neuronal mitochondria are contained in the perikaryon. Additionally, numerous proteins are turned over frequently in neuronal cell bodies as a function of their role in synaptic transmission. Some of these proteins are not metabolized entirely, and these nonmetabolized proteins are stored in structures known as *lysosomes*. Histologically, collections of these lysosomes are known as *lipofuscin granules*. Increased numbers of lipofuscin granules are evidence of normal metabolic wear and tear. As a consequence, they accumulate with age.

Microtubules, neurofilaments, and microfilaments are specialized structures that make up the neuronal cytoskeleton. Microtubules measure 20–30 nm, neurofilaments 10 nm, and microfilaments 5 nm in diameter. Microtubules are long, unbranched cylinders composed almost entirely of the protein tubulin (Vogel 1996). Many neurodegenerative processes cause abnormal aggregation or assembly of microtubule-associated proteins. This results in the formation of tangle inclusions in neuronal and glial cells.

The synapse is a specialized structure that permits the flow of information from one neuron to another neuron or to the end organ. The synapse is analogous to an electronic circuit so that the flow of information is from sensory to motor neurons, for example, but never the reverse. The synapse consists of the approximation of two membranes physically separated by approximately 20 nm. The contact between an axon and a cell body is termed an *axosomatic synapse*. Contact between an axon and a dendrite is termed an *axodendritic synapse*. The synaptic connection between two axons is known as an *axoaxonic synapse*, and the synapse between two dendrites is known as a *dendrodendritic synapse*. When an electrical impulse is transmitted from the nerve cell body through the axon or dendrite to the synapse, the neuron releases a substance known as a *neurotransmitter*. Each neuron releases only one neurotransmitter (Vogel 1996). Groups of neurons that are collected into nuclei generally release the same neurotransmitter. For example, the neurons in the nucleus basalis of Meynert release the neurotransmitter acetylcholine. Suppression or enhancement of neurotransmission is the pharmacological basis of most neuroactive compounds.

Normal Aging

We all recognize that as we age, our fund of knowledge and experience increases, but regrettably, we may not always recollect this information with the same speed as we did when we were younger. When the process of remembering is slightly slowed but still intact, this is recognized as normal aging. However, this normal slowing may progress in some individuals to mild cognitive impairment. In a further subgroup of individuals, this mild cognitive impairment and memory loss may follow an inexorable downhill decline into dementia. Subsequent sections of this chapter cover the changes observed in pathological aging. In this section, we discuss the neuropathological changes that are seen in persons who have aged normally.

Normal healthy aging is sometimes associated with no identifiable neuropathological changes. Approximately 30%–50% of normally aged individuals show no evidence of cortical atrophy, no evidence of cell loss, no evidence of senile neuritic plaques, and no evidence of neurofibrillary tangles. However, in most elderly individuals, some pathological changes are evident (Hulette et al. 1998). Both senile neuritic plaques and neurofibrillary tangles may be seen in cognitively intact aged individuals. Nevertheless, the frequency and distribution of these pathological changes in the elderly without dementia are generally much less extensive than those observed in individuals at the same age who have dementia.

Senile plaques first begin to appear in the cortex, where they are observed as round smudges on silver impregnation studies. Plaques at this stage are immunoreactive for β-amyloid, but there is no histological distortion of the surrounding neuropil. These are known as *diffuse plaques*. Diffuse plaques may occur quite early in individuals who are environmentally and genetically at risk for the development of Alzheimer's disease (Crain et al. 1995). Diffuse plaques are common in normally aged individuals and are considered to have no pathological significance. As the plaque matures, neurites that are filled with neurofibrillary tangles and other abnormally posttranslationally modified proteins begin to accumulate around a central amyloid core. At this point, these plaques are called *mature neuritic plaques*. A few mature neuritic plaques are common in normally aged individuals. Even frequent mature plaques may be seen. The distribution and frequency of mature neuritic plaques do not consistently correlate with cognitive function.

In contrast to this lack of correlation between neuritic plaques and cognition, neurofibrillary tangle frequency and distribution do predict cognitive status. Persons with neurofibrillary change limited to the entorhinal cortex and the inferior temporal lobe generally have functioned normally in their communities. Prior to death, they were able to live independently, to engage in conversation, and to be involved in all of the normal activities of daily living. However, when these persons are subjected to rigorous neuropsychological tests, they may show some slight slowing, especially on tests of frontal lobe function. Their ability to create trails is somewhat slowed compared with their counterparts who have absolutely no neuropathological changes. They also show some minor deficits in word list recall (Hulette et al. 1998; Welsh-Bohmer et al. 2001). When the neurofibrillary change has become more extensive, spreading to the neocortex, cognitive impairment develops (Markesberry et al. 2006; Mitchell et al. 2002). In a longitudinal study of patients with amnestic mild cognitive impairment, it was found that these patients showed pathological changes of early Alzheimer's disease (Markesberry et al. 2006). Further studies of normal aging may yield additional cognitive tests that are sensitive indicators of early decline. There is hope that in the future, individuals who begin to show cognitive decline may be subjects for cognitive or pharmacological intervention.

Alzheimer's Disease

Alzheimer's disease is, by definition, a dementing disorder that is associated with characteristic microscopic pathology. The diagnosis of Alzheimer's disease is a clinicopathological one, with definitive confirmation presently possible only with tissue examination, most commonly by brain autopsy. The macroscopic appearance of the brains of patients with Alzheimer's disease can be quite variable, ranging from nearly normal to severely atrophic. In general, patients with clinically evident Alzheimer's disease exhibit grossly noticeable brain atrophy with narrowing of gyri and widening of sulci (Figure 4–2). This cortical atrophy may be readily apparent in imaging studies that may have been performed years prior to death.

The atrophy associated with Alzheimer's disease results in a 200- to 500-g weight loss. The brain of a patient with Alzheimer's disease generally weighs less than 1,200 g and may be as small as 800 g. Typically, the atrophy is bilaterally symmetrical and eventually affects all lobes of the brain, with the occipital lobe being relatively spared until late in the disease. The cerebellum is generally uninvolved. The meninges are grossly normal. The cranial nerves usually are normal, and the large cerebral vessels in cases of uncomplicated Alzheimer's disease are not affected by atherosclerosis. When the brain is sectioned, moderate to severe ventricular dilation is grossly evident (Figure 4–3). In uncomplicated Alzheimer's disease, subcortical structures are grossly normal (Esiri et al. 1997).

When sections of the brain are stained and examined under the microscope, several characteristic features are seen. The *senile* or *neuritic plaque* is one of the most-studied pathological hallmarks of Alzheimer's disease. The senile plaque is a discrete globular structure ranging from 50 μm to 200 μm in diameter. The plaque consists of a dense amyloid core surrounded by swollen axonal and dendritic processes that contain abnormally assembled microtubule-associated proteins, extracellular amyloid deposits, reactive astrocytes, and microglial cells. Immunohistochemical studies of senile

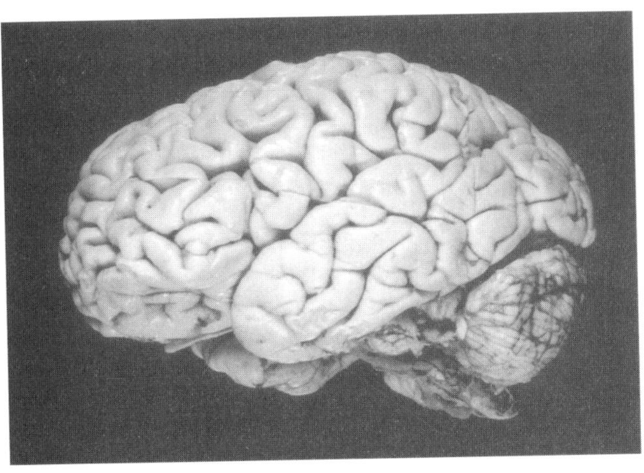
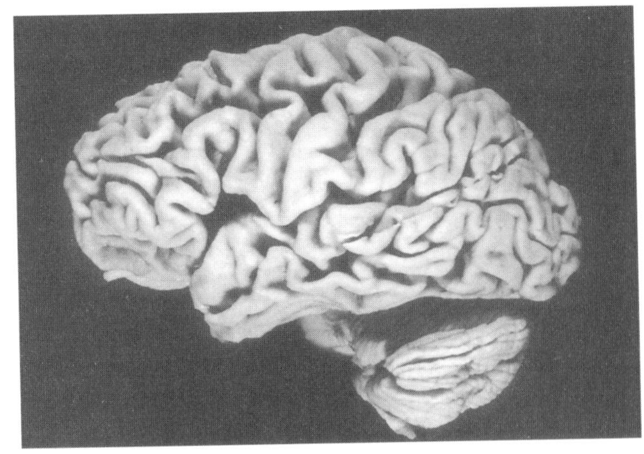

FIGURE 4–2. Normal brain: lateral view (*left*). Alzheimer's disease brain: lateral view (*right*).

In the Alzheimer's brain, moderate diffuse cortical atrophy is apparent. The gyri are narrowed, and the sulci are widened.

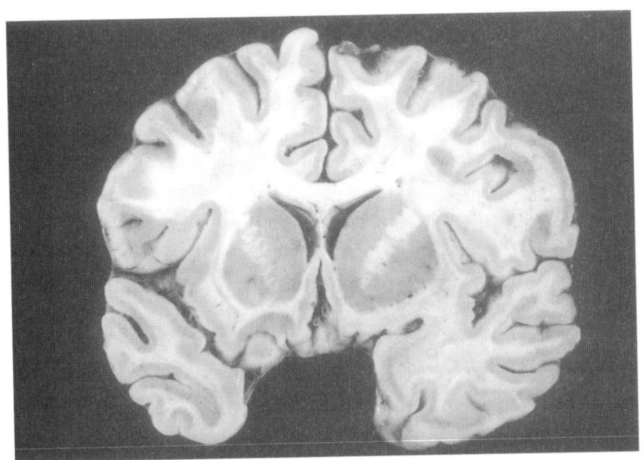
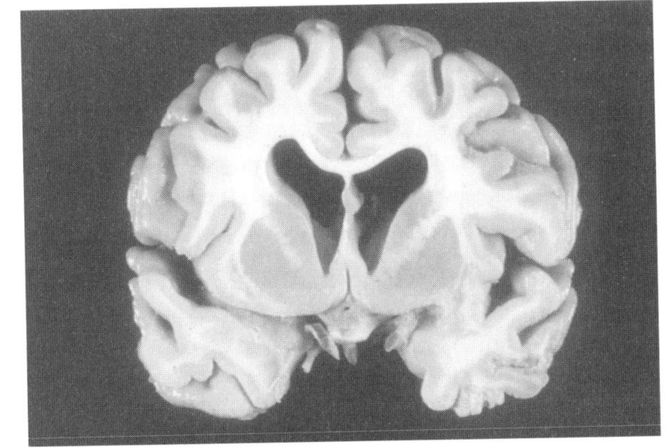

FIGURE 4–3. Normal brain: coronal section through the basal ganglia (*left*). Alzheimer's disease brain: coronal section through the basal ganglia (*right*).

In the normal brain, the lateral ventricles are small and there is no atrophy. In the Alzheimer's brain, the lateral ventricles are enlarged and dilated from neuronal loss and atrophy of the cortex.

plaques indicate that they are largely composed of β-amyloid protein. This fibrillar β-amyloid protein has a β-pleated sheet structure that binds to stains such as Congo red and thioflavine S, which allow for visualization of senile plaques at the light microscopic level using polarization and fluorescence optics, respectively. Senile neuritic plaques are also sometimes termed *amyloid plaques* to denote this characteristic feature.

Studies of the molecular composition of plaques have shown that the senile plaque also contains multiple proteins that are involved in the inflammatory cascade (Hulette and Walford 1987; McGeer et al. 1999). Reactive microglial cells, which are the resident immunocompetent cells of the CNS, are prominent. The presence of inflammatory mediators and immunocompetent cells in the vicinity of senile plaques has led some investigators to believe that the immune system plays a significant role in senile plaque formation (McGeer et al. 1999). Indeed, there are ever-increasing reports of use of nonsteroidal anti-inflammatory agents to slow progression and even prevent or delay the onset of Alzheimer's disease.

The *neurofibrillary tangle* is the second characteristic microscopic feature observed in Alzheimer's disease brain tissue. In contrast to the senile neuritic plaques, which are unique to Alzheimer's disease, neurofibrillary tangles occur in a wide variety of neurodegenerative

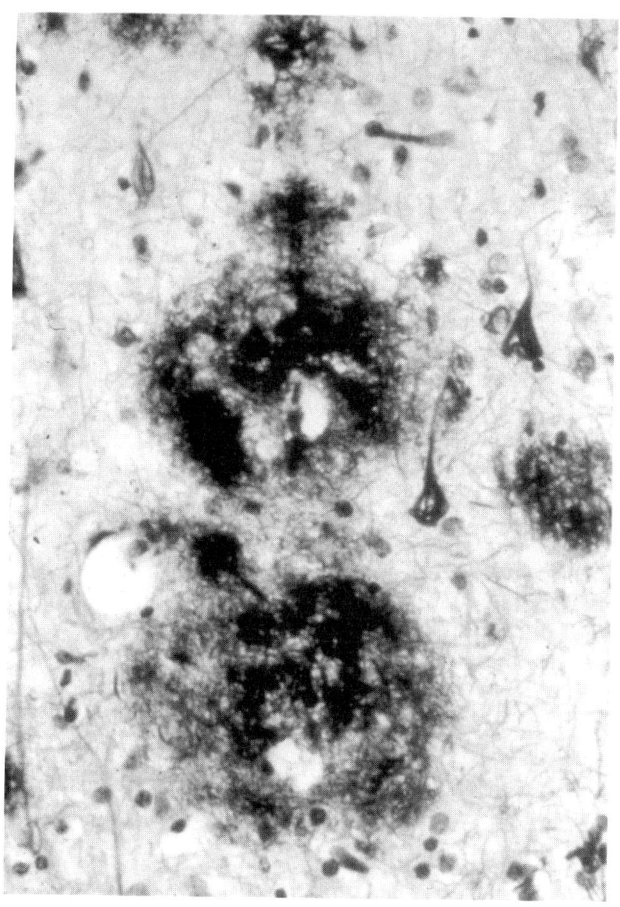

FIGURE 4–4. Alzheimer's disease brain.

The neocortex is filled with senile neuritic plaques and neurofibrillary tangles. (King's silver impregnation stain; original magnification ×400.)

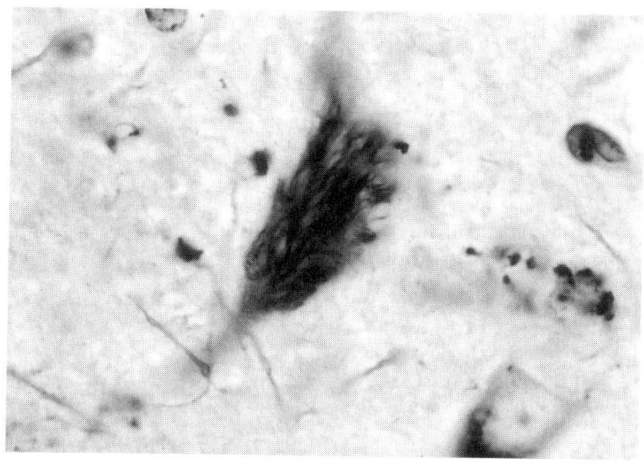

FIGURE 4–5. Alzheimer's disease brain: hippocampus, neurofibrillary tangle.

Note the fibrillary nature of this intraneuronal inclusion. The tangle is shaped like the neuron and fills the cell body. Tangle formation is due to abnormal assembly of phosphorylated microtubule-associated protein into paired helical filaments. (King's silver impregnation stain; original magnification ×1,000.)

disorders, such as frontotemporal lobar degeneration, progressive supranuclear palsy, corticobasal degeneration, postencephalitic parkinsonism, dementia pugilistica, amyotrophic lateral sclerosis–parkinsonism-dementia complex of Guam, subacute sclerosing panencephalitis, and Niemann-Pick disease (Hulette et al. 1991). Neurofibrillary tangles are neuronal inclusions composed of abnormally assembled low-molecular-weight microtubule-associated proteins known as *tau*. Their configuration is determined by the intrinsic shape of the neurons they affect, so tangles occurring in the hippocampal formation have a pyramidal or flame shape, and tangles occurring in subcortical structures may have a globoid shape (Figures 4–4 and 4–5).

Neurofibrillary tangles develop slowly. Early in the process of neurofibrillary degeneration, tangles may be difficult to discern. However, as disease progresses, intraneuronal tangles may be observed in routinely stained sections when examined by the skilled observer. These tangles are quite insoluble and persist as eosinophilic "ghost" tangles within the neuropil of regions of the brain, such as the entorhinal cortex and hippocampus, long after the affected neurons have died and been resorbed. Special stains that better demonstrate neurofibrillary tangles include the fluorescent thioflavine S stain, various silver impregnation procedures, and immunohistochemistry to visualize the various proteins implicated in tangle formation. The major components of neurofibrillary tangles are the low-molecular-weight microtubule-associated proteins tau, which are normal soluble cytoplasmic proteins that function in microtubule assembly and stabilization (Lantos and Cairns 2000). There are six normal isoforms of tau in the adult human brain. All of these isoforms are expressed, hyperphosphorylated, and abnormally assembled into insoluble filamentous inclusions in Alzheimer's disease. These inclusions are not confined to the neuronal cell bodies but also occur within neuronal cell processes or "neurites." When seen within a senile plaque, these neurites are referred to as *dystrophic neurites* and when seen in neuropil are called *neuropil threads*.

Electron microscopy shows neurofibrillary tangles to be composed of dense bundles of long filaments. These filaments occupy most of the neuron's cytoplasm. Each ribbonlike filament has a diameter of

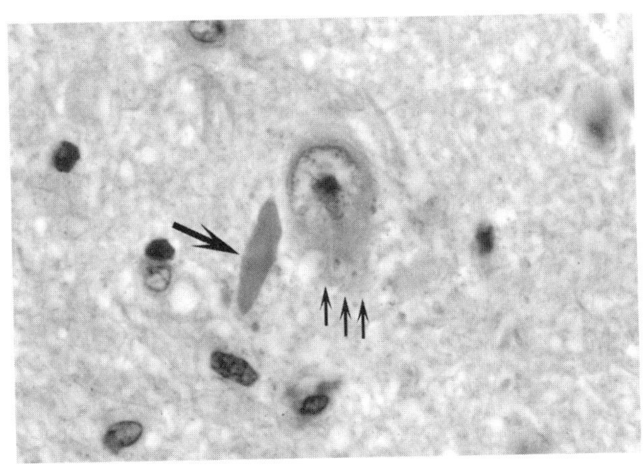

FIGURE 4–6. Alzheimer's disease brain: hippocampus.

This neuron has undergone granulovacuolar degeneration (*small arrows*). Granulovacuolar degenerations are seen almost exclusively in the hippocampal formation. The frequency of granulovacuolar degeneration increases as neurofibrillary change increases elsewhere in the neocortex. Also seen here is a Hirano body (*large arrow*). Hirano bodies are eosinophilic aggregates of actin protein. Hirano bodies are usually closely associated with granulovacuolar degeneration. (Hematoxylin-eosin stain; original magnification ×1,000.)

approximately 22 nm and exhibits a characteristic helical configuration that has been called *paired helical filaments*. These paired helical filaments displace normal cellular organelles and distort the nucleus.

Large population studies of young and old adults without Alzheimer's disease and elderly persons with dementia have found that neurofibrillary change follows a stereotypical progression (Braak and Braak 1991). Neurofibrillary tangles first begin to appear in the entorhinal cortex and the hippocampus. The first appearance of neurofibrillary tangles occurs during Braak Stages I and II. At these stages, persons, even elderly persons, with neurofibrillary change restricted to the entorhinal cortex, hippocampus, and inferior temporal lobe structures generally do not have significant cognitive impairment. At Braak Stage III or IV, tangles become more widespread, involving the inferior temporal lobe diffusely and parts of the neocortex. The individual may or may not develop significant cognitive impairment. However, when cognitive difficulties are present at this stage of neurofibrillary degeneration, they are frequently associated with other neuropathological processes known to cause dementia. Cognitive impairment at this stage of neurofibrillary tangle formation may actually be caused by the concurrence of several disorders, such as Alzheimer's disease plus cerebrovascular disease, Alzheimer's disease plus dementia with Lewy bodies, or Alzheimer's disease plus cardiovascular compromise. If neurofibrillary change progresses unimpeded to involve the cortex globally, including the primary sensory cortices, Braak Stage V or VI is reached. Individuals at this stage almost always have dementia.

Other histopathological changes that are invariably seen in Alzheimer's disease include granulovacuolar degeneration and Hirano bodies. Granulovacuolar degeneration is commonly found in pyramidal neurons of the hippocampus, appearing as distinct cytoplasmic inclusions composed of a central basophilic granule surrounded by a clear halo (Figure 4–6). It appears that these inclusions are derived from lysosomes and the central granule is composed of various cytoskeletal and, in particular, tau epitopes. Hirano bodies are refractile, eosinophilic, rod-shaped inclusions also composed of cytoskeletal proteins, in this instance actin and actin-associated proteins. These inclusions are intracellular structures that commonly involve pyramidal neurons in the CA1 subfield of the hippocampus. Ultrastructurally, Hirano bodies exhibit a very characteristic paracrystalline fine structure (Hirano 1994).

Neuronal and synaptic losses with subsequent chronic reactive astrogliosis are the essential pathological features of Alzheimer's disease and account for its characteristic atrophic changes. The neuronal loss accompanies the accumulation of senile plaques and neurofibrillary tangles that are seen pathologically in Alzheimer's disease. Neuronal loss would certainly result in loss of synapses, but it appears that synaptic loss may actually precede the loss of neuronal cells. This neuronal and synapse loss is nearly always accompanied by increased numbers and enlargement of astrocytic cells, the brain's version of a scar. This astrogliosis is readily observed on routine histological sections or by immunohistochemical preparations with an antibody to glial fibrillary acidic protein.

Vascular abnormalities are common in Alzheimer's disease brain tissue. Many, but not all, cases of Alzheimer's disease are associated with extracellular deposits of vascular amyloid and referred to as *cerebral amyloid angiopathy* (Schmechel et al. 1993). This vascular amyloid is essentially the same as the β-amyloid protein that is present in senile plaques. The severity of vascular amyloid deposition depends on many factors. Interestingly, we have determined that one of these factors is apolipoprotein E (apoE), a lipid transport molecule that occurs in three allelic forms: *APOE*E2*, *APOE*E3*, and *APOE*E4*. *APOE*E4* is a major genetic risk factor for the development of Alzheimer's disease in late life (Corder et al. 1993; Roses et al. 1995, 1996; Saunders et al. 1993, 1996).

Individuals who have inherited one copy of the *APOE*E4* allele have increased risk of vascular amyloid deposition, and individuals with two copies of the *APOE*E4* gene invariably have very severe vascular amyloid deposition. In a study comparing the neuropathological changes of *APOE*E3/APOE*E3*– and *APOE*E4/APOE*E4*–related Alzheimer's disease, it was discovered that *APOE*E4/APOE*E4* patients with severe vascular amyloid deposition also had markedly reduced smooth muscle actin in their cerebral vessels (Hulette et al. 1999). It would thus appear that vascular amyloid replaces smooth muscle actin in the blood vessels of persons with *APOE*E4/APOE*E4*–related Alzheimer's disease. Interestingly, apoE knockout mice have a leaky blood-brain barrier (Fullerton et al. 2001). This presents the intriguing possibility that vascular pathology may be an inciting event in *APOE*E4*-related Alzheimer's disease.

Abnormalities in the white matter are also common in Alzheimer's disease. Whether these abnormalities are a cause or a consequence of the basic neuropathological process is a matter of intense debate. Nevertheless, people with severe Alzheimer's-type pathology have myelin loss in the white matter and perivascular retraction of the neuropil. Frequently, increased numbers of macrophages are present in the perivascular space. Sometimes, areas of microinfarction develop.

Considerable effort has been expended to standardize the clinical and neuropathological assessment of patients with dementia (McKhann et al. 1984). Criteria based on neuritic plaque frequency and cognitive status, as well as criteria based on neurofibrillary tangle distribution and frequency, have been proposed (Braak and Braak 1991; Mirra et al. 1991). The National Institute on Aging (NIA), in cooperation with the Reagan Institute, proposed diagnostic guidelines that require the identification of both frequent senile neuritic plaques and frequent neurofibrillary tangles for a definitive diagnosis of Alzheimer's disease (Hyman and Trojanowski 1997). These criteria, known as NIA-Reagan criteria, have gained wide acceptance in research centers.

Dementia With Lewy Bodies

Lewy body disorders are a clinicopathological spectrum with Parkinson's disease at one end (clinically characterized by a hypokinetic movement disorder) and dementia with Lewy bodies at the other end. Dementia with Lewy bodies is the second most common neurodegenerative disorder manifesting as dementia (Ince et al. 2000). In some respects, dementia with Lewy bodies can be thought of as combined Alzheimer's disease and Parkinson's disease. Clinical and pathological features of both disorders are present. Patients may present for medical attention first complaining of a movement disorder, or they may present with a primary complaint of dementia. Patients who present with dementia often show subtle signs of extrapyramidal dysfunction when subjected to careful neurological examination. This form of dementia is frequently associated with psychotic features such as delusions, hallucinations, and bizarre behaviors (Hulette et al. 1995). The vast majority of cases of dementia with Lewy bodies are sporadic, although apparent familial cases have been reported.

Generally, the weight of the brain of the patient with dementia with Lewy bodies is greater than the weight of the brain of the patient with Alzheimer's disease and may closely approximate normal. Cortical atrophy occurs, but this atrophy is generally much less profound than that seen in Alzheimer's disease in its pure form. On sectioning of the brain, mild ventricular dilation is seen. The hippocampus is generally not grossly atrophic. Gross examination of the brain stem shows loss of normal pigmentation of the substantia nigra in the midbrain (Figure 4–7) and of the locus coeruleus in the pons.

Microscopic examination of the substantia nigra and locus coeruleus shows loss of normal pigmented neurons, presence of extraneuronal neuromelanin granules (so-called pigmentary incontinence), and presence of chronic reactive astrogliosis. Lewy bodies are readily identified (Figure 4–8). These are spherical, hyaline, lamellar, eosinophilic inclusions that are found in the cytoplasm of some of the surviving pigmented neurons. The frequency of these Lewy body inclusions in the substantia nigra of patients with dementia with Lewy bodies may be greater than in patients dying of idiopathic Parkinson's disease. In some patients with dementia, Lewy bodies may be confined to the brain stem and restricted subcortical and cortical regions, as is routinely seen in patients with idiopathic Parkinson's disease; however, these patients more commonly

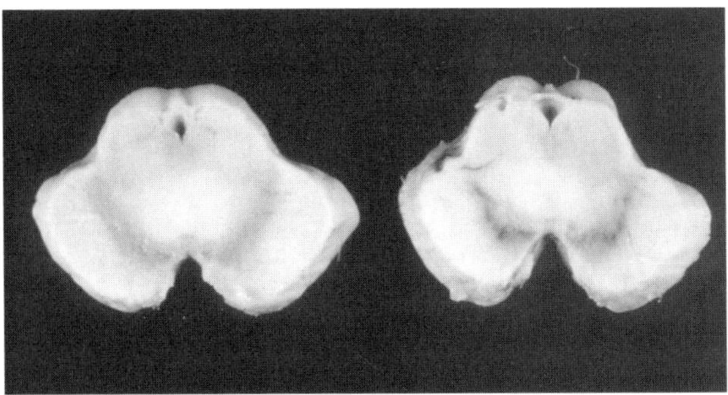

FIGURE 4–7. Dementia with Lewy bodies brain: section through the midbrain (*left*). Normal brain: section through the midbrain (*right*).

Note the loss of the black neuromelanin pigment in the substantia nigra of the patient with dementia with Lewy bodies. This degeneration of the substantia nigra may cause extrapyramidal symptoms such as tremor, rigidity, and bradykinesia.

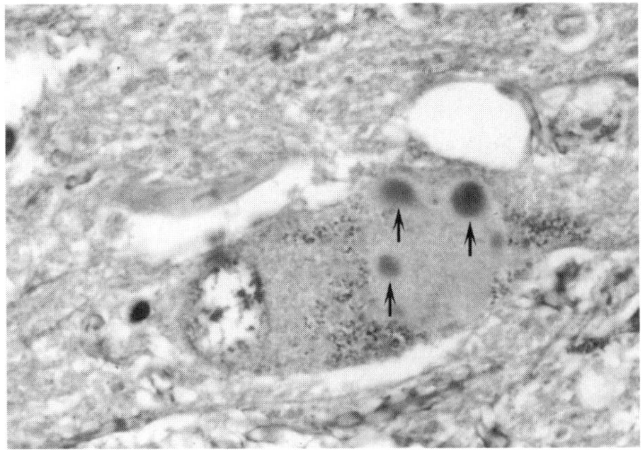

FIGURE 4–8. Dementia with Lewy bodies brain: pigmented neuron of the substantia nigra with several Lewy bodies (*arrows*).

Lewy bodies are intraneuronal cytoplasmic inclusions with a clear halo. (Hematoxylin-eosin stain; original magnification ×1,000.)

exhibit Lewy body pathology affecting the limbic system and the neocortex.

A number of proteins have been identified within Lewy bodies over the years, but neurofilament, ubiquitin, and, in particular, α-synuclein are the most important ones (Spillantini et al. 1997). Immunohistochemistry for α-synuclein has emerged as a sensitive and specific diagnostic tool for the evaluation of dementia with Lewy bodies (Hamilton 2000) (Figure 4–9). Alzheimer's-type pathology, which frequently, but not always, complicates the pathological picture, is generally mild in nature. Diffuse and neuritic plaques may be frequent, but neurofibrillary tangle pathology is generally less intense than in "pure" Alzheimer's disease. Braak stage neurofibrillary change of IV or less is very common in dementia with Lewy bodies (Rosenberg et al. 2001).

Consensus guidelines for the clinical and pathological diagnosis of dementia with Lewy bodies were proposed by the Consortium on Dementia With Lewy Bodies International Workshop (McKeith et al. 1996) and have provided researchers a method of scoring and describing the severity of the Lewy body pathology. The patterns of Lewy body pathology are divided into the following three descriptive categories: brain stem, limbic, and neocortical. In the brain stem category, Lewy body pathology is confined to the substantia nigra, locus coeruleus, and other brain stem nuclei, such as the dorsal motor nucleus of the vagus nerve. The limbic category is defined as disease involving the brain stem and limbic system structures, including amygdala, entorhinal cortex, insula, and cingulate gyrus. The neocortical category includes cases in which Lewy bodies are found throughout the neocortex, as well as in the midbrain and limbic system.

Vascular Dementia

Cerebrovascular disease is associated with a high risk of cognitive impairment and dementia (Brun 2000). Because vascular causes of cognitive impairment are common and potentially reversible, vascular dementia has received increasing attention in recent years. The risk factors for vascular dementia are identical to those for coronary atherosclerosis. These include arterial hypertension, atrial fibrillation, myocardial infarction, diabetes, systemic atherosclerosis, lipid abnormalities, and smoking.

Both small- and large-vessel disease may result in cognitive impairment (Meyer et al. 2000; Pasquier et al. 1999). Large-artery disease, particularly involving the anterior and posterior cerebral circulation, is likely to be associated with dementia. The pathological process may take the form of complete occlusion of the anterior or posterior cerebral artery with the evolution of complete infarcts. However, hypoperfusion syndromes due to severe nonocclusive cerebrovascular atheroscle-

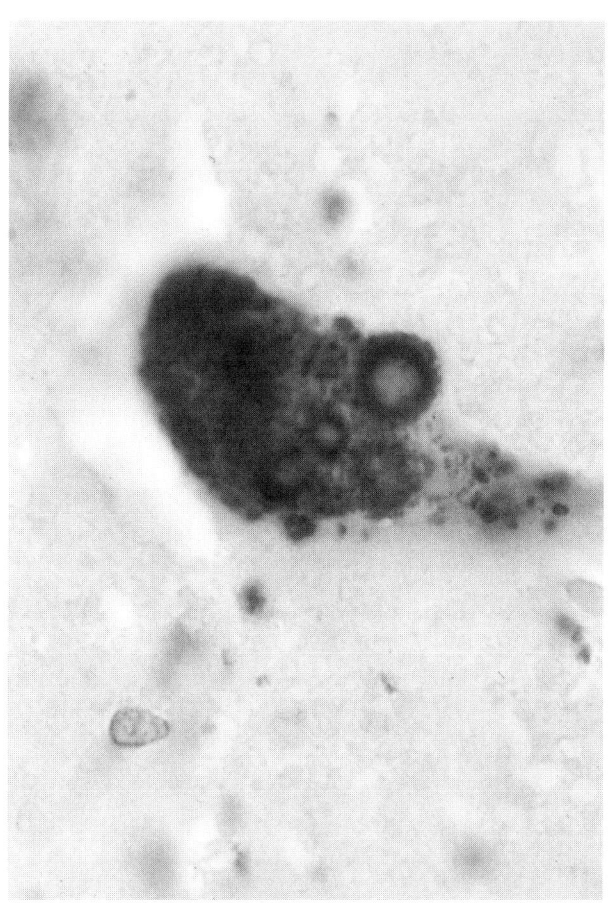

FIGURE 4–9. Dementia with Lewy bodies brain: pigmented neuron of the substantia nigra with numerous Lewy bodies.

Many more Lewy bodies are apparent with this α-synuclein immunostain than are seen in the routine preparation (Figure 4–8). (α-Synuclein immunostain; original magnification ×1,000.)

rosis are increasingly being recognized as a cause of dementia.

Small-vessel infarction or ischemia, especially when it occurs in a strategic location such as the dorsal medial nucleus of the thalamus or the hippocampal formation, also may be associated with cognitive impairment (Hulette et al. 1997). Lacunes and infarcts in the subcortical structures, especially the basal ganglia and thalamus, also may cause or contribute to dementia (Zekry et al. 2002) (Figure 4–10). Lacunes are seen pathologically as small defects in basal ganglia or cortex. Gliosis of the surrounding neuropil is seen, and the central infarcted tissue is gradually replaced by macrophages (Montine and Hulette 1997) (Figure 4–11).

Alternatively, chronic hypertension and atherosclerosis may cause widespread profound white matter ischemic injury without frank infarction. This is recognized pathologically as Binswanger's subcortical arteriosclerotic encephalopathy. In addition to atherosclerosis in the cerebral vasculature, coronary atherosclerosis and cardiovascular injury may result in hypoperfusion injury and contribute to the dementing process (Hulette et al. 2002).

A rare inherited form of vascular dementia is cerebral autosomal dominant arteriopathy with subcortical infarcts and leukoencephalopathy. These patients have strokes at an early age and subsequently may develop dementia. Characteristically, a vasculopathy without amyloid or atherosclerosis affects the arterioles of the white matter (Gray et al. 1994; Zhang et al. 1994). The genetic defect has been mapped to chromosome 19, with mutations in the Notch 3 gene (Tournier-Lasserve et al. 1993; reviewed in Kalimo et al. 2002).

Frontotemporal Lobar Degeneration

Frontotemporal lobar degeneration encompasses a group of disorders that have distinctive clinical, psychiatric, and pathological features (Hodges 2000; Kumar-Singh and Brockhoven 2007). Pick's disease is the prototypical example of these disorders and was first clinically described by Arnold Pick in 1892 and pathologically characterized by Alois Alzheimer in 1907. Macroscopically, there is typically asymmetric atrophy of the frontal and temporal lobes with sparing of the parietal and occipital lobes (Figures 4–12 and 4–13). Histologically, the involved cortex undergoes profound cell loss, which is much greater than that usually seen in Alzheimer's disease. In addition, characteristic Pick's bodies are found within the neurons of the involved areas of cortex. Pick's bodies are globular, intraneuronal inclusions that can be visualized with silver impregnation techniques (Figures 4–14 and 4–15). On immunohistochemical studies, they stain positively for tau epitopes.

Over the past few decades, a number of sporadic and familial disorders with clinical and pathological features similar to but not exactly like Pick's disease have been described. Through recent developments in the understanding of the pathology and genetics of many of these diseases, a pathology-based classification of frontotemporal lobar degeneration has been adopted (reviewed in Kumar-Singh and Brockhoven 2007). The classification is based on 1) the presence or absence

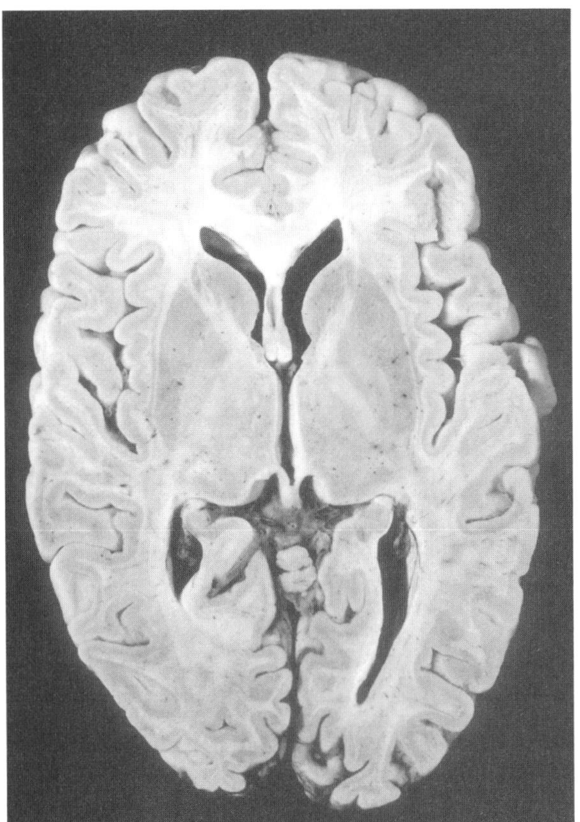

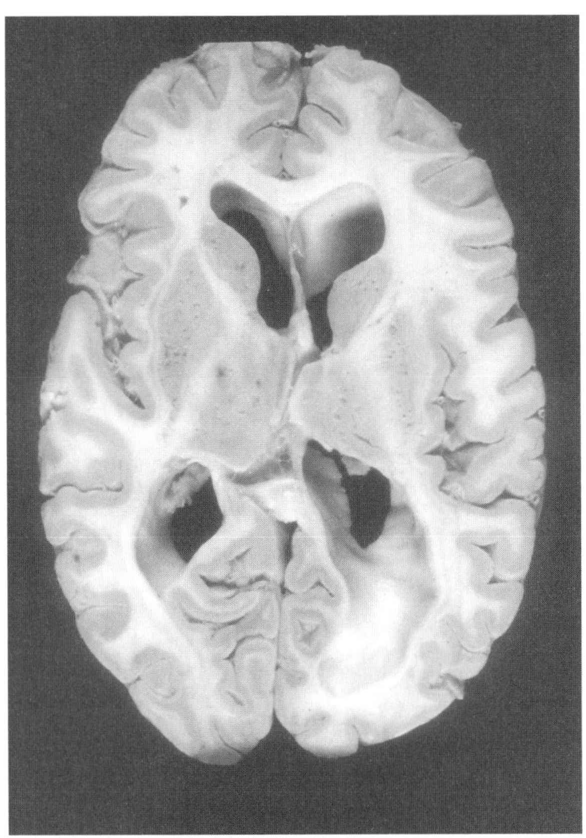

FIGURE 4–10. Normal brain: horizontal section through the basal ganglia (*left*). Vascular dementia, Binswanger's subcortical arteriosclerotic encephalopathy: horizontal section through the basal ganglia at the same level (*right*).

In the vascular dementia brain, the ventricles are dilated and the white matter is pitted and granular.

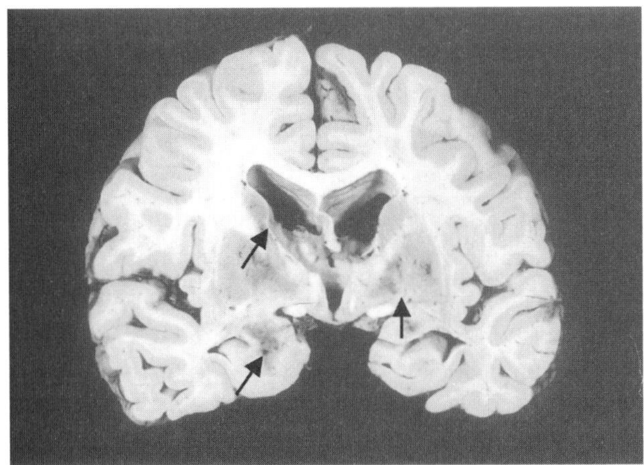

FIGURE 4–11. Vascular dementia with multiple lacunar infarcts (*arrows*): coronal section of brain.

Multiple lacunar infarcts are seen in the basal ganglia. These may cause strokes. Because the individual lesions may occur at different times, there is a stepwise progression of dementia.

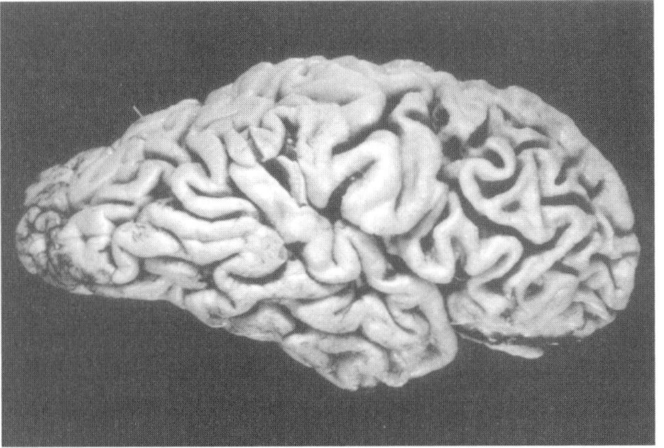

FIGURE 4–12. Pick's disease: lateral view of the brain.

Very severe atrophy ("knife blade") is most pronounced in the frontal and temporal lobes.

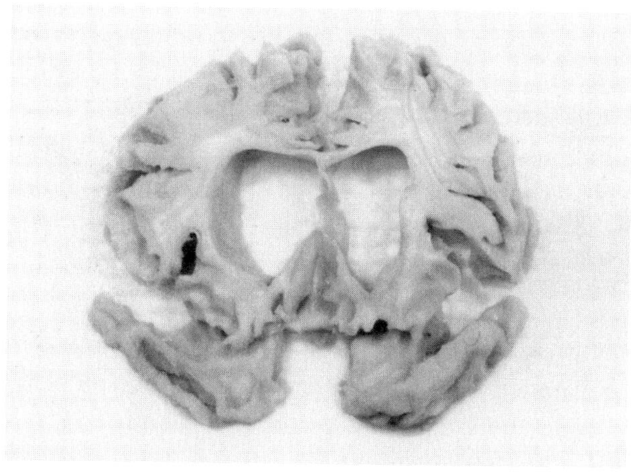

FIGURE 4–13. Pick's disease: coronal section through the basal ganglia.

This disease causes profound atrophy of the cortex. The ventricles are widely dilated. The caudate nucleus is flattened.

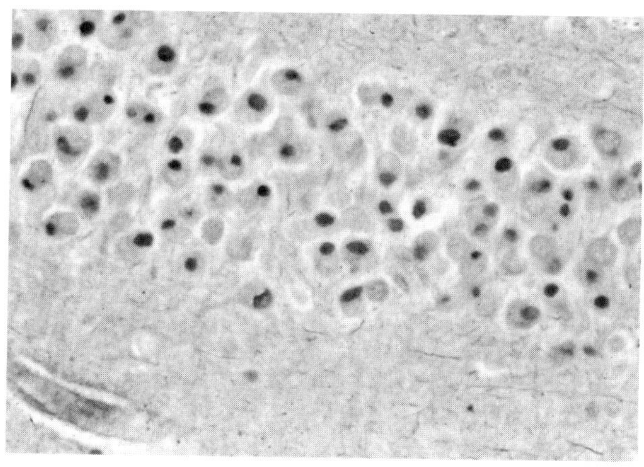

FIGURE 4–14. Pick's disease: hippocampal formation, fascia dentata.

Pick's bodies are round, densely homogeneous argyrophilic inclusions that fill the cytoplasm of virtually every neuron. Like neurofibrillary tangles, they contain abnormally assembled tau proteins. (Glees silver stain; original magnification ×400.)

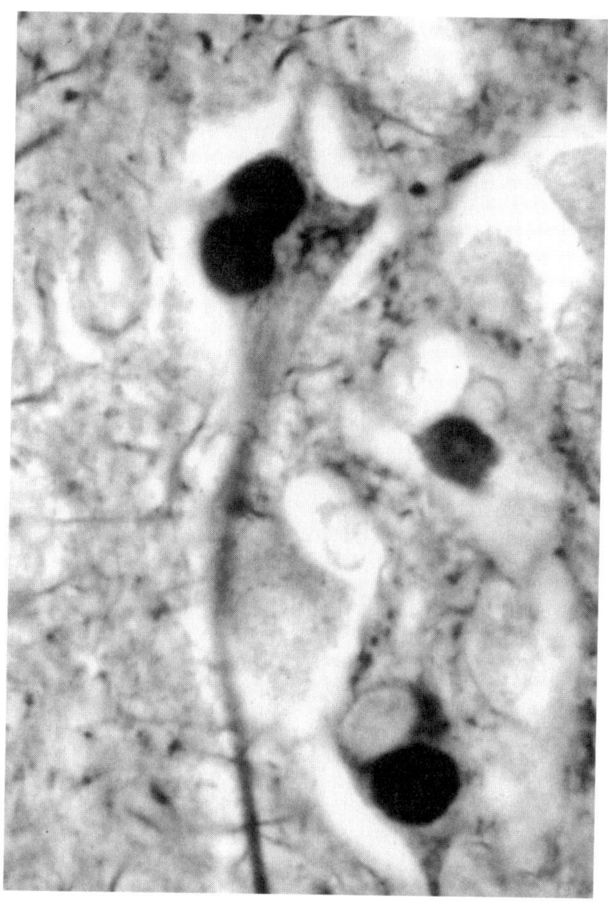

FIGURE 4–15. Pick's disease: hippocampal formation, Ammon's horn.

Pick's bodies are seen here within pyramidal neurons. (Glees silver stain; original magnification ×1,000.)

of neuronal inclusions, 2) the immunohistochemical and biochemical characteristics of inclusions in neuronal and glial cells, and 3) the anatomical distribution of the histopathological changes. The disorders of frontotemporal lobar degeneration are therefore subdivided into those that have tau inclusions; those that have tau-negative, ubiquitin-positive neuronal inclusions; and those that do not have identified protein inclusions. Frontotemporal lobar degeneration disorders with tau inclusions include Pick's disease, progressive supranuclear palsy, corticobasal ganglionic degeneration, and frontotemporal dementia and parkinsonism linked to chromosome 17. Approximately half of autopsy-confirmed cases of frontotemporal lobar dementia belong to the group with tau-negative, ubiquitin-positive neuronal inclusions (Figure 4–16). The latter inclusions are also known as motor neuron disease inclusions because they were first described in patients with amyotrophic lateral sclerosis. Mutations in the genes for valosin-containing protein, charged multivesicular body protein 2B, and progranulin have recently been identified in patients with tau-negative, ubiquitin-positive frontotemporal lobar degeneration (reviewed in Kumar-Singh and Brockhoven 2007). Another important finding has been that the inclusions also share a major common constituent, a nuclear protein called TDP-43. The third subtype of frontotemporal lobar degeneration is characterized by neuronal cell loss and

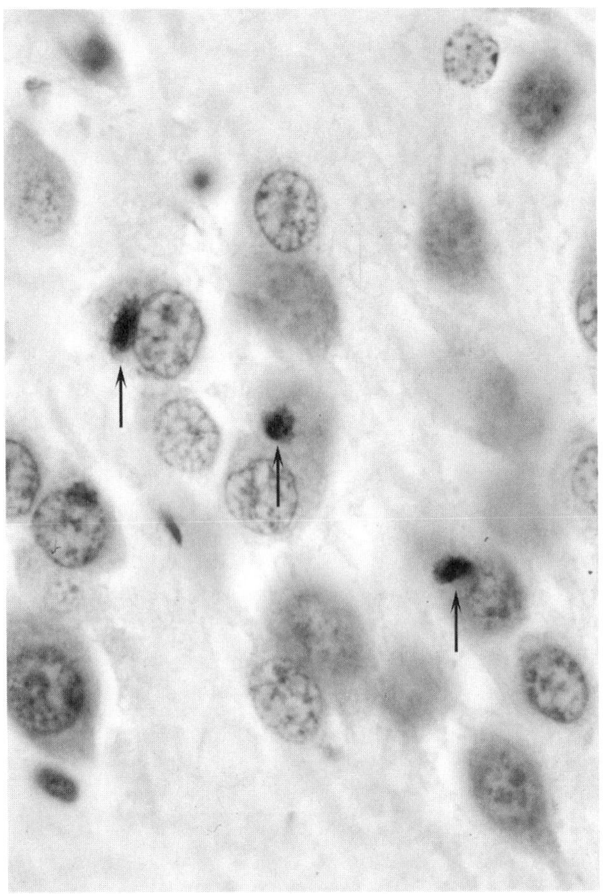

FIGURE 4–16. Frontotemporal lobar degeneration with tau-negative, ubiquitin-positive inclusions: hippocampal formation, fascia dentata.

Tau-negative, ubiquitin-positive inclusions (*arrows*) are small granular cytoplasmic inclusions that are best observed in the small neurons of the fascia dentata of the hippocampus. These inclusions cannot be seen on routine histological preparations. They stain positively only for ubiquitin. They lack tau, β-amyloid, α-synuclein, and other proteins that are present in the other major neurodegenerative disorders. (Ubiquitin immunostain; original magnification ×1,000.)

gliosis but lacks tau- or ubiquitin-positive inclusions, and the entity known as dementia lacking distinctive histopathology is the group's main representative.

Summary

The brain is a complex organ which, when functioning optimally, is a source of wonder. However, as people age, normal wear and tear results in some loss of cognition. This loss is manifested pathologically by the formation of a few plaques and tangles. At some point, synapse loss and the pathology of plaques and tangles reach a critical threshold and dementia ensues. Plaques and tangles, and therefore Alzheimer's disease, are the most common pathological substrate of dementia. Second most common in incidence is dementia with Lewy bodies, which may be considered the convergence of Alzheimer's disease and Parkinson's disease. The third and fourth most common causes of dementia are vascular dementias and frontotemporal dementia, respectively.

Genetic studies are beginning to unravel some of the genetic risk factors and autosomal dominant genes associated with the development of dementia and cognitive impairment. In the future, cognitive and therapeutic interventions will be aimed at persons who are genetically and behaviorally at risk for the insidious development of dementia.

Key Points

- Alzheimer's disease pathology is very common in the aging population and is the major neurodegenerative cause of cognitive impairment and dementia in the elderly.
- Senile plaques and neurofibrillary tangles are the hallmark pathological features of Alzheimer's disease.
- Dementia with Lewy bodies is the second most common cause of neurodegenerative dementias.
- Synaptic loss, neuronal cell loss, and brain atrophy are common pathological changes in all dementing disorders.
- Genetic factors, such as apolipoprotein E, play important roles in the development of various dementing disorders.
- Neuropathological examination of brain tissue is still the definitive way to confirm the nature of clinically diagnosed neurodegenerative and vascular dementias.

References

Adler G, Brassen S: Short-term rivastigmine treatment reduces EEG slow-wave power in Alzheimer patients. Neuropsychobiology 43:273–276, 2001

Anderer P, Pascual-Marqui RD, Semlitsch HV, et al: Electrical sources of P300 event-related brain potentials revealed by low resolution electromagnetic tomography, 1: effects of normal aging. Neuropsychobiology 37:20–27, 1998

APA Task Force on Quantitative Electrophysiological Assessment: Quantitative electroencephalography: a report on the present state of computerized EEG techniques. Am J Psychiatry 148:961–964, 1991

Braak H, Braak E: Neuropathological staging of Alzheimer-related changes. Acta Neuropathol 82:239–259, 1991

Brenner RP, Ulrich RF, Spiker DG, et al: Computerized EEG spectral analysis in elderly normal, demented and depressed subjects. Electroencephalogr Clin Neurophysiol 64:483–492, 1986

Brenner RP, Reynolds CF, Ulrich RF: EEG findings in depressive pseudodementia and dementia with secondary depression. Electroencephalogr Clin Neurophysiol 72:298–304, 1989

Bridgers SL, Ebersole JS: The clinical utility of ambulatory cassette EEG. Neurology 35:166–173, 1985

Brun A: Vascular dementia: pathological findings, in Dementia, 2nd Edition. Edited by O'Brien J, Ames D, Burns A. New York, Oxford University Press, 2000, pp 655–666

Claus JJ, Ongerboer De Visser BW, Bour LJ, et al: Determinants of quantitative spectral electroencephalography in early Alzheimer's disease: cognitive function, regional cerebral blood flow, and computed tomography. Dement Geriatr Cogn Disord 11:81–89, 2000

Cook IA, Leuchter AF: Synaptic dysfunction in Alzheimer's disease: clinical assessment using quantitative EEG. Behav Brain Res 78:15–23, 1996

Corder EH, Saunders AM, Strittmatter WJ, et al: Gene dose of apolipoprotein E type 4 allele and the risk of Alzheimer's disease in late onset families. Science 261:921–923, 1993

Crain BJ, Croom DW II, Hulette CM, et al: Argyrophilic plaques in children. Acta Neuropathol 89:42–49, 1995

Creutzfeldt OD, Watanabe S, Lux HD: Relations between EEG phenomena and potentials of single cortical cells, II: spontaneous and convulsoid activity. Electroencephalogr Clin Neurophysiol 20:19–37, 1966

Duffy FH, Albert MS, McAnulty G: Age-related differences in brain electrical activity in healthy subjects. Ann Neurol 16:430–438, 1984

Esiri MM, Hyman BT, Beyreuther K, et al: Aging and dementia, in Greenfield's Neuropathology, 6th Edition. Edited by Graham DI, Lantos PL. New York, Oxford University Press, 1997, pp 153–234

Fernández A, Hornero R, Mayo A, et al: MEG spectral profile in Alzheimer's disease and mild cognitive impairment. Clin Neurophysiol 117:306–314, 2006

Fullerton SM, Shirman GA, Strittmatter WJ, et al: Impairment of the blood-nerve and blood-brain barriers in apolipoprotein E knockout mice. Exp Neurol 169:13–22, 2001

Goodin DS, Aminoff MJ: Electrophysiological differences between subtypes of dementia. Brain 109 (pt 6):1103–1113, 1986

Goodin DS, Aminoff MJ: Electrophysiological differences between demented and nondemented patients with Parkinson's disease. Ann Neurol 21:90–94, 1987

Goodin D, Squires KC, Starr A: Age-related variations in evoked potentials to auditory stimuli in normal human subjects. Electroencephalogr Clin Neurophysiol 44:447–458, 1978a

Goodin D, Squires KC, Starr A: Long latency event-related components of the auditory evoked potential in dementia. Brain 101:635–648, 1978b

Gray F, Rober F, Labrecque R, et al: Autosomal dominant arteriopathic leuko-encephalopathy and Alzheimer's disease. Neuropathol Appl Neurobiol 20:22–30, 1994

Gustafson L: Physostigmine and tetrahydroaminoacridine treatment of Alzheimer's disease. Acta Neurol Scand Suppl 149:39–41, 1993

Hamilton RL: Lewy bodies in Alzheimer's disease: a neuropathological review of 145 cases using α-synuclein immunohistochemistry. Brain Pathol 10:378–384, 2000

Heyman RA, Brenner RP, Reynolds CF, et al: Age at initial onset of depression and waking EEG variables in the elderly. Biol Psychiatry 29:994–1000, 1991

Hirano A: Hirano bodies and related neuronal inclusions. Neuropathol Appl Neurobiol 20:3–11, 1994

Hodges J: Pick's disease: its relationship to progressive aphasia, semantic dementia and frontotemporal dementia, in Dementia, 2nd Edition. Edited by O'Brien J, Ames D, Burns A. New York, Oxford University Press, 2000, pp 747–758

Hogan MJ, Carolan L, Roche RAP, et al: Electrophysiological and information processing variability predicts memory decrements associated with normal age-related cognitive decline and Alzheimer's disease (AD). Brain Res 1119:215–226, 2006

Holschneider DP, Leuchter AF: Beta activity in aging and dementia. Brain Topogr 8:169–180, 1995

Holschneider DP, Leuchter AF: Clinical neurophysiology using electroencephalography in geriatric psychiatry: neurobiologic implications and clinical utility. J Geriatr Psychiatry Neurol 12:150–164, 1999

Hughes JR, Zialcita ML: EEG in the elderly: seizures vs. syncope. Clin Electroencephalogr 31:131–137, 2000

Hulette CM, Walford RL: Immunological aspects of Alzheimer's disease. Alzheimer Dis Assoc Disord 1:72–82, 1987

Hulette CM, Earl NL, Anthony DC, et al: Adult onset Niemann-Pick disease type C: a case presenting with dementia. Clin Neuropathol 11:293–297, 1991

Hulette CM, Mirra S, Heyman A, et al: A prospective clinical-neuropathological study of Parkinson's features in Alzheimer's disease: the CERAD experience, part IX. Neurology 45:1991–1995, 1995

Hulette CM, Mirra SS, Heyman A, et al: Clinical-neuropathologic findings in multi-infarct dementia: a report of six autopsied cases. Neurology 48:668–672, 1997

Hulette CM, Welsh-Bohmer K, MacIntyre L, et al: Neuropathological changes in normal aging. J Neuropathol Exp Neurol 57:1168–1174, 1998

Hulette CM, Van Eck M, Pannell C, et al: Vascular pathology in ApoE 3,3 and ApoE 4,4 dementia, in 1st International Congress on Vascular Dementia. Edited by Korczyn AD. Bologna, Italy, Monduzzi Editore, 1999, pp 45–49

Hulette CM, Huang H, Pan Y-P, et al: Cardiovascular disease in demented and non-demented elderly (abstract). J Neuropathol Exp Neurol 61:443, 2002

Hyman BT, Trojanowski JQ: Consensus recommendations for the postmortem diagnosis of Alzheimer disease from the National Institute on Aging and the Reagan Institute Working Group on Diagnostic Criteria for the Neuropathological Assessment of Alzheimer Disease. J Neuropathol Exp Neurol 56:1095–1097, 1997

Ince P, Perry R, Perry E: Pathology of dementia with Lewy bodies, in Dementia, 2nd Edition. Edited by O'Brien J, Ames D, Burns A. New York, Oxford University Press, 2000, pp 699–718

Jacobson SA, Leuchter AF, Walter DO, et al: Serial quantitative EEG among elderly subjects with delirium. Biol Psychiatry 34:135–140, 1993

Kalimo H, Ruchoux MM, Viitanen M, et al: CADASIL: a common form of hereditary arteriopathy causing brain infarcts and dementia. Brain Pathol 12:371–384, 2002

Knott V, Mohr E, Mahoney C, et al: Electroencephalographic coherence in Alzheimer's disease: comparisons with a control group and population norms. J Geriatr Psychiatry Neurol 13:1–8, 2000

Knott V, Mohr E, Mahoney C, et al: Quantitative electroencephalography in Alzheimer's disease: comparison with a control group, population norms and mental status. J Psychiatry Neurosci 26:106–116, 2001

Koenig T, Prichep L, Dierks T, et al: Decreased EEG synchronization in Alzheimer's disease and mild cognitive impairment. Neurobiol Aging 26:165–171, 2005

Koponen H, Partanen J, Paakkonen A, et al: EEG spectral analysis in delirium. J Neurol Neurosurg Psychiatry 52:980–985, 1989

Kumar-Singh S, Brockhoven CV: Frontotemporal lobar degeneration: current concepts in the light of recent advances. Brain Pathol 17:104–113, 2007

Lantos P, Cairns N: The neuropathology of Alzheimer's disease, in Dementia, 2nd Edition. Edited by O'Brien J, Ames D, Burns A. New York, Oxford University Press, 2000, pp 443–460

Leuchter AF, Jacobson SA: Quantitative measurement of brain electrical activity in delirium. Int Psychogeriatr 3:231–247, 1991

Leuchter AF, Spar JE, Walter DO, et al: Electroencephalographic spectra and coherence in the diagnosis of Alzheimer's-type and multi-infarct dementia. Arch Gen Psychiatry 44:993–998, 1987

Leuchter AF, Newton TF, Cook IA, et al: Changes in brain functional connectivity in Alzheimer-type and multi-infarct dementia. Brain 115:1543–1561, 1992

Leuchter AF, Cook IA, Newton TF, et al: Regional differences in brain electrical activity in dementia: use of spectral power and spectral ratio measures. Electroencephalogr Clin Neurophysiol 87:385–393, 1993a

Leuchter AF, Daly KA, Rosenberg-Thompson S, et al: Prevalence and significance of electroencephalographic abnormalities in patients with suspected organic mental syndromes. J Am Geriatr Soc 41:605–611, 1993b

Leuchter AF, Uijtdehaage SG, Cook IA, et al: Relationship between brain electrical activity and cortical perfusion in normal subjects. Psychiatry Res 90:125–140, 1999

Luhdorf K, Jensen LK, Plesner AM: Epilepsy in the elderly: incidence, social function, and disability. Epilepsia 27:135–141, 1986a

Luhdorf K, Jensen LK, Plesner AM: Etiology of seizures in the elderly. Epilepsia 27:458–463, 1986b

Marín-Padilla M: Prenatal development of fibrous (white matter), protoplasmic (gray matter), and layer I astrocytes in the human cerebral cortex: a Golgi study. J Comp Neurol 357:554–572, 1995

Markesberry WR, Schmitt FA, Kryscio RJ, et al: Neuropathologic substrate of mild cognitive impairment. Arch Neurol 63:38–46, 2006

McGeer PL, McGeer EG, Yasojima K: Alzheimer disease and neuroinflammation. J Neural Transm Suppl 59:53–57, 1999

McKeith IG, Galasko D, Kosaka K, et al: Consensus guidelines for the clinical and pathologic diagnosis of dementia with Lewy bodies (DLB): report of the Consortium on DLB international workshop. Neurology 47:1113–1124, 1996

McKhann G, Drachman D, Folstein M, et al: Clinical diagnosis of Alzheimer's disease: report of the NINCDS-ADRDA Work Group under the auspices of Department of Health and Human Services Task Force on Alzheimer's Disease. Neurology 34:939–944, 1984

Mendez MF, Catanzaro P, Doss RC, et al: Seizures in Alzheimer's disease: clinicopathologic study. J Geriatr Psychiatry Neurol 7:230–233, 1994

Meyer JS, Rauch G, Rauch RA, et al: Risk factors for cerebral hypoperfusion, mild cognitive impairment, and dementia. Neurobiol Aging 21:161–169, 2000

Minthon L, Gustafson L, Dalfelt G, et al: Oral tetrahydroaminoacridine treatment of Alzheimer's disease evaluated clinically and by regional cerebral blood flow and EEG. Dementia 4:32–42, 1993

Mirra SS, Crain BJ, Vogel FS, et al: The Consortium to Establish a Registry for Alzheimer's Disease (CERAD), part II: standardization of the neuropathologic assessment of Alzheimer's disease. Neurology 41:479–486, 1991

Mitchell TW, Mufson EJ, Schneider JA, et al: Parahippocampal tau pathology in healthy aging, mild cognitive impairment and early Alzheimer's disease. Ann Neurol 51:182–189, 2002

Montine TJ, Hulette CM: Pathology of ischemic cerebrovascular disease, in Neurosurgery, 2nd Edition. Edited by Wilkins RH, Rengachary SS. New York, McGraw-Hill, 1997, pp 2045–2052

Osipova D, Ahvenine J, Jensen O, et al: Altered generation of spontaneous oscillations in Alzheimer's disease. Neuroimage 27:835–841, 2005

Parent P: Carpenter's Human Neuroanatomy, 9th Edition. Philadelphia, PA, Williams & Wilkins, 1996

Pasquier F, Henon H, Leys D: Risk factors and mechanisms of poststroke dementia. Rev Neurol (Paris) 155:749–753, 1999

Pekkonen E, Jaaskelainen IP, Hietanen J, et al: Impaired preconscious auditory processing and cognitive functions in Alzheimer's disease. Clin Neurophysiol 110:1942–1947, 1999

Perryman KM, Fitten LJ: Quantitative EEG during a double-blind trial of THS and lecithin in patients with Alzheimer's disease. J Geriatr Psychiatry Neurol 4:127–133, 1991

Pfurtscheller G, Cooper R: Frequency dependence of the transmission of the EEG from cortex to scalp. Electroencephalogr Clin Neurophysiol 38:93–96, 1975

Polich J: P300 in the evaluation of aging and dementia. Electroencephalogr Clin Neurophysiol Suppl 42:304–323, 1991

Polich J: EEG and ERP assessment of normal aging. Electroencephalogr Clin Neurophysiol 104:244–256, 1997

Polich J, Kok A: Cognitive and biological determinants of P300: an integrative review. Biol Psychol 41:103–146, 1995

Polich J, Ehlers CL, Otis S, et al: P300 latency reflects the degree of cognitive decline in dementing illness. Electroencephalogr Clin Neurophysiol 63:138–144, 1986

Prichep LS, John ER, Ferris SH, et al: Prediction of longitudinal cognitive decline in normal elderly with subjective complaints using electrophysiological imaging. Neurobiol Aging 27:471–481, 2006

Reeve A, Rose DF, Weinberger DR: Magnetoencephalography: applications in psychiatry. Arch Gen Psychiatry 46:573–576, 1989

Rosenberg CK, Roses AD, Hulette CM, et al: Dementia with Lewy bodies and Alzheimer disease. Acta Neuropathol 102:621–626, 2001

Roses AD, Hulette C, Strittmatter WJ, et al: Influence of the susceptibility genes apolipoprotein E-4 and apolipoprotein E-2 on the rate of disease expressivity of late-onset Alzheimer's disease. Azneimittel-Forschung/Drug Research 45:413–417, 1995

Roses AD, Hulette CM, Strittmatter WJ, et al: Apolipoprotein E and Alzheimer disease. International Academy for Biomedical and Drug Research 11:187–197, 1996

Sander JW, Hart YM, Johnson AL, et al: National General Practice Study of Epilepsy: newly diagnosed epileptic seizures in a general population. Lancet 336:1267–1271, 1990

Saunders AM, Hulette CM, Roses AD, et al: Association of apolipoprotein E allele ε4 with late onset familial and sporadic Alzheimer's disease. Neurology 43:1467–1472, 1993

Saunders AM, Hulette CM, Roses AD, et al: Specificity, sensitivity and predictive value of apolipoprotein E genotyping in a consecutive autopsy series of sporadic Alzheimer disease patients. Lancet 348:90–93, 1996

Schmechel DE, Hulette CM, Roses AD, et al: Increased amyloid β-peptide deposition as a consequence of apolipoprotein E genotype in late-onset Alzheimer's disease. Proc Natl Acad Sci USA 90:9649–9653, 1993

Spillantini MG, Schmidt ML, Lee V M-Y, et al: Alpha-synuclein in Lewy bodies. Nature 388:839–840, 1997

Sunderman FW, Boerner F: Normal Values in Clinical Medicine. Philadelphia, PA, WB Saunders, 1949, pp 641–642

Tournier-Lasserve E, Joutel A, Melki J: Cerebral autosomal dominant arteriopathy with subcortical infarcts and leukoencephalopathy. Nat Genet 3:256–259, 1993

Visser SL, Van Tilburg W, Hooijer C, et al: Visual evoked potentials (VEPs) in senile dementia (Alzheimer type) and in non-organic behavioural disorders in the elderly: comparison with EEG parameters. Electroencephalogr Clin Neurophysiol 60:115–121, 1985

Vogel FS: Neuroanatomy and neuropathology of aging, in The American Psychiatric Press Textbook of Geriatric Psychiatry, 2nd Edition. Edited by Busse EW, Blazer DG. Washington, DC, American Psychiatric Press, 1996, pp 61–70

Welsh-Bohmer KA, Hulette C, Schmechel D, et al: Neuropsychological detection of preclinical Alzheimer's disease: results of a neuropathological series of "normal" controls, in Alzheimer's Disease: Advances in Etiology, Pathogenesis and Therapeutics: The Proceedings of the 7th International Conference on Alzheimer's Disease and Related Disorders. Edited by Iqbal K, Sisodia SS, Winblad B. London, Wiley, 2001, pp 111–122

Zekry D, Duyckaerts C, Moulias R, et al: Degenerative and vascular lesions of the brain have synergistic effects in dementia of the elderly. Acta Neuropathol 103:481–487, 2002

Zhang WW, Ma KC, Andersen O, et al: The microvascular changes in cases of hereditary multi-infarct disease of the brain. Acta Neuropathol 87:317–324, 1994

Suggested Readings

Esiri MM, Lee VMY, Trojanowski JQ (eds): The Neuropathology of Dementia, 2nd Edition. Cambridge, England, Cambridge University Press, 2004

Markesberry WR, Schmitt FA, Kryscio RJ, et al: Neuropathologic substrate of mild cognitive impairment. Arch Neurol 63:38–46, 2006

Parent P: Carpenter's Human Neuroanatomy, 9th Edition. Philadelphia, PA, Williams & Wilkins, 1996

CHAPTER 5

CHEMICAL MESSENGERS

Jason D. Kilts, Ph.D.
Jennifer C. Naylor, Ph.D.
Victoria M. Payne, M.D.
Jennifer L. Strauss, Ph.D.
Patrick S. Calhoun, Ph.D.
Christine E. Marx, M.D., M.A.

The clinical treatment of age-related diseases such as Alzheimer's disease (AD) has evolved from the initial challenges of simple recognition of the disorders, to attempts to delineate components important in the pathogenesis of those disorders, to attempts to define biomarkers that could be used for early detection of the onset of those disorders. Before attempting to determine which types of markers would be relevant for a given disease, however, one must be familiar with the molecules responsible for mediating the physiological responses that are being altered with age. The list of chemical messengers in the human body is extremely long, but many primary physiological functions can be attributed to the functions of a much smaller subset of messengers. In this chapter, we focus on specific receptor-mediated signaling systems, the molecules that transmit the cellular signals associated with them, and any compounds that have thus far appeared to be beneficial for the treatment of age-related disorders through these systems.

Many mental and physical disorders exhibit a clear association with age, and the ever-increasing life expectancy of the human population is creating an escalating need to understand these disorders and discover how to treat them. For example, AD is the most common age-related malady that results in severely impaired cognitive function, affecting approximately 10% of the population at age 65, and nearly 50% by age 85 (Hebert et al. 1995; Rose et al. 2005). AD is a progressive disorder, resulting in decline of cognitive function; deficits in memory, attention, and orientation; and changes in personality and consistency of mood. It appears that the neuropathological changes of AD generally begin well before the disease is recognized clinically, and that subtle changes in cognition and brain physiology are present and recognizable prior to clinical diagnosis. As research continues to progress and the pathophysiology of AD becomes more defined, earlier treatments designed to slow, stop, or even reverse the neuropathology of AD may become the norm. Before this research path can come to its most beneficial fruition, however, a complete understanding of the proteins involved in the biochemistry of AD must be obtained.

The primary groups of therapeutic targets within research on almost every age-related disorder are neurotransmitters that transmit signals between neurons in the brain. Many of these neurotransmitters have been recognized for decades and have been studied extensively, but the precise causes and consequences of their alteration by disease states remain to be determined in many instances. Along with the most widely recognized substances that act as neurotransmitters, recent discoveries of neurotransmitter roles for excitatory and inhibitory amino acids, neuropeptides, specific nucleotides, and diffusible gases have increased the breadth of possible chemical messengers involved in any degeneration-associated disorders such as AD. A detailed description of the pathophysiological findings associated with individual disorders is essential before one can appreciate the potential importance of each of these neurotransmitters; however, these descriptions can be found elsewhere in this volume, and inclusion here would be redundant. What follows in this chapter is an individual examination of many of these candidate neurotransmitter systems, including the biochemical actions, localization, associated functions, and age- and disease-related alterations in each. Discussion of the use of different facets of some of these neurotransmitters for diagnostics and treatment of age-related disorders is also included when current knowledge is sufficient to make those inclusions appropriate.

Muscarinic Acetylcholine Receptor System

Acetylcholine (ACh) was one of the first biochemicals recognized to be a neurotransmitter. It produces initiation of skeletal muscle contraction and mediates parasympathetic effects and preganglionic autonomic neurotransmission in the peripheral nervous system. ACh is found in cholinergic neurons as well as in the vicinity of cholinergic synapses. The rate of ACh synthesis by the enzyme choline acetyltransferase (which joins a choline molecule with an acetyl group from acetylcoenzyme A) is directly coupled to the firing rate of the cholinergic neuron. Hydrolysis of ACh is the primary control of the length of action and is performed by the enzymes acetylcholinesterase and butyrylcholinesterase.

ACh acts through the family of muscarinic ACh receptors, of which at least three subtypes (M_1, M_2, and M_3) of the five recognized (M_1–M_5) are involved in the modulation of neurotransmitter release (Caulfield 1993; Caulfield and Birdsall 1998; Raiteri et al. 1990; Starke et al. 1989). Muscarinic ACh receptors are members of the G-protein coupled receptor superfamily, with the M_1, M_3, and M_5 receptors coupling to the guanosine triphosphate binding proteins G_q and G_{11}, and the M_2 and M_4 receptors coupling to members of the inhibitory G_i subclass of G proteins. Three of these receptor subtypes (M_1, M_3, and M_5) have been associated with the phospholipase C-related phosphoinositide signaling pathway, whereas the others (M_2 and M_4) are generally thought to be negatively linked to adenylyl cyclase and the regulation of cyclic adenosine monophosphate (cAMP) levels (von Linstow Roloff and Platt 1999). Additionally, these receptors modulate Ca^{+2} influx, stimulation of guanylyl cyclase, and activation of K^+ channels (Allen and Brown 1993, 1996; Felder 1995).

M_2 and M_4 receptors are mainly located presynaptically, likely functioning as autoreceptors controlling the release of ACh from the presynaptic neuron terminal. They are found predominantly in the hippocampus and striatum (Levey 1996), where they are able to depress both inhibitory and excitatory neuronal responses. M_2 receptors are also found in the periphery and throughout the central nervous system (CNS), inhibiting norepinephrine release as an autoreceptor (Raiteri et al. 1990) and modulating bradycardia via membrane hyperpolarization in cardiomyocytes. Activation of these receptors also modulates the actions of several cytoplasmic and nuclear factors, including tyrosine kinases, focal adhesion kinase, mitogen-activated protein kinase, extracellular signal–related kinases, and c-Jun terminal kinases (Pratico et al. 2005).

M_1 receptors are the most abundant muscarinic receptors, representing 35%–60% of all muscarinic ACh receptors in neocortex and hippocampus tissue (Levey 1996). M_1 receptors increase norepinephrine release from noradrenergic terminals in the periphery (North et al. 1985; Raiteri et al. 1990), mediate slow excitatory postsynaptic potentials in the ganglions of postganglionic nerves (Xi-Moy et al. 1993), and activate a nitric oxide signal in submandibular glands (Perez Leiros et al. 1999) that may be relevant to memory and learning ability (Dawson and Dawson 1996). Stimulation of these receptors (as well as of M_3 and M_5) mobilizes phosphoinositides and generates IP_3 and diacylglycerol, resulting in increased intracellular Ca^{2+}, and also produces the opposite effect of M_2 and M_4 receptors in terms of initiation of the mitogen-activated protein kinase cascade, which is essential for cell proliferation and apoptosis (Felder 1995; Zhang and Liu 2002).

Age-related declines in ACh biosynthesis and release have been recognized from animal model systems for decades, with up to 75% deficits in advanced age (Gibson and Peterson 1981; Gibson et al. 1981). Additionally, several of the manifestations of the advancement of age-related diseases such as AD have been associated with alterations in signaling through muscarinic ACh receptors. Reduced activity of cholinergic projections to the hippocampus and cortex has been reported in AD, and the visual hallucinations reported by AD patients with dementia with Lewy bodies correlate with reduced neocortical ACh-related activity (Perry et al. 1999). It appears that the reduced response of these receptors through their related G proteins results from a downstream compound, because the levels of G proteins present are not altered in AD, but localized alterations in isoforms of phospholipase C (Shimohama and Matsushima 1995) and deficits in phosphoinositide (Stokes and Hawthorne 1987), phosphoinositide 3-kinase (Bothmer and Jolles 1994), and phosphoinositide 4-kinase (Wallace 1994) have been reported.

Severe degeneration of the cholinergic neurons projecting from basal forebrain to cortical and hippocampal areas is one of the most fundamental and consistent features of the advancement of AD, with up to 90% loss of these neurons (Coyle et al. 1983; Whitehouse et al. 1981, 1982). These reductions are far greater than those exhibited by many other neurotransmitter systems in these same patients (Coyle et al. 1983). Also, correlations with the severity of cognitive impairments and memory loss in patients with AD have been found for reductions in the enzymes controlling the synthesis of ACh (Perry et al. 1978), as well as for the degree of neuronal loss in basal forebrain (Perry 1986; Wilcock et al. 1982). Combined with the fact that ACh is known to be critically involved in the control of cognition (Everitt and Robbins 1997), findings such as these are the cornerstone of the widely recognized cholinergic hypothesis of AD.

Treatment strategies focused on the muscarinic ACh receptor signaling systems have fallen primarily within three distinct approaches, with varying degrees of success. The first approach attempted to increase ACh via loading of dietary precursors of ACh, such as choline salts and lecithin, but these studies failed to produce any clinical benefit (Higgins and Flicker 2000; Mohs et al. 1980). The second approach attempted to replace the decreased stimulation of postsynaptic muscarinic receptors (due to the decreased stimulation from the highly degenerated presynaptic neurons) with agonists of postsynaptic M_1 receptors. Although this approach enhances cholinergic transmission cognitive skills in animal models (Carey et al. 2001), the benefits in patients with AD have been inadequate at doses that are well tolerated (Bodick et al. 1997; Jones 2002). The third approach attempted to protect the endogenously produced ACh levels via inhibition of the actions of acetylcholinesterase and butyrylcholinesterase. Despite the failures of the approaches described in this paragraph to increase ACh neurotransmission, the use of cholinesterase inhibitors has become the most established treatment strategy in AD (Jones 2003).

Early acetylcholinesterase inhibitors had short half-lives and were poorly tolerated, but recently marketed compounds such as donepezil (Aricept), rivastigmine (Exelon), and galantamine (Reminyl) have produced greatly advanced selectivity, immunity to metabolism by the cytochrome P450 system, and low potential for drug interactions (Grossberg et al. 2000). In double-blind placebo-controlled studies, all three of these compounds have demonstrated positive effects on cognitive function and increased ability to perform activities of daily living (Burns et al. 1999; Raskind et al. 2000; Rogers et al. 1998; Rosler et al. 1999; Wilcock et al. 2000). Side effects from these treatments are generally mild and transient, but the length of time that patients can tolerate these treatments remains to be determined, as does the amount of benefit that can be achieved in severe AD.

Nicotinic Acetylcholine Receptor System

Nicotinic ACh receptors, unlike muscarinic ACh receptors, are members of the superfamily of ligand-gated ion channels. They are composed of five subunits arranged around a central pore that is permeable to cations. These subunits are encoded by nine α and three β subunit genes, with individual subunits capable of forming either homopentameric or heteropentameric complexes. Although these subtypes display a range of different functional and pharmacological properties, they also share some basic features. First, they exist in three primary functional states: closed at rest, open pore, and closed desensitized (Dani and Bertrand 2007). Stimulation with ACh results in opening of the pore and translocation of cations. Activation of presynaptic nicotinic ACh receptors enhances release of several neurotransmitters (Gray et al. 1996; Radcliffe and Dani 1998; Wonnacott 1997), whereas postsynaptic nicotinic ACh receptors control neuromuscular junction signal transmission and may have a role in fast excitatory neurotransmission, and nonsynaptic nicotinic ACh receptors modulate neuronal excitability (further modulating neurotransmitter release).

Nicotinic ACh receptors are located in several brain areas that receive significant cholinergic neuron innervation, including the thalamus, cortex, hippocampus, brain stem, olfactory tubercle, and cerebellum, as well as midbrain areas that are rich in dopaminergic innervations (Gotti and Clementi 2004). These receptors are present in both neural and nonneural cells in the brain and other organs, providing the receptor family as a whole a very pleiotropic role. Precise localization of all subtypes has not yet been determined in human brain, and some differences between distribution in humans and that found in animal models have been noted (Wada et al. 1989). Outside the brain, several nicotinic ACh receptor subtypes have been detected, in muscle (Corriveau et al. 1995; Maelicke et al. 2000; Sala et al. 1996), lymphoid tissue (Nordberg et al. 1990a), macrophages (Davies et al. 1982), skin (Grando et al. 1995), lung (Fu et al. 2003; Wang et al. 2001; Zia et al. 1997), vascular tissue (Bruggmann et al. 2003; Macklin et al. 1998), and astrocytes (Hosli et al. 1988). Given the extensive list of disparate locations and functions in which nicotinic ACh receptors are involved, the potential importance of age- or disease-dependent alterations is evident.

As might be expected when examining AD-related changes in the other receptor systems (muscarinic) responsive to ACh, selective decreases in nicotinic ACh receptors in brains of subjects with AD have been reported utilizing several biochemical methodologies (Burghaus et al. 2000; Martin-Ruiz et al. 1999; Mousavi et al. 2003; Nordberg and Winblad 1986; Perry et al. 1990, 1995; Shimohama et al. 1986; Sparks et al. 1998; Wevers and Schroder 1999). This reduction appears to be at the protein level, as messenger ribonucleic acid (mRNA) levels of different nicotinic ACh receptor subtypes are not different between patients with AD and controls (Mousavi et al. 2003; Terzano et al. 1998). Also, there is evidence that the loss of nicotinic ACh receptors is not a postmortem artifact; reductions in nicotinic ACh receptors have even been demonstrated in situ via positron emission topography (Nordberg et al. 1990b, 1995, 1997).

Extensive efforts to investigate the effects of nicotine administration on the amelioration of symptoms of AD and related measures have yielded little success to date. Although some studies report improved attention in patients with AD following both acute and chronic nicotine administration, none report any improvement on memory functions (Jones et al. 1992; Newhouse et al. 1988; Sahakian et al. 1989; White and Levin 1999; Wilson et al. 1995). Given the neuroprotective effects of nicotine (Yamashita and Nakamura 1996), the high expression of nicotinic ACh receptors in brain regions that develop AD neuropathology (Wevers and Schroder 1999), and the apparent relationship between nicotine and inhibition of amyloid β aggregation (Ono et al. 2002; Salomon et al. 1996), the rationale for using nicotinic agonists for the treatment of AD appears theoretically valid. However, human studies to date suggest little to no effect on memory. Possibly the development of subtype-selective agonists or the determination of nicotinic ACh receptor subtype turnover or expression increases in response to selective agonists will provide therapeutic benefit in the future.

γ-Aminobutyric Acid Receptors

The major inhibitory neurotransmitter in the mammalian CNS is γ-aminobutyric acid (GABA). GABA is one of the highest-concentration amino acids within the CNS and is synthesized from glutamate by the enzyme glutamic acid decarboxylase. GABA released into nerve terminals is metabolized by the enzyme GABA-transaminase to produce glutamate again and succinic semialdehyde. GABA, which has been recognized as a brain chemical messenger since the 1950s, was quickly determined to be the only inhibitory amino acid found exclusively in inhibitory neurons. GABA mediates the inhibitory actions of local interneurons in many areas of the brain (including cerebral cortex, cerebellum, olfactory bulb, cuneate nucleus, hippocampus, and lateral septal nucleus), as well as presynaptic inhibition in the spinal cord. GABA is also present in, and co-released by, about half of all brain neurons, and particularly those that release somatostatin, neuropeptide Y, vasopressin, vasoactive intestinal peptide, enkephalin, and substance P. Relatively high concentrations (micromolar) of GABA are detected in many brain regions, including the hypothalamus and striatum.

GABA acts through two receptor types in the CNS (a third has been detected in retina), designated $GABA_A$ and $GABA_B$ receptors. $GABA_A$ receptors are composed of five subunits, formed from combinations of any of six α subunits, four β subunits, four γ subunits, and four other subunits (δ, ε, θ, and π). Although a large array of possible combinations exists, it appears that a combination of at least one α, one β, and another subunit type is required for functionality. $GABA_A$ receptors are found both pre- and postsynaptically (although more are postsynaptic) and produce inhibition by hyperpolarization via an increase in the flux of chloride ions through their selective channels. When

GABA binds extracellularly between the α and β subunits, it acts as an agonist, inducing conformational changes that increase permeability of the central ion pore to chloride ions. When GABA is removed from the receptor, the channel returns to a closed state and the process can be repeated. Unlike $GABA_A$ receptors, $GABA_B$ receptors are linked to G proteins and second messenger systems that mediate the operation of calcium and potassium channels, producing slow inhibitory postsynaptic potentials in several brain regions. $GABA_B$ receptors are formed from two subunits and bind to almost completely different sets of compounds than $GABA_A$ receptors.

Alteration of GABA receptor function mediates actions of several drugs including anxiolytics, barbiturates, and ethanol, and it is believed that the GABA receptor interaction of each of these drugs is the physiological basis for their ability to potentiate each other's effects when they are administered concomitantly. The benzodiazepines, characterized by anxiolytic, anticonvulsant, sedative, muscle relaxant, and amnesic effects, enhance GABA function by acting primarily as positive allosteric modulators of $GABA_A$ receptors. They increase the affinity of GABA for the chloride channel opening and increase the frequency of channel open states. Barbiturates, on the other hand, produce a prolongation of the chloride channel open states, a more dangerous pharmacological state due to the ability of barbiturates to inhibit vital individual brain circuits above the level that can be achieved by natural GABAergic effects. Finally, GABA receptor modulation has also been implicated as a regulatory mechanism in several additional pathologies, including those associated with insomnia, epilepsy, depression, alcoholism, and schizophrenia, although comparatively little is known as to the precise role of GABA and its associated receptors in these disorders.

Although considerable effort has been expended in search of age-related alterations in GABAergic systems, physiological relevance from the changes found has not yet been clearly obtained. Many reports exist of age-related declines in GABA receptor expression and function in animal models, but comparisons between these studies and comparisons with studies performed in humans illuminate the fact that extrapolation from specific brain regions in animal models to other brain regions or other species may not provide accurate information. In humans, most age-related data on expression of GABA and GABA receptors have been collected with a focus on the advancement of AD and have revealed brain-region-specific alterations, just as animal studies have. Frontal cortex, temporal cortex, parietal cortex, amygdala, and thalamus all exhibit reduced GABA concentration in postmortem brains of patients with AD, whereas other regions such as hippocampus, caudate, putamen, and nucleus accumbens do not (Lanctot et al. 2004). GABA receptors in patients with AD demonstrate either moderate reductions (Chu et al. 1987; Vogt et al. 1991) or no change at all (Greenamyre et al. 1987; Jansen et al. 1990), but may be altered in terms of the subunit composition present (Mizukami et al. 1997, 1998a, 1998b). Additionally, it is notable that no changes in GABA uptake sites are detected in the frontal cortex due to advanced age (Sundman et al. 1997), and markers of GABA synthesis increase with age and have been hypothesized to lead to chronic depolarization of some axon terminals (Marczynski 1998).

Glutamate

Much like GABA is the major inhibitory neurotransmitter, glutamate (or glutamic acid) is the prototypical excitatory neurotransmitter in mammalian brain. Glutamate is also the most ubiquitous transmitter in the mammalian CNS, as nearly every excitatory neuron in the CNS is glutamatergic, and it is estimated that over half of all nerve endings release this amino acid. In addition to its own role as a neurotransmitter, glutamate is the metabolic precursor to GABA, so delineation of responses to glutamate itself has proven difficult in some instances.

Glutamate is released into the synaptic cleft in response to presynaptic depolarization, with glutamate-containing vesicles releasing their contents into the synapse via exocytosis. A release of glutamate in this fashion can cause a 1,000-fold change in the synaptic concentration of the amino acid, producing binding to postsynaptic receptors that causes a depolarization of the postsynaptic cell due to an influx of cations. Glutamate is then evacuated from the synaptic cleft by selective, high-affinity uptake transporters, then is subjected to a recycling system that converts it to glutamine and then back to glutamate for another round of vesicular compartmentalization. This ability of glutamate to stimulate target neurons has been exploited through the use of excitotoxic analogs of glutamate (including kainate and quisqualic acid) that can be used to create localized lesions of cell bodies by stimulating target neurons to which they are applied until those neurons die of exhaustion.

Receptors for glutamate are found on both neuronal and glial cell membranes and are divided into two classes: ionotropic (ligand-gated ion channels) and metabotropic (G-protein-coupled) glutamate receptors. Ionotropic glutamate receptors are generally thought to mediate fast glutamate transmission, but also contribute to synaptic plasticity and long-term potentiation; they include three classes of receptors, each named for its original selective agonist. The *N*-methyl-D-aspartate (NMDA) receptor, the best characterized of the ionotropic glutamate receptors, is responsible for controlling calcium influx, while also allowing transport of some monovalent cations. NMDA receptors are the ionotropic receptors most involved in the slower components of synaptic transmission and potentiation. Kainate and α-amino-3-hydroxy-5-methyl-4-isoxazole propionic acid (AMPA) receptors form channels permeable to sodium and potassium ions, and are responsible for the early peak of excitatory postsynaptic potentials. Unlike the ionotropic glutamate receptors, metabotropic glutamate receptors function through coupling to G proteins. There are eight known metabotropic receptors that can be arranged into three subfamilies based on associated second messengers and pharmacological profiles. Receptors in this class are known to activate the phospholipase C pathway, produce intracellular Ca^{2+} release, and modulate adenylyl cyclase activity, resulting in effects on a variety of functions, including neuronal excitability, synaptic transmission, and neuronal plasticity.

Given glutamate's ubiquitous expression and the wide-ranging presence of its target receptors, it is clear that glutamate plays significant roles in normal brain function and in brain development. Importantly, while normal glutamate signaling is crucial for normal plasticity, even minor perturbations of normal glutamate transmission can produce excitotoxicity. Increased activation of glutamate receptors, either via elevated glutamate presence in synapses or via increased receptor expression and/or stimulation, produces sustained depolarization of neurons, Na^+ and Ca^{2+} influx, and eventually necrosis. This type of response to glutamate toxicity has already been implicated in a number of brain disorders, including AD (Hynd et al. 2004; Tannenberg et al. 2004), Huntington's disease (Rego and de Almeida 2005), epilepsy (Fujikawa 2005), and amyotrophic lateral sclerosis (Pioro et al. 1999), as well as in traumatic brain injury (Yi and Hazell 2006).

Age-related changes in the glutamate system could logically be assumed based on the degree to which advanced age is a risk factor for many of the disorders with which alterations in the glutamate system have been associated. In addition to an ever-increasing collection of animal model data, studies in human brain also confirm this: advanced age correlates with declines in glutamate concentrations in the basal ganglia, parietal gray matter, and frontal white matter (Sailasuta et al. 2008), and glutamate receptors also decrease by 5%–9% per decade (Kornhuber et al. 1988, 1989). Given the generalized stimulatory effect demonstrated by glutamate and its subsequent interactions with almost all other neurotransmitter systems, it remains to be seen whether these age-related changes occur in response to alterations in other neurotransmitter systems or whether they occur independently and thus may contribute to the further loss of other neurotransmitters during the aging process.

Serotonin

The biogenic amine serotonin (5-hydroxytryptamine [5-HT]) is one of the most widely recognized neurotransmitters due to the recognition of its role in altering mood states. Serotonin is formed from the amino acid tryptophan by the enzyme tryptophan-5-hydroxylase and nonspecific aromatic L-amino acid decarboxylases and is taken up into secretory granules and stored. Based on the cell type in question, serotonin can be either formed within that cell or acquired from the cell's immediate environment. The vast majority of serotonin in humans is located in the gastrointestinal tract, with additional stores in both platelets and the CNS.

The primary function commonly associated with serotonin is its importance in the stabilization of mood. Pharmacological interventions to maintain serotonin levels in synaptic junctions are some of the most commonly accepted treatments for the prevention or amelioration of depression. Similar treatments are employed to treat anxiety disorders, obsessive-compulsive disorders, eating disorders, and even chronic pain. Interventions targeting serotonin, specifically the selective serotonin reuptake inhibitors (SSRIs), inhibit the reuptake of serotonin into the presynaptic cell, thereby increasing levels of serotonin in the synaptic cleft and allowing the serotonin present to stimulate the postsynaptic neuron for a longer period of time, thereby reducing any lack of stimulation of the recipient neuron in the synapse. The brain regions receiving the predominance of the serotonin-containing neuron projections lie in the midbrain dorsal raphe nucleus, the median raphe of the brain stem, and the spinal cord. Projections that innervate the entire cortex and limbic systems also lend credence to several hypotheses of serotonergic mediation of certain emotional states.

In addition to the role of serotonin in the maintenance of mood and prevention of depression, serotonin has been shown to serve multiple roles outside the CNS, including the regulation of gastrointestinal motility and the modulation of homeostasis when released from platelets, and it also may have roles in the vasospasm seen in some vascular diseases. In addition, serotonin can produce vasodilation, as well as positive inotropic and chronotropic effects, and contractions of bronchi.

The family of serotonin receptors comprises no fewer than 14 individual receptors, which can be effectively separated into seven subgroups based on their sequence identities and related functions. Most of these receptors have been shown to operate in a G-protein-coupled fashion, with certain subtypes opposing the effects of other subtypes. The 5-HT_1 group (5-HT_{1A}, 5-HT_{1B}, 5-HT_{1D}, 5-HT_{1E}, 5-HT_{1F}) is coupled through G_i/G_o proteins; decreases cellular levels of cAMP, and possesses varied physiological roles, including effects on anxiety, locomotion, and cerebral vasoconstriction. The 5-HT_2 group (5-HT_{2A}, 5-HT_{2B}, 5-HT_{2C}) is coupled through G_q/G_{11} proteins; increases production of inositol trisphosphate and diacylglycerol; and appears to mediate such responses as anxiety, behavior, learning, smooth muscle contraction, and platelet aggregation. 5-HT_3 receptors modulate the function of ligand-gated Na^+ and K^+ channels to produce membrane depolarization and neuronal excitation, and, like 5-HT_1 and 5-HT_2 receptors, may be important in the production and/or control of anxiety disorders. Because the 5-HT_4, 5-HT_5, 5-HT_6, and 5-HT_7 receptor types have been studied far less than the others, less is known about each. They are predominantly G-protein coupled (5-HT_4 and 5-HT_7 to G_s; 5-HT_5 to G_i/G_o), they have opposing effects on the activity of adenylyl cyclase due to their opposing G-protein activations, and their physiological importance is still relatively undiscovered.

While the use of serotonin reuptake inhibitors has proven beneficial in ameliorating the symptoms of depression, several other compounds that alter serotonergic neurotransmission also merit mention. First, hallucinogenic drugs such as lysergic acid diethylamide (LSD), mescaline, and psilocin/psilocybin all appear to function through modulation of serotonin-containing neuronal systems. Second, monoamine oxidase (MAO) inhibitors, although often not prescribed primarily for their effects on serotonergic systems, increase serotonin levels via inhibition of the primary method for enzymatic processing of serotonin. Finally, antagonists of serotonin receptors, based on their receptor subtype selectivity (or lack thereof), obviously block stimulation of serotonin receptors, producing effects on vascular smooth muscle contraction and blood pressure (especially via 5-HT_1 receptors), as well as helping in the reversal of migraine headache symptoms.

Aging-related changes in human serotonin neuronal systems include alterations in levels of specific receptor types and in serotonin transporters. 5-HT_{1A} receptors are decreased by 10% or more per decade in elderly people relative to young subjects (Moller et al. 2007). 5-HT_{2A} receptors are decreased to an even greater degree, with the predominant losses occurring prior to late life (Sheline et al. 2002). Serotonin transporter proteins also decrease with advancing age, with decreases of roughly 10% per decade in the thalamus and midbrain (Yamamoto et al. 2002) and decreases of approximately half that in the striatum (Pirker et al. 2000). Also, declines in neurons expressing specific receptor subtypes (5-HT_{2A} and 5-HT_6) have also been found in patients with Alzheimer's disease (Lai et al. 2005; Lorke et al. 2006).

Dopamine

Dopamine is one of three catecholamine neurotransmitters, the others being norepinephrine and epinephrine. Dopamine is the immediate metabolic precursor of norepinephrine and epinephrine and is formed by the decarboxylation of a previously hydroxylated tyrosine residue. Dopamine is a substrate for both MAO and catechol-*O*-methyltransferase (COMT), yielding the metabolic products homovanillic acid and dihydroxyphenylacetic acid. Due to its status as a substrate for both MAO and COMT, dopamine itself is ineffective when administered orally.

Despite dopamine's immediate relationship to norepinephrine metabolically, the distributions of these two messengers are markedly different. Dopamine represents greater than half of the CNS catecholamine content and is produced in highest concentrations in basal ganglia, nucleus accumbens, olfactory tubercle, amygdala, median eminence, and portions of the frontal cortex. Dopaminergic neurons arise primarily in the substantia nigra and the ventral tegmental area, but also within the retina and olfactory bulb. The longer projections from the substantia nigra to the striatum are among the most widely studied, based on their mediation of voluntary movement, whereas the projections from the ventral tegmental area to the forebrain are believed to mediate the emotional aspects of pleasure and reward.

The importance of dopamine is underscored by the number of primary physiological functions to which it has been integrally linked, including movement, neurocognition, motivation, and pleasure. Imbalance in dopamine production or availability in either direction can result in serious, harmful conditions that require prolonged medical care. Reduced dopamine concentrations and/or insufficient dopamine biosynthesis can produce Parkinson's disease, attention-deficit/hyperactivity disorder, and latent inhibition. Overproduction of dopamine or overstimulation of dopamine receptors can be equally detrimental, however, leading to psychoses and schizophrenia, as well as overly active reinforcing behaviors such as drug craving.

Dopamine acts through two classes of G-protein-coupled receptors, the D_1-like and the D_2-like. These two classes of receptors display different structures and couple to different regulatory G proteins. The D_1-like class includes D_1 and D_5 receptors in mammals (two additional subtypes exist in nonmammalian vertebrates), and these receptors are marked by a short third cytoplasmic loop and a long C-terminal tail. The D_2-like class includes D_2, D_3, and D_4 receptors, and exhibits a long third cytoplasmic loop and a short C-terminal tail. It is these portions of the receptors that interact with G proteins inside the cell and that provide the selectivity between the two classes, with D_1-like receptors coupling to stimulatory G_s/G_{olf} proteins and D_2-like receptors coupling to inhibitory G_i/G_o proteins. D_1-like receptors are predominantly postsynaptic and are generally thought to stimulate adenylyl cyclase activity and phosphoinositide turnover. D_2-like receptors are found both pre- and postsynaptically, as well as on the axons and dendrites of dopamine-producing neurons; these receptors inhibit adenylyl cyclase, Ca^{2+} channel activity, and potassium conductance. Given these rather contrary profiles, the two classes of dopamine receptors represent two very distinct groups, with their commonality being their ability to bind dopamine as a neurotransmitter.

Use of dopamine receptor agonists and antagonists has provided therapeutic benefit in debilitating disorders. Antagonism of D_2-like receptors is the mechanism providing the positive symptom relief seen with many successful antipsychotic medications. Also, precursor loading of dopamine or replacement of the dopamine deficit with another dopamine agonist following the death of dopaminergic neurons in Parkinson's disease has provided promising progress in returning muscle movement, although the continued loss of dopaminergic neurons with disease progression has not been overcome.

The amount of information regarding decreases in the function and protein expression within the dopamine system in animal models is considerable, and recent studies in humans have produced similar findings. D_2-like receptor levels decrease by 6%–12% per decade in thalamus, temporal cortex, and frontal cortex (Kaasinen et al. 2002); D_1-like receptors decrease by 7%–9% per decade in caudate, putamen, and occipital cortex (Wang et al. 1998); and dopamine transporter levels decrease in advanced age (Meng et al. 1999). The importance of changes such as these is highlighted by studies correlating decreased striatal D_2 receptor numbers with decreased cognitive function (Backman et al. 2000). Dopamine oxidative stress and its subsequent signaling have also been postulated as a contributor to the aging of the dopaminergic system, and possibly as a cause for some of the age-related deficits in locomotion, motivation, memory, and learning (Luo and Roth 2000).

Norepinephrine

Norepinephrine, the primary chemical messenger released by postganglionic adrenergic nerves, was originally recognized as a neurotransmitter in the peripheral sympathetic postganglionic fibers and only later found to be a component of the central nervous system. Norepinephrine differs from epinephrine only by lacking a methyl substitution in the amino group, and is produced by hydroxylation of dopamine by the enzyme dopamine β-hydroxylase. Like dopamine, norepinephrine is a substrate for both MAO and COMT, with the major degradative product being 3-methoxy-4-hydroxyphenylglycol.

Norepinephrine acts through two major classes of G-protein-linked adrenergic receptors (α and β), with several subtypes within each class. These receptors are generally associated with control of vascular smooth muscle contraction, cardiac contractile force and rate, and glycogenolysis in liver and skeletal muscle, as well as decreases in insulin secretion, control of platelet aggregation, and lipolysis in adipose tissue. Based on the receptor subtypes stimulated, norepinephrine can produce either stimulation or inhibition of adenylyl cyclase and phospholipase C, resulting in alterations in cellular levels of protein kinase A, protein kinase C, and Ca^{2+}, and consequently controlling cell-type-specific K^+ channels. After its release into the synaptic cleft and interaction with its target receptors, the actions of norepinephrine are terminated via three main mechanisms: reuptake into the nerve terminals, diffusion out of the synaptic cleft, and metabolic breakdown. Much like pharmacological agents that prolong serotonin half-life in the cleft, inhibitors of norepinephrine transporter proteins that prevent the reuptake of norepinephrine have proven somewhat effective in the amelioration of depressive symptoms in patients with major depressive disorder.

Norepinephrine-producing neurons reside predominantly in two distinct midbrain regions, the locus coeruleus and the dorsal tegmental nucleus. Neurons originating in the locus coeruleus innervate the hippocampus and many portions of the cerebral cortex surface. Control of release of norepinephrine from these neurons is an excellent example of the loops of multiple messenger systems that modulate each other in turn, as the triggering events in norepinephrine release are the liberation of ACh by preganglionic fibers and its subsequent interaction with nicotinic receptors that produces neuronal depolarization and release of stores of contents such as norepinephrine.

Norepinephrine circuits have not been widely recognized as primary targets for age-related signaling alterations, but some evidence indicates decreased potential responses. For example, β_1-adrenergic receptors in frontal cortex decline significantly from youth to advanced age (Sastre and Garcia-Sevilla 1994; Sastre et al. 2001). Furthermore, alterations in norepinephrine-sensitive receptor systems in age-related disease states such as AD have also been reported, including 33%–60% decreases in α_2-adrenergic receptors in frontal cortex, hypothalamus, and cerebellum (Meana et al. 1992), as well as significant losses in locus coeruleus noradrenergic neurons (Szot et al. 2006).

Histamine

Histamine is a low-molecular-weight amine that is generally recognized as a mediator of allergic reactions and inflammatory responses. However, histamine is also an important neurotransmitter, with histamine-producing neurons extending from the tuberomammilary nucleus of the posterior hypothalamus to virtually the entire brain, with extensive innervation of the frontal and temporal cortices. Histamine is synthesized from L-histidine by L-histidine decarboxylase, which is expressed solely in the posterior hypothalamus in the CNS, and also in gastric-mucosa parietal cells, mast cells, and basophils in the periphery.

The role of histamine in allergic responses as well as in immediate hypersensitivity is well established, as are the functional uses of histamine receptor antagonists to thwart anaphylaxis and allergy. However, in the CNS, histamine also produces release of stress hormones such as corticotropin-releasing factor and arginine vasopressin. Histamine-containing neurons may participate in the regulation of body temperature, signaling for increased fluid intake, and the secretion of antidiuretic hormone, as well as in the control of blood pressure and the perception of pain. Additionally, histamine may be important for the proper development of the brain, because animal studies indicate that it is one of the first neurotransmitters to appear, and the concentration of histamine is five times higher in prenatal brain than in adult brain.

Histamine acts through four distinct receptors, H_1–H_4, each with its own distribution pattern and associated functions. All four receptors are members of the seven-transmembrane-spanning family of G-protein-coupled receptors, with coupling to several different G proteins. H_1 receptors are widely distributed throughout neurons, smooth muscle cells, neutrophils, monocytes, hepatocytes, and many other cell types, and couple through $G_{q/11}$ proteins. H_1 receptors function primarily through modulation of free cytosolic calcium levels, but also have been reported to have effects on cAMP, cyclic guanosine monophosphate (cGMP), and phospholipases A2, C, and D, and they reportedly have CNS roles in such varied functions as sleep cycle, food intake, temperature regulation, aggression, locomotion, memory, and learning. H_2 receptors are also widespread, including high expression levels in gastric-mucosa parietal cells, smooth muscle, heart, and other cell types, and couple through G_s proteins. H_2 receptors produce cellular responses through elevations in cAMP production and are thought to play a part in neuroendocrine functions. Unlike H_1 and H_2 receptors, which are expressed both centrally and peripherally, it appears that H_3 and H_4 receptors are expressed exclusively inside or outside of the CNS, respectively. Both of these receptors couple to $G_{i/o}$ proteins, inhibit cAMP production, and affect intracellular Ca^{2+} levels and mitogen-activated protein kinase activity. It is believed that in the brain the H_3 receptor acts as a presynaptic heteroreceptor, decreasing release of many neurotransmitters, including histamine, dopamine, serotonin, norepinephrine, and ACh.

Compared with many other central neurotransmitter systems, little is known about histamine and histamine receptors with regard to the effects of age, especially in humans. An examination of Golgi apparatus and cell size indicated a lack of age-dependent change in the neuronal metabolic activity of histaminergic neurons in the tuberomamillary nucleus (Ishunina et al. 2003). Decreased histamine neuron function may play a role in the progression of AD, however, because the same study reported altered metabolic activity of histaminergic neurons in patients with AD (Ishunina et al. 2003). Also, positron emission topography revealed decreased binding potential of H_1 receptors in frontal and temporal regions of patients with AD (Higuchi et al. 2000), and levels of histamine, histidine, and histidine decarboxylase were all lower in postmortem brains of patients with AD (Schneider et al. 1997). Any cognitive deficits in subjects with AD are likely not from an increased input from H_2 receptors relative to other subtypes, because H_2 receptor antagonist administration fails to prevent AD symptom progression (Carlson et al. 2002).

Neurosteroids

Neurosteroids are a family of steroids synthesized in the CNS de novo from cholesterol or from peripheral steroid precursors. Many neurosteroids are neuroactive (sometimes termed *neuroactive steroids*), rapidly altering neuronal excitability via modulation of membrane-bound ligand-gated ion channel receptors such as inhibitory $GABA_A$ and excitatory NMDA receptors, among others. Neurosteroids are lipophilic and cross the blood-brain barrier readily in their unsulfated forms. The preponderance of knowledge obtained to date on the family of neurosteroids has focused on the neurosteroids allopregnanolone, pregnenolone and its sulfated derivative (pregnenolone sulfate), and dehydroepiandrosterone (DHEA) and its sulfated derivative, although many related enzymatic metabolism products and synthesis intermediates are also known to have significant physiological effects.

A growing body of evidence documents many potentially important roles for neurosteroids. For example, alterations in neuroactive steroid profiles have been reported in patients with major depression (Romeo et al. 1998; Uzunova et al. 1998), schizophrenia (Marx et al. 2006c; Ritsner et al. 2007), Alzheimer's disease (Bernardi et al. 2000; Marx et al. 2006d; Smith et al. 2006), bipolar disorder (Marx et al. 2006c), posttraumatic stress disorder (Rasmusson et al. 2006; Spivak et al. 2000), eating disorders (Monteleone et al. 2001), and attention-deficit/hyperactivity disorder (Strous et al. 2001). This extensive list is increased even further when one considers some of the beneficial actions of neurosteroids demonstrated in animal models, including anxiolytic (Wieland et al. 1991), anticonvulsant (Devaud et al. 1995; Kokate et al. 1996), and antiaggressive (Pinna et al. 2003) effects. Additionally, it appears that neurosteroids may be involved in the actions of both antidepressant drugs (Khisti et al. 2000; Marx et al. 2006b; Serra et al. 2001; Uzunov et al. 1996, 1998) and antipsychotic drugs (Barbaccia et al. 2001; Marx et al. 2000, 2003, 2006a, 2006b). Neurosteroid involvement in cellular functions relative to the treatment of neurodegenerative diseases and psychiatric disorders is also well established, including enhancement of myelination processes (Azcoitia et al. 2003; Ghoumari et al. 2003), neurogenesis (Brinton and Wang 2006; Mayo et al. 2005; Wang et al. 2005), and neuroprotection (Djebaili et al. 2005; Griffin et al. 2004; Labombarda et al. 2002; Lapchak et al. 2000).

The predominance of actions of neurosteroids has thus far been attributed to two opposing interactions with $GABA_A$ receptors. Some neurosteroids such as allopregnanolone act as positive allosteric modulators of $GABA_A$ receptors at locations separate from the benzodiazepine site, producing responses at nanomolar concentrations that are very robust, potentiating $GABA_A$ receptor responses 10 times more potently than the benzodiazepines diazepam and flurazepam, and approximately 200 times more potently than the barbiturate pentobarbital. Other neuroactive steroids, such as pregnenolone sulfate and DHEA sulfate, function in an opposite manner, acting as negative allosteric modulators of $GABA_A$ receptors. Additionally, pregnenolone sulfate and DHEA sulfate are both positive allosteric modulators of NMDA receptors, and pregnenolone sulfate demonstrates negative modulatory activities at both kainate and AMPA receptors. Additional evidence has indicated that various neurosteroids also may interact with serotonin, sigma, glycine, nicotinic ACh, and oxytocin receptors, but those interactions are less well characterized.

It is not yet known if advanced age alters the expression and/or function of all neurosteroids, but evidence to date indicates that average levels of a number of neurosteroids do indeed decrease with age (Berr et al. 1996; Mazat et al. 2001). Given the aforementioned protective effects of neurosteroids on several cellular functions important in advanced age, it is clear that maintenance of neurosteroid expression or replacement of already declining neurosteroid levels could potentially hold important therapeutic benefit for the cognitive well-being of elderly people.

Neuropeptides

The superfamily of neuropeptides comprises a large (and likely still growing) number of neurotransmitters, many of which fall into several subcategories based on sequence and function similarities. These small proteins are generally composed of fewer than 50 amino acids and are present in far lower concentrations than many of the previously discussed transmitters (often in only picomolar or femtomolar concentrations in brain). Neuropeptides are stored in presynaptic vesicles and released into the synaptic cleft much like more classical transmitters, and then the signal is halted via the actions of degradative peptidase enzymes. Because the recognition portion of a neuropeptide sequence typically comprises only a few of the amino acids present in the peptide's sequence, fragments of neuropeptides can retain partial or even full activity at the postsynaptic target receptor. Additionally, significant cross-reactivity at target receptors is possible due to the small recognition requirements at the receptor.

Several subfamilies of neuropeptides are present in the CNS, with some of those subfamilies having several members. Known neuropeptides now number nearly 100, with significant redundancy among the functions of many of them. Due to the sheer number of neuropeptides, we do not discuss each individual neuropeptide in this chapter, but rather more generally illuminate signaling via three of the larger, more intensively studied subfamilies. Tachykinins, which include substance P, neurokinin A, neurokinin B, and the endokinins, mediate smooth muscle responses and blood pressure modulation, among other functions; endogenous opioid peptides, including endorphins, enkephalins, and dynorphins, are primarily considered to produce analgesia; and the bradykinins, including bradykinin and kallidin, modulate inflammation and vascular responses following injury or infection. Finally, we discuss the releasing factors thyrotropin-releasing hormone (TRH) and corticotropin-releasing factor (CRF), two chemical messengers that are reportedly altered significantly in advanced age and/or neurodegenerative conditions.

Tachykinins

The tachykinin subfamily of neuropeptides is best known for the role of substance P in pain transmission. Substance P is present in the primary sensory afferent fibers, the dorsal root ganglia, and the dorsal horn of the spinal cord and has been recognized for decades to mediate the transmission of pain. In addition to the pain response, tachykinins have been linked to several other modulatory roles. They play a role in the induction and progression of inflammatory responses, elevated levels are associated with aggression, injection of them induces grooming and scratching in animal models, and they may mediate portions of the opioid withdrawal reaction. Blockade of their actions has even proven efficacious as an antidepressant treatment.

Members of the tachykinin family share a common C-terminal sequence (Phe-X-Gly-Leu-Met-NH_2) and are produced predominantly in the CNS, with the highest production in the hypothalamus. Receptors for the tachykinins belong to the G-protein-coupled superfamily and are generally divided into three subgroups, NK1, NK2, and NK3. Tachykinin receptors were initially recognized to couple through $G\alpha_q$ proteins to stimulate 1,4,5-inositol trisphosphate production and elevation of intracellular calcium levels, but were later found to also couple through $G\alpha_s$ proteins to activate adenylyl cyclase. Although substance P, neurokinin A, and neurokinin B all exhibit full agonist responses at all three receptor types in terms of intracellular calcium elevations, some selectivity among tachykinins and their receptors in terms of adenylyl cyclase stimulation has been reported. NK1 receptors are expressed most widely, including in neurons, the cardiovascular system, smooth muscle, gastrointestinal tract, genitourinary tract, pulmonary tissues, thyroid gland, and immune cells. NK2 receptors are expressed most abundantly in prostate, cerebellum, lung, trachea, uterus, and bronchus, whereas NK3 receptors are found in brain, kidney, lung, placenta, prostate, testis, muscle, intestine, and uterus.

As with many of the other neurotransmitter systems already described, age-dependent decreases have also been observed for the tachykinin system. NK1 receptor binding potential, as examined by positron emission topography, decreases by approximately 7% per decade, with decreases detected in temporal cortex, parietal cortex, frontal cortex, hippocampus, and parahippocampal formation (Nyman et al. 2007). The number of NK3 receptor-expressing neurons also decreases with age, although the expression of neurokinin B does not (Mileusnic et al. 1999). Interestingly, the effect of Alzheimer's disease on the tachykinin system is somewhat in question because AD has been associated both with striking depletions of substance P immunoreactive neurons in the cerebral cortex (Kowall et al. 1993) and with no change in the number of substance P–expressing cells in the hippocampus, frontal cortex, and occipital cortex (Yew et al. 1999), whereas the expression of NK1 receptors (for which substance P is the primary agonist) is unaltered in striatum and pallidum in patients with AD (Rioux and Joyce 1993).

Opioids

Endogenous opioids, also commonly known as endorphins or opioid peptides, are small molecules that are naturally produced both in the CNS and in various glands throughout the body, and are actually a class of compounds encompassing enkephalins and dynorphins as well as endorphins. They are peptides ranging from 5 to 31 amino acids in length, and primarily contain the sequence Tyr-Gly-Gly-Phe as a requirement for activity. These peptides function as both hormones and neuromodulators, and are effective as analgesics, prevent diarrhea, regulate cardiovascular function, and modulate brain reward systems from drugs of abuse. Endogenous opioids are secreted either by peripheral glands, producing hormone-type responses at distant target organs, or by central nerve cells, modulating the actions of other neurotransmitters. In peripheral tissues, their effects are similar to those of opioid alkaloids such as morphine, whereas in the brain, they are widely distributed and most often act via effects on other messenger systems, including GABAergic and dopaminergic pathways.

Opioid peptides act primarily through three types of opioid receptors, the μ, δ, and κ receptors, sharing extensive amino acid identity. These receptors are also members of the G-protein-coupled receptor superfamily and produce effects on adenylyl cyclase, Ca^{2+} channels, K^{+} channels, and phosphoinositide turnover. Endorphins exhibit the least selectivity between the receptor subtypes, but appear to show some preference for μ opioid receptors, the subtype that mediates the most potent antinociceptive effects. Enkephalins induce their effects mainly through activation of δ opioid receptors, which have lower analgesic efficacy but also appear to present a reduced addictive potential. Dynorphins have greater selectivity for κ opioid receptors, the subtype that may be most responsible for mediating pain relief in peripheral tissues.

It is presently unclear whether advancing age has any significant effect on opioid peptide signaling. Most but not all studies in animal models indicate that opioid peptide gene expression and the abundance of opioid peptides are increased with aging in organs such as the heart (Bhargava et al. 1988; Boluyt et al. 1993; Caffrey et al. 1994). This differs from findings in human brain that enkephalin content is decreased with age in both caudate nucleus and pallidum, while remaining unchanged in substantia nigra and putamen (Rinne et al. 1993). It should be noted, however, that these decreased levels produce no change in the total binding of opioid receptors in the caudate nucleus, possibly indicating a compensation with an increase in receptor number, a finding consistent with increased μ opioid receptor expression detected by positron emission topography in the anterior cingulate, prefrontal, temporal, and parietal cortices in advancing age (Ravert et al. 2004). In contrast to the effects seen solely with age, patients suffering from AD exhibit reductions in μ opioid receptor binding in the subiculum and hippocampus, as well as reductions in δ opioid receptor binding in amygdaloid complex and ventral putamen, but also exhibit increases in κ opioid receptor binding in the dorsal and ventral putamen and the cerebellar cortex (levels of binding to all three receptor types is unaltered by AD in the caudate, parahippocampal gyrus, and occipitotemporal gyrus) (Mathieu-Kia et al. 2001).

Bradykinins

The bradykinin subfamily consists primarily of two peptides differing by a single amino acid, the nonapeptide bradykinin (Arg-Pro-Pro-Gly-Phe-Ser-Pro-Phe-Arg) and the decapeptide kallidin (Lys-Arg-Pro-Pro-Gly-Phe-Ser-Pro-Phe-Arg). Both of these peptides appear to have roles in inflammation, pain, and vascular processes, and may be of increased importance in the CNS following injury, infection, or inflammation. Both are produced by enzymatic processing of low-molecular-weight kininogen by kallikrein, with the production of bradykinin following that of kalladin by the action of an aminopeptidase on the Lys-Arg bond. Interestingly, the degradation of these peptides by peptidases is very rapid, such that the half-life of bradykinins administered intravenously or intracerebroventricularly is only 30 seconds (Kariya et al. 1982).

Bradykinins generate actions through two major kinin receptors (B_1 and B_2). The B_2 receptor is more abundant in normal conditions and is involved in the acute phases of the response to pain and inflammation. Both bradykinin and kallidin exhibit higher affinity for the B_2 receptor than for the B_1 receptor. The B_1 receptor, although generally less abundant, is upregulated by tissue injury (Marceau et al. 1998; Siebeck et al. 1998) and appears to be more important in chronic phases of inflammation, as well as in the modulation of spinal cord plasticity in response to pain. However, it is possible that some redundancy in function or at least the ability of these receptors to take over the functions of the other subtype exists, as studies in knockout mice clearly indicate an upregulation and covering of function by the receptor still present (Duka et al. 2001).

Little is known about the effects of age and age-related diseases on the expression of bradykinin, kallidin, and their associated receptors. The studies of bradykinin-associated functions that are available indicate that age does not affect these transmitters significantly; bradykinin-induced vasodilation is unaltered in advanced age (Dachman et al. 1992), and bradykinin-induced alterations in cytosolic free calcium concentration do not differ between fibroblasts from young donors and fibroblasts from elderly donors (Huang et al. 1991). However, advanced age evidently does increase the stimulation of the phosphoinositide cascade in fibroblasts by bradykinin (Huang et al. 1991), and onset of AD may (McCoy et al. 1993) or may not (Huang et al. 1991) decrease the ability of bradykinin to increase cytosolic calcium in fibroblasts.

Thyrotropin-Releasing Hormone and Corticotropin-Releasing Factor

Thyrotropin-releasing hormone (TRH) is a tripeptide (Glu-His-Pro) and was the first of the hypothalamic-releasing hormones to be isolated and characterized. TRH is distributed throughout the extrahypothalamic nervous system, is rapidly metabolized to a cyclized His-Pro dipeptide that also has biological activity in the brain, and slowly penetrates the blood-brain barrier. TRH-containing neurons are found in highest concentration in the hypothalamus, as well as in anterior preoptic hypothalamus and septal nuclei, and TRH is also colocalized with other neurotransmitters such as serotonin, ACh, and the catecholamines. TRH produces a variety of effects, stimulating the release of pituitary hormones, modulating behavior, and controlling thermoregulation. Additionally, it appears to exhibit neuroprotective actions that could prove beneficial in the treatment of spinal cord trauma and AD (Hashimoto and Fukuda 1991).

TRH signals through two membrane-bound receptors in mammals (although only one has been found in humans) coupled through G proteins to the inositol trisphosphate/diacylglycerol system. Because reduced activity of TRH receptors has been associated with major depressive disorders, a great deal of effort has been put into the development of TRH analogs and receptor antagonists for clinical use. Subsequent to these efforts, the actions of TRH and its receptor have been linked to epilepsy, the reversal of anesthesia and narcotic overdoses, spinal trauma and brain injury, motor neuron disease, cerebral ischemia, and Alzheimer's disease. Although the progress in the development of TRH receptor ligands for these conditions has provided only incremental success to date, evidence showing decreased hypothalamic TRH activity in advanced age may indicate that TRH is a therapeutic target for many age-related deficits associated with the hypothalamic-pituitary-thyroid axis (such as reduced tolerance to temperature changes) (Monzani et al. 1996).

Corticotropin-releasing factor (CRF, also known as corticotropin-releasing hormone) is a peptide of 41 amino acids, most readily recognized for its role in regulating the stress response through modulation of the hypothalamic-pituitary-adrenal axis. CRF stimulates adrenocorticotropin hormone release from the pituitary gland, which in turn induces cortisol release. CRF is synthesized and released from multiple brain regions, including the paraventricular nucleus, hypothalamus, amygdala, and locus coeruleus. Production of CRF is stimulated through various neuronal peptides and transmitters such as ACh, histamine, and serotonin, with CRF-containing neurons projecting to the median eminence, lower brain stem, cerebral cortex, and spinal cord. CRF is also present peripherally in significant amounts in the stomach, pancreas, small intestine, lymphocytes, placenta, and testes, providing CRF with modulatory roles in immunity, digestion, and reproduction, in addition to its role in the stress response.

CRF exerts its actions through two G-protein-coupled receptors, CRF receptor 1 and CRF receptor 2. CRF receptor 1 is expressed at high levels throughout the brain in the neocortex, hippocampus, cerebellum, and amygdala, and in the pituitary. CRF receptor 2 is expressed centrally in the lateral septal nuclei and hypothalamic nuclei; in the bed nucleus of the stria terminalis; and peripherally in the heart, gastrointestinal tract, skeletal muscle, and lungs. The predominance of the known CRF functions results from stimulation of G_s proteins through CRF receptor 1, stimulating adenylyl cyclase, although coupling to G_q proteins has also been demonstrated in studies in cultured cells.

Evidence exists that advancing age decreases selective innervations of CRF, resulting in less CRF in gyrus cinguli but not in frontal cortex or hypothalamus (Arranz et al. 1996). Unlike the effects of age alone, however, age-related neurodegenerative diseases such as AD may result in significantly decreased CRF concentrations in frontal (and temporal, occipital, and parietal) cortex and caudate nucleus, but not in hypothalamus (Bissette et al. 1985; De Souza et al. 1986; Whitehouse et al. 1987). Reduced CRF in the cerebrospinal fluid of patients with AD has also been noted (Davis et al. 1999; May et al. 1987; Mouradian et al. 1986). Further, the number of CRF-immunoreactive neurons is decreased in individuals with AD (Bissette et al. 1985; Powers et al. 1987). In support of this correlation between decreased CRF and the advancement of diseases with cognitive components is the finding that administration of CRF or other molecules that produce increased free CRF levels in the brain may exert positive effects on learning and memory (Behan et al. 1995). When combined with demonstrations that CRF may be neuroprotective in certain settings (Elliott-Hunt et al. 2002; Fox et al. 1993; Lezoualc'h et al. 2000), it is clear that the continued examination of the role of CRF and its receptors in neurodegenerative diseases is warranted.

Other Chemical Messengers

Many other classes of neurotransmitters exist in numbers too great to describe here, but there are two additional classes that merit mention, if for no reason other than their reported alterations in advanced age and associated disorders. Growth factors, such as brain-derived neurotrophic factor (BDNF), nerve growth factor, insulin-like growth factor-1, and epidermal growth factor, comprise a family of neurotrophins that are small, basic, secreted proteins that aid in survival and maintenance of specific neuronal populations. Additionally, they promote regeneration of sensory neurons and retinal ganglion cells after injury, and stimulate choline acetyltransferase in developing motoneurons. These neurotrophins are found in many brain regions, including cortex, hippocampus, midbrain, hindbrain, cerebellum, olfactory bulb, spinal cord, and hypothalamus. As an example of the alterations discovered in advanced age and disease states, we consider brain-derived neurotrophic factor. BDNF mRNA levels decrease with advanced age in the temporal cortex (but not hippocampus), while the BDNF-associated receptor tyrosine kinase B decreases in the hippocampus (but not temporal cortex) (Webster et al. 2006). Advanced age also results in decreased plasma BDNF levels (Lommatzsch et al. 2005), similar to decreases in serum BDNF levels in age-related disorders such as AD (Yasutake et al. 2006).

Finally, it should be noted that nitric oxide (NO) and carbon monoxide (CO) also function as chemical messengers, regulating neuronal firing rates by activation of second messenger systems after diffusing into cells (Dawson and Snyder 1994). NO is synthesized from L-arginine by a Ca^{2+}/calmodulin-dependent nitric oxide synthase and diffuses independent of synaptic structures through cell membranes to adjacent neurons. NO activates soluble guanylyl cyclase, producing cGMP in target neurons, a response effected in conceivably larger populations of cells due to the lack of a need for specialized synapses when the transmitter is a diffusible gas. CO, produced from heme by the enzyme heme oxygenase, acts in much the same way, increasing guanylyl cyclase activity in a pathway shown to be important in the maintenance of vasodilation and neurotransmission. Although the toxicity of CO, the most abundant pollutant in the air in the lower atmosphere, is well recognized with regard to its reaction with hemoglobin, other neuroactive gases may play roles in the onset and progression of disease states as well. NO, for instance, has been hypothesized to contribute to oxidative damage during neurodegenerative changes in AD (Calabrese et al. 2000; Fernandez-Vizarra et al. 2004), a finding further supported by decreased levels of endogenous NO synthase inhibitors in AD (Abe et al. 2001).

Conclusion

The list of chemical messengers presented here is certainly not exhaustive, in view of the number of messengers already known and the amount of space it would take to do each of them justice. However, the recognition in this chapter of the major neurotransmitters, their localizations, and the physiological impact of each begins to provide an appreciation of the complexities involved and the level of interaction in each individual biochemical response (see Table 5–1 on the next page for a brief summary of the messengers highlighted in this chapter). More chemical messengers will undoubtedly be discovered as the tools available to researchers become more powerful and selective, and the melding of these findings with the knowledge already obtained will drive intelligent drug design for the foreseeable future. This is especially true for pharmaceutical intervention aimed at delaying or stopping age- and disease-mediated degenerative conditions as the population achieves enhanced longevity and introduces new age-related physiological challenges.

Key Points

- Acetylcholine, acting through G-protein-coupled M_1–M_5 muscarinic acetylcholine receptors, produces initiation of skeletal muscle contraction and mediates parasympathetic effects and preganglionic autonomic neurotransmission in the peripheral nervous system. Severe degeneration of specific acetylcholine-producing neurons is one of the most fundamental and consistent features of the advancement of Alzheimer's disease (AD), with up to 90% loss of these neurons. Correlations with the severity of cognitive impairments and memory loss in patients with AD have been found for reductions in the enzymes controlling the synthesis of acetylcholine.
- Nicotinic acetylcholine receptors (unlike muscarinic acetylcholine receptors) are members of the superfamily of ligand-gated ion channels and enhance release of several other neurotransmitters, control neuromuscular junction signal transmission, and modulate neuronal excitability. Despite the fact that nicotinic acetylcholine receptors are selectively decreased in brains of subjects with AD, extensive efforts to investigate the effects of nicotine administration on the amelioration of symptoms of AD and related measures have yielded little success to date.
- GABA (γ-aminobutyric acid) is the major inhibitory neurotransmitter in the mammalian central nervous system. GABA acts through two receptor types ($GABA_A$ and $GABA_B$) in the CNS to mediate the inhibitory actions of local interneurons in many areas of the brain, including cerebral cortex, cerebellum, olfactory bulb, cuneate nucleus, hippocampus, and lateral septal nucleus. Alteration of GABA receptor function mediates actions of several drugs, including anxiolytics and barbiturates.
- Glutamate (or glutamic acid) is the prototypical excitatory neurotransmitter in mammalian brain, and it is the most ubiquitous transmitter in the mammalian CNS. Receptors for glutamate are divided into two classes: ionotropic (ligand-gated ion channels), including NMDA and AMPA receptors, and metabotropic (G-protein-coupled) glutamate receptors. These receptors mediate fast glutamate transmission and contribute to synaptic plasticity and long-term potentiation via control of calcium influx, maintenance of sodium and potassium levels, activation of the phospholipase C pathway, and modulation of adenylyl cyclase activity. Overly increased activation of these receptors has already been implicated in a number of brain disorders, including AD, epilepsy, and amyotrophic lateral sclerosis.
- The biogenic amine serotonin (5-HT) is widely recognized for its role in the stabilization of mood. Pharmacological interventions to maintain serotonin levels in synaptic junctions are some of the most commonly utilized agents for the treatment of depression and anxiety disorders, among other conditions. Serotonin acts through a large family of G-protein-coupled receptors to decrease cellular levels of cAMP and increase production of inositol trisphosphate and diacylglycerol, and declines in various facets of human serotonin neuronal systems have been reported in aging as well as AD.
- Dopamine, the immediate metabolic precursor of norepinephrine and epinephrine, represents greater than half of the CNS catecholamine content and is

TABLE 5–1. Several of the primary signaling molecules, associated receptor types, and representative actions

Signaling molecules	Receptor types	Signal systems affected	Associated responses
Acetylcholine	Muscarinic M_1–M_5	Phospholipase C, Na^+ and K^+ channels, IP_3, adenylyl cyclase, guanylyl cyclase, diacylglycerol	Roles in bradycardia, memory, learning, cell proliferation, apoptosis; modulates actions of several tyrosine kinases, and inhibits norepinephrine release
	Nicotinic	Cation channels	Neurotransmitter release, neuromuscular junction signal transmission, neuronal excitability
γ-Aminobutyric acid (GABA)	$GABA_A$, $GABA_B$	Cl^- channels, Ca^{2+} and K^+ channels	Mediation of interneuron inhibitory action and of the actions of agents such as anxiolytics and barbiturates
Glutamate	NMDA, AMPA, kainate, mGluRs	Phospholipase C, Ca^{2+} channels, adenylyl cyclase, Na^+ and K^+ channels	Neuronal control and plasticity, both slow and fast synaptic transmission, long-term potentiation
Serotonin	5-HT groups 1–7	Adenylyl cyclase, IP_3, diacylglycerol	Regulation of mood, anxiety, learning, and depression; gastrointestinal motility; homeostasis; vasodilation; inotropy, chronotropy
Dopamine	D_1–D_5	Adenylyl cyclase, phospho-inositide turnover, Ca^{2+} channels, K^+ channels	Movement, neurocognition, motivation, pleasure, reward mechanisms
Norepinephrine	α-adrenergic β-adrenergic	Adenylyl cyclase, protein kinases A and C, Ca^{2+} and K^+ levels	Vascular smooth muscle contraction, cardiac contraction, glycogenolyis, lipolysis
Histamine	H_1–H_4	Ca^{2+} channels, adenylyl cyclase, guanylyl cyclase, phospholipases	Allergic responses, thermoregulation, pain perception, control of diuresis and blood pressure
Neurosteroids (allopregnanolone, pregnenolone, DHEA, others)	$GABA_A$, NMDA, others	Cl^- channels, Ca^{2+} channels, others	Roles in neurogenesis, neuroprotection, depression, stress, aggression, anxiety, and neurodegenerative diseases, among other areas
Neuropeptides (tachykinins, opioids, bradykinins, TRH, CRF, others)	NK1–3; μ, δ, κ opioids; B_1, B_2; TRH receptors; CRF receptors 1 and 2	IP_3, diacylglycerol, Ca^{2+} channels, K^+ channels, adenylyl cyclase	Smooth muscle control, blood pressure, analgesia, inflammation, response to injury/infection, reward mechanisms, cardiovascular function, thermoregulation
Growth factors (BDNF, NGF, IGF-I, EGF)	TrkA, TrkB, TrkC, IGF-I receptor, EGF receptor	Phospholipase C, diacylglycerol, Ca^{2+} channels, phosphoinositide turnover	Neuronal survival, regeneration of sensory neurons, other neurotrophic functions
Neuroactive gases (NO, CO)	—	Guanylyl cyclase	Regulation of neuronal firing, maintenance of vasodilation

Note. AMPA=α-amino-3-hydroxy-5-methyl-4-isoxazole propionic acid; BDNF=brain-derived neurotrophic factor; CRF=corticotropin-releasing factor; DHEA=dehydroepiandrosterone; EGF=epidermal growth factor; IGF-I=insulin-like growth factor 1; mGluR=metabotropic glutamate receptor; NGF=nerve growth factor; NMDA=*N*-methyl-D-aspartate; TRH=thyrotropin-releasing hormone; Trk=tyrosine kinase receptors.

involved in the mediation of voluntary movement and in the emotional aspects of pleasure and reward. Dopamine acts through two classes of G-protein-coupled receptors to control adenylyl cyclase activity, phosphoinositide turnover, Ca^{2+} channel activity, and potassium conductance.

- Norepinephrine is the primary chemical messenger released by postganglionic adrenergic nerves and acts through two major classes of G-protein-linked adrenergic receptors (α and β). These receptors are generally associated with control of vascular smooth muscle contraction, cardiac contractile force and rate, and glycogenolysis in liver and skeletal muscle, as well as decreases in insulin secretion, control of platelet aggregation, and lipolysis in adipose tissue.
- Histamine, a low-molecular-weight amine generally recognized as a mediator of allergic reactions and inflammatory responses, is also an important neurotransmitter, with roles in the release of stress hormones such as corticotrophin-releasing factor and arginine vasopressin, regulation of body temperature, signaling for increased fluid intake, secretion of antidiuretic hormone, and the control of blood pressure and the perception of pain. Histamine acts through four G-protein-coupled receptors, H_1–H_4, to modulate free cytosolic calcium levels, as well as cAMP, cGMP, and phospholipases A2, C, and D. Altered metabolic activity of histaminergic neurons has been noted in patients with AD, as have decreased binding potential of H_1 receptors in frontal and temporal regions and decreased levels of histamine, histidine, and histidine decarboxylase in postmortem brains of patients with AD.
- Neurosteroids are a family of steroids synthesized in the CNS de novo from cholesterol or from peripheral steroid precursors. A number of neurosteroids are also neuroactive, rapidly altering neuronal excitability via modulation of membrane-bound ligand-gated ion channel receptors such as inhibitory $GABA_A$ and excitatory NMDA receptors. Some of the more widely studied neurosteroids, such as allopregnanolone, pregnenolone and its sulfated derivative, and dehydroepiandrosterone and its sulfated derivative, appear to play important roles in major depression, schizophrenia, Alzheimer's disease, bipolar disorder, and posttraumatic stress disorder, among other conditions. Evidence to date suggests that the concentrations of many neurosteroids decrease with age.
- The superfamily of neuropeptides is a large and expanding list of neurotransmitters, many of them falling into several subcategories based on sequence and function similarities. These small proteins generally comprise fewer than 50 amino acids and are present in far lower concentrations than many other transmitters. Several subfamilies of neuropeptides are present in the CNS, with some of these subfamilies having several members. The total number of known neuropeptides is now nearly 100.

References

Abe T, Tohgi H, Murata T, et al: Reduction in asymmetrical dimethylarginine, an endogenous nitric oxide synthase inhibitor, in the cerebrospinal fluid during aging and in patients with Alzheimer's disease. Neurosci Lett 312:177–179, 2001

Allen TG, Brown DA: M_2 muscarinic receptor-mediated inhibition of the Ca^{2+} current in rat magnocellular cholinergic basal forebrain neurones. J Physiol 466:173–189, 1993

Allen TG, Brown DA: Detection and modulation of acetylcholine release from neurites of rat basal forebrain cells in culture. J Physiol 492 (pt 2):453–466, 1996

Arranz B, Blennow K, Ekman R, et al: Brain monoaminergic and neuropeptidergic variations in human aging. J Neural Transm 103:101–115, 1996

Azcoitia I, Leonelli E, Magnaghi V, et al: Progesterone and its derivatives dihydroprogesterone and tetrahydroprogesterone reduce myelin fiber morphological abnormalities and myelin fiber loss in the sciatic nerve of aged rats. Neurobiol Aging 24:853–860, 2003

Backman L, Ginovart N, Dixon RA, et al: Age-related cognitive deficits mediated by changes in the striatal dopamine system. Am J Psychiatry 157:635–637, 2000

Barbaccia ML, Affricano D, Purdy RH, et al: Clozapine, but not haloperidol, increases brain concentrations of neuroactive steroids in the rat. Neuropsychopharmacology 25:489–497, 2001

Behan DP, Heinrichs SC, Troncoso JC, et al: Displacement of corticotropin releasing factor from its binding protein as a possible treatment for Alzheimer's disease. Nature 378:284–287, 1995

Bernardi F, Lanzone A, Cento RM, et al: Allopregnanolone and dehydroepiandrosterone response to corticotropin-releasing factor in patients suffering from Alzheimer's disease and vascular dementia. Eur J Endocrinol 142:466–471, 2000

Berr C, Lafont S, Debuire B, et al: Relationships of dehydroepiandrosterone sulfate in the elderly with functional, psychological, and mental status, and short-term mortality: a French community-based study. Proc Natl Acad Sci U S A 93:13410–13415, 1996

Bhargava HN, Matwyshyn GA, Hanissian S, et al: Opioid peptides in pituitary gland, brain regions and peripheral tissues of spontaneously hypertensive and Wistar-Kyoto normotensive rats. Brain Res 440:333–340, 1988

Bissette G, Reynolds GP, Kilts CD, et al: Corticotropin-releasing factor-like immunoreactivity in senile dementia of the Alzheimer type: reduced cortical and striatal concentrations. JAMA 254:3067–3069, 1985

Bodick NC, Offen WW, Levey AI, et al: Effects of xanomeline, a selective muscarinic receptor agonist, on cognitive function and behavioral symptoms in Alzheimer disease. Arch Neurol 54:465–473, 1997

Boluyt MO, Younes A, Caffrey JL, et al: Age-associated increase in rat cardiac opioid production. Am J Physiol 265:H212–H218, 1993

Bothmer J, Jolles J: Phosphoinositide metabolism, aging and Alzheimer's disease. Biochim Biophys Acta 1225:111–124, 1994

Brinton RD, Wang JM: Preclinical analyses of the therapeutic potential of allopregnanolone to promote neurogenesis in vitro and in vivo in transgenic mouse model of Alzheimer's disease. Curr Alzheimer Res 3:11–17, 2006

Bruggmann D, Lips KS, Pfeil U, et al: Rat arteries contain multiple nicotinic acetylcholine receptor α-subunits. Life Sci 72:2095–2099, 2003

Burghaus L, Schutz U, Krempel U, et al: Quantitative assessment of nicotinic acetylcholine receptor proteins in the cerebral cortex of Alzheimer patients. Brain Res Mol Brain Res 76:385–388, 2000

Burns A, Rossor M, Hecker J, et al: The effects of donepezil in Alzheimer's disease: results from a multinational trial. Dement Geriatr Cogn Disord 10:237–244, 1999

Caffrey JL, Boluyt MO, Younes A, et al: Aging, cardiac proenkephalin mRNA and enkephalin peptides in the Fisher 344 rat. J Mol Cell Cardiol 26:701–711, 1994

Calabrese V, Bates TE, Stella AM: NO synthase and NO-dependent signal pathways in brain aging and neurodegenerative disorders: the role of oxidant/antioxidant balance. Neurochem Res 25:1315–1341, 2000

Carey GJ, Billard W, Binch H III, et al: SCH 57790, a selective muscarinic M_2 receptor antagonist, releases acetylcholine and produces cognitive enhancement in laboratory animals. Eur J Pharmacol 431:189–200, 2001

Carlson MC, Tschanz JT, Norton MC, et al: H_2 histamine receptor blockade in the treatment of Alzheimer disease: a randomized, double-blind, placebo-controlled trial of nizatidine. Alzheimer Dis Assoc Disord 16:24–30, 2002

Caulfield MP: Muscarinic receptors: characterization, coupling and function. Pharmacol Ther 58:319–379, 1993

Caulfield MP, Birdsall NJ: International Union of Pharmacology, XVII: Classification of muscarinic acetylcholine receptors. Pharmacol Rev 50:279–290, 1998

Chu DC, Penney JB Jr, Young AB: Quantitative autoradiography of hippocampal $GABA_B$ and $GABA_A$ receptor changes in Alzheimer's disease. Neurosci Lett 82:246–252, 1987

Corriveau RA, Romano SJ, Conroy WG, et al: Expression of neuronal acetylcholine receptor genes in vertebrate skeletal muscle during development. J Neurosci 15:1372–1383, 1995

Coyle JT, Price DL, DeLong MR: Alzheimer's disease: a disorder of cortical cholinergic innervation. Science 219:1184–1190, 1983

Dachman WD, Ford GA, Hoffman BB, et al: Bradykinin-induced venodilation is not impaired with aging in humans. J Gerontol 47:M166–M170, 1992

Dani JA, Bertrand D: Nicotinic acetylcholine receptors and nicotinic cholinergic mechanisms of the central nervous system. Annu Rev Pharmacol Toxicol 47:699–729, 2007

Davies BD, Hoss W, Lin JP, et al: Evidence for a noncholinergic nicotine receptor on human phagocytic leukocytes. Mol Cell Biochem 44:23–31, 1982

Davis KL, Mohs RC, Marin DB, et al: Neuropeptide abnormalities in patients with early Alzheimer disease. Arch Gen Psychiatry 56:981–987, 1999

Dawson TM, Dawson VL: Nitric oxide synthase: role as a transmitter/mediator in the brain and endocrine system. Annu Rev Med 47:219–227, 1996

Dawson TM, Snyder SH: Gases as biological messengers: nitric oxide and carbon monoxide in the brain. J Neurosci 14:5147–5159, 1994

De Souza EB, Whitehouse PJ, Kuhar MJ, et al: Reciprocal changes in corticotropin-releasing factor (CRF)–like immunoreactivity and CRF receptors in cerebral cortex of Alzheimer's disease. Nature 319:593–595, 1986

Devaud LL, Purdy RH, Morrow AL: The neurosteroid, 3α-hydroxy-5α-pregnan-20-one, protects against bicuculline-induced seizures during ethanol withdrawal in rats. Alcohol Clin Exp Res 19:350–355, 1995

Djebaili M, Guo Q, Pettus EH, et al: The neurosteroids progesterone and allopregnanolone reduce cell death, gliosis, and functional deficits after traumatic brain injury in rats. J Neurotrauma 22:106–118, 2005

Duka I, Kintsurashvili E, Gavras I, et al: Vasoactive potential of the B_1 bradykinin receptor in normotension and hypertension. Circ Res 88:275–281, 2001

Elliott-Hunt CR, Kazlauskaite J, Wilde GJ, et al: Potential signalling pathways underlying corticotrophin-releasing hormone-mediated neuroprotection from excitotoxicity in rat hippocampus. J Neurochem 80:416–425, 2002

Everitt BJ, Robbins TW: Central cholinergic systems and cognition. Annu Rev Psychol 48:649–684, 1997

Felder CC: Muscarinic acetylcholine receptors: signal transduction through multiple effectors. FASEB J 9:619–625, 1995

Fernandez-Vizarra P, Fernandez AP, Castro-Blanco S, et al: Expression of nitric oxide system in clinically evaluated cases of Alzheimer's disease. Neurobiol Dis 15:287–305, 2004

Fox MW, Anderson RE, Meyer FB: Neuroprotection by corticotropin releasing factor during hypoxia in rat brain. Stroke 24:1072–1075; discussion 1075–1076, 1993

Fu XW, Nurse CA, Farragher SM, et al: Expression of functional nicotinic acetylcholine receptors in neuroepithelial bodies of neonatal hamster lung. Am J Physiol Lung Cell Mol Physiol 285:L1203–L1212, 2003

Fujikawa DG: Prolonged seizures and cellular injury: understanding the connection. Epilepsy Behav 7 (suppl 3):S3–S11, 2005

Ghoumari AM, Ibanez C, El-Etr M, et al: Progesterone and its metabolites increase myelin basic protein expression in organotypic slice cultures of rat cerebellum. J Neurochem 86:848–859, 2003

Gibson GE, Peterson C: Aging decreases oxidative metabolism and the release and synthesis of acetylcholine. J Neurochem 37:978–984, 1981

Gibson GE, Peterson C, Sansone J: Neurotransmitter and carbohydrate metabolism during aging and mild hypoxia. Neurobiol Aging 2:165–172, 1981

Gotti C, Clementi F: Neuronal nicotinic receptors: from structure to pathology. Prog Neurobiol 74:363–396, 2004

Grando SA, Horton RM, Pereira EF, et al: A nicotinic acetylcholine receptor regulating cell adhesion and motility is expressed in human keratinocytes. J Invest Dermatol 105:774–781, 1995

Gray R, Rajan AS, Radcliffe KA, et al: Hippocampal synaptic transmission enhanced by low concentrations of nicotine. Nature 383:713–716, 1996

Greenamyre JT, Penney JB, D'Amato CJ, et al: Dementia of the Alzheimer's type: changes in hippocampal L-[^{3}H]glutamate binding. J Neurochem 48:543–551, 1987

Griffin LD, Gong W, Verot L, et al: Niemann-Pick type C disease involves disrupted neurosteroidogenesis and responds to allopregnanolone. Nat Med 10:704–711, 2004

Grossberg GT, Stahelin HB, Messina JC, et al: Lack of adverse pharmacodynamic drug interactions with rivastigmine and twenty-two classes of medications. Int J Geriatr Psychiatry 15:242–247, 2000

Hashimoto T, Fukuda N: Effect of thyrotropin-releasing hormone on the neurologic impairment in rats with spinal cord injury: treatment starting 24 h and 7 days after injury. Eur J Pharmacol 203:25–32, 1991

Hebert LE, Scherr PA, Beckett LA, et al: Age-specific incidence of Alzheimer's disease in a community population. JAMA 273:1354–1359, 1995

Higgins JP, Flicker L: Lecithin for dementia and cognitive impairment. Cochrane Database Syst Rev, CD001015, 2000

Higuchi M, Yanai K, Okamura N, et al: Histamine H_1 receptors in patients with Alzheimer's disease assessed by positron emission tomography. Neuroscience 99:721–729, 2000

Hosli L, Hosli E, Della Briotta G, et al: Action of acetylcholine, muscarine, nicotine and antagonists on the membrane potential of astrocytes in cultured rat brainstem and spinal cord. Neurosci Lett 92:165–170, 1988

Huang HM, Toral-Barza L, Thaler H, et al: Inositol phosphates and intracellular calcium after bradykinin stimulation in fibroblasts from young, normal aged and Alzheimer donors. Neurobiol Aging 12:469–473, 1991

Hynd MR, Scott HL, Dodd PR: Glutamate-mediated excitotoxicity and neurodegeneration in Alzheimer's disease. Neurochem Int 45:583–595, 2004

Ishunina TA, van Heerikhuize JJ, Ravid R, et al: Estrogen receptors and metabolic activity in the human tuberomamillary nucleus: changes in relation to sex, aging and Alzheimer's disease. Brain Res 988:84–96, 2003

Jansen KL, Faull RL, Dragunow M, et al: Alzheimer's disease: changes in hippocampal *N*-methyl-D-aspartate, quisqualate, neurotensin, adenosine, benzodiazepine, serotonin and opioid receptors: an autoradiographic study. Neuroscience 39:613–627, 1990

Jones GM, Sahakian BJ, Levy R, et al: Effects of acute subcutaneous nicotine on attention, information processing and short-term memory in Alzheimer's disease. Psychopharmacology 108:485–494, 1992

Jones R: A 12-week clinical trial of talsaclidine, a muscarinic agonist, in the treatment of mild to moderate Alzheimer's disease. Neurobiol Aging 23:122, 2002

Jones RW: Have cholinergic therapies reached their clinical boundary in Alzheimer's disease? Int J Geriatr Psychiatry 18:S7–S13, 2003

Kaasinen V, Kemppainen N, Nagren K, et al: Age-related loss of extrastriatal dopamine D_2-like receptors in women. J Neurochem 81:1005–1010, 2002

Kariya K, Yamauchi A, Hattori S, et al: The disappearance rate of intraventricular bradykinin in the brain of the conscious rat. Biochem Biophys Res Commun 107:1461–1466, 1982

Khisti RT, Chopde CT, Jain SP: Antidepressant-like effect of the neurosteroid 3α-hydroxy-5α-pregnan-20-one in mice forced swim test. Pharmacol Biochem Behav 67:137–143, 2000

Kokate TG, Cohen AL, Karp E, et al: Neuroactive steroids protect against pilocarpine- and kainic acid–induced limbic seizures and status epilepticus in mice. Neuropharmacology 35:1049–1056, 1996

Kornhuber J, Retz W, Riederer P, et al: Effect of antemortem and postmortem factors on [^{3}H]glutamate binding in the human brain. Neurosci Lett 93:312–317, 1988

Kornhuber J, Mack-Burkhardt F, Konradi C, et al: Effect of antemortem and postmortem factors on [^{3}H]MK-801 binding in the human brain: transient elevation during early childhood. Life Sci 45:745–749, 1989

Kowall NW, Quigley BJ Jr, Krause JE, et al: Substance P and substance P receptor histochemistry in human neurodegenerative diseases. Regul Pept 46:174–185, 1993

Labombarda F, Gonzalez SL, Gonzalez DM, et al: Cellular basis for progesterone neuroprotection in the injured spinal cord. J Neurotrauma 19:343–355, 2002

Lai MK, Tsang SW, Alder JT, et al: Loss of serotonin 5-HT_{2A} receptors in the postmortem temporal cortex correlates with rate of cognitive decline in Alzheimer's disease. Psychopharmacology 179:673–677, 2005

Lanctot KL, Herrmann N, Mazzotta P, et al: GABAergic function in Alzheimer's disease: evidence for dysfunction and potential as a therapeutic target for the treatment of behavioural and psychological symptoms of dementia. Can J Psychiatry 49:439–453, 2004

Lapchak PA, Chapman DF, Nunez SY, et al: Dehydroepiandrosterone sulfate is neuroprotective in a reversible spinal cord ischemia model: possible involvement of $GABA_A$ receptors. Stroke 31:1953–1956; discussion 1957, 2000

Levey AI: Muscarinic acetylcholine receptor expression in memory circuits: implications for treatment of Alzheimer disease. Proc Natl Acad Sci U S A 93:13541–13546, 1996

Lezoualc'h F, Engert S, Berning B, et al: Corticotropin-releasing hormone–mediated neuroprotection against oxidative stress is associated with the increased release of non-amyloidogenic amyloid beta precursor protein and with the suppression of nuclear factor-kappaB. Mol Endocrinol 14:147–159, 2000

Lommatzsch M, Zingler D, Schuhbaeck K, et al: The impact of age, weight and gender on BDNF levels in human platelets and plasma. Neurobiol Aging 26:115–123, 2005

Lorke DE, Lu G, Cho E, et al: Serotonin 5-HT_{2A} and 5-HT_6 receptors in the prefrontal cortex of Alzheimer and normal aging patients. BMC Neurosci 7:36, 2006

Luo Y, Roth GS: The roles of dopamine oxidative stress and dopamine receptor signaling in aging and age-related neurodegeneration. Antioxid Redox Signal 2:449–460, 2000

Macklin KD, Maus AD, Pereira EF, et al: Human vascular endothelial cells express functional nicotinic acetylcholine receptors. J Pharmacol Exp Ther 287:435–439, 1998

Maelicke A, Schrattenholz A, Albuquerque EX: Neuronal nicotinic acetylcholine receptors in non-neuronal cells, expression and renaturation of ligand binding domain and modulatory control by allosterically acting ligands, in Handbook of Pharmacology. Edited by Clementi F, Fornasari D, Cotti C. Berlin, Springer, 2000, pp 477–496

Marceau F, Hess JF, Bachvarov DR: The B_1 receptors for kinins. Pharmacol Rev 50:357–386, 1998

Marczynski TJ: GABAergic deafferentation hypothesis of brain aging and Alzheimer's disease revisited. Brain Res Bull 45:341–379, 1998

Martin-Ruiz CM, Court JA, Molnar E, et al: α_4 but not α_3 and α_7 nicotinic acetylcholine receptor subunits are lost from the temporal cortex in Alzheimer's disease. J Neurochem 73:1635–1640, 1999

Marx CE, Duncan GE, Gilmore JH, et al: Olanzapine increases allopregnanolone in the rat cerebral cortex. Biol Psychiatry 47:1000–1004, 2000

Marx CE, VanDoren MJ, Duncan GE, et al: Olanzapine and clozapine increase the GABAergic neuroactive steroid allopregnanolone in rodents. Neuropsychopharmacology 28:1–13, 2003

Marx CE, Shampine LJ, Duncan GE, et al: Clozapine markedly elevates pregnenolone in rat hippocampus, cerebral cortex, and serum: candidate mechanism for superior efficacy? Pharmacol Biochem Behav 84:598–608, 2006a

Marx CE, Shampine LJ, Khisti RT, et al: Olanzapine and fluoxetine administration and coadministration increase rat hippocampal pregnenolone, allopregnanolone and peripheral deoxycorticosterone: implications for therapeutic actions. Pharmacol Biochem Behav 84:609–617, 2006b

Marx CE, Stevens RD, Shampine LJ, et al: Neuroactive steroids are altered in schizophrenia and bipolar disorder: relevance to pathophysiology and therapeutics. Neuropsychopharmacology 31:1249–1263, 2006c

Marx CE, Trost WT, Shampine LJ, et al: The neurosteroid allopregnanolone is reduced in prefrontal cortex in Alzheimer's disease. Biol Psychiatry 60:1287–1294, 2006d

Mathieu-Kia AM, Fan LQ, Kreek MJ, et al: μ-, δ- and κ-opioid receptor populations are differentially altered in distinct areas of postmortem brains of Alzheimer's disease patients. Brain Res 893:121–134, 2001

May C, Rapoport SI, Tomai TP, et al: Cerebrospinal fluid concentrations of corticotropin-releasing hormone (CRH) and corticotropin (ACTH) are reduced in patients with Alzheimer's disease. Neurology 37:535–538, 1987

Mayo W, Lemaire V, Malaterre J, et al: Pregnenolone sulfate enhances neurogenesis and PSA-NCAM in young and aged hippocampus. Neurobiol Aging 26:103–114, 2005

Mazat L, Lafont S, Berr C, et al: Prospective measurements of dehydroepiandrosterone sulfate in a cohort of elderly subjects: relationship to gender, subjective health, smoking habits, and 10-year mortality. Proc Natl Acad Sci U S A 98:8145–8150, 2001

McCoy KR, Mullins RD, Newcomb TG, et al: Serum- and bradykinin-induced calcium transients in familial Alzheimer's fibroblasts. Neurobiol Aging 14:447–455, 1993

Meana JJ, Barturen F, Garro MA, et al: Decreased density of presynaptic α_2-adrenoceptors in postmortem brains of patients with Alzheimer's disease. J Neurochem 58:1896–1904, 1992

Meng SZ, Ozawa Y, Itoh M, et al: Developmental and age-related changes of dopamine transporter, and dopamine D_1 and D_2 receptors in human basal ganglia. Brain Res 843:136–144, 1999

Mileusnic D, Magnuson DJ, Hejna MJ, et al: Age and species-dependent differences in the neurokinin B system in rat and human brain. Neurobiol Aging 20:19–35, 1999

Mizukami K, Ikonomovic MD, Grayson DR, et al: Immunohistochemical study of $GABA_A$ receptor $\beta_{2/3}$ subunits in the hippocampal formation of aged brains with Alzheimer-related neuropathologic changes. Exp Neurol 147:333–345, 1997

Mizukami K, Grayson DR, Ikonomovic MD, et al: $GABA_A$ receptor β_2 and β_3 subunits mRNA in the hippocampal formation of aged human brain with Alzheimer-related neuropathology. Brain Res Mol Brain Res 56:268–272, 1998a

Mizukami K, Ikonomovic MD, Grayson DR, et al: Immunohistochemical study of $GABA_A$ receptor α_1 subunit in the hippocampal formation of aged brains with Alzheimer-related neuropathologic changes. Brain Res 799:148–155, 1998b

Mohs RC, Davis KL, Tinklenberg JR, et al: Choline chloride effects on memory in the elderly. Neurobiol Aging 1:21–25, 1980

Moller M, Jakobsen S, Gjedde A: Parametric and regional maps of free serotonin $5HT_{1A}$ receptor sites in human brain as function of age in healthy humans. Neuropsychopharmacology 32:1707–1714, 2007

Monteleone P, Luisi M, Colurcio B, et al: Plasma levels of neuroactive steroids are increased in untreated women with anorexia nervosa or bulimia nervosa. Psychosom Med 63:62–68, 2001

Monzani F, Del Guerra P, Caraccio N, et al: Age-related modifications in the regulation of the hypothalamic-pituitary-thyroid axis. Horm Res 46:107–112, 1996

Mouradian MM, Farah JM Jr, Mohr E, et al: Spinal fluid CRF reduction in Alzheimer's disease. Neuropeptides 8:393–400, 1986

Mousavi M, Hellstrom-Lindahl E, Guan ZZ, et al: Protein and mRNA levels of nicotinic receptors in brain of tobacco using controls and patients with Alzheimer's disease. Neuroscience 122:515–520, 2003

Newhouse PA, Sunderland T, Tariot PN, et al: Intravenous nicotine in Alzheimer's disease: a pilot study. Psychopharmacology 95:171–175, 1988

Nordberg A, Winblad B: Reduced number of [^{3}H]nicotine and [^{3}H]acetylcholine binding sites in the frontal cortex of Alzheimer brains. Neurosci Lett 72:115–119, 1986

Nordberg A, Adem A, Bucht G, et al: Alterations in lymphocyte receptor densities in dementia of Alzheimer type: a possible diagnostic marker, in Biological Markers in Dementia of Alzheimer Type. Edited by Fowler CJ. London: Smith-Gordon, 1990a, pp 149–159

Nordberg A, Hartvig P, Lilja A, et al: Decreased uptake and binding of ^{11}C-nicotine in brain of Alzheimer patients as visualized by positron emission tomography. J Neural Transm Park Dis Dement Sect 2:215–224, 1990b

Nordberg A, Lundqvist H, Hartvig P, et al: Kinetic analysis of regional (S)(-)^{11}C-nicotine binding in normal and Alzheimer brains: in vivo assessment using positron emission tomography. Alzheimer Dis Assoc Disord 9:21–27, 1995

Nordberg A, Lundqvist H, Hartvig P, et al: Imaging of nicotinic and muscarinic receptors in Alzheimer's disease: effect of tacrine treatment. Dement Geriatr Cogn Disord 8:78–84, 1997

North RA, Slack BE, Surprenant A: Muscarinic M_1 and M_2 receptors mediate depolarization and presynaptic inhibition in guinea-pig enteric nervous system. J Physiol 368:435–452, 1985

Nyman MJ, Eskola O, Kajander J, et al: Gender and age affect NK1 receptors in the human brain: a positron emission tomography study with [^{18}F]SPA-RQ. Int J Neuropsychopharmacol 10:219–229, 2007

Ono K, Hasegawa K, Yamada M, et al: Nicotine breaks down preformed Alzheimer's beta-amyloid fibrils in vitro. Biol Psychiatry 52:880–886, 2002

Perez Leiros C, Sterin-Borda L, Hubscher O, et al: Activation of nitric oxide signaling through muscarinic receptors in submandibular glands by primary Sjogren syndrome antibodies. Clin Immunol 90:190–195, 1999

Perry EK: The cholinergic hypothesis—ten years on. Br Med Bull 42:63–69, 1986

Perry EK, Tomlinson BE, Blessed G, et al: Correlation of cholinergic abnormalities with senile plaques and mental test scores in senile dementia. Br Med J 2:1457–1459, 1978

Perry EK, Smith CJ, Court JA, et al: Cholinergic nicotinic and muscarinic receptors in dementia of Alzheimer, Parkinson and Lewy body types. J Neural Transm Park Dis Dement Sect 2:149–158, 1990

Perry EK, Morris CM, Court JA, et al: Alteration in nicotine binding sites in Parkinson's disease, Lewy body dementia and Alzheimer's disease: possible index of early neuropathology. Neuroscience 64:385–395, 1995

Perry E, Walker M, Grace J, et al: Acetylcholine in mind: a neurotransmitter correlate of consciousness? Trends Neurosci 22:273–280, 1999

Pinna G, Dong E, Matsumoto K, et al: In socially isolated mice, the reversal of brain allopregnanolone down-regulation mediates the anti-aggressive action of fluoxetine. Proc Natl Acad Sci U S A 100:2035–2040, 2003

Pioro EP, Majors AW, Mitsumoto H, et al: ^{1}H-MRS evidence of neurodegeneration and excess glutamate + glutamine in ALS medulla. Neurology 53:71–79, 1999

Pirker W, Asenbaum S, Hauk M, et al: Imaging serotonin and dopamine transporters with ^{123}I-β-CIT SPECT: binding kinetics and effects of normal aging. J Nucl Med 41:36–44, 2000

Powers RE, Walker LC, DeSouza EB, et al: Immunohistochemical study of neurons containing corticotropin-releasing factor in Alzheimer's disease. Synapse 1:405–410, 1987

Pratico C, Quattrone D, Lucanto T, et al: Drugs of anesthesia acting on central cholinergic system may cause post-operative cognitive dysfunction and delirium. Med Hypotheses 65:972–982, 2005

Radcliffe KA, Dani JA: Nicotinic stimulation produces multiple forms of increased glutamatergic synaptic transmission. J Neurosci 18:7075–7083, 1998

Raiteri M, Marchi M, Paudice P: Presynaptic muscarinic receptors in the central nervous system. Ann N Y Acad Sci 604:113–129, 1990

Raskind MA, Peskind ER, Wessel T, et al: Galantamine in AD: a 6-month randomized, placebo-controlled trial with a 6-month extension. The Galantamine USA-1 Study Group. Neurology 54:2261–2268, 2000

Rasmusson AM, Pinna G, Paliwal P, et al: Decreased cerebrospinal fluid allopregnanolone levels in women with posttraumatic stress disorder. Biol Psychiatry 60:704–713, 2006

Ravert HT, Bencherif B, Madar I, et al: PET imaging of opioid receptors in pain: progress and new directions. Curr Pharm Des 10:759–768, 2004

Rego AC, de Almeida LP: Molecular targets and therapeutic strategies in Huntington's disease. Curr Drug Targets CNS Neurol Disord 4:361–381, 2005

Rinne JO, Lonnberg P, Marjamaki P: Human brain methionine- and leucine-enkephalins and their receptors during ageing. Brain Res 624:131–136, 1993

Rioux L, Joyce JN: Substance P receptors are differentially affected in Parkinson's and Alzheimer's disease. J Neural Transm Park Dis Dement Sect 6:199–210, 1993

Ritsner M, Maayan R, Gibel A, et al: Differences in blood pregnenolone and dehydroepiandrosterone levels between schizophrenia patients and healthy subjects. Eur Neuropsychopharmacol 17:358–365, 2007

Rogers SL, Farlow MR, Doody RS, et al: A 24-week, double-blind, placebo-controlled trial of donepezil in patients with Alzheimer's disease. Donepezil Study Group. Neurology 50:136–145, 1998

Romeo E, Strohle A, Spalletta G, et al: Effects of antidepressant treatment on neuroactive steroids in major depression. Am J Psychiatry 155:910–913, 1998

Rose GM, Hopper A, De Vivo M, et al: Phosphodiesterase inhibitors for cognitive enhancement. Curr Pharm Des 11:3329–3334, 2005

Rosler M, Anand R, Cicin-Sain A, et al: Efficacy and safety of rivastigmine in patients with Alzheimer's disease: international randomised controlled trial. BMJ 318:633–638, 1999

Sahakian B, Jones G, Levy R, et al: The effects of nicotine on attention, information processing, and short-term memory in patients with dementia of the Alzheimer type. Br J Psychiatry 154:797–800, 1989

Sailasuta N, Ernst T, Chang L: Regional variations and the effects of age and gender on glutamate concentrations in the human brain. Magn Reson Imaging 26:667–675, 2008

Sala C, Kimura I, Santoro G, et al: Expression of two neuronal nicotinic receptor subunits in innervated and denervated adult rat muscle. Neurosci Lett 215:71–74, 1996

Salomon AR, Marcinowski KJ, Friedland RP, et al: Nicotine inhibits amyloid formation by the β-peptide. Biochemistry 35:13568–13578, 1996

Sastre M, Garcia-Sevilla JA: Density of α_{2A} adrenoceptors and G_i proteins in the human brain: ratio of high-affinity agonist sites to antagonist sites and effect of age. J Pharmacol Exp Ther 269:1062–1072, 1994

Sastre M, Guimon J, Garcia-Sevilla JA: Relationships between β- and α_2-adrenoceptors and G coupling proteins in the human brain: effects of age and suicide. Brain Res 898:242–255, 2001

Schneider C, Risser D, Kirchner L, et al: Similar deficits of central histaminergic system in patients with Down syndrome and Alzheimer disease. Neurosci Lett 222:183–186, 1997

Serra M, Pisu MG, Muggironi M, et al: Opposite effects of short- versus long-term administration of fluoxetine on the concentrations of neuroactive steroids in rat plasma and brain. Psychopharmacology 158:48–54, 2001

Sheline YI, Mintun MA, Moerlein SM, et al: Greater loss of 5-HT_{2A} receptors in midlife than in late life. Am J Psychiatry 159:430–435, 2002

Shimohama S, Matsushima H: Signal transduction mechanisms in Alzheimer disease. Alzheimer Dis Assoc Disord 9 (suppl 2):15–22, 1995

Shimohama S, Taniguchi T, Fujiwara M, et al: Changes in nicotinic and muscarinic cholinergic receptors in Alzheimer-type dementia. J Neurochem 46:288–293, 1986

Siebeck M, Schorr M, Spannagl E, et al: B1 kinin receptor activity in pigs is associated with pre-existing infection. Immunopharmacology 40:49–55, 1998

Smith CD, Wekstein DR, Markesbery WR, et al: 3α,5α-THP: a potential plasma neurosteroid biomarker in Alzheimer's disease and perhaps non-Alzheimer's dementia. Psychopharmacology 186:481–485, 2006

Sparks DL, Beach TG, Lukas RJ: Immunohistochemical localization of nicotinic β_2 and α_4 receptor subunits in normal human brain and individuals with Lewy body and Alzheimer's disease: preliminary observations. Neurosci Lett 256:151–154, 1998

Spivak B, Maayan R, Kotler M, et al: Elevated circulatory level of $GABA_A$: antagonistic neurosteroids in patients with combat-related post-traumatic stress disorder. Psychol Med 30:1227–1231, 2000

Starke K, Gothert M, Kilbinger H: Modulation of neurotransmitter release by presynaptic autoreceptors. Physiol Rev 69:864–989, 1989

Stokes CE, Hawthorne JN: Reduced phosphoinositide concentrations in anterior temporal cortex of Alzheimer-diseased brains. J Neurochem 48:1018–1021, 1987

Strous RD, Spivak B, Yoran-Hegesh R, et al: Analysis of neurosteroid levels in attention deficit hyperactivity disorder. Int J Neuropsychopharmacol 4:259–264, 2001

Sundman I, Allard P, Eriksson A, et al: GABA uptake sites in frontal cortex from suicide victims and in aging. Neuropsychobiology 35:11–15, 1997

Szot P, White SS, Greenup JL, et al: Compensatory changes in the noradrenergic nervous system in the locus ceruleus and hippocampus of postmortem subjects with Alzheimer's disease and dementia with Lewy bodies. J Neurosci 26:467–478, 2006

Tannenberg RK, Scott HL, Westphalen RI, et al: The identification and characterization of excitotoxic nerve-endings in Alzheimer disease. Curr Alzheimer Res 1:11–25, 2004

Terzano S, Court JA, Fornasari D, et al: Expression of the α_3 nicotinic receptor subunit mRNA in aging and Alzheimer's disease. Brain Res Mol Brain Res 63:72–78, 1998

Uzunov DP, Cooper TB, Costa E, et al: Fluoxetine-elicited changes in brain neurosteroid content measured by negative ion mass fragmentography. Proc Natl Acad Sci U S A 93:12599–12604, 1996

Uzunova V, Sheline Y, Davis JM, et al: Increase in the cerebrospinal fluid content of neurosteroids in patients with unipolar major depression who are receiving fluoxetine or fluvoxamine. Proc Natl Acad Sci U S A 95:3239–3244, 1998

Vogt BA, Crino PB, Volicer L: Laminar alterations in $GABA_A$, muscarinic, and β adrenoceptors and neuron degeneration in cingulate cortex in Alzheimer's disease. J Neurochem 57:282–290, 1991

von Linstow Roloff E, Platt B: Biochemical dysfunction and memory loss: the case of Alzheimer's dementia. Cell Mol Life Sci 55:601–616, 1999

Wada E, Wada K, Boulter J, et al: Distribution of α_2, α_3, α_4, and β_2 neuronal nicotinic receptor subunit mRNAs in the central nervous system: a hybridization histochemical study in the rat. J Comp Neurol 284:314–335, 1989

Wallace MA: Effects of Alzheimer's disease-related β amyloid protein fragments on enzymes metabolizing phosphoinositides in brain. Biochim Biophys Acta 1227:183–187, 1994

Wang JM, Johnston PB, Ball BG, et al: The neurosteroid allopregnanolone promotes proliferation of rodent and human neural progenitor cells and regulates cell-cycle gene and protein expression. J Neurosci 25:4706–4718, 2005

Wang Y, Chan GL, Holden JE, et al: Age-dependent decline of dopamine D_1 receptors in human brain: a PET study. Synapse 30:56–61, 1998

Wang Y, Pereira EF, Maus AD, et al: Human bronchial epithelial and endothelial cells express α_7 nicotinic acetylcholine receptors. Mol Pharmacol 60:1201–1209, 2001

Webster MJ, Herman MM, Kleinman JE, et al: BDNF and trkB mRNA expression in the hippocampus and temporal cortex during the human lifespan. Gene Expr Patterns 6:941–951, 2006

Wevers A, Schroder H: Nicotinic acetylcholine receptors in Alzheimer's disease. J Alzheimers Dis 1:207–219, 1999

White HK, Levin ED: Four-week nicotine skin patch treatment effects on cognitive performance in Alzheimer's disease. Psychopharmacology 143:158–165, 1999

Whitehouse PJ, Price DL, Clark AW, et al: Alzheimer disease: evidence for selective loss of cholinergic neurons in the nucleus basalis. Ann Neurol 10:122–126, 1981

Whitehouse PJ, Price DL, Struble RG, et al: Alzheimer's disease and senile dementia: loss of neurons in the basal forebrain. Science 215:1237–1239, 1982

Whitehouse PJ, Vale WW, Zweig RM, et al: Reductions in corticotropin releasing factor-like immunoreactivity in cerebral cortex in Alzheimer's disease, Parkinson's disease, and progressive supranuclear palsy. Neurology 37:905–909, 1987

Wieland S, Lan NC, Mirasedeghi S, et al: Anxiolytic activity of the progesterone metabolite 5α-pregnan-3α-ol-20-one. Brain Res 565:263–268, 1991

Wilcock GK, Esiri MM, Bowen DM, et al: Alzheimer's disease: correlation of cortical choline acetyltransferase activity with the severity of dementia and histological abnormalities. J Neurol Sci 57:407–417, 1982

Wilcock GK, Lilienfeld S, Gaens E: Efficacy and safety of galantamine in patients with mild to moderate Alzheimer's disease: multicentre randomised controlled trial. Galantamine International-1 Study Group. BMJ 321:1445–1449, 2000

Wilson AL, Langley LK, Monley J, et al: Nicotine patches in Alzheimer's disease: pilot study on learning, memory, and safety. Pharmacol Biochem Behav 51:509–514, 1995

Wonnacott S: Presynaptic nicotinic ACh receptors. Trends Neurosci 20:92–98, 1997

Xi-Moy SX, Randall WC, Wurster RD: Nicotinic and muscarinic synaptic transmission in canine intracardiac ganglion cells innervating the sinoatrial node. J Auton Nerv Syst 42:201–213, 1993

Yamamoto M, Suhara T, Okubo Y, et al: Age-related decline of serotonin transporters in living human brain of healthy males. Life Sci 71:751–757, 2002

Yamashita H, Nakamura S: Nicotine rescues PC12 cells from death induced by nerve growth factor deprivation. Neurosci Lett 213:145–147, 1996

Yasutake C, Kuroda K, Yanagawa T, et al: Serum BDNF, TNF-α and IL-1β levels in dementia patients: comparison between Alzheimer's disease and vascular dementia. Eur Arch Psychiatry Clin Neurosci 256:402–406, 2006

Yew DT, Li WP, Webb SE, et al: Neurotransmitters, peptides, and neural cell adhesion molecules in the cortices of normal elderly humans and Alzheimer patients: a comparison. Exp Gerontol 34:117–133, 1999

Yi JH, Hazell AS: Excitotoxic mechanisms and the role of astrocytic glutamate transporters in traumatic brain injury. Neurochem Int 48:394–403, 2006

Zhang W, Liu HT: MAPK signal pathways in the regulation of cell proliferation in mammalian cells. Cell Res 12:9–18, 2002

Zia S, Ndoye A, Nguyen VT, et al: Nicotine enhances expression of the α_3, α_4, α_5, and α_7 nicotinic receptors modulating calcium metabolism and regulating adhesion and motility of respiratory epithelial cells. Res Commun Mol Pathol Pharmacol 97:243–262, 1997

Suggested Readings

Belelli D, Lambert JJ: Neurosteroids: endogenous regulators of the $GABA_A$ receptor. Nat Rev Neurosci 6:565–575, 2005

Eglen RM: Muscarinic receptor subtypes in neuronal and non-neuronal cholinergic function. Auton Autacoid Pharmacol 26:219–233, 2006

Gotti C, Clementi F: Neuronal nicotinic receptors: from structure to pathology. Prog Neurobiol 74:363–396, 2004

Green AR: Neuropharmacology of 5-hydroxytryptamine. Br J Pharmacol 147 (suppl 1):S145–S152, 2006

Greengard P: The neurobiology of dopamine signaling. Biosci Rep 21:247–269, 2001

Hallberg M, Nyberg F: Neuropeptide conversion to bioactive fragments: an important pathway in neuromodulation. Curr Protein Pept Sci 4:31–44, 2003

Michels G, Moss SJ: $GABA_A$ receptors: properties and trafficking. Crit Rev Biochem Mol Biol 42:3–14, 2007

Ramos BP, Arnsten AF: Adrenergic pharmacology and cognition: focus on the prefrontal cortex. Pharmacol Ther 113:523–536, 2007

Simons FE: Advances in H_1-antihistamines. N Engl J Med 351:2203–2217, 2004

Walton HS, Dodd PR: Glutamate-glutamine cycling in Alzheimer's disease. Neurochem Int 50:1052–1066, 2007

CHAPTER 6

GENETICS

Robert A. Sweet, M.D.
Patricia A. Wilkosz, M.D., Ph.D.

Genomics in Geriatric Psychiatry

The completion of the Human Genome Project (International Human Genome Sequencing Consortium 2004) provided 3 billion bases of reference nucleotides for comparative genetic studies that will fundamentally alter how diseases are defined, prevented, and treated (Guttmacher and Collins 2002). In addition to *Homo sapiens*, hundreds of other species have now had their genomes sequenced, with many more in progress (see National Center for Biotechnology Information 2008). In 2007, the first genetic sequences of living individuals were reported; personalized genomics is upon us (Levy et al. 2007). There is every reason to believe that this revolution will impact geriatric psychiatry. Family, twin, and adoption studies have demonstrated robust genetic influences in geriatric psychiatric disorders including schizophrenia, bipolar disorder, and Alzheimer's disease (AD). Conventional genetic approaches have advanced our understanding of the nature of the genetic contributions to these disorders. These gains have been hard won, and limited so far. However, the pace of discovery is notably quickening in this new postgenomics era. To prepare the reader for what lies ahead, we have therefore undertaken the task of summarizing key advances in genomic science and the current state of understanding of the genetics of mental disorders of aging.

Recent Advances in Genomic Science

Among the fundamental insights to arise from the sequencing of the human genome is that the number of genes, currently estimated as 20,000–25,000, was several-fold less than expected, encompassing only about 2% of all DNA. Both the number and function of genes are surprisingly conserved across mammalian species sequenced to date. These findings have caused investigators to look within and across species for other sources of variation, and thus complexity, within the genome. From this has emerged an awareness of the functional roles of the other approximately 98% of the genome, the so-called silent or noncoding DNA (ncDNA), which is never translated into protein. In addition, the search for sources of complexity has led to the realization that structural variation (deletions and replications of segments of chromosomes) makes up the largest proportion (at least in terms of numbers of DNA bases) of variation within humans and between humans and other primates (Cheng et al. 2005; Levy et al. 2007; Samonte and Eichler 2002). Finally, as a complement to these efforts to identify variation, the International HapMap Project has identified chromosomal regions of DNA sequence that are conserved across subjects, generating a powerful tool for finding regions that harbor sequences associated with disease (International HapMap Consortium 2007).

Functional Variation in the Human Genome: The Role of ncDNA

Increasingly, it has become apparent that a large degree of complexity results from regulation of gene transcription (the process of converting DNA to RNA) and gene splicing (affecting the isoform of the resulting translated protein) (Carninci et al. 2005). This regulation has been known to occur via sites within nontranscribed DNA sequences (e.g., promoter sequences) and within transcribed yet noncoding portions of the messenger RNA sequence (e.g., the splice sites at the boundaries of introns and exons). However, there has been a recent explosion of understanding regarding the extent to which ncDNA sequences are transcribed into noncoding RNA (ncRNA; sequences not functioning as messenger, transfer, or ribosomal RNA) (Carninci et al. 2005) and the breadth of cellular mechanisms under the control of ncRNA. ncRNA can regulate such diverse functions as chromosomal replication, gene expression, gene splicing, and even protein trafficking (Storz 2002; Storz et al. 2005).

Until very recently, the majority of known disease-causing mutations have been single DNA nucleotide changes (single-nucleotide polymorphisms [SNPs]) in coding DNA, resulting in altered amino acid sequence of the translated protein. Along with awareness of the diverse roles of ncDNA has come increasing recognition of the contribution to disease risk from SNPs in these sequences. For example, Koboldt and Miller (2007) mapped more than 9 million SNPs to gene sequences and ncDNA sequences of functional significance, including transcription factor binding sites, exon splicing enhancers or silencers, transcribed ncRNA, regulatory-potential sequences, and ncRNA binding sites. They found that those SNPs in coding DNA that altered protein structure had significantly decreased allele frequencies and increased population specificity (providing evidence of a functional effect subject to natural selection); however, they observed the same pattern among SNPs in ncDNA that map to transcription factor binding sites, ncRNA binding elements, regulatory-potential sequences, and splice sites. They found that substitutions in ncRNA binding sites or splice sites were more likely to show evidence of selection than coding SNPs. ncRNA has been implicated in diseases affecting the brain, including velocardiofacial syndrome, a disorder associated with high rates of schizophrenia (Han et al. 2004), and fragile X syndrome (Duan and Jin 2006).

Structural Variation in the Human Genome

Efforts to screen the human genome have shown that large segments of DNA have been deleted or duplicated (Inoue and Lupski 2002; Lupski 2007), resulting in changes in the number of genes within these regions and often disrupting gene structure at deletion or duplication breakpoints (Neumann et al. 2006). Diseases caused by those genomic rearrangements that result in an altered number of gene copies (copy-number variation [CNV]) are often referred to as *genomic disorders*. Work to map genomic variation in the complete human genome has identified CNV in 1,400 regions that overlap with 14.5% of the genes associated with human disease (Redon et al. 2006).

Although only very recently a subject of investigation, CNV has rapidly been shown to be associated with many neurodevelopmental and neurodegenerative disorders, including both sporadic and familial cases (Redon et al. 2006; Sebat et al. 2007). It is of note that familial early-onset cases of Alzheimer's disease and Parkinson's disease due to CNV have been described (see "Alzheimer's Disease" and "Other Neurodegenerative Illnesses of Late Life" sections later in this chapter). In many cases to date, reports have been limited to discovery of regions containing CNVs associated with disease, without identifying the specific DNA sequence resulting in illness. Identifying the underlying causative genetic effect remains an important need and area of development.

Genome-Wide Association Studies

The efforts of the International HapMap Project to identify contiguous blocks within the genome that are relatively invariant across individuals and populations have been critical to notable recent success in identifying genetic variation associated with several complex diseases, with the number of reports rapidly rising. The relative constancy of each haplotype block allows all the genetic sequence contained within it to be, in essence, represented by a single "tag" SNP. The result is that the entire genome can be rather thoroughly interrogated for association with disease (genome-wide association [GWA]) by about 10^5 tag SNPs, substantially smaller than the approximately 3 billion nucleotides within the genome.

Recently published, successful GWA studies are notable for several shared features (Coon et al. 2007; Parkes et al. 2007; Todd et al. 2007; Wellcome Trust Case Control Consortium 2007; Zeggini et al. 2007). Ultra-high-density genotyping chips, containing hundreds of thousands of SNPs, rendered GWA studies for thousands of cases and controls technically and financially possible. DNA samples were obtained from large and phenotypically well-characterized cohorts for many common diseases, and care was taken in the previously listed GWA studies to minimize bias stemming from possible population heterogeneity, genotyping errors, or DNA quality control issues. Replication of putative associations in independent sample populations is also essential.

Several important lessons can be gleaned from these early studies. Because these designs examine the entire genome, an important outcome is the discovery of new gene associations hitherto unrecognized as contributory to the disease being studied. In addition, often the associated SNPs are found in ncDNA that might not otherwise have been examined (Wellcome Trust Case Control Consortium 2007). Most variants identified contribute only modestly to disease risk, with odds ratios between 1.2 and 1.5. Detecting all effects of such small size will require many thousands of subjects, with reliably defined phenotypes. Finally, translating from an associated SNP to a genetic mechanism of a late-life mental disorder (as outlined below in the section "Finding Genetic Variants Contributing to Complex Diseases") is not straightforward.

Phenotypes Relevant to Mental Disorders of Aging

Stedman's Medical Dictionary (2005) defines *phenotype* as "The observable characteristics, at the physical, morphological, or biochemical level, of an individual, as determined by the genotype and environment." Phenotypes of interest to geriatric psychiatry that have been the subject of genetic investigation include early- and late-onset AD, other dementias, major depressive and bipolar disorders, and schizophrenia. Some of these phenotypes, such as early-onset familial AD, arise from single-gene disorders. However, the majority of these phenotypes, including late-onset AD, are complex disorders in that they are likely to be influenced by multiple genes, by environmental factors, and by their interactions.

Finding Genetic Variants Contributing to Complex Diseases: Challenges and Progress

Complex disorders have presented some of the greatest challenges in attempts to identify the underlying genetic variants that contribute to their development. In fact, until the recent advent of genome-wide association studies, the identification of an increased risk for late-onset AD in individuals carrying one or more copies of the apolipoprotein E (*APOE*) ε4 allele (*APOE*E4*) has been one of the few examples in all of medical genetics of successful identification of genetic variation underlying a complex disorder. This situation is now beginning to change. Nevertheless, it remains instructive to understand the reasons why identifying genes that lead to the development of a complex disorder is difficult. Many of the difficulties arise from the same underlying issues that impact how clinicians understand and use any newly emerging findings of genes associated with these disorders.

The flow of events that may lead from variation in the sequence of a gene to the development of the multiple cognitive, emotional, and behavioral criteria defining complex psychiatric disorders of late life is not straightforward. Genes encode proteins; therefore, a change in genetic sequence will have an effect via a change in level of expression or a change in function of the encoded protein. Proteins, however, act within extensive biochemical pathways, such that the effect of a change in any one protein may be amplified or compensated for by the effects of other proteins in the pathway, or by environmental manipulations (think, for instance, of altering diet in someone at genetic risk for atherosclerosis). In complex disorders, by definition, alteration in a single gene is insufficient to lead to the expression of disease; thus, alterations in multiple genes (proteins) impacting a pathway must contribute additive or interacting effects. In this scenario, individuals with the disorder will carry a subset of contributing genetic variations, but affected individuals may differ in the subsets they carry. Moreover, unaffected individuals will carry some of the contributing genetic variations, but not a complete set that would lead to disease. Finally, any given pathway may contribute directly to causing disease or may be more closely linked to a more narrowly defined biological component of disease (endophenotype) (Gottesman and Wolfgram 1991). For example, a genetic variation may affect a pathway leading to reduced working memory function or impaired affective regulation, which may contribute to schizophrenia or mood disorder, respectively (Egan et al. 2001a; Hariri and Holmes 2006). Such endophenotypes may be present in genetically related individuals without any evidence of the disease of interest (Egan et al. 2001a).

Adding to the difficulty in identifying genes associated with the development of a complex disorder in elderly individuals is the problem of competing causes of death. Individuals at genetic risk for the development of a disorder in late life may not express the disease symptoms during their lifetime. Late-onset AD can be used to illustrate this point. It has repeatedly been shown that the first-degree relatives of patients with AD have a 50% lifetime incidence rate of the disease. However, because of other causes of mortality, it is estimated that only about one-third of this theoretical familial predisposition to AD is realized in the usual life span (Breitner 1991; Breitner et al. 1988). This means that the actual predicted risk of developing AD in the first-degree relatives of individuals with AD is likely between 15% and 19%, compared with 5% in control subjects. Extrapolating from these findings, one could estimate that the risk to children of patients with AD is one in five or one in six (Liddell et al. 2001). In some cases, the same risk gene, *APOE*E4*, may lead to such competing processes, because the *APOE*E4* genotype predisposes an individual to both cardiovascular disease (Eichner et al. 2002) and AD (Farrer et al. 1997).

The net effect of the processes discussed previously in this section is that the magnitude of the observed increase in risk for a disorder due to any one genetic variation will most likely be relatively small. The result is both a limited ability to consistently detect such a genetic association and a reduced ability to predict an outcome for an individual even if one knows that he or she carries a genetic variation associated with the disease. It is not surprising, therefore, that the literature examining the association of genetic variations with complex diseases has had to struggle with how to identify replicable associations (Chanock et al. 2007). Recently, however, GWA studies have had success for complex disorders, including complex disorders of aging such as prostate cancer and macular degeneration (Couzin and Kaiser 2007). Whether similar success is around the corner for mental illnesses affecting elderly individuals remains to be determined.

Alzheimer's Disease

Alzheimer's disease is the predominant cause of dementia in the United States, with 3–4 million people affected. The etiology of AD is unknown, although significant strides have been made using gene mapping efforts. Consistent with the findings discussed previously in this chapter, success has been most notable for the single-gene disorders of early-onset familial AD, which comprises a minority (approximately 1%–2%) of the entire population of AD cases. Success in identifying genetic variants has led to a deepened understanding of the biology of AD, with potential therapeutic implications for both early-onset familial AD and late-onset AD.

Early-Onset Alzheimer's Disease

Identified Genes

Mutations at three genetic loci associated with early-onset AD have been identified. The first identified AD gene was the amyloid precursor protein (*APP*) gene located on chromosome 21 (Goate et al. 1991). Since this first report of a missense mutation (i.e., one amino acid is substituted for another) associated with AD on this gene, over 20 different missense mutations in *APP* that can cause AD have been identified (Alzheimer Disease and Frontotemporal Dementia Mutation Database 2008). Individuals with one of these *APP* mutations generally have onset of disease between ages 40 and 60 years, though occasionally later ages of onset can occur (Theuns et al. 2006). More recently, families with duplications of *APP*, leaving the mutation carrier with a total of three copies of the gene on their two chromosomes, have been reported (Rovelet-Lecrux et al. 2006; Sleegers et al. 2006). These families had early-onset AD associated with cerebral amyloid angiopathy and intracerebral hemorrhage. Although the identification of mutations in *APP* has been key to advancing our understanding of the genetic causes of AD, all *APP* mutations reported to date account for the disease in fewer than 100 families worldwide (Alzheimer Disease and Frontotemporal Dementia Mutation Database 2008).

A second AD locus was found on chromosome 14 (St. George-Hyslop et al. 1992; Schellenberg et al. 1992) and is now called presenilin-1 (*PS1*) (Sherrington et al. 1995). More than 160 mutations in the *PS1* locus have now been reported in several hundred families throughout the world (Alzheimer Disease and Frontotemporal Dementia Mutation Database 2008). Onset of symptoms for those with *PS1* mutations is often before age 50 years, but again, later ages are possible. Like the *APP* mutations, *PS1* mutations appear to act as autosomal dominant traits with nearly complete penetrance; that is, inheriting a single copy of the mutated gene is sufficient to cause disease in all individuals (Cruts et al. 1998). However, there has been at least one report of possible nonpenetrance of a *PS1* mutation in a healthy 68-year-old member of a pedigree with multiple affected members (Rossor et al. 1996).

A third AD gene has been localized to chromosome 1 and termed presenilin-2 (*PS2*) (Levy-Lahad et al. 1995a, 1995b). These mutations appear to be rare; only a few families of varying ethnicity have been identified with *PS2* mutations. Although the *PS2* mutations are autosomal dominant, they may not be fully penetrant. *PS2* mutations generally lead to onset of AD symptoms before age 65 years.

There has been conflicting information on the proportion of early-onset AD cases attributable to mutations in *APP*, *PS1*, and *PS2*. Some reports have suggested that *PS1* mutations may account for most early-onset familial AD cases (Campion et al. 1995, 1999; Hutton et al. 1996). Others have reported that a more realistic estimate is 20% or fewer of such cases, with *PS2* and *APP* accounting for 1% and 5%, respectively (Cruts et al. 1998). For the remainder of individuals with early-onset familial AD, it is unclear whether other causative single-gene mutations will be identified or whether these cases will prove to be multigenic in origin (Hardy 2007).

Implications for Mechanisms of Disease and Drug Target Identification

Although the postulate that overproduction of amyloid β protein (Aβ) would be causative of AD preceded the identification of AD genes (Glenner and Wong 1984), the identification of causative mutations in early-onset familial AD has confirmed the primacy of this mechanism. As noted, in some families AD results from simple duplication of *APP*. Similarly, AD pathology develops in individuals with Down syndrome, unless the trisomy of chromosome 21 occurs distal to the location of *APP* (Prasher et al. 1998). It is noteworthy that as assessed in animal and in vitro systems, the expressions of the identified mutations in *APP*, *PS1*, and *PS2* that lead to early-onset familial AD all result in overproduction of the toxic 42 amino acid species of Aβ, $A\beta_{42}$ (Hardy 2006; Selkoe 2004).

Perhaps more important for potential therapeutic implications are the contributions of these genetic findings to the development of an understanding regarding how *APP* is metabolized in the brain into $A\beta_{42}$. In brief, *APP* protein is cleaved by three enzymes, α-, β-, and γ-secretase. Cleavage by β-secretase and then γ-secretase generates Aβ, whereas cleavage by α-secretase yields the nontoxic p3 peptide. The identification of a mutation in *APP* that selectively enhanced metabolism of *APP* by β-secretase (known as the Swedish mutation) provided the assay necessary for the successful identification of β-secretase (Vassar et al. 1999). β-secretase inhibitors are now an active area of drug development in AD (Guo and Hobbs 2006). Similarly, the identification of AD-causing mutations in the novel proteins *PS1* and *PS2* led to a search for their function, ultimately converging on their identification as constituents of the proteolytic site in γ-secretase, which is now understood to be a complex of multiple proteins (Hardy 2006; Selkoe 2004). Efforts to identify effective γ-secretase inhibitors for the treatment of AD are also under way (Eder et al. 2007), although these are not as far advanced as the development of β-secretase inhibitors due to potential toxicity associated with inhibiting γ-secretase actions on proteins other than *APP*.

Late-Onset Alzheimer's Disease

Apolipoprotein E

The one gene with a clearly established relationship to late-onset AD is *APOE*, with increased risk of AD found in individuals carrying the ε4 allele (*APOE*E4*) in both familial and sporadic cases (Brousseau et al. 1994; Mayeux et al. 1993; Rebeck et al. 1993; Saunders et al. 1993; Schmechel et al. 1993). The risk for AD increases, and the mean age of onset of AD is earlier, as the number of ε4 alleles an individual carries increases from 0 to 2 (Corder et al. 1993). These findings were confirmed in a meta-analysis of more than 14,000 subjects who were recruited from clinical, community, and brain bank sources, representing multiple ethnic groups (Farrer et al. 1997). Importantly, although the effect of *APOE*E4* on increased risk of AD was evident in both sexes and in all age and ethnic groups, the magnitude of the risk associated with *APOE*E4* varied by age and ethnicity. Specifically, the risk appeared to be attenuated in older individuals and in African American and Hispanic individuals (relative to whites). In contrast, the risk conferred by *APOE*E4* was increased in individuals of Japanese ethnicity.

The strength of the relationship between *APOE*E4* and risk for late-onset AD cannot be overstated. *APOE*E4* accounts for up to 50% of the genetic contribution to late-onset AD (Pericak-Vance and Haines 1995). Nevertheless, carrying one or even two *APOE*E4* alleles does not translate into certain development of AD. It has been estimated that for those who are disease-free at age 65, at most 50% of the *APOE*E4* homozygotes will develop AD within their lifetimes (Henderson et al. 1995; Seshadri et al. 1997).

These uncertainties limit the use of the *APOE*E4* genotype as a clinical test. A number of studies have examined how *APOE*E4* genotyping impacts the sensitivity and specificity of diagnosing AD in individuals clinically diagnosed with cognitive symptoms consistent with a dementia. In general, the addition of *APOE*E4* testing to clinical assessment lowers the sensitivity of diagnosis of AD while enhancing specificity (reviewed in Ertekin-Taner 2007). That is, in combination with clinical evaluation, *APOE*E4* testing can reduce the rate of false-positive diagnoses. Similarly, in populations with normal or questionable cognitive impairment, *APOE*E4* testing may offer little improvement over cognitive testing in predicting subsequent AD (Cervilla et al. 2004; Klages et al. 2003), and may not be a sufficiently robust predictor of subsequent AD to use on its own (Devanand et al. 2005).

Other Putative Genes

As indicated in the previous section, best estimates suggest that at least half of the genetic contribution to late-onset AD is due to genes other than *APOE*E4*. A large number of linkage analyses of families with multiple individuals affected by late-onset AD have been conducted, with many regions throughout the genome implicated as possibly harboring risk genes, although no genes have been definitively identified using this approach (reviewed in Ertekin-Taner 2007).

Similarly, since 1994, hundreds of published reports comparing individuals with late-onset AD to normal controls have identified and/or refuted associations of candidate genes with late-onset AD (for a comprehensive listing, see http://www.alzgene.org). This large database has been recently subjected to a systematic meta-analysis, resulting in the identification of 20 variants in 13 genes that showed evidence for significant association with late-onset AD (Bertram et al. 2007). These results must be interpreted with caution at present and should be considered to be suggestive rather than confirmed associations. Importantly, for studies moving forward, this meta-analysis pointed out that most of the implicated genes were of small enough effect that reliable detection of significant associations in an individual study would typically require comparisons of greater (possibly far greater) than 1,000 individuals with AD and 1,000 individuals without cognitive impairment.

Behavioral and Psychotic Symptoms in Alzheimer's Disease

It has become increasingly recognized that nearly all individuals with AD will develop associated behavioral symptoms, including depression, psychosis, and aggression, over the course of the illness (Devanand et al. 1997; Swearer et al. 1988; Wragg and Jeste 1989). The presence of these symptoms can cause significant distress for the individuals experiencing them, as well as for the family members providing care to these patients (Kaufer et al. 1998).

We and others have been interested in whether psychosis and other behavioral disturbances in late-onset AD may result from the interaction of genetic variation with the neurodegenerative process. Tunstall et al. (2000) initially reported significant familial effects on mood state in AD, although they found evidence for familiality of psychosis in AD to be equivocal. In contrast, Sweet et al. (2002b) examined the familial aggregation of psychosis in a cohort of 371 subjects with AD and 461 of their siblings also diagnosed with AD, recruited and characterized as part of the National Institute of Mental Health AD Genetics Initiative. There was a significant association between the presence of psychotic symptoms in probands and in their siblings, resulting in an estimated heritability of psychosis in AD of 61% (Bacanu et al. 2005). This finding has since been confirmed in an independent sample (Hollingworth et al. 2007).

Identification of genes that may contribute to the familial risk of psychosis in late-onset AD is still in the early stages. Examination of genetic variation associated with depression or other behavioral syndromes is less well established. There is some replicated evidence from two analyses of psychosis in AD families, albeit conducted in overlapping samples, of linkage to a region on chromosome 6q (Bacanu et al. 2002; Hollingworth et al. 2007). Candidate gene association studies have largely focused on *APOE*E4*, which overall shows little indication of association with psychosis (Sweet et al. 2002a) or depression (Craig et al. 2005; Lopez et al. 1997). Although conclusions must necessarily be tentative because of the limited number of studied subjects and attempted replications, some recent evidence indicates that catechol-O-methyltransferase (*COMT*) and neuregulin 1 (*NRG1*), genes associated with increased risk of schizophrenic psychosis (see Table 6–1, later in this chapter), may also contribute to the risk for psychosis in AD (Borroni et al. 2004; Go et al. 2005; Sweet et al. 2005).

Other Neurodegenerative Illnesses of Late Life

Substantial progress has been made in identifying genetic variation that contributes to the risk of other common neurodegenerative diseases affecting elderly individuals. As seen for Alzheimer's disease, much of this progress has resulted from the identification of variants contributing to the risk of highly heritable, familial forms of these illnesses.

Frontotemporal Lobar Degeneration

Frontotemporal lobar degeneration (FTLD) defines a group of syndromes whose underlying pathology includes progressive degeneration of the prefrontal and anterior temporal lobes (Neary et al. 2005). Nearly all FTLD cases result from either of two major classes of neurodegenerative lesions: 1) cases with tau-positive inclusions and 2) cases with ubiquitin-positive inclusions, recently shown to contain TAR DNA-binding protein (TDP-43) (Neumann et al. 2006). Frontotemporal dementia, the most common clinical presentation of FTLD, is characterized by an insidious onset of progressive decline in personality, behavior, and social conduct, with typical onset between ages 45 and 65 (Neary et al. 1998). Other clinical manifestations of FTLD include primary progressive aphasia and semantic dementia. Which clinical manifestation predominates may relate more closely to the location of the preponderance of lesions than to whether TDP-43 inclusions or tauopathy is present (Neary et al. 2005). In contrast, FTLD neuropathological findings have a distinct pattern of overlap with several other neurodegenerative disorders. Thus, FTLD with tau-positive inclusions overlaps with the tauopathies progressive supranuclear palsy and corticobasal degeneration. FTLD with TDP-43-positive inclusions overlaps with motor neuron disease.

FTLD has been the subject of extensive genetic investigation. A family history is present in up to approximately 50% of FTLD cases, typically with an autosomal dominant pattern of transmission (Bird et al. 2003; Chow et al. 1999). Mutations in one of several genes can result in FTLD. The most commonly affected gene is progranulin (*GRN*) (Haugarvoll et al. 2007). Mutations resulting in loss of function of this gene result in the TDP-43 variant of FTLD and may account for up to 5%–10% of FTLD cases (Haugarvoll et al. 2007). The mechanism by which *GRN* mutations result in development of TDP-43 inclusions, however, is not known.

Mutations in microtubule-associated protein tau gene (*MAPT*) also can result in FTLD, although these mutations have been reported to account for disease in only slightly over 100 families worldwide (Alzheimer Disease and Frontotemporal Dementia Mutation Database 2008; Rademakers et al. 2004). Mutations in *MAPT* are associated with neuropathological findings of tau-positive inclusions in FTLD. Of interest, mutations in exons 1 and 10 and in intron 10 result in tau-positive inclusions in both neurons and glial cells, whereas mutations in exons 9, 11, 12, and 13 result in tau-positive inclusions confined to neurons (Haugarvoll et al. 2007). Though less commonly, FTLD has also been reported due to mutations in chromatin-modifying protein 2B (Skibinski et al. 2005) and valosin-containing protein (Watts et al. 2004).

Parkinson's Disease

Parkinson's disease (PD) is a common progressive neurodegenerative disorder affecting 1%–2% of the population ages 65 years and older (de Rijk et al. 1997). It is characterized by a combination of motor symptoms, including akinesia, rest tremor, rigidity, and disturbance of postural reflexes. The age at onset for PD ranges from the 20s through late life. Much of PD is thought to be sporadic. In fact, the risk for first-degree family members of patients with PD is increased only two- to threefold, and only in families where there is an early age of onset (Gasser 2005). In recent years, mutations in multiple genes have been identified that appear to cause PD via a Mendelian mode of inheritance. Just as with AD, however, all of these mutations combined account for a relatively small number of affected families and are primarily associated with onset of PD before age 50 or 60 years (for reviews, see Gasser 2005; Hardy et al. 2006).

Currently, mutations in two genes, alpha-synuclein (*SNCA*) (Polymeropoulos et al. 1997) and leucine-rich repeat kinase 2 (*LRRK2*) (Paisan-Ruiz et al. 2004), have been shown to result in autosomal dominant expression of PD. Variations in *SNCA* copy number are also associated with familial PD (Fuchs et al. 2007). Three additional genes, parkin (*PARK2*) (Kitada et al. 1998), PTEN-induced putative kinase 1 (*PINK1*) (Valente et al. 2004), and oncogene *DJ-1* (Bonifati et al. 2003), have been found to result in autosomal recessive transmission of PD. The role of the previously reported mutation in ubiquitin carboxy-terminal hydrolase L1 (*UCH-L1*) (Leroy et al. 1998) is now viewed as more controversial (Gasser 2005).

Linkages have also been reported to additional chromosomal loci for which the causative genetic variants have not yet been identified (Gasser 2005). In addition, there is evidence that mutations in genes causing other disorders may result in parkinsonian symptoms. For example, parkinsonism occurs in some individuals with FTLD due to mutations in *MAPT*. Similarly, parkinsonian symptoms can occur in spinocerebellar ataxia due to triplicate repeat expansions in *SCA3* and *SCA2* (Gwinn-Hardy 2002). In addition, it is possible that there are multiple susceptibility genes of small effect that may increase the risk of developing PD, possibly via interaction with as yet unspecified environmental factors (Gasser 2001). However, as with AD, replication studies have not consistently confirmed any of the candidate genes under study (for review, see Gasser 2001).

Schizophrenia

Recent findings that are highly likely to advance our understanding of psychoses have been the identification of genes demonstrating linkage and association with schizophrenia. A number of genes have been identified, with multiple replicated associations for seven of them, summarized in Table 6–1. These findings have been subject to several extensive reviews in the literature (Arnold et al. 2004; Craddock et al. 2006; Harrison and Weinberger 2005; O'Donovan et al. 2003; Shirts and Nimgaonkar 2004), so we focus on presenting an overview in this chapter. It should be noted that for all of the following genes, the identified associations have been with schizophrenia per se, and not specifically with late-life, or late-onset, schizophrenia.

Association of dystrobrevin binding protein 1 (*DTNBP1*, dysbindin) with schizophrenia was first described by Straub et al. (2002) using positional cloning within a linked region on 6p24–22 in a cohort of Irish families. At least 12 family-based and/or case-control studies in other populations, including multiple European populations, have confirmed this association with *DTNBP1*, although studies varied in the associated SNPs (Harrison and Weinberger 2005).

Stefansson et al. (2002) first identified a region of suggestive linkage on 8p12–21 in a cohort of Icelandic families, ultimately finding a core haplotype in the 5′ region of neuregulin1 (*NRG1*) that was strongly associated with schizophrenia risk. They then replicated this finding in an association study of Scottish subjects (Stefansson et al. 2003). Other replications in United Kingdom–wide, Irish, Chinese, and South African populations have been reported (Owen et al. 2005). There has also been identification of additional associated SNPs, including a coding SNP in exon 2 (Yang et al. 2003).

The gene "disrupted in schizophrenia 1" (*DISC1*) was initially identified after finding that a balanced translocation between chromosomes 1 and 11 (1;11) (q42.1;q14.3) cosegregated with schizophrenia and mood disorders in a large Scottish pedigree (St. Clair et al. 1990). The translocation breakpoint was ultimately mapped to within the *DISC1* gene, in which a variety of SNPs and haplotypes have been found to associate with schizophrenia across studies, including replication in European populations and in whites of European ancestry (Callicot et al. 2004; Hennah et al. 2003; Hodgkinson et al. 2004). A coding SNP in exon 11, yielding a cys704ser substitution, was found to be associated with schizophrenia and associated with intermediate phenotypes characterized by reduced hippocampal gray matter volume and integrity (Callicot et al. 2004).

The novel gene D-amino acid oxidase activator (*DAOA*, formerly known as *G72*, *G30*) was discovered by extensive SNP mapping of a region of linkage in schizophrenia on 13q32–34 (Chumakov et al. 2002). Initial attempted replications of the association of *DAOA* with schizophrenia were inconsistent, but more recently several replications have been reported in subjects with schizophrenia and psychotic disorder from populations including Europeans, whites of European ancestry, and individuals of Ashkenazi Jewish ancestry (Detera-Wadleigh and McMahon 2006).

AKT1 was initially pursued as a functional candidate gene, with reduced expression in lymphocytes and in frontal cortex reported in subjects with schizophrenia (Emamian et al. 2004). Follow-up family-based analyses revealed a significant association of *AKT1* with schizophrenia, with the SNPs showing the strongest associations in the intronic 5′ region (Emamian et al. 2004). The association of *AKT1* with schizophrenia was replicated in one of three Asian samples and in European and Iranian groups (Bajestan et al. 2006; Ikeda et al. 2004; Liu et al. 2006; Ohtsuki et al. 2004; Schwab et al. 2005).

COMT, an enzyme that inactivates dopamine (Axelrod and Tomchick 1958), has more recently been appreciated as a positional candidate gene in schizophrenia. *COMT* is located on chromosome 22q11.2, within the site of microdeletions found in patients with velocardiofacial syndrome, a disorder in which up to 30% of patients have schizophrenia (Carlson et al. 1997; Gross-

TABLE 6–1. Schizophrenia susceptibility genes: strength of evidence in schizophrenia and in psychosis in Alzheimer's disease

		Schizophrenia				Psychosis in AD	
Gene	Locus	Association[a]	Linkage to gene locus	Biological plausibility	Altered expression in schizophrenia	Association[b]	Linkage to gene locus
COMT	22q11	++++	++++	++++	Yes, +	++	
DTNBP1	6p22	+++++	++++	++	Yes, ++		
NRG1	8p12–21	+++++	++++	+++	Yes, ++	+	+
RGS4	1q21–22	+++	+++	+++	Yes, ++		
DISC1	1q42	+++	++	++	Yes,[c] +		
DAOA/G72	13q32–34	+++	++	++	Not known		
AKT1	14q22–32	+++	+	++	Yes, ++		

Note. *AKT1*=v-akt murine thymoma viral oncogene homolog 1; *COMT*= catechol-*O*-methyltransferase; *DAOA/G72*=D-amino acid oxidase activator; *DISC1*= disrupted in schizophrenia 1; *DTNBP1*=dystrobrevin binding protein 1; *NRG1*=neuregulin 1; *RGS4*= regulator of G-protein signaling 4;

[a]+++=at least three positive independent studies.

[b]Each +indicates an independent positive study.

[c]Altered expression of *DISC1* binding partners, not of *DISC1*.

Source. Adapted from Harrison and Weinberger 2005.

man et al. 1992; Lachman et al. 1996a; Murphy et al. 1999). *COMT* has been extensively studied in schizophrenia, with the most frequently examined SNP being RS4680, resulting in a final amino acid sequence containing either Val or Met. The Val variant has been shown to have three- to fourfold higher activity (Lachman et al. 1996b). A recent meta-analysis reviewed 14 case-control and five family studies of RS4680 in schizophrenia, concluding that there was a minor increase in risk for schizophrenia associated with the Val(G) allele in white populations of European ancestry (Glatt et al. 2003). The heterogeneity of findings may have resulted in part, however, from the failure of most studies to consider other variation within *COMT*. Recent studies have suggested that the contribution to schizophrenia risk due to *COMT* may be mediated through other variations. Shifman et al. (2002) examined 12 SNPs in *COMT* in a large case-control analysis of Ashkenazi Jews. They found the RS737865-RS4680-RS165599 haplotype to be the most strongly associated with schizophrenia. Two family-based studies provide further support for association of this haplotype with schizophrenia (Chen et al. 2004; Handoko et al. 2005). This haplotype may impact transcription of *COMT* (Bray et al. 2003). With regard to mechanism of increased psychosis risk, the *COMT* Val(G) allele is associated with a cognitive risk phenotype evident in subjects with schizophrenia, their unaffected family members, and normal controls (Egan et al. 2001b).

Regulator of G-protein signaling 4 (*RGS4*) was first identified for its potential association with schizophrenia by gene expression array analysis of prefrontal cortex of subjects with schizophrenia (Mirnics et al. 2001). Subsequent genetic analyses in two U.S. populations including white subjects of European ancestry and in one Asian-Indian family cohort found evidence for a modest association with schizophrenia, although the associated SNPs differed across studies (Chowdari et al. 2002). Several association studies have followed, replicating significant association with variation at some, but not all, of the previously associated SNPs and haplotypes in *RGS4* (Shirts and Nimgaonkar 2004). A more recent meta-analysis including 13,807 predominantly white subjects of European ancestry found evidence to support association of *RGS4* with schizophrenia, with two risk haplotypes (Talkowski et al. 2006).

Despite the convergence of genetic evidence, altered brain expression, and biological plausibility for the association of these genes with schizophrenia, it should also be noted that there are limitations to the data, which apply, to varying extents, to all of them. These include nonreplications and reported "replications" in which the associated variants or haplotypes, and populations, differ from the original report (but see discussion regarding *NRG1* in Gardner et al. 2006). Furthermore, in no case has one or more causal polymorphisms been clearly identified, although advances in understanding of mechanisms by which the disease variants may exert their effects are ongoing. For example, emerging data suggest that noncoding liability alleles may associate with altered brain mRNA expression levels of *NRG1* (Law et al. 2006), *DTNBP1* (Bray et al. 2005; Weickert et al. 2004), and *DISC1* binding partners (Lipska et al. 2006). Other proposed psychosis liability genes for which there is less current evidence or consistent replication include D-amino acid oxidase (*DAO*); protein phosphatase 3, catalytic subunit, gamma isoform (*PPP3CC*); alpha-7 nicotinic receptor (*CHRNA7*); metabotropic glutamate receptor 3 (*GRM3*); and proline dehydrogenase (*PRODH*) (Harrison and Weinberger 2005; O'Donovan et al. 2003; Shirts and Nimgaonkar 2004).

Bipolar Disorder

Bipolar disorder has long been recognized as having a substantial genetic component (Farmer et al. 2007). Rates of bipolar disorder are elevated in siblings of individuals with the disorder, markedly so in monozygotic twins (McGuffin et al. 2003), with an estimated heritability of well over 80% (Craddock et al. 2005). Despite this recognition, as well as the identification of multiple genomic regions with some evidence of linkage to bipolar disorder, progress has been slow (Kato 2007). As a result, there has been a focus on combining family data sets into larger samples in an effort to resolve discrepancies and improve the level of confidence in regions identified as linked to the illness (Farmer et al. 2007). Several studies using this approach have now been reported, with consistent evidence of a linkage region on chromosome 6q. Other implicated regions include chromosomes 4q and 8q (Lambert et al. 2005; McQueen et al. 2005; Schumacher et al. 2005). However, the causal variants in these loci have not been identified.

Perhaps more advances have recently resulted from heightened attention to the genetic overlap between bipolar disorder and schizophrenia. There is evidence from family and twin studies of aggregation of both disorders within the same families, and of families in which a spectrum of schizophrenia, schizoaffective disorder, and bipolar disorder are all present (Craddock et al. 2005). As a result, investigators have examined whether any of the genetic variants recently associated with schizophrenia also show evidence of association with bipolar disorder.

The best evidence for an association of putative schizophrenia risk genes with bipolar disorder exists for *DAOA* (Chen et al. 2004; Hattori et al. 2003). As described previously, the translocation in *DISC1* was first identified in a pedigree in which it cosegregated with both schizophrenia and bipolar disorder (St. Clair et al. 1990). Though less compelling, there is also some evidence for associations of *NRG1* and *COMT* with bipolar disorder (Craddock et al. 2005; Farmer et al. 2007).

Major Depression

Major depression appears to be heritable but with an estimated heritability of nearly 40%, substantially lower than the heritabilities reported for schizophrenia and bipolar disorder (Sullivan et al. 2000). Heritability may be greater when major depression occurs prior to age 30 and is recurrent (Camp and Cannon-Albright 2005). Not surprisingly, environmental factors play a significant role, and gene×environment interactions may be important (Kendler et al. 1995). Although major depression aggregates within families in which bipolar disorder is present, the converse may not be true (Levinson 2006).

Major depression is highly prevalent in elderly people, although the predominant environmental effects, such as medical comorbidity or bereavement, may differ from those of people at young or middle ages (Alexopoulos 2005; Reynolds and Kupfer 1999). Estimates of the heritability of depressive symptoms or syndromes in elderly people have been modest and appear to be lower than reported for major depression in people of young or middle ages (Jansson et al. 2004; Johnson et al. 2002), perhaps reflecting the greater diversity of risk factors. The lower overall heritability of major depression in elderly people may reflect an interaction between a more stable, and heritable, liability and occasion-specific occurrences such as psychosocial or biological stressors (McGue and Christensen 2003).

Despite these obstacles, some progress is being made in the genetics of major depression. The first large-scale family studies of linkage of major depression to chromosomal loci have been published, with some consistency of findings across studies (Camp and Cannon-Albright 2005). These studies have focused predominantly on early-onset, recurrent major depression; therefore, the ultimate relevance of these findings to depression with initial onset in late life may be reduced.

A moderate number of studies have evaluated whether the risk for major depression and/or depressive symptoms is associated with candidate genes, largely drawn from monoamine systems. There is some suggestion from these studies that short alleles of a 44 base pair insertion/deletion polymorphism in the serotonin transporter (*SLC6A4*), which may result in reduced transporter expression and function (Lesch et al. 1996), may associate with aspects of depressive symptomatology, if not with major depression per se (Levinson 2006).

A report that rightly garnered a great deal of interest found that *SLC6A4* short alleles moderated environmental effects on depression, increasing the risk for depression induced by stressful life events or childhood maltreatment (Caspi et al. 2003). The possibility that genetic variation in *SLC6A4* might influence stress reactivity has been supported by several smaller studies using differing approaches (see review in Levinson 2006). Subsequently, two large-scale studies have not replicated the interaction between short alleles and environmental stressors on depression risk (Gillespie et al. 2005; Surtees et al. 2006). Although these studies relied on analysis of the insertion/deletion polymorphism, there is evidence for a substantial amount of further genetic variation in *SLC6A4* that may well result in functional effects (Hahn and Blakely 2007). Clarifying the relationship of genetic variation in *SLC6A4* to depression risk will likely take further efforts to more comprehensively evaluate genetic variation within *SLC6A4* within the populations of interest.

Other candidate genes that have drawn a great deal of attention in major depression, as well as late-life depression, are brain-derived neurotrophic factor (*BDNF*), tryptophan hydroxylase 2 (*TPH2*), and *APOE*. As is often the case, promising initial reports of an association of major depression with genetic variation in *BDNF* have been followed by much more mixed results (Levinson 2006). *TPH2* has had a similar fate. It was identified by Walther et al. (2003) as the brain-specific isoform of the rate-limiting enzyme in serotonin synthesis. A loss-of-function mutation in *TPH2* was then reported to be present in 9 of 87 subjects with major depression and in none of 219 healthy controls (Zhang et al. 2005). This report generated a great deal of excitement but ultimately was not replicated in several large series of subjects with major depression (see, e.g., Zhou et al. 2005).

As described in the section "Late-Onset Alzheimer's Disease" earlier in this chapter, carrying one or more ε4 alleles of *APOE* (*APOE*E4*) is strongly associated with the risk of developing AD. There is also a substantial body of literature implicating major depression during late life as a risk factor for subsequent development of AD (Sweet et al. 2004). As a result, a number of investigations have evaluated whether *APOE*E4* was also a risk factor for late-life depression. Overall, there is little evidence for an association of *APOE*E4* with late-life depression, or with the risk for cognitive impairment during an episode of late-life depression (Butters et al. 2003).

Summary

We have now entered the postgenome era of medical genetics. Although the impact of this transition on practicing geriatric psychiatrists has been limited so far, it will soon be felt. The pace at which genetic variants have been found in neurodegenerative illness has noticeably quickened and is affecting treatment development. With the genomic approaches now available, untangling the genetic bases of some of the complex diseases in geriatric psychiatry should soon follow.

Key Points

- The completion of sequencing of the human genome has led to several profound insights regarding genetic mechanisms, with implications for mental disorders of late life.
- Discovery of rare disease-causing mutations has been instrumental in furthering understanding of the neurobiology of several mental disorders of late life, including Alzheimer's disease, frontotemporal dementia, and Parkinson's disease, and the pace of their discovery is accelerating.
- Most common mental disorders of late life, including the most common presentations of the dementias, are genetically complex diseases, resulting from the interaction of multiple genes and environmental factors; this complexity limits the definitive identification of contributing genes and reduces the ability to use genetic information for prediction of clinical outcome. Nevertheless, important strides have been made, particularly in the genetics of schizophrenia.

References

Alexopoulos GS: Depression in the elderly. Lancet 365:1961–1970, 2005

Alzheimer Disease and Frontotemporal Dementia Mutation Database. 2008. Available at http://www.molgen.ua.ac.be/ADMutations. Accessed February 13, 2008.

Arnold SE, Talbot K, Hahn CG: Neurodevelopment, neuroplasticity, and new genes for schizophrenia. Prog Brain Res 147:319–345, 2004

Axelrod J, Tomchick R: Enzymatic O-methylation of epinephrine and other catechols. J Biol Chem 233:702–705, 1958

Bacanu SA, Devlin B, Chowdari KV, et al: Linkage analysis of Alzheimer disease with psychosis. Neurology 59:118–120, 2002

Bacanu SA, Devlin B, Chowdari KV, et al: Heritability of psychosis in Alzheimer disease. Am J Geriatr Psychiatry 13:624–627, 2005

Bajestan SN, Sabouri AH, Nakamura M, et al: Association of AKT1 haplotype with the risk of schizophrenia in Iranian population. Am J Med Genet B Neuropsychiatr Genet 141:383–386, 2006

Bertram L, McQueen MB, Mullin K, et al: Systematic meta-analysis of Alzheimer disease genetic association studies: the AlzGene database. Nat Genet 39:17–23, 2007

Bird T, Knopman D, VanSwieten J, et al: Epidemiology and genetics of frontotemporal dementia/Pick's disease. Ann Neurol 54 (suppl 5):S29–S31, 2003

Bonifati V, Rizzu P, van Baren MJ, et al: Mutations in the DJ-1 gene associated with autosomal recessive early onset parkinsonism. Science 299:256–259, 2003

Borroni B, Agosti C, Archetti S, et al: Catechol-O-methyltransferase gene polymorphism is associated with risk of psychosis in Alzheimer disease. Neurosci Lett 370:127–129, 2004

Bray NJ, Buckland PR, Williams NM, et al: A haplotype implicated in schizophrenia susceptibility is associated with reduced COMT expression in human brain. Am J Hum Genet 73:152–161, 2003

Bray NJ, Preece A, Williams NM, et al: Haplotypes at the dystrobrevin binding protein 1 (DTNBP1) gene locus mediate risk for schizophrenia through reduced DTNBP1 expression. Hum Mol Genet 14:1947–1954, 2005

Breitner JC: Clinical genetics and genetic counseling in Alzheimer disease. Ann Intern Med 115:601–606, 1991

Breitner JC, Murphy EA, Silverman JM, et al: Age-dependent expression of familial risk in Alzheimer's disease. Am J Epidemiol 128:536–548, 1988

Brousseau T, Legrain S, Berr C, et al: Confirmation of the epsilon 4 allele of the apolipoprotein E gene as a risk factor for late-onset Alzheimer's disease. Neurology 44:342–344, 1994

Butters MA, Sweet RA, Mulsant BH, et al: APOE is associated with age-of-onset, but not cognitive functioning, in late-life depression. Int J Geriatr Psychiatry 18:1075–1081, 2003

Callicot J, Straub RE, Pezawas L, et al: Variation in DISC1 affects hippocampal structure and function and increases risk for schizophrenia. Neuropharmacology 29:S55–S56, 2004

Camp NJ, Cannon-Albright LA: Dissecting the genetic etiology of major depressive disorder using linkage analysis. Trends Mol Med 11:138–144, 2005

Campion D, Flaman JM, Brice A, et al: Mutations of the presenilin I gene in families with early onset Alzheimer's disease. Hum Mol Genet 4:2373–2377, 1995

Campion D, Dumanchin C, Hannequin D, et al: Early onset autosomal dominant Alzheimer disease: prevalence, genetic heterogeneity, and mutation spectrum. Am J Hum Genet 65:664–670, 1999

Carlson C, Sirotkin H, Pandita R, et al: Molecular definition of 22q11 deletions in 151 velo-cardio-facial syndrome patients. Am J Hum Genet 61:620–629, 1997

Carninci P, Kasukawa T, Katayama S, et al: The transcriptional landscape of the mammalian genome. Science 309:1559–1563, 2005

Caspi A, Sugden K, Moffitt TE, et al: Influence of life stress on depression: moderation by a polymorphism in the 5-HTT gene. Science 301:386–389, 2003

Cervilla J, Prince M, Joels S, et al: Premorbid cognitive testing predicts the onset of dementia and Alzheimer's disease better than and independently of APOE genotype. J Neurol Neurosurg Psychiatry 75:1100–1106, 2004

Chanock SJ, Manolio T, Boehnke M, et al: Replicating genotype-phenotype associations. Nature 447:655–660, 2007

Chen X, Wang X, O'Neill AF, et al: Variants in the catechol-O-methyltransferase (COMT) gene are associated with schizophrenia in Irish high-density families. Mol Psychiatry 9:962–967, 2004

Chen YS, Akula N, Detera-Wadleigh SD, et al: Findings in an independent sample support an association between bipolar affective disorder and the G72/G30 locus on chromosome 13q33. Mol Psychiatry 9:87–92, 2004

Cheng Z, Ventura M, She X, et al: A genome-wide comparison of recent chimpanzee and human segmental duplications. Nature 437:88–93, 2005

Chow TW, Miller BL, Hayashi VN, et al: Inheritance of frontotemporal dementia. Arch Neurol 56:817–822, 1999

Chowdari KV, Mirnics K, Semwal P, et al: Association and linkage analyses of RGS4 polymorphisms in schizophrenia. Hum Mol Genet 11:1373–1380, 2002

Chumakov I, Blumenfeld M, Guerassimenko O, et al: Genetic and physiological data implicating the new human gene G72 and the gene for D-amino acid oxidase in schizophrenia. Proc Natl Acad Sci U S A 99:13675–13680, 2002

Coon KD, Dunckley TL, Stephan DA: A generic research paradigm for identification and validation of early molecular diagnostics and new therapeutics in common disorders. Mol Diagn Ther 11:1–14, 2007

Corder EH, Saunders AM, Strittmatter WJ, et al: Gene dose of apolipoprotein E type 4 allele and the risk of Alzheimer's disease in late onset families. Science 261:921–923, 1993

Couzin J, Kaiser J: Genome-wide association: closing the net on common disease genes. Science 316:820–822, 2007

Craddock N, O'Donovan MC, Owen MJ: The genetics of schizophrenia and bipolar disorder: dissecting psychosis. J Med Genet 42:193–204, 2005

Craddock N, O'Donovan MC, Owen MJ: Genes for schizophrenia and bipolar disorder? Implications for psychiatric nosology. Schizophr Bull 32:9–16, 2006

Craig D, Hart DJ, McIlroy SP, et al: Association analysis of apolipoprotein E genotype and risk of depressive symptoms in Alzheimer's disease. Dement Geriatr Cogn Disord 19:154–157, 2005

Cruts M, van Duijn CM, Backhovens H, et al: Estimation of the genetic contribution of presenilin-1 and -2 mutations in a population-based study of presenile Alzheimer disease. Hum Mol Genet 7:43–51, 1998

de Rijk MC, Breteler MM, den Breeijen JH, et al: Dietary antioxidants and Parkinson disease: the Rotterdam Study. Arch Neurol 54:762–765, 1997

Detera-Wadleigh SD, McMahon FJ: G72/G30 in schizophrenia and bipolar disorder: review and meta-analysis. Biol Psychiatry 60:106–114, 2006

Devanand DP, Jacobs DM, Tang MX, et al: The course of psychopathologic features in mild to moderate Alzheimer disease. Arch Gen Psychiatry 54:257–263, 1997

Devanand DP, Pelton GH, Zamora D, et al: Predictive utility of apolipoprotein E genotype for Alzheimer disease in outpatients with mild cognitive impairment. Arch Neurol 62:975–980, 2005

Duan R, Jin P: Identification of messenger RNAs and microRNAs associated with fragile X mental retardation protein. Methods Mol Biol 342:267–276, 2006

Eder J, Hommel U, Cumin F, et al: Aspartic proteases in drug discovery. Curr Pharm Des 13:271–285, 2007

Egan MF, Goldberg TE, Gscheidle T, et al: Relative risk for cognitive impairments in siblings of patients with schizophrenia. Biol Psychiatry 50:98–107, 2001a

Egan MF, Goldberg TE, Kolachana BS, et al: Effect of COMT Val108/158 Met genotype on frontal lobe function and risk for schizophrenia. Proc Natl Acad Sci U S A 98:6917–6922, 2001b

Eichner JE, Dunn ST, Perveen G, et al: Apolipoprotein E polymorphism and cardiovascular disease: a HuGE review. Am J Epidemiol 155:487–495, 2002

Emamian ES, Hall D, Birnbaum MJ, et al: Convergent evidence for impaired AKT1-GSK3beta signaling in schizophrenia. Nat Genet 36:131–137, 2004

Ertekin-Taner N: Genetics of Alzheimer's disease: a centennial review. Neurol Clin 25:611–667, 2007

Farmer A, Elkin A, McGuffin P: The genetics of bipolar affective disorder. Curr Opin Psychiatry 20:8–12, 2007

Farrer LA, Cupples LA, Haines JL, et al: Effects of age, sex, and ethnicity on the association between apolipoprotein E genotype and Alzheimer disease: a meta-analysis. APOE and Alzheimer Disease Meta Analysis Consortium. JAMA 278:1349–1356, 1997

Fuchs J, Nilsson C, Kachergus J, et al: Phenotypic variation in a large Swedish pedigree due to SNCA duplication and triplication. Neurology 68:916–922, 2007

Gardner M, Gonzalez-Neira A, Lao O, et al: Extreme population differences across neuregulin 1 gene, with implications for association studies. Mol Psychiatry 11:66–75, 2006

Gasser T: Genetics of Parkinson's disease. J Neurol 248:833–840, 2001

Gasser T: Genetics of Parkinson's disease. Curr Opin Neurol 18:363–369, 2005

Gillespie NA, Whitfield JB, Williams B, et al: The relationship between stressful life events, the serotonin transporter (5-HTTLPR) genotype and major depression. Psychol Med 35:101–111, 2005

Glatt SJ, Faraone SV, Tsuang MT: Association between a functional catechol O-methyltransferase gene polymorphism and schizophrenia: meta-analysis of case-control and family-based studies. Am J Psychiatry 160:469–476, 2003

Glenner GG, Wong CW: Alzheimer's disease and Down's syndrome: sharing of a unique cerebrovascular amyloid fibril protein. Biochem Biophys Res Commun 122:1131–1135, 1984

Go RC, Perry RT, Wiener H, et al: Neuregulin-1 polymorphism in late onset Alzheimer's disease families with psychoses. Am J Med Genet B Neuropsychiatr Genet 139B:28–32, 2005

Goate A, Chartier-Harlin MC, Mullan M, et al: Segregation of a missense mutation in the amyloid precursor protein gene with familial Alzheimer's disease. Nature 349:704–706, 1991

Gottesman II, Wolfgram DL: Schizophrenia Genesis: The Origins of Madness. New York, WH Freeman, 1991

Grossman MH, Emanuel BS, Budarf ML: Chromosomal mapping of the human catechol-O-methyltransferase gene to 22q11.1–q11.2. Genomics 12:822–825, 1992

Guo T, Hobbs DW: Development of BACE1 inhibitors for Alzheimer's disease. Curr Med Chem 13:1811–1829, 2006

Guttmacher AE, Collins FS: Genomic medicine: a primer. N Engl J Med 347:1512–1520, 2002

Gwinn-Hardy K: Genetics of parkinsonism. Mov Disord 17:645–656, 2002

Hahn MK, Blakely RD: The functional impact of SLC6 transporter genetic variation. Annu Rev Pharmacol Toxicol 47:401–441, 2007

Han J, Lee Y, Yeom KH, et al: The Drosha-DGCR8 complex in primary microRNA processing. Genes Dev 18:3016–3027, 2004

Handoko HY, Nyholt DR, Hayward NK, et al: Separate and interacting effects within the catechol-O-methyltransferase (COMT) are associated with schizophrenia. Mol Psychiatry 10:589–597, 2005

Hardy J: A hundred years of Alzheimer's disease research. Neuron 52:3–13, 2006

Hardy J: Presenilin mutations directory. January 12, 2007. Available at http://www.alzforum.org/res/com/mut/pre/default.asp. Accessed February 13, 2008.

Hardy J, Cai H, Cookson MR, et al: Genetics of Parkinson's disease and parkinsonism. Ann Neurol 60:389–398, 2006

Hariri AR, Holmes A: Genetics of emotional regulation: the role of the serotonin transporter in neural function. Trends Cogn Sci 10:182–191, 2006

Harrison PJ, Weinberger DR: Schizophrenia genes, gene expression, and neuropathology: on the matter of their convergence. Mol Psychiatry 10:40–68, 2005

Hattori E, Liu C, Badner JA, et al: Polymorphisms at the G72/G30 gene locus, on 13q33, are associated with bipolar disorder in two independent pedigree series. Am J Hum Genet 72:1131–1140, 2003

Haugarvoll K, Wszolek ZK, Hutton M: The genetics of frontotemporal dementia. Neurol Clin 25:697–715, 2007

Henderson AS, Easteal S, Jorm AF, et al: Apolipoprotein E allele epsilon 4, dementia, and cognitive decline in a population sample. Lancet 346:1387–1390, 1995

Hennah W, Varilo T, Kestila M, et al: Haplotype transmission analysis provides evidence of association for DISC1 to schizophrenia and suggests sex-dependent effects. Hum Mol Genet 12:3151–3159, 2003

Hodgkinson CA, Goldman D, Jaeger J, et al: Disrupted in schizophrenia 1 (DISC1): association with schizophrenia, schizoaffective disorder, and bipolar disorder. Am J Hum Genet 75:862–872, 2004

Hollingworth P, Hamshere ML, Holmans PA, et al: Increased familial risk and genomewide significant linkage for Alzheimer's disease with psychosis. Am J Med Genet B Neuropsychiatr Genet 144:841–848, 2007

Hutton M, Busfield F, Wragg M, et al: Complete analysis of the presenilin 1 gene in early onset Alzheimer's disease. Neuroreport 7:801–805, 1996

Ikeda M, Iwata N, Suzuki T, et al: Association of AKT1 with schizophrenia confirmed in a Japanese population. Biol Psychiatry 56:698–700, 2004

Inoue K, Lupski JR: Molecular mechanisms for genomic disorders. Annu Rev Genomics Hum Genet 3:199–242, 2002

International HapMap Consortium: A second generation human haplotype map of over 3.1 million SNPs. Nature 449:851–861, 2007

International Human Genome Sequencing Consortium: Finishing the euchromatic sequence of the human genome. Nature 431:931–945, 2004

Jansson M, Gatz M, Berg S, et al: Gender differences in heritability of depressive symptoms in the elderly. Psychol Med 34:471–479, 2004

Johnson W, McGue M, Gaist D, et al: Frequency and heritability of depression symptomatology in the second half of life: evidence from Danish twins over 45. Psychol Med 32:1175–1185, 2002

Kato T: Molecular genetics of bipolar disorder and depression. Psychiatry Clin Neurosci 61:3–19, 2007

Kaufer DI, Cummings JL, Christine D, et al: Assessing the impact of neuropsychiatric symptoms in Alzheimer's disease: the Neuropsychiatric Inventory Caregiver Distress Scale. J Am Geriatr Soc 46:210–215, 1998

Kendler KS, Kessler RC, Walters EE, et al: Stressful life events, genetic liability, and onset of an episode of major depression in women. Am J Psychiatry 152:833–842, 1995

Kitada T, Asakawa S, Hattori N, et al: Mutations in the parkin gene cause autosomal recessive juvenile parkinsonism. Nature 392:605–608, 1998

Klages JD, Fisk JD, Rockwood K: APOE genotype, memory test performance, and the risk of Alzheimer's disease in the Canadian Study of Health and Aging. Dement Geriatr Cogn Disord 15:1–5, 2003

Koboldt DC, Miller RD: Identification of functional SNPs in noncoding regions of the human genome. 2007. Available at http://snp.wustl.edu/snp-and-fp-tdi-resources/abstracts/Koboldt-HUGO-Functional-SNPs.pdf. Accessed February 12, 2008.

Lachman HM, Morrow B, Shprintzen R, et al: Association of codon 108/158 catechol-O-methyltransferase gene polymorphism with the psychiatric manifestations of velo-cardio-facial syndrome. Am J Med Genet 67:468–472, 1996a

Lachman HM, Papolos DF, Saito T, et al: Human catechol-O-methyltransferase pharmacogenetics: description of a functional polymorphism and its potential application to neuropsychiatric disorders. Pharmacogenetics 6:243–250, 1996b

Lambert D, Middle F, Hamshere ML, et al: Stage 2 of the Wellcome Trust UK-Irish bipolar affective disorder sibling-pair genome screen: evidence for linkage on chromosomes 6q16-q21, 4q12-q21, 9p21, 10p14-p12 and 18q22. Molec Psychiatry 10:831–841, 2005

Law AJ, Lipska BK, Weickert CS, et al: Neuregulin 1 transcripts are differentially expressed in schizophrenia and regulated by 5′ SNPs associated with the disease. Proc Natl Acad Sci U S A 103:6747–6752, 2006

Leroy E, Boyer R, Auburger G, et al: The ubiquitin pathway in Parkinson's disease. Nature 395:451–452, 1998

Lesch KP, Bengel D, Heils A, et al: Association of anxiety-related traits with a polymorphism in the serotonin transporter gene regulatory region. Science 274:1527–1531, 1996

Levinson DF: The genetics of depression: a review. Biol Psychiatry 60:84–92, 2006

Levy S, Sutton G, Ng PC, et al: The diploid genome sequence of an individual human. PLoS Biol 5:e254, 2007

Levy-Lahad E, Wasco W, Poorkaj P, et al: Candidate gene for the chromosome 1 familial Alzheimer's disease locus. Science 269:973–977, 1995a

Levy-Lahad E, Wijsman EM, Nemens E, et al: A familial Alzheimer's disease locus on chromosome 1. Science 269:970–973, 1995b

Liddell MB, Lovestone S, Owen MJ: Genetic risk of Alzheimer's disease: advising relatives. Br J Psychiatry 178:7–11, 2001

Lipska BK, Peters T, Hyde TM, et al: Expression of DISC1 binding partners is reduced in schizophrenia and associated with DISC1 SNPs. Hum Mol Genet 15:1245–1258, 2006

Liu YL, Fann CS, Liu CM, et al: Absence of significant associations between four AKT1 SNP markers and schizophrenia in the Taiwanese population. Psychiatr Genet 16:39–41, 2006

Lopez OL, Kamboh MI, Becker JT, et al: The apolipoprotein E ε4 allele is not associated with psychiatric symptoms or extrapyramidal signs in probable Alzheimer's disease. Neurology 49:794–797, 1997

Lupski JR: Structural variation in the human genome. N Engl J Med 356:1169–1171, 2007

Mayeux R, Stern Y, Ottman R, et al: The apolipoprotein epsilon 4 allele in patients with Alzheimer's disease. Ann Neurol 34:752–754, 1993

McGue M, Christensen K: The heritability of depression symptoms in elderly Danish twins: occasion-specific versus general effects. Behav Genet 33:83–93, 2003

McGuffin P, Rijsdijk F, Andrew M, et al: The heritability of bipolar affective disorder and the genetic relationship to unipolar depression. Arch Gen Psychiatry 60:497–502, 2003

McQueen MB, Devlin B, Faraone SV, et al: Combined analysis from eleven linkage studies of bipolar disorder provides strong evidence of susceptibility loci on chromosomes 6q and 8q. Am J Hum Genet 77:582–595, 2005

Mirnics K, Middleton FA, Stanwood GD, et al: Disease-specific changes in regulator of G-protein signaling 4 (RGS4) expression in schizophrenia. Mol Psychiatry 6:293–301, 2001

Murphy KC, Jones LA, Owen MJ: High rates of schizophrenia in adults with velo-cardio-facial syndrome. Arch Gen Psychiatry 56:940–945, 1999

National Center for Biotechnology Information: NCBI Entrez Genome Project. February 12, 2008. Available at http://www.ncbi.nlm.nih.gov/genomes/static/gpstat.html. Accessed February 14, 2008.

Neary D, Snowden JS, Gustafson L, et al: Frontotemporal lobar degeneration: a consensus on clinical diagnostic criteria. Neurology 51:1546–1554, 1998

Neary D, Snowden J, Mann D: Frontotemporal dementia. Lancet Neurol 4:771–780, 2005

Neumann M, Sampathu DM, Kwong LK, et al: Ubiquitinated TDP-43 in frontotemporal lobar degeneration and amyotrophic lateral sclerosis. Science 314:130–133, 2006

O'Donovan MC, Williams NM, Owen MJ: Recent advances in the genetics of schizophrenia. Hum Mol Genet 12 (spec no 2): R125–R133, 2003

Ohtsuki T, Inada T, Arinami T: Failure to confirm association between AKT1 haplotype and schizophrenia in a Japanese case-control population. Mol Psychiatry 9:981–983, 2004

Owen MJ, Craddock N, O'Donovan MC: Schizophrenia: genes at last? Trends Genet 21:518–525, 2005

Paisan-Ruiz C, Jain S, Evans EW, et al: Cloning of the gene containing mutations that cause PARK8-linked Parkinson's disease. Neuron 44:595–600, 2004

Parkes M, Barrett JC, Prescott NJ, et al: Sequence variants in the autophagy gene IRGM and multiple other replicating loci contribute to Crohn's disease susceptibility. Nat Genet 39:830–832, 2007

Pericak-Vance MA, Haines JL: Genetic susceptibility to Alzheimer disease. Trends Genet 11:504–508, 1995

Polymeropoulos MH, Lavedan C, Leroy E, et al: Mutation in the alpha-synuclein gene identified in families with Parkinson's disease. Science 276:2045–2047, 1997

Prasher VP, Farrer MJ, Kessling AM, et al: Molecular mapping of Alzheimer-type dementia in Down's syndrome. Ann Neurol 43:380–383, 1998

Rademakers R, Cruts M, Van Broeckhoven C: The role of tau (MAPT) in frontotemporal dementia and related tauopathies. Hum Mutat 24:277–295, 2004

Rebeck GW, Reiter JS, Strickland DK, et al: Apolipoprotein E in sporadic Alzheimer's disease: allelic variation and receptor interactions. Neuron 11:575–580, 1993

Redon R, Ishikawa S, Fitch KR, et al: Global variation in copy number in the human genome. Nature 444:444–454, 2006

Reynolds CF III, Kupfer DJ: Depression and aging: a look to the future. Psychiatr Serv 50:1167–1172, 1999

Rossor MN, Fox NC, Beck J, et al: Incomplete penetrance of familial Alzheimer's disease in a pedigree with a novel presenilin-1 gene mutation. Lancet 347:1560, 1996

Rovelet-Lecrux A, Hannequin D, Raux G, et al: APP locus duplication causes autosomal dominant early onset Alzheimer disease with cerebral amyloid angiopathy. Nat Genet 38:24–26, 2006

Samonte RV, Eichler EE: Segmental duplications and the evolution of the primate genome. Nat Rev Genet 3:65–72, 2002

Saunders AM, Strittmatter WJ, Schmechel D, et al: Association of apolipoprotein E allele ε4 with late-onset familial and sporadic Alzheimer's disease. Neurology 43:1467–1472, 1993

Schellenberg GD, Bird TD, Wijsman EM, et al: Genetic linkage evidence for a familial Alzheimer's disease locus on chromosome 14. Science 258:668–671, 1992

Schmechel DE, Saunders AM, Strittmatter WJ, et al: Increased amyloid beta-peptide deposition in cerebral cortex as a consequence of apolipoprotein E genotype in late-onset Alzheimer disease. Proc Natl Acad Sci U S A 90:9649–9653, 1993

Schumacher J, Kaneva R, Jamra RA, et al: Genomewide scan and fine-mapping linkage studies in four European samples with bipolar affective disorder suggest a new susceptibility locus on chromosome 1p35–p36 and provides further evidence of loci on chromosome 4q31 and 6q24. Am J Hum Genet 77:1102–1111, 2005

Schwab SG, Hoefgen B, Hanses C, et al: Further evidence for association of variants in the AKT1 gene with schizophrenia in a sample of European sib-pair families. Biol Psychiatry 58:446–450, 2005

Sebat J, Lakshmi B, Malhotra D, et al: Strong association of de novo copy number mutations with autism. Science 316:445–449, 2007

Selkoe DJ: Alzheimer disease: mechanistic understanding predicts novel therapies. Ann Intern Med 140:627–638, 2004

Seshadri S, Wolf PA, Beiser A, et al: Lifetime risk of dementia and Alzheimer's disease: the impact of mortality on risk estimates in the Framingham study. Neurology 49:1498–1504, 1997

Sherrington R, Rogaev EI, Liang Y, et al: Cloning of a gene bearing missense mutations in early-onset familial Alzheimer's disease. Nature 375:754–760, 1995

Shifman S, Bronstein MSM, Pisante-Shalom A, et al: A highly significant association between a COMT haplotype and schizophrenia. Am J Hum Genet 71:1296–1302, 2002

Shirts BH, Nimgaonkar V: The genes for schizophrenia: finally a breakthrough? Curr Psychiatry Rep 6:303–312, 2004

Skibinski G, Parkinson NJ, Brown JM, et al: Mutations in the endosomal ESCRTIII-complex subunit CHMP2B in frontotemporal dementia. Nat Genet 37:806–808, 2005

Sleegers K, Brouwers N, Gijselinck I, et al: APP duplication is sufficient to cause early onset Alzheimer's dementia with cerebral amyloid angiopathy. Brain 129:2977–2983, 2006

St. Clair D, Blackwood D, Muir W, et al: Association within a family of a balanced autosomal translocation with major mental illness. Lancet 336:13–16, 1990

Stedman's Medical Dictionary, 28th Edition. Baltimore, MD, Lippincott Williams & Wilkins, 2005

Stefansson H, Sigurdsson E, Steinthorsdottir V, et al: Neuregulin 1 and susceptibility to schizophrenia. Am J Hum Genet 71:877–892, 2002

Stefansson H, Sarginson J, Kong A, et al: Association of neuregulin 1 with schizophrenia confirmed in a Scottish population. Am J Hum Genet 72:83–87, 2003

St. George-Hyslop P, Haines J, Rogaev E, et al: Genetic evidence for a novel familial Alzheimer's disease locus on chromosome 14. Nat Genet 2:330–334, 1992

Storz G: An expanding universe of noncoding RNAs. Science 296:1260–1263, 2002

Storz G, Altuvia S, Wassarman KM: An abundance of RNA regulators. Annu Rev Biochem 74:199–217, 2005

Straub RE, Jiang YX, MacLean CJ, et al: Genetic variation in the 6p22.3 gene DTNBP1, the human ortholog of the mouse dysbindin gene, is associated with schizophrenia. Am J Hum Genet 71:337–348, 2002

Sullivan PF, Neale MC, Kendler KS: Genetic epidemiology of major depression: review and meta-analysis. Am J Psychiatry 157:1552–1562, 2000

Surtees PG, Wainwright NW, Willis-Owen SA, et al: Social adversity, the serotonin transporter (5-HTTLPR) polymorphism and major depressive disorder. Biol Psychiatry 59:224–229, 2006

Swearer JM, Drachman DA, O'Donnell BF, et al: Troublesome and disruptive behaviors in dementia: relationships to diagnosis and disease severity. J Am Geriatr Soc 36:784–790, 1988

Sweet RA, Kamboh MI, Wisniewski SR, et al: Apolipoprotein E and alpha-1-antichymotrypsin genotypes do not predict time to psychosis in Alzheimer's disease. J Geriatr Psychiatry Neurol 15:24–30, 2002a

Sweet RA, Nimgaonkar VL, Devlin B, et al: Increased familial risk of the psychotic phenotype of Alzheimer disease. Neurology 58:907–911, 2002b

Sweet RA, Hamilton RL, Butters MA, et al: Neuropathologic correlates of late-onset major depression. Neuropsychopharmacology 29:2242–2250, 2004

Sweet RA, Devlin B, Pollock BG, et al: Catechol-O-methyltransferase haplotypes are associated with psychosis in Alzheimer disease. Mol Psychiatry 10:1026–1036, 2005

Talkowski ME, Seltman H, Bassett AS, et al: Evaluation of a susceptibility gene for schizophrenia: genotype based meta-analysis of RGS4 polymorphisms from thirteen independent samples. Biol Psychiatry 60:152–162, 2006

Theuns J, Marjaux E, Vandenbulcke M, et al: Alzheimer dementia caused by a novel mutation located in the APP C-terminal intracytosolic fragment. Hum Mutat 27:888–896, 2006

Todd JA, Walker NM, Cooper JD, et al: Robust associations of four new chromosome regions from genome-wide analyses of type 1 diabetes. Nat Genet 39:857–864, 2007

Tunstall N, Fraser L, Lovestone S, et al: Familial influence on variation in age of onset and behavioural phenotype in Alzheimer's disease. Br J Psychiatry 176:156–159, 2000

Valente EM, Abou-Sleiman PM, Caputo V, et al: Hereditary early onset Parkinson's disease caused by mutations in PINK1. Science 304:1158–1160, 2004

Vassar R, Bennett BD, Babu-Khan S, et al: Beta-secretase cleavage of Alzheimer's amyloid precursor protein by the transmembrane aspartic protease BACE. Science 286:735–741, 1999

Walther DJ, Peter JU, Bashammakh S, et al: Synthesis of serotonin by a second tryptophan hydroxylase isoform. Science 299:76, 2003

Watts GD, Wymer J, Kovach MJ, et al: Inclusion body myopathy associated with Paget disease of bone and frontotemporal dementia is caused by mutant valosin-containing protein. Nat Genet 36:377–381, 2004

Weickert CS, Straub RE, McClintock BW, et al: Human dysbindin (DTNBP1) gene expression in normal brain and in schizophrenic prefrontal cortex and midbrain. Arch Gen Psychiatry 61:544–555, 2004

Wellcome Trust Case Control Consortium: Genome-wide association study of 14,000 cases of seven common diseases and 3,000 shared controls. Nature 447:661–678, 2007

Wragg RE, Jeste DV: Overview of depression and psychosis in Alzheimer's disease. Am J Psychiatry 146:577–587, 1989

Yang JZ, Si TM, Ruan Y, et al: Association study of neuregulin 1 gene with schizophrenia. Mol Psychiatry 8:706–709, 2003

Zeggini E, Weedon MN, Lindgren CM, et al: Replication of genome-wide association signals in UK samples reveals risk loci for type 2 diabetes. Science 316:1336–1341, 2007

Zhang X, Gainetdinov RR, Beaulieu JM, et al: Loss-of-function mutation in tryptophan hydroxylase-2 identified in unipolar major depression. Neuron 45:11–16, 2005

Zhou Z, Peters EJ, Hamilton SP, et al: Response to Zhang et al. (2005): loss-of-function mutation in tryptophan hydroxylase-2 identified in unipolar major depression. Neuron 48:702–703, 2005

Suggested Readings

Ertekin-Taner N: Genetics of Alzheimer's disease: a centennial review. Neurol Clin 25:611–667, 2007

Guttmacher AE, Collins FS: Genomic medicine: a primer. N Engl J Med 347:1512-1520, 2002

Harrison PJ, Weinberger DR: Schizophrenia genes, gene expression, and neuropathology: on the matter of their convergence. Mol Psychiatry 10:40–68, 2005

Haugarvoll K, Wszolek ZK, Hutton M: The genetics of frontotemporal dementia. Neurol Clin 25:697–715, 2007

Subramanian G, Adams MD, Venter JC, et al: Implications of the human genome for understanding human biology and medicine. JAMA 286:2296–2307, 2001

CHAPTER 7

Psychological Aspects of Normal Aging

Ilene C. Siegler, Ph.D., M.P.H.
Leonard W. Poon, Ph.D.
David J. Madden, Ph.D.
Peggye Dilworth-Anderson, Ph.D.
K. Warner Schaie, Ph.D., Sc.D. (hon.), Dr.Phil.h.c.
Sherry L. Willis, Ph.D.
Peter Martin, Ph.D.

Research on psychological aspects of normal aging is now mature and middle-aged. Major longitudinal studies have collected data for up to 50 years of repeated observations, versions of the *Handbook of the Psychology of Aging* and chapters reviewing the psychology of normal aging have been written for up to 30 years, and the handbook is now in its 6th edition. In this chapter we take a life span approach that is focused on adult development and aging (Siegler 2007a). Thus, it is possible to cite previously published chapters on the normal psychology of aging for geriatric psychiatry (Poon and Siegler 1991; Siegler 1980; Siegler and Poon 1989; Siegler et al. 1996, 2004) and to focus here on the exciting data that recently have become available from mature longitudinal studies and from cross-sectional studies in cognition and neuropsychology, as well as personality and behavioral medicine, that routinely cross disciplinary boundaries. Since the last edition of this textbook, a series of edited volumes have presented reviews in areas of the psychology of normal aging (Birren and Schaie 2006; Carstensen and Hartel 2006; Costa and Siegler 2004) and of health and aging (Aldwin et al. 2007; Markides 2007); these reviews have updated the detailed information presented in the previously published chapters cited above. Attention to how ethnic factors may shape normal psychology of aging are now well recognized (Jackson et al. 2004), and ethnic variations in dementia are being considered (Dilworth-Anderson et al. 2005a, 2005b), as are discussions of cognitive changes with aging (integrated with neuroimaging and neurosciences [Madden and Whiting 2004; Pierce et al. 2004]), including work in motivation,

Dr. Siegler's work on this chapter was supported by grant R01-HL55356 from the National Heart, Lung and Blood Institute (NHLBI), with additional support by the National Institute on Aging (NIA) and by NHLBI grant P01-HL36587 and NIA grant AG19605 to Dr. Redford Williams and the Duke Behavioral Medicine Research Center. In addition, the authors received support for their work on this chapter from the following NIA grants: AG023113 (Dr. Dilworth-Anderson); R37-AG02163 and R01-AG011622 (Dr. Madden); P01-AG17533 (Dr. Martin and Dr. Poon); R01-AG0855 (Dr. Schaie); and R37-AG024102 (Dr. Willis).

The authors thank Dr. Redford Williams and Dr. Beverly Brummett for sharing prepublication copies of their work and Susan Boos for coordinating the chapter.

emotion, and social functioning (Carstensen et al. 2006). Summaries from these recent volumes are presented in this chapter.

These summaries will allow us to use the pages allotted to highlight new findings from ongoing research programs. We start with the Seattle Longitudinal Study (SLS) (Schaie 1996, 2005), which focuses on understanding adult intellectual development at its core with a much broader and more complete picture of multiple cohorts of aging persons ages 18–88. Next we discuss findings from the Georgia Centenarian Studies (Poon et al., in press), a series of studies of the extremely aged with comparison populations in their 60s and 80s, presenting data primarily on cognition, personality, coping, and the role of health status and psychological functioning. As we move to studies of personality, we present 40-year follow-up data from the UNC Alumni Heart Study (Brummett et al. 2006b; Siegler 2007b), which examine whether young adult measures predict midlife status and whether detailed measures during midlife help explain health and survival as members of the baby boom cohort reach their age 60 transition. We then look at personality predictors of midlife hypertension (Siegler 2007b) and review findings from the Maine-Syracuse Studies of the impact of hypertension on cognitive and neuropsychological measures (Dore et al. 2007; Elias et al. 2004). We also review some new findings in the coping literature and consider the major common stressor of caregiving as a way to illustrate important research in ethnic differences and models of stress that relate psychosocial variables to disease outcomes.

One might reasonably ask why such a chapter on normal psychology of aging is still needed in a modern 21st-century view of geriatric psychiatry. Clinicians will always need to know the limits of expectable behavior with age in terms of their own expectations as well as expectations of patients and their families. With the benefit of longitudinal findings and particular attention to what we have learned from centenarian studies, we hope to provide a useful set of benchmarks.

Intellectual and Cognitive Development

Course of Adult Intellectual Development

The development of intellectual competence in childhood and adolescence follows a fairly uniform path, with new stages of competence and differentiation of functioning occurring within a relatively narrow age band. By contrast, there are widely divergent individual trajectories over the life course of adult intelligence. However, over the 50-year course of the SLS (Schaie 1996, 2005), sufficient evidence has been gathered to reach some rather definitive conclusions on a number of core questions:

Does intelligence change uniformly through adulthood, or are there different life course ability patterns? The answer remains quite unambiguous: Uniform patterns of developmental change across the entire ability spectrum are not observed for the tests actually given or for the inferred latent ability constructs. Hence, it is only fair to warn those who would like to assess change in intellectual competence by means of an omnibus IQ-like measure that such an approach will not be very helpful to either thoughtful clinicians or basic researchers. Such global measures have little practical utility in monitoring changes (or differences) in intellectual competence for individuals or groups.

From the extensive longitudinal data on the primary mental abilities used in the SLS, it can be concluded that the abilities of verbal meaning (recognition vocabulary), spatial orientation, and inductive reasoning reach a peak plateau in midlife from the 40s to the early 60s, whereas number and word fluency peak earlier and show very modest decline beginning in the 50s. The steepness of late-life decline is greatest for number and least for the reasoning ability. Verbal meaning declines last but also shows steeper decline than the other abilities from the 70s to the 80s (see Figure 7–1). More limited data on the multiply marked latent construct estimates (obtained only in the fifth through seventh study cycles) suggest that a shift in peak ages of performance has been seen and is continuing, and that we now see these peaks occurring in the 50s for inductive reasoning and spatial orientation and in the 60s for verbal ability and verbal memory. By contrast, perceptual speed peaks in the 20s and numeric ability in the late 30s. Even by the late 80s, declines for verbal ability and inductive reasoning are modest, but they are severe in very old age for perceptual speed and numeric ability, with spatial orientation and verbal memory in between (see Figure 7–2).

At what age is there on average a reliably detectable decrement in ability, and what is its magnitude? For some ability markers, statistically significant but extremely modest average changes have been observed in the 50s. Nevertheless, it should be stressed that individual decline before age 60 is likely to represent a symptom of or a precursor to neuropathological age changes. On the

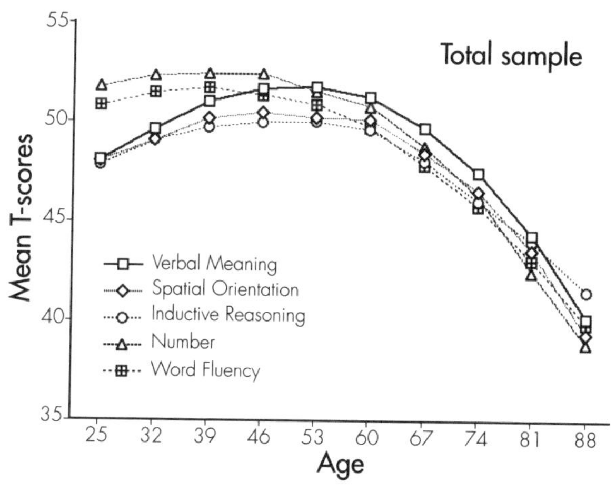

FIGURE 7–1. Longitudinal age changes for the primary mental abilities.

Source. Schaie KW: *Developmental Influences on Adult Intelligence: The Seattle Longitudinal Study.* New York, Oxford University Press, 2005, p. 116. Reprinted with permission.

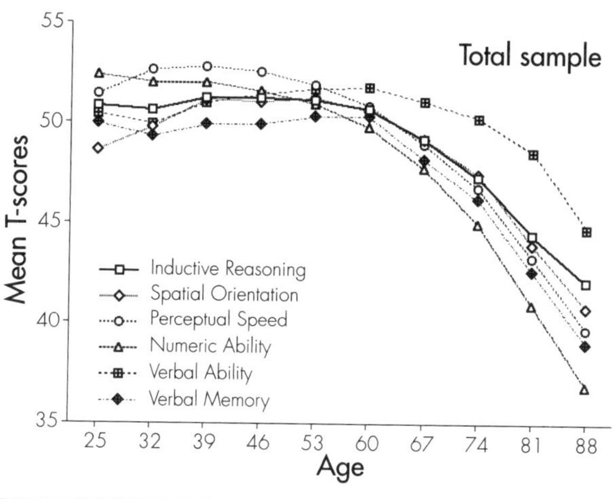

FIGURE 7–2. Longitudinal age changes for the latent ability constructs.

Source. Schaie KW: *Developmental Influences on Adult Intelligence: The Seattle Longitudinal Study.* New York, Oxford University Press, 2005, p. 127. Reprinted with permission.

other hand, it is clear that by the mid-70s significant *average* decrement can be observed for all abilities and that by the 80s average decrement is severe except for verbal ability. In the SLS, statistically significant decrement was found for number and word fluency by age 60 and for space and reasoning by age 67, but for verbal meaning only by age 81. At the latent construct level, statistically significant decrement is first observed by age 60 for spatial ability, numeric ability, and perceptual speed; by age 67 for inductive reasoning; and by age 74 for verbal ability and verbal memory.

The SLS data suggest that it is during the period of the late 60s and 70s that many people begin to experience noticeable ability declines. Even so, it is not until the 80s are reached that the average older adult will fall below the middle range of performance for young adults. Hence, it turns out that for decisions relating to the retention of individuals in the workforce, chronological age is not a useful criterion for groups and is certainly not useful for individuals. This conclusion has of course been the rationale for largely abandoning mandatory retirement in the United States.

What are the patterns of generational differences, and what is their magnitude? The facts of individual aging must also be considered within the context of profound changes over time in environmental and social support systems. In the SLS, the impact of these changes on intellectual development has been documented by charting cohort (generational) differences on the intellectual performance measures. These studies have clearly demonstrated that there are substantial generational trends in intellectual performance. The form of these generational trends has been positive for verbal meaning, space, and reasoning, but it is concave for number (with peak performance for the 1924 cohort and decline thereafter) and convex for word fluency (with lowest performance for the 1931 cohort and return to the 1889 baseline thereafter) (see Figure 7–3).

An understanding of cohort differences is important in order to account for the discrepancy between longitudinal (within-group) age changes and the cross-sectional (between-group) age differences. In general, it was found that cross-sectional findings will overestimate within-individual declines whenever there are positive cohort gradients and will underestimate decline in the presence of negative cohort gradients. Curvilinear cohort gradients will lead to temporary dislocations of age-difference patterns and will over- or underestimate age changes, depending on the direction of differences over a particular time period. The slowing of the cohort difference trend suggests that in the next 20 or 30 years concurrently measured age differences will become substantially smaller over that age range where there is little or no within-participant decline. This is fortunate, because there is a need to retain people to higher ages in the labor force because of the demographic reality of the aging of the baby boomers. Stereotypes about age decline will obviously be rein-

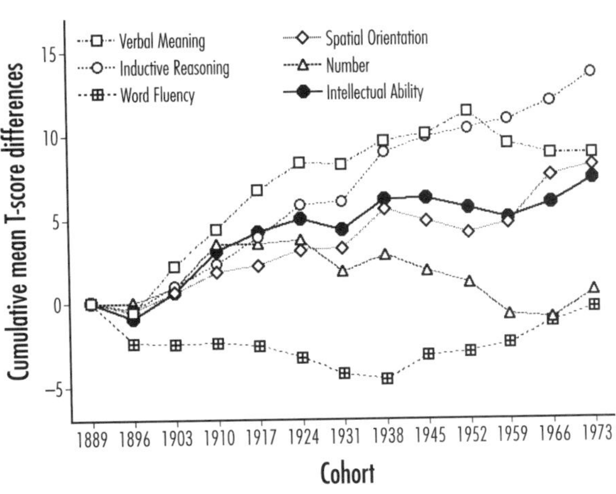

FIGURE 7–3. Cumulative cohort differences for the primary mental abilities.

Source. Schaie KW: *Developmental Influences on Adult Intelligence: The Seattle Longitudinal Study.* New York, Oxford University Press, 2005, p. 137. Reprinted with permission.

forced less in the absence of the dramatic shifts in ability base levels that were observed for cohorts entering adulthood in the first half of the twentieth century.

What accounts for individual differences in age-related change in adulthood? Some individuals, either because of the early onset of neuropathology or the experience of particularly unfavorable environments, begin to decline in their 40s, whereas a favored few maintain a full level of functioning into very advanced age. All individuals do not decline in lockstep. Although linear or quadratic forms of decline may best describe the average aging of large groups, individual decline occurs far more frequently in a stair-step fashion. Individuals may have unfavorable experiences, to which they respond with a modest decline in cognitive functioning but then tend to stabilize for some time, perhaps repeating this pattern repeatedly before their demise. Moreover, the sequence of decline of abilities is not uniform across individuals but may depend in any one individual on the circumstances of use and disuse of particular skills. Thus, in actuarial studies of the SLS core battery, it was observed that virtually all individuals had significantly declined on one ability by age 60, but virtually no one had declined on all five abilities even by age 88.

Genetic endowment, of course, will account for a substantial portion of individual differences (Schaie 2005, Chapter 16; Schaie and Zuo 2001). Nevertheless, there are many other important sources of individual differences in intellectual aging that have been implicated in our studies. To begin with, the onset of intellectual decline seems to be markedly affected by the presence or absence of a variety of chronic diseases; cardiovascular disease, diabetes, cancers, arthritis, and other inflammatory diseases have all been identified as risk factors for the occurrence of cognitive decline, as is a low level of overall health. On the other hand, high levels of cognitive functioning seem to be associated with survival after treated malignancies and with late onset of cardiovascular disease and arthritis. Those persons who function at high cognitive levels are also more likely to seek earlier and more competent medical intervention in the disabling conditions of late life. They also are more likely to comply effectively with preventive and ameliorative regimens that tend to stabilize their physiological infrastructure. Perhaps even more importantly, they are less likely to engage in high-risk lifestyles, and they will respond more readily to professional advice that maximizes their chances for survival and reduction of morbidity. On the other hand, there does not seem to be a high relation between cognitive competence and systematic adoption of effective health behaviors. However, the more able individuals tend to engage in more effective medication use. Findings from the UNC Alumni Heart Study suggest that some personality factors may also be at work, as discussed later in this chapter.

Can age-related ability change be modified through behavioral interventions? Since the 1970s, a number of cognitive training studies have examined the question of the modifiability of age-related decline in independent-living elders without dementia (Ball et al. 2007; Schaie and Willis 1986; Verhagen et al. 1992). The target of these interventions has been abilities (verbal memory, perceptual speed, inductive reasoning) showing early age-related decline in the mid-60s. On the basis of findings of small-scale training studies, the Advanced Cognitive Training in Vital Elders (ACTIVE) (Ball et al. 2002; Jobe et al. 2001) randomized, controlled clinical trial was conducted, and findings of the 5-year follow-up have been recently reported (Willis et al. 2006). Elders were randomly assigned to one of three interventions focusing on the abilities of inductive reasoning, verbal memory, or speed of processing or a control group. Booster training was provided to a random subset of each training intervention at 1 year and 3 years after training. Significant training effects for each of the interventions were found immediately after training and maintained at 5-year follow-up; effects were specific to the ability trained. Booster training significantly improved performance on the ability trained above the nonboosted intervention condition. At 5-year follow-up, those trained on reasoning reported significantly less difficulty performing instrumental tasks of daily living; those receiving booster training on speed of processing were faster at performing speeded tasks of daily living. Trainees in all interventions (compared with the control group) reported a higher level of quality of life 5 years after training (Wolinsky et al. 2006).

Cognitive Functioning Among the Oldest Old

Data on the oldest old come from the set of studies included in the Georgia Centenarian Studies (Poon et al. 2007). This section reviews three pertinent questions regarding cognitive functions in very old age: 1) Is dementia inevitable as one ages? 2) Is maintenance of high cognition an important contributor to longevity? and 3) What phenotypes of cognitive abilities can be employed to classify cognition among the oldest old?

Dementia

Prevalence of dementia is found to be about 1.5% in adults in their mid to late 60s. Both prevalence and incidence rise to as high as 25%–30% in the oldest old. If one lives to be very old, an interesting question is whether dementia is inevitable. If dementia is inevitable, then the development of dementia may be part of the normative process as one ages. If the development of dementia is found not to be universal, then one may conclude that the development of dementia is pathological and not normal aging.

Empirical data from centenarian studies do not support the assertion that dementia is inevitable in aging (Gondo and Poon 2007). The prevailing finding from centenarian studies is that dementia prevalence ranged from 42% to 80% (Akisaka 2000; Andersen-Ranberg et al. 2001; Asada et al. 1996; Beregi and Klinger 1989; Choi et al. 2003; Gondo et al. 2006; Hagberg et al. 2001; Inagaki 1995; Karasawa 1985; Poon et al., in press; Powell 1994; Ravaglia et al. 1999; Robine et al. 2003; Silver et al. 2001; Sobel et al. 1995). A lower prevalence of 27% was reported by the Swedish Centenarian Study; however, after considering nonparticipants, the investigators estimated that the prevalence could be as high as 42% (Samuelsson et al. 1997). It is interesting to note that only one study to date did report a 100% dementia rate in the assessment of community-dwelling centenarians (Blansjaar et al. 2000). Kliegel et al. (2004) found that about half of their centenarians in the Heidelberg Centenarian Study showed moderate to severe cognitive impairment but that one-quarter were cognitively intact. Results of the Heidelberg study also demonstrated that cognitive decline was slightly but significantly accelerated in the last 6 months before death. Finally, a recent Japanese study reported that 24.3% of their centenarian sample had no dementia, 13.8% were classified to "probably" have no dementia, and 61.8% were classified as having mild to severe dementia (Gondo et al. 2006). Gender effects were reported in the Japanese study, indicating that men were generally functioning cognitively better than women.

Issues surrounding factors contributing to the development of dementia in old age are controversial beyond whether dementia is inevitable. The wide range of reported dementia prevalence in different parts of the world could be due to the use of different criteria in diagnosing dementia, the use of nonrepresentative samples, and differential genetic and environmental factors affecting dementia in different geographic areas or cultures. Another potential contributor to the varying rates is that the female-to-male ratio among centenarians varied greatly, from 1:1 in Sardinia, Italy, to 12:1 in regions of South Korea. Because women tend to have a higher dementia prevalence (Andersen-Ranberg et al. 2001; Beregi and Klinger 1989; Choi et al. 2003; Gondo et al. 2006; Hagberg et al. 2001; Ravaglia et al. 1999; Robine et al. 2003; Sobel et al. 1995), the gender ratio could significantly affect the dementia prevalence of a sample or population. The time is ripe to better understand contributing factors to dementia prevalence within and between cultures and ethnicities.

Cognitive Function and Longevity

Does a high level of cognitive functioning contribute to longevity? A review by Gondo and Poon (in press) provided supportive evidence in both longitudinal and centenarian studies. A series of studies that collected intelligence test data among children showed a strong relationship between high childhood intelligence and low mortality in middle and old age (Batty et al. 2006; Deary et al. 2006; Hart et al. 2005; Shenkin et al. 2004; Whalley and Deary 2001; Whalley et al. 2000). Similarly, the Terman cohort study (Friedman and Martin 2007), which examined the life course of intellectually gifted children over seven decades, found that mortality rates of these gifted children were significantly lower than those of their birth cohorts in the general population (see also Siegler 1980 for a review of these studies).

Bosworth and Siegler (2002) reviewed nine studies that evaluated the relationship between terminal decline of cognitive function and death. Although they were not able to confirm this relationship in a consistent manner, they did verify that lower cognitive function is predictive of mortality. Ghisletta et al. (2006) and Rabbitt et al. (2006) reported similar relationship of cognitive functioning and mortality among well-controlled, representatively sampled longitudinal studies. Data from the Nun Study (Snowdon et al. 1999) showed that subjects with higher linguistic abilities tended to live 7 years longer than their cohorts with lower linguistic abilities. Wilson et al. (2007) provide data from the Rush Memory and Aging Project and found an increased rate of cognitive decline within the final 3.5 years of life.

The facilitative effect of higher cognitive function on longer survival among the very long lived (centenarians) was also demonstrated. Poon et al. (2000) examined predictors of number of days of survival beyond 100 years among 105 centenarians from the Georgia Centenarian Study. They found cognition was one of four significant predictors. The others were gender, father's age of death, and nutrition sufficiency. Cognitive status measured by the Short Portable Mental Status Questionnaire was one of five significant predictors of survival among 800 centenarians in the French Centenarian Study (Robine et al. 2003). The other predictors were residential condition, health status, activities of daily living, and instrumental activities of daily living. Similarly, data from the Tokyo Centenarian Study (Gondo et al. 2006) showed that Clinical Dementia Rating score had a significant influence on survival. Taken together, cognitive functioning is an important contributor to survival in the general population as well as in the oldest old.

Phenotypic Classification of Cognitive Functions Among the Oldest Old

There is large within- and across-subject variability in the cognitive performances of the oldest old (Hagberg et al. 2001). Although the progression of pathological changes is correlated with cognitive performances, recent studies reported a significant amount of variability in the concordance between pathology and performance (Gold et al. 2000; Haroutunian et al. 1998; Nagy et al. 1997). The seminal findings from these studies were that there were excellent correlations between normal and severe dementia with cognitive functions; however, the relationships were ambiguous in the moderate stages.

There are no commonly agreed-upon criteria for the classification of phenotypes of oldest old that take into account their cognitive ability and neuropathology (Gondo and Poon, in press). However, studies that examined premorbid cognitive performances and pathological diagnosis at postmortem autopsy may be helpful with the formulation of criteria. Mizutani and Shimada (1992) autopsied 27 centenarians, 11 of whom had not developed dementia. Some degree of brain degeneration was observed in 8 of the 11 centenarians without dementia, but there were no apparent anatomical changes in the brains of the remaining three. The researchers termed those neuropathologically and behaviorally dementia-free centenarians "supernormal." The autopsies performed with the New England Centenarian Study (Silver et al. 2002) and the Aichi Centenarian Study (Ding et al. 2006) reported, respectively, 4 out of 14 cases and 4 out of 6 cases of centenarians without dementia that met the criteria of supernormal, with the remaining centenarians, although dementia free at time of death, having brain neuropathology that pointed to pathological progression of dementia at autopsy. These centenarians could be classified as maintaining normal cognitive reserves.

The supernormal and "cognitive reserve" centenarians were both dementia free, although the second group presented some neuropathological degenerations. The second group could perform normally with everyday functions and communication; however, this group may have had difficulty with more complex tasks.

Finally, as noted earlier, 40%–80% of centenarians could be classified as having some degree of dementia. Most of these centenarians would have developed dementia at an advanced age, because early-onset dementia has been estimated to develop on average at 80 years. The final two phenotypes could be identified as "late-onset dementia" (defined as dementia with accompanying neuropathology developed at advanced age) and "early-onset dementia" (defined as dementia accompanying neuropathology developed at earlier age). In conclusion, although there is large individual diversity among the oldest old in both cognitive performance and neuropathological status, the four proposed phenotypes (supernormal, cognitive reserve, late-onset dementia, and early-onset dementia) could provide some guidelines in understanding the diversity.

Neuroimaging Data on Normal Aging

The rapidly developing field of neuroimaging can provide valuable data on the relation between pathological and normal aging. The identification of dementia and other brain disorders from neuroimaging has been described elsewhere (Buckner et al. 2004; Hoffman 1997; Marcus et al. 2007; Steffens 1997). Here we focus on the highlights of current neuroimaging research in normal aging and some implications for the practicing physician.

The goal of neuroimaging research in aging is to characterize structural and functional age-related changes in the brain as well as how these changes are manifest in cognitive performance. Behavioral studies of cognitive performance have yielded a complex pattern of age-related decline in many—but not all—abilities. The state of this field is represented in the recent editions of *The Handbook of Aging and Cognition* (Craik and Salthouse 2000). Within this broad area of cognition, relevant reviews are available in specific areas of perception (Baltes and Lindenberger 1997; Schneider and Pichora-Fuller 2000; Scialfa 2002), processing speed (Madden 2001; Salthouse 1996; Salthouse and Madden 2007), attention (Kramer and Madden 2008; Madden 2007; Madden and Whiting 2004), language (Burke and Shafto 2008), and memory (Pierce et al. 2004; Zacks et al. 2000). A general trend of this research is that cognitive abilities that depend on perceptual speed and contextual memory tend to decline significantly with age, even for healthy adults, whereas abilities that rely on semantic knowledge and highly overlearned patterns decline less or may even improve. This trend has been expressed as different types of distinctions, such as *crystallized* versus *fluid* abilities (Cattell 1971; Horn 1982), *aging-resilient* versus *aging-sensitive* abilities (Lindenberger 2001), and *pragmatics* versus *mechanics* (Baltes and Lindenberger 1997).

A specific illustration of the type of cognitive change to be expected during normal aging is a longitudinal study of Swedish twins, reported by Finkel et al. (2007). These authors obtained estimates of longitudinal change across several testing occasions that were up to 16 years apart from a sample of twins who were 50–88 years of age at initial testing. Participants performed a battery of cognitive tests representing four domains: verbal abilities, spatial abilities, memory, and processing speed, which were each defined by a composite of tests. The results indicated that although some longitudinal decline occurred for all four domains, the decline was most pronounced for the spatial and speed domains. In addition, speed was a leading statistical indicator of change in both the spatial and memory domains (fluid ability) but not of change in the verbal domain (crystallized ability).

Pierce et al. (2004) proposed that when interpreting these types of changes in cognitive ability, it is important to recognize that they represent an adaptation on the part of older adults to a changing neurological environment. These authors classified failures of memory as seven "sins," including three sins of omission—transience (forgetting over time), absent-mindedness, blocking (e.g., tip-of-the-tongue states)—and four sins of commission—misattribution, suggestibility, bias, and persistence. Pierce et al. emphasized that age-related increases that occur in these types of errors can be viewed as useful byproducts of otherwise adaptive features of memory. That is, the goal of memory is to support the encoding, retention, and retrieval of task-relevant information, not to preserve all incidental details of the environment. The neurological changes that occur with advancing age may lead to an increased reliance on adaptive strategies that maximize available cognitive resources but also leave older adults more vulnerable to the resulting loss of some forms of memory information (see also McDaniel et al. 2008).

Neuroimaging studies have characterized the age-related changes in brain structure and function relevant for the cognitive changes expressed in the behavioral measures. One edited volume summarizes current work in this area (Cabeza et al. 2005), as do several individual articles and book chapters (Cabeza 2001, 2002; Dennis and Cabeza 2008; Raz et al. 1998, 2005). Age-related change is prominent in both structural and functional imaging measures. Volumetric studies of gray matter have established that age-related decline occurs in cortical volume, with concomitant increase in ventricular size. A theme across many of these studies is that age-related volumetric decline is more pronounced for prefrontal regions than for more posterior cortical regions (Raz 2005; Raz et al. 2005). These findings have led to a frontal lobe hypothesis of cognitive aging (Dempster 1992; West 1996), which proposes that the cognitive changes associated with aging are the result of reduced frontal lobe efficiency. The degree to which reduced frontal lobe functioning can serve as an explanatory construct, however, is debated (Greenwood 2000; Tisserand and Jolles 2003). Age-related declines also occur, for example, in the volume and structure of posterior and sensory brain regions, such as gray matter near the primary visual cortex (Salat et al. 2004). In addition, although the division of the cerebral cortex into lobes is a useful pedagogical device, most cognitive tasks appear to rely on widely distributed cortical networks (Mesulam 1990; Tisserand et al. 2005).

Age-related decline in cerebral white matter volume is also observed, although it is not clear whether the trajectory of decline is comparable to that of gray matter. In addition, the magnitude of age-related decline in white matter appears to be sensitive to the proportion of study participants with hypertension or related cardiovascular disease. Increasing the proportion of these individuals tends to increase the degree of estimated age-related decline (Raz 2005). White matter hyperintensities, evident in T2-weighted structural magnetic resonance imaging (MRI), also increase in number and volume with age (Gunning-Dixon and Raz 2000; Raz et al. 2007; Yetkin et al. 1993). These hyperintensities are also correlated with hypertension and cardiovascular risk factors and represent decreased integrity of white matter (Oosterman et al. 2004; Raz et al. 2003; Soderlund et al. 2006; van den Heuvel et al. 2006).

Diffusion tensor imaging (DTI), in which the directionality and rate of molecular diffusion of water are measured (Mori and Zhang 2006), is a structural imaging method that is informative regarding age-related changes in white matter. This imaging modality is valuable because rather than relying on an ordinal-scale measure of pathology (e.g., number of hyperintensities), it provides an interval-scale measure of the range of white matter integrity throughout the brain. Studies using DTI have demonstrated that the integrity of white matter declines with age (Moseley 2002; Sullivan and Pfefferbaum 2006). This decline is also more prominent in the prefrontal regions but occurs posteriorly as well (Head et al. 2004; Salat et al. 2005).

Functional neuroimaging studies of aging complement these structural findings. Functional imaging has been conducted with both positron emission tomography (PET) and functional MRI, which measure cortical activation during task performance. Although many of the technological advances in neuroimaging have occurred in recent years, interest in the effects of normal aging dates to the first studies in the 1950s (Kety 1956). Neuroimaging of simple perceptual tasks, such as passively viewing checkerboards, has suggested that age-related decline occurs in both the amplitude (Buckner et al. 2000) and spatial extent (Huettel et al. 2001) of activation in primary visual (striate) cortex. By using appropriate control tasks, functional neuroimaging studies have identified age-related decline in brain regions associated with specific components of cognitive function. Many of these studies have found that age-related reduction of task-related activation in visual sensory regions is accompanied by age-related increased activation of prefrontal regions (Cabeza et al. 2004; Grady et al. 1994; Madden et al. 2005; McIntosh et al. 1999). This pattern has led to the suggestion that older adults compensate for deficiencies at a sensory/perceptual level by the recruitment of prefrontal regions associated with higher-order cognitive strategies. This type of theory is being investigated currently in a variety of task domains. One important issue is whether age-related increased activation is in fact compensatory, in which case better-performing older adults would exhibit relatively greater activation (Cabeza et al. 2002). In some instances, however, worse-performing older adults exhibit relatively greater activation, which may represent increased effort or task difficulty rather than compensation (Nielson et al. 2002). However this issue is resolved, current neuroimaging research suggests that 1) decline in activation is not the whole story, and 2) there is a high degree of plasticity of function in the aging brain (Craik 2006; Craik and Bialystok 2006; Grady 1998; Grady et al. 2006).

Ultimately, the contribution of neuroimaging will rely on relating the neuroimaging measures to behavioral measures. Although this may be intuitively obvious, the association of a particular brain structure or activation with a behavioral measure is still a correlational approach, and methodological and statistical care is required to identify causal relations in the data. Researchers are currently developing improved methods for analyzing the functional connectivity among brain regions in the context of specific task domains (Grady 2005; Ramnani et al. 2004). Structural imaging measures, such as white matter integrity from DTI, can be included in statistical models of age-related changes in cognitive function (Bucur et al. 2008; Colcombe et al. 2005; Madden et al. 2007). Functional imaging measures are being combined with behavioral measures in novel ways, for example, to distinguish remembered and forgotten items (Daselaar et al. 2006; Dennis et al. 2007).

For the practicing clinician, these theoretical developments are not always directly relevant but do lead to useful implications. First, cognitive change occurs throughout later adulthood; some decline in perceptual speed and fluid abilities will be evident even in healthy individuals. Second, significant changes in brain structure and function may also occur in individuals without noticeable cognitive impairment, although at some point impaired cognitive function will be reflected in the brain measures. Third, health status is a relevant variable, and to the degree that cardiovascular disease and other comorbidities can be avoided, age-related decline is likely to be minimized. Fourth, the brain and central nervous system are constantly adaptive, and this adaptation is expressed in measures of older adults' brain function as well as in behavioral measures of cognitive performance.

Work in psychology of aging is becoming integrated across traditional areas. Work in cognition generally reports some decrements, although typically there is maintenance of emotional functioning. Although this is not surprising to the practicing psychiatrist, it is a new approach in psychology that comes from attempts to understand the aging mind. Carstensen et al. (2006) review the relevant literature, and the nub of their argument is that older persons are motivated to be selective and use their cognitive processing resources to meet emotional needs. Carstensen et al. provide a framework that can accommodate gains as well as losses seen in cross-sectional aging studies.

Personality, Coping, and Behavioral Medicine Developments

Personality Developments

The unequivocal assertion that personality does not change over time is beginning to be challenged, particularly with the advent of more sophisticated statistical methods that allow for the test of individual growth curves and trajectories. A number of studies have pointed out that neuroticism appears to decline with age (Mroczek and Spiro 2003; Small et al. 2003) and that agreeableness and conscientiousness appear to increase over time (Helson et al. 2002; Small et al. 2003). Terracciano et al. (2005) reported that openness declined across adulthood, neuroticism declined up to age 80, and for extraversion there was first stability and then decline, whereas there was an increase in agreeableness and conscientiousness up to age 70.

Additional attention is being paid to possible cohort differences in personality. Twenge (2000), for example, reported an increase of neuroticism in more recent cohorts, but this has not been replicated in other studies (Terracciano et al. 2006). The Terracciano et al. (2006) study, however, did report cohort effects for personal relations, with later-born cohorts declining more than one T-score point per decade. In relation to this finding, Robinson and Jackson (2001) also reported a decline in trust among Americans born after the 1940s.

Continuity of personality and social preferences is expected across the adult life course; thus, changes have potential diagnostic significance and make knowledge about expected trajectories important. Although the work on cognitive development reviewed previously finds generally good patterns by domain of performance, individual differences in personality predict physical disease, which in turn has consequences for cognitive performance, which then leads to greater incidence of disease. This can be well illustrated with work on hypertension.

Findings from the UNC Alumni Heart Study indicate a relationship, dependent on covariates in the model, between personality in early middle age (approximately age 40) and incident hypertension 11–15 years later. The behavioral predictors of hypertension are well known and include age, education, exercise, family history, overweight, and obesity in the UNCAHS cohort. Hostility also predicted hypertension, but this effect was mediated only by overweight and obesity. This same pattern was seen for Neuroticism facet scale score findings of N5 (Impulsiveness) for overall N (Neuroticism). Because hypertension is a silent disease, it was also more likely in more conscientious persons and in Conscientiousness facets of C1 (Competence) and C3 (Dutifulness). Aside from Conscientiousness and its facets, only job strain and A4 (Anger) score predicted hypertension with all traditional covariates in the model. Because UNCAHS is a mail survey, hypertension was tested on 2 days—when first reported and when treatment first reported—to model how it would have been defined had we been able to measure blood pressure directly, where normal pressures with treatment are considered hypertension (Siegler 2007b). Midlife hypertension confers increased risk for later coronary heart disease and stroke and vascular dementia.

Elias et al. (2004) present 30 years of research on the impact of age and hypertension on normal cognitive functioning, a study that started in 1974. A summary of the findings is presented here. They found that almost all abilities are affected by hypertension and that antihypertensive treatments may not prevent this decline. After 30 years, questions remain about subtypes of disease and of treatments. Overall estimates of the impact of changes in blood pressure on summary indicators of Wechsler Adult Intelligence Scale performance and speed indicate that being hypertensive carried a 74% increased risk of poor performance, with a 67% increase in risk of poor speeded performance compared with estimates for 10 years of age at 58% and 85%, respectively, with a 20 mmHg increase in systolic blood pressure conferring 18% and 22% increases in risk. (Cross-sectional normative data are presented in Dore et al. 2007.) These are useful data derived from the Maine-Syracuse Longitudinal Study stratified by age and education showing level of mean –1.5 standard deviation of change, indicating an estimate of the level of performance that could be considered mild cognitive impairment, which may represent a heightened risk for Alzheimer's disease. Cognitive and neuropsychological measures in the battery were also evaluated by proportion of variance accounted for by age, education, and gender separately and together, as well as additional variance caused by disease indexed by depression and health indicators including risky behaviors like smoking and prevalent disease. On average, health variables added about 3%. These data underscore the importance of long-term chronic disease assessment and management for geriatric psychiatry.

Mroczek et al. (2006) cast traditional concerns of stability and change in personality with age into theoretical terms and note that the changes can be both positive and negative and respond to developing health conditions in adaptive ways. Work in this area still looks to see if nonnormative changes have medical consequences that should raise the level of suspicion in an insightful clinician. Theoretically, Hooker and McAdams (2003) have incorporated social processes into trait psychology, although empirical findings will take time to emerge. Latent growth curves are providing new techniques to evaluate sophisticated developmental patterns of change. Our own work on hostility (Siegler et al. 2003) finds the normative pattern of declining hostility with age is replicated longitudinally and cross-sectionally (Siegler 2007b) but reflects only 75% of the population; in a very small group (3.5%), hostility actually increases from age 18 to 60 years, whereas the remainder decline slowly. Differences in such trajectories have definite health consequences. At age 60, those who increased in hostility were more likely to be hypertensive,

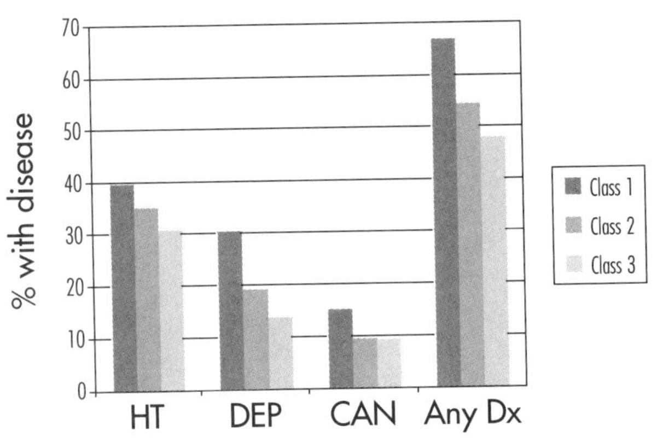

FIGURE 7–4. Classes of hostility and cumulative disease.

HT = hypertension; DEP = depression; CAN = cancer.

Source. Siegler IC: "Psychology of Aging and the Public Health." 2007 Developmental Health Award, Division 20 and Division 38. Invited address presented at the Annual Meeting of the American Psychological Association, San Francisco, CA, August 2007. Reprinted with permission.

to be depressed, and to have cancer (Siegler 2007b), as shown in Figure 7–4.

Work in behavioral medicine is based on a search for the biological and physiological mechanisms that relate psychosocial constructs such as personality to disease (Siegler 1989). All of these are variants of a stress model that involves neuroendocrine, immune, inflammatory, and cardiovascular reactivity paradigms. These are illustrated in a model by R.B. Williams (2007) (see Figure 7–5).

There are normative age differences in all of these biological indicators (see Hazzard et al. 1999; Markides 2007) and fewer longitudinal age change data to evaluate. Recent published chapters have worked to integrate aging data into these frameworks for cardiovascular and social risk domains (Berg et al. 2007), neuroendocrine parameters (Epel et al. 2007), and all of the systems that respond to chronic stressors such as caregiving (Young and Vitaliano 2007). Research is moving toward personalized medicine that will take genes and gene environment interactions into effect (R.B. Williams 2007).

A useful illustration of how this model works in an aging population is provided by emerging findings from our recently completed study of the impact of caregiving (Duke Caregiving Study: Brummett et al. 2005, 2006a, 2007b, 2008; Dilworth-Anderson et al. 2005a). The broad objectives of this research are to identify factors in the social (e.g., being a caregiver for a relative

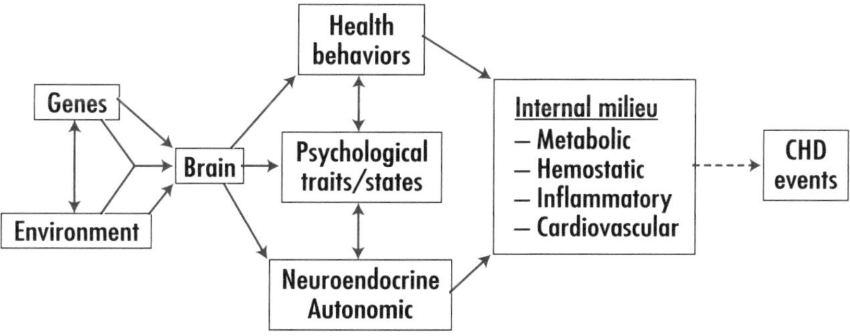

FIGURE 7–5. A model of psychosocial mediators of health events.

CHD = coronary heart disease.

Source. Williams RB: "Coping Skills Training in Different Cultures: The LifeSkills Experience." Poster presented at the First Conference of the Central Eastern European Society of Behavioral Medicine, Pecs, Hungary, August 20–22, 2007. Reprinted with permission.

with Alzheimer's disease) and physical (e.g., neighborhood characteristics) environments that interact to affect biological and behavioral characteristics that lead to poorer physical and mental health and to evaluate variants in genes that regulate function of the neurotransmitter serotonin as moderators of the impact of these environmental factors on health and disease.

We found that caregivers who expressed a higher level of concern about crime in their neighborhood had higher levels of fasting blood glucose and glycosylated hemoglobin (a measure of average blood glucose over the past 2–3 months) than either caregivers with low crime concerns or matched control subjects with high or low crime concerns. These findings suggest that among the millions of Americans with caregiving responsibilities for a relative with Alzheimer's disease, those who live in neighborhoods that engender concerns about crime are at higher risk for developing type 2 diabetes and the other diseases, such as heart disease, to which it leads (Brummett et al. 2005). In a structural equation model, we found that caregivers of a relative with Alzheimer's disease report poorer sleep quality indirectly through reduced social support and increased levels of negative emotions, compared with matched control subjects who do not have caregiving responsibilities (Brummett et al. 2006a) and that these differences in sleep quality are related to monoamine oxidase-A alleles associated with less transcriptional activity and with depression (Brummett et al. 2007b) in caregiving men. Poor sleep quality in women was associated with the S allele in the serotonin transporter gene (5-HTTLPR) (Brummett et al. 2007a). Gender effects in response to caregiving were seen in the UNCAHS, where for middle-aged caregivers, caregiving was associated with diabetes for men and depression for both men and women in models controlling for age and income. Age increased risk of disease, whereas income was protective (Siegler et al. 2006).

A literature is developing that finds consistent personality mortality associations. Not only does hostility in college predict premature mortality in the UNCAHS (Siegler 2007), we have also found that optimists compared with pessimists were more likely to survive 40 years after college entry (Brummett et al. 2006b). Friedman and Martin (2007) review conscientiousness as a critical construct in survival and an integrated way to think about personality as a system, whereas our own work is finding new implications for the facets of openness to experience in coronary patients (Jonassaint et al. 2007). The behavioral medicine literature focuses more on negative constructs (hostility, neuroticism, and pessimism), whereas survival studies focus more on the more positive traits. Whether the individual constructs or the broader domains prove more useful (R.B. Williams et al. 2003; Suls and Bunde 2005), the findings are starting to show the general trends seen above. What do long-term survivors actually look like?

Personality in Centenarians

In order to survive successfully into very old age, individuals appear to need a highly resilient or robust personality. Several centenarian studies appear to point this out. For example, the New England Centenarian Study noted that centenarians were very stress-resilient individuals (Perls and Silver 1999). Findings from the

Georgia Centenarian Study also noted that a particular cluster of personality traits was more likely to be found among centenarians: relatively high levels of extraversion, emotional stability, and conscientiousness (Martin et al. 2006). High ratings of emotional stability also were found in centenarian studies in Sweden (Samuelsson et al. 1997) and Japan (Shimonaka et al. 1996). A longitudinal follow-up showed that centenarians had decreased scores in sensitivity but higher scores in openness (Martin et al. 2002) after an 18-month follow-up testing. The results suggest that centenarians may compensate for physical and functional decline by having robust personality traits and by becoming less sensitive and more open-minded.

Coping Developments

There is considerable interest to study coping behaviors in centenarians. This group of "expert survivors" (Poon et al. 1992) faces accelerated changes in a number of functioning domains, such as activities of daily living, and considerable losses of peers and family members. How do individuals at such an advanced age cope with these changes? The results obtained so far suggest that centenarians are less likely to use "active behavioral" coping styles (Martin et al., in press). Active behavioral coping refers to all specific actions individuals take when being confronted with stressors or events. For example, seeking professional advice and talking with family and friends constitute active strategies. It is not surprising that centenarians are less likely to use active behavioral coping, because their resources are more limited. Although centenarians are restricted in their active behaviors, the level of active cognitive coping does not appear to diminish (Martin et al., in press). Centenarians may not be able to *do* something about a problem, but they surely can *think* about it as much as any other age group. Along the same lines, Martin et al. (2001) pointed out that it may not be the general coping modes (i.e., active behavioral, active cognitive, or avoidance) that play an important role. Rather, it may be specific "molecular" coping behaviors that distinguish the oldest old from other age groups. For example, centenarians are more likely to use religious coping and acceptance, whereas they are less like to worry about a problem (Martin et al. 2001). A centenarian study in Barbados also noted that successful adaptation and coping among centenarians were positively related to high levels of religiosity (Archer et al. 2005).

Coping With Caregiving in Diverse Populations

In the face of the growing numbers of people with Alzheimer's disease and related issues such as testing, assessment, and care, Peggye Dilworth-Anderson, Ramón Valle, Sam Fazio, and Teresa Radebaugh convened a conference in 2004 and published papers from this conference that address the 5 million Americans who have Alzheimer's disease. Of particular concern in the discussions and published papers is that what is known about aging and Alzheimer's disease is a function of the people studied, and currently little is known about diverse populations. It is important to further understand the heterogeneity of Alzheimer's disease, because heterogeneity may be within the disease as well as within the population. Including diverse populations in Alzheimer's disease research can provide opportunities for diagnosis, care, and treatment for everyone.

Further, despite many years of Alzheimer's disease research, our understanding of the effects of this disease on family caregivers is still limited for ethnic minorities. For example, we know, based on current evidence, that 1) the burden of Alzheimer's disease is greater among African Americans, among whom age-specific prevalence of dementia is 14%–100% higher than that found among European Americans; 2) first-degree relatives of African Americans who have Alzheimer's disease have a 43.7% cumulative risk of getting the disease compared with 26.9% for whites, and among blacks, spouses have an 18.5% cumulative risk of getting the disease compared with 10.4% for whites (Green et al. 2002); 3) African Americans are less likely to institutionalize relatives with dementia (43.7%), compared with whites (89.6%) (Stevens et al. 2004), and 29% of African American families provide care for their older family members compared with 24% of white families (Dilworth-Anderson et al. 2006); 4) African American caregivers are more likely to care for more than one dependent adult in their families, spending an average of 20.6 hours per week providing care; 5) African American caregivers tend to underutilize formal services; 6) 66% of African American caregivers are employed full- or part-time; and 7) African American caregivers are more likely to be middle-aged daughters rather than spouses, whereas white caregivers are as likely to be a spouse as an adult child (Hinrichsen and Ramirez 1992). These conditions would suggest that caregivers of African American elders are particularly vulnerable to poor emotional and physical health outcomes. Using data published from the Resources for Enhancing Alzheimer's Caregivers Health (REACH), investigators addressed these vulnerabilities, as well as those in other groups, through a multicomponent intervention (Belle et al. 2006). Their findings show that compared with minimal support provided in a control group, their multicomponent intervention statistically significantly improved the quality of life (as measured by indicators of depression, burden, social support, self-care, and patient problem behaviors) for white and Hispanic caregivers but not for African American caregivers. However, they found statistically significant quality-of-life changes with this intervention among African American spouse caregivers, in contrast to African American adult children in the caregiver role. Given that adult children provide the majority of care in black families (unlike in white and Hispanic families), additional research is needed to better identify and address their emotional and physical health vulnerabilities through interventions.

Limited information on psychological coping poses further concerns for understanding how diverse groups respond to and address the stress and strain of caregiving. Evidence shows that caregivers suffer emotionally from a variety of stressors because of the physical demands of assisting care recipients with daily activities (Alzheimer's Association and National Alliance for Caregiving 2004). Of particular concern is the type and degree of caregiver stress associated with caring for elders with dementia who often have behavioral and physical health problems (Haley et al. 2004; Hooker et al. 2002; Schulz and Martire 2004). Information on addressing emotional coping and well-being among dementia caregivers in diverse groups suggests that a sociocultural perspective is needed to understand the diversity issues that are involved. A sociocultural perspective takes into consideration an ethnic and cultural group's history, values, beliefs, and ways of thinking. It is also characterized by what is often described as the "historical memory" of a group as evidenced by customs, rituals, and ways of expressing themselves. Work from our Duke Caregiving Study found that African Americans have different cultural reasons for providing care for relatives with Alzheimer's disease and that this varies by educational level (Dilworth-Anderson et al. 2005a). Findings show that race and ethnicity appear to influence significantly the expression of depression, and depression is not always synonymous across cultures. Hence, it has been suggested that the application of standard mood inventories in African American groups may contribute to the observation of lower prevalence rates of depression in this group when compared with white samples (Harrelson et al. 2002). Studies of depression in caregivers of patients with Alzheimer's disease have also underscored the racial and ethnic differences in depressive symptomatology.

In some studies, it appears that African American caregivers of patients with Alzheimer's disease are often reported as less depressed when compared with white caregivers (Haley et al. 1996); however, both groups show other negative health outcomes from caregiving over time, such as increased physical symptoms (Roth et al. 2001). Findings by Dilworth-Anderson et al. (1999) show that very few African American caregivers experience depression assessed by the Center for Epidemiologic Studies Depression Scale (Radloff 1977); however, by using Derogatis's (1993) global index on distress, their findings did document that about 18% of the caregivers were emotionally distressed. These distressed caregivers received less social support, were in poorer physical health, and experienced more caregiving problems than caregivers who were not distressed (Dilworth-Anderson et al. 1999). Thus, to be appropriately sensitive to depression expression among African Americans and possibly other racial and ethnic groups, researchers need to rethink how best to measure depression with culture in mind. Both conceptual and methodological issues, therefore, will need to be revisited as we approach understanding emotional well-being among diverse groups of caregivers.

Behavioral Interventions

Research on the role of social factors in aging has benefited from the flowering of integrated theoretical work in emotion and motivation by Carstensen and her colleagues and has been the basis for behavioral intervention studies. Not only has there been great progress in basic research in the psychology of normal aging, but major intervention studies also have been completed and reported. Willis et al. (2006) present the results of a cognitive training intervention for normally aging persons (ACTIVE) that suggests that cognitive training can be beneficial; Gitlin et al. (2003) present REACH for interventions to reduce the stress of caregiving; and Berkman et al. (2003) and Lett et al. (2007) present ENRICHD, which attempted to modify depression and social support to reduce the impact of coronary heart disease. These three large clinical trials show the beginnings of applications of decades of findings in psychology to help mitigate the impact of age-related changes in the population. Williams LifeSkills (V.P. Williams and Williams 1999) teaches coping skills and has been found to reduce coronary heart disease risk indicators (Bishop et al. 2005). This approach is currently being tested as a framework to help caregivers. Randomized clinical trials with behavioral interventions are difficult to conduct because individuals who are randomly assigned to the control group can sometimes provide an intervention for themselves. The results of these behavioral interventions are less important than the fact that they are entering the realm of tested scientific practice. This represents an important acknowledgment of the role of psychosocial factors in disease as well as an optimism that something can be done to reduce the burden.

Implications for the Practice of Geriatric Psychiatry

The practice of geriatric psychiatry is healthy (Cohen 2005). There are still major gaps in our knowledge of how to define *normal* aging in frail institutionalized populations that have been defined as "abnormally" aging—however, this work is beginning (Buckman et al. 2007; Tyas et al. 2007; Welsh-Bohmer et al. 2006). Population-based national studies generally do not have sufficiently rich measurement batteries; thus, there is a growing group of older impaired persons and their caregivers who could benefit from more study. Similarly, we do not have a "psychology of aging with Alzheimer's disease" or "aging with multi-infarct dementia." If these disorders are soon cured, we will not need one. Until then, multiple generations of aging persons can be expected to live longer, more complex lives, and geriatric psychiatrists may have two or three generations in the same family as patients, needing to understand multiple trajectories of normal aging processes.

Key Points

- Individual decline in cognitive performance before age 60 generally is not normal aging. By the mid-70s, average decrement is observed for all abilities, and by the 80s this decrement is severe except for verbal ability.
- Empirical data from centenarian studies suggest that dementia is not inevitable.
- Cognitive abilities that depend on perceptual speed and contextual memory tend to decline with age, even for healthy adults, whereas abilities that rely on semantic knowledge and highly overlearned patterns decline less or may even improve.
- Continuity of personality and social preferences is expected across the adult life span; thus, changes have potential diagnostic significance.
- The effects of Alzheimer's disease and of caregiving for relatives with Alzheimer's disease vary in diverse populations.

References

Akisaka M: Study of Male Centenarians. Fukuoka, Japan, Kyushu University Press, 2000

Aldwin CM, Park CL, Spiro A (eds): Handbook of Health Psychology and Aging. New York, Guilford, 2007

Alzheimer's Association and National Alliance for Caregiving: Families care: Alzheimer's caregiving in the United States, 2004. Available at http://www.alz.org/national/documents/report_familiescare.pdf. Accessed October 11, 2007.

Andersen-Ranberg K, Vasegaard L, Jeune B: Dementia is not inevitable: a population-based study of Danish centenarians. J Geront Series B Psychol Sci Social Sci 56:P152–P15, 2001

Archer S, Brathwaite F, Fraser H: Centenarians in Barbados: the importance of religiosity in adaptive coping and life satisfaction in the case of extreme longevity. Journal of Religion, Spirituality and Aging 18:3–19, 2005

Asada T, Yamagata Z, Kinoshita T, et al: Prevalence of dementia and distribution of ApoE alleles in Japanese centenarians: an almost-complete survey in Yamanashi Prefecture, Japan. J Am Geriat Soc 44:151–155, 1996

Ball K, Berch DB, Helmers KF, et al: Effects of cognitive training interventions with older adults: a randomized controlled trial. JAMA 288:2271–2281, 2002

Ball K, Edwards JD, Ross LA: The impact of speed of processing training on cognitive and everyday function. J Gerontol Psychol Sci 62B (special issue I):19–31, 2007

Baltes PB, Lindenberger U: Emergence of a powerful connection between sensory and cognitive functions across the adult life span: a new window to the study of cognitive aging? Psychol Aging 12:12–21, 1997

Batty GD, Deary IJ, Macintyre S: Childhood IQ and life course socioeconomic position in relation to alcohol induced hangovers in adulthood: the Aberdeen children of the 1950s study. J Epidemiol Community Health 60:872–874, 2006

Belle SH, Burgio L, Burns R, et al: Enhancing the quality of life of dementia caregivers from different ethnic or racial groups: a randomized, controlled trial. Ann Intern Med 145:727–738, 2006

Beregi E, Klinger A: Health and living conditions of centenarians in Hungary. Int Psychogeriatr 1:195–200, 1989

Berg CA, Smith TW, Henry NJ, et al: A developmental approach to psychosocial risk factors and successful aging, in Handbook of Health Psychology and Aging. Edited by Aldwin CM, Park CL, Spiro A III. New York, Guilford, 2007, pp 30–53

Berkman LF, Blumenthal J, Burg M, et al: Effects of treating depression and low perceived social support on clinical events after myocardial infarction: the Enhancing Recovery in Coronary Heart Disease Patients (ENRICHD) randomized trial. JAMA 289:3106–3116, 2003

Birren JE, Schaie KW (eds): Handbook of the Psychology of Aging, 6th Edition. San Diego, CA, Academic Press, 2006

Bishop GD, Kaur D, Tan VLM: Effects of a psychosocial skills training workshop on psychophysiological and psychosocial risk in patients undergoing coronary artery bypass grafting. Am Heart J 150:602–609, 2005

Blansjaar BA, Thomassen R, Van Schaick HW: Prevalence of dementia in centenarians. Int J Geriatr Psychiatry 15:219–225, 2000

Bosworth HB, Siegler IC: Terminal change in cognitive function: an updated review of longitudinal studies. Exp Aging Res 28:299–315, 2002

Brummett BH, Siegler IC, Rohe WM, et al: Neighborhood characteristics moderate effects of caregiving on glucose metabolism. Psychosom Med 67:752–758, 2005

Brummett BH, Babyak MA, Siegler IC, et al: Associations among perceptions of social support, negative affect, and quality of sleep in caregivers and non-caregivers. Health Psychol 25:220–225, 2006a

Brummett BH, Helms MJ, Dahlstrom WG, et al: Prediction of all-cause mortality by the Minnesota Multiphasic Personality Inventory Optimism-Pessimism Scale Scores: study of a college sample during a 40-year follow-up period. Mayo Clin Proc 81:1541–1544, 2006b

Brummett BH, Krystal AD, Ashley-Koch A, et al: Sleep quality varies as a function of 5-HTTLPR genotype and stress. Psychosom Med 69:621–624, 2007a

Brummett BH, Krystal AD, Siegler IC, et al: Associations of a regulatory polymorphism of the monoamine oxidase-A gene promoter (MAOA-uVNTR) with symptoms of depression and sleep quality. Psychosom Med 69:396–401, 2007b

Brummett BH, Boyle SH, Siegler IC, et al: HPA axis function in male caregivers: effect of the monoamine oxidase-A gene promoter (MAOA-uVNTR). Biol Psychol 2008 Jul 1 [Epub ahead of print]

Buckman AS, Boyle PA, Wilson RS, et al: Frailty is associated with incident Alzheimer's disease and cognitive decline in the elderly. Psychosom Med 69:483–489, 2007

Buckner RL, Snyder AZ, Sanders AL, et al: Functional brain imaging of young, nondemented, and demented older adults. J Cogn Neurosci 12(suppl):24–34, 2000

Buckner RL, Head D, Parker J, et al: A unified approach for morphometric and functional data analysis in young, old, and demented adults using automated atlas-based head size normalization: reliability and validation against manual measurement of total intracranial volume. Neuroimage 23:724–738, 2004

Bucur B, Madden DJ, Spaniol J, et al: Age-related slowing of memory retrieval: contributions of perceptual speed and cerebral white matter integrity. Neurobiol Aging 29:1070–1071, 2008

Burke DM, Shafto MA: Language and aging, in The Handbook of Aging and Cognition, 3rd Edition. Edited by Craik FIM, Salthouse TA. New York, Psychology Press, 2008, pp 373–443

Cabeza R: Functional neuroimaging of cognitive aging, in Handbook of Functional Neuroimaging of Cognition. Edited by Cabeza R, Kingstone A. Cambridge, MA, MIT Press, 2001, pp 331–377

Cabeza R: Hemispheric asymmetry reduction in older adults: the HAROLD model. Psychol Aging 17:85–100, 2002

Cabeza R, Anderson ND, Locantore JK, et al: Aging gracefully: compensatory brain activity in high-performing older adults. Neuroimage 17:1394–1402, 2002

Cabeza R, Daselaar SM, Dolcos F, et al: Task-independent and task-specific age effects on brain activity during working memory, visual attention and episodic retrieval. Cereb Cortex 14:364–375, 2004

Cabeza R, Nyberg L, Park D (eds): Cognitive Neuroscience of Aging: Linking Cognitive and Cerebral Aging. Oxford, UK, Oxford University Press, 2005

Carstensen LL, Hartel CR (eds): When I'm 64. Washington, DC, National Academies Press, 2006

Carstensen LL, Mikels, JA, Mather M: Aging and the intersection of cognition, motivation, and emotion, in Handbook of the Psychology of Aging, 6th Edition. Edited by Birren JE, Schaie KW. Burlington, MA, Elsevier, 2006, pp 343–362

Cattell RB: Abilities: Their Structure, Growth, and Action. Boston, MA, Houghton Mifflin, 1971

Choi YH, Kim JH, Kim DK, et al: Distributions of ACE and APOE polymorphisms and their relations with dementia status in Korean centenarians. J Gerontol Series A Biol Sci Med Sci 58:227–231, 2003

Cohen GD: The Mature Mind. New York, Basic Books, 2005

Colcombe SJ, Kramer AF, Erickson KI, et al: The implications of cortical recruitment and brain morphology for individual differences in inhibitory function in aging humans. Psychol Aging 20:363–375, 2005

Costa PT Jr, Siegler IC (eds): Recent Advances in Psychology and Aging. San Diego, CA, Elsevier, 2004

Craik FI: Brain-behavior relations across the lifespan: a commentary. Neurosci Biobehav Rev 30:885–892, 2006

Craik FI, Bialystok E: Cognition through the lifespan: mechanisms of change. Trends Cogn Sci 10:131–138, 2006

Craik FIM, Salthouse TA (eds): The Handbook of Aging and Cognition, 2nd Edition. Mahwah, NJ, Erlbaum, 2000

Daselaar SM, Fleck MS, Dobbins IG, et al: Effects of healthy aging on hippocampal and rhinal memory functions: an event-related fMRI study. Cereb Cortex 16:1771–1782, 2006

Deary IJ, Spinath FM, Bates TC: Genetics of intelligence. Eur J Hum Genet 14:690–700, 2006

Dempster FN: The rise and fall of the inhibitory mechanism: toward a unified theory of cognitive development and aging. Dev Rev 12:45–75, 1992

Dennis NA, Cabeza R: Neuroimaging of Healthy Cognitive Aging, in The Handbook of Aging and Cognition, 3rd Edition. Edited by Craik FIM, Salthouse TA. New York, Psychology Press, 2008, pp 1–54

Dennis NA, Daselaar S, Cabeza R: Effects of aging on transient and sustained successful memory encoding activity. Neurobiol Aging 28:1749–1758, 2007

Derogatis LR: Brief Symptom Inventory: Administration, Scoring, and Procedures Manual, 3rd Edition. Minneapolis, MN, National Computer Systems, 1993

Dilworth-Anderson P, Williams SW, Cooper T: Family caregiving to elderly African Americans: caregiver types and structures. J Gerontol B Sci Soc Sci 54:S237–S241, 1999

Dilworth-Anderson P, Brummett BH, Goodwin P, et al: Effect of race on cultural justifications for caregiving. J Gerontol B Sci Soc Sci 60:S257–S262, 2005a

Dilworth-Anderson P, Valle R, Fazio S: Introduction. Alzheimer Dis Assoc Disord 19(suppl):249, 2005b

Dilworth-Anderson P, Gibson B, Burke JD: Working with African American families, in Ethnicity and the Dementias, 2nd Edition. Edited by Yeo G, Gallagher-Thompson D. New York, Routledge, 2006, pp 127–144

Ding ZT, Wang Y, Jiang YP, et al: Characteristics of alpha-synucleinopathy in centenarians. Acta Neuropathol 111:450–458, 2006

Dore GA, Elias MF, Robbins MA, et al: Cognitive performance and age: norms from the Maine-Syracuse Study. Exp Aging Res 33:205–271, 2007

Elias MF, Robbins MA, Budge MM, et al: Studies of aging, hypertension and cognitive functioning: with contributions from the Maine-Syracuse Study, in Advances in Cell Aging and Gerontology, Vol 15. Recent Advances in Psychology and Aging. Edited by Costa P, Siegler I. Amsterdam, Elsevier, 2004, pp 89–131

Epel ES, Burke HM, Wolkowitz OM: The psychoneuroendocrinology of aging: anabolic and catabolic hormones, in Handbook of Health Psychology and Aging. Edited by Aldwin CM, Park CL, Spiro A. New York, Guilford, 2007, pp 119–141

Finkel D, Reynolds CA, McArdle JJ, et al: Age changes in processing speed as a leading indicator of cognitive aging. Psychol Aging 22:558–568, 2007

Friedman HS, Martin LR: A lifespan approach to personality and longevity: the case of conscientiousness, in Handbook of Health Psychology and Aging. Edited by Aldwin CM, Park CL, Spiro A. New York, Guilford, 2007, pp 167–185

Ghisletta P, McArdle J, Lindenberger U: Longitudinal cognition-survival relations in old and very old age: 13-year data from the Berlin Aging Study. European Psychologist 11:204–223, 2006

Gitlin LN, Bell SH, Burgio LD, et al: Effect of multicomponent interventions on caregiver burden and depression in the REACH multisite initiative at 6-month follow-up. Psychol Aging 18:361–374, 2003

Gold G, Bouras C, Kövari E, et al: Clinical validity of Braak neuropathological staging in the oldest-old. Acta Neuropathol 99:579–582, 2000

Gondo Y, Poon LW: Biopsychosocial approaches to longevity, in Annual Review of Gerontology and Geriatrics. Edited by Poon LW, Perls T. New York, Springer, 2007, pp 129–149

Gondo Y, Hirose N, Arai Y, et al: Functional status of centenarians in Tokyo, Japan: developing better phenotypes of exceptional longevity. J Gerontol A Sci Biol Sci 61:305–310, 2006

Grady CL: Brain imaging and age-related changes in cognition. Exp Gerontol 33:661–673, 1998

Grady CL: Functional connectivity during memory tasks in healthy aging and dementia, in Cognitive Neuroscience of Aging: Linking Cognitive and Cerebral Aging. Edited by Cabeza R, Nyberg L, Park D. Oxford, UK, Oxford University Press, 2005, pp 286–308

Grady CL, Maisog JM, Horwitz B, et al: Age-related changes in cortical blood flow activation during visual processing of faces and location. J Neurosci 14 (pt 2):1450–1462, 1994

Grady CL, Springer MV, Hongwanishkul D, et al: Age-related changes in brain activity across the adult lifespan. J Cogn Neurosci 18:227–241, 2006

Green RC, Cupples LA, Go R, et al: Risk of dementia among White and African American relatives of patients with Alzheimer disease. JAMA 287:329–336, 2002

Greenwood PM: The frontal aging hypothesis evaluated. J Int Neuropsychol Soc 6:705–726, 2000

Gunning-Dixon FM, Raz N: The cognitive correlates of white matter abnormalities in normal aging: a quantitative review. Neuropsychology 14:224–232, 2000

Hagberg B, Alfredson B, Poon LW, et al: Cognitive functioning in centenarians: a coordinated analysis of results from three countries. J Gerontol Series B Psychol Sci Soc Sci 56:141–151, 2001

Haley WE, Roth DL, Coleton MI, et al: Appraisal, coping, and social support as mediators of well-being in black and white family caregivers of patients with Alzheimer's disease. J Consult Clin Psychol 64:121–129, 1996

Haley WE, Gitlin LN, Wisniewski SR, et al: Well-being, appraisal, and coping in African-American and Caucasian dementia caregivers: findings from the REACH study. Aging Ment Health 8:316–329, 2004

Haroutunian V, Perl D, Purohit D, et al: Regional distribution of neuritic plaques in the nondemented elderly and subjects with very mild Alzheimer disease. Arch Neurol 55:1185–1191, 1998

Harrelson TL, White TM, Regenberg AC, et al: Similarities and differences in depression among Black and White nursing home residents. Am J Geriatr Psychiatry 10:175–184, 2002

Hart CL, Taylor MD, Smith GD, et al: Childhood IQ and all-cause mortality before and after age 65: prospective observational study linking the Scottish Mental Survey 1932 and the Midspan studies. Br J Health Psychol 10:153–165, 2005

Hazzard WR, Blass JP, Ettinger WH, et al: Principles of Geriatric Medicine and Gerontology. New York, McGraw-Hill, 1999

Head D, Buckner RL, Shimony JS: Differential vulnerability of anterior white matter in nondemented aging with minimal acceleration in dementia of the Alzheimer type: evidence from diffusion tensor imaging. Cereb Cortex 14:410–423, 2004

Helson R, Jones CJ, Kwan SY: Personality, change over 40 years of adulthood: hierarchical linear modeling analysis of two longitudinal samples. J Pers Soc Psychol 83:752–766, 2002

Hinrichsen GA, Ramirez M: Black and White dementia caregivers: a comparison of their adaptation, adjustment, and service utilization. Gerontologist 32:375–381, 1992

Hoffman JM: Positron emission studies in dementia, in Brain Imaging in Clinical Psychiatry. Edited by Krishnan KRR, Doraiswamy PM. New York, Marcel Dekker, 1997, pp 533–573

Hooker K, McAdams DP: Personality reconsidered: a new agenda for aging research. J Gerontol B Sci Psychol Sci 58:P296–P304, 2003

Hooker K, Bowman SR, Coehlo DP, et al: Behavioral change in persons with dementia: relationships with mental and physical health of caregivers. J Gerontol B Sci Psychol Sci 57B:P453–P460, 2002

Horn JL: The theory of fluid and crystallized intelligence in relation to concepts of cognitive psychology and aging in adulthood, in Aging and Cognitive Processes. Edited by Craik F, Trehub S. New York, Plenum, 1982, pp 237–278

Huettel SA, Singerman JD, McCarthy G: The effects of aging upon the hemodynamic response measured by functional MRI. Neuroimage 13:161–175, 2001

Inagaki T: Socio-medical research of centenarian in Aichi prefecture. Bulletin of Kousei-in 21:59–70, 1995

Jackson J, Antonnucci TC, Brown E: A cultural lens on biopsychosocial models of aging, in Advances in Cell Aging and Gerontology, Vol 15: Recent Advances in Psychology and Aging. Edited by Costa P, Siegler I. New York, Elsevier, 2004, pp 221–241

Jobe JB, Smith DM, Ball K, et al: ACTIVE: a cognitive intervention trial to promote independence in older adults. Control Clin Trials 22:453–479, 2001

Jonassaint CR, Boyle SH, Williams RB, et al: Facets of the openness predict mortality in cardiac patients. Psychosom Med 68:319–322, 2007

Karasawa A: Declining of cognitive function in normal elderly. Brain Nerve 29:536–546, 1985

Kety SS: Human cerebral blood flow and oxygen consumption as related to aging. J Chronic Dis 3:478–486, 1956

Kliegel M, Zimprich D, Rott C: Life-long intellectual activities mediate the predictive effect of early education on cognitive impairment in centenarians: a retrospective study. Aging Ment Health 8:430–437, 2004

Kramer AF, Madden DJ: Attention, in The Handbook of Aging and Cognition, 3rd Edition. Edited by Craik FIM, Salthouse TA. New York, Psychology Press, 2008, pp 189–245

Lett HS, Blumenthal JA, Babyak MA, et al: Social support and prognosis in patients at increased psychosocial risk recovering from myocardial infarction. Health Psychol 26:418–427, 2007

Lindenberger U: Lifespan theories of cognitive development, in International Encyclopedia of the Social and Behavioral Sciences. Edited by Smelser, NJ, Baltes PB. Amsterdam, Netherlands, Elsevier, 2001, pp 8848–8854

Madden DJ: Speed and timing of behavioral processes, in Handbook of the Psychology of Aging, 5th Edition. Edited by Birren JE, Schaie KW. San Diego, CA, Academic Press, 2001, pp 288–312

Madden DJ: Aging and visual attention. Curr Dir Psychol Sci 16:70–74, 2007

Madden DJ, Whiting W: Age-related changes in visual attention, in Advances in Cell Aging and Gerontology, Vol 15: Recent Advances in Psychology and Aging. Edited by Costa P, Siegler I. New York, Elsevier, 2004, pp 41–88

Madden DJ, Whiting WL, Huettel SA: Age-related changes in neural activity during visual perception and attention, in Cognitive Neuroscience of Aging: Linking Cognitive and Cerebral Aging. Edited by Cabeza R, Nyberg L. Park D. Oxford, UK, Oxford University Press, 2005, pp 157–185

Madden DJ, Spaniol J, Whiting WL, et al: Adult age differences in the functional neuroanatomy of visual attention: a combined fMRI and DTI study. Neurobiol Aging 28:459–476, 2007

Markides K (ed): Encyclopedia of Health and Aging. Thousand Oaks, CA, Sage, 2007

Marcus D, Wang T, Parker J, et al: Open Access Series of Imaging Studies (OASIS): cross-sectional MRI data in young, middle aged, nondemented, and demented older adults. J Cogn Neurosci 19:1498–1507, 2007

Martin P, Rott C, Poon LW: A molecular view of coping behavior in older adults. J Aging Health 13:72–91, 2001

Martin P, Long MV, Poon LW: Age changes and differences in personality traits and states of the old and very old. J Gerontol B Sci Psychol Sci 57:P144–P152, 2002

Martin P, da Rosa G, Siegler I, et al: Personality and longevity: findings from the Georgia Centenarian Study. Age 28:343–352, 2006

Martin P, Kliegel M, Rott C, et al: Age differences and changes of coping behavior in three age groups: findings from the Georgia Centenarian Study. Int J Aging Hum Dev (in press)

McDaniel MA, Jacoby LL, Einstein GO: New considerations in aging and memory: the glass may be half full, in The Handbook of Aging and Cognition, 3rd Edition. Edited by Craik FIM, Salthouse TA. New York, Psychology Press, 2008, pp 251–310

McIntosh AR, Sekuler AB, Penpeci C, et al: Recruitment of unique neural systems to support visual memory in normal aging. Curr Biol 9:1275–1278, 1999

Mesulam MM: Large-scale neurocognitive networks and distributed processing for attention, language, and memory. Ann Neurol 28:597–613, 1990

Mizutani T, Shimada H: Neuropathological background of twenty-seven centenarian brains. J Neurol Sci 108:168–177, 1992

Mori S, Zhang J: Principles of diffusion tensor imaging and its applications to basic neuroscience research. Neuron 51:527–539 2006

Moseley M: Diffusion tensor imaging and aging—a review. NMR Biomed 15:553–560, 2002

Mroczek DK, Spiro A: Modeling intraindividual change in personality traits: findings from the Normative Aging Study. J Gerontol B Sci Psychol Sci 58:P153–P165, 2003

Mroczek DK, Spiro A III, Griffin PW: Personality and aging, in Handbook of the Psychology of Aging, 6th Edition. Edited by Birren JE, Schaie KW. New York, Academic, 2006, pp 363–377

Nagy Z, Vatter-Bittner B, Braak H, et al: Staging of Alzheimer-type pathology: an interrater-intrarater study. Dementia Geriatr Cogn Disord 8:248–251, 1997

Nielson KA, Langenecker SA, Garavan H: Differences in the functional neuroanatomy of inhibitory control across the adult life span. Psychol Aging 17:56–71, 2002

Oosterman JM, Sergeant JA, Weinstein HC, et al: Timed executive functions and white matter in aging with and without cardiovascular risk factors. Rev Neurosci 15:439–462, 2004

Perls TT, Silver MH: Living to 100: Lessons in Living to Your Maximum Potential at Any Age. New York, Basic Books, 1999

Pierce BH, Simons JS, Schacter DL: Aging and the seven sins of memory, in Advances in Cell Aging and Gerontology, Vol 15: Recent Advances in Psychology and Aging. Edited by Costa P, Siegler I. New York, Elsevier, 2004, pp 1–40

Poon LW, Siegler IC: Psychological aspects of normal aging, in Comprehensive Review of Geriatric Psychiatry. Edited by Sadavoy J, Lazarus LW, Jarvik LF. Washington, DC, American Psychiatric Press, 1991, pp 117–145

Poon LW, Clayton GM, Martin P, et al: The Georgia Centenarian Study. Int J Aging Hum Dev 34:1–17, 1992

Poon LW, Johnson M, Davey A, et al: Psycho-social predictors of survival among centenarians, in Autonomy Versus Dependence in the Oldest Old. Edited by Martin P, Rott C, Hagberg B, et al. New York, Springer, 2000, pp 77–89

Poon LW, Jazwinski SM, Green RC, et al: Methodological concerns and pitfalls in studying centenarians: lessons learned from the Georgia Centenarian Studies. Annual Review of Geriatrics and Gerontology, 2007, pp 231–264

Powell AL: Senile dementia of extreme aging: a common disorder of centenarians. Dementia 5:106–109, 1994

Rabbitt P, Lunn M, Wong D: Understanding terminal decline in cognition and risk of death: methodological and theoretical implications of practice and dropout effects. European Psychologist 11:164–171, 2006

Radloff LS: The CES-D scale: a self-report depression scale of research in the general population. Applied Psychological Measurement 1:385–401, 1977

Ramnani N, Behrens TE, Penny W, et al: New approaches for exploring anatomical and functional connectivity in the human brain. Biol Psychiatry 56:613–619, 2004

Ravaglia G, Forti P, De Ronchi D, et al: Prevalence and severity of dementia among northern Italian centenarians. Neurology 53:416–418, 1999

Raz N: The aging brain observed in vivo: Differential changes and their modifiers, in Cognitive Neuroscience of Aging: Linking

Cognitive and Cerebral Aging. Edited by Cabeza R, Nyberg L, Park D. Oxford, UK, Oxford University Press, 2005, pp 19–57

Raz N, Gunning-Dixon FM, Head D, et al: Neuroanatomical correlates of cognitive aging: evidence from structural magnetic resonance imaging. Neuropsychology 12:95–114, 1998

Raz N, Rodrigue KM, Acker JD: Hypertension and the brain: vulnerability of the prefrontal regions and executive functions. Behav Neurosci 117:1169–1180, 2003

Raz N, Lindenberger U, Rodrigue KM, et al: Regional brain changes in aging healthy adults: general trends, individual differences and modifiers. Cereb Cortex 15:1676–1689, 2005

Raz N, Rodrigue KM, Kennedy KM, et al: Vascular health and longitudinal changes in brain and cognition in middle-aged and older adults. Neuropsychology 21:149–157, 2007

Robine JM, Romieu I, Allard M: [French centenarians and their functional health status] (in French). Presse Med 32:360–364, 2003

Robinson RV, Jackson EF: Is trust in others declining in America? An age-period-cohort analysis. Soc Sci Res 30:117–145, 2001

Roth DL, Haley WE, Owen JE, et al: Latent growth models of the longitudinal effects of dementia caregiving: a comparison of African American and White family caregivers. Psychol Aging 16:427–436, 2001

Salat DH, Buckner RL, Snyder AZ, et al: Thinning of the cerebral cortex in aging. Cereb Cortex 14:721–730, 2004

Salat DH, Tuch DS, Greve DN, et al: Age-related alterations in white matter microstructure measured by diffusion tensor imaging. Neurobiol Aging 26:1215–1227, 2005

Salthouse TA: The processing-speed theory of adult age differences in cognition. Psychol Rev 103:403–428, 1996

Salthouse TA, Madden DJ: Information processing speed and aging, in Information Processing Speed in Clinical Populations. Edited by Deluca J, Kalmar J. New York, Psychology Press, 2007, pp 221–241

Samuelsson SM, Alfredson BB, Hagberg B, et al: The Swedish Centenarian Study: a multidisciplinary study of five consecutive cohorts at the age of 100. Int J Aging Hum Dev 45:223–253, 1997

Schaie KW: Intellectual Development in Adulthood: The Seattle Longitudinal Study. New York, Cambridge University Press, 1996

Schaie KW: Developmental Influences on Adult Intelligence: The Seattle Longitudinal Study. Oxford, UK, Oxford Press, 2005

Schaie KW, Willis SL: Can decline in adult intellectual functioning be reversed? Dev Psychol 22:223–232, 1986

Schaie KW, Zuo YL: Family environments and adult cognitive functioning, in Context of Intellectual Development. Edited by Sternberg RL, Grigorenko E. Hillsdale, NJ, Erlbaum, 2001, pp 337–361

Schneider BA, Pichora-Fuller MK: Implication of perceptual deterioration for cognitive aging research, in The Handbook of Aging and Cognition, 2nd Edition. Edited by Craik FIM, Salthouse TA. Mahwah, NJ, Erlbaum, 2000, pp 155–219

Schulz R, Martire LM: Family caregiving of persons with dementia. Am J Geriatr Psychiatry 12:240–249, 2004

Scialfa CT: The role of sensory factors in cognitive aging research. Can J Exp Psychol 56:153–163, 2002

Shenkin SD, Starr JM, Deary IJ: Birth weight and cognitive ability in childhood: a systematic review. Psychol Bull 130:989–1013, 2004

Shimonaka Y, Nakazato K, Homma A: Personality, longevity, and successful aging among Tokyo Metropolitan centenarians. Int J Aging Hum Dev 42:173–187, 1996

Siegler IC: The psychology of adult development and aging, in Handbook of Geriatric Psychiatry. Edited by Busse EW, Blazer DG. New York, Van Nostrand Reinhold, 1980, pp 169–221

Siegler IC: Developmental health psychology, in The Adult Years: Continuity and Change. Edited by Storandt MK, VandenBos GR. Washington, DC, American Psychological Association, 1989, pp 119–142

Siegler IC: Life course perspective on adult development, in Encyclopedia of Health and Aging. Edited by Markides K. Thousand Oaks, CA, Sage, 2007a, pp 324–326

Siegler IC: Psychology of aging and the public health. 2007 Developmental Health Award, division 20 and division 38. Invited Address presented at the Annual Meeting of the American Psychological Association, San Francisco, CA, [August] 2007b

Siegler IC, Poon LW: The psychology of aging, in Geriatric Psychiatry. Edited by Busse EW, Blazer DG. Washington, DC, American Psychiatric Press, 1989, pp 163–201

Siegler IC, Poon LW, Madden DJ, et al: Psychological aspects of normal aging, in The American Psychiatric Press Textbook of Geriatric Psychiatry, 2nd Edition. Edited by Busse EW, Blazer DG. Washington, DC, American Psychiatric Press, 1996, pp 105–127

Siegler IC, Costa PT, Brummett BH, et al: Patterns of change in hostility from college to midlife in the UNC Alumni Heart Study. Psychosom Med 65:738–745, 2003

Siegler IC, Poon LW, Madden DJ, et al: Psychological aspects of normal aging, psychological aspects of normal aging, in The American Psychiatric Press Textbook of Geriatric Psychiatry, 3rd Edition. Edited by Blazer DG, Steffens DC, Busse EW. Washington, DC, American Psychiatric Press, 2004, pp 121–138

Siegler IC, Vitaliano PP, Brummett BH, et al: Midlife caregiving, self-rated health and disease outcomes in middle aged caregivers in the UNC Alumni Heart Study. Abstract presented at 9th International Congress of Behavioral Medicine, Bangkok, Thailand, November 2006. Available at http://neuroscience.mahidol.ac.th/9icbm-2006/download/9ICBM_ProgramBook_6C.pdf. Accessed October 11, 2007.

Silver MH, Jilinskaia E, Perls TT: Cognitive functional status of age-confirmed centenarians in a population-based study. J Geront Series B Psychol Sci Soc Sci 56:134–140, 2001

Silver MH, Newell K, Brady C, et al: Distinguishing between neurodegenerative disease and disease-free aging: correlating neuropsychological evaluations and neuropathological studies in centenarians. Psychosom Med 64:493–501, 2002

Small BJ, Hertzog C, Hultsch DF, et al: Stability and change in adult personality over 6 years: findings from the Victoria Longitudinal Study. J Gerontol B Sci Psychol Sci 58:P166–P176, 2003

Snowdon DA, Greiner LH, Kemper SJ, et al: Linguistic ability in early life and longevity: findings from the Nun Study, in The Paradoxes of Longevity. Edited by Robine J, Forette B, Franceschi C, et al. Heidelberg, Germany, Springer, 1999, pp 103–113

Sobel E, Louhija J, Sulkava R, et al: Lack of association of apolipoprotein E allele epsilon 4 with late-onset Alzheimeŕs disease among Finnish centenarians. Neurology 45:903–907, 1995

Soderlund H, Nilsson LG, Berger K, et al: Cerebral changes on MRI and cognitive function: the CASCADE study. Neurobiol Aging 27:16–23, 2006

Steffens DC: MRI and MRS in dementia, in Brain Imaging in Clinical Psychiatry. Edited by Krishnan KRR, Doraiswamy PM. New York, Marcel Dekker, 1997, pp 503–532

Stevens A, Owen J, Roth D, et al: Predictors of time to nursing home placement in White and African American individuals with dementia. J Aging Health 16:375–397, 2004

Sullivan EV, Pfefferbaum A: Diffusion tensor imaging and aging. Neurosci Biobehav Rev 30:749–761, 2006

Suls J, Bunde J: Anger, anxiety, and depression as risk factors for cardiovascular disease: the problems and implications of overlapping affective dimensions. Psychol Bull 131:260–300, 2005

Terracciano A, McCrae RR, Brant LJ: Hierarchical linear modeling analyses of NEO-PI-R scales in the Baltimore Longitudinal Study of Aging. Psychol Aging 20:493–506, 2005

Terracciano A, McCrae RR, Costa PT: Longitudinal trajectories in Guilford-Zimmerman Temperament Survey data: results from the Baltimore Longitudinal Study of Aging. J Gerontol B Sci Psychol Sci 61:P108–P116, 2006

Tisserand DJ, Jolles J: On the involvement of prefrontal networks in cognitive ageing. Cortex 39:1107–1128, 2003

Tisserand DJ, McIntosh AR, van der Veen FM, et al: Age-related reorganization of encoding networks directly influences subsequent recognition memory. Brain Res Cogn Brain Res 25:8–18, 2005

Twenge JM: The age of anxiety? Birth cohort change in anxiety and neuroticism, 1952–1993. J Pers Soc Psychol 79:1007–1021, 2000

Tyas SL, Salazar JC, Snowdon DA, et al: Transitions to mild cognitive impairments, dementia, and death: findings from the Nun Study. Am J Epidemiol 165:1231–1238, 2007

van den Heuvel DM, ten Dam VH, de Craen AJ, et al: Increase in periventricular white matter hyperintensities parallels decline in mental processing speed in a non-demented elderly population. J Neurol Neurosurg Psychiatry 77:149–153, 2006

Verhagen P, Marcoen A, Goossens L: Improving memory performance in the aged through mnemonic training: a meta-analytic study. Psychol Aging 7:242–251, 1992

Whalley LJ, Deary IJ: Longitudinal cohort study of childhood IQ and survival up to age 76. Br Med J 322:819, 2001

Whalley LJ, Starr JM, Athawes R, et al: Childhood mental ability and dementia. Neurology 55:1455–1459, 2000

Welsh-Bohmer KA, Breitner JCS, Hayden KM, et al: Modifying dementia risk and trajectories of cognitive decline in aging: The Cache County Memory Study. Alzheimers Dement 2:257–260, 2006

West RL: An application of prefrontal cortex function theory to cognitive aging. Psychol Bull 120:272–292, 1996

Williams RB: Coping skills training in different cultures: the LifeSkills experience. Poster presented at the First Conference of the Central Eastern European Society of Behavioral Medicine, Pecs, Hungary, August 20–22, 2007

Williams RB, Barefoot JC, Schneiderman N: Psychosocial risk factors for cardiovascular disease: more than one culprit at work. JAMA 290:2190–2191, 2003

Williams VP, Williams RB: LifeSkills: 8 Simple Ways to Build Stronger Relationships, Communicate More Clearly, Improve your Health and Even the Health of Those Around You. New York, Times Books/Random House, 1999

Willis SE, Tennstedt SI, Marsiske M, et al: Long-term effects of cognitive training on everyday functional outcomes in older adults. JAMA 296:2805–2814, 2006

Wilson RS, Beck TL, Bienias JL, et al: Terminal cognitive decline: accelerated loss of cognition in the last years of life. Psychsom Med 69:131–137, 2007

Wolinsky F, Unverzagt F, Smith D, et al: The ACTIVE cognitive training trial and health-related quality of life: protection that lasts for 5 years. J Gerontol A Med Sci 61:1324–1329, 2006

Yetkin FZ, Fischer ME, Papke RA, et al: Focal hyperintensities in cerebral white matter or MR Images of asyptomatic volunteers: correlation with social and medical histories. American Journal of Reontgenology 161:855–858, 1993

Young H, Vitaliano P: Method in health psychology: relevance to aging, in Handbook of Health Psychology and Aging. Edited by Aldwin CM, Park CL, Spiro A. New York, Guilford, 2007, pp 54–74

Zacks RT, Hasher L, Li KZHL: Human memory, in The Handbook of Aging and Cognition, 2nd Edition. Edited by Craik FIM, Salthouse TA. Mahwah, NJ, Erlbaum, 2000, pp 293–357

Suggested Readings

Carstensen LL, Hartel CR (eds): When I'm 64. Washington, DC, National Academies Press, 2006

Costa PT Jr, Siegler IC (eds): Recent Advances in Psychology and Aging. Amsterdam, Elsevier, 2004

Dilworth-Anderson P, Valle R, Fazio S: Introduction. Alzheimer Dis Assoc Disord 19(suppl):249, 2005

Friedman HS, Martin LR: A lifespan approach to personality and longevity: the case of conscientiousness, in Handbook of Health Psychology and Aging. Edited by Aldwin CM, Park CL, Spiro A. New York, Guilford, 2007, pp 167–185

Gondo Y, Poon LW: Biopsychosocial approaches to longevity, in Annual Review of Gerontology and Geriatrics. Edited by Poon LW, Perls T. New York, Springer, 2007, pp 129–149

Schaie KW: Developmental Influences on Adult Intelligence: The Seattle Longitudinal Study. Oxford, UK, Oxford Press, 2005

Willis SE, Tennstedt SI, Marsiske M, et al: Long-term effects of cognitive training on everyday functional outcomes in older adults. JAMA 296:2805–2814, 2006

Wilson RS, Beck TL, Bienias JL, et al: Terminal cognitive decline: accelerated loss of cognition in the last years of life. Psychsom Med 69:131–137, 2007

CHAPTER 8

Social and Economic Factors Related to Psychiatric Disorders in Late Life

Linda K. George, Ph.D.

A comprehensive examination of geriatric psychiatry must include the perspectives of multiple disciplines. The authors of previous chapters addressed the physiological, neurological, and psychological changes that accompany the aging process. In this chapter, I examine the social and economic conditions of late life. (For the sake of convenience, henceforth the shorter term *social factors* will be used, although economic factors also are addressed.) Particular attention is paid to the ways that social conditions serve as risk factors for psychiatric disorders, as contingencies that affect the course and outcome of mental illness, and as determinants of mental health service utilization.

An adequate depiction of psychiatric disorders must include a dynamic perspective. The experience of psychiatric disorders varies over time as patients experience onset and remission of symptoms. Help-seeking and the course of care also are longitudinal phenomena. The distinctive features of geriatric psychiatry are affected by additional dynamic processes. The aging process itself leads to intraindividual changes that can affect the risk of developing psychiatric disorders and/or the use of mental health services. In addition, the effects of social change—generating cohort differences—also must be examined because, over time, social and economic factors change substantially across cohorts entering and traversing late life. These cohort differences have important implications for generalizing results across cohorts and for using current knowledge to plan for the future.

Given the importance of age changes versus cohort differences in drawing conclusions about the role of social factors in geriatric psychiatry, these terms merit closer examination. *Age changes* occur in organisms simply as a function of age. True age changes will be observed with considerable regularity across time and place because they are developmental. Most biological phenomena, as well as some psychological and social characteristics, that change with age appear to be driven by this kind of internal, developmental agenda. Other differences observed across age groups represent the effects of social changes that are external to the individual. The term *cohort* is used to refer to groups of people born at specific times—for example, the 1940 cohort consists of all persons born in 1940. Cohorts that experience different historical and environmental conditions often differ in ways that reflect those external conditions rather than developmental changes. Without longitudinal data from multiple cohorts, it is difficult to empirically distinguish between age changes and cohort differences. Moreover, some phenomena are affected by

This work was supported by a grant from the John Templeton Foundation.

both age changes and cohort differences (see, e.g., Lynch 2006).

Although it is difficult to separate age changes from cohort differences, this distinction is important for three reasons. First, the distinction is critical to attributions of etiology or causality. In their pure forms, age changes reflect developmental phenomena, and cohort differences reflect the effects of social or environmental conditions. Second, the distinction is relevant to the generalizability of research findings. If a risk factor for psychiatric disorders changes with age, the observed pattern will be broadly applicable across cohorts. If a risk factor differs across age groups because of differences in environmental exposure, the effects of that risk factor may be cohort specific. Third, the distinction between age changes and cohort differences is important for the design of interventions. If levels of a risk factor differ substantially across cohorts, interventions can be targeted to the environmental conditions that place certain cohorts at greatest risk. If, instead, a risk factor changes with age, interventions must be targeted toward alteration of a developmental trajectory.

In this chapter, then, I examine two dynamic phenomena simultaneously. First, I address the processes underlying the occurrence of psychiatric disorders and mental health service utilization from a social perspective. Second, I consider the degree to which social factors associated with psychiatric disorders and/or mental health service use change with age or differ across cohorts.

This chapter is organized in five sections. The first focuses on social characteristics as risk factors for psychiatric disorders in later life. The social factors examined include demographic variables (such as race and gender), indicators of social integration (such as social roles and the availability of social support), socioeconomic status, and the experience of acute and chronic stress. The second section examines the degree to which exposure to social risk factors for psychiatric disorders changes with age and varies across cohorts. A central issue here is whether current cohorts of younger and middle-aged adults have experienced or will confront environmental conditions that place them at more or less risk for psychiatric disorders than current cohorts of older adults. The third section focuses on the impact of social factors on the course and outcome of psychiatric disorders in later life. The central question of interest is whether social factors alter the probability or timing of recovery. The fourth section addresses social factors as determinants of mental health service use among older adults. An important distinction is made between help-seeking (which reflects the decisions and behaviors of individuals needing mental health services) and provider behavior (i.e., how clinicians respond to older persons presenting with psychiatric problems). The final section of the chapter examines the impact of social and economic policies on older adults. These policies and programs have both direct impact—by affecting the likelihood of help-seeking for psychiatric problems—and indirect impact—by affecting some social risk factors for mental illness, and thereby influencing the psychiatric status of the older population.

Social Risk Factors for Psychiatric Disorders

Theoretical Model

A consensual model of the precursors of psychiatric disorders has emerged in the social science, epidemiological, and social psychiatry literatures. The model remains flexible in terms of specific operationalizations and statistical estimation, but an overarching theoretical orientation has been forged. Table 8–1 presents the general conceptual model that emerges from previous research. It is a stage model in that each higher stage represents what are hypothesized to be increasingly proximate antecedents of psychiatric disorders.

The first stage consists of demographic variables that are associated with the risk of psychiatric disorders. Virtually all studies of social factors and psychiatric disorders include demographic factors, especially age, race/ethnicity, and sex. The causal mechanisms that underlie these relationships are unclear, however. One suggested explanation is that demographic factors serve as proxies for more mechanistic social factors. For example, the greater prevalence of depressive symptoms reported by women compared with men may be due to gender differences in other risk factors such as marital status, income, and exposure to stress. Alternatively, demographic variables may serve as proxies for biological mechanisms. In this review, I emphasize the social meanings of demographic variables. However, possible biological mechanisms should not be overlooked. Indeed, most research emphasizes the multiple types of risk factors that are implicated in the etiology of psychiatric morbidity.

Stages II and III of the model represent events and achievements relevant to mental health outcomes that are distinguished primarily by their timing and recency. Stage II consists of relatively early experiences that are

TABLE 8–1. Stage model of the social precursors of psychiatric disorders

Stage	Name	Illustrative indicators
I	Demographic variables	Age, sex, race/ethnicity
II	Early events and achievements	Education, childhood traumas
III	Later events and achievements	Occupation, income, marital status, fertility
IV	Social integration	Personal attachments to social structure (e.g., religious participation, community roles) Environmental context (e.g., neighborhood stability, economic climate)
V	Vulnerability and protective factors	Social support versus isolation, chronic stressors
VI	Provoking agents and coping efforts	Life events, coping strategies

hypothesized to have persistent effects on an individual's vulnerability to psychiatric disorders. Examples of such experiences include childhood traumas (e.g., the early death or marital disruption of parents) and educational attainment. Stage III consists of later events and experiences, including family relationships and economic achievements. In most studies, stage III indicators are based on the *current* status of individuals, reinforcing the temporal distinction between stage II and stage III. Causal interpretation of relationships between risk factors and psychiatric outcomes is uncertain. For example, some investigators view higher levels of education and income as resources that facilitate effective coping; others view them as tapping exposure to environments (e.g., occupational and residential settings) that directly affect psychiatric status. There are undoubtedly multiple mechanisms by which these factors affect mental health.

Stage IV consists of dimensions of social integration. Social integration occurs at two levels. At the *individual* level, social integration refers to personal attachments to formal aspects of the social structure (religious affiliation and participation in organizations are two examples). At the *aggregate* level, social integration refers to the extent to which a collectivity (e.g., a city, a country) is characterized by meaningful ties and a sense of collective identity among residents. Early studies of psychiatric epidemiology linked social integration at the aggregate level with lower rates of mental disorder (Leighton 1959). More recent research focuses exclusively on social integration at the individual level. The rationale for examining social integration as a risk factor for psychiatric disorders is that lack of social integration is believed to be psychologically stressful, restrict opportunities for social interaction and development of new social relationships, make informational support more difficult, and impede effective coping. Note that social integration is not synonymous with social support. Social support is a product of close, intimate relationships, whereas social integration involves more formal and less personal interactions.

Finally, the risk factors in stages V and VI have received the greatest empirical attention. *Vulnerability and protective factors* (stage V) refers to personal assets and liabilities that alter the probabilities of psychiatric problems. Chronic stressors are primary examples of vulnerability factors, and social support is an illustration of a protective factor. *Provoking agents and coping efforts* (stage VI) is more specific and proximate than vulnerability and protective factors. Life events have been the primary provoking agents examined in previous research and are viewed as sudden sources of stress that may be sufficiently severe to trigger the onset of psychiatric morbidity, especially in the presence of other risk factors. Coping efforts refer to the specific actions taken to confront a stressor. Effective coping may either prevent stresses from generating negative mental health outcomes or minimize their effects. Stages V and VI are distinguished primarily by specificity and immediacy. For example, although life events and chronic stressors both generate stress, life events are more discrete and bounded. Similarly, social support is a generalized resource for defusing stress, whereas coping efforts are specific to particular stressors.

The model in Table 8–1 should be viewed as a heuristic abstraction—as a useful way of summarizing the literature on social risk factors for psychiatric disorders. Undoubtedly, some researchers would classify the social precursors of psychiatric morbidity in somewhat different categories. Moreover, most studies do not include all the categories of risk factors included in this model. Nonetheless, most studies implicitly or explicitly adopt both the basic categories of risk factors and their ordering. Thus far, the conceptual framework depicted in Table 8–1 has been described in terms of direct effects—that is, the relationships, either bivariate or multivariate, between risk factors and psychiatric outcomes. An additional complexity is the possibility of interactive effects—that the effects of one risk factor are contingent on the presence or level of another risk factor.

In theory, any combination of risk factors may interact to alter the risk of psychiatric disorders. Evidence of such interactions is included in this chapter. I will use one illustration at this point to describe the potential importance of risk factor interactions: the frequently hypothesized interaction between life events and social support. Some investigators propose that life events and social support exert independent effects on mental health outcomes, with life events increasing the risk of psychiatric disorders and social support reducing the risk. This is a direct effects hypothesis. Other investigators suggest that social support buffers the effects of life events on psychiatric outcomes, maintaining that life events increase the risk of psychiatric disorders only (or primarily) among persons who lack adequate social support. This is an interactive hypothesis. Direct versus interactive effects are not mutually exclusive. It is possible, for example, that life events and social support directly affect mental health and that life events are especially damaging in the absence of social support. Thus, examination of the social precursors of psychiatric disorders includes consideration of not only multiple risk factors but also their interrelationships.

As presented here, there is nothing distinctively age related about the conceptual framework in Table 8–1. This general conceptual model can be used to examine age/cohort differences in the relationships between social risk factors and psychiatric disorders, age changes in those relationships, and variability within the older population with regard to those relationships. In this way, the distinctiveness of psychiatric disorders in later life can be empirically revealed.

Methodological Issues

Measurement of Psychiatric Disorders

Psychiatric disorders have been operationalized in a variety of ways. Two dimensions underlie most of this variability: 1) the use of diagnostic versus symptom measures and 2) the degree to which the measures tap general psychopathology versus specific diagnostic categories. With regard to the first dimension, some instruments are designed to measure psychiatric disorders using formal diagnostic criteria, typically DSM-III-R or DSM-IV-TR criteria (American Psychiatric Association 1987, 2000), Feighner diagnostic criteria (Feighner et al. 1972), or Research Diagnostic Criteria (Spitzer et al. 1978). Other measures are symptom scales in which higher numbers of symptoms are assumed to represent more severe morbidity. Examples include the Center for Epidemiologic Studies Depression Scale (Radloff 1977) and the Beck Depression Inventory (Beck et al. 1961, 1988). Diagnostic and symptom measures can yield different conclusions. For example, several studies suggest that older people report more depressive symptoms, on average, than middle-aged and younger adults (Adams et al. 2004) but that the prevalence of major depressive disorder is lower among older than younger adults (Blazer et al. 1994; Hopcroft and Bradley 2007; Steffens et al. 2000). (The identification of "cases" of depressive disorder is described in Chapter 15, "Mood Disorders.")

The second dimension applies primarily to symptom measures. Some scales include symptoms from a spectrum of disorders and generate measures of global psychopathology. Others measure symptoms within a single diagnostic category, such as depression or anxiety. The use of global psychopathology measures is problematic because some risk factors may be important for certain disorders but irrelevant to others. For example, there are substantial—and opposite—gender differences in the prevalence of alcohol abuse or dependence and depression, whereas gender differences are minimal for many other disorders (e.g., R. C. Kessler et al. 1994).

Differences in measurement strategies, as well as in the specific assessment tools used, complicate cross-study comparisons. When studies reach inconsistent conclusions about the effects of a given risk factor, part of the variability in findings may be due to differences in measurement. On the other hand, when studies reach similar conclusions despite the use of different measurement strategies, confidence in those conclusions is increased.

Sample Composition

Sampling variability also accounts for some of the inconsistencies observed across studies. Not surprisingly, samples vary widely in size and composition. Small samples often result in statistical analyses that are "underpowered," and therefore meaningful relationships remain undetected. Compositional differences across samples affect the distributions of both psychiatric disorders and social risk factors. Consequently, sample size and composition must be taken into account when synthesizing research findings across studies.

The age compositions of the samples used in previous research are especially relevant to this chapter. Some previous studies of the relationships between social risk factors and psychiatric outcomes relied exclusively on data from older adults. Other studies used data from samples covering much broader age ranges—typically, all adults ages 18 years and older. These two types of samples generate different, but valuable, information. Studies based on samples of older adults provide in-depth views of how social factors operate during later life; however, such designs cannot be used to identify risk factor effects that are specific to old age. In contrast, data from age-heterogeneous samples can be used to determine 1) how the role of age itself is a risk factor and 2) whether other risk factors vary in direction or magnitude across age groups.

Cross-Sectional Versus Longitudinal Studies

As noted previously, the onset and course of psychiatric disorders are dynamic. Much of the early research on social factors and mental illness was based on cross-sectional data; however, more recently, longitudinal studies appropriately dominate the field. Cross-sectional studies can be used to document the existence of hypothesized associations, but they cannot provide evidence of temporal order. Furthermore, cross-sectional data cannot provide information about the lag between exposure to a risk factor and the onset of mental illness. Evidence of temporal order and lagged effects can be obtained only from longitudinal data.

To fully understand the dynamics of psychiatric disorders in later life, other kinds of longitudinal data also are needed. Specifically, information is needed about the extent to which exposure to social risk factors for psychiatric disorders changes with age and varies across cohorts.

Evidence Bearing on the Theoretical Model

Evidence relevant to the model in Table 8–1 can be extracted from previous research. Overall, the model receives considerable support, although the amount and quality of evidence vary across specific risk factors. One limitation of the research base is that the vast majority of research focuses on geriatric depression. Consequently, this review focuses primarily on depression in late life; other disorders are discussed when possible.

Demographic Variables

Age is related to the risk of psychiatric disorders, but the associations are complex and often inconsistent across studies. Using symptom scales measuring global psychiatric symptoms, a few older studies found higher levels of symptoms among older adults, but most reported the absence of meaningful age differences. Evidence is most plentiful with regard to depressive symptoms. Older adults, especially the very old, usually report levels of depressive symptoms equal to or higher than those reported by younger and middle-aged adults (Blazer et al. 1991; Mirowsky and Ross 1992; Schieman et al. 2002). In studies of age differences within the older population, depressive symptoms are highest among the oldest old (see Cole and Dendukuri 2003 for a meta-analysis). In contrast, studies of psychiatric disorders (as opposed to symptom levels) demonstrate lower current and lifetime prevalence among older than among younger adults for all nonorganic psychiatric disorders (Robins and Regier 1991). Whether these age differences reflect cohort differences has not been definitively answered. Nonetheless, there is increasing consensus that there are significant cohort effects, as implied by the lower *lifetime* prevalence of depression among older adults. That is, it appears that every new generation exhibits higher rates of depressive disorder than its predecessors (Burke et al. 1991; R.C. Kessler et al. 1994; Levenson et al. 1998). The latter two studies report similar patterns for alcohol abuse and dependence.

Evidence concerning gender differences in psychiatric morbidity is also mixed. Older women report higher levels of psychiatric symptoms, especially depressive symptoms, than do men (Beekman et al. 1999; Hopcroft and Bradley 2007). The results of studies based on diagnoses, however, suggest that global symptom scales mask considerable variation across specific disorders. Affective and somatic disorders are more prevalent among women, alcohol and substance abuse are more common among men, and schizophrenia and most anxiety disorders are unrelated to gender (R.C. Kessler et al. 1994). Some evidence suggests that gender differences in depression narrow substantially in later life. Henderson et al. (1993) found higher rates of depressive symptoms among older women than among older men but no gender difference in rates of major depressive disorder. Similarly, gender was not a significant predictor of the onset of major depression among older adults in a prospective U.S. study (George 1992). In a prospective study in the Netherlands, however, Schoevers et al. (2000) found a higher incidence of major depression among older women than among older men.

Evidence concerning the relationship between race/ethnicity and psychiatric morbidity was mixed in earlier studies. Recent research, however, indicates that minority groups report levels of psychiatric symptoms comparable to those of whites (Blazer et al. 1998; Evans-Campbell et al. 2007) and have rates of psychiatric disorder that are no higher, and may be lower, than those of whites (Breslau et al. 2005, 2006). U.S. minority groups include higher proportions of immigrants than do whites. There is compelling evidence, however, that immigrants are less likely than their U.S.-born counterparts to have psychiatric disorders. This pattern has been observed for Latinos (Breslau et al. 2007a, 2007b), Asians (Breslau and Chang 2006), and Caribbean blacks (Neighbors et al. 2007). This issue is further complicated by substantial differences in education and income between whites and racial/ethnic minorities. When socioeconomic status is statistically controlled, the mental health advantage of racial/ethnic minorities is even larger.

Early Events and Achievements

Considerable evidence indicates that early events and achievements have persistent effects on psychiatric status throughout adulthood. Education is most strongly related to psychiatric morbidity in later life. (An advantage of examining education rather than income is that education is less likely to be affected by mental illness; thus, even in cross-sectional studies, causal direction can be assumed with some confidence.) High levels of depressive symptoms in late life are strongly related to low levels of education (Beekman et al. 1999; Cairney and Krause 2005; Ross and Mirowsky 2006). The strength of education as a risk factor for the onset of major depressive disorder is less clear. In a U.S. study, education was not significantly related to the onset of major depressive disorder in a community sample (George 1992). In contrast, in a recent study in the Netherlands, education was a significant predictor of incident cases of major depression among older adults (Koster et al. 2006).

Strong evidence shows that childhood traumas place individuals at increased risk of psychiatric morbidity. Parental divorce/separation, parental problem drinking, childhood physical and/or sexual abuse, and childhood poverty are significant risk factors for a variety of psychiatric disorders, especially depression, during adulthood (Brown and Harris 1978; R.C. Kessler et al. 1997; Landerman et al. 1991; Molnar et al. 2001; Ross and Mirowsky 1999), although only one study focused specifically on older adults (Kraaij and de Wilde 2001). Childhood adversities also appear to increase vulnerability to stressful life events during adulthood (Kraaij and de Wilde 2001; Landerman et al. 1991; Ross and Mirowsky 1999). That is, childhood adversities interact with recent stressors to increase the likelihood of depressive symptoms and disorder. This may be one of the mechanisms by which childhood problems exert persistent effects on adult mental health.

Later Events and Achievements

Current and/or recent life conditions also are related to the risk of psychiatric disorder. Income and—to a lesser extent—occupation are related to psychiatric disorder, with low income and low occupational prestige increasing risk during adulthood (R.C. Kessler et al. 1994; Robins and Regier 1991). Low income also is a risk factor for both depressive symptoms (Beekman et al. 1999; Harris et al. 2003; Kraaij and de Wilde 2001) and the onset of major depressive disorder (Koster et al. 2006) in late life. These relationships are observed using both symptom scales and diagnostic measures. Retirement is obviously a common transition in later life—a transition that removes individuals from the occupational structure and results in substantial income loss. Nonetheless, there is no evidence that retirement increases the risk of psychiatric disorders (Kim and Moen 2002; Midinik et al. 1995).

The relationship between marital status and psychiatric disorders remains ambiguous despite considerable research. In general, marital status appears to be weakly associated with psychiatric morbidity, regardless of whether symptom scales or diagnostic measures are used (Robins and Regier 1991). In studies of depression in community-dwelling older adults, the unmarried adults reported significantly more symptoms of depression than did the married adults (Blazer et al. 1991; Cairney and Krause 2005; Jones-Webb and Snowden 1993), with other risk factors statistically controlled. Two caveats, however, should be observed. First, undesirable changes in marital status appear to have negative effects on mental health, especially in the first year after marital disruption (typically widowhood in late life) (e.g., Adams et al. 2004; Choi and Bohman 2007). Changes in marital status, however, are typically examined as stressful life events rather than marital status changes. Second, the protective effects of marriage are confounded with measures of social support. Thus, in multivariate models, the effects of marital status are largely explained by stressful life events and social support.

Barrett (2000) examined the effects of marital *history* rather than marital status on psychiatric disorders. Marital history captures sources of heterogeneity that are ignored by measures of current marital status (e.g., among the currently married are individuals in first marriages as well as persons who have been married two or more times, and among the remarried, some previous marriages ended in divorce and others by widowhood). In general, Barrett found that marital history has significant effects on mental illness, over and above current marital status, but only for women. Regardless of the cause of the marital dissolution, remarried women were at significantly higher risk for depression than women married only once. Not surprisingly, perhaps, women who had been widowed more than once were at greater risk for depression than those widowed only once.

Social Integration

Although interest in social integration at the individual level as a risk factor for psychiatric morbidity is relatively recent, the research base is growing rapidly. Available evidence suggests that social integration plays a significant role in protecting individuals from psychiatric symptoms and disorders. Religious participation is the dimension of social integration that has received the most attention. A growing body of research suggests that attending religious services and participating in other religious activities are associated with a decreased risk of psychiatric morbidity, including alcohol abuse (Koenig et al. 1994; Neff and Husaini 1985), anxiety disorders (Koenig et al. 1993a, 1993b), and depression (Koenig et al. 1997; Mitchell et al. 1993). In a study based on data from six European countries, Braam et al. (2001) found that religious attendance was significantly associated with fewer depressive symptoms among older adults. In addition, at the population level, symptoms of depression were lower in countries with higher levels of religious involvement. Tepper et al. (2001) reported that among the chronically mentally ill, religious participants had fewer symptoms and higher functioning than their nonreligious peers.

Religious involvement has multiple dimensions (e.g., service attendance, denomination, private religious practices, religious coping—the latter is discussed below in the section "Provoking Agents and Coping Efforts"), and it is increasingly clear that 1) these dimensions are differentially important for mental health outcomes and 2) the multiple dimensions require systematic investigation to fully document the relationships between religious involvement and mental health. Kendler et al. (2003) reported that different dimensions of religious involvement are associated with internalizing versus externalizing psychiatric disorders. In an examination of depression and religious preference, Kennedy et al. (1996) found that both the prevalence and incidence of clinically significant depression are higher among Jews than among members of other religious denominations. There is much more to be learned about the complex relationships between religion and psychiatric morbidity, but it is clear that religion is a protective factor for many older adults.

Evidence suggests that participation in voluntary organizations has mental health benefits for adults of all ages (Grusky et al. 1985) and older adults in particular (Adams et al. 2004). Volunteering in community organizations is even more strongly related to lower levels of depressive symptoms (Morrow-Howell et al. 2003; Musick and Wilson 2003). In addition, the studies of volunteering are based on longitudinal data; as such, they are methodologically superior to the cross-sectional studies of organizational participation.

Vulnerability and Protective Factors

Chronic stress has been the most frequently examined vulnerability factor. Several investigative teams have reported a robust relationship between persistent financial problems and depressive symptoms in later life (Bruce and Hof 1994; Wilson et al. 2007)—an association also observed among all adults (Mirowsky and Ross 1999; Ross and Huber 1985).

Chronic illness, other health problems, and disability are especially strong risk factors for psychiatric disorder in later life, especially for depression. A large body of evidence indicates that chronic physical illness is strongly associated with both the prevalence of clinically significant depression (e.g., Adams et al. 2004; Blazer et al. 1991; Braam et al. 2005; Moldin et al. 1993; Roberts et al. 1997; see also the meta-analysis by Cole and Dendukuri 2003) and the incidence of major depressive disorder (George 1992; Harris et al. 2005). Increased risk of depression during late life is associated with other health indicators, including cognitive impairment

(Blazer et al. 1991) and perceived poor health (Henderson et al. 1993; see also the meta-analysis by Cole and Dendukuri 2003). Disability—measured in terms of impairment in activities of daily living and independent activities of daily living—is an especially powerful predictor of both the prevalence (Bruce 2001; Harris et al. 2003; Katsumata et al. 2005; Mitchell et al. 1993; Oxman and Hull 2001; Roberts et al. 1997) and incidence (George 1992; Kennedy et al. 1990) of depression. In cross-sectional studies, determining causal order is problematic: depression may be either a consequence or a cause of disability and perceptions of poor health, and cognitive impairment may be a part of the depressive episode rather than an independent phenomenon. Some investigators have examined the possible reciprocal relationships between disability and depression in late life. It appears that although there are significant reciprocal relationships, the dominant effect is from disability to depression (Ormel et al. 2002). It also is likely that genetic factors are related to both chronic physical illness and mental illness (see Chapter 6, "Genetics," in this text).

An extensive body of research indicates that caregiving for a mentally or physically ill elderly adult represents a chronic stressor that can lead to psychiatric problems for the caregiver. Large numbers of older adults have caregiving responsibilities—usually for spouses, but sometimes for very old parents or siblings. To date, research examining the effects of caregiver burden on psychiatric morbidity has focused on family caregivers of elderly adults with dementia. Studies suggest that 30%–50% of caregivers of patients with dementia meet the criteria for a DSM-III or DSM-IV diagnosis of major depression (Schulz and Williamson 1991; Schulz et al. 1995; Song et al. 1997). Two meta-analyses of studies of caregivers of relatives with a wide range of physical and mental illnesses estimate that 22%–35% of caregivers have major depressive disorder (Cuijpers 2005; Pinquart and Sorensen 2006). Even larger proportions of caregivers suffer high levels of psychiatric symptoms, albeit below the threshold for diagnosis.

The primary protective factor examined in previous research has been social support. There is consensus that social support is a multidimensional phenomenon. Most investigators recognize at least three major dimensions: 1) social network—the size and structure of the network of people available to provide support, 2) instrumental support—the specific tangible services provided by families and friends, and 3) perceptions of social support—subjective evaluations of satisfaction with the available support. Some investigators examine a fourth dimension: informational support, defined as the extent to which family and friends provide information that can be used when assessing options and confronting stress. The level of interaction with friends and family and the presence or absence of a confidant also have been examined as indicators of social support.

Overwhelming evidence shows that social support protects older adults from psychiatric morbidity, especially depressive symptoms and disorder. The protective power of social support has been reported in numerous cross-sectional and longitudinal investigations. Available evidence suggests that specific dimensions of social support may be differentially important in protecting against late-life depression. Accumulated evidence suggests that having small social networks increases the risk of depression among community-dwelling older adults (Adams et al. 2004; Blazer et al. 1991; Choi and McDougall 2007; Oxman and Hull 2001). Lack of a confidant also has been related to higher levels of symptoms (Hays et al. 1998; Oxman et al. 1992). Levels of social interaction have consistently distinguished between depressed and nondepressed elders (Henderson et al. 1986; Oxman and Hull 1997; Oxman et al. 1992) but have not been shown to predict the onset of disorder. Some investigators have found that instrumental and informational support decrease the risk of depression, but these effects appear to be highly specific and dependent on the particular stressor under examination (Krause 1986; Mitchell et al. 1993). There is general consensus that perceptions of social support are strongly related to depression—and, unlike other dimensions, this conclusion has strong support in both cross-sectional (Harris et al. 2003; Jongenelis et al. 2004) and longitudinal studies (Brummett et al. 1998; George 1992; Harris et al. 2005; C.K. Holahan and Holahan 1987; Koizumi et al. 2005; Krause et al. 1989; Oxman and Hull 1997, 2001; Oxman et al. 1992).

The strong relationships between perceived support and depression have raised interpretive questions. Henderson (1984), for example, worried that the dysphoria associated with depression might "contaminate" perceptions of social support among depressed persons. Several studies appear to resolve this concern, however. First, even in longitudinal studies in which perceptions of social support were measured *before* the onset of depressive disorder, perceived support had a significant protective effect (George 1992; Harris et al. 2005; Koizumi et al.

2005; Krause et al. 1989; Oxman et al. 1992). Second, results from other longitudinal studies indicated that although perceived support significantly predicted the onset of depression, baseline levels of depression did not predict subsequent levels of support (Cronkite and Moos 1984; Krause et al. 1989). Thus, the dominant direction of causal influence appears to be from perceived support to depression rather than the reverse.

Information illuminating the relationships between social support and psychiatric disorders other than depression among older adults is meager. Several studies involving large proportions of older persons have indicated that the social networks of persons with schizophrenia are unusually small (Link et al. 1987). Grusky et al. (1985) reported that older persons with schizophrenia in the community have even smaller networks than do younger ones. Grusky et al. also found that the composition of the support networks of persons with schizophrenia differed, depending on illness severity. Persons with mild symptoms relied primarily on family members for social support. Individuals with severe symptoms relied primarily on nonfamily—usually formal service providers—for assistance. In one study, researchers compared the social networks of older adults with and without late-onset alcohol problems. Dupree et al. (1984) found that those with alcohol problems had much smaller networks than did their peers. All of these studies were based on cross-sectional data; thus, causal order is unclear. In the one longitudinal study available, Hays et al. (1998) found that social support helped prevent the onset of a bipolar episode among older patients with a history of manic depression but was unrelated to first episodes of bipolar disorder in late life.

Provoking Agents and Coping Efforts

Life events are the major provoking agents implicated in the onset of psychiatric disorders. Two major strategies have been used to study the effects of life events: 1) studies of aggregated life events (summing the number of events that individuals experience in a given time period) and 2) studies of specific life events (e.g., widowhood or retirement). The results of research based on both strategies suggest that negative life events are strongly related to increased risk of both psychiatric symptoms and specific psychiatric disorders, especially depression, alcohol abuse, and generalized anxiety. These relationships have been observed in both age-heterogeneous samples and samples of older adults; only the latter are referenced here (Adams et al. 2004; Cutrona et al. 1986; Dupree et al. 1984; George 1992; Hays et al. 1998; Jongenelis et al. 2004; Katsumata et al. 2005; Lam et al. 1996; Lynch and George 2002; Neff and Husaini 1985; see also the meta-analysis by Kraaij et al. 2002).

Several studies offer important details about the relationship between life events and depression in later life. Devanand et al. (2002) reported a dose-response relationship of sorts between life events and depressive disorder: "doses" of life events are highest among persons with major depressive disorder, intermediate among those with dysthymia, and lowest among those with depressive symptoms that do not meet diagnostic thresholds. Brilman and Ormel (2001) compared the effects of life events and daily "hassles" on major depressive disorder in late life. They reported that stressful life events multiplied the odds of disorder 22 times, compared to a threefold increase for daily hassles. Because hassles are more common, however, they account for a larger proportion of new depressive episodes. Nolen-Hoekoema and Ahrens (2002) made an important distinction between the incidence of stressful life events and their effects. Older adults experience fewer life events than younger adults, on average, but the strength of the association between stressful life events and depression does not differ by age.

With regard to specific events, bereavement is a particularly strong predictor of both depressive symptoms and disorder in late life (see meta-analysis by Cole and Dendukuri 2003). In a review of previous studies, Onrust and Cuijpers (2006) estimated that 22% of older widows and widowers meet DSM criteria for major depressive disorder during the first year of bereavement. Estimates differ regarding the length of time before the depression associated with bereavement resolves: Mendes de Leon et al. (1994) reported that the widowed have no greater depression than their married counterparts a year after widowhood; Turvey et al. (1999) reported that it is 2 years before depression dissipates among the widowed. Several studies have reported that widowers experience larger increases in depressive symptoms than do widows. Lee et al. (2001) contend that this pattern is due to the fact that married men report substantially fewer depressive symptoms than married women rather than that widowers and widows experience different levels of depressive symptoms.

Although the evidence is scant in volume, research suggests that cessation of driving also places older adults at increased risk of depressive symptoms and disorder (Fonda et al. 2001; Ragland et al. 2005; Windsor et al. 2007). It is interesting that it has taken more than half a century of research to uncover that driving cessation is a stressful and consequential life event for older adults.

Both common sense and social science theory suggest that adequate coping will partially determine whether stress has negative effects on mental health. Scientific efforts to delineate the nature and effects of coping have been fraught with problems; valid methods for assessing coping effectiveness remain unavailable. Studying coping effects is particularly problematic because different stressors elicit, permit, and require different coping strategies. Limited evidence suggests that coping methods alter the probability that stress will have negative effects on mental health; some of that evidence is based on samples of older adults (Blanchard-Fields and Irion 1988; Freund and Baltes 1998). More recent studies have focused on cognitive coping styles (e.g., denial, avoidance); for example, Klein et al. (2007) examined the relationship between cognitive coping styles and depressive symptoms among heart failure patients. Nonetheless, investigations of general coping are uncommon.

One specific form of coping—religious coping—has received substantial attention. There are positive and negative dimensions of religious coping (Pargament et al. 2000). Positive religious coping involves turning to God or a "higher power" for support, strength, and reassurance. Typically, God is seen as one's partner and ally. Negative religious coping involves feelings that one is being punished or abandoned by God. Several studies indicate that religious coping buffers the effects of negative life events such that positive religious coping lessens distress and depressive symptoms and negative religious coping exacerbates the harmful effects of life events (Bjorck and Thurman 2007; Bosworth et al. 2003; Pargament et al. 1990).

Interactive Effects

Thus far, discussion of evidence bearing on the theoretical model shown in Table 8–1 has been restricted to main effects. Three kinds of interactive effects also merit comment: the stress-buffering hypothesis, age-related interactions, and several interactions unrelated to age.

The Stress-Buffering Hypothesis

Most studies support the stress-buffering hypothesis—that is, that stress has stronger negative effects on risk for psychiatric symptoms and disorder in the absence of social support. This conclusion applies both to studies of age-heterogeneous samples and to research restricted to older adults. Virtually all studies to date have addressed the stress-buffering hypothesis with regard to depressive symptoms and disorders. Several studies, both cross-sectional and longitudinal, have suggested that life events are moderated by the effects of social support (Cutrona et al. 1986; Krause 1986). Social support also has been shown to buffer the effects of chronic financial strain (Krause 1987) and disability (Arling 1987) during later life. Considerable complexity underlies the moderating effects of social support on stress. For example, Krause (1986, 1987) showed that stress-buffering effects are observed 1) for some but not all dimensions of social support, 2) for some but not all kinds of specific stressors, and 3) for some but not all dimensions of depressed affect.

Age-Related Interactions

Determining whether age interacts with other social precursors of psychiatric disorder is the best strategy for identifying distinctive age differences in the onset of depression. Unfortunately, few investigators have examined age interactions in the risk factors for psychiatric symptoms and disorders.

In perhaps the most comprehensive study to date, George (1992) explored age interactions of the predictors of the onset of major depression in a longitudinal study. Nine social factors were included in the study; six of them exhibited significant interactions with age. Three age groups were examined: young adults (ages 18–39), middle-aged adults (ages 40–64), and older adults (age 65 and older). The risk of onset of major depression was higher for women, African Americans, and urban residents—but all three of these relationships were significant only among young adults. Lower level of education and presence of chronic physical illness also increased the risk of depression only among younger adults. An interaction between marital status and age was shown to affect the risk of onset of major depression: being married was a significant protective factor only for the oldest respondents. Three risk factors did not interact with age. With other risk factors statistically controlled, income was unrelated to the risk of depression among all three age groups. In contrast, stressful life events and perceived social support were strongly related to risk of depression among all three age groups. Taken together, these findings suggest that the effects of social factors on the risk of depression tend to be weaker for older than for younger adults, although the strong effects of stress and social support for persons of all ages should not be overlooked.

Other Interactions

Some investigators have tested for gender and race interactions to better understand the role of these factors in psychiatric morbidity in later life. Using data from a sample of older African Americans, Husaini et al. (1991) found that the following social factors were associated with depression only among women: life events, level of social interaction, and perceived social support. Moldin et al. (1993) found that the effects of chronic physical illness on depression were significantly stronger for older women than for older men. Using data from an age-heterogeneous sample, Jones-Webb and Snowden (1993) found that several risk factors for depression were differentially important for whites and African Americans. Higher socioeconomic status was a significant protective factor only for African Americans; in contrast, younger age increased the risk of depression only among African Americans. Widowhood and unemployment increased the risk of depression only for whites. More recently, Schoevers et al. (2000) reported that both marital status and subjective social support moderate the effects of disability on the 3-year incidence of depressive disorder. Similarly, Choi and McDougall (2007) found that social network size moderated the effects of homebound versus ambulatory disability status on depressive symptoms. These findings require replication before firm conclusions can be drawn. It is clear, however, that increased attention should be paid to interactive effects in future research. Interactions provide a rigorous method for identifying the differential importance of social risk factors for specific subgroups of the older population.

Age Changes and Cohort Differences in Social Risk Factors

Thus far, I have discussed one set of dynamics affecting psychiatric disorder in later life—the impact of social factors on the risk of mental illness. A second set of dynamics also must be considered: age changes and cohort differences that affect *exposure* to social risk factors for psychiatric morbidity. To the extent that exposure to risk factors varies with age or differs across cohorts, the proportion of the older population at risk of psychiatric disorders also varies. Thus, the six categories of social risk factors are reexamined, with a focus on age changes and cohort differences that affect their prevalence and distribution during later life.

Demographic Variables

Age and gender are largely irrelevant in the context of age changes and cohort differences because gender is fixed and age changes are the focus of this discussion. Cohort differences in the age structure of society merit brief note, however. As is well documented, industrialized societies were aging throughout the twentieth century because of increasing life expectancy and declining fertility, and it is predicted that this trend will continue (U.S. Bureau of the Census 2003). Consequently, in the future, a larger proportion of the population of individuals with mental illness will consist of older adults. This does not mean that a larger proportion of the older population will experience mental illness—only that the number of mentally ill older adults will increase.

Race/ethnicity is a fixed characteristic. However, there are cohort differences in the ethnic compositions of societies. In the United States, current cohorts of older adults include substantial proportions of immigrants from Europe and Russia. Emigration from these countries declined precipitously after World War II, however, and future cohorts of elderly persons will differ in this regard. Currently, there is relatively little legal migration to the United States, with the majority of immigrants coming from Central America, South America, and the Far East. It is not clear how the size and composition of this new immigrant population will affect the prevalence of psychiatric disorders in later life.

Early Events and Achievements

Education typically is completed during early adulthood and does not change thereafter. There are substantial cohort differences in average levels of education, however. In comparison with their middle-aged and younger peers, current cohorts of older adults average relatively low levels of education (U.S. Bureau of the Census 2007). Given the evidence that education is negatively related to the prevalence of psychiatric disorders, higher levels of education may bode well for the mental health of future cohorts.

Childhood traumas become fixed experiences for individuals and do not change over time. Again, however, cohort differences are possible. Although there are few solid data on historical trends, cohort differences in the experience of specific childhood traumas are likely. Compared with their younger peers, current cohorts of older adults are more likely to have experienced parental death and severe poverty (because of the Great Depression) during childhood. Conversely, current cohorts of young adults are substantially more likely to have experienced parental separation or divorce during childhood (Casper and Bianchi 2001). Children in younger cohorts also have confronted unprecedented rates of parental drug abuse (Robins and Regier 1991). The implications of these cohort differences for mental health during later life remain unclear.

Later Events and Achievements

As with education, occupational attainment and income levels are higher among younger than among older cohorts. In light of the documented mental health benefits of higher socioeconomic status, future cohorts of older adults may be at lower risk for psychiatric disorders than are current cohorts. Family formation factors also differ substantially across cohorts. Compared with current cohorts of older adults, younger adults now are less likely to marry, more likely to marry for the first time at later ages, more likely to divorce, less likely to have children, and more likely to have fewer children (Casper and Bianchi 2001). These patterns generate major cohort differences in family size and structure. It is not clear whether or how these family changes will affect psychiatric outcomes during old age.

Social Integration

In U.S. society, personal attachments to community structures tend to change with age. Participation in religious, civic, and other organizations peaks during late middle age and declines thereafter as a result of health and mobility problems (Cutler and Hendricks 2000). Consequently, formal social attachments typically decrease, albeit modestly, during later life. Data concerning cohort differences in personal attachments to social structure are rare. Some authors suggest that there has been a trend away from community participation (Bellah et al. 1985; Putman 2000). Data supporting that conclusion, however, are scant and of questionable quality. Moreover, even if this trend exists, its meaning is ambiguous. It may be, for example, that recent cohorts invest greater personal commitment in fewer community structures. However, firm data exist concerning one facet of social integration: current cohorts of young and middle-aged adults attend religious services less frequently than have previous cohorts (Sherkat 2001).

Vulnerability and Protective Factors

Some chronic stressors are age related. Financial resources decrease and chronic illnesses increase during later life. Cohort differences also may operate. The economic climate of the larger society and the availability of income maintenance policies differ across time and can make financial strain more or less common during later life for specific cohorts. Similarly, medical advances affect both the health status of cohorts before old age and the ability to cure or manage chronic illnesses during later life. Policies that facilitate access to health care also affect the likelihood of impaired physical functioning during later life. Most evidence suggests that future cohorts will enter old age with better physical health and greater financial resources than their predecessors did. These trends should bode well for decreasing the risk of psychiatric disorders during later life among future cohorts.

Social networks tend both to decrease in size and to change in composition during later life (Fiori et al. 2006). These changes are largely a function of the death and impairment of age peers. Despite these changes, the vast majority of older adults are not socially isolated and report adequate levels of emotional and instrumental assistance from family and friends. Cohort differences in the size and structure of support networks are likely. Social trends in family formation strongly suggest that older persons in the future will be less likely to have spouses, children, siblings, and extended kin (Casper and Bianchi 2001). It is possible, however, that nonfamilial relationships will compensate for these changes.

Provoking Agents and Coping Efforts

Considerable evidence indicates that age is related to the occurrence of life events. Compared with their younger peers, older adults average fewer life events overall but are more likely to experience specific types of life events, especially widowhood, deaths of other family members and friends, and illness onset (Nolen-Hoekoema and Ahrens 2002; Turner et al. 1995). From a mental health perspective, these patterns have mixed implications. On the one hand, fewer life events should decrease the risk of psychiatric disorders. On the other hand, some events that are more common during later life are strongly related to psychiatric morbidity, especially depression. Neither empirical evidence nor theoretical speculation suggests major cohort differences in the frequency of life events during old age.

Information about the relationship between age and coping efforts is slim and ambiguous. This reflects both the limited research base and the difficulties inherent in studying coping. At this point, there is no evidence of age-related declines or cohort differences in coping effectiveness. These conclusions, however, are based on an absence of data rather than on empirical evidence.

Social Factors Affecting Recovery From Psychiatric Disorders

Given that social factors are substantially implicated in the onset and prevalence of psychiatric disorders during later life, it is plausible to expect that such factors might also influence the course of illness and the timing of recovery. To understand the effects of social factors on recovery, longitudinal data are required, preferably with multiple measurements, to provide an accurate picture of the dynamics of recovery and relapse. Fortunately, the number of studies of the course and outcome of psychiatric disorders has increased during the past two decades. Limitations continue to characterize this research base, however. One problem is the limited scope of many of these studies. Many studies exclude older adults and/or social factors. The scope of disorders that have been studied is limited as well. Most studies examine depression, and a few focus on bipolar disorder or alcohol abuse; other disorders have not been studied. Finally, most studies ignore treatment variables, despite the obvious relevance of treatment quality to the likelihood of recovery.

Recovery From Unipolar Depression and Bipolar Disorder

The results of most studies suggest that 40%–50% of depressed older patients receiving treatment from mental health professionals will recover from an episode of depression within the 1- to 3-year follow-up interval used in most investigations. Approximately half of the patients who recover will remain free of symptoms or below the diagnostic threshold for a major depressive episode. The remainder of the patients who recover will experience at least one relapse during the follow-up interval; a small proportion will cycle rapidly in and out of depressive episodes. Clearly, there is considerable variability in the prognosis and outcome of depressive disorder, and identification of factors that facilitate or impede recovery is an important research issue.

In addition to these older adults who receive treatment from mental health professionals, two other groups of depressed older adults have been studied: those who receive treatment in the general medical sector (i.e., from primary care rather than mental health professionals) and those who are untreated. Both groups fare substantially worse in terms of recovery from depression. Cole et al. (2006), for example, reported that 72% of patients treated in the general medical sector do not recover from depression within a year. Beekman et al. (2002) reported that a similar proportion of untreated older adults residing in the community remain depressed 1–3 years later. Both seeking treatment for depression in the general medical sector and obtaining no treatment for depression are common among adults of all age. But these patterns are more prevalent among older than middle-aged and younger adults, suggesting that older adults have disproportionately poorer odds of recovery from depression.

Whether the likelihood of recovery from a depressive episode is related to age remains unresolved. Most studies that compared older and younger depressed patients showed no age differences in the likelihood of recovery (Alexopoulos et al. 1996; Andrew et al. 1993; George et al. 1989; Hinrichsen and Hernandez 1993; Mueller et al. 2004). Other studies have demonstrated that older adults are less likely to recover than middle-aged and younger adults (Dew et al. 1997; Hughes et al. 1992); these differences, although statistically significant, are relatively modest. Age at onset also may be important, although the direction of effect is unclear. For example, Alexopoulos et al. (1996) observed lower rates of recovery among depressed older adults experiencing their first episodes of depression than among those with a history of depressive episodes. Dew et al. (1997), in contrast, observed the opposite pattern. This discrepancy may be due, in part, to different periods of observation. Mueller et al. (2004) reported no age differences in the odds of recovery over a year but also observed that older patients relapsed more quickly than younger ones.

Gender has been studied as a potential predictor of recovery by multiple investigators. Although some studies have found that men are more likely than women to recover from an episode of depression (George et al. 1989; Hughes et al. 1992; Winokur et al. 1993), other investigators have reported that gender is unrelated to recovery (Brugha et al. 1990b; Dew et al. 1997; Hinrichsen and Hernandez 1993; Zlotnick et al. 1996), and one study showed lower rates of recovery among older men than among older women (Baldwin and Jolley 1986).

Few studies have examined the role of socioeconomic status in recovery from depression. In the studies available, education—and, more broadly, socioeconomic status—did not affect the likelihood of recovery from depression (Andrew et al. 1993; George et al. 1989; Hinrichsen and Hernandez 1993). Despite the consistency of findings across studies, this issue requires additional attention.

The role of stress in impeding recovery from depression has received considerable attention, although results, again, are inconsistent. Four studies reported that the occurrence of life events was associated with a decreased likelihood of recovery (Brugha et al. 1990b; Dew et al. 1997; C.J. Holahan and Moos 1991; Murphy 1983); however, in two studies, life events were unrelated to the likelihood of recovery (George et al. 1989; Hinrichsen and Hernandez 1993). Baldwin et al. (1993) suggested that the relationship between life events and recovery from depression may be interactive rather than unidirectional. In their sample, life events reduced the likelihood of recovery among older patients without cerebral disease but not among those with cerebral disease. Investigators in two studies examined the effects of life events on recovery and relapse among patients with bipolar disorder. Again, the results were inconsistent. In one study, the occurrence of events increased the probability of relapse (Hunt et al. 1992); the other study showed no relationship between life events and recovery or relapse (McPherson et al. 1993).

Some investigators argue that a complicating factor in linking life events to recovery from mental illness is that life events are more strongly related to the onset of first episodes of mental illness than to recurrent episodes. A few studies, albeit not of older adults, have followed patients from first episode through subsequent episodes of depression and shown that life events are stronger predictors of first episodes than of relapses (e.g., Kendler et al. 2000). The "kindling" hypothesis has been suggested as an explanation for this pattern. Specifically, this hypothesis suggests that once an initial episode of mental illness is "kindled," the illness takes on a life of its own, becoming more autonomous from external provoking agents. In a superb review of the kindling hypothesis, Monroe and Harkness (2005) pointed out that the same pattern that is compatible with the kindling hypothesis is also compatible with the hypothesis that an episode of mental illness increases vulnerability to stressors. As a consequence, lower levels of stress are required to trigger recurrences than first episodes. Adjudicating these hypotheses will require very sophisticated additional research.

Chronic stress has been explored in relation to recovery from depression in multiple studies. Chronic physical illness has been examined frequently. Again, results have been mixed. Hinrichsen and Hernandez (1993) reported no relationship between chronic illness and recovery from depression. In contrast, Baldwin and Jolley (1986) and K.M. Harris et al. (2005) reported that chronic illness lowered the likelihood of recovery in their samples of older adults. Using data from a sample of middle-aged and older patients, Hughes et al. (1993) reported that physical illness reduced recovery from depression among middle-aged subjects but not among older participants.

The effects of functional disability on recovery from depression have also been studied as a chronic stressor. Evidence in these studies is consistent: rates of recovery from depression are lower among older adults with disabilities (Bosworth et al. 2002; Hays et al. 1997; Oxman and Hull 2001; Schoevers et al. 2003).

Social support has been the social factor most frequently studied in relation to recovery from depression during old age. Findings to date are consistent for some dimensions of social support and inconsistent for others. It is helpful to begin with objective dimensions of social support and to then move to subjective perceptions of support quality.

Results are contradictory with regard to the relationship between size of social network and probability of recovery from a depressive episode. Henderson and Moran (1983) observed no relationship between network size and recovery from depression in their sample of community-dwelling adults. In contrast, in their sample of middle-aged and older depressed patients, George et al. (1989) found larger network size to be associated with poorer prognosis. The direction of this relationship is counterintuitive and will be addressed shortly. More recently, Steffens et al. (2005) reported that larger social networks are associated with increased odds of recovery.

Presence versus absence of a confidant also is a structural property of the social network. To date, there is no evidence that the presence of a confidant affects the likelihood of recovery from depression (Andrew et al. 1993; Murphy 1983). Marital status is another characteristic of the social network. Three previous studies have scrutinized the relationship between marital status and recovery from depression. In two studies, marital status had no effect on recovery (Andrew et al. 1993; Hinrichsen and Hernandez 1993); in one study, married patients were less likely than unmarried patients to recover from an episode of depression (George et al. 1989). This result also is counterintuitive. We believe that the surprising effects of social network size and marital status on recovery from depression in this study reflect selectivity factors. In the community, undoubtedly a majority of social networks and marital relationships are of high quality; consequently, having larger social networks and being married are likely to have positive effects on mental health. In clinical samples, however, it is likely that patients disproportionately represent individuals whose social networks and marriages are problematic or of poor quality. If the quality of those relationships is poor, it is not surprising that their presence predicts a lower rather than a higher probability of recovery. It also should be noted that the negative effects of being married and having larger social networks are observed with the positive effects of subjective social support statistically controlled.

Only one study has addressed the effects of levels of social interaction with network members and receipt of instrumental support on recovery from depression (George et al. 1989). Although both measures were significant in bivariate analyses (with higher levels of interaction promoting recovery and high levels of instrumental assistance impeding recovery), the relationships were reduced to nonsignificance once the patients' perceptions of support were added in multivariate models.

Perceptions of support have received attention in many studies of the course and outcome of depressive disorder. Again, results have been mixed. Although a few studies have reported that perceptions of social support are unrelated to recovery (Andrew et al. 1993; Hinrichsen and Hernandez 1993; Hirschfeld et al. 1986), the vast majority of studies have reported that perceptions of the adequate availability of high-quality support strongly facilitate recovery per se and shorten time to recovery. All of the studies indicating that subjective support promotes recovery from depression are based on prospective designs, and most of them control on a wide range of potential confounding factors (Blazer et al. 1992; Bosworth et al. 2002; Brugha et al. 1990a; Dew et al. 1997; George et al. 1989; K.M. Harris et al. 2005; Hays et al. 1997; Henderson and Moran 1983; C.J. Holahan and Moos 1991; Hughes et al. 1993; Nasser and Overholser 2005; Oxman and Hull 2001; Sherbourne et al. 1995; Steffens et al. 2005; Vieil et al. 1992). Another study reports that perceptions of support quality are positively related to recovery from bipolar disorder (Stefos et al. 1996).

Thus far, this discussion has focused on the direct effects of social factors on the course and outcome of depression. A few investigators also have examined the interactive effects of social factors on recovery. First, the stress-buffering hypothesis, positing that social support is more important among persons experiencing stressful life events than among those without such stress, has been tested in two studies. The findings in one study supported the stress-buffering hypothesis (C.J. Holahan and Moos 1991), whereas data from the other study did not (George et al. 1989). Second, social support has been shown to interact with other factors to affect the likelihood of recovery. George et al. (1989) found that perceived social support interacted with both age and gender, such that it was more important for middle-aged than for older adults and more important for men than for women.

Social integration in the form of religious involvement has been shown to predict recovery from major depression. Several dimensions of religious involvement have been examined. Koenig et al. (1998) examined frequency of attending religious services, time devoted to private devotions (such as prayer and reading sacred texts), and intrinsic religious motivation (as opposed to participating for social rewards or escape from social pressures). Only intrinsic religiosity was a strong predictor of recovery itself and of time until recovery. Several studies have examined the effects of religious coping on recovery from depression. Koenig et al. (1992) and Bosworth et al. (2002) found that positive religious coping predicted a shorter time to recovery. Berg et al. (1995) found that negative religious coping was associated with a longer length of stay in a psychiatric inpatient facility for a sample of mixed affective disorder patients.

Recall from the discussion of social factors and the onset of depression that some investigators expressed concern that reports of perceived support by depressed persons may be contaminated by the dysphoria of their illness. This issue also has been raised with regard to the role of perceived support in recovery from depression (Henderson 1984). Results to date have failed to support the contamination hypothesis. First, as noted above, in one or more studies, perceived support has been shown to interact significantly with life events, age, and gender.

These complex interactions argue against the contamination hypothesis—it would be necessary to explain why the contamination disproportionately affected men, middle-aged adults, and persons who recently experienced stressful life events. Second, in studies in which bivariate correlations were reported, the relationships between perceived support and severity of depressive symptoms were quite modest (typically r=0.2–0.3), suggesting little overlap between the two concepts. Finally, two studies have demonstrated that perceived support is more stable over time than is the presence of depressive symptoms (Blazer et al. 1992; Brugha et al. 1990b), thereby arguing against the position that they reflect the same underlying phenomenon.

Ideally, one would like to know about the relative efficacy of social factors compared with the clinical features of the illness episode in predicting recovery from depression. To date, researchers in six studies have made such "head-to-head" comparisons. In four studies, the investigators reported that social factors were stronger predictors of outcome than were the clinical features of the index episode, although large proportions of variance remained unexplained (Alexopoulos et al. 1996; Andrew et al. 1993; George et al. 1989; Hays et al. 1997). Stefos et al. (1996) reported the same results with regard to predictors of recovery from bipolar disorder. In two of the studies, the investigators concluded that social factors and clinical features are equally important predictors of recovery from depression (Bosworth et al. 2002; Steffens et al. 2005). Examples of the clinical variables examined include previous episodes and hospitalizations, comorbid substance abuse, comorbid anxiety disorder, severity of symptoms at baseline, family history of disorder, and depressive subtype (e.g., melancholic vs. nonmelancholic).

Although firm conclusions about the relationships between social factors and recovery are generally premature because of inconsistencies across studies, it is clear that social factors are implicated in the course and outcome of depression. Research efforts on these issues are increasing, but considerable additional attention is warranted.

Recovery From Alcohol Abuse or Dependence

Compared with the work that has been done concerning depression, the amount of research on the course and outcome of alcohol abuse and dependence has been very limited, and the studies available are quite dated. Some researchers have studied age differences in alcohol abuse or dependence. Rates of alcohol abuse or dependence are lower among older adults than among any other age group (Compton et al. 2007; Hasin et al. 2007). However, a larger proportion of older adults seeks treatment for alcohol abuse or dependence than any other age group (Compton et al. 2007), perhaps because their excessive drinking has resulted in physical illness.

Available evidence suggests that the natural history associated with alcoholism is considerably different from that observed with depression. Using extensive longitudinal data, Vaillant (1983) described three major patterns of alcohol-related disorders: 1) a consistent pattern of occasional abuse that does not lead to dependence, 2) an atypical pattern of early and massive alcohol misuse that leads to dependence during early adulthood, and 3) the major pattern, in which "social drinking" on a regular basis leads to persistent heavy drinking and eventual dependence. The population of older alcoholic patients contains two groups: 1) persons who developed alcoholism earlier in life and who persist in alcohol abuse or dependence during old age and 2) late-onset alcoholic persons, for whom problem drinking emerged for the first time during late life (Helzer et al. 1991; Warheit and Auth 1985). Some investigators suggest that late-onset alcoholism is more strongly related to social risk factors than are early-onset alcohol problems (Dupree et al. 1984; Wattis 1983), but evidence for this assertion is scant.

A few researchers have investigated the possible role of social factors in the course of alcoholism, although most studies, unfortunately, are dated and/or rely on very small samples. Vaillant (1983) reported that social support and religious participation increased the probability of recovery from acute alcoholism, although these factors explain only a small proportion of the variance in illness duration. Similarly, Helzer et al. (1984) reported that social isolation—primarily the absence of a spouse or confidant—was a predictor of longer acute episodes of alcoholism and, interestingly, that social isolation was more strongly predictive of recovery for older than for younger persons. Helzer and colleagues also reported that among older alcoholic persons, more favorable outcomes were associated with female gender, white race, and higher socioeconomic status. Other studies have supported the conclusions that life events are related to poorer prognosis during later life (Finney et al. 1980; Wells-Parker et al. 1983) and that being married increases the likelihood of recovery, especially among older men (Bailey et al. 1965). Several investigators have also suggested that these social factors are more potent predictors of outcome for late-onset than for early-onset alcoholism (Abrahams and Patterson 1978–1979; Rosin and Glatt 1971; Schuckit et al. 1980). This topic clearly merits additional research.

Help-Seeking for Psychiatric Disorders

Social factors have been shown to play a meaningful—albeit not fully understood—role in the onset and course of psychiatric disorders. They also are related both to the likelihood that individuals will seek help for psychiatric problems and to the source from which help is sought.

Mental Health Service Use

The primary theory underpinning research on health service use was developed by Ronald Andersen and colleagues (Andersen 1968; Andersen et al. 1975); it remains the dominant theory in the field (Andersen 1995). This simple yet highly useful theory posited that health service use is a function of three generic classes of antecedents: predisposing variables, enabling factors, and need factors. *Predisposing variables* are social and attitudinal characteristics (such as gender, age, educational level, and attitudes toward physicians) that predispose certain individuals to seek help from medical providers. *Enabling factors* are resources that facilitate health service use (e.g., income level and insurance coverage). *Need factors* are the signs and symptoms of disease and disability that can trigger the decision to seek health care. Andersen developed this theory to identify predictors of differential access to health care. The theory has been used more broadly, however, to examine the major predictors of health service use.

The Andersen model has been used primarily in studies of health service use for physical illnesses, both acute and chronic. However, it also has proven useful for understanding the role of social and economic factors in help-seeking for psychiatric disorders. Those studies suggest that mental health treatments, especially in the mental health specialty sector, are viewed as more discretionary than are treatments for physical complaints—both by the public and by administrators of reimbursement programs (e.g., insurance coverage is less likely to exist at all and is more limited for mental health treatments than for services sought for physical illness). Research confirms that this pattern has been stable for at least 25 years (Sturm and Sherbourne 2001). As one would hope in a health care system that strives for equity, need factors are the strongest predictors of service use for psychiatric disorders (Katz et al. 1997; Leaf et al. 1985). Nonetheless, predisposing and enabling factors are stronger predictors of service use for psychiatric disorders than they are for physical illnesses. Having lower education and income levels, being a member of a racial or ethnic minority, being male, and being old are all associated with lower probability of receiving mental health treatment in the presence of psychiatric disorder (Katz et al. 1997; Leaf et al. 1985; Wang et al. 2006).

The relationship between race and utilization of mental health services is especially troubling because race remains a significant predictor of service use after socioeconomic factors are taken into account. Padgett et al. (1994) examined patterns of mental health service use in a well-insured, nonpoor population—federal employees. No racial differences were found for inpatient psychiatric care. However, large differences in outpatient treatment between whites and African Americans were observed for adults of all ages and for the elderly in particular. In the older population, African Americans and other minorities are substantially less likely to receive mental health services than are whites (K.M. Harris et al. 2005; Neighbors et al. 2007). Indeed, despite the fact that racial and ethnic minorities have lower rates of mental illness than whites, their underutilization of mental health services produces higher levels of unmet need for services among racial and ethnic minorities (K.M. Harris et al. 2005).

Interestingly, research on help-seeking by older adults has identified an enabling factor that was omitted from the original Andersen model—that is, social support. Adding social support to the Andersen model requires professionals to address the interface between formal services provided by physicians and other professional providers and informal services provided by family and friends. Two competing hypotheses have been raised to explain the relationship between formal and informal service use by older adults with impairments (Noelker and Bass 1989). The first hypothesis suggests that formal services typically are used as substitutes for informal services. Thus, the *substitution hypothesis* posits that formal services will be used primarily by persons without informal sources of assistance. In contrast, the *supplementation hypothesis* posits that formal services are used most often to supplement the contributions of family and friends. Indeed, the supplementation hypothesis suggests that health professionals and informal providers complement and reinforce one another—for example, by working together to ensure the impaired older adult's maximum compliance with treatment plans. (More recently, these hypotheses have been labeled as the *compensatory hypothesis* [Griffith 1985; Jorm 2005] and the *hierarchical compensatory hypothesis* [Crabb and Hunsley 2006; Litwin 1997], respectively.) Tests of these competing hypotheses have seldom been performed with regard to mental health service use. The limited evidence available from research focused on physical illness primarily supports the supplementation hypothesis (Edelman and Hughes 1990; Murdock and Schwartz 1978; Noelker and Bass 1989; Smith 1985; Wan 1987), although some studies support the substitution hypothesis (Krause 1988). Given evidence that 1) mental health care is viewed as more discretionary than treatment for physical illness and 2) the role of social support strongly affects the course and outcome of psychiatric disorders, investigation of these hypotheses in the context of mental health problems is a high-priority issue for future research. In the one study available, lack of social support increased volume of outpatient care among persons with high levels of psychiatric symptoms (Kouzis and Eaton 1998).

Another issue needs to be addressed with regard to predictors of mental health service use. As applied in most research, the Andersen model has been used to predict both receipt of any medical care and volume of care received. However, evidence suggests that these indicators of service use must be examined separately, using different models. The decision to seek or not seek treatment is largely in the control of the individual; thus, receipt of any care versus no care measures help-seeking. In contrast, volume of treatment is largely determined by the physician or service provider. A study by Leaf et al. (1985) clearly demonstrated the importance of this distinction. Although need factors were the strongest predictor of any care, they were not significant predictors of volume of care received. Similarly, women were more likely to seek care for psychiatric problems, but gender was unrelated to volume of care received. Interestingly, only age was a significant predictor of both receipt and volume of care. Both older (age 65 and older) and younger adults (ages 18–24) were less likely to seek mental health treatment than those ages 25–64, and when treatment was received, the older and younger adults obtained less care.

Although the Andersen model has dominated research on health service use, there are other useful theories. Two major alternatives are the *health belief models* (Strecher et al. 1997) and the *congruence theories* (Berkanovic and Telesky 1982). These theories focus on the beliefs, attitudes, and modes of symptom recognition and attribution that underlie decisions to seek medical care. Research based on these theories adds a useful psychological and interpretive dimension to the social determinism of the Andersen model. In general, research based on these models is compatible with findings generated by use of the Andersen model. Of particular interest is the fact that the same subgroups found to be less likely to seek help in research based on the Andersen model (i.e., men, elderly people, and racial and ethnic minorities) are identified in research based on health belief and/or congruence models to be less likely to recognize symptoms, to make accurate attributions about their cause, and to believe that medical care would be beneficial. More recent research focuses on the implications of patients' symptom attributions for the identification and treatment of psychiatric problems by their physicians. Results of these studies indicate that when patients attribute their psychiatric symptoms to physical health problems, physicians are especially unlikely to identify psychiatric disorders (Greer et al. 2004; D. Kessler et al. 1999).

Sector Choice for Treatment of Psychiatric Problems

It is widely recognized that the general medical sector provides the majority of care to persons with psychiatric disorders (R.C. Kessler et al. 1999; Regier et al. 1993). There also is considerable concern that persons with mental illness may receive lower quality care when treated in the general medical sector. These concerns are supported by evidence that general medical sector providers often 1) fail to identify psychiatric disorders; 2) fail to treat mental disorders, even when identified; and 3) do not provide the most efficacious treatments to the patients they treat. Indeed, there is compelling evidence that both the identification and treatment of psychiatric disorders in the general health sector are poor; consequently, patient outcomes are poor as well (Rost et al. 1998; Simon et al. 1999; Wang et al. 2006). These patterns are stronger for older adults than for middle-aged and younger adults (Callahan 2001; Klapp et al. 2003; Ohayon 2007). Inappropriate use of psychotropic drugs is of particular concern, especially for older patients. Thus, it is important to understand the determinants of sector choice for treatment of psychiatric disorders.

Most older adults seeking outpatient care for mental health problems are diagnosed and treated in the general medical sector. Using data from three community samples, George et al. (1988) found that older adults were two times more likely to receive mental health treatments from general medical providers than from specialty mental health providers. Leaf et al. (1989) reported similar distributions across general medical and mental health sectors. Using data from the National Ambulatory Medical Care Surveys, Schurman et al. (1985) reported that 80% of all older adults with primary or secondary psychiatric diagnoses were treated by primary care physicians. Wang et al. (2006) reported that older adults were more likely to present psychiatric symptoms to their primary care physicians in 2001–2003 than they were in 1991–1992.

There are multiple reasons that the majority of psychiatric disorders among older adults are treated in the general medical sector. First, most older persons prefer to present psychiatric problems to and receive treatment from primary care physicians (Robb et al. 2003). Second, primary care physicians typically do not refer patients with psychiatric disorders to mental health professionals (Gallo et al. 1999). This is especially true for older patients. Schurman et al. (1985), for example, reported that primary care physicians refer only 5% of older patients with psychiatric problems to psychiatrists, although the most severely ill are the most likely to be referred. Rates of referral to mental health specialists were lower for older than for young and middle-aged patients. This pattern also has been observed in a health maintenance organization setting in which psychiatrists were located in the same building as the primary care physicians (Goldstrom et al. 1987). More recently, Fischer et al. (2003) reported that primary care physicians were only one-fourth as likely to refer an older patient with significant psychiatric symptoms to a mental health professional as to refer a young or middle-aged patient. It also should be noted, however, that older adults report greater unwillingness to be referred to mental health professionals (Robb et al. 2003).

Sector choice is important, however, because general medical providers treat psychiatric disorders differently than do mental health professionals. Both the amount of time spent with patients and the types of treatments used differ between general medical and mental health providers. Schurman et al. (1985) reported that the average outpatient visit for treatment of psychiatric problems was 19.6 minutes for general medical providers compared with 44.3 minutes for mental health providers. The major factor accounting for this difference is that primary care physicians are unlikely to provide psychotherapy. Psychotherapy is provided in 96% of office visits to mental health professionals but in only 25% of visits to general medical providers (Schurman et al. 1985). Ironically, there is strong evidence that older adults prefer psychotherapy to other treatment modalities (Choi and Morrow-Howell 2007; Gum et al. 2006; Landreville et al. 2001).

In contrast, general medical providers are far more likely to prescribe psychotropic drugs than are mental health professionals. Schurman et al. (1985) reported that 78% of the office visits to primary care physicians for mental health problems included the prescription of psychotropic medications, as compared with 25% of the visits to mental health providers. Studies restricted to samples of older adults have revealed the same pattern. For example, Burns and Taube (1990) estimated that older adults with psychiatric disorders who are treated in the general medical sector are four times more likely to receive psychotropic drugs than to receive psychotherapy. More recently, Unutzer et al. (2003) reported that the vast majority of older patients receiving treatment in the general health sector are prescribed psychotropic medications. Even more sobering are the results of another study: only 30% of patients treated by mental health professionals obtained accurate psychotropic medication management (Young et al. 2001). This suggests serious medication mismanagement. Moreover, this 30% rate of accurate medication management is nearly twice as high as the rate of accurate psychotropic medication management (17%) observed among primary care providers.

Another barrier to the use of mental health professionals by older adults with mental illness may be resistance by the older adults who need care. Despite decades of public education, the stigma associated with having mental illness and receiving care from mental health professionals remains a concern among many Americans (Link et al. 1997). Also, evidence suggests that older adults have more negative attitudes toward mental health professionals than do their younger peers (Robb et al. 2003; Sirey et al. 2001). This barrier is especially disconcerting in light of evidence that, in the abstract, older adults report that psychotherapy is greatly preferred over psychotropic medications for emotional problems (Landreville et al. 2001).

Public Policies and Programs

This chapter would not be complete without consideration of the role of public policies and programs. Public policies and programs are interventions. Not all public policies are intended to affect the risk of psychiatric disorder in later life or to assist with help-seeking for such problems. Indeed, most policies and programs are intended to achieve very different goals. Nonetheless, because public policies and programs alter distributions of social and economic characteristics of the elderly, they frequently affect—either directly or indirectly—the prevalence and distribution of psychiatric disorders during later life.

In the United States, federal programs for the elderly are concentrated in two areas: income maintenance and health care financing. Social Security retirement benefits are the major income transfers to older Americans, but such income is augmented by other programs such as disability benefits and food stamps. Other policies ensure that older Americans are taxed at lower rates than their younger peers, permitting them to retain larger portions of their incomes. There is substantial heterogeneity in levels of income and assets among older adults. Nonetheless, on the whole, older Americans are less likely than younger citizens to live in poverty (U.S. Bureau of the Census 2007). As noted earlier, socioeconomic status is related both to the risk of psychiatric disorders in later life and to the likelihood that mental health services will be obtained. Thus, federal income maintenance programs undoubtedly affect the prevalence and distribution of psychiatric disorders in later life.

Medicare and Medicaid, the major public health care financing programs in the United States, were designed to serve the elderly and the poor, respectively. Medicare coverage is nearly universal among current cohorts of older adults, and a sizable minority of older Americans is covered by Medicaid. There is indisputable evidence that Medicare and Medicaid have increased accessibility to health services for older adults and the poor. Despite the beneficial effects of Medicare and Medicaid, however, mental health benefits—especially for Medicare—are much lower than those for physical illnesses. Indeed, even a change in the regulations that govern those programs can alter the availability and quality of health care. For example, enactment of Medicare Part D, providing subsidies for prescription medications, may greatly benefit older persons with psychiatric disorders—although it is too early to tell.

Space limitations preclude a review of other, less universal policies and programs targeted in whole or in part toward older adults—programs ranging from veterans' benefits to senior centers to subsidized housing. All of these programs, as well as many others, however, have the potential to favorably affect risk factors for psychiatric disorders in later life and/or patterns of help-seeking for mental health problems. Conversely, reductions in or elimination of these programs may increase risk factors for subgroups that are affected by the changes.

One issue emphasized throughout this chapter has been the degree to which risk factors vary across cohorts. Awareness of cohort differences is especially relevant for generalizing over time and anticipating future trends. The public policy arena, however, is one area in which speculation is very difficult because programs are often changed rapidly as a result of shifting political climates and priorities. Anticipation of the future is further complicated by the fact that the psychiatric status of future cohorts will be affected by the policies and programs to which they are exposed during earlier stages of the life course. Thus, I can only note that major policy changes have the potential to generate cohort differences in the prevalence and distribution of psychiatric disorders and in patterns of help-seeking and service utilization for mental health problems during later life.

Conclusion

Social and economic factors play complex and substantial roles in psychiatric disorders in later life. There is excellent evidence that some factors, such as stress and social support, are strongly related to the risk of psychiatric disorders in later life. For other potential risk factors, the links are less well documented, and additional research is needed. Strong evidence also indicates that social factors are implicated in both the course of psychiatric disorders and the likelihood of recovery from these disorders, although additional research is required to resolve the inconsistencies observed in previous studies. Social factors also are strongly related to the likelihood that older adults with psychiatric disorders will seek help for them and to the sources from which treatment will be obtained. Federal income maintenance and health care financing programs directly affect distributions of social and economic risk factors and thus indirectly affect the prevalence and patterns of help-seeking for psychiatric disorders in later life. The greatest and most interesting challenge in this area is monitoring the multiple dynamic processes that intersect and intertwine to affect the risk of experiencing psychiatric disorders, the likelihood of recovering from those illnesses, and the receipt of appropriate treatment for psychiatric disorders in later life.

Key Points

- Social factors, including stressors, social support, social integration, and socioeconomic achievements, are strong and consistent risk and protective factors for the onset of psychiatric disorders.
- Social factors, especially social support, also strongly predict both the likelihood of recovery from mental illness and the time required for recovery.
- Social factors, especially socioeconomic status and social support, are strong predictors of help-seeking for psychiatric symptoms and of the specific sources from which help is sought.
- Most public policies affect the distributions of social and economic risk and protective factors and, therefore, indirectly affect rates of mental illness.
- Tracing processes over time is essential to understanding the pathways by which social and economic factors affect mental health, as well as understanding the onset, course, and outcome of psychiatric disorders.

References

Abrahams R, Patterson P: Psychological distress among community elderly: prevalence, characteristics, and implications for service. Int J Aging Hum Dev 9:1–19, 1978–1979

Adams KB, Sanders S, Auth EA: Loneliness and depression in independent living retirement communities: risk and resilience factors. Aging Ment Health 8:475–485, 2004

Alexopoulos GS, Meyers BS, Young RC, et al: Recovery in geriatric depression. Arch Gen Psychiatry 53:305–312, 1996

American Psychiatric Association: Diagnostic and Statistical Manual of Mental Disorders, 3rd Edition, Revised. Washington, DC, American Psychiatric Association, 1987

American Psychiatric Association: Diagnostic and Statistical Manual of Mental Disorders, 4th Edition, Text Revision. Washington, DC, American Psychiatric Association, 2000

Andersen R: A Behavioral Model of Families' Use of Health Services. Chicago, IL, University of Chicago Center for Health Administration, 1968

Andersen RM: Revisiting the behavioral model and access to medical care: does it matter? J Health Soc Behav 36:1–10, 1995

Andersen R, Kravits J, Anderson O: Equity in Health Services. Cambridge, MA, Ballinger, 1975

Andrew B, Hawton K, Fagg J, et al: Do psychological factors influence outcome in severely depressed female psychiatric inpatients? Br J Psychiatry 163:747–754, 1993

Arling G: Strain, social support, and distress in old age. J Gerontol 42:107–113, 1987

Bailey M, Haberman P, Alksne H: The epidemiology of alcoholism in an urban residential area. Q J Stud Alcohol 26:19–40, 1965

Baldwin RC, Jolley DJ: The prognosis of depression in old age. Br J Psychiatry 149:574–583, 1986

Baldwin RC, Benbow SM, Marriott A, et al: Depression in old age: a reconsideration of cerebral disease in relation to outcome. Br J Psychiatry 163:82–90, 1993

Barrett AE: Marital trajectories and mental health. J Health Soc Behav 41:451–464, 2000

Beck AT, Ward CH, Mendelson M, et al: An inventory for measuring depression. Arch Gen Psychiatry 4:561–571, 1961

Beck AT, Steer RA, Garbin MG: Psychometric properties of the Beck Depression Inventory: twenty-five years of evaluation. Clin Psychol Rev 8:77–100, 1988

Beekman AT, Copeland JR, Prince MJ: Review of community prevalence of depression in later life. Br J Psychiatry 174:307–311, 1999

Beekman AT, Gerlings TF, Deeg SW, et al: The natural history of late life depression: a 6-year prospective study in the community. Arch Gen Psychiatry 59:605–611, 2002

Bellah RN, Madsen R, Sullivan WM, et al: Habits of the Heart. Berkeley, CA, University of California Press, 1985

Berg GE, Fonss N, Reed AJ, et al: The impact of religious faith and practice on patients suffering from a major affective disorder: a cost analysis. J Pastoral Care 49:359–363, 1995

Berkanovic E, Telesky C: Social networks, beliefs, and the decision to seek medical care: an analysis of congruent and incongruent patterns. Med Care 20:1018–1026, 1982

Bjorck JP, Thurman JW: Negative life events, patterns of positive and negative religious coping, and psychological functioning. J Sci Study Relig 46:159–167, 2007

Blanchard-Fields F, Irion JC: The relation between locus of control and coping: age as a moderator variable. Psychol Aging 3:197–203, 1988

Blazer DG, Burchett B, Service C, et al: The association of age and depression among the elderly: an epidemiologic exploration. J Gerontol 46:M210–M215, 1991

Blazer DG, Hughes DC, George LK: Age and impaired subjective support: predictors of symptoms at one-year follow-up. J Nerv Ment Dis 180:172–178, 1992

Blazer DG, Kessler RC, McGonagle KA, et al: The prevalence and distribution of major depression in a national community sample: the National Comorbidity Survey. Am J Psychiatry 151:979–986, 1994

Blazer DG, Landerman LR, Hays JC, et al: Symptoms of depression among community-dwelling elderly African-American and white older adults. Psychol Med 28:1311–1320, 1998

Bosworth HB, Hays JC, George LK, et al: Psychosocial and clinical predictors of unipolar depression outcome in older adults. Int J Geriatr Psychiatry 17:238–246, 2002

Bosworth HB, Park K, McQuoid DR, et al: The impact of religious practice and religious coping on geriatric depression. Int J Geriatr Psychiatry 18:905–914, 2003

Braam AW, Van den Eeden P, Prince MJ, et al: Religion as a cross-cultural determinant of depression in elderly Europeans: results from the EURODEP collaboration. Psychol Med 31:803–814, 2001

Braam AW, Prince MJ, Beekman AT, et al: Physical health and depressive symptoms in older Europeans: results from EURODEP. Br J Psychiatry 187:35–42, 2005

Breslau J, Chang D: Psychiatric disorders among foreign-born and U.S.-born Asian-Americans in a U.S. national survey. Soc Psychiatry Psychiatr Epidemiol 41:943–950, 2006

Breslau J, Kendler KS, Su M, et al: Lifetime risk and persistence of psychiatric disorders across ethnic groups in the United States. Psychol Med 35:317–327, 2005

Breslau J, Aguillar-Gaxiola S, Kendler KS, et al: Specifying race-ethnic differences in risk for psychiatric disorder in a USA national sample. Psychol Med 36:57–68, 2006

Breslau J, Aguillar-Gaxiola S, Borges G, et al: Mental disorders among English-speaking Mexican immigrants to the U.S. compared to a national sample of Mexicans. Psychiatry Res 151:115–122, 2007a

Breslau J, Aguillar-Gaxiola S, Borges G, et al: Risk for psychiatric disorder among immigrants and their U.S.-born descendents: evidence from the National Comorbidity Survey Replication. J Nerv Ment Dis 195:189–195, 2007b

Brilman EI, Ormel J: Life events, difficulties and onset of depressive episodes in later life. Psychol Med 31:859–869, 2001

Brown GW, Harris T: Social Origins of Depression: A Study of Psychiatric Disorder in Women. London, Tavistock, 1978

Bruce ML: Depression and disability in late life: Directions for future research. Am J Geriatr Psychiatry 9:99–101, 2001

Bruce ML, Hoff RA: Social and physical health factors for first-onset major depressive disorder in a community sample. Soc Psychiatry Psychiatr Epidemiol 29:165–171, 1994

Brugha TS, Bebbington PE, MacCarthy B, et al: Gender, social support, and recovery from depressive disorders: a prospective clinical study. Psychol Med 20:147–156, 1990a

Brugha TS, Bebbington PE, Sturt E, et al: The relation between life events and social support networks in a clinically depressed cohort. Soc Psychiatry Psychiatr Epidemiol 25:308–312, 1990b

Brummett BH, Babyak MA, Barefoot JC, et al: Social support and hostility as predictors of depressive symptoms in cardiac patients one month after hospitalization: a prospective study. Psychosom Med 60:707–713, 1998

Burke KC, Burke JD Jr, Rae DS, et al: Comparing age at onset of major depression and other psychiatric disorders by birth cohorts in five US community populations. Arch Gen Psychiatry 48:789–795, 1991

Burns B, Taube C: Mental health services in general medical care and in nursing homes, in Mental Health Policy for Older Americans: Protecting Minds at Risk. Edited by Fogel BS, Furino A, Gottleib GL. Washington, DC, American Psychiatric Press, 1990, pp 63–84

Cairney J, Krause N: The social distribution of psychological distress and depression in older adults. J Aging Health 17:807–835, 2005

Callahan CM: Quality improvement research on late life depression in primary care. Med Care 39:756–759, 2001

Casper LM, Bianchi SM: Continuity and Change in the American Family. Century Oaks, CA, Sage, 2001

Choi NG, Bohman TH: Predicting the changes in depressive symptomatology in later life: how much do changes in health status, marital and caregiving status, work and volunteering, and health related behaviors contribute? J Aging Health 19:152–177, 2007

Choi NG, McDougall GJ: Comparison of depressive symptoms between homebound older adults and ambulatory older adults. Aging Ment Health 11:310–322, 2007

Choi NG, Morrow-Howell N: Low-income older adults' acceptance of depressive treatments: examination of within-group differences. Aging Ment Health 11:423–433, 2007

Cole MG, Dendukuri N: Risk factors for depression among elderly community subjects: a systematic review and meta-analysis. Am J Psychiatry 160:1147–1156, 2003

Cole MG, McCusker J, Ciampi A, et al: The prognosis of major and minor depression in older medical inpatients. Am J Geriatr Psychiatry 14:966–975, 2006

Compton WM, Thomas YF, Stinson FS, et al: Prevalence, correlates, disability, and comorbidity of DSM-IV drug abuse and dependence in the United States: results from the National Epidemiologic Survey on alcohol and related conditions. Arch Gen Psychiatry 64:566–576, 2007

Crabb R, Hunsley J: Utilization of mental health services among older adults with depression. J Clin Psychol 62:299–312, 2006

Cronkite RC, Moos RH: The role of predisposing and moderating factors in the stress-illness relationship. J Health Soc Behav 25:372–393, 1984

Cuijpers P: Depressive disorders in caregivers of dementia patients: a systematic review. Aging Ment Health 9:325–330, 2005

Cutler SJ, Hendricks J: Age differences in voluntary association memberships: fact or artifact? J Gerontol B Psychol Sci Soc Sci 55:S98–S107, 2000

Cutrona C, Russell D, Rose J: Social support and adaptation to stress by the elderly. Psychol Aging 1:47–54, 1986

Devanand DP, Kim MK, Paykina N, et al: Adverse life events in elderly patients with major depression or dysthymic disorder and in healthy-control subjects. Am J Geriatr Psychiatry 10:265–274, 2002

Dew MA, Reynolds CF III, Houck PR, et al: Temporal profiles of the course of depression during treatment: predictors of pathways toward recovery in the elderly. Arch Gen Psychiatry 54:1016–1024, 1997

Dupree LW, Broskowski H, Schonfeld L: The gerontology alcohol project: a behavioral treatment program for elderly alcohol abusers. Gerontologist 24:510–516, 1984

Edelman P, Hughes S: The impact of community care on provision of informal care to homebound elderly persons. J Gerontol 45:S74–S84, 1990

Evans-Campbell T, Lincoln KD, Takeuchi DT: Race and mental health: past debates, new opportunities, in Mental Health, Social Mirror. Edited by Avison WR, McLeod JD, Pescosolido BA. New York, Springer, 2007

Feighner JP, Robins E, Guze SB, et al: Diagnostic criteria for use in psychiatric research. Arch Gen Psychiatry 26:57–63, 1972

Finney J, Moos R, Mewborn CR: Posttreatment experiences and treatment outcome of alcoholic patients six months and two years after hospitalization. J Consult Clin Psychol 48:17–29, 1980

Fiori KL, Antonucci TC, Cortina KS: Social network typologies and mental health among older adults. J Gerontol B Psychol Sci Soc Sci 61:P25–P32, 2006

Fischer LR, Wei F, Solberg LJ, et al: Treatment of elderly and other adult patients for depression in primary care. J Am Geriatr Soc 51:1554–1562, 2003

Fonda SJ, Wallace RB, Herzog AR: Changes in driving patterns and worsening depressive symptoms among older adults. J Gerontol B Psychol Sci Soc Sci 56:S343–S351, 2001

Freund AM, Baltes PB: Selection, optimization, and compensation as strategies of life management: correlations with subjective indicators of successful aging. Psychol Aging 13:531–543, 1998

Gallo JJ, Ryan SD, Ford DE: Attitudes, knowledge, and behavior of family physicians regarding depression in late life. Arch Fam Med 8:249–256, 1999

George LK: Social factors and the onset and outcome of depression, in Aging, Health Behaviors, and Health Outcomes. Edited by Schaie KW, House JS, Blazer DG. Hillsdale, NJ, Erlbaum, 1992, pp 137–159

George LK, Blazer DG, Winfield-Laird I, et al: Psychiatric disorders and mental health service use in later life: evidence from the Epidemiologic Catchment Area program, in Epidemiology and Aging. Edited by Brody J, Maddox GL. New York, Springer, 1988, pp 189–219

George LK, Blazer DG, Hughes DC, et al: Social support and the outcome of major depression. Br J Psychiatry 154:478–485, 1989

Goldstrom ID, Burns BJ, Kessler LG, et al: Mental health services use by elderly adults in a primary care setting. J Gerontol 42:147–153, 1987

Greer J, Halgin R, Harvey E: Global versus specific symptom attribution: predicting the recognition and treatment of psychological distress in primary care. J Psychosom Res 57:521–527, 2004

Griffith J: Social support providers: who are they? where are they? and the relationship of network characteristics to psychological distress. Basic Appl Soc Psych 6:41–60, 1985

Grusky O, Tierney K, Manderscheid RW, et al: Social bonding and community adjustment of chronically mentally ill adults. J Health Soc Behav 26:49–63, 1985

Gum AM, Arean PA, Hunkeler E, et al: Depression treatment preferences in older primary care patients. Gerontologist 46:14–22, 2006

Harris KM, Edlund MJ, Larson S: Racial and ethnic differences in mental health problems and use of mental health care. Med Care 43:775–784, 2005

Harris T, Cook DG, Victor C, et al: Predictors of depressive symptoms in older people: a survey of two general practice populations. Age Ageing 32:510–518, 2003

Hasin DS, Stinson FS, Ogburn E, et al: Prevalence, correlates, disability, and comorbidity of DSM-IV alcohol abuse and dependence: results from the National Epidemiologic Survey on Alcohol and Related Conditions. Arch Gen Psychiatry 64:830–842, 2007

Hays JC, Krishnan KR, George LK, et al: Psychosocial and physical correlates of chronic depression. Psychiatry Res 72:149–159, 1997

Hays JC, Landerman LR, George LK, et al: Social correlates of the dimensions of depression in the elderly. J Gerontol B Psychol Sci Soc Sci 53:P31–P39, 1998

Helzer JE, Carey KE, Miller RH: Predictors and correlates of recovery in older versus younger alcoholics, in Nature and Extent of Alcohol Problems Among the Elderly. Edited by Maddox G, Robins LN, Rosenberg N. Rockville, MD, National Institute on Alcohol Abuse and Alcoholism, 1984, pp 83–99

Helzer JE, Burnam A, McEvoy LT: Alcohol abuse and dependence, in Psychiatric Disorders in America. Edited by Robins LN, Regier DA. New York, Free Press, 1991, pp 81–115

Henderson AS: Interpreting the evidence on social support. Soc Psychiatry 19:49–52, 1984

Henderson AS, Moran PAP: Social relationships during the onset and remission of neurotic symptoms: a prospective community study. Br J Psychiatry 143:467–472, 1983

Henderson AS, Grayson DA, Scott R, et al: Social support, dementia, and depression among the elderly in the Hobart community. Psychol Med 16:379–390, 1986

Henderson AS, Jorm AF, MacKinnon A, et al: The prevalence of depressive disorders and the distribution of depressive symptoms in later life: a survey using draft ICD-10 and DSM-III-R. Psychol Med 23:719–729, 1993

Hinrichsen GA, Hernandez NA: Factors associated with recovery from and relapse into major depressive disorder in the elderly. Am J Psychiatry 150:1820–1825, 1993

Hirschfeld RMA, Klerman GL, Andreasen N, et al: Psychosocial predictors of chronicity in depressed patients. Br J Psychiatry 148:648–654, 1986

Holahan CJ, Moos RH: Life stressors, personal and social resources, and depression: a 4-year structural model. J Abnorm Psychol 100:31–38, 1991

Holahan CK, Holahan CJ: Self-efficacy, social support, and depression in aging: a longitudinal analysis. J Gerontol 42:65–68, 1987

Hopcroft RL, Bradley DB: The sex difference in depression across 28 countries. Soc Forces 85:1483–1507, 2007

Hughes DC, Turnbull JE, Blazer DG: Family history of psychiatric disorder and low self-confidence: predictors of depressive symptoms at 12-month follow-up. J Affect Disord 25:197–212, 1992

Hughes DC, DeMallie D, Blazer DG: Does age make a difference in the effects of physical health and social support on the outcome of a major depressive episode? Am J Psychiatry 150:728–733, 1993

Hunt N, Bruce-Jones W, Silverstone T: Life events and relapse in bipolar affective disorder. J Affect Disord 25:13–20, 1992

Husaini BA, Moore ST, Castor RS, et al: Social density, stressors, and depression: gender differences among the black elderly. J Gerontol 46:P236–P242, 1991

Jones-Webb RJ, Snowden LR: Symptoms of depression among blacks and whites. Am J Public Health 83:240–244, 1993

Jongenelis K, Pot AM, Eisses AMH: Prevalence and risk indicators of depression in elderly nursing home patients: the AGED study. J Affect Disord 83:135–142, 2004

Jorm AF: Social networks and health: it's time for an intervention trial. J Epidemiol Community Health 59:537–539, 2005

Katsumata Y, Arai A, Ishida K, et al: Gender differences in the contributions of risk factors to depressive symptoms among the elderly persons dwelling in a community, Japan. Int J Geriatr Psychiatry 20:1084–1089, 2005

Katz SJ, Kessler RC, Frank RG, et al: Mental health use, morbidity, and socioeconomic status in the United States and Ontario. Inquiry 34:38–49, 1997

Kendler KS, Thornton LM, Gardner CO: Stressful life events and previous episodes of major depression in women: an evaluation of the "kindling" hypothesis. Am J Psychiatry 157:1243–1251, 2000

Kendler KS, Liu XQ, Gardner CO, et al: Dimensions of religiosity and their relationship to lifetime psychiatric and substance use disorders. Am J Psychiatry 160:496–503, 2003

Kennedy GJ, Kelman HR, Thomas C: The emergence of depressive symptoms in late life: the importance of declining health and increasing disability. J Community Health 15:93–104, 1990

Kennedy GJ, Kelman HR, Thomas C, et al: The relation of religious preference and practice to depressive symptoms among

1,855 older adults. J Gerontol B Psychol Sci Soc Sci 51:P301–P308, 1996

Kessler D, Lloyd K, Lewis G, et al: Cross-sectional study of symptom attribution and recognition of depression and anxiety in primary care. BMJ 318:436–439, 1999

Kessler RC, McGonagle KA, Zhao S, et al: Lifetime and 12-month prevalence of DSM-III-R psychiatric disorders in the United States: results from the National Comorbidity Survey. Arch Gen Psychiatry 51:8–19, 1994

Kessler RC, Davis CG, Kendler KS: Childhood adversity and adult psychiatric disorder in the US National Comorbidity Survey. Psychol Med 27:1101–1119, 1997

Kessler RC, Zhao S, Katz SJ, et al: Past-year use of outpatient services for psychiatric problems in the National Comorbidity Survey. Am J Psychiatry 156:115–123, 1999

Kim J, Moen P: Retirement transitions, gender, and psychological well-being: a life-course, ecological model. J Gerontol B Psychol Sci Soc Sci 57:P212–P222, 2002

Klapp R, Unroe KT, Unutzer J: Caring for mental illness in the United States: a focus on older adults. Am J Geriatr Psychiatry 11:517–524, 2003

Klein DM, Turvey CL, Pies CJ: Relationship of coping styles with quality of life and depressive symptoms in older heart failure patients. J Aging Health 19:22–38, 2007

Koenig HG, Cohen HJ, Blazer DG, et al: Religious coping and depression among elderly, hospitalized medically ill men. Am J Psychiatry 149:1693–1700, 1992

Koenig HG, Ford SM, George LK, et al: Religion and anxiety disorder: an examination and comparison of associations in young, middle-aged, and elderly adults. J Anxiety Disord 7:321–342, 1993a

Koenig HG, George LK, Blazer DG, et al: The relationship between religion and anxiety in a sample of community-dwelling older adults. J Geriatr Psychiatry 26:65–93, 1993b

Koenig HG, George LK, Meador KG, et al: The relationship between religion and alcoholism in a sample of community-dwelling adults. Hosp Community Psychiatry 45:225–231, 1994

Koenig HG, Hays JC, George LK, et al: Modeling the cross-sectional relationships between religion, physical health, social support, and depressive symptoms. Am J Geriatr Psychiatry 5:131–144, 1997

Koenig HG, George LK, Peterson BL: Religiosity and remission of depression in medically ill older patients. Am J Psychiatry 155:536–542, 1998

Koizumi Y, Awata S, Kuriysms S, et al: Association between social support and depression status in the elderly: results of a 1-year community-based prospective cohort study in Japan. Psychiatry Clin Neurosci 59:563–569, 2005

Koster A, Bosma H, Kempen GLM, et al: Socioeconomic differences in incident depression in older adults: the role of psychological factors, physical health status, and behavioral factors. J Psychosom Res 61:619–627, 2006

Kouzis AC, Eaton WW: Absence of social networks, social support, and health services utilization. Psychol Med 28:1301–1310, 1998

Kraaij V, de Wilde EJ: Negative life events and depressive symptoms in the elderly: a life span perspective. Aging Mental Health 5:84–91, 2001

Kraaij V, Arensman E, Spinhoven P: Negative life events and depression in elderly persons: a meta-analysis. J Gerontol B Psychol Sci Soc Sci 57:P67–P94, 2002

Krause N: Social support, stress, and well-being among older adults. J Gerontol 41:512–519, 1986

Krause N: Chronic financial strain, locus of control, and depressive symptoms among older adults. Psychol Aging 2:375–382, 1987

Krause N: Stressful life events and physician utilization. J Gerontol 43:S53–S61, 1988

Krause N, Liang J, Yatomi N: Satisfaction with social support and depressive symptoms: a panel analysis. Psychol Aging 4:88–97, 1989

Lam DH, Green B, Power MJ, et al: Dependency, matching adversities, length of survival and relapse in major depression. J Affect Disord 37:81–90, 1996

Landerman R, George LK, Blazer DG: Adult vulnerability for psychiatric disorders: interactive effects of negative childhood experiences and recent stress. J Nerv Ment Dis 179:656–663, 1991

Landreville P, Landry J, Baillargeon L, et al: Older adults' acceptance of psychological and pharmacological treatments for depression. J Gerontol B Psychol Sci Soc Sci 56:P285–P291, 2001

Leaf PJ, Livingston MM, Tischler GL, et al: Contact with health professionals for treatment of psychiatric and emotional problems. Med Care 23:1322–1337, 1985

Leaf PJ, Bruce ML, Tischler GL, et al: Factors affecting the utilization of specialty and general medical mental health services. Med Care 26:9–26, 1989

Lee GR, DeMaris A, Bavin S, et al: Gender differences in the depressive effect of widowhood in later life. J Gerontol B Psychol Sci Soc Sci 56B:S536–S561, 2001

Leighton AH: My Name Is Legion: Foundations for a Theory of Man in Relation to Culture. New York, Basic Books, 1959

Levenson MR, Aldwin CM, Spiro A III: Age, cohort, and period effects on alcohol consumption and problem drinking: findings from the Normative Aging Study. J Stud Alcohol 59:712–722, 1998

Link BG, Cullen FT, Frank J, et al: The social rejection of former mental patients: understanding why labels matter. Am J Sociol 92:1461–1500, 1987

Link BG, Struening E, Rahav M, et al: On stigma and its consequences: evidence from a longitudinal study of men with dual diagnoses of mental illness and substance abuse. J Health Soc Behav 38:117–190, 1997

Litwin H: Support network type and health service utilization. Res Aging 19:274–300, 1997

Lynch SM: Explaining life course and cohort variations in the relationship between education and health: the role of income. J Health Soc Behav 47:324–338, 2006

Lynch SM, George LK: Interlocking trajectories of loss-related events and depressive symptoms among elders. J Gerontol B Psychol Sci Soc Sci 57:S117–S125, 2002

McPherson H, Herbison P, Romans S: Life events and relapse in established bipolar affective disorder. Br J Psychiatry 163:381–385, 1993

Mendes de Leon CE, Kasl SV, Jacobs S: A prospective study of widowhood and changes in symptoms of depression in a community sample of the elderly. Psychol Med 24:613–624, 1994

Midinik LT, Soghikian K, Ransom LJ, et al: The effect of retirement on mental health and health behaviors: the Kaiser Permanente Retirement Study. J Gerontol B Psychol Sci Soc Sci 50:S59–S61, 1995

Mirowsky J, Ross CE: Age and depression. J Health Soc Behav 33:187–205, 1992

Mirowsky J, Ross CE: Economic hardship across the life course. Am Sociol Rev 64:548–569, 1999

Mitchell J, Mathews HF, Yesavage JA: A multidimensional examination of depression among the elderly. Res Aging 15:198–219, 1993

Moldin SO, Scheftner WA, Rice JP, et al: Association between major depressive disorder and physical illness. Psychol Med 23:755–761, 1993

Molnar BE, Buka SL, Kessler RC: Child sexual abuse and subsequent psychopathology: results from the National Comorbidity Survey. Am J Public Health 91:753–760, 2001

Monroe SM, Harkness KI: Stress, the "kindling" hypothesis, and the recurrence of depression: considerations from a life stress perspective. Psychol Rev 112:417–445, 2005

Morrow-Howell N, Hinterlong J, Rozario PA, et al: Effects of volunteering on the well-being of older adults. J Gerontol B Psychol Sci Soc Sci 58:S137–S145, 2003

Mueller TI, Kohn R, Leventhal N, et al: The course of depression in elderly patients. Am J Geriatr Psychiatry 12:22–29, 2004

Murdock SH, Schwartz DF: Family structure and the use of agency services: an examination of patterns among elderly Native Americans. Gerontologist 18:475–481, 1978

Murphy E: The prognosis of depression in old age. Br J Psychiatry 142:111–119, 1983

Musick MA, Wilson J: Volunteering and depression: the role of psychological and social resources in different age groups. Soc Sci Med 56:259–269, 2003

Nasser EH, Overholser JC: Recovery from major depression: the role of support from family, friends, and spiritual beliefs. Acta Psychiatr Scand 111:125–132, 2005

Neff JA, Husaini BA: Stress-buffer properties of alcohol consumption: the role of urbanicity and religious identification. J Health Soc Behav 26:207–221, 1985

Neighbors HW, Caldwell C, Williams DR, et al: Race, ethnicity, and use of services for mental disorders: results from the National Survey of American Life. Arch Gen Psychiatry 64:485–494, 2007

Noelker LS, Bass DM: Home care for elderly persons: linkages between formal and informal caregivers. J Gerontol 44:S63–S70, 1989

Nolen-Hoekoema S, Ahrens C: Age differences and similarities in the correlates of depressive symptoms. Psychol Aging 17:116–124, 2002

Ohayon MM: Epidemiology of depression and its treatment in the general population. J Psychiatr Res 41:207–213, 2007

Onrust SA, Cuijpers P: Mood and anxiety disorders in widowhood: a systematic review. Aging Ment Health 10:327–234, 2006

Ormel J, Rijsdijk FV, Sullivan M, et al: Temporal and reciprocal relationship between IADL/ADL disability and depressive symptoms in late life. J Gerontol B Psychol Sci Soc Sci 57:P338–P347, 2002

Oxman TE, Hull JG: Social support, depression, and activities of daily living in older heart surgery patients. J Gerontol B Psychol Sci Soc Sci 52:P1–P14, 1997

Oxman TE, Hull JG: Social support and treatment response in older depressed primary care patients. J Gerontol B Psychol Sci Soc Sci 56:P35–P45, 2001

Oxman TE, Berkman LF, Kasl S, et al: Social support and depressive symptoms in the elderly. Am J Epidemiol 135:356–368, 1992

Padgett DK, Patrick C, Burns BJ, et al: Ethnicity and the use of outpatient mental health services in a national insured population. Am J Public Health 84:222–226, 1994

Pargament KI, Ensing DS, Falgout K, et al: God help me: religious coping efforts as predictors of the outcomes to significant negative life events. Am J Community Psychol 56:519–543, 1990

Pargament KI, Koenig HG, Perez LM: The many methods of religious coping: development and initial validation of the RCOPE. J Clin Psychol 56:519–543, 2000

Pinquart M, Sorensen S: Gender differences in caregiver stressors, social resources, and health: an updated meta-analysis. J Gerontol B Psychol Sci Soc Sci 61:P33–P45, 2006

Putman RD: Bowling Alone: The Collapse and Renewal of American Community. New York, Simon & Schuster, 2000

Radloff LS: The CES-D: a self-report depression scale for research in the general population. Applied Psychological Measurement 1:385–401, 1977

Ragland DR, Satariano WA, MacLeod KE: Driving cessation and increased depressive symptoms. J Gerontol A Biol Sci Med Sci 60:M399–M403, 2005

Regier DA, Narrow WE, Rae DS, et al: The de facto U.S. mental and addictive disorders service system: Epidemiologic Catchment Area prospective 1-year prevalence rates of disorders and services. Arch Gen Psychiatry 50:85–94, 1993

Robb C, Haley WE, Becker MA, et al: Attitudes toward mental health care in younger and older adults: similarities and differences. Aging Ment Health 7:142–152, 2003

Roberts RE, Kaplan GA, Shema SJ, et al: Prevalence and correlates of depression in an aging cohort: the Alameda County study. J Gerontol B Psychol Sci Soc Sci 52:S252–S258, 1997

Robins LN, Regier DA (eds): Psychiatric Disorders in America. New York, Free Press, 1991

Rosin A, Glatt M: Alcohol excess in the elderly. Q J Stud Alcohol 32:53–59, 1971

Ross CE, Huber J: Hardship and depression. J Health Soc Behav 26:312–327, 1985

Ross CE, Mirowsky J: Parental divorce, life-course disruption, and adult depression. J Marriage Fam 61:1034–1045, 1999

Ross CE, Mirowsky J: Sex differences in the effects of education on depression: resource multiplication or resource substitution? Soc Sci Med 63:1400–1413, 2006

Rost K, Zhang M, Fortney J, et al: Persistently poor outcomes of undetected major depression in primary care. Gen Hosp Psychiatry 20:12–20, 1998

Schieman S, Van Gundy K, Taylor J: The relationship between age and depressive symptoms: a test of competing explanatory and suppression influences. J Aging Health 14:260–285, 2002

Schoevers RA, Beekman AT, Deeg DJ, et al: Risk factors for depression in later life: results of a prospective community based study. J Affect Disord 59:127–137, 2000

Schoevers RA, Beekman AT, Deeg DJ, et al: The natural history of late-life depression: results from the Amsterdam Study of the Elderly. J Affect Disord 76:5–14, 2003

Schuckit MA, Atkinson JH, Miller PL, et al: A three-year follow-up of elderly alcoholics. J Clin Psychiatry 41:412–416, 1980

Schulz R, Williamson GM: A two-year longitudinal study of depression among Alzheimer's caregivers. Psychol Aging 6:569–578, 1991

Schulz R, O'Brien AT, Bookwala J, et al: Psychiatric and physical morbidity effects in Alzheimer's disease caregiving: prevalence, correlates, and causes. Gerontologist 35:771–791, 1995

Schurman RA, Kramer PD, Mitchell JB: The hidden mental health network: treatment of mental illness by non-psychiatrist physicians. Arch Gen Psychiatry 42:88–94, 1985

Sherbourne CD, Hays RD, Wells KB: Personal and psychosocial risk factors for physical and mental health outcomes and course of depression among depressed patients. J Consult Clin Psychol 63:345–355, 1995

Sherkat DE: Tracking the restructuring of American religions: religious affiliation and patterns of religious mobility. Soc Forces 79:1459–1493, 2001

Simon GE, Goldberg D, Tiemens BG, et al: Outcomes of recognized and unrecognized depression: an international primary care study. Hosp Psychiatry 21:97–105, 1999

Sirey JA, Bruce ML, Alexopoulos GS, et al: Perceived stigma as a predictor of treatment discontinuation in young and old outpatients with depression. Am J Psychiatry 158:479–481, 2001

Smith K: Sex differences in benzodiazepine use among the elderly: effects of social support. Doctoral dissertation, Duke University, Durham, NC, 1985

Song LY, Biegel DE, Milligan SE: Predictors of depressive symptomatology among lower class caregivers of persons with chronic mental illness. Community Ment Health J 33:269–286, 1997

Spitzer RL, Endicott J, Robins E: Research Diagnostic Criteria (RDC) for a Selected Group of Functional Disorders, 3rd Edition. New York, New York State Psychiatric Institute, 1978

Steffens DC, Skoog I, Norton MC, et al: Prevalence of depression and its treatment in an elderly population: the Cache County study. Arch Gen Psychiatry 57:601–607, 2000

Steffens DC, Pieper CF, Bosworth HB, et al: Biological and social predictors of long-term geriatric depression outcome. Int Psychogeriatr 17:41–56, 2005

Stefos G, Bauwens F, Pardoen D, et al: Psychosocial predictors of major affective recurrences in bipolar disorder: a 4-year longitudinal study of patients on prophylactic treatment. Acta Psychiatr Scand 93:420–426, 1996

Strecher VJ, Champion VL, Rosenstock IM: The health belief model and health behavior, in Handbook of Health Behavior Research, Volume 1: Personal and Social Determinants. Edited by Gochman DS. New York, Plenum, 1997, pp 71–91

Sturm R, Sherbourne CD: Are barriers to mental health and substance abuse care still rising? J Behav Health Serv Res 28:81–88, 2001

Tepper L, Rogers SA, Coleman EM, et al: The prevalence of religious coping among persons with persistent mental illness. Psychiatr Serv 52:660–665, 2001

Turner RJ, Wheaton B, Lloyd D: The epidemiology of social stress. Am Sociol Rev 60:104–125, 1995

Turvey CL, Carney C, Arndt S, et al: Conjugal loss and syndromal depression in a sample of elders aged 70 years or older. Am J Psychiatry 156:1596–1601, 1999

Unutzer J, Caton W, Callahan CM, et al: Depression treatment in a sample of 1,801 depressed older adults in primary care. J Am Geriatr Soc 51:505–514, 2003

U.S. Bureau of the Census: The older population in the United States: March 2002. Current Population Reports. April 2003. Available at http://www.census.gov/population/www/socdemo/age.html. Accessed February 14, 2008.

U.S. Bureau of the Census: Historical poverty tables: Table 3: poverty status of people, by age, race, and Hispanic origin, 1959–2006. 2007. Available at http://www.censusbureau.biz/hhes/www/poverty/histpov/hstpov3.html. Accessed February 14, 2008.

Vaillant GE: The Natural History of Alcoholism. Cambridge, MA, Harvard University Press, 1983

Vieil HO, Kuhner C, Brill G, et al: Psychosocial correlates of clinical depression after psychiatric inpatient treatment: methodological issues and baseline differences between recovered and non-recovered patients. Psychol Med 22:415–427, 1992

Wan TH: Functionally disabled elderly: health status, social support, and use of health services. Res Aging 9:61–78, 1987

Wang PS, Demler O, Olfson M, et al: Changing profiles of service sectors used for mental health care in the United States. Am J Psychiatry 163:1187–1198, 2006

Warheit GL, Auth JB: Epidemiology of alcohol abuse in adulthood, in Psychiatry, Vol 3. Edited by Cavenar JL. Philadelphia, PA, JB Lippincott, 1985, pp 512–537

Wattis JP: Alcohol and old people. Br J Psychiatry 143:306–307, 1983

Wells-Parker E, Miles S, Spencer B: Stress experiences and drinking histories of elderly drunken driving offenders. J Stud Alcohol 44:429–437, 1983

Wilson K, Mottram P, Sixsmith A: Depressive symptoms in the very old living alone: prevalence, incidence and risk factors. Int J Geriatr Psychiatry 22:361–366, 2007

Windsor TD, Anstey KJ, Butterworth P, et al: The role of perceived control in explaining depressive symptoms associated with driving cessation in a longitudinal study. Gerontologist 47:215–223, 2007

Winokur G, Coryell W, Keller M, et al: A prospective follow-up of patients with bipolar and primary unipolar affective disorder. Arch Gen Psychiatry 50:457–465, 1993

Young AS, Klap R, Sherbourne CD, et al: The quality of care for depressive and anxiety disorders in the United States. Arch Gen Psychiatry 58:55–61, 2001

Zlotnick C, Shea MT, Pikonis PA, et al: Gender, type of treatment, dysfunctional attitudes, social support, life events, and depressive symptoms over naturalistic follow-up. Am J Psychiatry 153:1021–1027, 1996

Suggested Readings

Bosworth HB, Hays JC, George LK, et al: Psychosocial and clinical predictors of unipolar depression outcome in older adults. Int J Geriatr Psychiatry 17:238–246, 2002

Brown GW, Harris T: Social Origins of Depression: A Study of Psychiatric Disorder in Women. London, Tavistock, 1978

Choi NG, Bohman TH: Predicting the changes in depressive symptomatology in later life: how much do changes in health status, marital and caregiving status, work and volunteering, and health related behaviors contribute? J Aging Health 19:152–177, 2007

Cole MG, Dendukuri N: Risk factors for depression among elderly community subjects: a systematic review and meta-analysis. Am J Psychiatry 160:1147–1156, 2003

Fiori KL, Antonucci TC, Cortina KS: Social network typologies and mental health among older adults. J Gerontol B Psychol Sci Soc Sci 61:P25–P32, 2006

Kendler KS, Thornton LM, Gardner CO: Stressful life events and previous episodes of major depression in women: an evaluation of the "kindling" hypothesis. Am J Psychiatry 157:1243–1251, 2000

Koster A, Bosma H, Dempen GLM, et al: Socioeconomic differences in incident depression in older adults: the role of psychological factors, physical health status, and behavioral factors. J Psychosom Res 61:619–627, 2006

Kraaij V, Arensman E, Spinhoven P: Negative life events and depression in elderly persons: a meta-analysis. J Gerontol B Psychol Sci Soc Sci 57:P67–P94, 2002

Neighbors HW, Caldwell C, Williams DR, et al: Race, ethnicity, and use of services for mental disorders: results from the National Survey of American Life. Arch Gen Psychiatry 64:485–494, 2007

Oxman TE, Hull JG: Social support and treatment response in older depressed primary care patients. J Gerontol B Psychol Sci Soc Sci 56:P35–P45, 2001

PART II

The Diagnostic Interview in Late Life

CHAPTER 9

The Psychiatric Interview of Older Adults

Dan G. Blazer, M.D., Ph.D.

The foundation of the diagnostic workup of the older adult experiencing a psychiatric disorder is the diagnostic interview. Unfortunately, in this age of increasing technology in the laboratory and standardization of interview techniques, the art of the clinical interview has suffered. Also, time pressures limit clinicians' ability to perform a thorough diagnostic workup. Nevertheless, such a workup will save valuable time over the course of an older adult's illness. In fact, there is no substitute, even with modern technologies, for a thorough initial assessment of the older adult. In this chapter, I review the core of the psychiatric interview, including history taking, assessment of the family, and the mental status examination; describe structured interview schedules and rating scales that are of value in the assessment of older adults; and outline techniques for communicating effectively with older adults.

History

The elements of a diagnostic workup of the elderly patient are presented in Table 9–1. To obtain historical information, the clinician should first interview the patient, if that is feasible, and then ask the patient's permission to interview family members. Members from at least two generations, if available for interview, can expand the perspective on the older adult's impairment. If the patient has difficulty providing an accurate or understandable history, the clinician should concentrate especially on eliciting the symptoms or problems that the patient perceives as being most disabling, then fill the historical gap with data from the family.

Present Illness

DSM-IV-TR (American Psychiatric Association 2000) provides the clinician with a useful catalogue of symptoms and behaviors of psychiatric interest that are relevant to the diagnosis of the present illness. Symptoms are bits of data—the most visible part of the clinical picture and generally the part most easily agreed on among clinicians. Symptoms should be defined in such a way that if multiple clinicians each obtain equivalent information, they would have minimal disagreement about the presence or absence of a symptom. The decision about whether those symptoms form a syndrome or derive from a particular etiology must be determined independently of the data collection on symptoms.

Even so, the clinical interaction may be confounded by bias when a clinician communicates with an older adult about psychiatric symptoms. As many insightful clinicians, such as Eisenberg (1977), have recognized, physicians diagnose and treat diseases—that is, abnormalities in the structure and function of body organs and systems. Patients have illnesses—experiences of disvalued changes in states of being and in social function. Disease and illness do not maintain a one-to-one relationship. Factors that determine who becomes a patient and who does not can be understood only by expanding horizons beyond symptoms. In other words, patienthood is a social state (Eisenberg and Kleinman

TABLE 9–1. Diagnostic workup of the elderly patient

History
Present illness
Past history
Family history
Context
Medication history
Medical history
Family assessment
Mental status examination

1981). During the process of becoming a patient, the older adult, usually with the advice of others, forms a self-diagnosis of his or her problem and makes a judgment about the degree of ill-being perceived. For some, illness is perceived when a specific discomfort is experienced. For others, illness reflects a general perception of physical or social alienation and despair. Given that few uniform, satisfactory definitions of illness (or ill-being) exist, it is not surprising that terms for wellness (or well-being) also mean different things to different people. The historical background and the values of the older adult in a social class and culture contribute to the formation of constructs regarding the nature of the problem, the cause, and the possibility for recovery.

For these reasons, the clinician must take care to avoid accepting the patient's explanation for a given problem or set of problems. Statements such as "I guess I'm just getting old and there's nothing really to worry about" or "Most people slow down when they get to be my age" can lull the clinician into complacency about what may be a treatable psychiatric disorder. On the other hand, the advent of new and disturbing symptoms in an older adult between office visits can exhaust the clinician's patience, thereby derailing pursuit of the problem. For example, the older adult with hypochondriasis whose awakenings during the night are increasing may insist that this symptom be treated with a sedative and plead with the clinician not to allow continual suffering. In the clinician's view, however, the symptom is a normal accompaniment of old age and therefore should be accepted. Distress over changes in functioning, such as sexual functioning, may overwhelm the older adult patient and, especially if the clinician is perceived as unconcerned, may precipitate self-medication or even a suicide attempt.

To prevent attitudinal biases when eliciting reports by the older adult (which may result in missing the symptoms and signs of a treatable psychiatric disorder), the clinician must include in the initial interview a review of the more important psychiatric symptoms in a relatively structured format. Common symptoms that should be reviewed include excessive weakness or lethargy; depressed mood or "the blues"; memory problems; difficulty concentrating; feelings of helplessness, hopelessness, and uselessness; isolation; suspicion of others; anxiety and agitation; sleep problems; and appetite problems and weight loss. Critical symptoms that should be reviewed include the presence or absence of suicidal thoughts, profound anhedonia, impulsive behavior ("I can't control myself"), confusion, and delusions and hallucinations.

The review of symptoms is most valuable when considered in the context of symptom presentation: When did the symptoms begin? How long have they lasted? Has their severity changed over time? Are there physical or environmental events that precipitate the symptoms? What steps, if any, have been taken to try to correct the symptoms? Have any of these interventions proved successful? Do the symptoms vary during the day (diurnal variation)? Do they vary during the week or with seasons of the year? Do the symptoms form clusters—that is, are they associated with one another? Which symptoms appear ego-syntonic, and which appear ego-dystonic? As symptoms are reviewed, a specific time frame facilitates focus on the present illness. Having a 1-month or 6-month window enables the patient to review symptoms and events temporally—an approach not usually taken by distressed elders, who tend to concentrate on immediate sufferings.

Critical to the assessment of the present illness is an assessment of function and change in function. The two parameters that are most important (and not included in usual assessments of physical and psychiatric illness) are social functioning and activities of daily living (ADLs). Questions should be asked about the social interaction of the older adult, such as the frequency of his or her visits outside the home, telephone calls, and visits from family and friends. Many scales have been developed to assess ADLs; however, in the interview, the clinician can simply ask about the patient's ability to get around (e.g., walk inside and outside the house), to perform certain physical activities independently (e.g., bathe, dress, shave, brush teeth, and select clothes), and to do instrumental activities (e.g., cook, maintain a bank account, shop, and drive). It is also important to assess how often the elder actually engages in these activities; for example, the ability to walk outside does not always translate to outside exercise.

Past History

Next, the clinician must review the past history of symptoms and episodes. Has the patient had similar episodes in the past? How long did the episodes last? When did they occur? How many times in the patient's lifetime have such episodes occurred? Unfortunately, the older adult may not equate present distress with past episodes that are symptomatically similar, so the perspective of the family is especially valuable in the attempt to link current and past episodes.

Other psychiatric and medical problems should be reviewed as well, especially medical illnesses that have led to hospitalization and the use of medication. Not infrequently, an older adult has experienced a major illness or trauma in childhood or as a younger adult but views this information as being of no relevance to the present episode and therefore dismisses it. Probes to elicit these data are essential. Older adults may ignore or even forget past psychiatric difficulties, especially if these difficulties were disguised. For example, mood swings in early or middle life may have occurred during periods of excessive and productive activity, episodes of excessive alcohol intake, or periods of vague, undiagnosed physical problems. Previous periods of overt disability in usual activities may flag those episodes. An older person sometimes becomes angry or irritated when the clinician continues to probe. Reassurance regarding the importance of obtaining this information will generally suffice, except when dealing with a patient who cannot tolerate the discomfort and distress, even for brief periods. Older persons who have chronic and moderately severe anxiety or a histrionic personality style, as well as distressed Alzheimer's patients, tolerate their symptoms poorly.

Family History

The distribution of psychiatric symptoms and illnesses in the family should be determined next. The older person with symptoms consistent with senile dementia or primary degenerative dementia is highly likely to have a family history of dementia. The genogram can be valuable for charting the distribution of mental illness and other relevant behaviors throughout the family tree. This genogram should include parents, blood-related aunts and uncles, brothers and sisters, spouse(s), children, grandchildren, and great-grandchildren (recognizing that data from many family members will not be complete). A history should be obtained about institutionalization, significant memory problems in family members, hospitalization for a nervous breakdown or depressive disorder, suicide, alcohol abuse and dependence, electroconvulsive therapy, long-term residence in a mental health facility (and possibly a diagnosis of schizophrenia), and use of mental health services by family members (Blazer 1984).

Of relevance to the pharmacological treatment of certain disorders—especially depression—in older adults is the tendency of individuals in a family to respond therapeutically to the same pharmacological agent. If the older adult has a depressive disorder and if biological relatives have been treated effectively for depression, the clinician should determine what pharmacological agent was used to treat the depression. For example, a positive response to sertraline in a family member of the depressed older patient could make sertraline the drug of choice in treating that patient, assuming side effects are not at issue (Ayd 1975).

Mendlewicz et al. (1975) discussed that accurate genetic information can be better obtained when family members from more than one generation are interviewed. Many psychiatric disorders are characterized by a variety of symptoms, so asking the patient or one family member for a history of depression is insufficient. Research on the genetic expression of psychiatric disorders in families requires the psychiatric investigator to interview directly as many family members as possible to determine accurately the distribution of disorders throughout the family. Such detailed family assessment is not feasible for clinicians, yet a telephone call to a relative with permission from the patient may become a standard of clinical assessment as the genetics of psychiatric disorders are clarified.

Context

Psychiatric disorders occur in a biomedical and psychosocial context. Although the clinician will try to determine what medical problems the patient has experienced, it is possible to overlook a variation in the relative contribution of these medical disorders to psychopathology or to overlook the psychosocial contribution to the onset and continuance of the problem. Has the spouse of the older adult undergone a change? Are the middle-aged children managing high stress, such as simultaneously caring for an emotionally disturbed child and the loss of employment? Are the grandchildren placing emotional stress on the elderly patient, perhaps by requesting money? Has the economic status of the older adult deteriorated? Has the availability of medical care changed? Although many psychiatric disorders are biologically driven, they do not occur in a psychosocial vacuum. Environmental precipitants remain important in the web of causation leading to the onset of an episode of emotional distress and are critical to the assessment of the older adult.

Medication History

It is essential to evaluate the medication history of the older adult. A careful review of current and past medications by the clinician, a nurse, or a physician's assistant is essential. The older person should be asked to bring to the appointment all pill bottles, a list of medications taken, and the dosage schedule. A comparison between the written schedule and the pill containers will frequently expose some discrepancy. Both prescription and over-the-counter drugs, such as laxatives and vitamins, should be recorded. The clinician can then identify the medications that are potentially critical in terms of drug-drug interactions and ask about them during subsequent patient visits.

Most elderly persons take a variety of medicines simultaneously, and the potential for drug-drug interaction is high. For example, concomitant use of fluoxetine and warfarin has been associated with an increase in the half-life of warfarin, which could lead to severe bruising (although this finding is not well documented). Some medications prescribed for older persons—such as the beta-blocker propranolol and the antihypertensive drug alpha-methyldopa—can exacerbate or produce depressive symptoms.

Older persons are less likely than younger persons to abuse alcohol, but a careful history of alcohol intake is essential to the diagnostic workup. Although older persons do not usually volunteer information about their alcohol intake, they are generally forthcoming when asked about their drinking habits. Substance abuse beyond alcohol and prescription drugs is rare in older adults but not entirely absent.

Medical History

Given the high likelihood of comorbid medical problems associated with psychiatric disorders in late life, a comprehensive medical history is essential. Most older persons see a primary care physician regularly (although decreasing payments from Medicare render this assumption less accurate each year). The geriatric psychiatrist should obtain medical records, if possible. Major illnesses should be recorded. A brief phone call to the primary care physician can be extremely useful.

Family Assessment

Clinicians working with older adults must be equipped to evaluate the family—both its functionality and its potential as a resource for the older adult. Geriatric psychiatry, almost by definition, is family psychiatry. Just as an elevated white blood cell count is not pathognomonic for a particular infectious agent yet is critical to the diagnosis, the complaint that "my family no longer loves me" does not reveal the specific problems in the family yet does highlight the need to assess the potential of that family for providing care and support for the older adult (Blazer 1984). The purpose of a comprehensive diagnostic family workup is to determine the nature of the family structure in interaction, the presence or absence of a crisis in the family, and the type and amount of support available to the older adult.

A primary goal of the clinician, as advocate for the older adult with psychiatric disturbance, is to facilitate family support for the elder during a time of disability. At least four parameters of support are important for the clinician to evaluate as the treatment plan evolves: 1) the availability of family members to the older person over time; 2) the tangible services provided by the family to the older person; 3) the perception of family support by the older patient (and therefore the willingness of the patient to cooperate and accept support); and 4) tolerance by the family of specific behaviors that derive from the psychiatric disorder.

The clinician should ask the older person, "If you become ill, is there a family member who will take care of you for a short period of time?" Next, the availability of family members who can care for the older adult over an extended period should be determined. If a particular member is designated as the primary caregiver, plans for respite care should be discussed. Given the increased focus on short hospital stays and the documented higher levels of impairment on discharge, the availability of family members becomes essential to the effective care of the older adult after hospitalization for a psychiatric disorder or a combined medical and psychiatric disorder.

What specific, tangible services can be provided to the older adult by family members? Even the most devoted spouse can be limited in the delivery of certain services because, for example, he or she does not drive a car, and therefore cannot provide transportation, or is not physically strong enough to provide certain types of nursing care. Generic services of special importance in at-home support of the older adult with psychiatric impairment include transportation; nursing services (e.g., administering medications at home); physical therapy; checking on or continuous supervision of the patient; homemaker and household services; meal preparation; administrative, legal, and protective services; financial assistance; living quarters; and coordination of the delivery of services. These services are considered generic because they can be defined in terms of their activities, regardless of who provides each service. Assessing the range and extent of service delivery by the family to the older person with functional impairment provides a convenient barometer of the economic, social, and emotional burdens placed on the family.

Regardless of the level and types of services provided by the family to the older person, if these services are to be effective, it is beneficial for the older person to perceive that he or she lives in a supportive environment. Intangible supports include the perception of a dependable network, participation or interaction in the network, a sense of belonging to the network, intimacy with network members, and a sense of usefulness to the family (Blazer and Kaplan 1983). The sense of usefulness may be of less importance to some older adults who believe they have contributed to the family for many years and therefore deserve reciprocal services in their waning years. Unfortunately, family members, frequently stressed across generations, may not recognize this reciprocal responsibility.

Family tolerance of specific behaviors may not correlate with overall support. Every person has a level of tolerance for specific behaviors that are especially difficult. Sanford (1975) found that the following behaviors were tolerated by families of older persons with impairments (in decreasing percentages): incontinence of urine (81%), personality conflicts (54%), falls (52%), physically aggressive behavior (44%), inability to walk unaided (33%), daytime wandering (33%), and sleep disturbance (16%). This frequency may appear counterintuitive, since incontinence is generally considered particularly aversive to family members. However, although the outcome of incontinence can be corrected easily enough, a few nights of no sleep can easily extend family members beyond their capabilities for serving a parent, sibling, or spouse.

The Mental Status Examination

Physicians and other clinicians are at times hesitant to perform a structured mental status examination, fearing that the effort will insult or irritate the patient or that the patient will view the examination as a waste of time. Nevertheless, the mental status examination of the older psychiatric patient is central to the diagnostic workup. Many aspects of this examination can be assessed during the history-taking interview.

Appearance may be affected by the older patient's psychiatric symptoms (e.g., the depressed patient may neglect grooming), cognitive status (e.g., the patient with dementia may not be able to match clothes or even put on clothes appropriately), and environment (e.g., a nursing home patient may not be groomed as well as a patient living at home with a spouse).

Affect and mood can usually be assessed by observing the patient during the interview. *Affect* is the feeling tone that accompanies the patient's cognitive output (Linn 1980). Affect may fluctuate during the interview; however, the older person is more likely to demonstrate a constriction of affect. *Mood*, the state that underlies overt affect and is sustained over time, is usually apparent by the end of the interview. For example, the affect of a depressed older adult may not reach the degree of dysphoria seen in younger persons (as evidenced by crying spells or protestations of uncontrollable despair), yet the depressed mood is usually sustained and discernible from beginning to end.

Psychomotor activity may be agitated or retarded. Psychomotor retardation or underactivity is characteristic of major depression and severe schizophreniform symptoms, as well as of some variants of primary degenerative dementia. Psychiatrically impaired older persons, except some who have advanced dementia, are more likely to exhibit hyperactivity or agitation. Those who are depressed will appear uneasy, move their hands frequently, and have difficulty remaining seated through the interview. Patients with mild to moderate dementia, especially those with vascular dementia, will be easily distracted, rise from a seated position, and/or walk around the room or even out of the room. Pacing is often observed when the older adult is admitted to a hospital ward. Agitation can usually be distinguished from anxiety, for the agitated individual does not complain of a sense of impending doom or dread. In patients with psychomotor dysfunction, movement generally relieves the immediate discomfort, although it does not correct the underlying disturbance. Occasionally, the older adult with motor retardation may actually be experiencing a disturbance in consciousness and may even reach an almost stuporous state. The patient may not be easily aroused, but when aroused, he or she will respond by grimacing or withdrawal.

Perception is the awareness of objects in relation to each other and follows stimulation of peripheral sense organs (Linn 1980). Disturbances of perception include hallucinations—that is, false sensory perceptions not associated with real or external stimuli. For example, a paranoid older person may perceive invasion of his or her house at night by individuals who disarrange belongings and abuse him or her sexually. Hallucinations often take the form of false auditory perceptions, false perceptions of movement or body sensation (e.g., palpitations), and false perceptions of smell, taste, and touch. The older patient who is severely depressed may have frank auditory hallucinations that condemn or encourage self-destructive behavior.

Disturbances in thought content are the most common disturbances of cognition noted in older patients with psychosis. The depressed patient often develops beliefs that are inconsistent with the objective information obtained from family members about the patient's abilities and social resources. In a series of studies, Meyers and colleagues (Meyers and Greenberg 1986; Meyers et al. 1985) found delusional depression to be more prevalent among older depressed patients than among middle-aged adults. Of 161 patients with endogenous depression, 72 (45%) were found to be delusional as determined by Spitzer et al.'s (1978) Research Diagnostic Criteria (RDC). These delusions included beliefs such as "I've lost my mind," "My body is disintegrating," "I have an incurable illness," and "I have caused some great harm." Even after elderly persons recover from depression, they may still experience periodic recurrences of delusional thoughts, which can be most disturbing to otherwise rational older adults. Older patients appear less likely to experience delusional remorse, guilt, or persecution.

Even if delusions are not obvious, preoccupation with a particular thought or idea is common among depressed elderly persons. Such preoccupation is closely associated with obsessional thinking or irresistible intrusion of thoughts into the conscious mind. Although the older adult rarely acts on these thoughts compulsively, the guilt-provoking or self-accusing thoughts may occasionally become so difficult to bear that the person considers, attempts, or succeeds in committing suicide.

Disturbances of thought progression accompany disturbances of content. Evaluation of the content and process of cognition may uncover disturbances such as problems with the structure of associations, the speed of associations, and the content of thought. Thinking is a goal-directed flow of ideas, symbols, and associations initiated in response to environmental stimuli, a perceived problem, or a task that requires progression to a logical or reality-based conclusion (Linn 1980). The older adult who is compulsive or has schizophrenia may pathologically repeat the same word or idea in response to a variety of probes, as may the patient who has primary degenerative dementia. Some older adults with dementia exhibit circumstantiality—that is, the introduction of many apparently irrelevant details to cover a lack of clarity and memory problems. Interviews with patients who have this problem can be most frustrating because they proceed at a very slow pace. On other occasions, elderly patients may appear incoherent, with no logical connection to their thoughts, or they may produce irrelevant answers. The intrusion of thoughts from previous conversations into a current conversation is a prime example of the disturbance in association found in patients with primary degenerative dementia (e.g., Alzheimer's disease). This symptom is not typical of other dementias, such as the dementia of Huntington's disease. However, in the absence of dementia, even paranoid older adults do not generally demonstrate a significant disturbance in the structure of associations.

Suicidal thoughts are critical to assess in the elderly patient with psychiatric impairment. Although thoughts of death are common in late life, spontaneous revelations of suicidal thoughts are rare. A stepwise probe is the best means of assessing the presence of suicidal ideation (Blazer 1982). First, the clinician should ask the patient if he or she has ever thought that life was not worth living. If so, has the patient considered acting on that thought? If so, how would the patient attempt to inflict such harm? If definite plans are revealed, the clinician should probe to determine whether the implements for a suicide attempt are available. For example, if a patient has considered shooting himself, the clinician should ask, "Do you have a gun available and loaded at home?" Suicidal ideation in an older adult is always of concern, but intervention is necessary when suicide has been considered seriously and the implements are available.

Assessment of memory and cognitive status is most accurately performed through psychological testing. However, the psychiatric interview of the older adult must include a reasonable assessment. Although older adults may not complain of memory dysfunction, they are more likely than younger patients to have problems with memory, concentration, and intellect. There are brief, informal means of testing cognitive functioning that should be included in the diagnostic workup. The clinician proceeding through an evaluation of memory and intellect must also remember that poor performance may reflect psychic distress or a lack of education, as opposed to mental retardation or dementia. In addition, to rule out the potential confounding of agitation and anxiety, testing can be performed on more than one occasion.

Testing of memory is based on three essential processes: 1) registration (the ability to record an experience in the central nervous system), 2) retention (the persistence and permanence of a registered experience), and 3) recall (the ability to summon consciously the registered experience and report it) (Linn 1980). *Registration*, apart from recall, is difficult to evaluate directly. Occasionally, events or information that the older adult denies remembering will appear spontaneously during other parts of the interview. Registration usually is not impaired except in patients with one of the more severely dementing illnesses.

Retention, on the other hand, can be blocked by both psychic distress and brain dysfunction. Lack of retention is especially relevant to the unimportant data often asked for on a mental status examination. For example, requesting the older adult to remember three objects for 5 minutes will frequently reveal a deficit if the older adult has little motivation to attempt the task.

Disturbances of *recall* can be tested directly in a number of ways. The most common are *tests of orientation* to time, place, person, and situation. Most persons continually orient themselves through radio, television, and reading material, as well as through conversations with others. Some elderly persons may be isolated through sensory impairment or lack of social contact; poor orientation in these patients may represent deficits in the physical and social environment rather than brain dysfunction. *Immediate recall* can be tested by asking the older person to repeat a word, phrase, or series of numbers, but it can also be tested in conjunction with cognitive skills by requesting that a word be spelled backward or that elements of a story be recalled.

During the mental status examination, intelligence can be assessed only superficially. Tests of simple arithmetic calculation and fund of knowledge, supplemented by portions of well-known psychiatric tests, are helpful. The classic test for calculation is to ask a patient to subtract 7 from 100 and to repeat this operation on the succession of remainders. Usually, five calculations are sufficient to determine the older adult's ability to complete this task. If the older adult fails the task, a less exacting test is to request the patient to subtract 3 from 20 and to repeat this operation on the succession of remainders until 0 is reached. These examinations must not be rushed, for older persons may not perform as well when they perceive time pressure. A capacity for *abstract thinking* is often tested by asking the patient to interpret a well-known proverb, such as "A rolling stone gathers no moss." A more accurate test of abstraction, however, is classifying objects in a common category. For example, the patient is asked to state the similarity between an apple and a pear. Whereas naming objects from a category (such as fruits) is retained despite moderate and sometimes marked declines in cognition, the opposite process of classifying two different objects in a common category is not retained as well.

Rating Scales and Standardized Interviews

Rating scales and standardized or structured interviews have progressively been incorporated into the diagnostic assessment of the elderly psychiatric patient. Such rating procedures have increased in popularity as the need has increased for systematic, reproducible diagnoses for third-party carriers (part of the impetus for the dramatic change in nomenclature evidenced in DSM-IV-TR) and for a standard means of assessing change in clinical status. A thorough review in this chapter of all instruments that are used is not possible. Therefore, selected instruments are presented and evaluated in this section, chosen either because they have special relevance to the geriatric patient or because they are widely used.

Cognitive Dysfunction and Dementia Schedules

A number of standardized assessment methods for delirium have emerged. Perhaps the best and the most easily used is the Confusion Assessment Method (Inouye 1990). The scale assesses nine characteristics of delirium, including acute onset (evidence of such onset), fluctuating course (behavior change during the day), inattention (trouble in focusing), disorganized thinking (presence of rambling or irrelevant conversations and illogical flow of ideas), and altered level of consciousness (rated from alert to comatose). Diagnosis of delirium according to DSM-IV-TR criteria can be derived from the scale.

Two interviewer-administered cognitive screens for dementia have been popular in both clinical and community studies. The first is the Short Portable Mental Status Questionnaire (SPMSQ) (Pfeiffer 1975), a derivative of the Mental Status Questionnaire developed by Kahn et al. (1960). The SPMSQ consists of 10 questions designed to assess orientation, memory, fund of knowledge, and calculation. For most community-dwelling older adults, two or fewer errors indicate intact functioning; three or four errors, mild impairment; five to seven errors, moderate impairment; and eight or more errors, severe impairment. The ease of administration of this instrument and its reliability as supported by accumulated epidemiological data make it useful for both clinical and community screens.

The Mini-Mental State Examination (Folstein et al. 1975) is a 30-item screening instrument that assesses orientation, registration, attention and calculation, recall, and language. It requires 5–10 minutes to administer and includes more items of clinical significance than does the SPMSQ. Seven to 12 errors suggest mild to moderate cognitive impairment, and 13 or more errors indicate severe impairment. This instrument is perhaps the most frequently used standardized screening instrument in clinical practice.

A number of clinical assessment procedures for dementia have emerged. The most widely used, and one of the first to appear, is the scale suggested by Blessed et al. (1968), usually referred to as the Blessed Dementia Index. In contrast to what can be gleaned through use of the screening scales described above, clinical judgment is required in using the Blessed Dementia Index to assess changes in performance of everyday activities, such as handling money, household tasks, and shopping; changes in eating and dressing habits; changes in personality, interests, and drive; tests of information (orientation and recognition of persons); memory of past information, such as occupation, place of birth, and town where the individual worked; and concentration (calculation task). A score is assigned to each of these tasks, and a summary score is tabulated. The score has been shown to correlate well with the cerebral changes of primary degenerative dementia.

A dementia scale for assessing the probability that dementia is a vascular dementia was suggested by Hachinski et al. (1975). In the study, cerebral blood flow in patients with primary degenerative dementia was compared with that of patients who had vascular dementia. Certain clinical features were determined to be more associated with multi-infarct dementia, and each of these features was assigned a score. Those clinical features, along with their scores, are as follows: abrupt onset=2, stepwise deterioration=1, fluctuating course=2, nocturnal confusion=1, relative preservation of personality=1, depression=1, somatic complaints=1, emotional incontinence=1, history of hypertension=1, history of strokes=2, evidence of associated atherosclerosis=1, focal neurological symptoms=2, and focal neurological signs=2. A score of 7 or greater was highly suggestive of multi-infarct dementia. However, given the frequent overlap of multiple small infarcts and primary degenerative dementia, as well as the difficulty of assessing these items effectively, most investigators have ceased to rely on the Hachinski scale for clinical use.

Depression Rating Scales

A number of self-rating depression scales have been used to screen for depression in patients at all stages of the life cycle; most of these scales have been studied in older populations. The most widely used of the current instruments in community studies is the Center for Epidemiologic Studies Depression Scale (CES-D) (Radloff 1977). The scale consists of 20 behaviors and feelings, and the patient indicates how frequently each was experienced over the past week (from no days to most days). In a factor-analytic study of the CES-D in a community population, four factors were identified: somatic symptoms, positive affect, negative affect, and interpersonal relationships (Ross and Mirowsky 1984). The disaggregation of these factors and the exploration of their interaction are significant steps forward in understanding the results derived from symptom scales such as the CES-D in older populations. For example, the somatic items (e.g., loss of interest, poor appetite) are more likely to be associated with a course of depressive episodes similar to that described for major depression with melancholia, and the positive-affect items are more likely to be associated with life satisfaction scores.

A scale that has been widely used in clinical studies, although less studied in community populations, is the Beck Depression Inventory (BDI) (Beck et al. 1961). The reliability of the BDI has been shown to be good in both depressed and nondepressed samples of older people (Gallagher et al. 1982). The instrument consists of 21 symptoms and attitudes, rated on a scale of 0–3 in terms of intensity. In another study by Gallagher et al. (1983), the BDI misclassified only 16.7% of subjects who had been diagnosed on the basis of Spitzer et al.'s (1978) RDC as having major depression.

The Geriatric Depression Scale (GDS) was developed because the scales discussed above present problems for older persons who have difficulty in selecting one of four forced-response items (Yesavage et al. 1983). The GDS is a 30-item scale that permits patients to rate items as either present or absent; it includes questions about symptoms such as cognitive complaints, self-image, and losses. Items selected were thought to have relevance to late-life depression. The GDS has not been used extensively in community populations and is not as well standardized as the CES-D, but its yes/no format is preferred to the CES-D by many clinicians.

Of the scales used by interviewers to rate patients, the Hamilton Rating Scale for Depression (Ham-D) (Hamilton 1960) is by far the most commonly used. The advantage of having ratings based on clinical judgment has made the Ham-D a popular instrument for rating outcome in clinical trials. For example, a reduction in the score to one-half the initial score or to a score below a certain value would indicate partial or complete recovery from an episode of depression.

A scale that has received considerable attention clinically, having been standardized in clinical but not community populations, is the Montgomery-Åsberg Rating Scale for Depression (Montgomery and Åsberg 1979). This scale follows the pattern of the Hamilton scale and concentrates on 10 symptoms of depression; the clinician rates each symptom on a scale of 0–6 (for a range of scores between 0 and 60). The symptoms include apparent sadness, reported sadness, inattention, reduced sleep, reduced appetite, concentration difficulties, lassitude, inability to feel, pessimistic thoughts, and suicidal thoughts. Theoretically, this scale is an improvement over the Ham-D in that it appears to better differentiate between responders and nonresponders to intervention for depression. The instrument does not include many somatic symptoms that tend to be more common in older adults, and therefore it may be of greater value in tracking the symptoms of depressive illness that would be expected to change with therapy.

General Assessment Scales

A number of general assessment scales of psychiatric status (occasionally combined with functioning in other areas) have been found to be useful in both community and clinical populations. One of the more frequently used scales is the Global Assessment of Functioning Scale (American Psychiatric Association 2000). Using this scale, the rater makes a single rating, from 0 to 100, that best describes—on the basis of his or her clinical judgment—the lowest level of the subject's functioning in the week before the rating. The scale has not been standardized for older adults, but its common use in psychiatric studies suggests the need for standardization. The scale was incorporated as Axis V in DSM-IV (American Psychiatric Association 1994) to measure overall functioning.

The Geriatric Mental State Schedule (Copeland et al. 1976), an adaptation of the Present State Exam (Wing et al. 1974) and the Psychiatric Status Schedule (Spitzer et al. 1968), is a semistructured interviewing guide that allows the rater to inventory symptoms associated with psychiatric disorders. More than 500 ratings are made on the basis of information obtained by a highly trained interviewer, who elicits reports of symptoms from the month preceding the evaluation. Data are computerized to derive psychiatric diagnoses (Copeland et al. 1986). The instrument measures depression, impaired memory, selected neurological symptoms such as aphasia, and disorientation.

The Comprehensive Assessment and Referral Evaluation (CARE) (Gurland et al. 1977) is a hybridized assessment procedure developed for older adults. Dimensional scores are obtained in these areas: Memory–Disorientation, Depression–Anxiety, Immobility–Incapacity, Isolation, Physical–Perceptual Difficulty, and Poor Housing–Income. The goal of CARE is to provide a comprehensive assessment of the older adult that bridges the professional disciplines. The instrument has not been used extensively, although it has been used in cross-national studies. For example, Herbst and

Humphrey (1980) used CARE in a study examining how hearing impairment relates to mental status. The investigators found a relationship between deafness and depression that was independent of age and socioeconomic status.

The Older Americans Resources and Services (OARS) Multidimensional Functional Assessment Questionnaire (Duke University Center for the Study of Aging and Human Development 1978), administered by a lay interviewer, produces functional impairment ratings in five dimensions: mental health, physical health, social functioning, economic functioning, and activities of daily living. In one community survey using OARS (Blazer 1978a), 13% of persons in the community were found to have mental health impairment. The OARS instrument was developed to integrate functional measures across a series of parameters relevant to older adults; it has been used widely in both community and clinical surveys. With the recent emphasis on discrete psychiatric disorders, however, the instrument has not been as widely used by mental health workers as it might otherwise have been.

Any discussion of clinical rating scales is not complete without a discussion of the Abnormal Involuntary Movement Scale (AIMS) (National Institute of Mental Health 1975). There has been an increased incidence of tardive dyskinesia among older adults, coupled with the need for better documentation of this outcome of prolonged use of antipsychotic agents. Regular ratings of patients on the AIMS by clinicians have therefore become essential to the practice of inpatient and outpatient geriatric psychiatry. The scale consists of seven movement disorders; the presence and severity of each is rated from "none" to "severe." Three items require a global judgment: severity of abnormal movements, incapacitation due to abnormal movements, and the patient's awareness of abnormal movements. Current problems with teeth or dentures are also assessed. Procedures are described to increase the reliability of this rating scale.

Structured Diagnostic Interviews

A number of structured interview schedules are available for both clinical and community diagnosis. These interview schedules have allowed increased reliability of the identification of particular symptoms and psychiatric diagnoses; however, if one adheres closely to the structured interview, the richness inherent in the unstructured interview tends to be lost. Comments made by the patient during the evaluation that could be used to trace relevant associations must be ignored to push through the interview schedule. Most of these interviews require more time than the traditional unstructured first session with the patient.

The most frequently used instrument in the United States is the Structured Clinical Interview for DSM-IV (SCID) (First et al. 1997). This instrument is easily adaptable to the RDC, DSM-IV, and DSM-IV-TR. Although specific questions are suggested for probing most areas of interest, the interviewer using the SCID has the flexibility to ask additional questions and can use any available data to assign a diagnosis. The interviewer must have clinical training but does not have to be a psychiatrist. Many of the symptoms may not be relevant to older adults (especially the extensive probes for psychotic symptoms), and the interview frequently takes 2.5–3 hours to administer. Nevertheless, the experience gained by the clinician in using this instrument can contribute to a more effective clinical practice.

The Diagnostic Interview Schedule (DIS) (Robins et al. 1981) is a highly structured, computer-scored interview that can be administered by a lay interviewer and allows psychiatric diagnoses to be made according to DSM-IV criteria, Feighner criteria (Feighner et al. 1972), and RDC. The DIS questions probe for the presence or absence of symptoms or behaviors relevant to a series of psychiatric disorders, the severity of the symptoms, and the putative cause of the symptoms. Diagnoses of cognitive impairment, schizophrenia or schizophreniform disorder, major depression, generalized anxiety disorder, panic disorder, agoraphobia, obsessive-compulsive disorder, dysthymic disorder, somatization disorder, alcohol abuse and/or dependence, and other substance abuse and/or dependence can be made from Axis I of DSM-IV. A diagnosis of antisocial personality disorder (Axis II) can also be made. The instrument has proved reasonably reliable in clinical populations for both current and lifetime diagnoses.

The range of disorders probed by the DIS questions, coupled with the instrument's relative ease of administration (it generally takes 45–90 minutes to administer to an older adult), has made it popular for use in clinical studies. In addition, community-based comparative data are available on a large sample from the Epidemiologic Catchment Area study (Myers et al. 1984; Regier et al. 1984). The DIS can be supplemented with additional questions to probe for specific symptoms, such as melancholic symptoms, and additional data on sleep disorders for depressed older adults. No problems have arisen when the instrument is used among older adults in the community. In general, the memory decay that occurs in elderly persons causes no more of a performance problem on this instrument than on others. Nevertheless, the DIS is of less value in the study of institutional populations and in reconstruction of lifetime history regardless of setting, because memory problems cannot be circumvented by clinical judgment. Supplementary data can be added to the instrument for developing a standardized diagnosis. A shortened version of the DIS, which has been used in recent epidemiological surveys, is the Composite International Diagnostic Interview (World Health Organization 1989).

Effective Communication With the Older Adult

The clinician who works with the older adult should be cognizant of factors relating to both the patient and the clinician that may produce barriers to effective communication (Blazer 1978b). Many older persons experience a relatively high level of anxiety yet do not complain of this symptom. Stress deriving from a new situation, such as visiting a clinician's office or being interviewed in a hospital, may intensify such anxiety and subsequently impair effective communication. Perceptual problems, such as hearing and visual impairment, may exacerbate disorientation and complicate the communication of problems to the clinician. Elderly persons are more likely to withhold information than to hazard answers that may be incorrect—in other words, older persons tend to be more cautious. Elderly persons frequently take longer to respond to inquiries and resist the clinician who attempts to rush through the history-taking interview.

The elderly patient may perceive the physician unrealistically, on the basis of previous life experiences (i.e., transference may occur). Although the older patient will sometimes accept the role of child, viewing the physician as parent, the patient is initially more likely to view the clinician as the idealized child who can provide reciprocal care to the previously capable but now impaired parent. Splitting between the physician (idealized) and the children of the patient (devalued) may subsequently occur. Also, the clinician may perceive the older adult patient incorrectly because of fears of aging and death or because of previous negative experiences with his or her own parents. In order for a clinician to work effectively with older adults, these personal feelings should be discussed during training—and afterward.

Once physician and patient attitudes have been recognized and acknowledged, certain techniques have generally proved to be valuable in communicating with the elderly patient. These techniques should not be implemented indiscriminately, however, for the variation in the population of older adults is significant. First, the older person should be approached with respect. The clinician should knock before entering a patient's room and should greet the patient by surname (e.g., Mr. Jones, Mrs. Smith) rather than by a given name, unless the clinician also wishes to be addressed by a given name.

After taking a position near the older person—near enough to reach out and touch the patient—the clinician should speak clearly and slowly and use simple sentences in case the person's hearing is impaired. Because of hearing problems, older patients may understand conversation better over the telephone than in person. By placing the receiver against the mastoid bone, the patient with otosclerosis can take advantage of preserved bone conduction.

The interview should be paced so that the older person has enough time to respond to questions. Most elders are not uncomfortable with silence, because it gives them an opportunity to formulate their answers to questions and elaborate certain points they wish to emphasize. Nonverbal communication is frequently a key to effective communication with elderly persons, because they may be reticent about revealing affect verbally. The patient's facial expressions, gestures, postures, and long silences may provide clues to the clinician about issues that are unspoken.

One key to successful communication with an older adult is a willingness to continue working as a professional with that person. Older adults—possibly unlike some of their children and grandchildren—place a great deal of stress on loyalty and continuity. Most elderly patients do not require large amounts of time from clinicians, and those who are more demanding can usually be controlled through structure in the interview.

Key Points

- The diagnostic interview is the cornerstone of assessment and treatment assignment for the older adult with psychiatric impairment.

- A thorough medication history, although it takes time to obtain, saves valuable time and complications in the treatment of psychiatric disorders in older adults.
- Functional status (i.e., the ability to perform usual activities of daily living) is often as important as diagnosis in tracking the progress of treatment of psychiatric disorders in older adults.
- Geriatric psychiatry is family psychiatry.
- What is gained in reliability by using a structured diagnostic interview is offset by the loss of valuable information about the subjective feelings of the older adult and the context of the emergence of symptoms.
- Speak clearly and slowly but not in a patronizing way to the older adult, who might have a hearing impairment.

References

American Psychiatric Association: Diagnostic and Statistical Manual of Mental Disorders, 4th Edition. Washington, DC, American Psychiatric Association, 1994

American Psychiatric Association: Diagnostic and Statistical Manual of Mental Disorders, 4th Edition, Text Revision. Washington, DC, American Psychiatric Association, 2000

Ayd FJ: Treatment-resistant patients: a moral, legal and therapeutic challenge, in Rational Psychopharmacotherapy and the Right to Treatment. Edited by Ayd FJ. Baltimore, MD, Ayd Medical Communications, 1975, pp 3–15

Beck AT, Ward CH, Mendelson M, et al: An inventory for measuring depression. Arch Gen Psychiatry 4:561–571, 1961

Blazer DG: The OARS Durham surveys: description and application, in Multidimensional Functional Assessment: The OARS Methodology—A Manual, 2nd Edition. Durham, NC, Duke University Center for the Study of Aging and Human Development, 1978a, pp 75–88

Blazer DG: Techniques for communicating with your elderly patient. Geriatrics 33:79–80, 83–84, 1978b

Blazer DG: Depression in Late Life. St Louis, MO, CV Mosby, 1982

Blazer DG: Evaluating the family of the elderly patient, in A Family Approach to Health Care in the Elderly. Edited by Blazer D, Siegler IC. Menlo Park, CA, Addison-Wesley, 1984, pp 13–32

Blazer DG, Kaplan BH: The assessment of social support in an elderly community population. Am J Soc Psychiatry 3:29–36, 1983

Blessed G, Tomlinson BE, Roth M: The association between quantitative measures of dementia and of senile change in the cerebral gray matter of elderly subjects. Br J Psychiatry 114:797–811, 1968

Copeland JRM, Kelleher MJ, Kellet JM, et al: A semi-structured clinical interview for the assessment and diagnosis of mental state in the elderly: the Geriatric Mental State Schedule, I: development and reliability. Psychol Med 6:439–449, 1976

Copeland JRM, Dewey ME, Griffiths-Jones HM, et al: A computerized psychiatric diagnostic system and case nomenclature for elderly subjects: GMS and AGECAT. Psychol Med 16:89–99, 1986

Duke University Center for the Study of Aging and Human Development: Multidimensional Functional Assessment: The OARS Methodology—A Manual, 2nd Edition. Durham, NC, Duke University Center for the Study of Aging and Human Development, 1978

Eisenberg L: Disease and illness: distinctions between professional and popular ideas of sickness. Cult Med Psychiatry 1:9–23, 1977

Eisenberg L, Kleinman A: Clinical social science, in The Relevance of Social Science for Medicine. Edited by Eisenberg L, Kleinman A. Boston, MA, D Reidel, 1981, pp 1–26

Feighner JP, Robins E, Guze SB, et al: Diagnostic criteria for use in psychiatric research. Arch Gen Psychiatry 26:57–63, 1972

First MB, Spitzer RL, Gibbon M: Structured Clinical Interview for DSM-IV. Washington, DC, American Psychiatric Press, 1997

Folstein MF, Folstein SE, McHugh PR: "Mini-Mental State": a practical method for grading the cognitive state of patients for the clinician. J Psychiatr Res 12:189–198, 1975

Gallagher D, Nies G, Thompson LW: Reliability of the Beck Depression Inventory with older adults. J Consult Clin Psychol 50:152–153, 1982

Gallagher D, Breckenridge J, Steinmetz J, et al: The Beck Depression Inventory and Research Diagnostic Criteria: congruence in an older population. J Consult Clin Psychol 51:945–946, 1983

Gurland B, Kuriansky J, Sharpe L, et al: The Comprehensive Assessment and Referral Evaluation (CARE)—rationale, development and reliability. Int J Aging Hum Dev 8:9–42, 1977

Hachinski VC, Iliff LD, Zilhka E, et al: Cerebral blood flow in dementia. Arch Neurol 32:632–637, 1975

Hamilton M: A rating scale for depression. J Neurol Neurosurg Psychiatry 23:56–62, 1960

Herbst KG, Humphrey C: Hearing impairment and mental state in the elderly living at home. BMJ 281:903–905, 1980

Inouye SK: Clarifying confusion: the Confusion Assessment Method—a new method for detection of delirium. Ann Intern Med 113:941–950, 1990

Kahn RL, Goldfarb AI, Pollack M, et al: Brief objective measures for the determination of mental status in the aged. Am J Psychiatry 117:326–328, 1960

Linn L: Clinical manifestations of psychiatric disorders, in Comprehensive Textbook of Psychiatry, 3rd Edition, Vol 1. Edited by Kaplan HI, Freedman AM, Sadock BJ. Baltimore, MD, Williams and Wilkins, 1980, pp 990–1034

Mendlewicz J, Fleiss JL, Cataldo M, et al: Accuracy of the family history method in affective illness: comparison with direct interviews in family studies. Arch Gen Psychiatry 32:309–314, 1975

Meyers BS, Greenberg R: Late-life delusional depression. J Affect Disord 11:133–137, 1986

Meyers BS, Greenberg R, Varda M: Delusional depression in the elderly, in Treatment of Affective Disorders in the Elderly. Edited by Shamoian CA. Washington, DC, American Psychiatric Press, 1985, pp 37–63

Montgomery SA, Åsberg M: A new depression scale designed to be sensitive to change. Br J Psychiatry 134:382–389, 1979

Myers JK, Weissman MM, Tischler GL, et al: Six-month prevalence of psychiatric disorders in three communities: 1980 to 1982. Arch Gen Psychiatry 41:959–967, 1984

National Institute of Mental Health: Development of a Dyskinetic Movement Scale (Publ No 4). Rockville, MD, National Institute of Mental Health, Psychopharmacology Research Branch, 1975

Pfeiffer E: A Short Portable Mental Status Questionnaire for the assessment of organic brain deficit in elderly patients. J Am Geriatr Soc 23:433–441, 1975

Radloff LS: The CES-D Scale: a self-report depression scale for research in the general population. Applied Psychological Measurement 1:385–401, 1977

Regier DA, Myers JK, Kramer M, et al: The NIMH Epidemiologic Catchment Area program: historical context, major objectives, and study population characteristics. Arch Gen Psychiatry 41:934–941, 1984

Robins LN, Helzer JE, Croughan J, et al: National Institute of Mental Health Diagnostic Interview Schedule: its history, characteristics, and validity. Arch Gen Psychiatry 38:381–389, 1981

Ross CE, Mirowsky J: Components of depressed mood in married men and women: the CES-D. Am J Epidemiol 119:997–1004, 1984

Sanford JRA: Tolerance of debility in elderly dependents by supporters at home: its significance for hospital practice. BMJ 3:471–473, 1975

Spitzer RL, Endicott J, Cohen GM: Psychiatric Status Schedule, 2nd Edition. New York, New York State Department of Mental Hygiene, Evaluation Unit, Biometrics Research, 1968

Spitzer RL, Endicott J, Robins E: Research Diagnostic Criteria: rationale and reliability. Arch Gen Psychiatry 35:773–782, 1978

Wing JK, Cooper JE, Sartorius N: The Measurement and Classification of Psychiatric Symptoms. London, Cambridge University Press, 1974

World Health Organization: Composite International Diagnostic Interview. Geneva, Switzerland, World Health Organization, 1989

Yesavage JA, Brink TL, Rose TL, et al: Development and validation of a geriatric depression screening scale: a preliminary report. J Psychiatr Res 17:37–49, 1983

Suggested Readings

Blazer DG: Techniques for communicating with your elderly patient. Geriatrics 33:79–80, 83–84, 1978

Folstein MF, Folstein SE, McHugh PR: "Mini-Mental State": a practical method for grading the cognitive state of patients for the clinician. J Psychiatr Res 12:189–198, 1975

Inouye SK: Clarifying confusion: the Confusion Assessment Method: a new method for detection of delirium. Ann Intern Med 113:941–950, 1990

Othmer E, Othmer SC, Othmer JP: Psychiatric interview, history and mental status examination, in Kaplan and Sadock's Comprehensive Textbook of Psychiatry, Vol 1. Edited by Sadock BJ, Sadock VA. Philadelphia, PA, Lippincott Williams & Wilkins, 2005, pp 794–826

CHAPTER 10

Use of the Laboratory in the Diagnostic Workup of Older Adults

Mugdha Thakur, M.D.
P. Murali Doraiswamy, M.D.

Laboratory testing is an essential component of the psychiatric evaluation of elderly individuals, who often present with comorbid medical illnesses. The laboratory does not replace the clinician; there is no test that is pathognomonic for a primary psychiatric illness. However, laboratory testing does aid in the evaluation of comorbidities that complicate or contribute to a psychiatric diagnosis.

There has been significant growth in the number and quality of diagnostic tools available. Progress in research and technology, particularly in imaging technology and genetic testing, has advanced rapidly over the past decade. Regardless of the tools available, however, we must balance what we *can* do with what we *should* do, as guided by our clinical judgment, relative risk to the patient, and cost expenditure. When all risks are considered, the decision to proceed with a test should be based on the clinical presentation and on how the test results may change a treatment plan.

The following discussion of specific diagnostic tests is not an exhaustive review. We focus on tests currently being used or being considered for clinical use. We hope this chapter will assist the clinician in selecting laboratory tests that are appropriate for the individual patient.

Serologic Tests

Basic clinical chemistry and hematologic screens are routine for all hospital admissions and many outpatient evaluations. Although these screens infrequently identify causes of primary psychiatric disorders, they are critical for identifying previously undiagnosed or poorly controlled medical illnesses that may contribute to mental status changes, such as in dementia or delirium. These tests should also be monitored when patients are on medications that may result in potentially dangerous abnormalities. For most of these tests, the only risks are associated with blood draws, which may result in transient pain, bruising, and occasional bleeding or fainting. These risks are reduced, but not totally eliminated, by skilled phlebotomists.

Hematologic Tests

A complete blood cell count (CBC) is a standard part of any evaluation. It screens for multiple problems, including infections and anemia. It also provides a platelet count, a value important to monitor in psychiatric medications associated with thrombocytopenia, such as divalproex sodium or carbamazepine. This concern is particularly important in elderly patients, because there is some evidence that the risk of drug-induced thrombocytopenia may increase with age (Trannel et al. 2001). Lithium, in contrast, may result in mild leukocytosis. Due to the risk of agranulocytosis, CBC testing is required weekly or biweekly for patients on clozapine and may be needed more frequently if the patient develops signs of infection. Mirtazapine can also rarely lead to agranulocytosis, and although routine CBC monitoring is not indicated, it should be pursued if a patient develops sore throat, fever, stomatitis, or other signs of infection.

Chemistry Tests

Most general chemistry panels have a variety of values that may be helpful in medical evaluations. Blood glucose values may reveal hyperinsulinemia and hypoglycemia, which may produce anxiety and weakness; more commonly it shows hyperglycemia, which may be associated with diabetes and result in lethargy or, in severe cases, delirium, diabetic coma, or ketoacidosis. This testing is critical for the diagnosis of diabetes, which can be diagnosed with 1) an overnight fasting glucose greater than 126 mg/dL, 2) a random plasma glucose greater than 200 mg/dL with symptoms of diabetes, or 3) an oral glucose tolerance test resulting in a plasma glucose over 200 mg/dL 2 hours after a 75-g glucose load (Dagogo-Jack 2001).

Kidney function tests are equally important. Blood urea nitrogen and creatinine will be elevated in kidney failure and in hypovolemic states such as dehydration. These tests also must be performed before initiating lithium therapy because of lithium's potential for nephrotoxicity.

General chemistry panels also measure serum sodium, potassium, and other electrolytes. Hyponatremia—commonly defined as a serum sodium concentration less than 135 mEq/L—has been reported with selective serotonin reuptake inhibitors (SSRIs), particularly in the elderly (Jacob and Spinler 2006). The signs and symptoms of hyponatremia result from neurological dysfunction secondary to cerebral edema. Acute hyponatremia can start with nausea and malaise when the plasma sodium concentration falls below 125–130 mEq/L and progresses rapidly to coma and respiratory arrest if the plasma sodium concentration falls below 115–120 mEq/L. In chronic hyponatremia, the brain cells adapt to the edema, and symptoms are much less severe. Patients may be asymptomatic despite a plasma sodium concentration that is persistently as low as 115–120 mEq/L. When symptoms do occur in patients with such low sodium concentrations, they are relatively nonspecific (e.g., fatigue, nausea, dizziness, gait disturbances, forgetfulness, confusion, lethargy, muscle cramps). The clinician should be vigilant to this risk in older adults started on SSRIs. Of all the electrolyte abnormalities, potassium disorders may be the most crucial to identify. These rarely cause psychiatric symptoms but may result in severe cardiac arrhythmias. Although not always included in routine chemistry screens, calcium and magnesium levels are also important to consider, as abnormal levels may result in paranoid ideation or frank psychosis. Any or all of these results may be abnormal in patients on hemodialysis.

Because second-generation antipsychotic drugs can lead to weight gain and diabetes, a new set of guidelines has been proposed to screen and monitor patients started on these drugs for risk of metabolic dysregulation (American Diabetes Association et al. 2004) (Table 10–1). These guidelines should be routinely incorporated into clinical practice by all geropsychiatrists. Additionally, in patients who develop abdominal pain while being treated with atypical antipsychotics or valproic acid, amylase and lipase levels should be checked to rule out pancreatitis because several cases have been reported. Liver function tests should be monitored periodically in patients on valproic acid. There have been case reports of both venlafaxine and duloxetine causing elevated hepatic enzymes and even hepatic failure. Liver function tests should be obtained in patients on these drugs who develop symptoms of liver disease.

Serologic Tests for Syphilis

Since the early 1980s, there have been no reported cases of tertiary syphilis in any of the incidence or prevalence studies conducted in North America (Knopman et al. 2001). There are only a few areas in the United States, mainly in the South and in some regions of the Midwest, with high numbers of syphilis cases. According to the American Academy of Neurology's guidelines for diagnosis of dementia, unless the patient has some specific risk factor (e.g., another sexually transmitted disease) or evidence of prior syphilitic infection or unless the patient resides in one of the few areas in the United States with high numbers of syphilis cases, screening for the disorder in patients with dementia is not justified (Knopman et al. 2001). If a clinician suspects syphilis infection, the Venereal Disease Research Laboratory and the rapid plasmin reagin tests are screening tools for infection with *Treponema pallidum*, the cause of syphilis. These tests are unfortunately nonspecific; false-positive results may occur in acute infections and chronic illnesses such as systemic lupus erythematosus. More specific tests, the fluorescent treponemal antibody and the

TABLE 10–1. Guidelines for screening and monitoring of patients started on second-generation antipsychotic agents[a]

Assessment	Frequency
Personal and family history[b]	At baseline and annually
Weight	At baseline, every 4 weeks for 12 weeks, then quarterly
Waist circumference[c]	At baseline and annually
Blood pressure	At baseline, at 12 weeks, and annually
Fasting plasma glucose	At baseline, at 12 weeks, and annually
Fasting lipid profile	At baseline, at 12 weeks, and every 5 years

[a]More frequent assessments may need to be done based on clinical status.
[b]Personal and family history includes obesity, diabetes, dyslipidemia, hypertension, or cardiovascular disease.
[c]Waist circumference is measured at umbilicus.

Source. American Diabetes Association, American Psychiatric Association, American Association of Clinical Endocrinologists, North American Association for the Study of Obesity: "Consensus Development Conference on Antipsychotic Drugs and Obesity and Diabetes." *Diabetes Care* 27:596–601, 2004.

microhemagglutination–*Treponema pallidum*, may distinguish false-positive from true-positive results and may aid in diagnosing late syphilis when blood and even cerebrospinal fluid (CSF) reagin tests are negative.

Human Immunodeficiency Virus Testing

From 1990 to the end of 2001, the cumulative number of acquired immunodeficiency syndrome (AIDS) cases reported to the Centers for Disease Control and Prevention in adults age 50 years or older increased fivefold, from 16,288 to 90,513 (Mack and Ory 2003). A higher prevalence of human immunodeficiency virus (HIV) infection has been reported in older individuals in specific states, such as Florida (13%) and Hawaii (20%).

The diagnosis of AIDS in the elderly is complicated; like syphilis, AIDS has been described as the "great imitator" because its clinical presentation may mimic that of other diseases (Sabin 1987). AIDS may mimic not only medical illnesses but also neuropsychiatric disorders, because AIDS may result in dementia.

There is no evidence that HIV treatment for elderly AIDS patients should differ from that for younger patients. It is thus the role of the geriatric psychiatrist to assist the internist by screening for risk factors, such as a history of sexually transmitted diseases, intravenous drug use, risky sexual behavior, or a history of blood transfusions, particularly if they occurred prior to the early 1990s. We recommend HIV testing in individuals who have these risk factors or those who present with atypical neuropsychiatric symptoms. For patients for whom testing is warranted, the geriatric psychiatrist will also play an important role in counseling the patients about the reasons behind testing, and then providing further counseling as the test results are reported.

Thyroid Function Tests

To understand the significance of thyroid test results, one must first understand the hormones themselves. Secretion of the thyroid hormones thyroxine (T_4) and triiodothyronine (T_3) is regulated by pituitary gland secretion of thyroid-stimulating hormone (TSH). TSH secretion, in turn, is controlled through negative feedback by thyroid hormones. Both T_4 and T_3 are reversibly bound to the plasma protein thyroxine-binding globulin (TBG), and only the small unbound fraction exerts its physiological effects.

A serum TSH test is the most frequently used screen for thyroid disease; it is an excellent screening test because of its high negative predictive value (Klee and Hay 1997). However, many medications may result in increased TSH levels (amiodarone, estrogens) or decreased TSH levels (glucocorticoids, phenytoin) (Kaplan 1999), and altered TSH levels may also be seen in patients with acute nonthyroidal illness or systemic stress. A physical examination and measurement of T_4, T_3, and TBG may be required for a definitive diagnosis of thyroid disease (Table 10–2). TSH testing should be done in all older adults presenting with neuropsychiat-

TABLE 10–2. Patterns of thyroid function tests

TSH	Free T_4	T_3	Suggested diagnosis
Normal	Normal	Normal	Euthyroid
High	Low	Low or normal	Primary hypothyroidism
High	Normal	Normal	Subclinical hypothyroidism
Low	High or normal	High	Hyperthyroidism

Note. TSH=thyroid-stimulating hormone; T_4=thyroxine; T_3=triiodothyronine.

ric symptoms because hypothyroidism may cause symptoms of depression, fatigue, and impaired cognition, and hyperthyroidism can cause symptoms of anxiety or even psychosis. Older women in particular have a high prevalence of hypothyroidism. Patients on lithium treatment should have their TSH checked every 6 months.

Vitamin B_{12}, Folate, and Homocysteine

Measurement of serum vitamin B_{12} and folate levels is an integral part of the laboratory evaluation. The prevalence of B_{12} deficiency increases with age; the deficiency is present in up to 15% of the elderly population (Stabler et al. 1997). Although macrocytic anemia is a well-known sign of B_{12} deficiency, it is a later presentation in most cases, with neuropsychiatric symptoms presenting much earlier.

B_{12} and folate deficiencies may result in neuropsychiatric disturbances, including depression, psychosis, or cognitive deficits. Studies in populations with dementia demonstrate that B_{12} deficiencies often result in delirium or disorientation (Carmel et al. 1995; Cunha et al. 1995). Low levels of these vitamins may also result in visuospatial and word fluency deficits (Robins Wahlin et al. 2001) and even greater behavioral disturbances in Alzheimer's disease (Meins et al. 2000).

However, B_{12} and folate levels may not tell the entire story; there is also considerable interest in homocysteine. Serum homocysteine levels may serve as a functional indicator of B_{12} and folate status (Selhub et al. 2000), because both vitamins are needed to convert homocysteine to methionine in one-carbon metabolism in brain tissue. Hyperhomocysteinemia is prevalent in elderly persons, and high serum levels of homocysteine can be attributed to an inadequate supply of B_{12} and folate, even in the presence of low normal serum levels (Selhub et al. 2000). High levels of homocysteine have also been associated with increased risk of occlusive vascular disease, thrombosis, and stroke (Boushey et al. 1995). Hyperhomocysteinemia is further associated with cognitive dysfunction (Leblhuber et al. 2000; Selhub et al. 2000), although not all authors have found this association (Ravaglia et al. 2000). In a longitudinal study of 965 older individuals, a lower incidence of Alzheimer's disease was noted among those subjects in the highest quartile of total folate intake, after adjustments for age, sex, education, ethnicity, and other comorbidities. Neither vitamin B_6 nor vitamin B_{12} intake was associated with risk of Alzheimer's disease (Luchsinger et al. 2007). Results on whether vitamin supplementation to reduce plasma homocysteine levels also leads to improved cognition are mixed, with some studies showing benefit (Durga et al. 2007; Nilsson et al. 2001) and others showing no benefit despite lowered homocysteine levels (McMahon et al. 2006).

Toxicology

When there is an acute change in an individual's mental status, an investigation of the cause of the change must include ingestion of a substance. This consideration is particularly important in individuals with a history of substance abuse or with a history of depression in which there is the risk of medication overdose.

When mental status changes in an individual who is taking medications such as lithium, phenytoin, tricyclic antidepressants (TCAs), or any medication that requires monitoring of blood levels, those levels should be checked. Toxic levels of many pharmacological agents may cause a variety of psychiatric or life-threatening medical conditions. Likewise, levels for common over-the-counter medications such as acetaminophen and salicylates can be tested. Concomitantly, a serum alcohol level should also be drawn. Depending on the individual's history, even a negative result may be critical if there is the possibility of withdrawal. Finally, urine can be tested for prescription medications, such as benzodiazepines, barbiturates, and opioids, as well as illicit substances, such as cocaine and marijuana. Advanced age does not preclude addiction.

Urinalysis

A urinalysis is an inexpensive, noninvasive test that provides a significant amount of information. It determines the urine's specific gravity, which may indicate dehydration, and also tests for glucose and ketones, important in the evaluation of diabetic patients. In the elderly population, the most important use of urinalysis may be as a screening tool for urinary tract infections (UTIs). A UTI is suggested by a microscopic examination showing high levels of white blood cells, bacteria, positive leukocyte esterase and nitrite, and possibly red blood cells; high numbers of epithelial cells make the results difficult to interpret, because they suggest contamination. A urine culture is a definitive means of diagnosing a UTI and will identify the infecting organism and its susceptibility to antimicrobial treatments. Approximately 20% of admissions from the community to a geropsychiatry unit may have UTIs, and many cases of UTI result in a delirium that improves with appropriate antibiotic treatment (Levkoff et al. 1991; Manepalli et al. 1990).

Cerebrospinal Fluid Analysis

Although the lumbar puncture is known to be useful in the workup of suspected central nervous system infections, such as meningitis, CSF analysis has only recently become part of the assessment of patients with dementia. Patients with Alzheimer's disease show lower levels of β-amyloid$_{1-42}$ and higher levels of tau protein than do healthy older adults (Galasko et al. 1998; Hulstaert et al. 1999). However, because the utility of these tests over clinical diagnosis is not yet established, they are not recommended in routine clinical practice.

Hsich et al. (1996) described an immunoassay for the detection of the 14-3-3 protein in CSF that had a specificity of 99% and a sensitivity of 96% for the diagnosis of Creutzfeldt-Jakob disease (CJD) among patients with dementia. CSF 14-3-3 protein assay has been found to be superior to electroencephalography or magnetic resonance imaging in identifying cases of CJD (Poser et al. 1999). However, other acute neurological conditions such as stroke, viral encephalitis, and paraneoplastic neurological disorders can provide false-positive results. Nevertheless, the American Academy of Neurology recommends testing for CSF 14-3-3 protein for confirming or rejecting the diagnosis of CJD in clinically appropriate circumstances (Knopman et al. 2001).

Electrocardiogram

An electrocardiogram (ECG) provides a graphic representation of the heart's electrical activity, obtained via surface electrodes placed in specific locations on the patient's chest. This placement makes possible a graph of electrical activity from a variety of spatial perspectives. In psychiatry, the most important roles of the ECG include screening for cardiovascular disease that may preclude the use of specific medications and monitoring for drug-induced electrocardiographic changes either from standard doses or from overdose. Electrocardiographic changes associated with specific psychotropic medications are summarized in Table 10–3.

The tricyclic antidepressants are well known to be cardiotoxic in overdose; even at therapeutic doses, their use is considered unsafe in patients with cardiovascular disease, particularly ischemic disease (Roose 2000). Although the most common cardiovascular complication of TCAs is orthostatic hypotension (Glassman and Bigger 1981), TCAs have the same pharmacological properties as type IA antiarrhythmics, such as quinidine and procainamide. TCAs slow conduction at the bundle of His; individuals with preexisting bundle branch block who take TCAs are at increased risk for atrioventricular

TABLE 10–3. Common electrocardiographic abnormalities associated with psychotropic medications

Medication	Electrocardiographic change
Antipsychotics (typical or atypical agents)	Increased QTc interval Potential for torsades de pointes
β-blockers	Bradycardia
Lithium	Sick sinus syndrome Sinoatrial block
Tricyclic antidepressants	Increased PR, QRS, or QT intervals Atrioventricular block

block. Even therapeutic levels are associated with prolonged PR intervals and QRS complexes; these results may be more pronounced in elderly individuals because the incidence and severity of adverse drug reactions increase with age (Pollock 1999). If TCAs are used, baseline and frequent follow-up ECGs should be obtained.

Lithium may also result in electrocardiographic changes, and an ECG is recommended prior to starting lithium treatment and regularly while on therapy. Lithium appears to most affect the sinus node, and even at therapeutic levels it may result in sick sinus syndrome or sinoatrial block, either of which may occur early or later in treatment. At higher levels, there have been reports of sinus arrest and asystole.

Antipsychotics also result in electrocardiographic changes; about 25% of individuals receiving antipsychotics exhibit electrocardiographic abnormalities (Thomas 1994). Although many of these changes have historically been considered benign, there is increased concern that prolongation of the QT interval (when corrected for heart rate, the QTc interval) may contribute to potentially fatal ventricular arrhythmias, particularly torsades de pointes. QTc values are typically around 400 milliseconds in duration; values lower than this are considered normal. Because the greater the duration, the greater the risk of torsades, 500 milliseconds is frequently used as a cutoff (Glassman and Bigger 2001). It is important to note that other medications also affect the QTc interval and produce an additive effect when combined with an antipsychotic. This phenomenon may be seen with almost any antipsychotic agent but is most likely to be associated with thioridazine and haloperidol among typical antipsychotics and with ziprasidone among atypical antipsychotics (Glassman and Bigger 2001). Unfortunately, there are currently concerns about QTc prolongation for all atypical antipsychotic agents.

Routine ECGs for all patients receiving antipsychotics are not currently recommended, but it is wise to be prudent. A careful history for cardiac illness, family history, or syncope should be obtained for all patients. ECGs should be considered more carefully in patients with other risk factors, such as heart failure, bradycardia, electrolyte imbalance, female sex, old age, hepatic or renal impairment, and slow metabolizer status.

With few exceptions, an ECG should always be obtained in cases of potential medication overdose, even in cases where the medication used is not associated with arrhythmias. ECGs are important because some medications may affect heart rhythm in overdose when they would not do so at usual doses. Also, suicidal patients often do not report all the medications that they have used to overdose; suicide attempts may be impulsive, and patients who have an altered mental status may not be able to provide a complete report.

Imaging Studies

Plain film radiographs remain an integral piece of the diagnostic imaging performed in geriatric psychiatry. Such techniques are most commonly used to detect lung pathology that may contribute to mental status changes or to detect bone fractures. Plain film radiographs are critical for individuals who have both severe dementia and either a recent history of falls or newly developed limb immobility.

A number of more recently developed imaging techniques have greatly enhanced our diagnostic abilities. These techniques are costly, so they should not be used without a good rationale that includes why they are needed and how the specific findings may affect a patient's treatment plan. The following discussion focuses on two commonly used structural imaging techniques: computed tomography and magnetic resonance imaging. Because these techniques are also discussed in other chapters of this book, we focus on the scientific basis behind these tools and provide information to support their clinical use, particularly in brain imaging, and to facilitate providing informed consent.

This section does not discuss functional imaging techniques, such as positron emission tomography (PET) and single-photon emission computed tomography (SPECT), which play a role in examining brain metabolic rates or regional blood flow. These imaging procedures have a limited clinical use and are used primarily in research.

Computed Tomography

Computed tomography (CT) is a general term for several radiographic techniques that result in the computer-assisted generation of a series of images showing slices of an organ or body region, such as the brain or abdomen. The CT scanner uses a small X-ray device that rotates around the body region of interest in a fixed plane; these signals are sent to a computer that produces the corresponding cross-sectional slice for that plane. The computer can create sections in axial, coronal, and sagittal alignments. More recent advances in software and display systems have led to many useful clinical applications, including virtual CT colonoscopy or angiography.

When used to examine brain structure, CT can allow for the ready identification of many structures, although it does have limitations. By measuring differences in density, it can distinguish among CSF, blood, bone, gray matter, and white matter. CT is particularly useful for demonstrating bone abnormalities (such as skull fractures), areas of hemorrhage (such as a subdural hematoma), and the mass effect from various lesions. It can also display atrophy or ventricular enlargement. However, CT is not very useful for visualizing posterior fossa or brain stem structures because of surrounding bone.

A typical concern of patients is radiation exposure. CT scans require the use of a limited amount of radiation; any given CT procedure results in a radiation exposure, but that exposure is well below governmental recommendations for individuals who work around radiation. However, these recommendations do not consider multiple CT scans (thus multiple radiation exposures) or CT studies that overlap scanned regions, a technique that increases the radiation dose (Nickoloff and Alderson 2001). CT imaging should be used when appropriate, but other assessment techniques that may result in lower radiation exposure should also be considered.

Magnetic Resonance Imaging

Whereas CT scanners rely on radiation, in magnetic resonance imaging (MRI), the scanner creates a magnetic field that is 3,000–25,000 times the strength of the earth's natural magnetic field. The underlying principle behind MRI is that the nuclei of identifiable endogenous isotopes (such as hydrogen or phosphorous) behave like tiny spinning magnets. Strong magnetic fields alter this behavior, and an MRI scanner can identify the resultant change.

When a patient is put into the strong, static magnetic field generated by the MRI scanner, his or her nuclei align parallel to the field. Because the nuclei are also spinning, they wobble randomly around the field; different molecules can be identified because their nuclei wobble at different frequencies. A second, oscillating magnetic field is then applied at a right angle to the first. This field affects only the nuclei that are in resonance with it—that is, the nuclei that wobble at the field's frequency. This second field forces those resonant nuclei to wobble in unison. When this field is deactivated, the nuclei return to their original positions, and the synchronized movement creates a voltage that can be measured and displayed. Measurements taken at various times during the procedure produce the different magnetic resonance images.

MR imaging has advantages and disadvantages when compared with CT imaging. MRI produces higher-resolution images and can obtain good detail in regions (such as the posterior fossa) that are poorly visualized on CT. Additionally, no radiation is involved. Unfortunately, the procedure is more grueling than CT because the patient must remain motionless for a longer period of time in a smaller, enclosed space. This may be difficult for claustrophobic individuals. Additionally, the magnetic device must be housed in an area devoid of iron, and staff and patients must not carry or wear certain metals or have them embedded in their bodies. Moreover, MRI tends to be more costly than CT imaging in most institutions.

In the psychiatric workup of a geriatric patient (Table 10–4), MRI should be considered when the clinician suspects small lesions in regions difficult to visualize—for example, to obtain evidence of midbrain hemorrhage in a patient with suspected Wernicke's encephalopathy, or to confirm a suspected pituitary tumor in a patient with hyperprolactinemia, which may be seen

TABLE 10–4. Neuroimaging in geriatric psychiatry

Suspected condition	Indicated neuroimaging study
Sudden loss of consciousness	Noncontrast CT scan
Pituitary tumor (hyperprolactinemia)	MRI
Old vs. new lacunar infarct	Diffusion weighted imaging
Hippocampal atrophy	Coronal thin slice MRI
Wernicke's encephalopathy	MRI to rule out midbrain hemorrhage

Note. CT=computed tomography; MRI=magnetic resonance imaging.

in association with risperidone and other high-potency antipsychotic agents. Hyperprolactinemia carries risks of osteopenia, sexual dysfunction, amennorhea, breast enlargement, and possibly cardiac disease and breast cancer. Switching from high-potency to low-potency antipsychotic drugs such as quetiapine or aripiprazole has been shown not only to normalize prolactin but also in some instances to reverse menstrual function or other symptoms (Shim et al. 2007). MRI can also easily identify vascular pathology, including lacunar infarcts, and it is better than CT for defining exact anatomical localization.

A limitation of both CT and MRI is that they cannot differentiate between acute and chronic lesions. Diffusion-weighted imaging (DWI) overcomes this difficulty. DWI is based on the capacity of fast MRI to detect a signal related to the movement of water molecules between two closely spaced radiofrequency pulses (diffusion). This technique can detect abnormalities due to ischemia within 3–30 minutes of onset, while conventional MRI and CT images would still appear normal. Therefore, DWI is helpful in defining the clinically appropriate infarct when multiple subcortical infarcts of various ages are present.

The American Academy of Neurology recommends routine use of structural neuroimaging (noncontrast head CT or MRI) in the initial evaluation of all patients with dementia (Knopman et al. 2001).

Electroencephalography

Electroencephalography is a technique in which scalp electrodes allow the measurement of cortical electrical activity. A skilled reader can interpret the electroencephalographic (EEG) waveforms to identify the presence of epileptic activity, the slowing of electrical activity, or a patient's sleep stage. EEG testing is most useful in a psychiatric evaluation of individuals with known or suspected seizure disorders. Although a history of brain injury or trauma with mental status changes or psychosis may be an important indication for an EEG evaluation, imaging studies are generally preferred for diagnostic clarification in these situations.

In elderly patients, EEG changes occur in both delirium and dementia, but these changes are not specific to a given diagnosis. In delirium, except that caused by alcohol or sedative-hypnotic withdrawal, electroencephalograms typically display slowing of the posterior dominant rhythm and increased generalized slow-wave activity (Jacobson and Jerrier 2000). Electroencephalography has limited clinical use in this area because the diagnosis of delirium is typically made clinically, increased slow-wave activity is seen in other disorders, and the electroencephalogram provides minimal information about the causes of delirium. However, EEG testing is useful for distinguishing between depression and "quiet" delirium because no EEG changes are seen in depression, whereas generalized slowing is seen in delirium.

Likewise, there are EEG changes in dementia. Alzheimer's disease results in multiple changes in EEG parameters (Kowalski et al. 2001; Stevens et al. 2001). Although Kowalski et al. (2001) reported that the degree of EEG change (slowing of normal background activity) is correlated with cognitive impairment, there are also reports that worsening of EEG results does not always parallel the clinical deterioration. Various treatments, including cholinesterase inhibitors, may mitigate EEG changes in individuals with mild dementia (Kogan et al. 2001). However, significant negative correlations have been found between frontal theta activity and hippocampal volumes (Grunwald et al. 2001). Apparently, electroencephalography has limited clinical utility in most dementing syndromes.

EEG testing may be useful, however, when Creutzfeldt-Jakob disease is a consideration in the differential diagnosis. CJD is a rare, rapidly progressive prion disease characterized by dementia and neurological signs that may include gait disturbances and myoclonus. Electroencephalography may play an important role in diagnosing this disease: periodic sharp-wave complexes are strongly associated with CJD, with a sensitivity of 67% and a specificity of 86% (Steinhoff et al. 1996). Although electroencephalography is an important diagnostic tool when considering CJD, it is important to remember that periodic sharp-wave complexes may also occur in Alzheimer's disease and dementia with Lewy bodies (Tschampa et al. 2001).

Genetic Testing

Genetics in geriatric psychiatry is covered in more detail in Chapter 6, "Genetics." This brief section is intended to serve as an introduction to genetic testing, including a discussion of a well-researched test examining for alleles of apolipoprotein E (*APOE*).

APOE Testing

Extensive research has attempted to identify genetic markers for Alzheimer's disease. Mutations on chromosomes 1, 14, and 21 have been linked to rare forms of early-onset familial Alzheimer's disease; such findings may help families make decisions about pregnancies (Verlinsky et al. 2002). One of the most studied genes for Alzheimer's disease is *APOE*. This gene encodes for an astrocyte-secreted plasma protein that is involved in cholesterol transport. *APOE* may also play a role in the regeneration of injured nerve tissue. There are three possible alleles (ε2, ε3, ε4) of the *APOE* gene that may be combined in a heterozygous (ε2/ε3, ε2/ε4, ε3/ε4) or homozygous (ε2/ε2, ε3/ε3, ε4/ε4) fashion.

Multiple epidemiological studies have documented that the presence of the ε4 allele is a risk factor for Alzheimer's disease (Roses 1997). Additionally, the presence of ε4 alleles increases the specificity of the diagnosis of Alzheimer's disease. Despite these associations, the presence of an ε4 allele, even a homozygous ε4/ε4 genotype, is not diagnostic for Alzheimer's disease. Other causes of dementia would have to be explored as clinically indicated. *APOE* testing is not currently recommended to predict dementia risk in asymptomatic individuals. Arguments against routine testing include the lack of an effective treatment to modify the disease course and the lack of evidence that *APOE* status may influence current supportive treatments.

Ethical and Psychological Concerns in Genetic Testing

The results of genetic testing may have significant psychological, social, and personal repercussions. These possible effects are likely to be of less concern for a patient already diagnosed with dementia than for his or her family members faced with their own risk for inheriting the disease. Adverse psychological effects may include stigmatization or worry because of increased risk of Alzheimer's disease. The offspring of a patient with Alzheimer's disease are at increased risk for the disease based on family history alone. If a parent with Alzheimer's disease is found to be homozygous for *APOE*E4*, the children, who will have at least one copy of *APOE*E4*, have at least two to three times the average risk of developing Alzheimer's disease. Unfortunately, this knowledge does not allow offspring to anticipate with certainty whether and when they will develop Alzheimer's disease. Also, no treatment is available to *APOE*E4* carriers to prevent the disease.

Beyond personal and psychological concerns, there are also financial concerns. Genetic testing should be confidential. The inappropriate release of such information could result in job loss or lack of insurability. Medical and life insurance in particular might be exceedingly difficult to obtain if insurance agencies had access to this information.

In the end, however, genetic testing is yet another tool at our disposal. It is a tool with much untapped potential. It also carries significant risks that are different from the risks associated with other laboratory tests described in this chapter. As with other procedures, clinicians must make sure that patients or patients' families understand clearly not only the benefits but also the risks before they proceed with testing.

Future Directions

There is currently great interest in how metabolomics may improve our understanding of disease in various body systems, including the brain. *Metabolomics* is the term that describes defining and quantifying metabolites that result from various cell processes in a single organism. *Metabolome* refers to the complete set of small-molecule metabolites (such as metabolic intermediates, hormones and other signaling molecules, and secondary metabolites) found within a single organism. The metabolome reflects not only the genotype of the organism but also the interaction between the genotype and the environment, as well as the interaction between the genotype and the unique physiology of the organism. In January 2007, the first draft of the human metabolome was completed, containing 2,500 metabolites as well as food and drug components that can be found in the human body (Wishart et al. 2007).

There is evidence that metabolite and protein biomarkers for brain disorders can potentially be detected in bodily fluids (Karrenbauer et al. 2006; Marchi et al. 2003), suggesting that noninvasive metabolomics can be applied even to the study of complex neurological disorders. In the future, metabolomics may help advance our understanding of psychiatric disease mechanisms and risk factors and may aid in tailoring treatment to individual patients.

Key Points

- Laboratory testing is an essential component of the psychiatric evaluation in elderly individuals, who often present with comorbid medical illnesses.

- Laboratory tests are also useful in monitoring medication side effects. New guidelines have been proposed to monitor patients on atypical antipsychotics.
- Neuroimaging is useful in evaluation of a variety of neuropsychiatric illnesses including, but not limited to, dementia.
- Genetic testing has great potential in geriatric psychiatry but currently has limited clinical utility. Important ethical issues should be considered when using genetic testing.

References

American Diabetes Association, American Psychiatric Association, American Association of Clinical Endocrinologists, North American Association for the Study of Obesity: Consensus Development Conference on Antipsychotic Drugs and Obesity and Diabetes. Diabetes Care 27:596–601, 2004

Boushey CJ, Beresford SAA, Omenn GS, et al: A quantitative assessment of plasma homocysteine as a risk factor for vascular disease: probable benefits of increasing folic acid intakes. JAMA 274:1049–1057, 1995

Carmel R, Gott PS, Waters CH, et al: The frequently low cobalamin levels in dementia usually signify treatable metabolic, neurologic and electrophysiologic abnormalities. Eur J Haematol 54:245–253, 1995

Cunha UG, Rocha FL, Peixoto JM, et al: Vitamin B_{12} deficiency and dementia. Int Psychogeriatr 7:85–88, 1995

Dagogo-Jack S: Diabetes mellitus and related disorders, in The Washington Manual of Medical Therapeutics. Edited by Ahya SN, Flood K, Paranjothi S. Philadelphia, PA, Lippincott Williams & Wilkins, 2001, p 455

Durga J, van Boxtel MP, Schouten EG, et al: Effect of 3-year folic acid supplementation on cognitive function in older adults in the FACIT trial: a randomised, double blind, controlled trial. Lancet 369:208–216, 2007

Galasko D, Chang L, Motter R, et al: High cerebrospinal fluid tau and low amyloid beta42 levels in the clinical diagnosis of Alzheimer disease and relation to apolipoprotein E genotype. Arch Neurol 55:937–945, 1998

Glassman AH, Bigger JT: Cardiovascular effects of therapeutic doses of tricyclic antidepressants: a review. Arch Gen Psychiatry 38:815–820, 1981

Glassman AH, Bigger JT: Antipsychotic drugs: prolonged QTc interval, torsade de pointes, and sudden death. Am J Psychiatry 158:1774–1782, 2001

Grunwald M, Busse F, Hensel A, et al: Correlation between clinical theta activity and hippocampal volumes in health, mild cognitive impairment, and dementia. J Clin Neurophysiol 18:178–184, 2001

Hsich G, Kenney K, Gibbs CJ, et al: The 14-3-3 brain protein in cerebrospinal fluid as a marker for transmissible spongiform encephalopathies. N Engl J Med 335:924–930, 1996

Hulstaert F, Blennow K, Ivanoiu A, et al: Improved discrimination of AD patients using beta-amyloid(1–42) and tau levels in CSF. Neurology 52:1555–1562, 1999

Jacob S, Spinler SA: Hyponatremia associated with selective serotonin-reuptake inhibitors in older adults. Ann Pharmacother 40:1618–1622, 2006

Jacobson S, Jerrier H: EEG in delirium. Semin Clin Neuropsychiatry 5:86–92, 2000

Kaplan MM: Clinical perspectives in the diagnosis of thyroid disease. Clin Chem 45:1377–1383, 1999

Karrenbauer VD, Leoni V, Lim ET, et al: Plasma cerebrosterol and magnetic resonance imaging measures in multiple sclerosis. Clin Neurol Neurosurg 108:456–460, 2006

Klee GG, Hay ID: Biochemical testing of thyroid function. Endocrinol Metab Clin North Am 26:763–775, 1997

Knopman, DS, DeKosky ST, Cummings JL, et al: Practice parameter: diagnosis of dementia (an evidence-based review). Report of the Quality Standards Subcommittee of the American Academy of Neurology. Neurology 56:1143–1153, 2001

Kogan EA, Korczyn AD, Virchovsky RG, et al: EEG changes during long-term treatment with donepezil in Alzheimer's disease patients. J Neural Transm 108:1167–1173, 2001

Kowalski JW, Gawel M, Pfeffer A, et al: The diagnostic value of EEG in Alzheimer disease: correlation with the severity of mental impairment. J Clin Neurophysiol 18:570–575, 2001

Leblhuber F, Walli J, Artner-Dworzak E, et al: Hyperhomocysteinemia in dementia. J Neural Transm 107:1469–1474, 2000

Levkoff S, Cleary P, Liptzin B, et al: Epidemiology of delirium: an overview of research issues and findings. Int Psychogeriatr 3:149–167, 1991

Luchsinger JA, Tang MX, Miller J, et al: Relation of higher folate intake to lower risk of Alzheimer disease in the elderly. Arch Neurol 64:86–92, 2007

Mack KA, Ory MG: AIDS and older Americans at the end of the twentieth century. J Acquir Immune Defic Syndr 1 (suppl 2):S68–S75, 2003

Manepalli J, Grossberg GT, Mueller C: Prevalence of delirium and urinary tract infection in a psychogeriatric unit. J Geriatr Psychiatry Neurol 3:198–202, 1990

Marchi N, Rasmussen P, Kapural M, et al: Peripheral markers of brain damage and blood-brain barrier dysfunction. Restor Neurol Neurosci 21:109–121, 2003

McMahon JA, Green TJ, Skeaff CM, et al: A controlled trial of homocysteine lowering and cognitive performance. N Engl J Med 354:2764–2772, 2006

Meins W, Muller-Thomsen T, Meier-Baumgartner H-P: Subnormal serum vitamin B_{12} and behavioural and psychological symptoms in Alzheimer's disease. Int J Geriatr Psychiatry 15:415–418, 2000

Nickoloff EL, Alderson PO: Radiation exposures to patients from CT: reality, public perception, and policy. AJR Am J Roentgenol 177:285–287, 2001

Nilsson K, Gustafson L, Hultberg B: Improvement of cognitive functions after cobalamin/folate supplementation in elderly patients with dementia and elevated plasma homocysteine. Int J Geriatr Psychiatry 16:609–614, 2001

Pollock BG: Adverse reactions of antidepressants in elderly patients. J Clin Psychiatry 60:4–8, 1999

Poser S, Mollenhauer B, Kraubeta A, et al: How to improve the clinical diagnosis of Creutzfeldt–Jakob disease. Brain 122: 2345–2351, 1999

Ravaglia G, Forti P, Mailoi F, et al: Elevated plasma homocysteine levels in centenarians are not associated with cognitive impairment. Mech Ageing Dev 121:251–261, 2000

Robins Wahlin TB, Wahlin A, Winblad B, et al: The influence of serum vitamin B12 and folate status on cognitive functioning in very old age. Biol Psychol 56:247–265, 2001

Roose SP: Considerations for the use of antidepressants in patients with cardiovascular disease. Am Heart J 140:S84–S88, 2000

Roses AD: A model for susceptibility polymorphisms for complex diseases: apolipoprotein E and Alzheimer disease. Neurogenetics 1:3–11, 1997

Sabin TD: AIDS: the new "great imitator." J Am Geriatr Soc 35:460–464, 1987

Selhub J, Bagley LC, Miller J, et al: B vitamins, homocysteine, and neurocognitive function in the elderly. Am J Clin Nutr 71(suppl):614S–620S, 2000

Shim J, Shin JK, Kelly DL, et al: Adjunctive treatment with a dopamine partial agonist, aripiprazole, for antipsychotic-induced hyperprolactinemia: a placebo-controlled trial. Am J Psychiatry 164:1404–1410, 2007

Stabler SP, Lindenbaum J, Allen RH: Vitamin B_{12} deficiency in the elderly: current dilemmas. Am J Clin Nutr 66:741–749, 1997

Steinhoff BJ, Racker S, Herrendorf G, et al: Accuracy and reliability of periodic sharp wave complexes in Creutzfeldt-Jakob disease. Arch Neurol 53:162–166, 1996

Stevens A, Kircher T, Nickola M, et al: Dynamic regulation of EEG power and coherence is lost early and globally in DAT. Eur Arch Psychiatry Clin Neurosci 251:199–204, 2001

Thomas SHL: Drugs, QT interval abnormalities, and ventricular arrhythmias. Adverse Drug React Toxicol Rev 13:77–102, 1994

Trannel TJ, Ahmed I, Goebert D: Occurrence of thrombocytopenia in psychiatric patients taking valproate. Am J Psychiatry 158:128–130, 2001

Tschampa HJ, Neumann M, Zerr I, et al: Patients with Alzheimer's disease and dementia with Lewy bodies mistaken for Creutzfeldt-Jakob disease. J Neurol Neurosurg Psychiatry 71:33–39, 2001

Verlinsky Y, Rechitsky S, Verlinsky O, et al: Preimplantation diagnosis for early-onset Alzheimer disease caused by V717L mutation. JAMA 287:1018–1021, 2002

Wishart DS, Tzur D, Knox C, et al: HMDB: The Human Metabolobe Database. Nucleic Acids Res 35 (database issue) D521–D526, 2007. Available at http://www.hmdb.ca.

Suggested Readings

Knopman DS, DeKosky ST, Cummings JL, et al: Practice parameter: diagnosis of dementia (an evidence-based review). Report of the Quality Standards Subcommittee of the American Academy of Neurology. Neurology 56:1143–1153, 2001

Townsend BA, Petrella, JR, Murali Doraiswamy P: The role of neuroimaging in geriatric psychiatry. Curr Opin Psychiatry 15:427–432, 2002

CHAPTER 11

NEUROPSYCHOLOGICAL ASSESSMENT OF DEMENTIA

KATHLEEN A. WELSH-BOHMER, PH.D.
DEBORAH K. ATTIX, PH.D.

Alzheimer's disease is by far the most common disorder of aging that causes dementia. Affecting nearly 10% of the population over age 65, Alzheimer's disease is estimated to have a prevalence of 25%–40% in those age 85 years or older (Brayne 2007; Breitner 2006). Because of its slow and insidious onset, the early stages of the illness can be confused with relatively benign memory impairments associated with normal aging.

Neuropsychological assessment plays a central role in the diagnosis of early dementing disorders, in the detection of mild cognitive impairment that may transition to dementia (Petersen and Morris 2005; Petersen et al. 2001), and in the differentiation between the plethora of cognitive disorders that can interfere with functional ability and quality of life (Knopman et al. 2001). The neuropsychological assessment offers a sensitive, reliable, and noninvasive approach to early symptom verification as well as a potentially cost-effective means for managing patients with memory disorders (Welsh-Bohmer et al. 2003).

The goals of this chapter are 1) to describe in detail the instances in which neuropsychological assessment can be most useful in geriatric settings, 2) to describe in detail the neuropsychological examination process, and 3) to summarize the neurobehavioral presentations of common disorders in geriatric practices, specifically the profiles of normal aging, various common dementias, and depression.

Neuropsychological Assessment in Geriatric Settings

In geriatric practices, the neuropsychological evaluation finds utility in four common situations, none of which are mutually exclusive. First, and by far the most frequent use of the examination, is to assist in the diagnosis of a cognitive disorder. Specifically, the examination is used to verify the presence or absence of a cognitive syndrome (e.g., dementia) and to determine the likely differential diagnostic possibilities based on the behavioral profile (e.g., Alzheimer's disease versus vascular dementia). Second, neuropsychological testing commonly is also used as an objective baseline for purposes of tracking changes in mentation over time. This is useful in clarifying diagnostic assignments of dementia caused by Alzheimer's disease and similar disorders in which the establishment of progression is essential. The neuropsychological examination in this context can also be used to monitor treatment response. A third common referral scenario is the request for testing to guide clinical care decisions, including the determination of functional capacities and competency (see Koltai and Welsh-Bohmer 2000 for review). Issues typically confronted by a geriatric evaluation are a patient's ability to live independently, financial capacity, medication management, and driving safety. Finally, the neuropsychological evaluation can be used to guide appropriate therapeutic interventions. Based on the results of testing, identified cognitive strengths and weaknesses can be used for designing appropriate rehabilitation approaches, such as those involving compensatory strategies or psychotherapy (for full discussion, see Attix and Welsh-Bohmer 2006).

The actual neuropsychological evaluation process itself can vary in its form across clinical practices, depending in part on the populations typically served (e.g., a Spanish-speaking population versus native English speakers) and in part on the training emphasis of the neuropsychologist administering the examination. The approach can use a fixed battery or may use more flexible methods tailored to the referral issue. Regardless, there are standard features that uniformly are applied across neuropsychological settings to ensure that all testable areas of cognition are assessed (Lezak et al. 2004). The evaluation typically begins with a diagnostic interview to identify the major referral issues and obvious symptoms. In this interview, a patient's orientation to situation, language, behavioral organization, memory, mood, and affect are observed within a naturalistic context. With patient consent, family members generally are also interviewed separately to determine changes in functional ability and to clarify historical and medical information. In the formal testing session, 10 central domains of cognition and behavior are generally assessed: orientation, intelligence, language expression and comprehension, memory, attention/concentration, higher executive functions, visuoperception/spatial abilities, sensorimotor integration, personality, and mood. The tests commonly used to assess these various functional domains are listed in Table 11–1. From the battery of tests, a profile of performance can be constructed, examined in reference to normative standards, and then interpreted relative to the established behavioral profiles of known neurobehavioral syndromes.

Simplifying the geriatric assessment are several neuropsychological batteries designed for use with the elderly and the availability of appropriate normative information (see Strauss et al. 2006 for a review). Among these are the Mattis Dementia Rating Scale (Mattis et al. 2002) and the neuropsychological battery from the Consortium to Establish a Registry for Alzheimer's Disease (Morris et al. 1989). Both are relatively brief and sensitive to early stages of Alzheimer's disease dementia. Additionally, they offer presentation formats, such as the use of large print and an oral format, to minimize the influences of sensory confounding (see Welsh-Bohmer and Mohs 1997).

It must be emphasized that the neuropsychological examination is not simply a process of actuarial comparisons to normative tables. The neuropsychological evaluation, as with other forms of clinical diagnosis, rests on an inferential process. The neuropsychological diagnosis is an iterative process that incorporates multiple sources of information to arrive at diagnostic impressions (see Potter and Attix 2006). In assessing the geriatric patient, the psychologist must first determine likely premorbid ability to determine whether any observed changes are newly acquired for that individual or reflect longstanding weaknesses. Once this has been established, the presence of cognitive impairment is determined in reference to appropriate normative values from similarly aged individuals with comparable education level or intellectual function (Steinberg and Bieliauskas 2005). Consideration is given to any potential confounding influences to test performance, including subject motivation factors, extra-test factors (such as interruptions), and other test behaviors that might interfere with optimal function (e.g., anxiety). The interpretation of the likely medical and psychological contributions to the cognitive profile requires a good appreciation of brain-behavior organization. The neuropsychologist must consider whether the results obtained make sense from a functional anatomical perspective and then analyze the profile to determine its conformity to known neurobehavioral syndromes, such as normal aging, mild cognitive impairment, Alzheimer's disease, and depression. Before final diagnostic determination, consideration is given to other attendant data, such as medical history, ancillary studies (including imaging data), and informant report of functional change. Based on the combined information, the designations of normal aging or early dementia can be more comfortably supported and diagnostic accuracy improved (Tschanz et al. 2000). The next sections of this chapter summarize the neuropsychology of normal aging and the differentiation of various common forms of late-life dementia. Separately from this, we also consider in some detail the neuropsychology of geriatric depression and the contribution of mood disorders to the presentation of dementing disorders.

Neuropsychology of Normal Aging

Cognitive change after age 50 is common and is a reflection of the aging nervous system (Drachman 2006; Ebly et al. 1994). Compared with young adults, older

TABLE 11–1. Common neuropsychological tests used in geriatric assessment

Domain	Tests commonly used	References
Orientation/global mental status	Temporal Orientation Test Mini-Mental State Examination Alzheimer's Disease Assessment Scale–Cognitive	Benton et al. 1964 Folstein et al. 1975 Mohs and Cohen 1988
Intellect	Wechsler Adult Intelligence Scale, 3rd Edition (WAIS-III)	Wechsler 1997a
Language	Multilingual Aphasia Examination Category Fluency Boston Naming Test	Benton and Hamsher 1983 Strauss et al. 2006 Kaplan et al. 1978
Memory	Wechsler Memory Scale, 3rd Edition (WMS-III) California Verbal Learning Test, 2nd Edition Selective Reminding Test Consortium to Establish a Registry for Alzheimer's Disease Word List Memory Test Rey Auditory Verbal Learning Test	Wechsler 1997b Delis et al. 1987 Buschke and Fuld 1974 Welsh-Bohmer and Mohs 1997 Ivnik et al. 1992
Attention/ concentration	Subtests from the WMS-III and WAIS-III	Lezak et al. 2004
Executive function	Trail Making Test Symbol Digit Modalities Test Short Category Test Wisconsin Card Sorting Test	Reitan 1958 Smith 1968 Wetzel and Boll 1987 Berg 1948
Visuoperception	Benton Facial Recognition Test Judgment of Line Orientation Test Tests of Constructional Praxis	Benton et al. 1983 Benton et al. 1981 Lezak et al. 2004
Sensorimotor abilities	Grooved Pegboard Finger Oscillation	Strauss et al. 2006 Heaton et al. 1991
Personality and mood	Minnesota Multiphasic Personality Inventory–2 (MMPI-2) Geriatric Depression Scale Beck Depression Inventory–II	Hathaway and McKinley 1951 Yesavage et al. 1983 Beck et al. 1996

individuals show selective losses in functions related to speed and efficiency of information processing. Particularly vulnerable are memory retrieval abilities, attentional capacity, executive skills, and divergent thinking such as working memory and multitasking (Cullum et al. 1990; Salthouse et al. 1996; van Hooren et al. 2007). On formal neuropsychological testing, memory measures involving delayed free recall are typically affected (Craik 1984), although not to the pronounced extent found in Alzheimer's disease (Welsh et al. 1991). Unlike in individuals with Alzheimer's disease, performance on other memory procedures, such as cued recall or delayed recognition, is typically intact in the normal older adult. This profile of performance suggests different mechanisms underlying the memory loss of aging and Alzheimer's disease. In Alzheimer's disease, it is suggested that the problem resides in the consolidation or storage of new information into long-term memory stores. In normal aging, the principal problem appears to be primarily in the efficient accessing of recently stored information. Therefore, procedures providing structural support for recall (e.g., recognition) facilitate the retrieval process. Beyond memory, normal older adults also show some decrements compared with younger cohorts on tests of visuoperceptual, visuospatial, and constructional functions (Eslinger et al. 1985; Howieson et al. 1993; Koss et al. 1991). These modest declines are seen on tests involving visual analysis and integration, such as the Block Design test of the Wechsler Adult Intelligence Scale, 3rd Edition (WAIS-III), and similar tests involving visual integration. Performance on measures of executive control (e.g., Trail Making), language retrieval (e.g., verbal fluency), and divided attention (e.g., Digit Span from WAIS-III) also tend to be lower in older groups compared with their younger counterparts (Salthouse et al. 1996).

A number of explanations for age-related cognitive change have been suggested, none of which are mutually exclusive. All basically support a premise of a broad explanatory mechanism for age-related cognitive change rather than unique and specific changes in restricted cognitive domains. Speed of central processing has been one popular unifying notion, given that the majority of tasks affected in aging involve motor responses or reaction times (Salthouse 2005). Empirical studies support slowed central processing as a leading explanation for cognitive change with aging (Finkel et al. 2007). Another explanation posits that the profile of cognitive change in normal aging is the result of a loss in "fluid" abilities, skills that require novel problem solving and flexible thought (Botwinick 1977; Horn 1982). Well-rehearsed verbal abilities, so-called crystallized skills, by contrast are less susceptible to age-associated change. More contemporary refinements of this hypothesis conceptualize normal aging as a selective vulnerability in frontal, dysexecutive processes (Daigneault and Braun 1993; Mittenberg et al. 1989; Van Gorp and Mahler 1990). This notion is consistent with the behavioral difficulties observed, suggesting subtle impairments in integrative and retrieval functions, and is also supported by neuroimaging (Coffey et al. 1992; Gur et al. 1987; Langley and Madden 2000; Tisserand 2003) and histopathological findings (Haug et al. 1983) within the frontal-subcortical brain connections. Although this hypothesis is conceptually appealing and capable of explaining much of the observed change with aging, some work suggests that the deficits may not be localizable in their entirety to a single brain system (Finkel et al. 2007; Salthouse et al. 1996). A significant problem in the interpretation of any of the earlier studies is that many did not routinely screen for nervous system disorders or operationalize their criteria for normal aging. Work continues to identify the nature of the mechanisms that underlie age-related cognitive change and the association of these mechanisms with brain diseases common to aging, specifically Alzheimer's disease (Finch 2005).

Differentiation of Alzheimer's Dementia

Alzheimer's disease is the leading cause of dementia in the elderly, contributing to 50%–75% of all dementia cases identified within community-based cohort and population-based series (Breitner 2006; Breitner et al. 1999; Ebly et al. 1995; Fratiglioni et al. 1999; Gascon-Bayarri et al. 2007). Vascular dementia occurs either alone or in combination with Alzheimer's disease in 12%–30% of the cases (Lobo et al. 2000; Roman 2003), whereas dementia with Lewy bodies accounts for 3%–26% of the cases (Lippa et al. 2007; McKeith et al. 2005; Zaccai et al. 2005). Rare dementias of late life, such as frontotemporal dementia, account for an additional 3%–5% of the reported cases (Cairns et al. 2007; Johnson et al. 2005). Illnesses such as hydrocephalus, metabolic disorders, and infectious dementias are etiologically tied to the remaining cases (Holman et al. 1995; Savolainen et al. 1999). The cognitive profiles of the various dementing disorder subtypes are to some extent overlapping, but there are unique features to many of them that can be of diagnostic utility. These characteristics are summarized in Table 11–2.

The presentation of Alzheimer's disease dementia is dominated by a pronounced impairment in recent memory processing, which remains the most affected area of mentation in the majority of cases. This difficulty is now understood to arise from the selective involvement of the medial temporal lobe early in the illness (Braak and Braak 1991; Hyman et al. 1984), giving rise to impaired consolidation of newly learned information into more permanent memory stores located across interconnected neocortical structures. On formal neuropsychological testing, the memory problem of Alzheimer's disease is manifest as a rapid forgetting of new information after very brief delays of 5 minutes or more (Welsh et al. 1991). Patients in the mild prodrome of the illness often show the characteristic memory disorder of more fully expressed disease and may show other mild deficits in executive function, language expression, visuoperception, and attention (Bäckman et al. 2005; Hayden et al. 2005; Twamley et al. 2006). At this early symptomatic stage, a diagnosis of mild cognitive impairment is often made (see Petersen and Morris 2005 for review). A diagnosis of amnesic mild cognitive impairment or multidomain mild cognitive impairment is often considered synonymous with early Alzheimer's disease (Petersen and Morris 2005).

As the disease progresses, other areas of cognition become progressively more involved, reflecting the specific spread of neuropathological involvement to the lateral temporal areas, parietal cortex, and frontal neocortical areas (Small et al. 2000; Storandt et al. 2006; Welsh et al. 1992). Prototypical changes occur in expressive language, visuospatial function, higher executive control, and semantic knowledge (Locasio et al.

TABLE 11–2. Clinical cognitive syndromes and associated neuropsychological profiles

Cognitive syndrome and characteristics	Neuropsychological profile
Normal aging	
Subjective memory complaints	Impaired fluid abilities (novel problem solving)
Annoying but not disabling problems	Deficiencies in memory retrieval
Frequent problems with name retrieval	Decreased general speed of processing
Minor difficulties in recalling detailed events	Lowered performance on executive tasks and visuospatial skills/ visuomotor speed
Mild cognitive impairment–amnesic form	
Subjective memory complaints	Memory performance 1.5 standard deviations below age-matched peers
Noticeable change in memory as noted by informants	Otherwise intact neurocognitive function or only minimal losses (<1.5 SD)
Clinical Dementia Rating score of 0.5 (mild, questionable dementia) (Hughes et al. 1982)	Functional disorder limited to mild interference from the memory difficulty
Problem not disabling	
Alzheimer's disease	
Insidious onset	Impaired memory consolidation with rapid forgetting
Progressive impairment	Diminished executive skills
Prominent memory impairment	Impaired semantic fluency and naming
Possible disorders: aphasia, apraxia, agnosia	Impaired visuospatial analysis and praxis
Frontotemporal dementia	
Prominent personality/behavioral change	Pronounced executive impairments
Disinhibition or apathy	–Cognitive inflexibility
Impaired judgment/insight	–Impaired sequencing
Normal mental status initially	–Perseverative, imitative, utilization behaviors
	–Poor use of feedback
	–Prone to interference
	Less obvious memory impairments
Lewy body dementia	
Fluctuations in alertness/acute confusional state	Memory impairment of Alzheimer's disease but with some partial saving
Visual hallucinations	Pronounced apraxia, visuospatial difficulties
Memory impairment	Rapidly increasing quantifiable deficits in many cases
Parkinsonian signs	
Neuroleptic sensitivity	
Falls resulting from orthostatic hypotension	
Vascular dementia	
Variation of symptoms with subtype	Language/memory retrieval difficulties common
Focality on examination	Benefit from structural support/cueing
Abrupt onset	Asymmetric motor speed/dexterity
In multi-infarct dementia, stepwise progression	Executive inefficiencies
Parkinson's disease dementia	
Extrapyramidal motor disturbance	Slowed performance
Gait dysfunction and frequent falls	Retrieval memory deficit
Bradykinesia	Executive deficiencies (slowed sequencing, impaired lexical fluency)
Bradyphrenia	Impaired fine motor speed (asymmetry common)
	Constructional deficits

TABLE 11–2. Clinical cognitive syndromes and associated neuropsychological profiles *(continued)*

Cognitive syndrome and characteristics	Neuropsychological profile
Huntington's disease	
Early age at onset (midlife)	Slowed performance
Choreiform movements	Memory difficulty in retrieval
Dementia	Benefit from retrieval supports (recognition OK)
Bradyphrenia	Executive compromises
	Poor verbal fluency/preserved naming
Progressive supranuclear palsy	
Extrapyramidal syndrome but no tremor	Mild dysexecutive symptoms: impaired sequencing, fluency, flexibility
Ophthalmic abnormalities (limited downgaze)	Motor slowing
Axial rigidity	Memory weakness characterized as inefficiencies in storage and retrieval
Pseudobulbar palsy	
Frequent falls	
Hydrocephalus	
Memory impairment	Slowed information processing
Gait disturbance	Memory retrieval problems
Incontinence	Benefit from retrieval supports
Creutzfeldt-Jakob disease	
Rare	Rapidly evolving dementia
Typically, rapid onset and course	Subtypes with a profile akin to Alzheimer's disease or a pronounced complex visuospatial disorder (Balint's syndrome)
Dementia with pyramidal and extrapyramidal signs	
Transient spikes on electroencephalogram	
Dementia of geriatric depression	
Affective disorder	Impaired performance on tasks involving effortful processing
Psychomotor slowing	Impaired attention, concentration, sequencing, cognitive flexibility, and executive control
Memory complaints	Retrieval memory difficulty
Cognitive complaints linked temporally to the depressive disorder	Memory improvement with cueing/recognition
	Behavioral tendencies to abandon tasks, poor motivation

1995; Mickes et al. 2007; Storandt et al. 2006). At these latter stages of the illness, anomia with impaired semantic fluency (e.g., generation of names of animals) is generally seen on examination. Word search and circumlocution tendencies are common in conversational speech, whereas speech comprehension itself is better preserved, as are all other fundamental elements of communication (Bayles et al. 1989). Visuospatial problems become more prominent in later stages of illness, resulting in dressing apraxia, difficulty in recognizing objects or people, and problems in performing familiar motor acts (Benke 1993). Subtle problems in spatial processing can occur early and may be detectable only on formal examination. The problem can be illuminated by tests of spatial judgment and visual organization (Rizzo et al. 2000). In everyday settings, the problem may manifest as intermittent topographical disorientation, leading to difficulties in finding familiar routes while driving (Rizzo et al. 1997). An example of the profound memory loss characterizing Alzheimer's disease and mild cognitive impairment from normal aging appears in Figure 11–1.

Vascular Dementia

The neuropsychological profile of vascular dementia differs in many respects from that of Alzheimer's disease, the largest difference being the absence of the profound memory impairment that is a hallmark of the latter disorder (Tierney et al. 2001). The presentation of vascular dementia will vary according to the type and extent of the vascular disorder—multiple infarctions, a single strategic stroke, microvascular disease, cerebral hypoperfusion, hemorrhage, or combinations of these etiologies (Cohen et al. 2002). Multi-infarct dementia, arising from multiple large and small vessel strokes, will

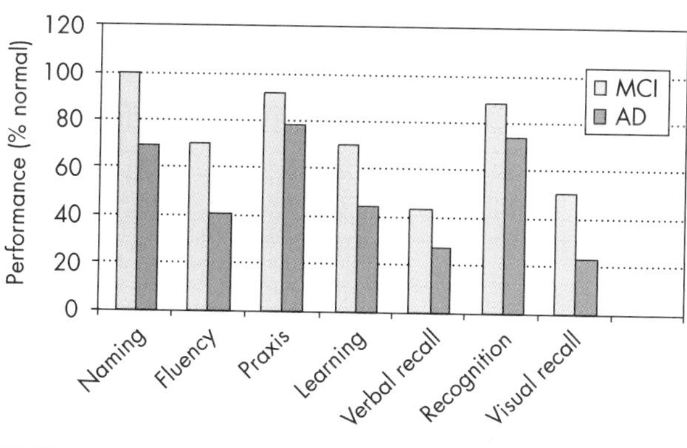

FIGURE 11–1. Profiles of neuropsychological test performance by patients with mild cognitive impairment and by patients with moderate Alzheimer's disease.

Bars indicate the performance of patients with mild cognitive impairment (*n*=153; MCI in figure) and moderately impaired Alzheimer's disease patients (*n*=277; AD in figure) on the subtests of the Consortium to Establish a Registry for Alzheimer's Disease (CERAD; Tariot 1996) neuropsychological battery, compared to the performance of normal elderly control subjects (*n*=158) of similar age, sex, and education. The overall neuropsychological test performance of the Alzheimer's disease patients is well below that of both subjects having mild cognitive impairment and subjects experiencing normal aging. Patients with mild cognitive impairment perform at normal levels on naming and praxis. Learning and verbal fluency are mildly affected in this group, falling at 71% of normal. Memory is particularly affected in both Alzheimer's disease and mild cognitive impairment. Verbal recall on the CERAD Word List Memory test was 45% of normal in the sample with mild cognitive impairment and only 28% for the Alzheimer's disease patients. Visual memory was 51% of normal in mild cognitive impairment and 23% in Alzheimer's disease.

MCI=moderate cognitive impairment; AD=Alzheimer's disease.

Source. Data are derived from the Cache County Study of Memory sample (K.A. Welsh-Bohmer, unpublished).

demonstrate a pattern of multifocal impairments on testing that respect the cerebral territories involved by the infarctions (Chui et al. 1992; Roman et al. 1993). In dementias attributable to diffuse small vessel disease (e.g., Binswanger's disease), the pattern shown on testing reflects the disruption in the dorsolateral prefrontal and subcortical circuitry (Kramer et al. 2002). Memory is involved, but the deficits are often patchy in nature. Patients may show impaired recollection of some recent event but show a surprising memory of some other occurrence transpiring within the same time frame. On formal neuropsychological testing, the pattern on memory testing is one of inefficient acquisition of new information leading to a flattened learning curve over repeating trials (Looi and Sachdev 1999; Padovani et al. 1995). Recall performance can be quite low, similar to that seen in Alzheimer's disease and mild cognitive impairment, but rapid forgetting is not a typical feature (Hayden et al. 2005; Matsuda et al. 1998). The information acquired, albeit limited, is generally retained so that savings scores between a final learning trial and a later delayed recall trial generally are high. Finally, recognition improves dramatically with a recognition format, suggesting a primary difficulty in retrieval rather than in storage or consolidation of new information (Hayden et al. 2005). Beyond memory, dysexecutive functions are typically involved, leading to slowed sequencing, cognitive inflexibility, and decreased verbal fluency (Kertesz and Clydesdale 1994). Asymmetries on sensory motor function or deficits in coordination also are frequently demonstrated.

Frontotemporal Lobar Dementia

Frontotemporal lobar dementia (FTLD) refers to a heterogeneous group of neurodegenerative conditions that are now recognized as a major non–Alzheimer's disease dementia. Typically the onset of disease is in the presenium, distinguishing it from Alzheimer's disease, in which the typical age at onset appears to occur later (i.e., after age 65). The exact prevalence of FTLD in late old age has not been conclusively established, but several studies suggest that it accounts for approximately 10%–20% of the early-onset dementias (Ratnavalli et al. 2002; Snowden et al. 2002). The neuropathological features of FTLD are heterogeneous, but uniformly the histological changes and atrophy are confined to the frontal and anterior temporal cortices. Clinically, from the outset, the disorders are distinct from Alzheimer's disease and other forms of dementia. Typically there are prominent early changes in behavior, personality, or language as opposed to impairments in memory and other aspects of cognition. As a consequence of impaired judgment and social inappropriateness, patients may have tremendous difficulties in their everyday lives, but on formal psychometric screening they may score entirely within normal limits. A number of investigations have delineated the cognitive profile of these disorders (Pachana et al. 1996) and indicate double dissociations between FTLD and Alzheimer's disease. In Alzheimer's disease, there is classic rapid forgetting; in FTLD, there is impairment in executive function. The dysexecutive syndrome of FTLD is characterized by slowed information processing, cognitive rigidity, diminished abstract reasoning, poor response inhibition, and impaired planning. At the neurobehavioral level, there are major changes in personality and general social decorum. Disinhibition, or its converse, behavioral apathy and inertia, frequently occurs. Insight into impairment and into personality change is also affected, and this capacity commonly is disturbed early in the course of FTLD (Rankin et al. 2005). This behavior pattern contrasts with Alzheimer's disease, in which insight is generally lost later in the Alzheimer's disease dementia process (Salmon et al. 2007). In fact, appreciation of memory impairment and other symptoms may be quite acute early in the disease and be a harbinger of the progressive disorder (Geerlings et al. 1999).

There is considerable clinical variability in the presentation of FTLD (McKhann et al. 2001; Snowden et al. 2002), and at least three different subtypes of FTLD are now described based on common clinical and neuropsychological features (see Hodges 2001). These subtypes are described behaviorally as 1) a so-called frontal variant with the prominent behavioral disorder, 2) a semantic variant with primary progressive aphasia (Weintraub et al. 1990), and 3) a rare form with behavioral inertia and mutism (Hodges 2001). The disorder can also be segregated into two subtypes based on regional brain involvement of predominantly the frontal or temporal neocortices (e.g., Seeley et al. 2005). Beyond this, the neuropathological features of FTLD appear heterogeneous (Brun et al. 1994; Cairns et al. 2007; Jackson and Lowe 1996). Microvacuolation, neuronal loss, cortical thinning, and gliosis are often observed on gross and histological examination. With immunohistochemisty, some cases show the spherical Pick bodies with tau-positive inclusions. However, the majority of cases stain positive for ubiquitin, not tau, and invariably are without these Pick bodies. Clinicopathological studies are beginning to emerge suggesting that the clinical expression of the various forms of FTLD may be related to the underlying neuropathology. Progressive aphasia has shown a relationship to the tauopathies, semantic dementia to ubiquitin, and behavioral FTLD to tau and ubiquitin pathology (Cairns et al. 2007). Work continues in this area, having implications for the work to identify biomarkers that would help distinguish the early clinical expression of FTLD from primary psychiatric and other neurological disorders.

It should be underscored that the subtypes do not always present distinctly and that there can be a combination of symptoms. Additionally, there are other types of frontal lobe dementia, which can include presenile dementia associated with motor neuron disease, such as amyotrophic lateral sclerosis with dementia. There are also a variety of degenerative conditions with "secondary" frontal lobe effects. Vascular conditions such as subcortical ischemic vascular dementia or Binswanger's disease (described previously in the "Vascular Dementia" section) often present with frontal lobe impairments, which are likely secondary to the disruption of subcortical white matter pathways.

Parkinson's Disease and Lewy Body Dementias

Patients with Parkinson's disease commonly have cognitive complaints, and many go on to develop dementia. Although the cumulative prevalence estimates of Parkinson's disease dementia (PDD) remain unclear, some estimates suggest that 10%–30% of patients newly diagnosed with Parkinson's disease develop dementia within 3 years (Reid et al. 1996; Williams-Gray et al. 2007). Related to PDD is dementia with Lewy bodies (DLB), a progressive neurological condition that is heralded by cognitive, behavioral, and functional impairments, as opposed to extrapyramidal motor symptoms, and is associated with a disorder of α-synuclein metabolism. The disorder has been referred to by a variety of different names—diffuse Lewy body dementia, senile dementia of the Lewy body type, and the Lewy body variant of Alzheimer's disease—depending in large measure on what the regional distribution of the neuropathology is and whether amyloid plaques co-occur (McKeith et al. 2005; Zaccai et al. 2005). The recognition that DLB and PDD share a common biology has led to their being grouped together and referred to collectively as *Lewy body dementias* (LBDs) (Lippa et al. 2007).

Clinically, PDD and DLB present differently, as described later, but they share a core symptom complex that allows their recognition and distinction from Alzheimer's disease (Geser et al. 2005). In LBD, the prevailing features are parkinsonism, akinetic rigidity, and generalized slowing in motor movement/initiation and thought processes (bradykinesia and bradyphrenia, respectively). DLB, in contrast, is characterized by early fluctuations in cognition and attention, recurrent and persistent visual hallucinations, and extrapyramidal motor symptoms. Diagnosing the conditions rests on the relative occurrence of dementia with respect to the extrapyramidal motor symptoms. In PDD, symptoms of dementia emerge in the context of a previously established diagnosis of Parkinson's disease, whereas in DLB the symptoms of cognitive and functional impairments either predate or follow the onset of parkinsonian symptoms within a 1-year time interval.

On neuropsychological evaluation, the cognitive impairments of PDD and DLB are similar, but the profiles can be differentiated from those typically observed in Alzheimer's disease (for reviews, see Tröster and Woods 2007; Welsh-Bohmer and Warren 2006). Both PDD and DLB are characterized by a pattern of memory retrieval problems and mild dysexecutive disturbances, which early in the course are less dramatic and globally impairing than the cognitive deficits of Alzheimer's disease (Hamilton et al. 2004). Visuospatial disturbances are commonly observed early in the course of the LBDs (Ballard et al. 1999; Hanson et al. 1990; Salmon et al. 1996), but expressive language such as naming tends to be better preserved than in Alzheimer's disease (Ballard et al. 1999; Heyman et al. 1999). Despite these differences on neuropsychological testing, making a solid differential diagnosis based solely on the cognitive profile alone will be difficult (Monza et al. 1998; Soliveri et al. 2000; Testa et al. 2001). The integration of the clinical examination findings (which includes history and review of systems, motor examination, cognitive findings, behavioral ratings, psychiatric interview, and supportive laboratory studies such as neuroimaging) is really necessary to clarify these disorders from one another. In this context, particular attention to the history of symptoms (e.g., fluctuations in ability throughout the day) and to the presence or absence of defined behavioral impairments is crucial to the diagnosis (Geser et al. 2005; Pillon et al. 1991). Cognitively impaired patients with Parkinson's disease can be differentiated from patients with Alzheimer's disease by the comparatively increased apathy observed in the former group and memory impairment within the latter (Cahn-Weiner et al. 2002), whereas presence of visual hallucinations not associated with treatment can help distinguish LBD from PDD (Aarsland et al. 2001). Visual hallucinations can occur in Alzheimer's disease but are uncommon in the earliest stages; hence, their presence early in an early dementia signals another etiological cause such as LBD.

Geriatric Depression and Mood Disorders

Among the most common uses of neuropsychological assessment in the elderly are for evaluating memory disorders and determining the role of depression. By itself, serious mood depression in the elderly can result in disabling cognitive impairment, or what has been called the dementia of depression or "pseudodementia" (see Breitner and Welsh 1995). The problem of geriatric depression is fairly common, with some epidemiologically based studies suggesting that nearly one-third (28%) of elderly populations over the age of 65 exhibit prominent affective syndromes (Lyketsos et al. 2001). Depression also frequently co-occurs in the context of a range of medical disorders, including Alzheimer's disease, stroke, and Parkinson's disease, complicating the diagnosis of these disorders and exacerbating functional loss associated with each (Ballard et al. 1996; Krishnan 2000; Migliorelli et al. 1995; Reichman and Coyne 1995). Distinguishing between depression and other conditions in the elderly can be challenging but is assisted by a thorough screening of both depressive symptoms and cognitive status.

When screening fails to give a clear picture of the contribution of depression to the cognitive picture, neuropsychological examination can assist. It must be noted that depression in late life is clinically heterogeneous, with variable concordance between severity of depressive symptoms and level of cognitive impairment (Alexopoulus et al. 2002; Krishnan 1993). Despite the heterogeneity, there are some distinctive neurocognitive and behavioral changes that appear ascribable to the condition of late-life depression and that are characteristic of a rather large subgroup of patients who present without neurological disease (Beats et al. 1996; Lockwood et al. 2002). The neurocognitive profile tends to be one of a dysexecutive syndrome with impairments residing in planning, organization, initiation, sequencing, working memory, and behavioral shifting in response to feedback. Short-term memory and visuospatial skills are also disturbed, in part because of the attentional and organizational compromises. Behaviorally, these patients show apathy and psychomotor retardation as opposed to prominent mood dysphoria of younger counterparts.

On formal neuropsychological testing, these patients show impairments on tests sensitive to frontal lobe function. Difficulties can be readily seen on tests of selective and sustained attention, verbal fluency, inhibitory control, and set shifting (Boone et al. 1994, 1995; Lockwood et al. 2002). Memory is impaired on both acquisition and recall, leading to a profile characterized by a flattened learning curve and impaired free recall of previously learned information after brief delays (Hart et al. 1987). Recognition memory is better preserved but can be characterized by false-negative tendencies (not recognizing previous target material). The memory disturbance of depression is distinguished from Alzheimer's disease by the impaired acquisition and recognition elements. In Alzheimer's disease, acquisition is relatively better preserved, whereas recognition is characterized by false-positive tendencies (recognizing foils incorrectly as previously presented targets). The profile of impairment in depression leads to the impression of generalized cognitive inefficiency and suppression of performance. Other qualitative differences also may be seen in the performance of these two groups; in depressed patients there is often a heightened tendency to abandon effortful tests.

Importantly, even with treatment, not all of the cognitive impairments associated with geriatric depression remit. In the older patient, this may be due to the co-occurrence of another disease process, such as Alzheimer's disease or cerebrovascular disease. Although far from conclusive, a number of studies report that depression in the elderly exerts a discernible additional effect on cognition and functional independence and may be a risk factor for later cognitive decline (Steffens et al. 2006). Neuropsychological evaluation of the elderly patient can provide clinically useful information regarding the nature of the cognitive failures, differential diagnostic information, and a baseline for future comparisons. The information is useful in diagnosis and management, regardless of whether all of the cognitive change detected is reversible.

Conclusion

The neuropsychological evaluation provides a useful and cost-effective management approach for diagnosis and management of the growing geriatric population with memory complaints. A neuropsychological evaluation is not needed in the majority of dementia cases in which symptoms are obvious and the diagnosis is secure. It can be enormously useful, however, in more complex, less straightforward diagnostic situations, such as in early Alzheimer's disease detection or in geriatric depression. By its objective nature, the neuropsychological examination has strong applications in medical management, providing information regarding patient capacities and deficits that is important for choosing intervention approaches and for guiding future decision making with respect to competency and safety.

Key Points

- The neuropsychological presentation of Alzheimer's disease is characterized by a pronounced deficit in the consolidation of new information from short-term, immediate memory to a more permanent store. Thus, the deficit early in the disorder is a problem of rapid forgetting of newly learned information.
- The profile of normal cognitive aging is characterized by modest declines on executive function tests, in large measure because of inefficiencies in multitask processing and declines in perceptual motor speed.
- The neuropsychological deficits associated with Parkinson's disease dementia are clinically very similar to those of a closely aligned condition, dementia with Lewy bodies. However, the neuropsychological profiles of these conditions can be distinguished from Alzheimer's disease dementia. Visuospatial deficits are common early in the PDD and DLB conditions, and the memory disorders are less severe than those of Alzheimer's disease.
- Frontotemporal lobar dementia is characterized by profound functional and behavioral changes. The neurocognitive deficits associated with the disorder, particularly in the early stages, may be difficult to discern with mental status instruments. Neuropsychological testing targeting executive functions can tease out the impairments in behavioral regulation, disinhibition, perseveration, judgment, and abstraction.
- Geriatric depression can cause significant impairments in the efficiency of cognitive processing, leading to selective problems in sustained attention, concentration, and memory. It is a risk factor for cognitive decline to dementia. When co-occurring with progressive neurological disorders, such as Alzheimer's disease or vascular dementia, depression can lead to excess disability and an overall reduction in the quality of life that might otherwise be achieved.

References

Aarsland D, Cummings JL, Larsen JP: Neuropsychiatric differences between Parkinson's disease with dementia and Alzheimer's disease. Int J Geriatr Psychiatry 16:184–191, 2001

Alexopoulos GS, Kiosses DN, Klimstra S, et al: Clinical presentation of the "depression-executive dysfunction syndrome" of late life. Am J Geriatr Psychiatry 10:98–106, 2002

Attix DK, Welsh-Bohmer KA: Geriatric Neuropsychology: Assessment and Intervention. Edited by Attix DK, Welsh-Bohmer KA. New York, Guilford, 2006

Bäckman L, Jones S, Berger A, et al: Cognitive impairment in preclinical Alzheimer's disease: a meta-analysis. Neuropsychology 19:520–531, 2005

Ballard C, Bannister C, Solis M, et al: The prevalence, associations and symptoms of depression amongst dementia sufferers. J Affect Disord 36:135–144, 1996

Ballard C, Ayre G, O'Brien J: Simple standardized neuropsychological assessment aid in the differential diagnosis of dementia with Lewy bodies and Alzheimer's disease and vascular dementia. Dement Geriatr Cogn Disord 10:104–108, 1999

Bayles KA, Boone DR, Tomoeda CK, et al: Differentiating Alzheimer's patients from the normal elderly and stroke patients with aphasia. J Speech Hear Disord 54:74–87, 1989

Beats BC, Sahakian BJ, Levy R: Cognitive performance in tests sensitive to frontal lobe dysfunction in the elderly depressed. Psychol Med 26:591–603, 1996

Beck AT, Steer RA, Brown GK: Beck Depression Inventory, II. San Antonio, TX, Psychological Corporation, 1996

Benke T: Two forms of apraxia in Alzheimer's disease. Cortex 29:715–725, 1993

Benton AL, Hamsher K: Multilingual Aphasia Examination. Iowa City, IA, AJA Associates, 1983

Benton AL, Van Allen MW, Fogel ML: Temporal orientation in cerebral disease. J Nerv Ment Dis 139:110–119, 1964

Benton AL, Eslinger PJ, Damasio AR: Normative observations on neuropsychological test performance in old age. J Clin Neuropsychol 3:33–42, 1981

Benton AL, Hamsher K, Varney NR, et al: Contributions to Neuropsychological Assessment. New York, Oxford University Press, 1983

Berg EA: A simple objective treatment for measuring flexibility in thinking. Journal of General Psychology 39:15–22, 1948

Boone KB, Lesser I, Miller B, et al: Cognitive functioning in a mildly to moderately depressed geriatric sample: relationship to chronological age. J Neuropsychiatry Clin Neurosci 6:267–272, 1994

Boone KB, Lesser I, Miller B, et al: Cognitive functioning in older depressed outpatients: relationship of presence and severity of depression on neuropsychological test scores. Neuropsychology 9:390–398, 1995

Botwinick J: Intellectual abilities, in The Handbook of the Psychology of Aging. Edited by Birren JE, Schaie KW. New York, Van Nostrand Reinhold, 1977, pp 508–605

Braak H, Braak E: Neuropathological staging of Alzheimer-related changes. Acta Neuropathol 82:239–259, 1991

Brayne C: The elephant in the room: healthy brains in later life, epidemiology and public health. Nat Rev Neurosci 8:233–239, 2007

Breitner JCS: Dementia: epidemiological considerations, nomenclature, and a tacit consensus definition. J Geriatr Psychiatry Neurol 19:129–136, 2006

Breitner JCS, Welsh KA: An approach to diagnosis and management of memory loss and other cognitive syndromes of aging. Psychiatr Serv 46:29–35, 1995

Breitner JC, Wyse BW, Anthony JC, et al: APOE-epsilon4 count predicts age when prevalence of AD increases, then declines: the Cache County Study. Neurology 53:321–331, 1999

Brun A, Englund B, Gustafson L, et al: Consensus statement: clinical and neuropathological criteria for frontotemporal dementia: the Lund and Manchester groups. J Neurol Neurosurg Psychiatry 57:416–418, 1994

Buschke H, Fuld PA: Evaluation of storage, retention and retrieval in disordered memory and learning. Neurology 11:1019–1025, 1974

Cahn-Weiner DA, Grace J, Ott BR, et al: Cognitive and behavioral features discriminate between Alzheimer's and Parkinson's disease. Neuropsychiatry Neuropsychol Behav Neurol 15:79–87, 2002

Cairns NJ, Bigio EH, Mackenzie IR, et al: Neuropathologic diagnostic and nosologic criteria for frontotemporal lobar degeneration: consensus of the Consortium for Frontotemporal Lobar Degeneration. Acta Neuropathol 114:5–22, 2007

Chui HC, Victoroff JI, Margolin D, et al: Criteria for the diagnosis of ischemic vascular dementia proposed by the State of California Alzheimer's Disease Diagnostic and Treatment Centers. Neurology 42 (part 1):473–480, 1992

Coffey CE, Wilkinson WE, Parashos IA, et al: Quantitative cerebral anatomy of the aging human brain: a cross-sectional study using magnetic resonance imaging. Neurology 43:527–536, 1992

Cohen RA, Paul RH, Ott BR, et al: The relationship of subcortical MRI hyperintensities and brain volume to cognitive function in vascular dementia. J Int Neuropsychol Soc 8:743–752, 2002

Craik FIM: Age differences in remembering, in Neuropsychology of Memory. Edited by Squire L, Butters N. New York, Guilford, 1984, pp 3–12

Cullum CM, Butters N, Troster AL, et al: Normal aging and forgetting rates on the Wechsler Memory Scale–Revised. Arch Clin Neuropsychol 5:23–30, 1990

Daigneault S, Braun CM: Working memory and the Self-Ordered Pointing Task: further evidence of early prefrontal decline in normal aging. J Clin Exp Neuropsychol 15:881–895, 1993

Delis DC, Kramer JH, Kaplan E, et al: California Verbal Learning Tests: Adult Version. San Antonio, TX, Psychological Corporation, 1987

Drachman DA: Aging of the brain, entropy, and Alzheimer disease. Neurology 67:1340–1352, 2006

Ebly EM, Parhad IM, Hogan DB, et al: Prevalence and types of dementia in the very old: results from the Canadian Study of Health and Aging. Neurology 44:1593–1600, 1994

Ebly EM, Hogan DB, Parhad IM: Cognitive impairment in the nondemented elderly: results from the Canadian Study of Health and Aging. Arch Neurol 52:612–619, 1995

Eslinger PJ, Damasio AR, Benton AL, et al: Neuropsychologic detection of abnormal mental decline in older persons. JAMA 253:670–674, 1985

Finch CE: Developmental origins of aging in brain and blood vessels: an overview. Neurobiol Aging 26:281–291, 2005

Finkel D, Reynolds CA, McArdle JJ, et al: Age changes in processing speed as a leading indicator of cognitive aging. Psychol Aging 22:558–568, 2007

Folstein MF, Folstein SE, McHugh PR: "Mini-mental state": a practical method for grading the cognitive state of patients for the clinician. J Psychiatr Res 12:189–198, 1975

Fratiglioni L, De Ronchi D, Aguero-Torres H: Worldwide prevalence and incidence of dementia. Drugs Aging 15:365–375, 1999

Gascon-Bayarri J, Rene R, Del Barrio JL, et al: Prevalence of dementia subtypes in El Prat de Llobregat, Catalonia, Spain: the PRATICON study. Neuroepidemiology 28:224–234, 2007

Geerlings MI, Jonker C, Bouter LM, et al: Association between memory complaints and incident Alzheimer's disease in elderly people with normal baseline cognition. Am J Psychiatry 156:531–537, 1999

Geser F, Wenning GK, Poewe W, et al: How to diagnose dementia with Lewy bodies: state of the art. Mov Disord 20:S11–S20, 2005

Gur RC, Gur RE, Obrist WD, et al: Age and regional cerebral blood flow at rest and during cognitive activity. Arch Gen Psychiatry 44:617–621, 1987

Hamilton JM, Salmon DP, Galasko D, et al: A comparison of episodic memory deficits in neuropathologically confirmed Dementia with Lewy bodies and Alzheimer's disease. J Int Neuropsychol Soc 10:689–697, 2004

Hanson L, Salmon D, Galasko D, et al: The Lewy body variant of Alzheimer's disease: a clinical and pathological entity. Neurology 40:1–8, 1990

Hart RP, Kwentus JA, Taylor JR, et al: Rate of forgetting in dementia and depression. J Consult Clin Psychol 55:101–105, 1987

Hathaway SR, McKinley JC: Minnesota Multiphasic Personality Inventory: Manual (Revised). San Antonio, TX, Psychological Corporation, 1951

Haug H, Barmwater U, Eggers R, et al: Anatomical changes in aging brain: morphometric analysis of the human proscencephalon, in Neuropharmacology, Vol 21: Aging. Edited by Cervos-Navarro J, Sarkander HI. New York, Raven, 1983, pp 1–12

Hayden KM, Warren LH, Pieper CF, et al: Identification VaD and AD prodromes: the Cache County Study. Alzheimers Dement 1:19–29, 2005

Heaton RK, Grant I, Matthews CG: Comprehensive Norms for an Expanded Halstead-Reitan Battery: Demographic Corrections, Research Findings, and Clinical Applications. Odessa, FL, Psychological Assessment Resources, 1991

Heyman A, Fillenbaum GG, Gearing M, et al: Comparison of Lewy body variant of Alzheimer's disease with pure Alzheimer's disease: Consortium to Establish a Registry for Alzheimer's Disease, Part XIX. Neurology 52:1839–1844, 1999

Hodges JR: Frontotemporal dementia (Picks disease): clinical features and assessment. Neurology 56:S6–S10, 2001

Holman RC, Khan AS, Kent J, et al: Epidemiology of Creutzfeldt-Jakob disease in the United States 1979–1990: analysis of national mortality data. Neuroepidemiology 14:174–181, 1995

Horn J: The theory of fluid and crystallized intelligence in relation to concepts of cognitive psychology and aging in adulthood, in Aging and Cognitive Processes. Edited by Craik F, Trehub S. New York, Plenum, 1982, pp 237–278

Howieson D, Holm L, Kaye J, et al: Neurologic function in the optimally healthy oldest old: Neuropsychological evaluation. Neurology 43:1882–1886, 1993

Hughes CP, Berg L, Danziger WL, et al: A new clinical scale for the staging of dementia. Br J Psychiatry 140:566–572, 1982

Hyman BT, Van Hoesen GW, Damasio AR, et al: Alzheimer's disease: cell-specific pathology isolates the hippocampal formation. Science 225:1168–1170, 1984

Ivnik RJ, Malec JF, Smith GE, et al: Mayo's older Americans normative studies: updated AVLT norms for ages 56–97. Clin Neuropsychol 6:83–104, 1992

Jackson M, Lowe J: The new neuropathology of degenerative frontotemporal dementias. Acta Neuropathol 91:127–134, 1996

Johnson JK, Diehl J, Mendez MF, et al: Frontotemporal lobar degeneration: demographic characteristics of 353 patients. Arch Neurol 62:925–930, 2005

Kaplan EF, Goodglass H, Weintraub S: The Boston Naming Test, 2nd Edition. Philadelphia, PA, Lea & Febiger, 1978

Kertesz A, Clydesdale S: Neuropsychological deficits in vascular dementia vs Alzheimer's disease: frontal lobe deficits prominent in vascular dementia. Arch Neurol 51:1226–1231, 1994

Knopman DS, DeKosky ST, Cummings JL, et al: Practice parameter: diagnosis of dementia (an evidence based review). Report of the Quality Standards Subcommittee of the American Academy of Neurology. Neurology 56:1143–1153, 2001

Koltai DC, Welsh-Bohmer KA: Geriatric neuropsychological assessment, in Clinician's Guide to Neuropsychological Assessment, 2nd Edition. Edited by Vanderploeg RD. Mahwah, NJ, Erlbaum Associates, 2000, pp 383–415

Koss E, Haxby JV, DeCarli C, et al: Patterns of performance preservation and loss in healthy aging. Dev Neuropsychol 7:99–113, 1991

Kramer JH, Reed BR, Mungas D, et al: Executive dysfunction in subcortical ischaemic vascular disease. J Neurol Neurosurg Psychiatry 72:217–220, 2002

Krishnan KR: Neuroanatomic substrates of depression in the elderly. J Geriatr Psychiatry Neurol 6:39–58, 1993

Krishnan KR: Depression as a contributing factor in cerebrovascular disease. Am Heart J 140:70–76, 2000

Langley LK, Madden DJ: Functional neuroimaging of memory: implications for cognitive aging. Microsc Res Tech 51:75–84, 2000

Lezak MD, Howieson DB, Loring DW: Neuropsychological Assessment, 4th Edition. New York, Oxford University Press, 2004

Lippa CF, Duda JE, Grossman M, et al: DLB and PDD boundary issues: diagnosis, treatment, molecular pathology, and biomarkers. Neurology 68:812–819, 2007

Lobo A, Launer LJ, Fratiglioni L, et al: Prevalence of dementia and major subtypes in Europe: a collaborative study of population-based cohorts. Neurologic Diseases in the Elderly Research Group. Neurology 54 (suppl 5):S4–S9, 2000

Locascio JJ, Growdon JH, Corkin S: Cognitive test performance in detecting, staging, and tracking Alzheimer's disease. Arch Neurol 52:1087–1099, 1995

Lockwood KA, Alexopoulos GS, van Gorp WG: Executive dysfunction in geriatric depression. Am J Psychiatry 159:1119–1126, 2002

Looi J, Sachdev PS: Differentiation of vascular dementia from AD on neuropsychological tests. Neurology 53:670–678, 1999

Lyketsos CG, Sheppard JM, Steinberg M, et al: Neuropsychiatric disturbance in Alzheimer's disease clusters into three groups: the Cache County study. Int J Geriatr Psychiatry 16:1043–1053, 2001

Matsuda O, Saito M, Sugishita M: Cognitive deficits of mild dementia: a comparison between dementia of the Alzheimer's type and vascular dementia. Psychiatr Clin Neurosci 52:87–91, 1998

Mattis S, Jurica PJ, Leitten CL: Dementia Rating Scale-2TM (DRS-2TM). Professional Manual. Odessa, FL, Psychological Assessment Resources, 2002

McKeith IG, Dickson DW, Lowe J, et al: Diagnosis and management of dementia with Lewy bodies: third report of the DLB Consortium. Neurology 65:1863–1872, 2005

McKhann GM, Albert MS, Grossman M, et al: Clinical and pathological diagnosis of frontotemporal dementia: report of the Work Group on Frontotemporal Dementia and Pick's Disease. Arch Neurol 58:1803–1809, 2001

Mickes L, Wixted JT, Fennema-Notestine C, et al: Progressive impairment on neuropsychological tasks in a longitudinal study of preclinical Alzheimer's disease. Neuropsychology 21:696–705, 2007

Migliorelli R, Teson A, Sabe L, et al: Prevalence and correlates of dysthymia and major depression among patients with Alzheimer's disease. Am J Psychiatry 152:37–44, 1995

Mittenberg W, Seidenberg M, O'Leary DS, et al: Changes in cerebral functioning associated with normal aging. J Clin Exp Neuropsychol 11:918–932, 1989

Mohs RC, Cohen L: Alzheimer's Disease Assessment Scale (ADAS). Psychopharmacol Bull 24:627–628, 1988

Monza D, Soliveri P, Radice D, et al: Cognitive dysfunction and impaired organization of complex motility in degenerative parkinsonism syndromes. Arch Neurol 55:372–378, 1998

Morris JC, Heyman A, Mohs RC, et al: The Consortium to Establish a Registry for Alzheimer's Disease (CERAD). Part I: clinical and neuropsychological assessment of Alzheimer's disease. Neurology 39:1159–1165, 1989

Pachana NA, Boone KB, Miller BL, et al: Comparison of neuropsychological functioning in Alzheimer's disease and frontotemporal dementia. J Int Neuropsychol Soc 2:505–510, 1996

Padovani A, Di Piero V, Bragoni M, et al: Patterns of neuropsychological impairment in mild dementia: a comparison between Alzheimer's disease and multi-infarct dementia. Acta Neurol Scand 92:433–442, 1995

Petersen RC, Morris JC: Mild cognitive impairment as a clinical entity and treatment target. Arch Neurol 62:1160–1163, 2005

Petersen RC, Stevens JC, Ganguli M, et al: Practice parameter: early detection of dementia: mild Cognitive impairment (an evidence based review). Report of the Quality Standards Subcommittee of the American Academy of Neurology. Neurology 56:1133–1142, 2001

Pillon B, Dubois B, Agid Y: Severity and specificity of cognitive impairment in Alzheimer's, Huntington's, and Parkinson's diseases and Progressive Supranuclear Palsy. Ann N Y Acad Sci 640: 224–227, 1991

Potter GG, Attix DK: An integrated model for geriatric neuropsychological assessment, in Geriatric Neuropsychology: Assessment and Intervention. Edited by Attix DK, Welsh-Bohmer KA. New York, Guilford, 2006, pp 5–26

Rankin KP, Baldwin E, Pace-Savitsky C, et al: Self awareness and personality change in dementia. J Neurol Neurosurg Psychiatry 76:632–639, 2005

Ratnavalli E, Brayne C, Dawson K, et al: The prevalence of frontotemporal dementia. Neurology 58:1615–1621, 2002

Reichman WE, Coyne AC: Depressive symptoms in Alzheimer's disease and multi-infarct dementia. J Geriatr Psychiatry Neurol 8:96–99, 1995

Reid WG, Hely MA, Morris JG, et al: A longitudinal study of Parkinson's disease: clinical and neuropsychological correlates of dementia. J Clin Neurosci 3:327–333, 1996

Reitan RM: Validity of the Trail Making Test as an indicator of organic brain damage. Percept Mot Skills 8:271–276, 1958

Rizzo M, Reinach S, McGehee D, et al: Simulated car crashes and crash predictors in drivers with Alzheimer disease. Arch Neurol 54:545–551, 1997

Rizzo M, Anderson SW, Dawson J, et al: Vision and cognition in Alzheimer's disease. Neuropsychologia 38:1157–1169, 2000

Roman GC: Vascular dementia: distinguishing characteristics, treatment, and prevention. J Am Geriatr Soc 51:S296–S304, 2003

Roman GC, Tatemichi TK, Erkinjuntti T, et al: Vascular dementia: diagnostic criteria for research studies. Report of the NINDS-AIREN International Workshop. Neurology 43:250–260, 1993

Salmon DP, Galasko D, Hansen LA, et al: Neuropsychological deficits associated with diffuse Lewy body disease. Brain Cogn 31:148–165, 1996

Salmon E, Perani D, Collette F, et al: A comparison of unawareness in frontotemporal dementia and Alzheimer's disease. J Neurol Neurosurg Psychiatry 79:176–179, 2007

Salthouse TA: Relations between cognitive abilities and measures of executive functioning. Neuropsychology 19:532–545, 2005

Salthouse TA, Fristoe N, Rhee SH: How localized are age-related effects on neuropsychological measures? Neuropsychology 10:272–285, 1996

Savolainen S, Palijarvi L, Vapalahti M: Prevalence of Alzheimer's disease in patients investigated for presumed Normal Pressure Hydrocephalus: a clinical and neuropathological study. Acta Neurochir (Wien) 141:849–853, 1999

Seeley WW, Bauer AM, Miller BL, et al: The natural history of temporal variant frontotemporal dementia. Neurology 64:1384–1390, 2005

Small BJ, Fratiglioni L, Viitanen M, et al: The course of cognitive impairment in preclinical Alzheimer disease: three- and 6-year follow-up of a population-based sample. Arch Neurol 57:839–844, 2000

Smith A: The Symbol Digit Modalities Test: a neuropsychologic test for economic screening of learning and other cerebral disorders. Learning Disorders 3:83–91, 1968

Snowden JS, Neary D, Mann DM: Frontotemporal dementia. Br J Psychiatry 180:140–143, 2002

Soliveri P, Monza D, Paridi D, et al: Neuropsychological follow up in patients with Parkinson's disease, striatonigral degeneration type multisystem atrophy and progressive supranuclear palsy. J Neurol Neurosurg Psychiatry 69:313–318, 2000

Spreen O, Strauss E: A Compendium of Neuropsychological Tests: Administration, Norms, and Commentary, 2nd Edition. New York, Oxford University Press, 1996

Steffens DC, Otey E, Alexopoulos GS, et al: Perspectives on depression, mild cognitive impairment, and cognitive decline. Arch Gen Psychiatry 63:130–138, 2006

Steinberg B, Bieliauskas L: Introduction to the special edition: IQ-based MOANS norms for multiple neuropsychological instruments. Clin Neuropsychol 19:277–279, 2005

Storandt M, Grant EA, Miller JP, et al: Longitudinal course and neuropathologic outcomes in original vs revised MCI and in pre-MCI. Neurology 67:467–473, 2006

Strauss E, Sherman EM, Spreen O: A Compendium of Neuropsychological Tests: Administration, Norms, and Commentary, 3rd Edition. New York, Oxford University Press, 2006

Tariot PN: CERAD behavior rating scale for dementia. Int Psychiogeriatr 8 (suppl 3):317–320, 1996

Testa D, Monza D, Ferrarini M, et al: Comparison of natural histories of progressive supranuclear palsy and multiple system atrophy. Neurol Sci 22:247–251, 2001

Tierney MC, Black SE, Szalai JP, et al: Recognition memory and verbal fluency differentiate probable Alzheimer disease from subcortical ischemic vascular dementia. Arch Neurol 58:1654–1659, 2001

Tisserand DJ: Structural and Functional Changes Underlying Cognitive Aging. Maastricht, The Netherlands, Maastricht University, 2003

Tröster AI, Woods SP: Neuropsychological aspects, in Handbook of Parkinson's Disease, 4th Edition. Edited by Pahwa R, Lyons KE. New York, Informa, 2007, pp 109–131

Tschanz JT, Welsh-Bohmer KA, West N, et al: Identification of dementia cases derived from a neuropsychological algorithm: comparisons with clinically derived diagnoses. Neurology 54:1290–1296, 2000

Twamley EW, Ropacki S, Bondi MW: Neuropsychological and neuroimaging changes in preclinical Alzheimer's disease. J Int Neuropsychol Soc 12:707–735, 2006

Van Gorp WG, Mahler ME: Subcortical features of normal aging, in Subcortical Dementia. Edited by Cummings JL. New York, Oxford University Press, 1990, pp 231–250

van Hooren SA, Valentijn AM, Bosma H, et al: Cognitive functioning in healthy older adults aged 64–81: a cohort study into the effects of age, sex, and education. Neuropsychol Dev Cogn B Aging Neuropsychol Cogn 14:40–54, 2007

Wechsler D: Wechsler Intelligence Scale, 3rd Edition. San Antonio, TX, Psychological Corporation, 1997a

Wechsler D: Wechsler Memory Scale, 3rd Edition. San Antonio, TX, Psychological Corporation, 1997b

Weintraub S, Rubin NP, Mesulam MM: Primary progressive aphasia: longitudinal course, profile and language features. Arch Neurol 47:1329–1335, 1990

Welsh KA, Butters N, Hughes JP, et al: Detection of abnormal memory decline in mild Alzheimer's disease using CERAD neuropsychological measures. Arch Neurol 48:278–281, 1991

Welsh KA, Butters N, Hughes JP, et al: Detection and staging of dementia in Alzheimer's disease: use of the neuropsychological measures developed for the Consortium to Establish a Registry for Alzheimer's Disease (CERAD). Arch Neurol 49:448–452, 1992

Welsh-Bohmer KA, Mohs RC: Neuropsychological assessment of Alzheimer's disease. Neurology 49:S11–S13, 1997

Welsh-Bohmer KA, Warren LH: Neurodegenerative dementias, in Geriatric Neuropsychology: Assessment and Intervention. Edited by Attix DK, Welsh-Bohmer KA. New York, Guilford, 2006, pp 56–88

Welsh-Bohmer KA, Koltai DC, Mason DJ: The clinical utility of neuropsychological evaluation of patients with known or suspected dementia, in Demonstrating Utility and Cost Effectiveness in Clinical Neuropsychology. Edited by Prigatano G, Pliskin N. Philadelphia, PA, Psychology Press-Taylor and Francis Group, 2003, pp 177–200

Wetzel L, Boll TJ: Short Category Test, Booklet Format. Los Angeles, CA, Western Psychological Services, 1987

Williams-Gray CH, Foltynie T, Brayne CE, et al: Evolution of cognitive dysfunction in an incident Parkinson's disease cohort. Brain 130 (pt 7):1787–1798, 2007

Yesavage J, Brink TL, Rose TL, et al: Development and validation of a geriatric depression scale: a preliminary report. J Psychiatr Res 17:37–49, 1983

Zaccai J, McCracken C, Brayne C: A systematic review of prevalence and incidence studies of dementia with Lewy bodies. Age Ageing 34:561–566, 2005

Suggested Readings

Attix DK, Welsh-Bohmer KA (eds): Geriatric Neuropsychology: Assessment and Intervention. New York, Guilford, 2006

Strauss E, Sherman EM, Spreen O: A Compendium of Neuropsychological Tests: Administration, Norms, and Commentary, 3rd Edition. New York, Oxford University Press, 2006

Tröster AI, Woods SP: Neuropsychological aspects, in Handbook of Parkinson's Disease, 4th Edition. Edited by Pahwa R, Lyons KE. New York, Informa, 2007, pp 109–131

PART III

Psychiatric Disorders in Late Life

CHAPTER 12

DELIRIUM

Michael A. Fearing, Ph.D.
Sharon K. Inouye, M.D., M.P.H.

Delirium, defined as an acute and sudden change in attention and overall cognitive function, is a substantial medical problem for older persons—and one that may be preventable. Patients ages 65 years and older account for almost half (49%) of all days of hospital care, and although delirium is the most frequent complication affecting this population, it often goes unrecognized. In fact, delirium affects over 2.5 million patients ages 65 and older during hospitalization annually (Inouye et al. 1999; U.S. Department of Health and Human Services 2004). Delirium is a costly condition, leading to increased costs per hospital stay of at least $2,500 per patient, which translates to $6.9 billion (values in U.S. dollars in 2004) of annual excess Medicare hospital expenditures directly related to delirium and its complications. Patients with delirium have a worse prognosis than patients without delirium and are at an increased risk of developing long-term cognitive and functional decline (Inouye 2006; Jackson et al. 2004), which in turn leads to additional posthospitalization treatment costs, such as for institutionalization, rehabilitation services, and home health care (Inouye 2006). Total health care costs related to delirium are estimated at $38 billion to $152 billion annually (Leslie et al. 2008).

Definition and Epidemiology

The diagnostic criteria for delirium that appear in DSM-IV-TR (American Psychiatric Association 2000) are generally accepted as the current diagnostic standard (see Table 12–1). Expert consensus was used to develop the DSM-IV-TR criteria, and sensitivity and specificity estimates of the criteria have not been reported. The Confusion Assessment Method (CAM) (Inouye et al. 1990) provides a simple diagnostic algorithm that has become widely used as a practical means for identification of delirium (see Table 12–1). The CAM diagnosis of delirium is based on an assessment of the clinical features of acute onset and fluctuating course, inattention, disorganized thinking, and altered level of consciousness. The CAM algorithm has a sensitivity of 94%–100%, specificity of 90%–95%, positive predictive accuracy of 91%–94%, and negative predictive accuracy of 90%–100% compared with the ratings of geropsychiatrists, as well as high interrater reliability (Inouye et al. 1990).

Delirium is often the only sign of an acute and serious medical condition affecting a patient, and it most commonly occurs in frail older persons with an underlying disease process. Occurrence estimates suggest that delirium affects 14%–56% of hospitalized elderly patients (Cole 2004). Delirium is a symptom in up to 30% of older patients presenting to the emergency department (Agostini and Inouye 2003; Inouye 2006). Delirium following surgery is common in patients ages 65 and older, occurring in 15%–53% postoperatively (Balasundaram and Holmes 2007; Inouye 2006; Olin et al. 2005). Not surprisingly, incidence rates increase to 70% –80% of older patients in intensive care (Pisani et al. 2003) and to over 50% of those in nursing home or post–acute care settings (Kiely et al. 2004, 2006). Following hospitalization, the estimated 1-year mortality rate for patients with delirium is 35%–40% (Moran and Dorevitch 2001).

TABLE 12–1. Diagnostic criteria for delirium

DSM-IV-TR diagnostic criteria

A. Disturbance of consciousness (i.e., reduced clarity of awareness of the environment) with reduced ability to focus, sustain, or shift attention.

B. A change in cognition (such as memory deficit, disorientation, language disturbance) or the development of a perceptual disturbance that is not better accounted for by a preexisting, established, or evolving dementia.

C. The disturbance develops over a short period of time (usually hours to days) and tends to fluctuate during the course of the day.

D. There is evidence from the history, physical examination, or laboratory findings that the disturbance is caused by the direct physiological consequences of a general medical condition.

The Confusion Assessment Method (CAM) diagnostic algorithm[a]

Feature 1. Acute onset and fluctuating course

This feature is usually obtained from a reliable reporter, such as a family member, caregiver, or nurse, and is shown by positive responses to these questions: Is there evidence of an acute change in mental status from the patient's baseline? Did the (abnormal) behavior fluctuate during the day, that is, tend to come and go, or did it increase and decrease in severity?

Feature 2. Inattention

This feature is shown by a positive response to this question: Did the patient have difficulty focusing attention, for example, being easily distractible, or have difficulty keeping track of what was being said?

Feature 3. Disorganized thinking

This feature is shown by a positive response to this question: Was the patient's thinking disorganized or incoherent, such as rambling or irrelevant conversation, unclear or illogical flow of ideas, or unpredictable switching from subject to subject?

Feature 4. Altered level of consciousness

This feature is shown by any answer other than "alert" to this question: Overall, how would you rate this patient's level of consciousness (alert [normal], vigilant [hyperalert], lethargic [drowsy, easily aroused], stupor [difficult to arouse], or coma [unarousable])?

[a]The CAM ratings should be completed following brief cognitive assessment of the patient, for example, with the Mini-Mental State Examination. The diagnosis of delirium by CAM requires the presence of features 1 and 2 and of either 3 or 4.

Source. Diagnostic criteria for delirium reprinted from American Psychiatric Association: *Diagnostic and Statistical Manual of Mental Disorders*, 4th Edition, Text Revision. Washington, DC, American Psychiatric Association, 2000. Used with permission.
CAM diagnostic algorithm adapted from Inouye SK, Vandyck CH, Alessi CA, et al.: "Clarifying Confusion: The Confusion Assessment Method—A New Method for Detection of Delirium. *Annals of Internal Medicine* 113:941–948, 1990. Used with permission.

Clinical Features and Course of Delirium

Sudden and acute onset, alteration in attention, and fluctuating course are the central features of delirium. Therefore, it is important to establish a patient's level of baseline cognitive functioning and the course of cognitive change when evaluating for the presence of delirium. A detailed and in-depth background interview with a proxy informant, such as a family member, caregiver, or medical professional who knows the patient, proves invaluable when documenting change in a patient's mental status. It is important to differentiate between 1) cognitive changes that increase and decrease in severity over a period of days, which is indicative of delirium, and 2) changes that are more chronic and progressive over a period of months to years, which is indicative of dementia. To fulfill the criteria for delirium, the change in cognitive status must occur in the context of a medical illness, a metabolic disorder, drug toxicity, or drug withdrawal.

The cognitive evaluation for delirium should encompass the following domains: global cognitive changes, impairment in attention, disorganized thought process, and altered level of consciousness. Global cognitive changes associated with delirium can be assessed through simple cognitive testing and close clinical observation during test administration and the patient's completion of tasks. It is important not to underestimate the waxing and waning periods of delirium, because periods of lucidity and reversal of symptoms can often be deceiving. Impairment in attention, a hallmark feature of delirium, is clinically manifested through the patient's difficulty focusing on the task at hand, maintaining or following a conversation, and/or shifting attention, often leading to perseveration on a previous topic or task. Disorganized thought is present when the patient's speech is incoherent or jumbled and when the patient lacks a clear or logical presentation of ideas; this problem can be similar to the "word salad" phenomenon seen in schizophrenia and other formal thought disorders. Alteration in consciousness is highly variable and can range from an agitated or aggressive state to one of lethargy or stupor. Other clinical features commonly associated with delirium that are not included in the diagnostic criteria are psychomotor agitation, paranoid delusions, sleep-wake cycle disruption, emotional lability, and perceptual disturbances or hallucinations.

Clinically, delirium typically presents in one of two major forms: hypoactive or hyperactive (Table 12–2). The hypoactive form, which is more common in older patients, is characterized by lethargy and reduced psychomotor functioning. It is important to note that the hypoactive form of delirium is associated with an overall poorer prognosis and often goes unrecognized by clinicians and caregivers (Liptzin and Levkoff 1992; Sandberg et al. 1999). The reduced level of patient activity associated with hypoactive delirium is often attributed to low mood or fatigue, which may contribute to its misdiagnosis or underrecognition. The hyperactive form of delirium is characterized by agitation, increased vigilance, and often concomitant hallucinations. The hyperactive form rarely goes unnoticed by caregivers or clinicians. Clinicians should be aware of a mixed form of delirium, in which patients fluctuate between the hypoactive and the hyperactive forms. The mixed form creates a challenge in distinguishing symptoms of delirium from symptoms of other psychotic or mood disorders.

Pathophysiology of Delirium

The fundamental pathophysiological mechanisms of delirium remain unclear, most likely because many different etiologies may result in delirium through different mechanisms or pathways (Flacker and Lipsitz 1999). Historically, delirium was thought to result from a functional rather than a structural lesion; electroencephalographic findings demonstrated global functional impairments and generalized slowing of alpha wave activity (Pro and Wells 1977). Several studies of cerebral blood flow using positron emission tomography (PET) or single-photon emission computed tomography (SPECT) have found that delirium is associated mostly with decreased blood flow, especially in the prefrontal cortex, thalamus, basal ganglia, temporoparietal cortex, and lingual gyri (Burns et al. 2004; Fong et al. 2006; Trzepacz and van der Mast 2002). However, results from previous imaging studies have been highly variable.

Other neuroimaging studies, using either computed tomography (CT) or magnetic resonance imaging (MRI), have demonstrated structural abnormalities in the brains of patients with delirium, especially in the splenium of the corpus callosum, thalamus, and right temporal lobe (Bogousslavsky et al. 1988; Doherty et al. 2005; Naughton et al. 1997; Ogasawara et al. 2005; Takanashi et al. 2006). Results from neuropsychological testing also suggest that delirium is related to disruptions in higher cortical function, especially in the frontal lobe region (Rudolph et al. 2006). The leading current hypotheses view delirium as the final common pathway of many different pathogenic mechanisms, including imbalances in neurotransmission, inflammation, and chronic stress.

The most frequently considered mechanism of delirium is dysfunction in the cholinergic system. Acetylcholine plays a key role in mediating consciousness and attentional process. Given that delirium is manifested by an acute confusional state, often with alterations of consciousness, it is likely to have a cholinergic basis. Evidence for the cholinergic connection includes findings that anticholinergic drugs can induce delirium in humans and animals and that serum anticholinergic activity is increased in patients with delirium (Marcantonio et al. 2006). Also, cholinesterase inhibitors have been found to reduce symptoms of delirium in some studies (Gleason 2003; Wengel et al. 1998). An excess of dopaminergic neurotransmitters has also been cited as a mechanism of delirium and is most likely related to the role they play in regulating the release of acetylcholine (Trzepacz and van der Mast 2002). Elevated serotonin, such as that seen in hepatic encephalopathy and "serotonin syndrome," is another proposed mechanism of delirium (Marcantonio et al. 2006).

Other neurotransmitters, including norepinephrine, glutamate, and melatonin, have also been implicated in the development of delirium, most likely due to their interactions with cholinergic and dopaminergic path-

TABLE 12–2. Features of hypoactive and hyperactive delirium

Feature	Hypoactive delirium	Hyperactive delirium
Consciousness, behavior	Fatigue, lethargy	Hallucinations, vigilance, combativeness
Psychomotor functioning	Reduced activity and functioning	Increased activity, agitation
Clinical diagnosis	Often goes unrecognized	Rarely missed

ways; however, support for their involvement is less substantiated (Cole 2004; Inouye 2006). Chronic stress induced by severe illness, trauma, or surgery involves sympathetic and immune system activation that may lead to delirium; this activation may include increased activity of the hypothalamic-pituitary-adrenal axis with hypercortisolism, release of cerebral cytokines that alter neurotransmitter systems, alterations in the thyroid axis, and modification of blood-brain barrier permeability.

Assessment Tools for Delirium

The Confusion Assessment Method (introduced in "Definition and Epidemiology" earlier in this chapter) is a widely used assessment tool that has been adapted for use in many settings, such as the intensive care unit (CAM-ICU; Ely et al. 2001) and nursing home (MDS Version 3.0; Centers for Medicare and Medicaid Services, n.d.). For use with nonverbal or intubated patients, the CAM-ICU applies the same four diagnostic criteria as the CAM for the diagnosis of delirium (Ely et al. 2001). In addition to the CAM, several other instruments are used to identify the presence or absence of delirium, including the Delirium Rating Scale—Revised–98 (Trzepacz et al. 2001) and the Delirium Symptom Interview (Albert et al. 1992). In validation studies, each instrument has been found to have a sensitivity of 0.83 or greater and a specificity of 0.75 or greater. In reliability studies, each instrument was found to have a kappa coefficient (κ) or a correlation coefficient (*r*) of 0.90 or greater. Both the Delirium Rating Scale—Revised–98 and the Memorial Delirium Assessment Scale (MDAS; Breitbart et al. 1997) are used to rate delirium severity.

Neuropsychological Assessment of Delirium

Administering neuropsychological tests during an acute delirium phase can prove to be difficult, due to the patient's alteration in basic attention capabilities, and may provide minimal useful information beyond that obtained from global cognitive screening tools such as the Mini-Mental State Examination (Folstein et al. 1975) followed by the CAM. Given that the hallmark of delirium is alteration in attention, additional neuropsychological instruments that target attention should be used when assessing delirium if possible.

Deficits in attention can be measured using tasks such as Digit Span forward and backward (Wechsler 1989); backward reciting of the days of the week or the months of the year; Trail Making Test A (Reitan 1958); and the visual search and attention task, which is a cancellation task that requires the patient to cross out letters and symbols that are identical to a target (Trenerry et al. 1990). In one previous study, postoperative delirium was found to be associated with preoperative deficits in attention and executive function (Rudolph et al. 2006), both of which are useful to evaluate in delirium. Executive function measures that are both brief and informative include the following: Trail Making Test B (Reitan 1958), Digit Symbol Modalities Test (Wechsler 1997), Stroop Neuropsychological Screening Test (Trenerry et al. 1989), and Controlled Oral Word Association Test (Benton et al. 1983). A study of the Clock Drawing Test found that although this instrument was a good detector of overall cognitive impairment, it is not suitable for detection of delirium (Adamis et al. 2005). Identification of cognitive measures that predict delirium onset has received some attention in the literature. For example, a study of the Mini-Mental State Examination demonstrated that four items (i.e., year, date, "sword" spelled backwards, and design copying) of the original 20 items are accurate screening measures for delirium (Fayers et al. 2005).

Risk Factors for Delirium

Delirium usually occurs as a result of multifactorial causes (Inouye and Charpentier 1996). Although it can be caused by a single factor, delirium more typically develops due to the interrelationship between patient vulnerability at hospital admission and noxious insults or precipitating factors occurring during the course of hospitalization. For example, a single dose of a sedative given to a patient who is cognitively impaired or severely ill may lead to delirium. However, a patient without severe illness or cognitive impairment has greater resistance to developing delirium unless he or she is repeatedly exposed to multiple insults such as surgery, anesthesia, and psychoactive medications (Gleason 2003). The observant clinician will recognize that addressing only a single noxious insult or factor may not aid in improving delirium but that all predisposing and precipitating factors need to be addressed for resolution of delirium.

Existing cognitive impairment and dementia are the leading risk factors for the development of delirium. In fact, patients with dementia have a two- to fivefold increased risk for developing delirium, and nearly two-thirds of cases of delirium occur in patients with dementia (Cole 2004; Inouye 2006; Trzepacz and van der Mast 2002). Other predisposing factors include advanced age, chronic or severe underlying illness, number and severity of comorbid conditions, functional impairment, male gender, dehydration, vision or hearing impairments, chronic renal insufficiency, history of alcohol abuse or dependence, and malnutrition (see Table 12–3) (Elie et al. 1998; Francis 1992; Rockwood 1989; Rogers et al. 1989).

Various chronic medical illnesses also serve as predisposing factors to delirium, including neurological disorders (e.g., Parkinson's disease, cerebrovascular disease, mass lesions, trauma, infection, collagen vascular disease); systemic or nonneurological infections; metabolic alterations; and cardiac, pulmonary, endocrine, renal, and neoplastic conditions. A validated predictive model for development of delirium (Inouye et al. 1993) at the time of hospital admission identified several independent risk factors, including severe underlying illness, vision impairment, baseline cognitive impairment, and a high blood urea nitrogen to creatinine ratio (used as an index of dehydration).

Predictive risk models that identify predisposing factors for delirium have been developed in specific medical populations, such as surgical patients, cancer patients, and nursing home patients (Boyle 2006; Hamann et al. 2005). A validated model for prediction of persistent delirium in hospitalized older patients at discharge has identified five risk factors: dementia, vision impairment, functional impairment, high comorbidity, and use of physical restraints during delirium (Inouye et

TABLE 12–3. Predisposing and precipitating factors for delirium

Predisposing factors	
Demographic characteristics	*Sensory impairment*
Age of 65 years or older	Visual impairment
Male sex	Hearing impairment
Cognitive status	*Functional status*
Dementia	Functional dependence
Cognitive impairment	Immobility
History of delirium	Low level of activity
Depression	History of falls
Drugs	*Decreased oral intake*
Treatment with psychoactive drugs	Dehydration
Treatment with many drugs	Malnutrition
Alcohol abuse	
Coexisting medical conditions	
Severe illness	Metabolic derangements
Multiple coexisting conditions	Neurological disease
Chronic renal or hepatic disease	Terminal illness
History of stroke	Fracture or trauma
Infection with HIV	
Precipitating factors	
Drugs	*Surgery*
Sedative-hypnotics	Orthopedic surgery
Narcotics	Cardiac surgery
Anticholinergic drugs	Prolonged cardiopulmonary bypass
Treatment with multiple drugs	Noncardiac surgery
Alcohol or drug withdrawal	
Sensory impairment	*Primary neurological disease*
Visual impairment	Stroke, particularly nondominant hemispheric
Hearing impairment	Intracranial bleeding
	Meningitis or encephalitis
Intercurrent illnesses	*Environment*
Infections	Admission to intensive care unit
Iatrogenic complications	Use of physical restraints
Severe acute illness	Use of bladder catheter
Hypoxia	Use of multiple procedures
Shock	Pain
Fever or hypothermia	Admission to intensive care unit
Anemia	Emotional stress
Dehydration	
Poor nutritional status	
Low serum albumin level	
Metabolic derangements (e.g., electrolytes)	

Source. Adapted from Inouye SK: "Current Concepts: Delirium in Older Persons." *New England Journal of Medicine* 354:1157–1165, 2006. Used with permission.

al. 2007). Overall, the development of these risk models aids in understanding the contribution of patient characteristics to delirium risk.

Precipitating factors for delirium include medications, immobilization, use of indwelling bladder catheters, use of physical restraints, dehydration, malnutrition, iatrogenic events, medical illnesses, organ insufficiency or failure (particularly renal or hepatic), infections, electrolyte or metabolic derangement, alcohol or drug intoxication or withdrawal, environmental influences, and psychosocial factors (see Table 12–3) (Agostini and Inouye 2003; Inouye 2006). Decreased mobility, including that associated with the use of medical devices (e.g., indwelling bladder catheters and physical restraints), greatly increases the risk of delirium and functional decline (Lazarus et al. 1991). Environmental factors (e.g., inadequate lighting, increased noise levels), psychosocial factors (e.g., depression, pain, anxiety), and iatrogenic events (e.g., transfusion reactions, allergic reactions) can also precipitate delirium.

With the introduction of oxygen-saturation monitoring (and subsequent decline of arterial blood gas determination), occult respiratory failure has emerged as an increasing problem for the development of delirium in elderly patients. Acute myocardial infarction and congestive heart failure commonly present with delirium as well. Metabolic disorders, such as hyper- or hyponatremia, hyper- or hypoglycemia, hypercalcemia, and thyroid or adrenal dysfunction, may also contribute to the development of delirium. Occult infection due to a variety of medical conditions (e.g., pneumonia, urinary tract infection, abdominal abscess) is a precipitating cause of delirium that is worth noting because older patients may not present with leukocytosis or the typical febrile response. A validated model of precipitating factors for the development of delirium in hospitalized older patients includes five factors: the use of physical restraints, malnutrition, more than three medications added during the previous day (over 70% of these were psychoactive drugs), indwelling bladder catheter, and any iatrogenic event (Inouye and Charpentier 1996).

TABLE 12–4. Drugs associated with delirium

Sedatives/hypnotics
Benzodiazepines (especially flurazepam, diazepam)
Barbiturates
Sleeping medications (diphenhydramine, chloral hydrate)
Narcotics (especially meperidine)
Anticholinergics
Antihistamines (diphenhydramine, hydroxyzine)
Antispasmodics (belladonna, Lomotil)
Heterocyclic antidepressants (amitriptyline, imipramine, doxepin)
Neuroleptics (chlorpromazine, haloperidol, thioridazine)
Incontinence (oxybutynin, hyoscyamine)
Atropine/Scopolamine
Cardiac
Digitalis glycosides
Antiarrhythmics (quinidine, procainamide, lidocaine)
Antihypertensives (β-blockers, methyldopa)
Gastrointestinal
Histamine H_2 receptor antagonists (cimetidine, ranitidine, famotidine, nizatidine)
Proton pump inhibitors
Metoclopramide (Reglan)
Herbal remedies (valerian root, St. John's wort, kava kava)

Source. Reprinted from Hazzard WR, Blass JP, Halter JB, et al. (eds.): *Principles of Geriatric Medicine and Gerontology*, Fifth Edition. New York, McGraw-Hill, 2003. Used with permission.

Medications and Delirium

The role of medications in the development of delirium deserves special attention (Table 12–4). Medication use contributes to delirium in more than 40% of cases (Inouye 1994; Inouye and Charpentier 1996). The medications most frequently associated with delirium are those with psychoactive effects, such as sedative-hypnotics, anxiolytics, narcotics, and histamine H_2 blockers. Drugs with anticholinergic effects, including antipsychotics, antihistamines, antidepressants, antiparkinsonian agents, and anticonvulsants, are also commonly associated with delirium. Previous studies have demonstrated that the use of psychoactive medication results in a 4-fold increased risk of delirium, whereas the use of two or more psychoactive medications is associated with a 5-fold increased risk (Inouye and Charpentier 1996). Sedative-hypnotic drugs are associated with a 3- to 12-fold increased risk of delirium, narcotics with a 3-fold risk, and anticholinergic drugs with a 5- to 12-fold risk (Agostini and Inouye 2003; Foy et al. 1995; Inouye 2006; Marcantonio et al. 1994; Schor et al. 1992).

A greater number of medications prescribed leads to a proportionately greater increased risk for developing delirium. This is related to the direct toxicity of the medications themselves, as well as the increased risk of drug-drug and drug-disease interactions. Previous studies suggest that overuse of psychoactive drugs and poor management of medications commonly occur in hospitalized geriatric patients, providing support for the preventable nature of many cases of delirium (Bates et al. 1995; Lindley et al. 1992). Some homeopathic or herbal therapies, especially those used for mood disorders (e.g., St. John's wort, kava kava), may increase the risk of delirium, especially when used in combination with prescribed psychoactive medications.

Given the role of medications in contributing to the development of delirium, it is essential to conduct a complete review of all prescription and over-the-counter medications a patient is taking. The majority of older patients take several prescribed medications during hospitalization, increasing the risk for drug-drug and disease-drug interactions. Medications with known psychoactive effects should be discontinued or minimized whenever possible. At the very least, steps should be taken to reduce dosage or to substitute medications with less toxic potential. In aging adults, medications may cause adverse effects even when given at the recommended dosages and with serum drug levels that are within the "therapeutic range." Determining if the patient has a history of chronic medication use or alcohol dependence is critical in assessing for withdrawal risk.

Diagnosis and Differential Diagnosis of Delirium

The diagnosis of delirium is based on clinical observation and relies on a thorough cognitive assessment, a detailed history from an informant close to the patient, and a comprehensive physical and neurological examination. The goal of a thorough background history interview is to establish that a change in cognition has occurred from the patient's baseline functioning. Acute alterations in cognition, representing abrupt deteriorations in mental status, may occur over hours or weeks, although it is important to keep in mind that these alterations may be superimposed on an underlying dementia as well. Delirium goes unrecognized by clinicians in up to 70% of patients who develop this condition (Rockwood et al. 1994); therefore, careful clinical assessment for this condition is imperative. To facilitate immediate and effective diagnosis and treatment of delirium, it is important to identify all multifactorial contributors. Identification of these factors relies on insightful clinical judgment combined with a thorough medical evaluation. Guidelines have been established by the American Psychiatric Association (1999) and the Royal College of Physicians (2006), both of which outline approaches to diagnosis and management of delirium in the older population.

The initial step during evaluation for delirium should be to determine the extent of change from the patient's baseline cognitive status by a careful history with a reliable proxy informant. The importance of obtaining a complete history that focuses on the patient's baseline cognitive status and chronology of recent mental status changes cannot be underestimated. The clinician should also assess recent changes or updates in medication regimen, new infections, or recent development of medical illnesses that may contribute to delirium.

The next step involves conducting a careful assessment of the patient's cognitive status (see "Neuropsychological Assessment of Delirium" section above). Assessment of vital signs often aids in identifying factors such as fever, tachycardia, or tachypnea, each of which may provide important etiological clues. Physical examination for signs of medical illnesses or occult infections such as pneumonia, urinary tract infection, or acute abdominal processes should also be conducted. Often, delirium may be the initial and only sign of a serious and life-threatening underlying illness, such as sepsis, pneumonia, or myocardial infarction. Additionally, a detailed neurological examination assessing for focal changes or evidence of head trauma, infection, or cerebrovascular disease should be performed during the evaluation.

The clinician's most important and difficult task is to differentiate delirium from dementia. Traditionally, delirium has been conceptualized as a brief and transient condition; however, many recent studies have shown that delirium symptoms may persist for months or years (Levkoff et al. 1994; Marcantonio et al. 2003; McCusker et al. 2003). Previous studies have indicated that dementia is the leading risk factor for delirium and that nearly two-thirds of cases of delirium occur in patients with dementia (Cole 2004; Inouye 2006). Patients with dementia who develop a superimposed delirium experience a more rapid progression of cognitive dysfunction and worse long-term prognosis (Fick and Foreman 2000; Jackson et al. 2004).

The key diagnostic feature that aids in distinguishing these two conditions is that delirium has an acute and rapid onset, whereas dementia is much more gradual in progression. Alterations in attention and changes in level of consciousness also point to a diagnosis of delirium. However, establishing the occurrence of those changes can be difficult in the face of missing baseline cognitive data or if preexisting cognitive deficits are reported by an informant. If the differentiation cannot be made with certainty, then given the life-threatening nature of delirium, the patient should be treated as delirious until proven otherwise.

Other important diagnoses that must be differentiated from delirium include psychiatric conditions such as depression, mania, and nonorganic psychotic disorders including schizophrenia. In general, these conditions do not develop suddenly in the context of a medical illness. Although hallucinations and perceptual disturbances can occur within the context of delirium, alterations in attention and global cognitive impairment are the key features that help to identify delirium. Differentiating among diagnoses is critical because delirium carries a more serious prognosis without proper evaluation and management. For example, treatment for certain conditions such as depression or affective disorders may involve the use of drugs with anticholinergic activity, which in turn could exacerbate an unrecognized case of delirium. Establishing the diagnosis can be difficult when the clinician is faced with symptoms that are subtle, when a background history is unavailable, or when the clinician is faced with an uncooperative patient. Again, given the seriousness of delirium and the fact that certain medical treatments may actually worsen symptoms, it is best for the clinician to assume that delirium is present until further diagnostic information is available.

No specific laboratory tests currently exist that will aid in the definitive identification of delirium. The laboratory evaluation for delirium is intended to identify contributing factors that will need to be addressed, and the approach should be guided by astute clinical judgment and tailored to the individual situation. Laboratory tests that should be considered in the delirium evaluation include complete blood count, electrolytes, kidney and liver function, oxygen saturation, and glucose levels. Evaluation of occult infection can be obtained through blood cultures, urinalysis, and urine culture. Other laboratory tests, such as thyroid function, arterial blood gas, vitamin B_{12} level, cortisol level, drug levels, toxicology screen, and ammonia levels, are also helpful in identifying factors that contribute to delirium. An electrocardiogram and/or chest radiograph may prove useful in patients with cardiac or respiratory diseases.

Brain imaging, using CT, PET, SPECT, or MRI, is indicated in the cases of head trauma or injury, evaluation of new focal neurological symptoms, evaluation for suspected encephalitis, or development of fever of unknown origin. Electroencephalography serves a limited role in the diagnosis of delirium—it has a false-negative rate of 17% and a false-positive rate of 22% (Pisani et al. 2003; Trzepacz et al. 1988)—and is most useful for detecting an occult seizure disorder. Cerebrospinal fluid examination, accomplished through lumbar puncture, may be useful in cases of febrile delirium or to exclude meningitis or encephalitis. Overall, the routine use of neuroimaging in delirium is not recommended, because the overall diagnostic yield is low, and the findings from neuroimaging change the management of patients in less than 10% of cases (Hirao et al. 2006).

Prevention and Management of Delirium

Prevention

Primary prevention—that is, preventing delirium before it develops—is the most effective strategy to alleviate symptoms associated with delirium. The Hospital Elder Life Program (HELP) (http://www.hospitalelderlifeprogram.org) utilizes a multidisciplinary team approach to aid in preventing delirium. HELP is a hospital-wide program that was designed to implement delirium prevention strategies and to promote an overall increase in quality of medical care.

Several controlled clinical trials have also identified successful strategies to help prevent delirium. A targeted multicomponent strategy resulted in a 40% reduction in the risk of delirium in patients following hip fractures (Marcantonio et al. 2001). The targeted multifactorial strategy focused on 10 domains: adequate brain oxygen delivery, fluid and electrolyte balance, pain management, reduction in psychoactive medications, bowel and bladder function, nutrition, early mobilization, prevention of postoperative complications, appropriate environmental stimuli, and treatment of delirium (Marcantonio et al. 2001). Controlled trials of educational strategies targeted toward training staff to assess, prevent, and treat delirium have demonstrated positive results in reducing episodes and duration of delirium (Milisen et al. 2001; Tabet et al. 2005). Controlled trials of multifactorial interventions, which usually consist of a combination of staff education and treatments tailored to meet the individual needs of patients, have demonstrated reductions in delirium rate and/or duration (Bergmann et al. 2005; Lundstrom et al. 2005; Naughton et al. 2005; Pitkala et al. 2006). A recent controlled trial found that compared with rehabilitation in the hospital setting, home rehabilitation of elderly patients after acute hospitalization was associated with lower risk of delirium and greater patient satisfaction (Caplan et al. 2006). Overall, results from these controlled trials suggest that 30%–40% of cases of delirium may be preventable and support the idea that prevention strategies should begin as soon as possible after hospital admission.

Management

In general, nonpharmacological approaches should be implemented as the first-line treatment of delirium. Nonpharmacological treatment approaches include reorientation (e.g., using orientation boards, clocks, calendars), behavioral interventions, encouraging the presence of family members, and transferring a disruptive patient to a private room or closer to the nurse's station for increased supervision. Consistent and compassionate staff are essential in facilitating contact and communication with the patient through frequent verbal reorienting strategies, clear instructions, frequent eye contact, and the inclusion of patients as much as possible in all decision making regarding their daily and medical care. Sensory deficits should be assessed and then corrected by ensuring that all assistive devices, such as eyeglasses and hearing aids, are readily available, functioning, and being used properly by the patient. The use of physical restraints should be minimized due to their role in prolonging delirium, worsening agitation, and increasing complications such as strangulation (Inouye et al. 2007). Strategies that increase the patient's mobility, self-care, and independence should be promoted.

Other environmental interventions include limiting room and staff changes as well as providing a quiet patient care setting with low-level lighting at night, allowing for an uninterrupted period for sleep. In fact, improving sleep in the patient with delirium is a highly effective and important intervention. McDowell et al. (1998) developed and tested a nonpharmacological sleep protocol that included treatment strategies such as a back massage, a warm drink, relaxation techniques, and soothing music. Use of the sleep protocol was highly effective, reducing reliance on sleeping medications from 54% to 31% ($P<0.002$) in a hospital environment (McDowell et al. 1998). Implementation of this type of sleep enhancement program may require unitwide changes in the coordination and scheduling of nursing and medical procedures. Hospital-wide changes may also be warranted to ensure a low level of noise at night by, for example, minimizing hallway noise and staff conversations.

Pharmacological management of delirium (see Table 12–5) should be used only in patients who have severe agitation that interferes with application of medical treatments (e.g., intubation) or in patients who pose a danger to themselves, other patients, or staff. It is important to remember that the lowest dose of medication should be prescribed for the shortest period of time possible, because drugs used to treat delirium can also lead to an increase in acute confusion. The goal for drug management should be an alert and manageable patient, not one who is lethargic and sedated.

If required, neuroleptics are the first line of pharmacological treatment. Haloperidol is the most widely used agent with documented efficacy to decrease agitation associated with delirium (Breitbart et al. 1996). Although haloperidol can be administered orally, intramuscularly, or intravenously, the oral route appears to be the most optimal due to favorable pharmacokinetics. Even though rapid onset of action is present during intravenous administration of haloperidol, this route should be avoided because of the short duration of treatment effects. The average geriatric patient who has not received prior treatment with a neuroleptic should require a total loading dose not exceeding 3–5 mg of haloperidol. Subsequently, a maintenance dose consisting of one-half of the loading dose should be administered over the next 24-hour period, with doses tapered during the next several days. It is important that vital signs be monitored before each additional dose is administered. Side effects that may occur following treatment with haloperidol include sedation, hypotension, extrapyramidal side effects, acute dystonias, and anticholinergic effects (e.g., dry mouth, constipation, urinary retention, increased confusion).

Atypical antipsychotics that have been used in the treatment of delirium include risperidone, olanzapine, and quetiapine; however, these agents have been tested

TABLE 12–5. Pharmacological treatment of delirium

Class and drug	Dose	Adverse effects	Comments
Antipsychotic			
Haloperidol	0.5–1.0 mg twice daily orally, with additional doses every 4 hr as needed (peak effect, 4–6 hr)	Extrapyramidal symptoms, especially if dose is >3 mg per day	Usually agent of choice
	0.5–1.0 mg intramuscularly; observe after 30–60 min and repeat if needed (peak effect, 20–40 min)	Prolonged corrected QT interval on electrocardiogram	Effectiveness demonstrated in randomized controlled trials (American Psychiatric Association 1999; Breitbart et al. 1996)
		Avoid in patients with withdrawal syndrome, hepatic insufficiency, neuroleptic malignant syndrome	Avoid intravenous use because of short duration of action
Atypical antipsychotic			
Risperidone	0.5 mg twice daily	Extrapyramidal effects equivalent to or slightly less than those with haloperidol	Tested only in small uncontrolled studies
Olanzapine	2.5–5.0 mg once daily	Prolonged corrected QT interval on electrocardiogram	Associated with increased mortality rate among older patients with dementia
Quetiapine	25 mg twice daily		
Benzodiazepine			
Lorazepam	0.5–1.0 mg orally, with additional doses every 4 hr as needed[a]	Paradoxical excitation, respiratory depression, oversedation	Second-line agent
			Associated with prolongation and worsening of delirium symptoms demonstrated in clinical trial (Breitbart et al. 1996)
			Reserve for use in patients undergoing sedative and alcohol withdrawal, those with Parkinson's disease, and those with neuroleptic malignant syndrome
Antidepressant			
Trazodone	25–150 mg orally at bedtime	Oversedation	Tested only in uncontrolled studies

[a]Intravenous use of lorazepam should be reserved for emergencies.

Source. Adapted from Inouye SK: "Current Concepts: Delirium in Older Persons." *New England Journal of Medicine* 354:1157–1165, 2006. Used with permission.

in only small, uncontrolled studies and may be associated with a higher mortality rate among older patients with dementia (Inouye 2006). Extrapyramidal effects of atypical neuroleptics may be equivalent to or slightly less than those associated with haloperidol. Olanzapine in particular has fewer extrapyramidal properties but greater anticholinergic properties when compared with haloperidol. Olanzapine is generally less effective than haloperidol for controlling delirium symptoms and poses the risk of inducing increased levels of confusion. Benzodiazepines typically lead to oversedation and exacerbation of confusion and are therefore not recommended in treating most forms of delirium (Breitbart et al. 1996). However, benzodiazepines still remain the treatment of choice in treating alcohol or sedative-hypnotic drug withdrawal symptoms. For geriatric patients, lorazepam is the preferred agent for treating alcohol or sedative-hypnotic withdrawal symptoms because of its shorter half-life, lack of active metabolites, and availability in parenteral form.

Key Points

- Delirium is a common problem for older persons that may be preventable.
- Delirium is the most frequent complication affecting older persons and often goes unrecognized.
- Patients with delirium have a worse prognosis than patients without delirium and an increased risk of developing long-term cognitive and functional decline.
- It is important to establish a patient's level of baseline cognitive functioning and course of cognitive change when evaluating for delirium.
- The Confusion Assessment Method provides a simple diagnostic algorithm and has become widely used for identification of delirium.
- Although delirium can be caused by a single factor, it is usually multifactorial.
- Existing cognitive impairment and/or dementia are the leading risk factors for development of delirium.
- Nonpharmacological approaches should be implemented as the first line of treatment for delirium.
- Pharmacological management of delirium should be used only in patients with severe agitation.

References

Adamis D, Morrison C, Treloar A, et al: The performance of the Clock Drawing Test in elderly medical inpatients: does it have utility in the identification of delirium? J Geriatr Psychiatry Neurol 18:129–133, 2005

Agostini JV, Inouye SK: Delirium, in Principles of Geriatric Medicine and Gerontology, 5th Edition. Edited by Hazzard WR, Blass JP, Halter JB, et al. New York, McGraw-Hill, 2003, pp 1503–1515

Albert MS, Levkoff SE, Reilly C, et al: The Delirium Symptom Interview: an interview for the detection of delirium symptoms in hospitalized patients. J Geriatr Psychiatry Neurol 5:14–21, 1992

American Psychiatric Association: Practice guideline for the treatment of patients with delirium. Am J Psychiatry 156(suppl):1–20, 1999. Available at http://www.guideline.gov/summary/summary.aspx?doc_id=2180. Accessed February 20, 2008.

American Psychiatric Association: Diagnostic and Statistical Manual of Mental Disorders, 4th Edition, Text Revision. Washington, DC, American Psychiatric Association, 2000

Balasundaram B, Holmes J: Delirium in vascular surgery. Eur J Vasc Endovasc Surg 34:131–134, 2007

Bates DW, Cullen DJ, Laird N, et al: Incidence of adverse drug events and potential adverse drug events: implications for prevention. ADE Prevention Study Group. JAMA 274:29–34, 1995

Benton AL, Hamsher K, Sivan AB: Multilingual Aphasia Examination, 3rd Edition. Iowa City, IA, AJA Associates, 1983

Bergmann MA, Murphy KM, Kiely DK, et al: A model for management of delirious postacute care patients. J Am Geriatr Soc 53:1817–1825, 2005

Bogousslavsky J, Ferrazzini M, Regli F, et al: Manic delirium and frontal-like syndrome with paramedian infarction of the right thalamus. J Neurol Neurosurg Psychiatry 51:116–119, 1988

Boyle DA: Delirium in older adults with cancer: implications for practice and research. Oncol Nurs Forum 33:61–78, 2006

Breitbart W, Marotta R, Platt MM, et al: A double-blind trial of haloperidol, chlorpromazine, and lorazepam in the treatment of delirium in hospitalized AIDS patients. Am J Psychiatry 153:231–237, 1996

Breitbart W, Rosenfeld B, Roth A, et al: The Memorial Delirium Assessment Scale. J Pain Symptom Manage 13:128–137, 1997

Burns A, Gallagley A, Byrne J: Delirium. J Neurol Neurosurg Psychiatry 75:362–367, 2004

Caplan GA, Coconis J, Board N, et al: Does home treatment affect delirium? A randomised controlled trial of rehabilitation of elderly and care at home or usual treatment (the REACH-OUT trial). Age Ageing 35:53–60, 2006

Centers for Medicare and Medicaid Services: Minimum Data Set (MDS) 3.0. n.d. Available at http://www.cms.hhs.gov/NursingHomeQualityInits/25_NHQIMDS30.asp. Accessed July 7, 2008.

Cole MG: Delirium in elderly patients. Am J Geriatr Psychiatry 12:7–21, 2004

Doherty MJ, Jayadev S, Watson NF, et al: Clinical implications of splenium magnetic resonance imaging signal changes. Arch Neurol 62:433–437, 2005

Elie M, Cole MG, Primeau FJ, et al: Delirium risk factors in elderly hospitalized patients. J Gen Intern Med 13:204–212, 1998

Ely EW, Margolin R, Francis J, et al: Evaluation of delirium in critically ill patients: validation of the Confusion Assessment Method for the Intensive Care Unit (CAM-ICU). Crit Care Med 29:1370–1379, 2001

Fayers PM, Hjermstad MJ, Ranhoff AH, et al: Which Mini-Mental State Exam items can be used to screen for delirium and cognitive impairment? J Pain Symptom Manage 30:41–50, 2005

Fick D, Foreman M: Consequences of not recognizing delirium superimposed on dementia in hospitalized elderly individuals. J Gerontol Nurs 26:30–40, 2000

Flacker JM, Lipsitz LA: Neural mechanisms of delirium: current hypotheses and evolving concepts. J Gerontol A Biol Sci Med Sci 54:239–246, 1999

Folstein MF, Folstein SE, McHugh PR: "Mini-Mental State": a practical method for grading cognitive state of patients for clinicians. J Psychiatr Res 12:189–198, 1975

Fong TG, Bogardus ST Jr, Daftary A, et al: Cerebral perfusion changes in older delirious patients using 99mTc HMPAO SPECT. J Gerontol A Biol Sci Med Sci 61:1294–1299, 2006

Foy A, O'Connell D, Henry D, et al: Benzodiazepine use as a cause of cognitive impairment in elderly hospital inpatients. J Gerontol A Biol Sci Med Sci 50:M99–M106, 1995

Francis J: Delirium in older patients. J Am Geriatr Soc 40:829–838, 1992

Gleason OC: Donepezil for postoperative delirium. Psychosomatics 44:437–438, 2003

Hamann J, Bickel H, Schwaibold H, et al: Postoperative acute confusional state in typical urologic population: incidence, risk factors, and strategies for prevention. Urology 65:449–453, 2005

Hazzard WR, Blass JP, Halter JB, et al: Principles of Geriatric Medicine and Gerontology, 5th Edition. New York, McGraw-Hill, 2003

Hirao K, Ohnishi T, Matsuda H, et al: Functional interactions between entorhinal cortex and posterior cingulate cortex at the very early stage of Alzheimer's disease using brain perfusion single-photon emission computed tomography. Nucl Med Commun 27:151–156, 2006

Inouye SK: The dilemma of delirium: clinical and research controversies regarding diagnosis and evaluation of delirium in hospitalized elderly medical patients. Am J Med 97:278–288, 1994

Inouye SK: Current concepts: delirium in older persons. N Engl J Med 354:1157–1165, 2006

Inouye SK, Charpentier PA: Precipitating factors for delirium in hospitalized elderly persons: predictive model and interrelationship with baseline vulnerability. JAMA 275:852–857, 1996

Inouye SK, Vandyck CH, Alessi CA, et al: Clarifying confusion: the Confusion Assessment Method—a new method for detection of delirium. Ann Intern Med 113:941–948, 1990

Inouye SK, Viscoli CM, Horwitz RI, et al: A predictive model for delirium in hospitalized elderly medical patients based on admission characteristics. Ann Intern Med 119:474–481, 1993

Inouye SK, Schlesinger MJ, Lydon TJ: Delirium: a symptom of how hospital care is failing older persons and a window to improve quality of hospital care. Am J Med 106:565–573, 1999

Inouye SK, Zhang Y, Jones RN, et al: Risk factors for delirium at discharge: development and validation of a predictive model. Arch Intern Med 167:1406–1413, 2007

Jackson JC, Gordon SM, Hart RP, et al: The association between delirium and cognitive decline: a review of the empirical literature. Neuropsychol Rev 14:87–98, 2004

Kiely DK, Bergmann MA, Jones RN, et al: Characteristics associated with delirium persistence among newly admitted postacute facility patients. J Gerontol A Biol Sci Med Sci 59:344–349, 2004

Kiely DK, Jones RN, Bergmann MA, et al: Association between delirium resolution and functional recovery among newly admitted postacute facility patients. J Gerontol A Biol Sci Med Sci 61:204–208, 2006

Lazarus BA, Murphy JB, Coletta EM, et al: The provision of physical activity to hospitalized elderly patients. Arch Intern Med 151:2452–2456, 1991

Leslie DL, Marcantonio ER, Zhang Y, et al: One-year health care costs associated with delirium in the elderly population. Arch Intern Med 168:27–32, 2008

Levkoff SE, Liptzin B, Evans DA, et al: Progression and resolution of delirium in elderly patients hospitalized for acute care. Am J Geriatr Psychiatry 2:230–238, 1994

Lindley CM, Tully MP, Paramsothy V, et al: Inappropriate medication is a major cause of adverse drug reactions in elderly patients. Age Ageing 21:294–300, 1992

Liptzin B, Levkoff SE: An empirical study of delirium subtypes. Br J Psychiatry 161:843–845, 1992

Lundstrom M, Edlund A, Karlsson S, et al: A multifactorial intervention program reduces the duration of delirium, length of hospitalization, and mortality in delirious patients. J Am Geriatr Soc 53:622–628, 2005

Marcantonio ER, Goldman L, Mangione CM, et al: A clinical-prediction rule for delirium after elective noncardiac surgery. JAMA 271:134–139, 1994

Marcantonio ER, Flacker JM, Wright RJ, et al: Reducing delirium after hip fracture: a randomized trial. J Am Geriatr Soc 49:516–522, 2001

Marcantonio ER, Simon S, Bergmann M, et al: Delirium symptoms in post-acute care: prevalent, persistent, and associated with poor functional recovery. J Am Geriatr Soc 51:4–9, 2003

Marcantonio ER, Rudolph JL, Culley D, et al: Serum biomarkers for delirium. J Gerontol A Biol Sci Med Sci 61:1281–1286, 2006

McCusker J, Cole M, Dendukuri N, et al: The course of delirium in older medical inpatients: a prospective study. J Gen Intern Med 18:696–704, 2003

McDowell JA, Mion LC, Lydon TJ, et al: A nonpharmacologic sleep protocol for hospitalized older patients. J Am Geriatr Soc 46:700–705, 1998

Milisen K, Foreman MD, Abraham IL, et al: A nurse-led interdisciplinary intervention program for delirium in elderly hip-fracture patients. J Am Geriatr Soc 49:523–532, 2001

Moran JA, Dorevitch MI: Delirium in the hospitalized elderly. Australian Journal of Hospital Pharmacy 31:35–40, 2001

Naughton BJ, Moran M, Ghaly Y, et al: Computed tomography scanning and delirium in elder patients. Acad Emerg Med 4:1107–1110, 1997

Naughton BJ, Saltzman S, Ramadan F, et al: A multifactorial intervention to reduce prevalence of delirium and shorten hospital length of stay. J Am Geriatr Soc 53:18–23, 2005

Ogasawara K, Komoribayashi N, Kobayashi M, et al: Neural damage caused by cerebral hyperperfusion after arterial bypass surgery in a patient with moyamoya disease: case report. Neurosurgery 56:E1380; discussion E1380, 2005

Olin K, Eriksdotter-Jönhagen M, Jansson A, et al: Postoperative delirium in elderly patients after major abdominal surgery. Br J Surg 92:1559–1564, 2005

Pisani MA, McNicoll L, Inouye SK: Cognitive impairment in the intensive care unit. Clin Chest Med 24:727–737, 2003

Pitkala KH, Laurila JV, Strandberg TE, et al: Multicomponent geriatric intervention for elderly inpatients with delirium: a randomized, controlled trial. J Gerontol A Biol Sci Med Sci 61:176–181, 2006

Pro JD, Wells CE: The use of the electroencephalogram in the diagnosis of delirium. Dis Nerv Syst 38:804–808, 1977

Reitan R: Validity of the Trail Making Test as an indicator of organic brain damage. Percept Mot Skills 8:271–276, 1958

Rockwood K: Acute confusion in elderly medical patients. J Am Geriatr Soc 37:150–154, 1989

Rockwood K, Cosway S, Stolee P, et al: Increasing the recognition of delirium in elderly patients. J Am Geriatr Soc 42:252–256, 1994

Rogers MP, Liang MH, Daltroy LH, et al: Delirium after elective orthopedic surgery: risk factors and natural history. Int J Psychiatry Med 19:109–121, 1989

Royal College of Physicians: Concise Guidance to Good Practice: A Series of Evidence-Based Guidelines for Clinical Management. London, Royal College of Physicians, 2006. Available at http://www.rcplondon.ac.uk/pubs/books/pdmd/DeliriumConciseGuide.pdf. Accessed February 20, 2008.

Rudolph JL, Jones RN, Grande LJ, et al: Impaired executive function is associated with delirium after coronary artery bypass graft surgery. J Am Geriatr Soc 54:937–941, 2006

Sandberg O, Gustafson Y, Brannstrom B, et al: Clinical profile of delirium in older patients. J Am Geriatr Soc 47:1300–1306, 1999

Schor JD, Levkoff SE, Lipsitz LA, et al: Risk factors for delirium in hospitalized elderly. JAMA 267:827–831, 1992

Tabet N, Hudson S, Sweeney V, et al: An educational intervention can prevent delirium on acute medical wards. Age Ageing 34:152–156, 2005

Takanashi J, Barkovich AJ, Shiihara T, et al: Widening spectrum of a reversible splenial lesion with transiently reduced diffusion. AJNR Am J Neuroradiol 27:836–838, 2006

Trenerry MR, Crosson B, DeBoe J, et al: Stroop Neuropsychological Screening Test (SNST). Odessa, FL, Psychological Assessment Resources, 1989

Trenerry MR, Crosson B, DeBoe J, et al: Visual Search and Attention Test (VSAT). Odessa, FL, Psychological Assessment Resources, 1990

Trzepacz PT, van der Mast R: The neuropathophysiology of delirium, in Delirium in Old Age. Edited by Lindesay J, Rockwood K, MacDonald AJ. New York, Oxford University Press, 2002, pp 51–90

Trzepacz PT, Brenner RP, Coffman G, et al: Delirium in liver transplantation candidates: discriminant analysis of multiple test variables. Biol Psychiatry 24:3–14, 1988

Trzepacz PT, Mittal D, Torres R, et al: Validation of the Delirium Rating Scale—Revised-98: comparison with the Delirium Rating Scale and the Cognitive Test for Delirium. J Neuropsychiatry Clin Neurosci 13:229–242, 2001

U.S. Department of Health and Human Services: 2004 CMS statistics. Washington, DC, Centers for Medicare and Medicaid Services, 2004

Wechsler D: Wechsler Adult Intelligence Scale—Revised. New York: Psychological Corporation, 1989

Wengel SP, Roccaforte WH, Burke WJ: Donepezil improves symptoms of delirium in dementia: implications for future research. J Geriatr Psychiatry Neurol 11:159–161, 1998

Suggested Readings

Breitbart W, Marotta R, Platt MM, et al: A double-blind trial of haloperidol, chlorpromazine, and lorazepam in the treatment of delirium in hospitalized AIDS patients. Am J Psychiatry 153:231–237, 1996

Inouye SK: Current concepts: delirium in older persons. N Engl J Med 354:1157–1165, 2006

Inouye SK, Vandyck CH, Alessi CA, et al: Clarifying confusion: the confusion assessment method—a new method for detection of delirium. Ann Intern Med 113:941–948, 1990

Inouye SK, Bogardus ST, Charpentier PA, et al: A multicomponent intervention to prevent delirium in hospitalized older patients. N Engl J Med 340:669–676, 1999

Inouye SK, Zhang Y, Jones RN, et al: Risk factors for delirium at discharge: development and validation of a predictive model. Arch Intern Med 167:1406–1413, 2007

Marcantonio ER, Flacker JM, Wright RJ, et al: Reducing delirium after hip fracture: a randomized trial. J Am Geriatr Soc 49:516–522, 2001

Naughton BJ, Saltzman S, Ramadan F, et al: A multifactorial intervention to reduce prevalence of delirium and shorten hospital length of stay. J Am Geriatr Soc 53:18–23, 2005

CHAPTER 13

Dementia and Milder Cognitive Syndromes

Constantine G. Lyketsos, M.D., M.H.S.

Dementia is a clinical syndrome that can be caused by a range of diseases or injuries to the brain. Although it can affect young people, it is most commonly seen in older individuals because dementia prevalence increases with age. Given the aging of the population worldwide, dementia is already epidemic and one of the top 10 causes of disability in developed countries (Murray and Lopez 1997). As shown in Figure 13–1, by 2040 an estimated 81 million new cases of dementia will occur worldwide, mostly in the developing world (Ferri et al. 2005). In the United States, as many as 15 million new cases of dementia are expected in the next several decades (Hebert et al. 2003). Given that dementia is a chronic disease, with estimates of its duration ranging from 3–4 years in community settings (Graham et al. 1997) to 10–12 years in clinical settings (Rabins et al. 2006), it poses a unique public health problem with serious effects on its victims, their families, and society at large. In the United States alone, it is estimated that by 2050, the annual cost of dementia will be close to $400 billion in direct and indirect expenses (Murman 2001; Murman et al. 2007).

In this chapter, I discuss definitions, clinical presentation, evaluation, and differential diagnosis of dementia and related cognitive disorders; describe specific dementia syndromes according to their etiology; and discuss how to approach treatment. For an in-depth discussion of the clinical management of dementia, the reader is referred to the book *Practical Dementia Care* by Rabins et al. (2006).

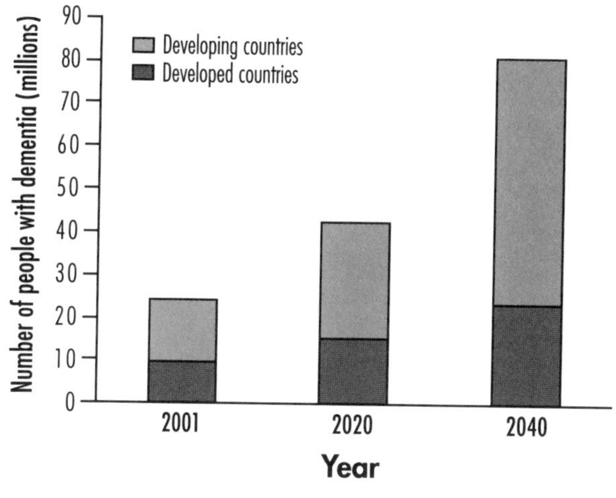

FIGURE 13–1. Projected prevalence of dementia worldwide.

Source. Adapted from Ferri CP, Prince M, Brayne C, et al.: "Global Prevalence of Dementia: A Delphi Consensus Study." *Lancet* 366:2112–2117, 2005.

Definitions

Table 13–1 provides definitions espoused by the American Association for Geriatric Psychiatry (Lyketsos et al. 2006). Cognitive syndromes (dementia and cognitive impairment not dementia) are differentiated from "subsyndromes" associated with specific diseases such as mild cognitive impairment. Finally, the table clarifies that Alzheimer's disease refers to a process in the brain whose pathology is fairly well known and whose etiol-

TABLE 13–1. Definitions related to dementia

Cognitive impairment not dementia (CIND): A clinical syndrome consisting of a measurable or evident decline in memory or other cognitive abilities, with little effect on day-to-day functioning; does not meet criteria for dementia.

Mild cognitive impairment: A clinical subsyndrome of CIND, most likely the prodrome to Alzheimer's dementia. Can be amnestic (having memory deficits) or nonamnestic.

Dementia: A clinical syndrome not entirely due to delirium, consisting of global cognitive decline, with memory plus one other area of cognition affected, and significant effect on day-to-day functioning.

Alzheimer's dementia: A dementia syndrome that has gradual onset and slow progression and is best explained as caused by Alzheimer's disease.

Alzheimer's disease: A brain disease characterized by plaques, tangles, and neuronal loss.

Source. Adapted from Lyketsos CG, Colenda CC, Beck C, et al: "Position Statement of the American Association for Geriatric Psychiatry Regarding Principles of Care for Patients With Dementia Resulting From Alzheimer Disease." *American Journal of Geriatric Psychiatry* 14:561–572, 2006. Used with permission.

ogy is under investigation. Although these definitions are important to the clinical world, one should recognize that uncertainty remains about linking cognitive syndrome to brain pathology. For example, in the environments of Alzheimer's centers, most patients diagnosed with Alzheimer's dementia usually have the Alzheimer's pathology as the unique cause, whereas in community settings, many patients at autopsy are found to have extensive Alzheimer's disease pathology despite having had no cognitive changes before death (Neuropathology Group, Medical Research Council Cognitive Function and Aging Study 2001). Furthermore, in community settings, most patients with dementia who come to autopsy have mixed brain pathologies including Alzheimer's disease, micro infarcts, lacunar infarcts, and Lewy bodies (Neuropathology Group, Medical Research Council Cognitive Function and Aging Study 2001; White and Launer 2006).

Clinical Presentation, Evaluation, and Differential Diagnosis

Clinical Presentation of the Dementia Syndrome

Dementia, being a syndrome, is defined entirely on clinical grounds. Table 13–2 lists the four critical elements of the definition. Dementia is a condition that affects *cognition,* which is defined as the mental processes used to obtain knowledge or to become aware of and interact with the environment. These processes include perception, imagination, judgment, memory, and language, as well as the processes people use to think, organize, and learn. For the dementia syndrome to be present, *several* areas of cognition must be affected

TABLE 13–2. The four key elements of the dementia syndrome

1. Global
2. Cognitive
3. Decline
4. Absence of delirium

(*global*). To differentiate dementia from mental retardation, the cognitive symptoms must represent a cognitive *decline* for the individual. The decline must be significant, typically sufficient to affect the person's daily functioning, operationalized as instrumental or basic daily living activities. Finally, because delirium can cause the full range of cognitive symptoms associated with dementia, it is critical that the cognitive syndrome be present in the *absence of delirium.* This broad definition has been operationalized in several criteria, with those of DSM-IV-TR (American Psychiatric Association 2000) being the most commonly used.

Traditionally, dementia is differentiated into cortical and subcortical "subsyndromes." Although these terms are misnomers because the subsyndromes do not strictly involve cortical and subcortical brain areas, they have important clinical implications (Table 13–3). The cortical subsyndrome refers to losses of cognitive *abilities,* whereas the subcortical subsyndrome refers to losses in the *coordination* of these abilities—sometimes referred to as executive functioning or executive control. The cortical subsyndrome is characterized by the four A's of impairment, and the subcortical subsyndrome by the four D's (Table 13–3); these are discussed in greater detail in *Practical Dementia Care* (Rabins et al. 2006).

TABLE 13–3. Cortical versus subcortical subsyndromes of dementia

Cortical	Subcortical
Abilities:	Coordination:
The four A's	The four D's
Amnesia	Dysmnesia
Apraxia	Delay
Aphasia	Dysexecutive
Agnosia	Depletion

Although the dementia syndrome is defined around cognitive disturbances, patients with dementia have a wider range of impairments that are of relevance to themselves, their daily life, and their caregivers. These include functional, neuropsychiatric (behavioral), and neurological impairments. In the functional realm, patients with dementia have problems in their social and interpersonal functioning and in their ability to live independently. Patients with milder dementia have difficulties with instrumental abilities, whereas patients with more severe dementia develop impairments in their basic abilities of daily living.

Dementia has been associated also with several neuropsychiatric symptoms. These are generally grouped into four types: 1) affective and motivational symptoms, such as apathy, depression, anxiety, and irritability; 2) perceptual disturbances, such as delusions and hallucinations; 3) disturbances of basic drives, including sleep, sexuality, and feeding; and 4) disturbances typically arising in more severe dementia, representing unexpected, socially inappropriate, or disinhibited behaviors. These inappropriate behaviors, which include spontaneous violence, intrusiveness, wandering, and the like, represent behavioral manifestations of loss of executive control, sometimes referred to as executive dysfunction syndrome (Lyketsos et al. 2004). Recent research has found that over the course of a progressive dementia, essentially all patients develop one or more of these behavioral symptoms (Steinberg et al. 2008).

Finally, patients with dementia develop a range of neurological findings. Depending on the cause of dementia, specifically on the parts of the brain affected over time, a range of neurological symptoms may occur. Most common are gait disorders, especially unstable, ataxic, or labored gait. Other neurological symptoms include incontinence, focal findings, seizures, and, less commonly, cranial nerve findings.

Clinical Presentation of Milder Cognitive Syndromes

Epidemiological studies have found that large numbers of older people have cognitive impairments that are troubling to them or family members but not sufficiently severe or broad to meet criteria for dementia. The prevalence of these impairments might be as high as 18% among people older than age 65 (Lopez et al. 2003). Several terms have evolved to refer to these: age-associated memory impairment, age-associated cognitive decline, cognitive impairment not dementia, and mild cognitive impairment (MCI). Long-term follow-up studies suggest that about one-third of these individuals improve so that their cognitive impairments are no longer detectable in the next few years; the majority go on to develop dementia (Rosenberg et al. 2006). These findings are consistent with the idea that most patients who develop progressive dementia do so in stages and typically go through a prodromal period of cognitive impairment, most often with memory symptoms, that is characteristic of the specific cause of the dementia. Thus, for example, it appears that amnestic MCI is a prodrome to Alzheimer's disease. Pathological studies have confirmed that after long-term follow-up, large numbers of patients who meet MCI criteria have Alzheimer's disease pathology. The term *vascular cognitive impairment* (VCI) (Hachinski 2007) has been coined to refer to nondementia disturbances associated with brain vascular disease, likely the prodrome of vascular dementia. Whereas the prodrome of Alzheimer's disease, MCI, appears to have primarily cortical features, the prodrome of vascular dementia, VCI, typically affects executive functions (Hayden et al. 2006).

Conducting an Evaluation

Although a detailed discussion of how to evaluate a patient with suspected dementia is beyond the scope of this chapter, this section highlights critical aspects of the evaluation, with a focus on taking a history, conducting a cognitive assessment, and using diagnostic tests. A thorough discussion of the evaluation of the patient with suspected dementia, including reasons for doing an evaluation, the setting for the evaluation, and ways to communicate the diagnosis to the patient, can be found in *Practical Dementia Care* (Rabins et al. 2006).

History Taking

The patient's medical history is critical to a good dementia evaluation. Because a patient with suspected dementia may have difficulty providing history due to language problems, memory disturbance, or nosoagnosia (lack of insight), the inclusion of an informant is critical during history taking. Informants need to be people who know the patient well, such as spouses, children, friends, neighbors, or other family members. Because informants themselves can be influenced by their own mental states, such as depression or denial of the situation, it is often useful to have additional informants to confirm or disconfirm discrepancies between the history and the evaluation of the patient.

Dating the onset of cognitive symptoms is critical. Often, comparing the severity of the patient's current impairment with its duration via history influences the differential diagnosis. Slowly progressive dementias evolve over many years; therefore, discrepancies in reports of severity and duration need to be resolved because they portend different prognoses and recommendations. It is important to spend a lot of time trying to determine when the patient was last well as opposed to when the first symptom started. Many times, informants minimize early symptoms by attributing them to "normal aging." It is also important to remember that the history should systematically survey for the presence or absence of the broader dementia syndrome presentation, as discussed in the earlier section "Clinical Presentation of the Dementia Syndrome." Therefore, the history should survey for cortical and subcortical cognitive symptoms; functional losses in social, interpersonal, and daily functioning; the full range of neuropsychiatric symptoms; and neurological deficits.

Cognitive Assessment

Conducting a cognitive assessment is the central aspect of the evaluation. Many specialists tend to use the Mini-Mental State Examination (MMSE) (Folstein et al. 1975) as their primary tool. The MMSE may be appropriate in more severe dementia but is inefficient in evaluating patients with milder cognitive symptoms or mild dementia because the MMSE has ceiling effects, especially for premorbidly well-educated and intelligent individuals, and has limitations in evaluating executive control function. Specialists in geriatric psychiatry and other clinicians who work with patients who have dementia are behooved to broaden their bedside standardized assessments. The Modified Mini-Mental State (3MS) provides a broader assessment of cognition (Teng and Chui 1987). The 3MS has many advantages: several translations exist; it has been validated in Spanish, Chinese, and other languages; it assesses abstract thinking, delayed recall, and verbal fluency better than the MMSE; and it has well-known population norms. In addition, for closer assessments of executive functioning, geriatric psychiatrists should consider incorporating these three measures in every dementia evaluation: the Clock Drawing test (van der Burg et al. 2004), the Frontal Assessment Battery (Dubois et al. 2000), and the Mental Alternation Test (Jones et al. 1993).

Differential Diagnosis and Diagnostic Testing

The establishment of a careful differential diagnosis is a key aspect of the dementia evaluation. The first step is to develop a differential diagnosis of the syndrome. Figure 13–2 provides a useful flowchart for this purpose. The first decision is whether any cognitive changes seen are disproportionate to aging. This can be determined by reviewing the patient's history or by assessing the patient's performance against well-known norms for age and education. If the cognitive changes are beyond age appropriate, the next question is whether the patient meets criteria for dementia such as those found in DSM-IV-TR. If the patient does not meet these criteria, then either cognitive impairment not dementia (which might be further subtyped as MCI or VCI) or delirium is present. If dementia is present, the geriatric psychiatrist will determine whether it is cortical or subcortical, progressive or nonprogressive, and its severity (typically labeled mild, moderate, or severe, often guided by the MMSE), as well as the severity of functional impairments, the presence or absence of neuropsychiatric symptoms and their specific phenomenology, the presence or absence of motor symptoms, and the presumptive cause of the dementia.

Neuropsychological testing is often useful in differentiating dementia from milder cognitive syndromes or normal aging, especially in investigating profiles of cognitive impairment that suggest specific etiologies. However, neuropsychological testing is not needed in every case, assuming that the geriatric psychiatrist conducts standardized assessment using tools similar to those discussed in the previous section on cognitive assessment. When conducted, neuropsychological testing should be requested with specific questions in mind such as clarifying the differential diagnosis or helping set the stage for monitoring the prognosis or treatment response.

Further workup using laboratory studies is needed in most cases of dementia. Blood tests and brain imaging are typically used in all cases. The American Acad-

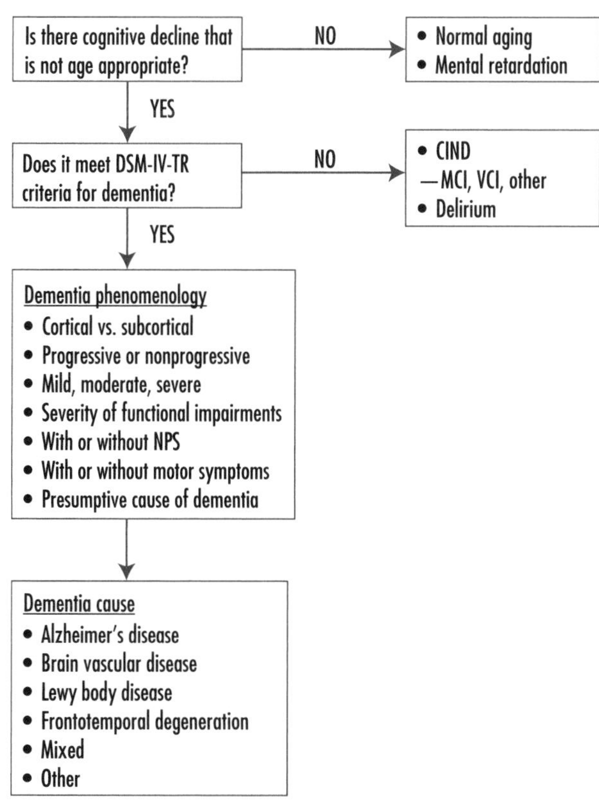

FIGURE 13–2. Flowchart in the diagnosis of dementia.

CIND=cognitive impairment not dementia; MCI=mild cognitive impairment; NPS=neuropsychiatric symptoms; VCI=vascular cognitive impairment.

emy of Neurology (Knopman et al. 2001) recommends thyroid studies, liver tests, metabolic panel, complete blood count, and vitamin B_{12} and folate levels. Additional tests, such as heavy metal screen, syphilis serology, toxicology, electrocardiogram, and chest X ray, should be considered to determine possible underlying causes. The type of brain imaging to be used is somewhat controversial. Most clinicians suggest that computed tomography (CT) of the head is adequate, but others feel that it is important to perform magnetic resonance imaging (MRI), especially when brain vascular disease may be involved. In the near future, quantification of specific MRI components, such as hippocampal volume, will provide information that is important to differential diagnosis, prognosis, and treatment targeting. Functional brain imaging using positron emission tomography (PET) or single-photon emission computed tomography (SPECT) has come into broader use and is reimbursed by Medicare under specific circumstances (Kulasingam et al. 2003). This imaging is most useful in the differential diagnosis of dementia caused by Alzheimer's disease or by frontotemporal degeneration, if the rest of the clinical picture is inconclusive.

Other biomarkers, such as cerebrospinal fluid tau and amyloid-β levels, continue to be used in research and likely will have clinical applications in the future. The same is true for genetic testing. Apolipoprotein E (*APOE*) genotyping, although not of universal utility in clinical settings, might in the near future have greater utility for treatment targeting: some studies suggest that certain medications may be more effective in different *APOE* subgroups (Petersen et al. 2005; Watson et al. 2005). Testing for specific genetic mutations associated with Alzheimer's disease also has its place in the rare instances in which a clear familial autosomal dominant case of Alzheimer's dementia is being evaluated and those in which knowledge of the specific genetic mutation involved might be useful to the patient or the patient's progeny after appropriate counseling.

Over 100 different disease processes have been associated with dementia (Rabins et al. 2006). Most cases can be assessed adequately using the patient history and the diagnostic testing approach discussed previously in this section. In the past, reference was made to treatable and nontreatable dementias. This differentiation is no longer useful for two reasons. First, reversibility of a "treatable dementia" depends on the severity of brain damage that has occurred. For example, dementia resulting from moderate to severe vitamin B_{12} deficiency, hypothyroidism, or normal pressure hydrocephalus does not reverse when treated. Second, the implication that Alzheimer's disease, vascular dementia, and other dementias are not treatable is also incorrect. Although these cases tend to be progressive despite available treatments, the application of treatments makes a big difference to patients, caregivers, and families, because treatments may attenuate progression, reduce symptoms, and improve quality of life.

Specific Dementias

Dementia Due to Alzheimer's Disease

Alzheimer's dementia is the most common form of dementia. Depending on the population series, 50%–70% of people with dementia are diagnosed clinically as having dementia due to Alzheimer's disease (Ranginwala et al. 2008), sometimes referred to as possible or probable Alzheimer's disease by the National Institute of Neurological Disorders and Stroke criteria (McKhann et al. 1984). Although experts can make the clinical diagnosis with high reliability, in population series, the pathological changes seen in the brains of people with Alzheimer's dementia are varied. The vast majority of patients meet pathological criteria for Alzheimer's disease; a significant number of patients have other pathological findings as well, such as infarcts, Lewy bodies, and lacunes.

The prevalence of Alzheimer's dementia is closely tied to age, which is the primary risk factor. Other risk factors include head or traumatic brain injury, reduced reserve capacity of the brain, limited educational or occupational attainment, brain vascular disease, hyperlipidemia, hypertension, atherosclerosis, coronary heart disease, atrial fibrillation, smoking, obesity, and diabetes. A possible risk factor is homocysteinemia. Some but not other epidemiological studies have suggested that dietary intake of folate and vitamin B_{12}, antioxidants (especially vitamins C and D), moderate alcohol (especially red wine), nonsteroidal anti-inflammatory agents, and estrogen during the perimenopausal period are associated with reduced risk of Alzheimer's disease.

A major risk factor is genetic, however, with 70%–80% of the disease being heritable, as supported by twin studies (Blennow et al. 2006). Alzheimer's disease is a heterogeneous genetic disorder with familial and polygenic forms. The familial forms follow classical autosomal dominant inheritance and typically have onset before age 65. Several mutations have been associated with the familial conditions; all involve mutations in genes associated with the amyloid precursor protein on chromosome 21 and also include the presenilin 1 and 2 genes (on chromosomes 14 and 1, respectively). Taken together, these familial genes account for one-half to two-thirds of the familial cases, suggesting that many autosomal dominant genes are unknown.

Most cases of Alzheimer's disease are polygenic. Several genes, most unknown, likely increase risk but do not absolutely determine the occurrence of the disease. The most well-known gene is the *APOE* gene whose ε4 allele is a risk factor for Alzheimer's dementia. Heterozygous ε4 carriers have 3 times and homozygous ε4 carriers have 15 times the risk of non-ε4 carriers. *APOE*E4* probably operates mainly by modifying age of onset through uncertain molecular mechanisms (Breitner et al. 1999). The sortilin 1 gene, probably involved in amyloid clearance, has also been identified as a risk factor (Rogaeva et al. 2007). Several other candidate genes have been investigated, although none have been consistently supported as risk factors for the disease.

The current hypothesis is that Alzheimer's dementia is a heterogeneous condition representing a range of etiologies involving different interactions between different sets of genetic and environmental risk factors (Blennow et al. 2006). At one end of the spectrum are individuals who have familial disease, for whom genes such as *APOE* influence the age of onset, and who will develop the disease if they live long enough. At the other end of the spectrum are individuals with a weak predisposition, perhaps carriers of few or no risk genes, but in whom the occurrence of environmental risk factors is critical to the onset of Alzheimer's pathology and the later dementia. As an example of gene-environment interactions, individuals with traumatic brain injury appear to be at increased risk of progressive dementia if they also carry one or more ε4 alleles (Isoniemi et al. 2006).

The natural history of Alzheimer's dementia has been well described from tertiary clinical centers. Time from diagnosis to death in these settings is on the order of 10–12 years, with considerable variability around this median estimate. Population studies from Canada and the United States suggest that a significant proportion of patients with dementia do not make it to clinical centers and that if all of the latter group are included, the median time from onset of symptoms to death in patients with dementia in the broader population is on the order of 3–5 years (Larson et al. 2004; Wolfson et al. 2001). The variability in time to death is also reflected in the variability of the cognitive and functional progression of Alzheimer's dementia. Significant numbers of patients (as noted, for example, in placebo-controlled trials of anti-Alzheimer drugs) exhibit slow progression after the onset of dementia. In one population-based study in Cache County, Utah, 25%–30% of patients exhibited limited to no progression from milder stages of Alzheimer's dementia even 3–5 years after onset (Isoniemi et al. 2006; Jellinger et al. 2001).

Factors that influence progression in Alzheimer's dementia are poorly known. The *APOE* genotype does not appear to affect the rate of progression. The presence of psychosis and of extrapyramidal symptoms is associated with faster progression, as is the presence of hypertension and atrial fibrillation. Despite the variability in rate, patients who progress show a typical pattern, with loss of memory occurring fairly early, followed by the development of agnosia, apraxia, and aphasia. Patients also follow predictable progression in functional impairments and, in later stages, universally develop problems with mobility and continence. In terminal stages, patients with Alzheimer's disease may live a long time, sometimes years, in near-vegetative states if they are in good general health and receive good care.

Neuropsychiatric symptoms are nearly universal. Several cohort studies suggest that affective, psychotic, and sleep symptoms relapse and remit through the course of Alzheimer's dementia and are very troubling for patients and caregivers (Rabins et al. 2006; Steinberg et al. 2008). Apathy, in contrast, appears to be a steadily accumulating symptom in that many but not all patients gradually develop persistent and pervasive apathy (Onyike et al. 2007; Steinberg et al. 2008).

The brain changes seen in Alzheimer's dementia are well known. Even in early stages of the disease, brain imaging studies show volume reduction in the hippocampus bilaterally, and this reduction appears to progress with the illness. In early stages of the disease, brain imaging using fluorodeoxyglucose PET typically shows bitemporoparietal and often frontal hypoperfusion. This hypoperfusion eventually spreads throughout the brain as the disease progresses. PET or SPECT of neurotransmitters involving the cholinergic, dopaminergic, and serotonergic systems shows neurotransmitter loss even in living patients in early stages of Alzheimer's dementia (Sabbagh et al. 2006). More recently, imaging of amyloid deposition in the brain is becoming possible using Pittsburgh Compound B, FDDNP, and other PET or SPECT ligands (Lockhart 2006). Using these ligands, researchers have found that by the time dementia begins, there is abundant deposition of amyloid, which does not increase over time and is not necessarily specific to Alzheimer's dementia (Engler et al. 2006; Lockhart et al. 2007). Thus, the deposition of amyloid may be fairly extensive by the time early symptoms appear, suggesting a time course of many years of brain changes before symptom onset. Other lines of evidence also support a long delay, perhaps decades, between pathological onset and clinical expression of Alzheimer's dementia (Blennow et al. 2006).

Pathologically, the characteristic lesions of Alzheimer's disease include senile or neuritic plaques and neurofibrillary tangles, with associated loss of neurons in several neurotransmitter systems: cholinergic, serotonergic, and dopaminergic. These changes typically occur early in the disease and affect both the nuclei and the cortical projections of neurons. The current hypothesis about etiopathogenesis suggests a cascade (Blennow et al. 2006). Genetic and environmental risk factors interact to increase the production or to decrease the clearance of amyloid derived from the amyloid precursor protein (APP); APP is present on most neurons, and its function is unknown. APP may be processed through cleavage by β-secretase preferentially over α-secretase, leading to the formation of a form of amyloid beta ($A\beta_{1-42}$). The latter is prone to dimerization, oligomerization, and deposition in the extracellular space. The deposition of this toxic form of Aβ, as opposed to less toxic forms (e.g., $A\beta_{1-40}$) that are produced when α-secretase cleaves before β-secretase, accumulates close to the synaptic cleft and is thought to lead over time to synaptic disconnection, the loss of neurotransmitter systems, and the emergence of symptoms.

The manifestation of the several Alzheimer's dementia symptoms probably depends more on the brain location and neurotransmitter systems affected than on the cause of the pathology present (Lyketsos 2006). How amyloid deposition leads to neuronal toxicity remains uncertain. A range of downstream factors have been implicated in the disease cascade, including activation of microglia that might injure neurons through several mechanisms (Rosenberg 2005). Other downstream factors involved in progression include glutamatergic toxicity, lipid peroxidation products, and the loss of trophic factor.

The Alzheimer's pathology likely begins many years and perhaps decades before the onset of symptoms; therefore, there is an opportunity for prevention once future advances make it possible to diagnose the disease through the use of biomarkers before symptom onset. Also, the distribution of the neuropathology appears to change with the course of the disease such that it begins in the mesial temporal lobe and then disseminates widely throughout the brain. The tissue loss that follows can become extensive so that patients dying with advanced Alzheimer's disease have atrophic brains and significantly enlarged ventricles. These changes during the course of the disease may mean that different treatments will have differential efficacy at different phases of the disease.

Dementia Due to Brain Vascular Disease (Vascular Dementia)

Vascular dementia continues to be a controversial nosological entity, in part because of the absence of clear neuropathological agreement about it. Also, it is difficult to differentiate on clinical grounds those patients who have Alzheimer's dementia from those who have vascular dementia (Groves et al. 2000). Further complicating the differentiation, recent evidence suggests that cerebrovascular risk factors and diseases influence the progression of Alzheimer's dementia (Mielke et al. 2007) and the emergence of Alzheimer's pathology in the brain (Beach et al. 2007; Roher et al. 2006). Most patients with vascular dementia who come to autopsy have mixed pathology, often with significant Alzheimer's disease pathology (Jellinger and Attems 2006).

Vascular dementia, therefore, is best understood as a heterogeneous group of dementias. On one end of the spectrum are pure genetic forms, such as 1) cerebral autosomal dominant arteriopathy with subcortical infarcts and leukoencephalopathy and 2) mitochondrial encephalopathy with lactic acidosis and strokelike episodes. At the other end are patients who develop dementia after multiple strokes in which significant portions of the brain are damaged. Between those two endpoints are patients with mixtures of pathologies and clinical presentations that impact one another (e.g., smaller strokes or chronic subcortical hypoxia might both damage brain tissue and lead to the onset and progression of Alzheimer's pathology).

In addition to genetic conditions such as those mentioned in the previous paragraph, genes that predispose to cerebrovascular disorders are risk factors for vascular dementia (Meschia et al. 2005; Schneider et al. 2007). The following are some of the risk factors for cerebrovascular disease that are also risk factors for vascular dementia: disease of the large and small vessels of the brain, diabetes, hypertension, and atrial fibrillation and other cardiac disease.

The clinical presentation of vascular dementia is variable. Typically, it presents in fits and spurts, often with acute or subacute onset after a cerebrovascular event. A mix of symptoms usually presents, often including apathy, depression, and motor symptoms. Of patients with vascular dementia or Alzheimer's dementia who have similar MMSE scores, those with vascular dementia are usually more functionally impaired. Gait disorders, parkinsonism, and incontinence are early features of vascular dementia.

The diagnosis of vascular dementia is based on a typical clinical history and associated physical examination findings. The diagnosis requires brain imaging that shows completed infarcts or lacunes in brain areas associated with the cognitive changes. A temporal relationship between the brain vascular disease and the cognitive changes should be demonstrable, but this might be difficult. Radiological findings of white matter change alone, with no evidence of completed strokes or associated examination findings (e.g., motor focality or gait disorder), are not supportive of a diagnosis of vascular dementia. White matter changes, as evident on MRI, are common in older people who are cognitively normal (Longstreth 1998; Longstreth et al. 2005). The diagnosis becomes more complex when patients with established Alzheimer's dementia develop strokes; many such patients also meet criteria for a diagnosis of vascular dementia. Results from the Nun Study (Snowdon et al. 1997) and the Religious Order Study (Bennett 2006; Schneider et al. 2004) suggested that for a given degree of Alzheimer's pathology, dementia is more severe in the presence of comorbid cerebrovascular disease.

Little is known about the progression of clinically diagnosed vascular dementia. Therefore, only speculative comments can be made here. Clinical anecdotes suggest that many patients with vascular dementia can have a nonprogressive condition for many years as long as they do not have other strokes. However, other patients decline rather precipitously, and most patients have various slower rates of progressive decline.

Dementias Due to Lewy Body Disease

A recent consensus panel (Lippa et al. 2007) has proposed the term *Lewy body disorders* as an umbrella term for Parkinson's disease (PD), Parkinson's disease dementia (PDD), and dementia with Lewy bodies (DLB). This proposal appropriately recognizes the existence of a spectrum of dementias associated with Lewy body disease of the brain whose shared pathology involves impairments in alpha synuclein metabolism. The hypothesis is that these three conditions, which can also be termed *synucleinopathies*, represent brain diseases in which abnormal synuclein metabolism leads to dementia. The sequence of events involved is poorly known. One of the complicating factors in determining a diagnosis is that many patients with Lewy body pathologies have coexisting pathologies, in particular Alzheimer's and vascular pathology. Additionally, the clinical presentations of PDD and DLB can be similar, with motor parkinsonism, gait imbalance, visual hallucinations, and dementia being the unifying clinical features. The discussion that follows focuses on each of these conditions separately.

Parkinson's Disease Dementia

With the advent of the use of L-dopa to help control Parkinson's motor symptom, it has become apparent that some of the most common and impairing symptoms of PD are in the cognitive realm. Patients with PD typically show impairments in executive functioning, including delays in problem solving, difficulties in set shifting, and poor fluency. They also have memory impairments characteristic of dysmnesia, affecting working memory and the organization of explicit memory. Some have visuospatial difficulties arising out of difficulty with set shifting and the need for high executive demand to complete visuospatial tests. In early to midstage PD, 16%–20% of patients develop dementia, in contrast to as many as 80% in later PD. In early stages, a further 15%–30% have milder cognitive symptoms. These cognitive impairments have been associated with deficits in several neurotransmitter systems, including dopaminergic, cholinergic, serotonergic, and noradrenergic. Also, although high rates of Alzheimer's pathology appear to be present in patients with PD and dementia, this linkage remains controversial because of the different findings in different autopsy series. For more information, see Metzler-Baddeley (2007) and Rippon and Marder (2005).

The term *Parkinson's disease dementia* (PDD) refers to patients who have had PD for many years and then develop dementia most likely caused by the PD itself. PDD can be quite impairing of daily functioning and adversely affects caregivers (Mehta 2005). PDD has become a therapeutic target, leading to the U.S. Food and Drug Administration's approval of the cholinesterase inhibitor rivastigmine for treatment of PDD.

Dementia With Lewy Bodies

The Consortium on Dementia With Lewy Bodies continues to systematically update diagnostic and management recommendations for DLB. The most recent revision of the DLB diagnostic criteria (McKeith et al. 2005) presents central, core, suggestive, and supportive features. The central feature is a progressive dementia with primary persistent memory impairment and deficits in attention, executive, and visuospatial abilities. Core features, at least one of which is necessary for the diagnosis of DLB, include fluctuating cognition with pronounced variations in attention and alertness, visual hallucinations, or spontaneous parkinsonism. Suggestive features include REM (rapid eye movement) sleep behavior disorder, severe neuroleptic sensitivity, and low dopamine transporter uptake in the basal ganglia demonstrated on PET or SPECT imaging. The long list of supportive features includes falls and syncope, unexplained loss of consciousness, autonomic dysfunction, nonvisual hallucinations, delusions, depression, and brain imaging or electroencephalographic findings consistent with the diagnosis.

If dementia and parkinsonism coexist, the differential diagnosis is sorted out by examining the relative course of the cognitive and motor symptoms. The emergence of dementia after many years of motor symptoms supports a diagnosis of PDD. In contrast, the early presence of dementia in a patient with motor parkinsonism supports a diagnosis of DLB. It should be noted that many patients with Alzheimer's dementia develop a DLB picture, which is reflected in the neuropathology, and many DLB patients have concurrent Alzheimer's dementia pathology. It is difficult to clinically distinguish Alzheimer's dementia patients with and without DLB pathology (Lopez et al. 2000).

Although the progression of DLB tends to be similar overall to that of Alzheimer's dementia, the course of DLB is more variable. Because many patients have a more fulminant course, some experts believe that DLB has a worse prognosis than Alzheimer's dementia (McKeith et al. 2003, 2004). DLB is associated with considerable suffering for patients, particularly because of the very common, persistent, and hard-to-treat neuropsychiatric symptoms, especially hallucinations, delusions, and affective symptomatology (Ballard et al. 1999; McKeith and Cummings 2005). Patients also tend to become affected early with balance, sleep, and motor disorders and to become confined in their mobility.

Dementia Due to Frontotemporal Degeneration

Frontotemporal degeneration (FTD) is in many ways the paradigmatic non-Alzheimer's dementia and has recently become a major focus of interest because of the appreciation that in individuals under age 65, FTD is the second most common form of dementia, with a rate of occurrence that is close to that of Alzheimer's dementia (Neary et al. 2005). Previously referred to as Pick's disease, FTD is heterogeneous both clinically and pathologically (Kertesz 2005; Neary et al. 2005). The clinical syndrome typically begins with changes in behavior, affect, and personality, which result in disinhibition, hyperorality, social inappropriateness, apathy, and related symptoms of loss of executive control. Cognitive changes leading to difficulties in attention, memory, set shifting, and organization occur early in the disease (Kertesz et al. 2005). The phenotype, however, is variable because many patients develop progressive expressive aphasia, whereas others develop semantic dementia early on (Shinagawa et al. 2006). As the condition progresses, disinhibited behaviors and apathy—often at the same time—worsen, leading to admixtures of productive-type and deficit-type loss of executive control. Further complicating the picture is the co-occurrence of FTD with amyotrophic lateral sclerosis (ALS). Some patients with FTD develop ALS presentations later in the course of their condition, whereas some ALS patients develop FTD dementia as their disease progresses (Chow et al. 1999; Grossman et al. 2007; Murphy et al. 2007).

Pathologically, FTD is characterized by knife-edge lobar atrophy, typically in the anterior temporal and posterior inferior areas of the frontal lobes. Microscopically, neurons appear enlarged and vacular, with extensive gliosis. Revised consensus neuropathological criteria take into account advances in both genetics and biochemistry and reflect the diversity of pathological pictures (Cairns et al. 2007a). Most of these conditions appear to be tauopathies and include the pathologies of FTD with Pick bodies, corticobasal degeneration, progressive supranuclear palsy, hippocampal sclerosis, and other less common pathologies. TDP-43 proteinopathy appears to be the most frequent histological finding in FTD. FTD is familial in a considerable number of patients; mutations in the tau, progranulin, and ubiquitin genes have been associated with the condition. Familial TDP-43 proteinopathy is associated with defects in multiple genes and several neuropathological types (Cairns et al. 2007b).

FTD is almost invariably progressive, especially if language symptoms occur early on. In clinical settings, the time from an FTD diagnosis to death is on the order of 3–5 years, shorter than the periods associated with Alzheimer's dementia (Chow et al. 2006). Also, compared with Alzheimer's dementia, FTD is a greater burden to caregivers, given the disinhibited behaviors that are hard to treat and require aggressive supervision to manage.

Less Common Dementias

Dementia Due to Normal Pressure Hydrocephalus

The dementia of normal pressure hydrocephalus is a subcortical dementia associated with a characteristic magnetic-like gait disorder and incontinence. Little is known about its epidemiology and progression. It is estimated to have an annual incidence of 0.5–2 per million (Wilson and Williams 2006). Much interest has focused on efforts to diagnose and treat normal pressure hydrocephalus using shunts (see discussion in "Disease Therapies" later in this chapter). The condition is suspected when patients present with the classic triad of findings and brain imaging reveals enlarged ventricles disproportionate to cortical atrophy. The diagnosis is confirmed by a high-volume lumbar puncture cannulation of the cerebrospinal fluid for continuous monitoring of pressure waves (Pfisterer et al. 2007). Although this remains an active area of investigation, uncertainty continues regarding how to diagnose and optimally treat patients who present with this syndrome.

Dementia Due to Prion Diseases (Spongiform Encephalopathies)

Recent knowledge regarding prion protein transmission across species has led to concerns about animal-to-human transmission of these proteins through the diet, followed by incurable, rapidly progressive dementias. The annual incidence of Creutzfeldt-Jakob dementia (CJD), the most common human prion dementia, is on the order of 1 per million per year worldwide, with a few hundred cases presenting every year in the United States (Caramelli et al. 2006). Until recently, the prevalence was higher in the United Kingdom because of transmission of a variant form of this disease from eating affected beef; however, this epidemic appears to have subsided (Collee et al. 2006).

All mammals, including humans, carry the prion protein on the short arm of chromosome 20. Several mutations in this protein have been reported and are associated with a familial progressive dementia (Michalczyk and Ziman 2007) that is sometimes referred to as Gerstmann-Sträussler-Scheinker syndrome (GSS). CJD and GSS have variable clinical presentations, although the most characteristic presentation is that of a rapidly progressive dementia, prominent gait disorder, and motor findings early on. The typical time from onset to death is 6–9 months. Patients become disabled rapidly and may experience difficulty in obtaining a diagnosis because they often present with psychiatric symptoms such as depression, apathy, and executive dysfunction. Although the time course of CJD is almost invariably rapid, cases in the literature have been reported with longer courses, sometimes lasting years. The familial cases, in particular, tend to run longer courses, as long as a decade in younger persons (Lyketsos 1999).

The basic pathophysiology of the disease, partly worked out by Stanley Prusner (who won the Nobel Prize in Medicine for this work), is thought to involve transformation of human prion protein from its alpha-helical form to a beta-sheet form (Michalczyk and Ziman 2007). How this is brought about is uncertain. It might occur spontaneously or result from interactions with mutant prion proteins or those of other species that make their way into the human brain. Some cases of the disease have been the result of transplantation with affected organs (Ironside 2006). Beta-sheet prion proteins tend to transform other prion proteins from alpha-helix to beta-sheet form, leading to a snowball cascade with widespread dissemination of these proteins, which become clumpy and toxic and lead to the classic spongiform appearance of the nervous system. Little is known about factors that initiate or accelerate these transitions, although some of the familial cases appear to have been initiated by biological stress to the brain through stroke, hypoxia, or traumatic brain injury (Lyketsos 1999). At present, this disease is incurable. The familial forms are a target of genetic counseling.

Treatment

Treatment for Milder Cognitive Syndromes

Given the increased public awareness of dementia, memory clinics and primary care physicians anecdotally report that patients are presenting with increasingly milder cognitive symptoms to request diagnosis and treatment. At present, there is little empirical knowledge about how to manage these patients clinically; most experts recommend continued observation, the use of nonpharmacological therapies such as exercise and mental activity, and possibly cognitive rehabilitation. The results of at least one randomized trial suggest that the cholinesterase inhibitor donepezil may delay progression to dementia, especially in patients who are *APOE*E4* carriers (Petersen et al. 2005), but this has not been replicated or supported by other trials (Rosenberg et al. 2006). Initiation of pharmacological therapy is reserved for cases for which there is strong evidence of likely benefit—for example, when the patient appears to be about to transition to Alzheimer's dementia. For more a detailed approach to this issue, see Rosenberg et al. (2006).

The Four Pillars of Dementia Care

Dementia care has four basic elements or pillars (Lyketsos et al. 2006). The first pillar relates to management of key aspects of the disease with the goal of reversing its effects or delaying its progression in the brain. Although few disease therapies exist at present, several therapies are being developed for different types of dementia targeted at underlying pathophysiological mechanisms. The second pillar of dementia care relates to the management of its symptoms, whether they are cognitive, neuropsychiatric, or functional. The final two pillars involve providing supportive care to patients and caregivers in ways that are systematic and evidence based.

The overall premise of this approach is that an affective, systematic care model exists for patients with dementia resulting from Alzheimer's disease (Lyketsos et al. 2006). This care model also has implications for patients suffering from other forms of dementia. The remainder of this chapter deals with critical aspects of the implementation of dementia care. It should be noted that even a decade ago, dementia care interventions were few and provided on faith, with limited evidence of effectiveness. Evidence from randomized trials now indicates that the "package" of dementia care as currently conceived provides significant benefits to patients and caregivers by reducing symptoms, improving disability and quality of life, and reducing caregiver effects. Based on results from a randomized trial, Callahan et al. (2006) reported that in primary care settings, guideline-based dementia care leads to better patient and caregiver outcomes, likely related to more appropriate use of medications and of interventions targeting both caregivers and patients. Similarly, long-term follow-up (Drentea et al. 2006; Mittelman et al. 2006) found that caregiver-targeted intervention prolonged the time patients spent in the community. These findings have been supported by an observational cohort (Lyketsos et al. 2007) from the Maryland Assisted Living Study, which suggested that treatment for dementia might delay discharge by as much as 7 months.

Disease Therapies

Alzheimer's Disease

As articulated in the American Association for Geriatric Psychiatry's principles of care (Lyketsos et al. 2006), estrogen, anti-inflammatory agents, and ginkgo biloba are not effective treatments for Alzheimer's dementia.

High doses of the antioxidant vitamin E were found, in one large randomized, controlled trial, to delay progression of Alzheimer's dementia, lengthening the time before onset of the next phase (Sano et al. 1997). Given safety concerns about dosing, the American Association for Geriatric Psychiatry recommended that vitamin E be considered for Alzheimer's dementia but that doses above 400 IU/day should be avoided. Similarly, although 3-hydroxy-3-methylglutaryl coenzme A (HMG-CoA) reductase inhibitors (i.e., statins) have shown some promise as treatments for Alzheimer's dementia in observational studies and a randomized clinical trial, it is premature to think of these as disease therapies for Alzheimer's dementia.

Probably the most effective therapy for Alzheimer's disease is management of associated vascular risk factors—blood pressure in particular—and treatment with the glutamatergic antagonist memantine. Reduction of blood pressure that is above 160 systolic, weight loss, exercise, management of diabetes, and a healthy diet all probably constitute effective therapy for Alzheimer's disease. For patients with moderate or more severe Alzheimer's dementia, memantine titrated to 10 mg twice daily has very small but measurable effects, especially in patients with more severe disease.

A better understanding of the pathology and etiopathogenesis of Alzheimer's dementia has led to the development of a series of therapies that target amyloid precursor protein metabolism, $A\beta_{1-42}$ deposition or clearance, or ways by which amyloid injures neurons. For example, inhibition of β-secretase and γ-secretase targets the metabolism of amyloid precursor protein. Immunotherapies, through either injection of amyloid to create host immunity (active immunization) or injection of antibodies to clear amyloid from the brain (passive immunization), are under investigation. Also under investigation are medications that influence the deposition or clearance of amyloid in in vitro or animal models. Treatments that target other mechanisms—that is, treatments such as anti-inflammatories, prednisone, and estrogen—have not been successful in clinical trials, although some remain under investigation as preventative efforts. The use of folate to reduce hypercystinemia, the use of antioxidants (vitamins D and C), and dietary modifications also continue under investigation.

Other Diseases

Management of stroke risk typically with anticoagulation as well as vascular risk factors is fully indicated in treating patients with vascular dementia or possibly Alzheimer's dementia with relevant vascular comorbidities. Use of L-dopa is probably effective for treating patients with PDD; some patients with DLB also may have partial response.

Shunting is indicated for some patients with normal pressure hydrocephalus, but this treatment remains controversial. Indicators of positive response to shunting are improvement in gait after a high-volume lumbar puncture or high cerebrospinal fluid flow pressure on continuous monitoring (Bergsneider et al. 2005; Marmarou et al. 2005; Meier et al. 2006; Poca et al. 2005; Tisell et al. 2006). The size of ventricle or the severity of gait disorder is not a good predictor of outcome (Meier et al. 2006). Up to 40%–50% of shunt patients experience complications from shunting. In a Dutch study (Vanneste et al. 1992), also the largest outcome study to date, notable mortality was noted after shunt placement, with the risks of shunting outweighing the benefits. No randomized, controlled trial has been conducted to evaluate the issue. Many patients have favorable outcomes that can be enduring after shunt placement; the beneficial effects typically involve gait and continence but not cognition (Aygok et al. 2005; Savolainen et al. 2002; Tisell et al. 2006).

Therapies for Cognitive Symptoms

The cholinesterase inhibitors huperzine, tacrine, donepezil, rivastigmine, and galantamine are all approved by the U.S. Food and Drug Administration (FDA) or otherwise available in the United States for treatment of the cognitive symptoms of Alzheimer's dementia. Most of these medications have been approved for the treatment of mild to moderate Alzheimer's dementia; donepezil has been approved for the treatment of severe Alzheimer's dementia. They are available in a variety of formulations as pills, delayed-release pills, and patch form (rivastigmine only). Huperzine, an over-the-counter nutraceutical that is currently under study and whose safety is poorly known, and tacrine, which has hepatotoxicity concerns, are used very infrequently. Although clinical trials have suggested that these medications may be of value in treating vascular dementia, none of them has been approved by the FDA for that purpose. The results of one study suggest that donepezil is associated with increased mortality in vascular dementia relative to placebo. Rivastigmine has been approved for the treatment of PDD and has also been found in randomized trials to be effective in DLB.

These agents share the property of being inhibitors of acetylcholinesterase, thus effectively increasing brain levels of acetylcholine. They benefit some patients for 6–9 months and in 10%–15% of cases lead to notable, albeit temporary, symptomatic improvements. Rivastigmine also has biological activity against butyrylcholinesterase. Galantamine is also an allosteric modulator of the nicotinic receptors. Despite differences in biological activity, in the absence of solid relevant clinical data, the choice of agent continues to be driven by ease of use and ease of titration, because they appear to have comparable efficacy. Prior to the development of the patch delivery form of rivastigmine, approved in the United States in 2007, and the extended-release form of galantamine, there were important differences in toxicity that also entered into the clinical decision about which medication to use first.

Currently, most experts recommend, and the data support, initiation of one of these medications titrated to the highest approved and tolerated dose and assessment of response over 6–12 months (Rabins et al. 2006). There is debate, however, about whether patients should stay on a cholinesterase inhibitor for a longer period of time. In primary care settings in the United States, most patients who start a prescription do not stay on it for more than a few months. Nevertheless, many experts recommend continuation of therapy once it is started because discontinuation studies suggest that patients may get worse when a cholinesterase inhibitor is stopped. However, other experts point out that some patients do well after a discontinuation trial and that many benefit from switching to another agent when they do not respond to an earlier one (Tariot et al. 2006). I have followed one patient who benefited from sequential use of four of the cholinesterase agents (huperzine, donepezil, rivastigmine, and galantamine). Although clearly that was an extreme case, which is probably quite rare, it points out that the issue of long-term therapy is not a settled matter.

Therapies for Neuropsychiatric Symptoms

Neuropsychiatric symptoms are nearly universal over the course of dementia. They have severe adverse effects for patients and caregivers and are a frequent target of treatment. Nevertheless, there continues to be uncertainty about how to manage these symptoms. Detailed discussion of the evaluation and management of neuropsychiatric symptoms in dementia is beyond the scope of this chapter (see Rabins et al. 2006 for an in-depth discussion); however, a few principles are articulated here.

A useful approach to the management of neuropsychiatric symptoms employs, once again, a mnemonic of four D's: define, decode, devise, and determine. *Define* refers to an evaluation phase in which the patient, caregivers, and other relevant informants (e.g., charts and professional caregivers in long-term care facilities and hospitals) provide the history, which is used to describe in detail the phenomenology of the patient's disturbance. Then, the patient undergoes an examination, which sometimes involves laboratory studies. This information is used to decide what type of disturbance is present: delirium, affective disorder, psychotic disorder, sleep disturbance, apathy, executive dysfunction, and so on (Lyketsos, 2007).

Subsequently, the clinician, working as part of a team, seeks contributing factors to the disorder; this is the *decode* phase. Contributing causes to neuropsychiatric symptoms are listed in Table 13–4. In general, most disturbances are multifactorial; therefore, it is best to address several factors at once. The *devise* phase, which derives from the decoding process, consists of pharmacological, behavioral, environmental, and educational approaches that target the causes identified and are often delivered through the patient's caregiver. For example, a patient's urinary tract infection or constipation might be treated while teaching the caregiver how not to rush the patient during toileting. In early

TABLE 13–4. Contributing causes of neuropsychiatric symptoms

- Biological stress or delirium that accompanies a recurrent or new medical condition (e.g., constipation, urinary or upper respiratory infection, pain, poor dentition, headaches, hunger, thirst)
- Identifiable psychiatric syndrome that is either recurrent or associated with the dementia
- Aspects of the cognitive disturbance itself (catastrophic reaction due to inability to express oneself vocally
- Environmental stressor (e.g., too much noise, not enough heat)
- Unmet needs (e.g., hunger, thirst, feeling lonely)
- Unsophisticated or intrusive caregiving (e.g., poor communication, being rushed)
- Medication side effects, whether from new medications or previously prescribed medications

dementia, psychotherapy might be attempted with patients who are anxious, depressed, or demoralized. Occasionally, management with psychotropics is needed, especially if nonpharmacological approaches have failed. Although extensive effort has been put into the development of nonpharmacological approaches, there is little controlled evidence to suggest that they work, and they are often hard to implement in real-world settings, especially in primary and institutional care (Livingston et al. 2005). The interventions with the best evidence to support their use are outlined in Table 13–5. Finally, the *determine* phase refers to setting reasonable goals for assessing the effect of the intervention and readjusting the plan if the intervention is not successful.

If medication treatments are indicated, it is important to follow an approach similar to the one outlined in Table 13–6. Several different classes of medications have been studied, but for some of them, safety concerns exist and efficacy remains uncertain. The use of antipsychotics, especially the atypical antipsychotics, is controversial because their efficacy is modest (Schneider et al. 2005, 2006) and they have been associated with a higher risk of cerebrovascular or cardiovascular conditions and mortality in patients with dementia specifically (Schneider et al. 2005). Both conventional and atypical antipsychotics carry this risk in dementia, whereas other psychotropics, such as antidepressants and anticonvulsants, do not (Kales et al. 2007). Although these antipsychotics are not contraindicated in dementia, the risk-benefit threshold has recently been raised, and they should be used with caution (Rabins and Lyketsos 2005). Evidence is limited regarding the efficacy of cholinesterase inhibitors and memantine for behavior. In general, although these medications may delay the emergence of neuropsychiatric symptoms or treat very mild symptoms, they should not be considered first-line agents in managing acute neuropsychiatric symptoms of moderate or greater severity until better evidence of their efficacy emerges (Weintraub and Katz 2005). Similarly, there is evidence to suggest that selective serotonin reuptake inhibitors, such as citalopram (Pollock et al. 2002) and sertraline (Lyketsos et al. 2003), have efficacy for the treatment of agitation and depression in patients with Alzheimer's dementia. Putting this information together, a widely used algorithm for use of medications to treat neuropsychiatric symptoms in dementia has been published (Sink et al. 2005).

TABLE 13–5. Evidence-based nonpharmacological treatments for neuropsychiatric symptoms

- Cognitive stimulation and behavioral management techniques centered on patient behavior or caregiver behavior are effective treatments whose benefits last for months.
- Music therapy and controlled multisensory stimulation (snoezelen) are useful during the treatment session but have no longer-term effects.
- Specific education for caregiving staff about managing neuropsychiatric symptoms is very beneficial, but other educational interventions are not.
- Changing the visual environment (e.g., painting doors to disguise them) is promising, but more research is needed.

TABLE 13–6. Guidelines for use of medications to treat neuropsychiatric symptoms

- Differentiate which disturbance is present; they are not all the same.
- Consider possible contributing causes and the need for medical workup.
- Implement nonpharmacological interventions.
- Decide whether to treat with medications.
- Use medications cautiously, with defined targets and close monitoring.
- Be mindful that select *isolated* disturbances are unlikely to respond to medications.
- Have in place a backup plan and a plan to deal with after-hours crisis.

Supportive Care for Patients

The provision of systematic supportive care to patients with dementia is critical. This care is typically tailored to individual patients and is implemented in collaboration with caregivers and other team members. Table 13–7 lists areas that should be addressed in every case (Lyketsos et al. 2006). In addition, where appropriate, patients should be educated as much as possible about their condition and their prognosis.

Supportive Care for Caregivers

Because caregivers are greatly affected by dementia and are the lifeline of the patient, They should be involved intimately in the development and implementation of any

TABLE 13–7. Supportive care for patients

- Comfort and emotional support
- Safety in regard to driving, living alone, medications, falls
- Proper approach and communication
- A safe, predictable place to live with support for independent activities of daily living and activities of daily living
- Structure, activity, and stimulation in day-to-day life
- Planning and assistance with decision making
- Aggressive management of medical comorbidity
- Good nursing care in advanced stages

TABLE 13–8. Supportive care for the caregiver

- Comfort and emotional support
- Education about dementia and caregiving
- Instruction in the skills of caregiving
- Support with problem solving
- Availability of an expert clinician, especially for crisis intervention
- Respite from caregiving
- Attention to general and mental health
- Maintenance of social network

dementia care program. Table 13–8 lists key intervention areas involving caregivers (Lyketsos et al. 2006; Rabins et al. 2006; Selwood et al. 2007). The importance of the delivery of interventions to caregivers is supported by the work of Mittelman and colleagues (2006), which suggests that caregiver interventions can have effect sizes as large as or larger than medications in delaying out-of-home placement for patients with dementia. In particular, making sure that caregivers are educated about dementia, have an understanding of the diagnosis, are able to access resources, use respite appropriately, and have an expert available around the clock to help them in times of crisis are central to good dementia care.

Key Points

- Dementia is a clinical syndrome that can be accurately diagnosed and differentiated from CIND and MCI.
- The evaluation and differential diagnosis of dementia, and of milder cognitive syndromes, involves an initial focus on defining the phenomenology of the syndrome and its associated features, followed by a workup for a putative clause.
- The concept of treatable and nontreatable dementias is no longer relevant; all dementias are treatable, albeit not necessarily curable.
- The four pillars of dementia treatment are disease treatment, symptom treatments, supportive care for the patient, and supportive care for the caregiver. All of these areas must be addressed in contemporary dementia care.
- Nonpharmacological interventions, in the context of carefully orchestrated dementia care, can be as effective as currently available medications (and in some cases more effective) in helping patients and caregivers.

References

American Psychiatric Association: Diagnostic and Statistical Manual of Mental Disorders, 4th Edition, Text Revision. Washington, DC, American Psychiatric Association, 2000

Aygok G, Marmarou A, Young HF: Three-year outcome of shunted idiopathic NPH patients. Acta Neurochir Suppl 95:241–245, 2005

Ballard C, Holmes C, McKeith I, et al: Psychiatric morbidity in dementia with Lewy bodies: a prospective clinical and neuropathological comparative study with Alzheimer's disease. Am J Psychiatry 156:1039–1045, 1999

Beach TG, Wilson JR, Sue LI, et al: Circle of Willis atherosclerosis: association with Alzheimer's disease, neuritic plaques and neurofibrillary tangles. Acta Neuropathol 113:13–21, 2007

Bennett DA: Postmortem indices linking risk factors to cognition: results from the religious order study and the memory and aging project. Alzheimer Dis Assoc Disord 20 (suppl 2):S63–S68, 2006

Bergsneider M, Black PM, Klinge P, et al: Surgical management of idiopathic normal-pressure hydrocephalus. Neurosurgery 57(suppl):S29–S39; discussion ii–v, 2005

Blennow K, de Leon MJ, Zetterberg H: Alzheimer's disease. Lancet, 368:387–403, 2006

Breitner JC, Wyse BW, Anthony JC, et al: APOE-epsilon4 count predicts age when prevalence of AD increases, then declines: the Cache County study. Neurology 53:321–331, 1999

Cairns NJ, Bigio EH, Mackenzie IR, et al: Neuropathologic diagnostic and nosologic criteria for frontotemporal lobar degeneration: consensus of the Consortium for Frontotemporal Lobar Degeneration. Acta Neuropathol 114:5–22, 2007a

Cairns NJ, Neumann M, Bigio EH, et al: TDP-43 in familial and sporadic frontotemporal lobar degeneration with ubiquitin inclusions. Am J Pathol 171:227–240, 2007b

Callahan CM, Boustani MA, Unverzagt FW, et al: Effectiveness of collaborative care for older adults with Alzheimer disease in primary care: a randomized controlled trial. JAMA 295:2148–2157, 2006

Caramelli M, Ru G, Acutis P, et al: Prion diseases: current understanding of epidemiology and pathogenesis, and therapeutic advances. CNS Drugs 20:15–28, 2006

Chow TW, Miller BL, Hayashi VN, et al: Inheritance of frontotemporal dementia. Arch Neurol 56:817–822, 1999

Chow TW, Hynan LS, Lipton AM: MMSE scores decline at a greater rate in frontotemporal degeneration than in AD. Dement Geriatr Cogn Disord 22:194–199, 2006

Collee JG, Bradley R, Liberski PP: Variant CJD (vCJD) and bovine spongiform encephalopathy (BSE): 10 and 20 years on, part 2. Folia Neuropathol 44:102–110, 2006

Drentea P, Clay OJ, Roth DL, et al: Predictors of improvement in social support: five-year effects of a structured intervention for caregivers of spouses with Alzheimer's disease. Soc Sci Med 63:957–967, 2006

Dubois B, Slachevsky A, Litvan I, et al: The FAB: a frontal assessment battery at bedside. Neurology 55:1621–1626, 2000

Engler H, Forsberg A, Almkvist O, et al: Two-year follow-up of amyloid deposition in patients with Alzheimer's disease. Brain 129 (pt 11):2856–2866, 2006

Ferri CP, Prince M, Brayne C, et al: Global prevalence of dementia: a Delphi consensus study. Lancet 366:2112–2117, 2005

Folstein MF, Folstein SE, McHugh PR: "Mini-Mental State": a practical method for grading the cognitive state of patients for the clinician. J Psychiatr Res 12:189–198, 1975

Graham JE, Rockwood K, Beattie BL, et al: Prevalence and severity of cognitive impairment with and without dementia in an elderly population. Lancet 349:1793–1796, 1997

Grossman AB, Woolley-Levine S, Bradley WG, et al: Detecting neurobehavioral changes in amyotrophic lateral sclerosis. Amyotroph Lateral Scler 8:56–61, 2007

Groves WC, Brandt J, Steinberg M, et al: Vascular dementia and Alzheimer's disease: is there a difference? A comparison of symptoms by disease duration. J Neuropsychiatry Clin Neurosci 12:305–315, 2000

Hachinski V: The 2005 Thomas Willis lecture: stroke and vascular cognitive impairment: a transdisciplinary, translational and transactional approach. Stroke 38:1396, 2007

Hayden KM, Zandi PP, Lyketsos CG, et al: Vascular risk factors for incident Alzheimer disease and vascular dementia: the Cache County study. Alzheimer Dis Assoc Disord 20:93–100, 2006

Hebert LE, Scherr PA, Bienias JL, et al: Alzheimer disease in the U.S. population: prevalence estimates using the 2000 census. Arch Neurol 60:1119–1122, 2003

Ironside JW: Variant Creutzfeldt-Jakob disease: risk of transmission by blood transfusion and blood therapies. Haemophilia 12 (suppl 1):8–15; discussion 26–28, 2006

Isoniemi H, Tenovuo O, Portin R, et al: Outcome of traumatic brain injury after three decades: relationship to ApoE genotype. J Neurotrauma 23:1600–1608, 2006

Jellinger KA, Attems J: Prevalence and impact of cerebrovascular pathology in Alzheimer's disease and parkinsonism. Acta Neurol Scand 114:38–46, 2006

Jellinger KA, Paulus W, Wrocklage C, et al: Traumatic brain injury as a risk factor for Alzheimer disease: comparison of two retrospective autopsy cohorts with evaluation of ApoE genotype. BMC Neurol 1:3, 2001

Jones BN, Teng EL, Folstein MF, et al: A new bedside test of cognition for patients with HIV infection. Ann Intern Med 119:1001–1004, 1993

Kales HC, Valenstein M, Kim HM, et al: Mortality risk in patients with dementia treated with antipsychotics versus other psychiatric medications. Am J Psychiatry 164:1568–1576, 2007

Kertesz A: Frontotemporal dementia: one disease, or many? Probably one, possibly two. Alzheimer Dis Assoc Disord 19 (suppl 1):S19–S24, 2005

Kertesz A, McMonagle P, Blair M, et al: The evolution and pathology of frontotemporal dementia. Brain 128 (pt 9):1996–2005, 2005

Knopman DS, DeKosky ST, Cummings JL, et al: Practice parameter: diagnosis of dementia (an evidence-based review): report of the Quality Standards Subcommittee of the American Academy of Neurology. Neurology 56:1143–1153, 2001

Kulasingam SL, Samsa GP, Zarin DA, et al: When should functional neuroimaging techniques be used in the diagnosis and management of Alzheimer's dementia? A decision analysis. Value 6:542–550, 2003

Larson EB, Shadlen MF, Wang L, et al: Survival after initial diagnosis of Alzheimer disease. Ann Intern Med 140:501–509, 2004

Lippa CF, Duda JE, Grossman M, et al: DLB and PDD boundary issues: diagnosis, treatment, molecular pathology, and biomarkers. Neurology 68:812–819, 2007

Livingston G, Johnston K, Katona C, et al, for the Old Age Task Force of the World Federation of Biological Psychiatry: Systematic review of psychological approaches to the management of neuropsychiatric symptoms of dementia. Am J Psychiatry 162:1996–2021, 2005

Lockhart A: Imaging Alzheimer's disease pathology: one target, many ligands. Drug Discov Today 11:1093–1099, 2006

Lockhart A, Lamb JR, Osredkar T, et al: PIB is a non-specific imaging marker of amyloid-beta (Abeta) peptide-related cerebral amyloidosis. Brain 130:2607–2615, 2007

Longstreth WT Jr, for the Cardiovascular Health Study Collaborative Research Group: Brain abnormalities in the elderly: frequency and predictors in the United States (the Cardiovascular Health Study). J Neural Transm 53(suppl):9–16, 1998

Longstreth WT Jr, Arnold AM, Beauchamp NJ Jr, et al: Incidence, manifestations, and predictors of worsening white matter on serial cranial magnetic resonance imaging in the elderly: the Cardiovascular Health Study. Stroke 36:56–61, 2005

Lopez OL, Wisniewski S, Hamilton RL, et al: Predictors of progression in patients with AD and Lewy bodies. Neurology 54:1774–1779, 2000

Lopez OL, Jagust WJ, DeKosky ST, et al: Prevalence and classification of mild cognitive impairment in the Cardiovascular Health Study Cognition Study, part 1. Arch Neurol 60:1385–1389, 2003

Lyketsos C: The prion dementias. Md Med J 48:18–22, 1999

Lyketsos CG: Lessons from neuropsychiatry. J Neuropsychiatry Clin Neurosci 18:445–449, 2006

Lyketsos CG: Neuropsychiatric symptoms (behavioral and psychological symptoms of dementia) and the development of dementia treatments. Int Psychogeriatr 19:409–420, 2007

Lyketsos CG, DelCampo L, Steinberg M, et al: Treating depression in Alzheimer disease: efficacy and safety of sertraline therapy, and the benefits of depression reduction: the DIADS. Arch Gen Psychiatry 60:737–746, 2003

Lyketsos CG, Rosenblatt A, Rabins P: Forgotten frontal lobe syndrome or "executive dysfunction syndrome." Psychosomatics 45:247–255, 2004

Lyketsos CG, Colenda CC, Beck C, et al: Position statement of the American Association for Geriatric Psychiatry regarding principles of care for patients with dementia resulting from Alzheimer disease. Am J Geriatr Psychiatry 14:561–572, 2006

Lyketsos CG, Samus QM, Baker A, et al: Effect of dementia and treatment of dementia on time to discharge from assisted living facilities: the Maryland Assisted Living Study. J Am Geriatr Soc 55:1031–1037, 2007

Marmarou A, Young HF, Aygok GA, et al: Diagnosis and management of idiopathic normal-pressure hydrocephalus: a prospective study in 151 patients. J Neurosurg 102:987–997, 2005

McKeith I, Cummings J: Behavioural changes and psychological symptoms in dementia disorders. Lancet Neurol 4:735–742, 2005

McKeith IG, Burn DJ, Ballard CG, et al: Dementia with Lewy bodies. Semin Clin Neuropsychiatry 8:46–57, 2003

McKeith I, Mintzer J, Aarsland D, et al: Dementia with Lewy bodies. Lancet Neurol 3:19–28, 2004

McKeith IG, Dickson DW, Lowe J, et al: Diagnosis and management of dementia with Lewy bodies: third report of the DLB consortium. Neurology 65:1863–1872, 2005

McKhann G, Drachman D, Folstein M, et al: Clinical diagnosis of Alzheimer's disease: report of the NINCDS-ADRDA Work Group under the auspices of Department of Health and Human Services Task Force on Alzheimer's Disease. Neurology 34:939–944, 1984

Mehta KK: Stress among family caregivers of older persons in Singapore. J Cross Cult Gerontol 20:319–334, 2005

Meier U, Lemcke J, Neumann U: Predictors of outcome in patients with normal-pressure hydrocephalus. Acta Neurochir Suppl 96:352–357, 2006

Meschia JF, Brott TG, Brown RD Jr: Genetics of cerebrovascular disorders. Mayo Clin Proc 80:122–132, 2005

Metzler-Baddeley C: A review of cognitive impairments in dementia with Lewy bodies relative to Alzheimer's disease and Parkinson's disease with dementia. Cortex 43:583–600, 2007

Michalczyk K, Ziman M: Current concepts in human prion protein (prp) misfolding, prnp gene polymorphisms and their contribution to Creutzfeldt-Jakob disease (CJD). Histol Histopathol 22:1149–1159, 2007

Mielke MM, Rosenberg PB, Tschanz J, et al: Vascular factors predict rate of progression in Alzheimer disease. Neurology 69:1850–1858, 2007

Mittelman MS, Haley WE, Clay OJ, et al: Improving caregiver well-being delays nursing home placement of patients with Alzheimer disease. Neurology 67:1592–1599, 2006

Murman DL: The costs of caring: medical costs of Alzheimer's disease and the managed care environment. J Geriatr Psychiatry Neurol 14:168–178, 2001

Murman DL, Von Eye A, Sherwood PR, et al: Evaluated need, costs of care, and payer perspective in degenerative dementia patients cared for in the United States. Alzheimer Dis Assoc Disord 21:39–48, 2007

Murphy J, Henry R, Lomen-Hoerth C: Establishing subtypes of the continuum of frontal lobe impairment in amyotrophic lateral sclerosis. Arch Neurol 64:330–334, 2007

Murray CJ, Lopez AD: Global mortality, disability, and the contribution of risk factors: global burden of disease study. Lancet 349:1436–1442, 1997

Neary D, Snowden J, Mann D: Frontotemporal dementia. Lancet Neurol 4:771–780, 2005

Neuropathology Group, Medical Research Council Cognitive Function and Aging Study: Pathological correlates of late-onset dementia in a multicentre, community-based population in England and Wales. Lancet 357:169–175, 2001

Onyike CU, Sheppard JM, Tschanz JT, et al: Epidemiology of apathy in older adults: the Cache County study. Am J Geriatr Psychiatry 15:365–375, 2007

Petersen RC, Thomas RG, Grundman M, et al: Vitamin E and donepezil for the treatment of mild cognitive impairment. N Engl J Med 352:2379–2388, 2005

Pfisterer WK, Aboul-Enein F, Gebhart E, et al: Continuous intraventricular pressure monitoring for diagnosis of normal-pressure hydrocephalus. Acta Neurochir (Wien) 149:983–990, 2007

Poca MA, Mataro M, Matarin M, et al: Good outcome in patients with normal-pressure hydrocephalus and factors indicating poor prognosis. J Neurosurg 103:455–463, 2005

Pollock BG, Mulsant BH, Rosen J, et al: Comparison of citalopram, perphenazine, and placebo for the acute treatment of psychosis and behavioral disturbances in hospitalized, demented patients. Am J Psychiatry 159:460–465, 2002

Rabins PV, Lyketsos CG: Antipsychotic drugs in dementia: what should be made of the risks? JAMA 294:1963–1965, 2005

Rabins PV, Lyketsos CG, Steele CD: Practical Dementia Care, 2nd Edition. New York, Oxford University Press, 2006

Ranginwala NA, Hynan LS, Weiner MF, et al: Clinical criteria for the diagnosis of Alzheimer disease: still good after all these years. Am J Geriatr Psychiatry 16:384–388, 2008

Rippon GA, Marder KS: Dementia in Parkinson's disease. Adv Neurol 96:95–113, 2005

Rogaeva E, Meng Y, Lee JH, et al: The neuronal sortilin-related receptor SORL1 is genetically associated with Alzheimer disease. Nat Genet 39:168–177, 2007

Roher AE, Kokjohn TA, Beach TG: An association with great implications: vascular pathology and Alzheimer disease. Alzheimer Dis Assoc Disord 20:73–75, 2006

Rosenberg PB: Clinical aspects of inflammation in Alzheimer's disease. Int Rev Psychiatry 17:503–514, 2005

Rosenberg PB, Johnston D, Lyketsos CG: A clinical approach to mild cognitive impairment. Am J Psychiatry 163:1884–1890, 2006

Sabbagh MN, Shah F, Reid RT, et al: Pathologic and nicotinic receptor binding differences between mild cognitive impairment, Alzheimer disease, and normal aging. Arch Neurol 63:1771–1776, 2006

Sano M, Ernesto C, Thomas RG, et al: A controlled trial of selegiline, alpha-tocopherol, or both as treatment for Alzheimer's disease: the Alzheimer's Disease Cooperative Study. N Engl J Med 336:1216–1222, 1997

Savolainen S, Hurskainen H, Paljarvi L, et al: Five-year outcome of normal pressure hydrocephalus with or without a shunt: predictive value of the clinical signs, neuropsychological evaluation and infusion test. Acta Neurochir (Wien) 144:515–523, 2002

Schneider JA, Wilson RS, Bienias JL, et al: Cerebral infarctions and the likelihood of dementia from Alzheimer disease pathology. Neurology 62:1148–1155, 2004

Schneider JA, Arvanitakis Z, Bang W, et al: Mixed brain pathologies account for most dementia cases in community-dwelling older persons. Neurology 69:2197–2204, 2007

Schneider LS, Dagerman KS, Insel P: Risk of death with atypical antipsychotic drug treatment for dementia: meta-analysis of randomized placebo-controlled trials. JAMA 294:1934–1943, 2005

Schneider LS, Tariot PN, Dagerman KS, et al: Effectiveness of atypical antipsychotic drugs in patients with Alzheimer's disease. N Engl J Med 355:1525–1538, 2006
Selwood A, Johnston K, Katona C, et al: Systematic review of the effect of psychological interventions on family caregivers of people with dementia. J Affect Disord 101:75–89, 2007
Shinagawa S, Ikeda M, Fukuhara R, et al: Initial symptoms in frontotemporal dementia and semantic dementia compared with Alzheimer's disease. Dement Geriatr Cogn Disord 21:74–80, 2006
Sink KM, Holden KF, Yaffe K: Pharmacological treatment of neuropsychiatric symptoms of dementia: a review of the evidence. JAMA 293:596–608, 2005
Snowdon DA, Greiner LH, Mortimer JA, et al: Brain infarction and the clinical expression of Alzheimer disease: the Nun Study. JAMA 277:813–817, 1997
Steinberg M, Shao H, Zandi P, et al: Point and 5-year period prevalence of neuropsychiatric symptoms in dementia: the Cache County study. Int J Geriatr Psychiatry 23:170–177, 2008
Tariot P, Cummings J, Ismael S, et al: New paradigms in the treatment of Alzheimer's disease. J Clin Psychiatry 67:2002–2013, 2006
Teng EL, Chui HC: The Modified Mini-Mental State (3MS) examination. J Clin Psychiatry 48:314–318, 1987
Tisell M, Hellstrom P, Ahl-Borjesson G, et al: Long-term outcome in 109 adult patients operated on for hydrocephalus. Br J Neurosurg 20:214–221, 2006
van der Burg M, Bouwen A, Stessens J, et al: Scoring Clock Tests for dementia screening: a comparison of two scoring methods. Int J Geriatr Psychiatry 19:685–689, 2004
Vanneste J, Augustijn P, Dirven C, et al: Shunting normal-pressure hydrocephalus: do the benefits outweigh the risks? A multicenter study and literature review. Neurology 42:54–59, 1992
Watson GS, Cholerton BA, Reger MA, et al: Preserved cognition in patients with early Alzheimer disease and amnestic mild cognitive impairment during treatment with rosiglitazone: a preliminary study. Am J Geriatr Psychiatry 13:950–958, 2005
Weintraub D, Katz IR: Pharmacologic interventions for psychosis and agitation in neurodegenerative diseases: evidence about efficacy and safety. Psychiatr Clin North Am 28:941–983, ix–x, 2005
White L, Launer L: Relevance of cardiovascular risk factors and ischemic cerebrovascular disease to the pathogenesis of Alzheimer disease: a review of accrued findings from the Honolulu-Asia Aging Study. Alzheimer Dis Assoc Disord 20 (suppl 2):S79–S83, 2006
Wilson RK, Williams MA: Normal pressure hydrocephalus. Clin Geriatr Med 22:935–951, viii, 2006
Wolfson C, Wolfson DB, Asgharian M, et al: A reevaluation of the duration of survival after the onset of dementia. N Engl J Med 344:1111–1116, 2001

Suggested Readings

Blennow K, de Leon MJ, Zetterberg H: Alzheimer's disease. Lancet 368:387–403, 2006
Ferri CP, Prince M, Brayne C, et al: Global prevalence of dementia: a Delphi consensus study. Lancet 366:2112–2117, 2005
Livingston G, Johnston K, Katona C, et al, for the Old Age Task Force of the World Federation of Biological Psychiatry: Systematic review of psychological approaches to the management of neuropsychiatric symptoms of dementia. Am J Psychiatry 162:1996–2021, 2005
Lyketsos CG: Lessons from neuropsychiatry. J Neuropsychiatry Clin Neurosci 18:445–449, 2006
Metzler-Baddeley C: A review of cognitive impairments in dementia with Lewy bodies relative to Alzheimer's disease and Parkinson's disease with dementia. Cortex 43:583–600, 2007
Neary D, Snowden J, Mann D: Frontotemporal dementia. Lancet Neurol 4:771–780, 2005
Rosenberg PB, Johnston D, Lyketsos CG: A clinical approach to mild cognitive impairment. Am J Psychiatry 163:1884–1890, 2006
Sink KM, Holden KF, Yaffe K: Pharmacological treatment of neuropsychiatric symptoms of dementia: a review of the evidence. JAMA 293:596–608, 2005
Steinberg M, Shao H, Zandi P, et al: Point and 5-year period prevalence of neuropsychiatric symptoms in dementia: the Cache County study. Int J Geriatr Psychiatry 23:170–177, 2008
White L, Launer L: Relevance of cardiovascular risk factors and ischemic cerebrovascular disease to the pathogenesis of Alzheimer disease: a review of accrued findings from the Honolulu-Asia Aging Study. Alzheimer Dis Assoc Disord 20 (suppl 2):S79–S83, 2006

CHAPTER 14

Movement Disorders

Burton Scott, Ph.D., M.D.

As people age, a variety of movement disorders can either appear for the first time or progress after onset earlier in life. Arthritis, bursitis, tendonitis, and other non–central nervous system conditions can in some ways mimic neurological conditions by causing stooped posture and overall slowing of movement. In this chapter, I discuss central nervous system–based movement disorders that occur in elderly individuals and result in impaired or abnormal movement.

Movement disorders in the elderly population can be divided into *hypokinetic* conditions (in which the ability to move decreases because of a neurological condition) and *hyperkinetic* conditions (in which there is excessive abnormal movement). Hypokinetic movement disorders encompass a variety of parkinsonian disorders, in which there is some combination of the following signs and symptoms: tremor at rest, rigidity, slowness of movement (bradykinesia), and balance difficulty (postural instability). Parkinsonian disorders include Parkinson's disease (PD), several "Parkinson's plus" syndromes, and normal pressure hydrocephalus (NPH). Hyperkinetic movement disorders include tremors, tics, dystonia, myoclonus, chorea, stereotypies, and other dyskinesias, including tardive dyskinesia and tardive dystonia. Tremor disorders are represented in both groups of movement disorders: tremor at rest is a cardinal feature of parkinsonism, which is a hypokinetic condition, and postural and kinetic tremor are common features of essential tremor, which is a hyperkinetic movement disorder.

Hypokinetic Movement Disorders

Parkinsonism

The term *parkinsonism* refers to a condition characterized by a combination of at least two of the following clinical signs: resting tremor, rigidity, bradykinesia, and postural instability; no specific etiology is implied by the term (Table 14–1). The term *Parkinson's disease* refers to levodopa-responsive, idiopathic parkinsonism associated with the presence of Lewy bodies and neuronal degeneration in the substantia nigra pars compacta. *Secondary parkinsonism* refers to parkinsonism caused by other lesions of the basal ganglia, such as tumors, strokes (vascular parkinsonism), encephalitis, hypoxic or ischemic insult, and toxins (e.g., manganese, carbon monoxide, carbon disulfide). NPH can cause a parkinsonian-like gait disorder, urinary incontinence, and dementia (Table 14–2).

Parkinsonism is well known to be associated with use of dopamine receptor–blocking agents, including antipsychotic medications and antiemetics. Classic antipsychotic medications typically exhibit strong antagonism at dopamine D_2 receptors (Mendis et al. 1994), whereas the newer atypical antipsychotics have less affinity for dopamine D_2 receptors. The newer agents have fewer parkinsonian side effects but are not totally free of them (Chouinard et al. 1993). Based on clinical experience with PD patients who have levodopa-related psychosis, my colleagues and I have determined that of these newer agents, risperidone has the greatest

TABLE 14–1. Clinical features of parkinsonism

- Rigidity to passive movement of the limbs, neck
- Bradykinesia (slowing of voluntary limb movement)
- Resting tremor (in contrast to tremor with action or with movement)
- Postural instability (balance difficulty, falling)
- Hypomimia (decreased facial expression, masked facies)
- Hypophonia (soft speech)
- Stooped posture (flexion at neck, hips, knees)
- Shuffling gait

TABLE 14–2. Differential diagnosis of parkinsonism

- Parkinson's disease (idiopathic parkinsonism)
  - Tremor-dominant Parkinson's disease
  - Akinetic-rigid Parkinson's disease
- Vascular (stroke)
- Tumor involving the basal ganglia
- Medication related (dopamine receptor–blocking agents including metoclopramide, phenothiozines)
- Communicating hydrocephalus (normal pressure hydrocephalus; NPH)
- Toxins (carbon monoxide, carbon disulfide, manganese)
- "Parkinson's plus" syndromes
  - Progressive supranuclear palsy (PSP)
  - Multiple system atrophy–parkinsonism (MSA-P)
  - Multiple system atrophy–cerebellar (MSA-C)
  - Multiple system atrophy–autonomic (MSA-A)
  - Cortical-basal ganglionic degeneration (CBGD)

number of parkinsonian side effects, followed by olanzapine and then quetiapine. Clozapine exhibits a lower relative affinity for dopamine D_2 receptors compared with conventional antipsychotics (Meltzer 1992) and suppresses levodopa-related psychosis in PD while minimizing exacerbation of PD symptoms; however, clozapine can suppress bone marrow such that blood counts must be monitored. Antiemetic agents such as metoclopramide, promethazine, and prochlorperazine can also produce parkinsonism as an acute side effect, and patients who take these medications for prolonged periods can develop tardive movement disorders. Older antidepressants that contain a phenothiazine derivative also have side effects of parkinsonism and tardive dyskinesia or tardive dystonia.

Parkinson's Disease

PD is a chronic, progressive neurodegenerative illness that produces rigidity, slowness of movement (bradykinesia), postural instability, and, often, tremor at rest. It affects up to 1 million individuals in North America and is newly diagnosed in up to 50,000 people each year. The prevalence of PD increases with age, with estimates of 1% at age 60 and up to 2.6% at age 85 or older (Mutch et al. 1986; Sutcliffe et al. 1985). PD results from progressive loss of dopamine-containing neurons in the substantia nigra pars compacta of the midbrain and is characterized pathologically by abnormal collections of proteins, called Lewy bodies, in the cytoplasm of degenerating neurons (Forno 1996; Golbe 1999). The diagnosis is made clinically (Suchowersky et al. 2006b). Although no laboratory test is diagnostic, scans using positron emission tomography and single-photon emission computed tomography may demonstrate loss of postsynaptic dopamine uptake in PD.

Other common clinical features of PD include hypomimia (masked facies or facial masking), micrographia (small handwriting), stooped posture, retropulsion, and shuffling and festinating gait. Symptoms typically begin gradually on one side of the body, and patients may ignore the initial symptoms when the nondominant arm is the one affected first, particularly in the absence of tremor. The typical resting tremor in PD has a frequency of 4–6 Hz. When resting tremor occurs in the hand, it may have the classic pill-rolling appearance—a combination of flexion-extension tremor of the fingers and thumb, giving the appearance of rolling a marble or pill between the thumb and fingertips. The resting tremor of PD typically attenuates at least transiently during voluntary movement of the affected extremity, such as when the patient picks up an object. Resting tremor is to be distinguished from the postural antigravity tremor observed in essential tremor. Usually, treatment with levodopa, a precursor of the neurotransmitter dopamine, results in significant clinical benefit in PD.

PD can be divided into two clinical forms: 1) tremor-dominant PD, in which there is prominent tremor at rest, and 2) postural instability and gait disorder, or akinetic-rigid PD, in which resting tremor is minimal, if present at all, and patients exhibit earlier balance difficulty. Both tremor-dominant PD and akinetic-rigid PD respond to levodopa treatment, at least initially; however, tremor-dominant PD tends to progress more slowly and thus has a more favorable prognosis than akinetic-rigid PD.

The stiffness or rigidity of PD is detected clinically by testing for involuntary resistance to passive movement of the extremities. This resistance can manifest as lead-pipe rigidity—that is, a steady resistance to passive movement. In patients with resting tremor, the combination of rigidity and tremor results in cogwheel rigidity—that is, a jerky resistance to passive movement. In addition, active, voluntary movement of the contralateral extremity (synkinetic movement) can bring out subtle rigidity in an ipsilateral limb. For example, rapid, repetitive opening and closing of the contralateral hand in early PD may result in slightly increased tone in the ipsilateral arm; similarly, repetitive flexion-extension at the contralateral elbow can bring out abnormally increased tone in the ipsilateral leg in PD.

Slowed movement, or bradykinesia, is tested in the clinic by observing the ease with which the patient performs repetitive movements such as tapping the index finger and thumb together, opening and closing the hand, twisting the hand clockwise and counterclockwise (like turning a doorknob), and tapping the heel on the ground. In a patient with PD, the clinician looks for decreasing size (i.e., decrementing amplitude) of a repeated movement. Micrographia can be a manifestation of bradykinesia. Early in PD, handwriting might be of normal size at the beginning of a sentence and then become progressively smaller by the end of the sentence.

Postural instability usually occurs later than other clinical signs of PD and can be very disabling. Patients fall because of an inability to keep their feet under their center of gravity, and these patients exhibit retropulsion (inability to maintain balance when suddenly displaced backward) and anteropulsion (inability to maintain balance when suddenly displaced forward). Freezing of gait occurs when the feet appear to become stuck to the floor during attempted walking. Sometimes, a patient can overcome this freezing by performing a motor trick such as kicking his or her walking cane to initiate gait. Festination occurs in an upright, walking PD patient whose feet are lagging behind his or her center of gravity. This clinical sign manifests as rapid, tiny steps taken to keep from falling. Other motor complications that occur in PD as the disease progresses are medication-related dyskinesias (involuntary writhing, twisting, and/or head bobbing movements associated with levodopa replacement therapy), motor fluctuations, and on-off phenomena in which the patient experiences "on" time when medications are working and the patient can move better but experiences "off" times when medication effects wear off (Pahwa et al. 2006) (Table 14–3).

Nonmotor complications of PD are common and, in some patients, can become even more disabling than the motor symptoms (Miyasaki et al. 2006) (Table 14–4). Depression, dementia, urinary incontinence, constipation, hallucinations, impulse dyscontrol behaviors, sweating, and excessive drowsiness can result from progression of the disease itself, as well as from side effects of medications used to treat the motor symptoms of PD. Successful recognition and treatment of these conditions can result in significant improvement of quality of life for patients.

The onset of PD symptoms is usually recognized earlier in individuals with tremor-dominant PD, because even mild tremor is likely to bring a patient into

TABLE 14–3. Motor complications of Parkinson's disease

- Dyskinesias
- Dystonia
- Motor fluctuations
- On-off phenomena
- Freezing of gait
- Festination

TABLE 14–4. Nonmotor features of Parkinson's disease

- Hallucinations (mostly visual, very rarely auditory)
- Dementia (bradyphrenia or slowness of thinking)
- Depression
- Urinary incontinence
- Constipation
- Sexual dysfunction
- Impulse dyscontrol (pathological gambling; punding or useless repetitive behaviors)
- Excessive, unintended sleep episodes during activities of daily living

clinic earlier. In PD patients who have resting tremor, walking may be associated with increased tremor amplitude. In addition, patients with PD often exhibit decreased arm swing when walking, even early in the disease course. A reduction or absence of arm swing noticed by others may be the first indication of PD in a patient who does not have much resting tremor. Other patients may present with gradual loss of fine coordination of an extremity. The posture in a PD patient is often stooped, with flexion at the neck, upper back, shoulders, hips, and knees. The gait is typically narrow based and shuffling. Symptom onset is usually noticed earlier in patients affected first on the dominant side (i.e., the right hand in a right hand–dominant individual). By several years after the onset of symptoms, it is expected that both sides of the body will be affected, although the side affected first usually remains the side most affected, even in late-stage PD.

Medications used to treat PD can be divided into drugs for treating symptoms (levodopa, dopamine agonists, etc.; see Table 14–5), putative neuroprotective agents, and possible restorative agents (growth factors, neuroimmunophilins). There are no medications that clearly slow progression of PD and provide neuroprotection (Suchowersky et al. 2006a); however, several medications are being investigated to determine if they may have neuroprotective, disease-altering effects.

PD results from a deficiency of the neurotransmitter dopamine in the brain, and administration of levodopa, a precursor of dopamine, is the most effective treatment for PD symptoms. Although levodopa is the mainstay of therapeutic treatment in PD, oral or intravenous dopamine itself is not an effective medication in PD because of its poor ability to cross the blood-brain barrier. However, levodopa effectively crosses the blood-brain barrier and is taken up by any remaining dopaminergic neurons throughout the PD patient's brain, including the desired target—the substantia nigra. Levodopa is converted to dopamine within these neurons and is stored in synaptic vesicles for subsequent use in neurotransmission. In the United States, the usual formulation of levodopa (Sinemet) consists of a combination of levodopa and carbidopa, a peripheral decarboxylase inhibitor that reduces destruction of levodopa before it has a chance to cross the blood-brain barrier and reach the brain.

Selegiline is a relatively selective monoamine oxidase B inhibitor that delays the need for therapeutic treatment with levodopa in early PD by several months. However, selegiline's modest effect on parkinsonian symptoms appears to be due to the drug's metabolism to an amphetamine-like metabolite that blocks synaptic dopamine reuptake, rather than to a true neuroprotective effect. Entacapone and tolcapone are catechol O-methyltransferase (COMT) inhibitors that reduce the breakdown of levodopa before it reaches the brain. Some COMT inhibitors may also slow the breakdown of dopamine in the brain. Because of rare, fulminant hepatotoxicity, tolcapone is not used much clinically. Anticholinergic medications (trihexyphenidyl, benztropine) are also sometimes used to treat early PD symptoms. Amantadine, an antiviral medication with anticholinergic and antiglutamate effects, produces mild improvement of parkinsonism early in the disease course, in part because of enhanced release of endogenous dopamine stores from the substantia nigra.

Dopamine agonists are useful adjuncts in the symptomatic treatment of PD. These agents act directly on dopamine receptors and are particularly useful in smoothing the therapeutic response to levodopa by reducing motor fluctuations ("on-off" phenomena) and by increasing the period of benefit obtained from each dose of levodopa. The side effects of dopamine agonists are similar to those of levodopa; hallucinations, dyskinesias (involuntary head bobbing and involuntary writhing and twisting movements of the extremities), and dystonia (muscle spasms) are most common. The dopamine agonists that have been available in the United States are bromocriptine, pergolide, pramipexole, and ropinirole; however, bromocriptine and pergolide are ergot-derived dopamine agonists and are no longer commonly used in PD treatment due to concern for cardiac valve fibrosis. For a time, a newer dopamine agonist, rotigotine, was available in patch form (discontinued in April 2008).

Surgical treatments for PD include 1) ablative surgery, in which destructive lesions are precisely placed in basal ganglia targets; 2) deep brain stimulator implantation, in which deep brain stimulation (DBS) is applied to similar basal ganglia targets; and 3) potentially restorative procedures, such as transplantation of dopaminergic tissue (fetal tissue transplantation) (Lang and Lozano 1998a, 1998b). Ablative surgeries consist of thalamotomy, in which lesioning is performed at the ventral intermediate nucleus (VIM) of the contralateral thalamus; pallidotomy, in which the target is the internal segment of the globus pallidus (GPi); and, less commonly, subthalamotomy, in which the target is the subthalamic nucleus (STN). In deep brain stimulation, the

TABLE 14–5. Medical treatment of Parkinson's disease

Drug class and generic name	Trade name	Daily dose
Endogenous dopamine releaser		
Amantadine	Symmetrel	100–300 mg
Anticholinergics		
Trihexyphenidyl	Artane	2–10 mg
Benztropine	Cogentin	0.5–8 mg
MAO-B inhibition		
Selegiline	Eldepryl	5–10 mg
Rasagiline	Azilect	0.5–1 mg
Dopamine agonists		
Bromocriptine	Parlodel	2.5–40 mg
Pergolide	Permax	0.25–4.5 mg
Pramipexole	Mirapex	0.25–4.5 mg
Ropinirole	Requip	1–24 mg
Apomorphine	Apokyn	1–6 mg
Rotigotine patch	Neupro	2–2.4 mg
Dopamine precursor		
Carbidopa/levodopa	Sinemet	100–1,500 mg as levodopa
	Sinemet CR	100–1,500 mg as levodopa
	Parcopa	100–1,500 mg as levodopa
COMT inhibitor		
Entacapone	Comtan	200–1,200 mg
Tolcapone	Tasmar	100–300 mg[a]
Peripheral decarboxylase inhibitor		
Carbidopa	Lodosyn	25–150 mg
Combination		
Carbidopa/levodopa/entacapone	Stalevo	100–1,500 mg as levodopa

[a]Monitor liver function tests.

neurosurgeon places a thin stimulating electrode at the target. The electrode is connected to an implantable pulse generator that can be adjusted to provide electrical pulses of appropriate energy and frequency to alter output from the targeted nuclei, thereby reducing contralateral PD symptoms. Although no proven restorative surgeries are yet available, researchers are exploring several potential interventions, including intracerebral transplantation of dopaminergic tissue and injection of adenovirus-linked genes coding for brain-derived neurotrophic factor.

The differential diagnosis of PD involves considering a host of disorders that can mimic aspects of PD, including essential tremor, drug-induced parkinsonism (see "Parkinsonism" earlier in this chapter), and other secondary parkinsonian syndromes (tumors and other mass lesions of the basal ganglia, vascular parkinsonism). Additional conditions that can have parkinsonian features are NPH; primary gait ignition failure, which may represent early parkinsonism; and other atypical parkinsonian syndromes, such as progressive supranuclear palsy, multiple system atrophy, and cortical-basal ganglionic degeneration or corticobasal degeneration (see "'Parkinson's Plus' Syndromes" discussed below).

Normal Pressure Hydrocephalus

Normal pressure hydrocephalus, also known as communicating hydrocephalus, is more common in elderly persons than in younger adults and can result in a progressive gait disorder, urinary incontinence, and memory decline. It can be caused by a slowed flow of cerebrospinal fluid (CSF) across the arachnoid villi and out of the brain via the superior sagittal sinus. NPH can develop after meningitis or a subarachnoid bleed but more commonly develops in the absence of these relatively rare conditions. Individuals with NPH may take small steps and exhibit a "magnetic gait," in which they experience difficulty lifting their feet to walk because of a sense that their feet are stuck to the ground. The triad of gait disorder, urinary incontinence, and memory loss suggests a diagnosis of NPH. Brain imaging demonstrates enlarged intraventricular spaces that are out of proportion to the size of the sulci, the CSF-filled spaces between cortical gyri. A diagnosis of NPH is supported by observation of clinical improvement after a large-volume lumbar puncture or by observation of reversed CSF flow, identified by introducing a tracer into the CSF and performing a cisternography to visualize the flow of tracer in the brain. Reduction of CSF during a single diagnostic lumbar puncture may not result in immediate clinical benefit; however, placement of a lumbar drain for up to several days in the hospital may help determine whether a patient might benefit from surgical placement of a shunt to treat NPH.

"Parkinson's Plus" Syndromes

Progressive Supranuclear Palsy

Progressive supranuclear palsy (PSP), also called Steele-Richardson-Olszewski syndrome, is a progressive, neurodegenerative condition consisting of parkinsonism without prominent tremor, vertical gaze palsy, axial (midline) more than appendicular (arm and leg) rigidity, early postural instability, and poor response to levodopa (Golbe and Davis 1993; Litvan 1998; Litvan et al. 1996). The syndrome was first described by Steele et al. (1964). The Society for Progressive Supranuclear Palsy estimates that 20,000 people in the United States have PSP—only 3,000–4,000 of whom have received a diagnosis—yielding an estimated known prevalence in the United States of 1.39 per 100,000. PSP is often associated with frequent falling, lack of eye contact, monotonous speech, sloppy eating, and slowed mentation (Jankovic et al. 1990). Patients may have a surprised or worried facial expression, with raised eyebrows resulting from bradykinesia and increased tone in facial musculature, and may have difficulty opening their eyes because of eyelid apraxia (Jankovic 1984). There is early suppression of vertical optokinetic nystagmus and voluntary vertical saccadic eye movements. Later in the illness, horizontal saccades and horizontal optokinetic nystagmus are also suppressed. Impairment of voluntary downgaze is more specific to PSP, whereas impairment of voluntary upgaze is nonspecific in older adults. As is expected with a supranuclear gaze palsy, passive head movement overcomes the compromised voluntary eye movements in PSP.

PSP has an insidious onset. Often, the first symptom is a decrease in balance, which results in falls. The usual age at symptom onset is 55–70 years, with a mean age in the early 60s (in contrast to the late 50s for the onset of PD). In PSP, the posture is upright and rigid, not stooped as in PD, and the gait is typically stiff, with the legs extended at the knees, not flexed as in PD. In addition, patients with PSP tend to pivot when turning rather than exhibit en bloc shuffling as in PD.

Cognitive decline can begin in the first year of PSP symptoms and may manifest as apathy, impaired abstract thinking, decreased verbal fluency, utilization or imitative behavior, and frontal release signs. Visual symptoms, including diplopia, blurry vision, burning eyes, and light sensitivity, appear in about 60% of cases during the first year, dysarthria in about 40% of cases, and bradykinesia in 20%.

Supranuclear gaze palsy has also been observed in other neurodegenerative disorders, including diffuse Lewy body disease (dementia with Lewy bodies) (de Bruin et al. 1992), cortical-basal ganglionic degeneration (Gibb et al. 1990), and other parkinsonian syndromes. Atypical parkinsonian syndromes other than PSP may be suggested by a recent history of encephalitis, alien hand syndrome (in which one hand seems to have a mind of its own and behaves as if it no longer belongs to the patient), cortical sensory deficits, focal frontal or temporoparietal atrophy, early cerebellar signs, early dysautonomia, severely asymmetric parkinsonism, or a relevant structural injury visualized by an imaging study.

Early in the course of PSP, visual pursuits may become saccadic (jerky), and voluntary saccades may become slow despite preserved range of extraocular movements. Saccades become smaller (hypometric), and there is decreased convergence of the eyes when they follow a target brought in toward the patient's nose. The ability to voluntarily suppress the vestibulo-ocular reflex during passive head movement decreases or disappears. Later, there is progression of eye-associated abnormalities, including slowing of eyelid opening and closing and slowing of eyelid movement during attempted vertical gaze saccades. In addition, patients often lose the ability to suppress blinks in response to a bright light.

Another common eye-related sign seen in PSP is an excessive frequency and amplitude of square-wave jerks (small involuntary saccadic or jerky eye movements that intrude on midline ocular fixation). In addition, patients may have difficulty performing the antisaccade task, which involves looking rapidly in the direction opposite that of a novel visual stimulus. A typical pattern in a patient with early PSP is to 1) make an increased number of errors while performing the antisaccade task, 2) exhibit hypometric saccades with normal latencies, and 3) exhibit impaired visual pursuits. Also, during vestibular and optokinetic nystagmus testing, initiation of the quick phase of nystagmus may be compromised, leading to tonic eye deviation to one side.

Another finding that supports a diagnosis of PSP is the presence of symmetric limb akinesia or rigidity, usually more in the proximal than distal portions of limbs. In contrast, akinesia or rigidity in PD is typically asymmetric at first, occurring initially on one side of the body, with the other side expected to become affected within a few years. Abnormal neck posture, especially retrocollis, is commonly seen in PSP, as are early dysphagia and dysarthria.

Unlike in PD, in PSP there is little or no response to levodopa therapy because of degeneration of secondary neurons downstream from the dopaminergic substantia nigra pars compacta. Response to other medical treatment is usually poor as well; however, some patients with PSP have at least a transient response to treatment with amantadine, levodopa, or dopamine agonists. There is no known effective neurosurgical intervention for PSP.

After symptom onset, the course of PSP is typically 5–10 years. Death may result from infections such as aspiration pneumonia or from complications of falls.

Neuropathology is the gold standard for diagnosis of PSP, a syndrome that can be confused clinically with PD, cortical-basal ganglionic degeneration, multiple system atrophy, Alzheimer's disease, or dementia with Lewy bodies. Pathological changes in PSP include development of neurofibrillary tangles and neuropil threads (filamentous structures in neuronal cytoplasm). PSP pathology is primarily found in the pallidum, subthalamic nucleus, substantia nigra, and pons. Abnormalities in tau protein, an important component of intracellular microtubules, have been implicated in some cases of PSP, and tau-positive astrocytes or astrocytic processes have been found in affected areas of the brain.

Multiple System Atrophy

Multiple system atrophy (MSA) encompasses several "Parkinson's plus" conditions that are characterized by bilateral, symmetric parkinsonism that is poorly responsive to levodopa therapy, as well as the absence or near absence of tremor (Quinn 1994; Shulman and Weiner 1997; Wenning et al. 1994). MSA can be divided into three main clinical types: MSA-parkinsonism (MSA-P), in which parkinsonism is the main clinical feature; MSA-cerebellar (MSA-C), in which cerebellar ataxia is the main clinical feature; and MSA-autonomic (MSA-A), in which autonomic dysfunction such as severe orthostatic hypotension is a major clinical feature. MSA-P represents a majority of cases.

MSA-P cases were formerly diagnosed as striatonigral degeneration, a diagnostic term that is now less frequently used. Clinical features that may help distinguish MSA-P from other parkinsonian disorders include falls occurring early in the illness, severe dysarthria and dysphonia, sleep apnea and excessive snoring, anterocollis, respiratory stridor, and pyramidal signs (brisk reflexes and extensor plantar responses). Development of parkinsonism and gait disturbance is expected as well. Treatment of orthostatic symptoms includes liberalizing dietary salt, elevation of the head of the bed, and the use of fludrocortisone, midodrine, and sometimes indomethacin and yohimbine. Although the clinical response to treatment is usually poor, trials of levodopa (up to 1,500 mg/day in divided doses) with or without a dopamine agonist (pramipexole, ropinirole) are sometimes temporarily beneficial. The clinical course is approximately 10 years. Brain magnetic resonance imaging (MRI) may demonstrate decreased (dark) T2 signal laterally in the putamen portion of the basal ganglia (Kraft et al. 1999).

MSA-C, or sporadic olivopontocerebellar atrophy, often presents with gait ataxia. Other features that may develop are limb ataxia, breakdown of visual smooth pursuit, and cerebellar dysarthria (ataxic dysarthria). Autonomic dysfunction, parkinsonism, and pyramidal signs can also occur, but the cerebellar findings are usually most prominent. Brain MRI can demonstrate cerebellar and brain stem atrophy, particularly in the pons and medulla.

MSA-A, formerly known as Shy-Drager syndrome, presents with early autonomic impairment, including orthostatic hypotension or syncope, impotence in males, and bowel and bladder dysfunction (Shy and Drager 1960).

The neuropathological changes in MSA include neuronal loss and iron deposition in the substantia nigra and putamen (striatum). In addition, glial cytoplasmic inclusions, particularly in oligodendrocytes, are characteristic of all forms of MSA, and cell loss and gliosis can be found in the striatum, substantia nigra, locus coeruleus, pontine nuclei, middle cerebellar peduncles, Purkinje cells of the cerebellum, inferior olives, and intermediolateral columns of the spinal cord. Lewy bodies and neurofibrillary tangles are not common in MSA.

Cortical-Basal Ganglionic Degeneration

Cortical-basal ganglionic degeneration (CBGD), also referred to as corticobasal degeneration, causes marked asymmetric parkinsonism and dystonia (Litvan et al. 1997; Riley and Lang 2000; Schneider et al. 1997). Resting tremor is uncommon in this condition. CBGD can result in jerky (myoclonic), apraxic, rigid, akinetic movements and alien hand syndrome. There may be early dementia, cortical sensory findings (such as hemineglect to double simultaneous tactile stimulation), and unilateral agraphesthesia (manifested as the inability to identify a number written on the palm of one's hand). Stimulus-sensitive myoclonus and action tremor may also occur. Response to levodopa therapy is poor, but administration of up to 1,500 mg/day in divided doses can provide transient benefit. The disease course is typically 5–10 years from the time of symptom onset.

Neuropathological changes include swollen (ballooned) neurons in substantia nigra and basal ganglia, as well as tau-positive inclusion bodies. Brain MRI often demonstrates asymmetric atrophy in posterior frontal and parietal cortex contralateral to the more affected side of the body (Savoiardo et al. 2000).

Frontotemporal Dementia and Parkinsonism Linked to Chromosome 17

In the degenerative condition of frontotemporal dementia and parkinsonism linked to chromosome 17 (FTDP-17), insidious onset of behavioral and motor changes occurs. Cognitive impairment typically leads to dementia, parkinsonism, nonfluent aphasia, a change in personality, and/or psychosis (Foster et al. 1997; Lund and Manchester Groups 1994). Onset is generally in the fifth decade of life and can be as late as the sixth decade. Duration is usually longer than 10 years but can be as short as 3 years. Behavioral changes range from aggressiveness to apathy and may include hyperorality, hyperphagia, obsessive stereotyped behavior, psychosis, delusions, and muteness. Common motor findings include parkinsonism—particularly rigidity, bradykinesia, and postural instability, but not resting tremor. Hyperreflexia, clonus, and extensor plantar responses may be present. Levodopa treatment results in no significant response. Autonomic function is spared early in the course until dementia becomes severe. Neuropsychological testing demonstrates disturbed executive functioning, with relative preservation of visual-spatial functioning, orientation, and memory until late in the disease course. Electroencephalographic findings are often normal until late in the disease, and functional imaging suggests frontal and anterior temporal hypoperfusion and hypometabolism.

Hyperkinetic Movement Disorders

Essential Tremor

Tremor consists of rhythmic oscillations across a joint resulting from involuntary, alternating activation of agonist and antagonist muscles. For example, wrist tremor is caused by alternating activation and relaxation of forearm flexor and extensor muscles. Essential tremor (ET) is the most prevalent movement disorder among adults, affecting up to 2% of the general population. The prevalence of ET increases with age; estimates range up to more than 10% in individuals older than age 70 years. Also called benign essential tremor and familial tremor, ET may not be benign and can result in severe impairment in activities of daily living in some individuals. ET manifests as postural and kinetic tremor at the arms and hands; the head and voice are often involved (Benito-Leon and Louis 2007; Jankovic 2000).

Postural tremor is tremor that appears when a posture is held against gravity. This tremor is distinguished from the tremor at rest that is characteristic of tremor-dominant PD. Kinetic tremor is tremor that occurs with action or when approximating a target, such as during finger-to-nose testing. Kinetic tremor can be prominent and interfere with eating and drinking; the tremor may interfere with bringing food to the mouth, holding a soup spoon, or carrying a tray. Patients may need to use two hands to hold a cup or to write.

The frequency of the hand tremor in ET is typically 6–8 Hz; however, it can decrease with age. Progression may be more rapid in patients whose age at onset is greater than 60 years and in patients who do not have head tremor. The tremor in ET is commonly symmetric in the upper extremities; however, one arm may be more involved than the other, and even unilateral tremor may occur. Patients may exhibit a "yes-yes," "no-no," or mixed head titubation and may have a tremulous voice as well. A key feature of ET, at least early on, is that the tremor is absent at rest, occurring only during action or when holding a posture. Later in the course, some resting tremor may appear, but it is always less prominent than the postural or kinetic tremor. There is usually a clear family history of tremor, and often the tremor attenuates with alcohol use, a phenomenon that can contribute to alcoholism in susceptible individuals.

The mainstays of medical treatment for ET are propranolol therapy and primidone therapy. Deep brain stimulation targeting the ventral intermediate nucleus of the contralateral thalamus can be therapeutic in medically refractory cases. Other tremor-related disorders seen in the elderly population include enhanced physiological tremor (characterized by postural or kinetic tremor that is more prominent than normal physiological tremor but not as prominent as essential tremor) and orthostatic tremor (a high-frequency, low-amplitude tremor that develops in the legs while the patient is standing still and that responds to clonazepam therapy) (Myers and Scott 2003).

Dystonia

Dystonia is a movement disorder that usually begins by middle age and may persist in elderly individuals (Scott 2000; Tarsy and Simon 2006). In dystonia, involuntary muscle spasms result in bizarre, sustained postures. These postures initially occur during attempted voluntary movement and may persist at rest. Dystonia can be idiopathic (associated with no identifiable structural abnormality) or secondary (associated with a known structural lesion demonstrated by an imaging study) and can have delayed onset, appearing after a previous injury (Scott and Jankovic 1996). Dystonia may be focal (affecting one body part), segmental (affecting two or more adjacent body parts), multifocal (affecting two or more nonadjacent body parts), generalized (affecting most of the body, including at least one leg), or hemidystonic (affecting one side of the body). Common examples of focal dystonia include writer's cramp (involuntary, sometimes painful cramping during writing), blepharospasm (eyelid spasms resulting in exaggerated, forceful blinking), spasmodic torticollis or cervical dystonia (a disorder in which there is sustained, involuntary twisting or turning of the neck), and oromandibular dystonia (muscle contractions producing involuntary grinding of the teeth or opening of the jaw while eating or talking). An example of segmental dystonia is craniofacial dystonia, in which both blepharospasm and jaw-closing spasms may occur. Hemidystonia most commonly results from a stroke or structural lesion, such as a mass in the contralateral basal ganglia, often involving the putamen.

In adults, dystonia tends to stay localized in the part of the body first affected and is less likely to affect other body parts. Medical treatments include anticholinergic agents such as trihexyphenidyl; however, this class of medication is poorly tolerated by elderly adults. Other medications used are muscle relaxants such as baclofen and benzodiazepines such as clonazepam. The most effective treatment is often botulinum toxin injections. In individuals exposed to dopamine receptor–blocking medications such as neuroleptics and antiemetics, dystonia can also be a tardive condition, similar to tardive dyskinesia (see the following section, "Tardive Movement Disorders").

Tardive Movement Disorders

The term *tardive movement disorder* refers to hyperkinetic movements that develop in individuals subjected to prolonged exposure to dopamine receptor–blocking medications such as phenothiazine-containing antiemetics and antipsychotic medications (DeLeon and Jankovic 2004). Elderly women taking these medications appear to be most susceptible to tardive movement disorders. *Tardive dyskinesia* typically manifests as semivoluntary, repetitive oro-bucco-lingual movements. The movements often attenuate temporarily with concentration and disappear during sleep. The movements can also involve the head, face, and limbs. They can be choreiform in appearance, although they are often more stereotypic and repetitive than the more random movements characteristic of classic chorea. Tardive dyskinesia can affect muscles involved in breathing, resulting in respiratory dyskinesia. The term *tardive dystonia* refers to dystonic movements that are associated with chronic use of dopamine receptor–blocking agents that can be difficult to treat. The sustained abnormal posturing of tardive dystonia can affect the neck in the form of retrocollis (backward displacement of the neck) and limb dystonia. *Akathisia* refers to inner restlessness in an individual treated with dopamine receptor–blocking agents. It manifests as constant squirming and fidgeting, such as when the person is sitting.

Treatment for tardive movement disorders involves, whenever possible, first tapering the dose of the offending medication and then discontinuing the drug. Tetrabenazine, a dopamine-depleting agent available outside the United States, is often helpful in suppressing tardive movement disorders, particularly tardive dyskinesia. A newer, atypical antipsychotic medication such as quetiapine can be tried if tetrabenazine is not an option. Botulinum toxin injections are helpful in some patients with bothersome focal dyskinesias.

Chorea

Chorea refers to involuntary, dancelike movements that consist of continuous, random, unpredictable, often twitchlike motions that flow from one body part to another. Chorea can be hard to distinguish from tardive dyskinesia in the absence of a complete history; however, movements in chorea are more random, and movements in tardive dyskinesia tend to be repetitive and stereotyped. Chorea can occur in elderly individuals in association with Huntington's disease (Walker 2007), neuroacanthocytosis, overdose of drugs such as amphetamines or stimulants, alcohol intoxication, and metabolic abnormalities such as hyperthyroidism, hypo- or hypernatremia, hypo- or hyperglycemia, hypocalcemia, and hypomagnesemia. The term *hemiballismus* is applied to choreiform throwing or flinging movements that affect one side of the body. This condition is often associated with a lesion in the contralateral subthalamic nucleus, most commonly due to a stroke. Therapy consists of treating any underlying toxic or metabolic condition and using a dopamine-depleting agent such as tetrabenazine or an atypical antipsychotic such as quetiapine.

Tics

Tics are brief, repetitive, semivoluntary, jerklike movements. Vocal tics consist of audible vocalizations, and motor tics consist of rapid movements of the head, face, limbs, and other body parts. Tics can be simple or complex. They can usually be suppressed for a short time. During voluntary suppression of tics, patients may feel unpleasant sensations building up in an involved body part and experience transient relief from the unpleasant sensation by performing the tic once again. Tourette's syndrome, a tic disorder that begins in childhood but can persist in adults (Sheppard et al. 1999), is often associated with obsessive-compulsive disorder, a condition that can become more disabling than the tics themselves. Other causes of tic disorders in elderly individuals include use of stimulants or other drugs, encephalitis, carbon monoxide poisoning, head trauma, and stroke. Treatments include administration of antipsychotic medications; however, the clinician must be aware of the associated risk of producing a tardive movement disorder, especially in elderly patients. Treatment with tetrabenazine or clonazepam is also helpful in some patients.

Myoclonus

The term *myoclonus* refers to sudden jerklike or shocklike movements caused by involuntary activation of affected muscles (positive myoclonus) or to sudden loss of activation of affected muscles (negative myoclonus) (Vercueil 2006). The movements can occur randomly or with regular frequency. Myoclonus can arise from dysfunction at multiple levels of the central nervous system, from cortex to brain stem to spinal cord. For example, spinal inflammation from a dermatomal herpes infection (shingles) can result in persistent focal myoclonus in the same dermatome. Negative myoclonus can manifest as asterixis (flapping movements of the hands when the arms are held outstretched with the wrists extended), as is seen in hepatic failure. Also, disabling negative myoclonus affecting the legs and trunk upon standing can be a consequence of hypoxic or ischemic brain stem injury in elderly patients. Benzodiazepines such as clonazepam, anticonvulsants such as levetiracetam, and piracetam are sometimes beneficial in the treatment of this condition.

Hemifacial Spasm

Hemifacial spasm is another movement disorder that occurs in the elderly population. The disorder consists of simultaneous, involuntary, rapid, jerklike movements of facial muscles on one side of the face. The movements are not painful. Typically, the patient experiences blinking of one eye and synchronous drawing up of the same side of the face. No sensory deficit on the affected side of the face should be present, because this disorder affects only the facial nerve (cranial nerve VII), which provides motor but not sensory innervation to the face.

Hemifacial spasm can be caused by irritation of the facial nerve. The disorder is sometimes associated with an ectatic, tortuous basilar artery at the level of the pons in the brain stem. Physical contact between the basilar artery and the point where the facial nerve emerges from the pons is thought to produce aberrant, ephaptic nerve transmission in the facial nerve, resulting in transient activation of facial muscles on one side of the face. An ectatic basilar artery can be identified by brain MRI and magnetic resonance angiography. Anticonvulsants such as carbamazepine and phenytoin are sometimes helpful, and botulinum toxin injections are often effective (Papapetropoulos and Singer 2007). If medical treatment is insufficient, a neurosurgical procedure to insulate the facial nerve from the basilar artery can be considered.

Psychogenic Movement Disorders

Psychogenic movement disorders are diagnoses of exclusion and most commonly take the form of waxing and waning tremor, dystonia, or myoclonus that attenuates with distraction (Hallett et al. 2006). The onset of these conditions is often abrupt, and it is often possible to identify periods of normal function between periods of dysfunction. Psychogenic tremor (Koller et al. 1989) is characterized by tremor that speeds up or slows down in synchrony with repetitive movements of the opposite limb. The movements often respond to positive or negative suggestion, and successful treatment may require intensive psychiatric or psychological intervention.

Restless Legs Syndrome

Restless legs syndrome, which can occur in elderly persons, is characterized by unpleasant sensations in the legs when the individual is sitting or lying down, particularly during periods of fatigue (Patrick 2007). The individual experiences creeping, crawling sensations under the skin of the calves, and these sensations attenuate only when the patient stands up and walks. No visible abnormal movement is necessarily present, but the unpleasant leg sensations interfere with sleep and can be disabling for that reason. The condition sometimes results from renal failure or from iron deficiency anemia, in which case symptoms improve with successful treatment of the underlying medical condition. A sleep study (polysomnography) may identify periodic leg movements in sleep, which are commonly associated with restless legs syndrome. Use near bedtime of a dopamine agonist, clonazepam, levodopa, or sometimes a narcotic such as codeine may be beneficial. Prolonged use of levodopa and sometimes dopamine agonists, however, has been associated with intrusion of uncomfortable sensations into the daytime in some patients, a phenomenon known as augmentation.

Conclusion

Movement disorders in the elderly population are to be distinguished from changes associated with normal aging, in which mobility may become somewhat more limited because of a lifetime of wear and tear on muscles, ligaments, bones, and joints. Normal aging includes some slowing of movement, aches and pains, and perhaps stooping. However, clinical experience enables one to distinguish these phenomena of aging from neurodegenerative movement disorders. Excessive poverty of movement is indicative of a hypokinetic movement disorder such as PD or another parkinsonian condition. Development of a hyperkinetic movement disorder such as tremor, tics, chorea, or myoclonus cannot be attributed to normal aging and is worthy of further evaluation for the purpose of identifying an underlying, treatable condition.

Key Points

- Movement disorders are common and often treatable in elderly persons.
- Movement disorders are defined as *hypokinetic* (too little movement) and *hyperkinetic* (too much movement).
- Hypokinetic movement disorders include the various forms of parkinsonism (rigidity, bradykinesia, with or without resting tremor); hyperkinetic movement disorders include the majority of remaining movement disorders, including essential tremor, tics, myoclonus, dystonia, tardive movement disorders, and chorea.
- Parkinson's disease is a common, progressive neurodegenerative illness that causes disability from both motor and nonmotor dysfunction.

- Hypokinetic movement disorders may respond to dopamine replacement; hyperkinetic movement disorders may respond to dopamine reduction (reduction of brain dopamine levels or blockade of dopamine receptors).
- Essential tremor is the most common movement disorder. It is distinguished clinically from tremor-dominant Parkinson's disease by the fact that in essential tremor, tremor occurs when the person is holding a posture and moving, whereas in tremor-dominant Parkinson's disease, the tremor occurs when the person is at rest.
- Dystonia can affect a variety of body parts and can result from structural lesions (strokes, tumors) as well as from primary disease processes. Botulinum toxin injections are often partially therapeutic.
- Tardive movement disorders (tardive dyskinesia, tardive dystonia) are recognizable and sometimes avoidable. To limit development of tardive movement disorders, avoid prolonged use of metoclopramide and other dopamine receptor–blocking agents in elderly patients as much as possible.
- Psychogenic movement disorders are fairly common and present as atypical, nonphysiological patterns of abnormal movements, such as distractible tremor of variable frequency, and the presence of periods of normalcy in the case of psychogenic tremor.
- Restless legs syndrome is a treatable condition that adversely affects quality of life due to poor sleep. Patients with this condition should be screened for iron deficiency and, if present, should be worked up for the etiology of the iron deficiency.

References

Benito-Leon J, Louis ED: Clinical update: diagnosis and treatment of essential tremor. Lancet 369:1152–1154, 2007

Chouinard G, Jones B, Remington G, et al: Canadian multicenter placebo-controlled study of fixed doses of risperidone and haloperidol in the treatment of chronic schizophrenic patients. J Clin Psychopharmacol 13:25–40, 1993

de Bruin VMS, Lees AJ, Daniel SE: Diffuse Lewy body disease presenting with supranuclear gaze palsy, parkinsonism, and dementia: a case report. Mov Disord 7:355–358, 1992

DeLeon ML, Jankovic J: Clinical features and management of tardive dyskinesias, tardive myoclonus, tardive tremor, and tardive tourettism, in Drug Induced Movement Disorders. Edited by Sethi K. New York, Marcel Dekker, 2004, pp 77–109

Forno LS: Neuropathology of Parkinson's disease. J Neuropathol Exp Neurol 55:259–272, 1996

Foster NL, Wilhelmsen K, Sima AAF, et al: Frontotemporal dementia and parkinsonism linked to chromosome 17: a consensus conference. Participants of the Chromosome 17–Related Dementia Conference. Ann Neurol 41:706–715, 1997

Gibb WRG, Luthert PJ, Marsden CD: Clinical and pathological features of corticobasal degeneration. Adv Neurol 53:51–54, 1990

Golbe LI: Alpha-synuclein and Parkinson's disease. Mov Disord 14:6–9, 1999

Golbe LI, Davis PH: Progressive supranuclear palsy, in Parkinson's Disease and Movement Disorders, 2nd Edition. Edited by Jankovic J, Tolosa E. Baltimore, MD, Williams & Wilkins, 1993, pp 145–161

Hallett M, Fahn S, Jankovic J, et al (eds): Psychogenic Movement Disorders: Neurology and Neuropsychiatry. Philadelphia. Lippincott Williams & Wilkins, 2006

Jankovic J: Progressive supranuclear palsy: clinical and pharmacologic update. Neurol Clin 2:473–486, 1984

Jankovic J: Essential tremor: clinical characteristics. Neurology 54:S21–S25, 2000

Jankovic J, Friedman DI, Pirozzolo FJ, et al: Progressive supranuclear palsy: motor, neurobehavioral, and neuro-ophthalmic findings. Adv Neurol 53:293–304, 1990

Koller WC, Lang A, Vetere-Overfield B, et al: Psychogenic tremors. Neurology 39:1094–1099, 1989

Kraft E, Schwarz J, Trenkwalder C, et al: The combination of hypointense and hyperintense signal changes on T2-weighted magnetic resonance sequences: a specific marker for multiple system atrophy? Arch Neurol 56:225–228, 1999

Lang AE, Lozano AM: Parkinson's disease: first of two parts. N Engl J Med 339:1044–1053, 1998a

Lang AE, Lozano AM: Parkinson's disease: second of two parts. N Engl J Med 339:1130–1143, 1998b

Litvan I: Progressive supranuclear palsy revisited. Acta Neurol Scand 98:73–84, 1998

Litvan I, Agid Y, Calne D, et al: Clinical research criteria for the diagnosis of progressive supranuclear palsy (Steele-Richardson-Olszewski syndrome): report of the NINDS-SPSP international workshop. Neurology 47:1–9, 1996

Litvan I, Agid Y, Goetz C, et al: Accuracy of the clinical diagnosis of corticobasal degeneration: a clinicopathologic study. Neurology 48:119–125, 1997

Lund and Manchester Groups: Clinical and neuropathological criteria for frontotemporal dementia. J Neurol Neurosurg Psychiatry 57:416–418, 1994

Meltzer HY: The mechanism of action of clozapine in relation to its clinical advantages, in Novel Antipsychotic Drugs. Edited by Meltzer HY. New York, Raven, 1992, pp 1–13

Mendis T, Mohr E, George A, et al: Symptomatic relief from treatment-induced psychosis in Parkinson's disease: an open-label pilot study with remoxipride. Mov Disord 9:197–200, 1994

Miyasaki JM, Shannon K, Voon V, et al: Practice parameter: evaluation and treatment of depression, psychosis, and dementia in Parkinson disease (an evidence-based review). Neurology 66:996–1002, 2006

Mutch WJ, Dingwall-Fordyce I, Downie AW, et al: Parkinson's disease in a Scottish city. Br Med J (Clin Res Ed) 292:534–536, 1986

Myers BH, Scott BL: A case of combined orthostatic tremor and primary gait ignition failure. Clin Neurol Neurosurg 105:277–280, 2003

Pahwa R, Factor SA, Lyons KE, et al: Practice parameter: Treatment of Parkinson disease with motor fluctuations and dyskinesia (an evidence-based review). Neurology 66:983–995, 2006

Papapetropoulos S, Singer C: Botulinum toxin in movement disorders. Semin Neurol 27:183–194, 2007

Patrick LR: Restless legs syndrome: pathophysiology and the role of iron and folate. Altern Med Rev 12:101–112, 2007

Quinn NP: Multiple system atrophy, in Movement Disorders 3 (Butterworth-Heinemann International Medical Reviews. Neurology 12). Edited by Marsden CD, Fahn S. Boston, MA, Butterworth-Heinemann, 1994, pp 262–281

Riley DE, Lang AE: Clinical diagnostic criteria, in Corticobasal Degeneration (Advances in Neurology, Vol 82). Edited by Litvan I, Goetz CG, Lang AE. Philadelphia, PA, Lippincott Williams & Wilkins, 2000, pp 29–34

Savoiardo M, Grisoli M, Girotti F: Magnetic resonance imaging in CBD, related atypical parkinsonian disorders, and dementias, in Corticobasal Degeneration (Advances in Neurology, Vol 82). Edited by Litvan I, Goetz CG, Lang AE. Philadelphia, PA, Lippincott Williams & Wilkins, 2000, pp 197–208

Schneider JA, Watts RL, Gearing M, et al: Corticobasal degeneration: neuropathologic and clinical heterogeneity. Neurology 48:959–969, 1997

Scott BL: Evaluation and treatment of dystonia. South Med J 93:746–751, 2000

Scott BL, Jankovic J: Delayed-onset progressive movement disorders after static brain lesions. Neurology 46:68–74, 1996

Sheppard DM, Bradshaw JL, Purcell R, et al: Tourette's and comorbid syndromes: obsessive compulsive and attention deficit hyperactivity disorder: a common etiology? Clin Psychol Rev 19:531–552, 1999

Shulman LM, Weiner WJ: Multiple-system atrophy, in Movement Disorders: Neurologic Principles and Practice. Edited by Watts RL, Koller WC. New York, McGraw-Hill, 1997, pp 297–306

Shy GM, Drager GA: A neurological syndrome associated with orthostatic hypotension. Arch Neurol 2:511–527, 1960

Steele JC, Richardson JC, Olszewski J: Progressive supranuclear palsy: a heterogeneous degeneration involving the brain stem, basal ganglia and cerebellum, with vertical gaze and pseudobulbar palsy, nuchal dystonia and dementia. Arch Neurol 10:333–359, 1964

Suchowersky O, Gronseth G, Perlmutter J, et al: Practice parameter: neuroprotective strategies and alternative therapies for Parkinson disease (an evidence-based review). Neurology 66:976–982, 2006a

Suchowersky O, Reich S, Perlmutter J, et al: Practice parameter: diagnosis and prognosis of new onset Parkinson disease (an evidence-based review). Neurology 66:968–975, 2006b

Sutcliffe RL, Prior R, Mawby B, et al: Parkinson's disease in the district of the Northampton Health Authority, United Kingdom: a study of prevalence and disability. Acta Neurol Scand 72:363–379, 1985

Tarsy D, Simon DK: Dystonia. N Engl J Med 355:818–829, 2006

Vercueil L: Myoclonus and movement disorders. Neurophysiol Clin 36:327–331, 2006

Walker FO: Huntington's disease. Semin Neurol 27:143–150, 2007

Wenning GK, Ben Shlomo Y, Magalhaes M, et al: Clinical features and natural history of multiple system atrophy: an analysis of 100 cases. Brain 117:835–845, 1994

Suggested Readings

DeLeon ML, Jankovic J: Clinical features and management of tardive dyskinesias, tardive myoclonus, tardive tremor, and tardive tourettism, in Drug Induced Movement Disorders. Edited by Sethi K. New York, Marcel Dekker, 2004, pp 77–109

Hallett M, Fahn S, Jankovic J, et al (eds): Psychogenic Movement Disorders: Neurology and Neuropsychiatry. Philadelphia, Lippincott Williams & Wilkins, 2006

Pahwa R, Factor SA, Lyons KE, et al: Practice parameter: treatment of Parkinson disease with motor fluctuations and dyskinesia (an evidence-based review). Neurology 66:983–995, 2006

Stacy MA (ed): Handbook of Dystonia. New York, Informa Healthcare, 2007

Suchowersky O, Reich S, Perlmutter J, et al: Practice parameter: diagnosis and prognosis of new onset Parkinson disease (an evidence-based review). Neurology 66:968–975, 2006

CHAPTER 15

Mood Disorders

Dan G. Blazer, M.D., Ph.D.
David C. Steffens, M.D., M.H.Sc.
Harold G. Koenig, M.D., M.H.Sc.

Questions regarding depression in old age are frequently posed: Do persons become more depressed as they grow older? Does depression become more difficult to treat with increased age? Is depression more difficult to identify in the older adult? The answers to these questions rest in part with the definition of late-life depression. Depression in late life is not a unitary construct. Depending on how depression is defined, the answers to questions regarding late-life depression vary.

Depression can be construed in at least three ways, each of which has clinical relevance for older adults. First, depression can be viewed as a unitary phenomenon, with the various manifestations of depression forming a continuum. Depression symptom checklists, such as the Center for Epidemiologic Studies Depression Scale (CES-D; Radloff 1977) and the Geriatric Depression Scale (GDS; Yesavage et al. 1983), are useful in determining the degree to which an individual suffers from depression in late life.

Most modern investigators, however, find it difficult to conceive of depression as phenomenologically homogeneous. A categorical approach, as exemplified in DSM-IV-TR (American Psychiatric Association 2000), has been of more interest to modern clinicians. If one views the mood disorders as a group of distinct entities or independent syndromes, with each of the categories being mutually exclusive, diagnosis and management of depression are allied with the traditional medical model. Given the availability of excellent, but potentially dangerous, biological therapies for depressed older adults, the categorical approach has been adopted by most geriatric psychiatrists. Specific therapies can be prescribed for distinct diagnostic entities.

The third approach to the conceptualization of the depressed elder is a functional approach: when depressive symptoms become so severe that functioning is impaired, the case is considered worthy of clinical attention. Social functioning, especially the performance of role responsibilities, has been targeted as a critical variable in monitoring treatment. Examples of the functional approach can be found in many surveys of community subjects, such as the Older Adults Resources and Services assessment (Fillenbaum 1988; Shulman 1986). Functional capacity is a critical element for family members, who do not view symptom remission alone as an essential marker of improvement but, rather, consider a return to social involvement and improved life satisfaction as critical signs. An older adult who sleeps better, has a better appetite, and ceases to be suicidal may be determined to be improved by the clinician but little improved by the family, if the patient's social isolation and disinterest in the social environment persist after appropriate therapy. The clinician can use Axis V of DSM-IV-TR to partially assess the effect of a disorder on social functioning. Clinical entities listed under the mood disorders in DSM-IV-TR relevant to depression in elderly patients include 1) bipolar disorder, 2) major depressive disorder (with or without psychotic features), 3) dysthymic disorder, and 4) minor or subsyndromal depression (found in Appendix B of DSM-IV-TR). Depressive symptoms are likewise present in other DSM-IV-TR disorders, such as bereavement, adjustment disorder with depressed mood, and mood disorder due to a general medical condition (see Table 15–1.)

Manic episodes in later life also may present with a mixture of manic, dysphoric, and cognitive symptoms, with euphoria being less common (Post 1978). When mania is associated with significant changes in cognitive function—so-called manic delirium—it may be difficult to distinguish from organic conditions or schizophrenia (Shulman 1986).

TABLE 15–1. Subtypes of depression in later life

- Bipolar disorder
- Major depression, single episode or recurrent
- Psychotic depression
- Dysthymic disorder
- Minor or subsyndromal depression
- Bereavement
- Adjustment disorder with depressed mood
- Depression associated with medical illness

Epidemiology

An overview of the epidemiology of psychiatric disorders in late life is presented in Chapter 2, "Demography and Epidemiology of Psychiatric Disorders in Late Life"; this chapter includes information relevant to mood disorders. Using a community survey, investigators at Duke University Medical Center attempted to untangle the different subtypes of depression in late life (Blazer et al. 1987b). More than 1,300 older adults in urban and rural communities who were age 60 or older were screened for depressive symptomatology. Of the 27% reporting depressive symptoms, 19% had mild dysphoria only. Persons with symptomatic depression—that is, subjects with more severe depressive symptoms—made up 4% of the population. These individuals were primarily experiencing stressors, such as physical illness and stressful life events. Only 2% had a dysthymic disorder, and 0.8% were experiencing a current major depressive episode. No cases of current manic episode were identified. Finally, 1.2% had a mixed depression and anxiety syndrome. These data suggest that the traditional DSM-IV-TR depression categories do not apply to most depressed older adults in the community. Recent surveys have confirmed the lower frequency of major depression in the community (Kessler et al. 2005).

In hospital and long-term care settings, the frequency of major depression among older adults is much higher than in community settings. Up to 21% of hospitalized elders meet criteria for a major depressive episode, and an additional 20%–25% have a minor depression (Koenig et al. 1988). Rates of major depression among elderly nursing home patients are even higher, exceeding 25% in some studies (Parmelee et al. 1989).

How does one reconcile these seemingly disparate results? *Depression in late life* remains a generic term that captures many constructs, some of which are well defined and others of which are ill defined. The burden of depression in the elderly, as indicated by the just-described frequency of significant depressive symptoms in community populations, is unquestioned. Many older persons with atypical presentations of depression do not meet criteria for major depression yet have clinically significant depressive symptoms (Hybels et al. 2001).

The Epidemiologic Catchment Area surveys identified bipolar disorder in 9.7% of nursing home patients, which suggests that nursing homes may have become a dumping ground for such patients (Weissman et al. 1991). In clinical settings, about 10%–25% of geriatric patients with mood disorder have bipolar disorder, and 3%–10% of all older psychiatric patients have this disorder (Wylie et al. 1999; Young and Klerman 1992). About 5% of all individuals admitted as geropsychiatry inpatients present with mania (Yassa et al. 1988).

Clinical Course

Episodes of depression across the life cycle, especially episodes of more severe major depression, almost always remit or at least partially remit. Nevertheless, depression is a chronic and recurrent illness. Data from a community study from the Netherlands illustrate this chronicity. Among subjects with clinically significant depressive symptoms, 23% improved, 44% experienced an unfavorable but fluctuating course, and 33% experienced a severe and chronic course. In a second group of subjects with less severe depression, 25% experienced a chronic course. Overall, 35% of those subjects diagnosed with major depression and 52% of the subjects diagnosed with dysthymic disorder experienced a chronic course (Beekman et al. 2002).

Studies that have focused on older adults in clinical settings have found similar chronicity (Alexopoulos et al. 1996; Baldwin and Jolley 1986; Murphy 1983; Post 1962). In an early study, Post (1962) followed a clinical sample for 6 years and found that 31% recovered and remained well over the follow-up, 28% experienced at least one relapse but later recovered, and 23% only partially recovered, whereas 17% remained depressed throughout the period of follow-up. Murphy (1983) followed a group of elderly depressed subjects (many of whom were medically ill) over 1 year. Of those subjects, 35% experienced a good outcome, 48% experienced a fluctuating course or remained continuously ill, and 14% died. In an Australian study of a group of elderly patients who were followed for 25 years after experiencing severe depression earlier in life, only 12% fully remitted and experienced no recurrences over the period of follow-up (Brodaty et al. 2001). The prognosis from clinical studies of depressed older adults with late-life depression, however, is similar to that found among younger adults if the older adult is not plagued with comorbid medical illness, functional impairment, or cognitive impairment (Keller et al. 1982a, 1982b). Comorbid depression is associated with a less favorable prognosis. For example, when major depression is comorbid with dysthymic disorder, the prognosis is poor. Factors predicting partial remission were similar to those predicting no remission, and poor social support and functional limitations increased the risk for poor outcome in these subjects (Hybels et al. 2005).

Cognitive impairment is often associated with depressive symptoms. When the depression improves, the cognitive impairment often improves as well. Nevertheless, comorbid depression and cognitive impairment are a risk for the later emergence of Alzheimer's disease (Alexopoulos et al. 1993). Therefore, early depressive symptoms associated with mild cognitive impairment may represent a preclinical sign and should be considered a risk for impending Alzheimer's disease or vascular dementia (Li et al. 2001). Depression can further complicate Alzheimer's disease over time by increasing disability and physical aggression, thereby contributing to depression among caregivers (Gonzalez-Salvador et al. 1999). Depressive symptoms in patients with Alzheimer's disease resolve spontaneously at a greater frequency without requiring intensive therapy (such as medication therapy) than among older adults experiencing depression and vascular dementia, where depressive symptoms tend to be persistent and refractory to drug treatment (Li et al. 2001).

Depression and medical problems are frequently comorbid, and the causal pathway may be bidirectional (Blazer and Hybels 2005). Depression, for example, is a frequent and important contributing cause of weight loss in late life (Morley and Kraenzle 1994). Frailty, leading to profound weight loss, can in turn contribute to clinically important depressive symptoms (Fried 1994). Many chronic medical illnesses are associated with depression, including cardiovascular disease, diabetes, osteoporosis, and hip fracture, to name a few (Blazer et al. 2002b; Lenze et al. 2007; Lyles 2001; Williams et al. 2002). The mechanisms that explain the close association between depression and physical illness in older adults are for the most part not well documented. Clues, however, have emerged. For example, platelet activation is increased in older depressed patients, especially those with a specific polymorphism in the serotonin transporter–linked promoter region. This polymorphism leads to higher levels of platelet aggregation and β-thromboglobulin, both pathophysiological changes that increase the risk for myocardial infarction (Whyte et al. 2001).

Perhaps the best-established association between depression and physical problems is the association between depression and functional impairment (Blazer et al. 1991; Bruce 2001). For example, in one study, older adults who were depressed were 67% more likely to experience impairment in activities of daily living and 73% more likely to experience mobility restrictions 6 years following initial evaluation than those not depressed (Penninx et al. 1999b). Disability, in turn, can increase the risk for depressive symptoms (Kennedy et al. 1990; Roberts et al. 1997). Explanations for this bidirectional association include the following: the propensity for physical disability to lead to a higher frequency of negative life events, which in turn increases the risk for depression; the loss of independence and concomitant need to depend on others; restricted social and leisure activities secondary to physical disability; and the isolation and reduced quality of social support often inherent with physical disability (Blazer 1983). Functional decline, however, is not inevitable when the older adult becomes depressed. For example, the instrumental support provided to older adults, such as help in tasks necessary for daily living, can be protective against the worsening of performance on instrumental abilities, which in turn buffers against the onset of depression (Hays et al. 2001).

Despite the frequency and clinical importance of late-life depression, long-term psychiatric follow-up investigations involving survivors of severe episodes of this disorder have been relatively scarce. The typical course of major depression throughout the life cycle is remission and relapse. In patients who have a history of recurrent episodes, new episodes tend to be associated with similar symptoms and to last about as long as prior episodes. Classic studies of depression suggest that the duration of major depression throughout the life cycle is approximately 9 months if untreated (Dunner 1985). As individuals age, however, they may experience episodes more frequently, and these episodes can merge into a chronic condition.

Most clinicians and clinical investigators report that more than 70% of elderly patients with major depression who are treated with antidepressant medication (at an adequate dose for a sufficient time) recover from the index episode of depression if the depression is uncomplicated by comorbid factors. Reynolds et al. (1992) reported that treatment of physically healthy depressed elders with combined interpersonal psychotherapy and nortriptyline was associated with response rates nearing 80%. In a long-term outcome study of treatment-resistant depression in older adults, 47% of patients were clinically improved 15 months after treatment with an antidepressant or electroconvulsive therapy (ECT); at 4-year follow-up, the percentage had increased to 71% (Stoudemire et al. 1993). These optimistic results are tempered by the fact that physical illness and impaired cognition may complicate both the course of depression and the response to treatment (Baldwin and Jolley 1986; Koenig et al. 1989a; Murphy et al. 1988). Once an older patient has experienced one or more moderate to severe episodes of major depression, he or she may need to continue antidepressant therapy permanently to minimize the risk of relapse (Reynolds et al. 2006).

Persons with a dysthymic disorder (depressive neurosis) experience a more chronic clinical course than do persons with major depression. By DSM-IV-TR definition, an individual's depressive symptoms must last at least 2 years for a dysthymic disorder diagnosis to be made. An undetermined percentage (as high as 4%–8%) of community-dwelling (and possibly institutionalized) elders experience moderately severe depressive symptoms for more than 2 years, although they report intermittent periods, lasting longer than a few days, of relative freedom from depressive symptoms. The severity of their symptoms is not great enough to meet the criteria for major depression, and the intermittent symptom-free periods disqualify them from the diagnosis of dysthymic disorder. Nevertheless, these individuals experience chronic depression. Other older adults experience chronic depression secondary to medical or even psychiatric disease (e.g., alcoholism and anxiety disorders such as obsessive-compulsive disorder). Each of these disorders contributes to residual depression in ambulatory elderly individuals.

Factors associated with improved outcome in late-life depression include a history of recovery from previous episodes, a family history of depression, female gender, extroverted personality, current or recent employment, absence of substance abuse, no history of major psychiatric disorder, less severe depressive symptomatology, and absence of major life events and serious medical illness (Baldwin and Jolley 1986; Cole et al. 1999; Post 1972). The results of a number of studies suggest a relationship between social support during an index episode and outcome in psychological distress and depression. Intuition suggests that adequate support should enhance recovery from a severe or moderately severe psychiatric disorder such as major depression. In a study involving 493 community respondents, Holahan and Moos (1981) found that decreases in social support of family and in work environments were related to increases in psychological maladjustment over a 1-year follow-up period.

Coping behavior may also affect the prognosis of late-life depression. One of the coping behaviors most commonly used by this generation of older adults is religious involvement. In a study involving 100 middle-aged or elderly adults, one-third of men and nearly two-thirds of women used religious cognitions or behaviors to help them cope with a stressful period (Koenig et al. 1988). A number of investigators have reported inverse associations between religious coping and depressive symptoms in older adults with or without medical illness (Braam et al. 1997b; Idler 1987; Koenig 2007a; Koenig et al. 1992; Pressman et al. 1990). A study involving 850 hospitalized medically ill older adults found that those using religion to cope were less likely to be depressed and more likely to experience improvement in depressive symptoms over time (Koenig et al. 1992). Religious involvement also appears to be a predictor of faster recovery from depression in both community-dwelling and clinical samples of older adults (Braam et al. 1997a; Koenig 2007b; Koenig et al. 1998).

Personality pathology is another measurable phenomenon that is known to affect the outcome of major depression (Weissman et al. 1978). Unfortunately, there are no published reports of personality as a predictor of major depression outcome in elderly patients. In addition, studies with mixed-age samples have generally been confounded by the interaction of depressive symptomatology and personality variables at baseline assessment—that is, a depressed affect may influence the underlying personality. Given the stability of personality in late life, longitudinal studies of relationships between personality and both onset and outcome of major depression would be most helpful.

The outcome of bipolar disorder in elderly patients remains virtually unknown. In a long-term follow-up study involving 500 patients in Iowa, Winokur (1975) found that bipolar disorder tended to occur in clusters over time and speculated that early-onset bipolar illness may "burn itself out" in time. Shulman and Post (1980) studied elderly patients with bipolar disorder and found that only 8% had their first episode of mania before age 40. In a review of records of a small number of untreated patients with severe and prolonged bipolar disorder, Cutler and Post (1982) found a tendency toward more rapid recurrences late in the illness, with decreasing periods of remission. In other words, if bipolar disorder reemerges in the later years, the episodes of mania—or mania mixed with depression—may once again cluster, just as the disorder typically clusters at earlier periods of life. Most clinicians who have worked with patients with bipolar disorder in late life recognize the tendency of these disorders to recur frequently for a time, only to remit for an extended period.

Ambelas (1987) emphasized a relationship between life events and onset of mania, noting that stressful events were more likely to precede early-onset mania than late-onset mania. Likewise, Shulman (1989) stressed that increased cerebral vulnerability due to organic insults (stroke, head trauma, other brain insults) played a stronger role than life events in precipitating late-onset mania (a factor that may also play a role in treatment resistance). Young and Klerman (1992) emphasized the low rates of familial affective disorder and the increased frequency of certain diseases and drug use associated with late age at onset.

Controversy exists over whether age at onset of first manic episode affects response to treatment. Glasser and Rabins (1984) described no significant age-related differences in presentation or treatment response. Young and Falk (1989) reported that late-onset mania was associated with lower activity level, lower sexual drive, and less-disturbed thought processes; however, they also found that older age was associated with longer hospitalization, greater residual psychopathology, and poorer response to pharmacotherapy. Eastham et al. (1998) suggested that elderly patients with bipolar disorder often require lithium doses that are 25%–50% lower than those used in younger patients. Data on the use of valproic acid in elderly patients with this disorder are limited but encouraging. There is almost no information on the use of carbamazepine or other drugs in late-life bipolar disorder. ECT has been reported to be well tolerated and effective in the treatment of these patients (Eastham et al. 1998).

All-cause mortality is a significant adverse outcome resulting from late-life depression. In one review of multiple reports, 72% of the studies demonstrated a positive association between depression and mortality in elderly people (Schulz et al. 2002). In another review of 23 outcome studies of depression in subjects ages 65 years and older, the pooled odds of dying if subjects were depressed were 1.75 (Geerlings et al. 2002). A longer follow-up predicted smaller effect size. Both severity and duration of depressive symptoms predicted mortality in the elderly population in these studies (Geerlings et al. 2002). For example, investigators from the Epidemiologic Catchment Area study found a fourfold increase in the odds of dying over a follow-up of 15 months if persons over 55 years of age experienced a mood disorder (Bruce and Leaf 1989). Also, community-dwelling persons in the Netherlands who experienced both major and minor depression were at increased risk for cardiac mortality (Penninx et al. 1999a).

The association between depression and mortality holds in many of these studies, despite the addition of potentially confounding variables. In studies from North Carolina and New York, however, investigators failed to find an association (Blazer et al. 2001; Thomas et al. 1992).

One reason for the lack of association in some studies may be the selection of specific control variables, especially chronic disease and functional impairment. For example, in a study of the North Carolina Established Populations for Epidemiologic Study of the Elderly cohort, the unadjusted relative odds of mortality among depressed subjects at baseline was 1.98 (Blazer et al. 2001). These odds moved toward unity when other risk factors, such as chronic disease, were controlled, and when health habits, cognitive impairment, functional impairment, and social support were added to the model. Therefore, the specific control variables used in mortality studies may determine the association between depression and mortality.

The effect of depression on mortality may vary by sex. In elderly Japanese American men but not women, depressive symptoms were a risk for mortality in the physically healthy (Takeshita et al. 2002). In another study, depressive symptoms were a significant risk factor for cardiovascular but not cancer mortality in older women (Whooley and Browner 1998). In a controversial report, investigators found that subthreshold depression, as indicated by CES-D scores of 12–16, was not associated with mortality in men but was negatively related to 3-year mortality in women (odds ratio 0.56) (Hybels et al. 2002). In other words, mild depressive symptoms were protective in this highly controlled analysis of community-based data.

Murphy et al. (1988) examined all-cause mortality in a 4-year follow-up study involving 120 depressed elderly psychiatric inpatients, comparing them with 197 age- and gender-matched control subjects. Among the depressed women, mortality was twice the expected rate; among the men, it was three times the expected rate. Older men with physical health problems and depression were significantly more likely to die than were similarly aged, physically ill, nondepressed men. A study involving elderly veterans hospitalized with medical illness found a significantly higher mortality rate during hospitalization for 41 patients who were depressed, compared with 41 nondepressed patients matched for age, gender, and severity and type of medical illness (Koenig et al. 1989b). Rovner et al. (1991) also found greater death rates among elderly nursing home patients with depression. Several other studies involving medically ill elderly patients likewise found greater mortality rates among those with depression than among those without (Arfken et al. 1999; Black 1999; Covinsky et al. 1999).

These studies indicate higher rates of mortality for depressed elderly patients (men in particular) with concurrent physical health problems; in clinical samples, this relationship persisted after important covariates were controlled. The association between late-life depression and mortality is intuitively attractive, because older persons are thought to experience loss of meaningful roles and emotional support through retirement, death of friends or a spouse, decreased economic and material well-being, and increased isolation and loneliness (Atchley 1989; Fassler and Gaviria 1978). When poor physical health compounds these age-related changes, depression may be particularly prone to affect health outcomes.

Etiology[1]

Biological Origins

Genetics

The etiology of late-life affective disorders is undoubtedly multifactorial (see Table 15–2). Twin and family studies, along with studies focusing on molecular genetics, provide strong evidence for a heritable contribution to the etiology of major depression and bipolar disorder (Gatz et al. 1992). Evidence that these genetic factors weigh heavily in the etiology of bipolar disorders in late life is virtually nonexistent, although the biological nature of this disorder would suggest some genetic contribution. Evidence from studies of unipolar depression in late life suggests that the genetic contribution is weaker in late-life depression than in depression at earlier stages of the life cycle. In a study of elderly twins in Sweden, genetic influences accounted for 16% of the variance in total depression scores on the CES-D and 19% of the somatic symptoms. In contrast, genetic influences minimally contributed to the variance of symptoms of depressed mood and positive affect (Gatz et al. 1992).

Hypothesized genetic markers for late-life depression have usually not stood the test of well-controlled studies, yet some studies present intriguing possibilities. Many candidate genes, such as genes encoding enzymes for serotonin synthesis, the norepinephrine transporter,

[1]The discussion on etiology is abstracted, with permission, from Blazer D, Hybels C: "Origins of Depression in Later Life." *Psychological Medicine* 35:1241–1252, 2005.

TABLE 15–2. Origins of late-life depression

Biological risks

Genetics (e.g., abnormalities in the serotonin transporter gene)

Female sex

Neurotransmitter dysfunction (e.g., underactivity of serotonergic neurotransmission)

Endocrine changes (e.g., long-standing elevated blood levels of cortisol)

Vascular changes (e.g., vascular depression secondary to subcortical vascular changes)

Medical illness (e.g., cardiovascular disease)

Other psychiatric disorders (e.g., long-standing anxiety disorder)

Psychological risks

Personality attributes (e.g., hopelessness and ambivalence)

Neuroticism

Cognitive distortions (e.g., feelings of abandonment when left alone for short periods)

Social origins

Stressful life events (e.g., the death of a close friend or a change of residence)

Chronic stress/strain (e.g., residence in an unsafe neighborhood)

Low socioeconomic status

and even the neurotrophic factor, have been hypothesized and explored in animal studies. As yet, however, these hypotheses await further testing in older adults with depression (Smith et al. 2007). Some pharmacological studies with depressed elders have shown associations between speed of response and antidepressant side effects with the serotonin transporter promoter polymorphism (Pollock 2000).

Despite many studies of the ε4 allele of the apolipoprotein E gene, no association was found in a community sample between the ε4 allele and depressive symptoms (Blazer et al. 2002a). Investigators have also concentrated on genes that may be associated with cerebrovascular lesions that are associated with depression. In one study, subjects with late-onset major depression exhibited a higher frequency of *C677T* mutation of the methylene tetrahydrofolate reductase enzyme compared to control subjects. This mutation may place older persons at risk for major depression associated with cerebrovascular lesions (vascular depression) (Hickie et al. 2001).

Neurotransmitter Dysfunction

Decreased activity of serotonergic neurotransmission has been the focus of much research on the pathophysiology of depression in younger adults. Dysfunctions in the transmission of norepinephrine and dopamine have also been implicated. Serotonin activity, specifically 5-HT_{2A} receptor binding, decreases dramatically in a variety of brain regions through midlife, yet there is less decrease from midlife to late life. 5-HT_{2A} receptors in normal subjects decreased markedly from young adulthood to midlife (70% from the levels at age 20 years through the fifth decade) and then leveled off as age advanced (Sheline et al. 2002). Activity of these receptors, however, may vary with age.

Endocrine Changes

Hypersecretion of corticotropin-releasing factor (CRF) has been associated with depression for many years across the life cycle. CRF is thought to mediate sleep and appetite disturbances, reduced libido, and psychomotor changes (Arborelius et al. 1999) and is diminished with normal aging (Gottfries 1990). Aging is associated with an increased responsiveness of dehydroepiandrosterone sulfate to CRF (Luisi et al. 1998).

Serum testosterone levels decline with aging (Liverman and Blazer 2004) and have been found to be even lower in elderly men with dysthymic disorder than in men without depressive symptoms (Seidman et al. 2002). The efficacy of testosterone treatment for major depression in men, however, has not been established (Liverman and Blazer 2004). In women, improvement of mood has resulted from hormone replacement (Sherwin and Gelfand 1985).

Endocrine dysregulation over time has been associated with anatomical changes related to late-life depressive symptoms, suggesting a vicious cycle downward to chronic and moderately severe depressive symptoms. Depressive symptoms have been hypothesized to cause atrophy of the hippocampus (Sapolsky 1996, 2001; Sheline et al. 1996; Steffens et al. 2002). Stress that accumulates over the life cycle may lead to a sustained increase in secretion of cortisol, leading to loss of preexisting hippocampal neurons (Sapolsky 1996). This loss may be prevented in part by use of antidepressant medications (Czéh et al. 2001).

Vascular Depression

Vascular risk factors have been known to be associated with depressive symptoms for many years (Post 1962). Because major depression is a frequent outcome of stroke (Robinson and Price 1982) and hypertension (Rabkin et al. 1983), investigators have proposed a vascular-based depression among elderly individuals (Coffey et al. 1990; Krishnan et al. 1988; Kumar et al. 2002; Olin et al. 2002; Post 1962). In a study of 139 depressed older adults, 54% met neuroimaging criteria for subcortical ischemic vascular depression. Age was most strongly associated with the increased prevalence of subcortical changes; also associated were lassitude, a history of hypertension, and poorer outcome (Krishnan et al. 2004; Taylor et al. 2003). Vascular depression is associated with white matter hyperintensities (Guttmann et al. 1998; Krishnan et al. 1997). These lesions probably contribute to the disruption of neural circuits associated with depression (Taylor et al. 2003).

Clinical symptoms and signs associated with these vascular impairments resemble impairments found in frontal lobe syndromes. Magnetic resonance imaging (MRI) of depressed patients has revealed structural abnormalities in areas related to limbic-cortical-striatal-pallidal-thalamic-cortical pathways (M.S. George et al. 1994), including the frontal lobes (Krishnan et al. 1993), caudate (Krishnan et al. 1992), and putamen (Husain et al. 1991; Sheline 2003). In MRI studies of mood disorders, structures that make up this tract show volume loss or structural abnormalities (Sheline 2003).

Medical and Psychiatric Comorbidity

Myocardial infarction and other heart conditions often lead to late-life depression (Sullivan et al. 1997), as do diabetes (Blazer et al. 2002b), hip fracture (Magaziner et al. 1990), and stroke (Robinson and Price 1982). In a survey of community-dwelling Mexican Americans, depressive symptoms were found to be associated with diabetes, arthritis, urinary incontinence, bowel incontinence, kidney disease, and ulcers (Black et al. 1998). Poor functional status secondary to physical illness and dementing disorders are the most important causes of depressive symptoms in older adults (Bruce 2001; Hays et al. 1997). For example, in one longitudinal study, depressive symptoms increased the risk for activities of daily living disability and mobility disability by 67% and 73%, respectively, over 6 years (Penninx et al. 1999b). Depressive symptoms are consistently associated with health status in cross-sectional studies of older adults (Kraaij et al. 2002); however, the association is not always clear-cut (Fiske et al. 2003). In one study, for example, health status was associated with depressive symptoms, but new illnesses in the previous 3 years did not consistently predict increases in depressive symptoms (Fiske et al. 2003).

Late-life depression is frequently comorbid with other biologically driven psychiatric disorders (although comorbidity with other disorders, except dementia, is less frequent in late life than earlier in the life cycle), and these other disorders may contribute to the depressive symptoms. Alcohol use and major depression frequently co-occur, as would be expected, in community studies of older adults (Devanand 2002). Anxiety is a common symptom comorbid with depressive symptoms, whether or not the depressive symptoms meet criteria for a depressive disorder (Blazer et al. 1989).

Biological vulnerability to depressive symptoms and disorders appears to be greater in late life than in midlife. Brain changes coupled with the increased frequency of diseases known to be associated with depression are typical of the aging process, especially as the individual advances into the era of the oldest old (Blazer 2000). Some biological protective mechanisms may increase with age, but these remain unknown at present.

Psychological Origins

Psychological factors, such as personality attributes, neuroticism, cognitive distortions, and emotional control, may contribute to the onset of late-life depression yet are not specific to the origins of depression in older adults. Therefore, we briefly address examples of recent studies.

In a study comparing older patients with and without personality disorder, Morse and Lynch (2004) found that those with a personality disorder were four times more likely to continue with or experience a reemergence of depressive symptoms. Specific personality traits were not correlated with clinical features of depression, such as age at onset and number of previous episodes. Nevertheless, some of the traits were associated with depressive symptoms such as hopelessness. Basic personality attributes often underlie the origin and expression of depressive symptoms in older adults.

Neuroticism—a construct rarely studied by psychiatrists in North America though popular in Europe and

Australia—is consistently associated with late-life depressive symptoms in cross-sectional and longitudinal studies of community samples (Henderson et al. 1993, 1997; Lyness et al. 2002) and older adults in residential homes (Eisses et al. 2004). Cognitive distortions (Beck 1987) are among the most studied psychological origins of depression across the life cycle. Depressed individuals may overreact to life events or misinterpret these events and exaggerate their adverse outcome. For example, in a study of the experience and impact of adverse life events, older patients with major depression reported more adverse life events in the recent past and a greater negative impact of these events (particularly for interpersonal conflicts) than did comparison groups of elderly patients with dysthymia and healthy control subjects (Devanand et al. 2002). It is not clear whether the reported impact reflects an increased vulnerability to events or a bias in reporting due to current depressed mood. In another study from a community sample, elderly persons with more frequent depressive symptoms used acceptance, rumination, and catastrophizing (maladaptive cognitive distortions) to a higher extent and positive reappraisal to a lower extent than did those with fewer symptoms (Kraaij and de Wilde 2001).

Beekman and colleagues, in the Longitudinal Aging Study Amsterdam (Beekman et al. 1995), found that major and minor depression, as well as the persistence and emergence of depressive symptoms over 3 years, were predicted by external locus of control (Beekman et al. 2001). Higher levels of mastery, that is, a perception of being able to accomplish tasks and having control over one's life, have been shown to have a direct association with fewer depressive symptoms in older adults and to buffer the adverse impact of disability on depression (Jang et al. 2002). Self-efficacy may have a direct effect and also may work indirectly through its effect on social support to prevent depressive symptoms, as indicated in a sample of older adults followed for 1 year (Holahan and Holahan 1987).

Social Origins

In addition to having biological and psychological origins, late-life depression derives from social origins, including stressful life events, bereavement, chronic stress or strain, low socioeconomic status, and impaired social support. The relative contribution of these factors appears to vary across the life cycle.

Some years ago, Murphy (1982) found a strong association between both severe life events (e.g., bereavement, life-threatening illness of someone else, major personal illness) and social difficulties (e.g., difficulties in health of someone close to subject, housing issues, marital and family relationships) with the onset of late-life depression. Elders lacking a confidant were especially vulnerable to the effects of life stress. Social support may therefore buffer the effect of a stressful event. The association, however, may not be straightforward. Based on a meta-analysis of 25 studies of the relationship between negative life events and depression in late life, Kraaij et al. (2002) reported that the total number of life events and the total number of daily hassles were strongly associated with depressive symptoms, as would be expected. In contrast, sudden unexpected events were not related to depression.

Compared with younger adults, older adults are at greater risk for depressive symptoms secondary to stressful life events. At least three factors, however, modify this risk. First, ongoing problems may have a smaller effect on the risk for depression in older adults than in younger adults (Bruce 2002). For example, in one study, the onset of depressive symptoms was not associated with baseline psychosocial stressors but was associated with factors that changed through time (Kennedy et al. 1990). Second, stressful events that are predictable or "on-time" events often cause less depression in older adults than in younger adults. For example, death of a spouse is a severe and at times catastrophic event leading to depression. For young or middle-aged adults, this event is unexpected and the adjustment is especially difficult. Older adults, in contrast, recognize that death of a spouse is frequent (by observing their peers) and have actually rehearsed the event, such as by considering what they might do if a spouse dies. Third, many events that can lead to depression, such as divorce and difficulties with the law, are more frequent early in life than in late life. In one study, significant difficulty with the law (something more serious than a traffic violation) was reported during the preceding year by 9% of younger adults but less than 1% of older adults (Hughes et al. 1988). Bereavement is a common cause of depressive symptoms in late life (Clayton 1990; de Beurs et al. 2001; Prigerson et al. 1994). In a study of 1,810 community-dwelling older adults, onset of clinically significant depressive symptoms over a 3-year follow-up was predicted by death of a partner or other relatives (Prigerson et al. 1994). Although some studies have found bereavement to predict depressive symptoms, others have not (Prince et al. 1998).

Yet another common cause of depression in later life is chronic strain. For example, the prevalence of depressive symptoms in caregivers of people with dementia is 43%–47% (Livingston et al. 1996; Waite et al. 2004). Therefore, providing support for caregivers is important to prevent the onset and progression of depression in this vulnerable group of elders. In cross-sectional analyses using data from a community study of older Mexican Americans, financial strain was associated with level of depressive symptoms (Black et al. 1998).

Lower socioeconomic status has been associated with depression across the life cycle. Both the frequency of depressive symptoms and their persistence over 2–4 years were associated with socioeconomic disadvantage in a sample of community-dwelling adults age 50 years or older who originally met criteria for major depression (Mojtabai and Olfson 2004). In another study, although the level of education did not predict emergence of depressive symptoms over 1 year, emergence of depression over a 3-year period was predicted by lower level of education (Beekman et al. 2001).

Social support is a multifactorial construct that includes perception, structure of the social network, and tangible help and assistance (Turner and Turner 1999). Perceived social support has proved to be the most robust predictor of late-life depressive symptoms (Bruce 2002). Investigators from Hong Kong, in a community study, found that depressive symptoms were associated with impaired social support (including network size, network composition, social contact frequency, satisfaction with social support, and instrumental-emotional support) (Chi and Chou 2001). Findings from another longitudinal study substantiated that poor social support predicted depressive symptoms at follow-up after 3–6 years (Henderson et al. 1997). The impact of social support on depression may vary by sex. In one study of middle-aged and older patients, impaired social support was associated with poorer outcome of major depression in older men but not older women (L.K. George et al. 1989).

The clinician must not assume that older adults in general experience a deficit in social support. Social support is perceived to be adequate in older adults, even among clinical samples (Blazer 1982). Old social networks thin out, but new ones emerge for many people. Most older people believe that they have enough contact with both family and friends and assess the relationships that they have with their social networks as positive (Cornoni-Huntley et al. 1990). Even so, when the social network is depleted suddenly, either through loss of someone close to the older adult (such as a spouse or child) or through a change in the quality of the relationship (such as a dispute within the family), impaired social support may emerge as a most important contributor to late-life depression.

How does the clinician or investigator resolve the discrepancy between a relatively lower frequency of major depression in the older adult community with increased biological vulnerability, and perhaps only slightly better social resources, compared to younger adults? Psychological factors may modify the biological and social risks for depression. Most older adults, for example, who experience a significant physical illness do not become depressed. Older people may in general possess psychological strengths that actually protect them from the onset of clinically significant depressive symptoms. Two such potential strengths are described below.

Socioemotional selectivity theory may explain differences across the life cycle in the experience of events that lead to depression (Carstensen et al. 2000). The theory focuses on the perception by older persons of time left in life, rather than on past experiences. Younger adults have much to learn and relatively long futures over which to learn. They are motivated by pursuit of knowledge, even when this requires that they suppress emotional well-being. In contrast, elders perceive that they have lived longer than they should live and therefore deemphasize negative experience and prioritize emotionally meaningful goals. In one study, negative emotional experiences (e.g., the perception of stressors) declined from young adulthood until around age 60 (Carstensen et al. 2000). Periods of highly positive emotional experience endured as meaningful among older adults compared with younger adults.

Adults are also thought to acquire increased wisdom as they age. Wisdom is a nebulous concept. Investigators with the Berlin Aging Group, however, have operationalized wisdom and studied it in community samples (Baltes and Staudinger 2000). Wisdom is an expert knowledge system concerning the fundamental pragmatics of life, including knowledge and judgment about the meaning and conduct of life and the orchestrating of human development toward excellence while attending conjointly to personal and collective well-being. Five criteria can be used to assess wisdom: rich factual knowledge; rich procedural knowledge (e.g., the ability to develop strategies for addressing problems); life span contextualization (e.g., integrating life experiences); relativism of values and life priorities (e.g., tolerance for differences in society); and recognition and management of uncertainty (accepting that the future cannot be known with certainty and that the ability to assess one's sociocultural environment is inherently constrained). Wisdom is thought to accumulate over the life cycle if severe physical illness and cognitive impairment do not intervene. Cumulative wisdom over time should protect older adults from spiraling down into depression when confronted with a complex of negative experiences.

Diagnosis and Differential Diagnosis of Late-Life Mood Disorders

Clinical entities listed under the mood disorders in DSM-IV-TR that are relevant to depression in elderly patients are listed in Table 15–1, presented earlier in this chapter. Depressive symptoms are likewise present in other DSM-IV-TR disorders, such as bereavement and mood disorder due to a general medical condition (Blazer 2002, 2003).

Bipolar Disorder

To meet criteria for a manic episode, an older adult must exhibit three or more (four or more if the mood is only irritable) of the following symptoms: 1) inflated self-esteem or grandiosity; 2) decreased need for sleep; 3) more talkativeness than usual; 4) flight of ideas; 5) distractibility; 6) psychomotor agitation; and 7) excessive involvement in pleasurable activities (such as unrestricted buying episodes). Yet bipolar disorder varies somewhat with aging. Post (1978) found that most elderly patients with bipolar disorder exhibited a depressive admixture with manic symptomatology. Spar et al. (1979) reported that manic elders are atypical in presentation, with dysphoric mood and denial of classic manic symptoms. Shulman (1986) described the special problem of manic delirium. When an individual is experiencing a full-blown manic episode, cognitive function is difficult to test, yet perseverative behavior, catatonia-like symptoms, and even negativistic symptoms may emerge. The patient in manic delirium may demonstrate the delirium-like symptom of picking at imaginary objects. Differentiating a manic episode from an agitated depressive episode is often not possible without a thorough examination of the longitudinal course and therapeutic response to medications. In fact, more and more evidence suggests that mixed episodes (with both manic and depressive symptoms) may be the rule rather than the exception (American Psychiatric Association 2000, p. 363).

Major Depressive Disorder

The diagnosis of a major depressive episode is made when the older adult exhibits one or both of two core symptoms (depressed mood and lack of interest), as well as four or more of the following symptoms, for at least 2 weeks: feelings of worthlessness or inappropriate guilt, diminished ability to concentrate or make decisions, fatigue, psychomotor agitation or retardation, insomnia or hypersomnia, significant decrease or increase in appetite, and recurrent thoughts of death or suicidal ideation. First-onset episodes of major depression after age 60 (referred to as *late onset*) are common, making up about one-half of all episodes in older adults. Personality abnormalities and a family history of psychiatric illness are more common if the depression is *early onset* (i.e., the first episode occurs before age 60), but for the most part, the phenomenology is no different between early-onset and late-onset major depression (Brodaty et al. 2001).

In a study involving hospitalized patients with a diagnosis of major depressive episodes with melancholia but without comorbid physical impairment or cognitive impairment, the criterion symptoms of depression and symptoms specifically associated with melancholia (or endogenous depression) did not differ between individuals in midlife and those in late life (Blazer et al. 1987a). Nevertheless, there may be subtle changes with age, because melancholia (symptoms of noninteractiveness and psychomotor retardation or agitation) emerges at a later age than nonmelancholic symptoms. Psychomotor disturbances are the most distinct in older persons (Parker et al. 2001).

Psychotic Depression

Late-onset psychotic depression deserves special attention. Meyers et al. (1984) studied the prevalence of delusions in 50 patients hospitalized for endogenous major depression. Depressed patients with illness onset at age 60 or later had delusions more frequently than did those with earlier onset. Individuals with delusional depression tended to be older and to respond to ECT, as opposed to tricyclic antidepressants (TCAs). Delusions of persecution or of having an incurable illness are more common than delusions associated with guilt. If guilt predominates the delusional picture, it usually involves some relatively trivial episode that occurred many years before the onset of the depressive episode, was forgotten over time, but is presently viewed as a major problem (Bridges 1986). For example, a one-time sexual liaison, forgotten or forgiven by the spouse, is resurrected by a patient with a fear of an ongoing venereal disease or cancer or is associated with chronic and severe pain. Nihilistic delusions (delusions of nothingness) may occur more commonly in late life. Focus on the abdomen is common in an elderly patient with a delusional or psychotic depression. Hallucinations are uncommon, however.

Thakur et al. (1999) compared the clinical, demographic, and social characteristics of psychotic and nonpsychotic depression in a tertiary care sample of 674 elderly and younger patients. In this study, younger age, psychomotor retardation, guilt, feelings of worthlessness, a history of delusions in the past, and increased suicidal ideation and intent were found more commonly in psychotic than in nonpsychotic patients, and these associations were largely confirmed when sociodemographic variables were controlled. Psychotic depression also tended to be associated with poor social support and, not surprisingly, bipolar illness. Cerebrovascular risk factors did not differ significantly between psychotic and nonpsychotic patients. The weakness of this study is that it dealt with hospitalized patients, not a population-based sample.

Dysthymic Disorder

Every clinician who has worked with elderly patients has observed dysthymic disorder, characterized by significant and unremitting depressive symptoms associated with apparently psychosocial causes. Like major depressive disorder, dysthymic disorder is diagnosed across the life cycle. Although dysthymic disorder requires fewer criteria symptoms than does major depressive disorder, these symptoms must last 2 years or more. Dysthymia and major depression often coexist, leading to a "double depression." Results of some research suggest that dysthymic disorder in older persons may differ from that in younger persons. Devanand et al. (2000) examined 76 outpatients, ages 60 and older, who had dysthymic disorder based on DSM-IV-TR criteria. They found that less than one-third of the patients had a diagnosable personality disorder. Personality disorder was associated with an earlier age at onset of depressive illness, a greater lifetime history of comorbid Axis I disorders, greater severity of depressive symptoms, and lower socioeconomic status. The most common personality disorders were the obsessive-compulsive and avoidant types—the personality disorders most commonly found in elderly patients with major depression. The late onset of dysthymia in many of the patients in the study, as well as the lack of psychiatric comorbidity, caused the authors to conclude that dysthymia in elderly individuals is different from dysthymia in younger persons.

Minor or Subsyndromal Depression

Minor, subsyndromal, or subthreshold depression is diagnosed, according to Appendix B of DSM-IV-TR, when one of the core symptoms of major depression is present along with one to three additional symptoms (American Psychiatric Association 2000). Another definition is a score of less than 16 on the CES-D (Radloff 1977), which does not meet the CES-D criteria for clinically significant depression. Associations with subsyndromal depression are similar to those for major depression, including impaired physical functioning, disability days, poorer self-rated health, use of psychotropic medications, perceived low social support, female gender, and unmarried status (Beekman et al. 1995; Hybels et al. 2001). Other investigators have suggested a syndrome of depression without sadness, thought to be more common in older adults (Gallo et al. 1997).

Bereavement

Bereavement in late life is usually characterized by a symptom picture of major depression, yet the syndrome is recognized by the older adult as normal following the death of a loved one and does not seriously interfere with necessary functioning. In DSM-IV-TR, the category of bereavement is designated for virtually all symptoms of depression experienced during the first 2 months after the loss, with the possible exception of extreme feelings of worthlessness or active suicidal ideation. Any person exhibiting the full symptom picture of major depression at least 2 months after the death is considered to have a major depressive disorder warranting treatment.

Adjustment Disorder With Depressed Mood

The DSM-IV-TR category of adjustment disorder with depressed mood is reserved for those individuals who exhibit a maladaptive reaction to an identifiable stressor. The relationship of the syndrome to the stressful event is clear. Typical stressors for older adults include life events such as marital problems, difficulty with children, loss of a social role, and an ill-advised change of residence. Retirement is usually not a source of excessive stress for the older adult. Therefore, the onset of significant depressive symptomatology and withdrawal from activities after retirement may indicate a true adjustment disorder. Of much greater frequency is the development of depressive symptomatology secondary to a physical illness. When an episode of depression accompanies a physical illness and the level of symptoms dramatically exceeds the expected level, a diagnosis of either adjustment disorder or depression associated with medical illness (discussed below) is indicated.

Depression Associated With Medical Illness

Depressive disorders have been associated with a variety of physical illnesses, including cardiovascular disease (Glassman and Shapiro 1998; Musselman et al. 1998), endocrine disturbances (Blazer et al. 2002b), Parkinson's disease (Zesiewicz et al. 1999), stroke (Robinson and Price 1982), and cancer (Spiegel 1996). Depressive symptoms and disorders are common findings in surveys of general medical inpatients (Koenig et al. 1988). Controversy continues over the degree to which acute or chronic medical illnesses cause depression because of direct physiological effects on the brain or because of a psychological reaction to the disability and other life changes evoked by these illnesses.

Physical functioning is highly correlated with depression in cancer patients. In one study (Bukberg et al. 1984), among patients with a Karnofsky score of 40 or less (i.e., patients who were most disabled), almost 80% had major depression, whereas only 23% of those who scored 60 or better (i.e., had moderate to good function) had major depression. Lower rates of depression (5%–13%) were found among ambulatory outpatients with cancer (Koenig and Blazer 1992). Many studies documenting high rates of depression in patients with cancer are controversial because they often involve patients referred for treatment of cancer, who may have more advanced or complicated illness. It is important that myths about depression and cancer be dispelled. One myth is that all cancer patients are depressed; another is that physicians should not bother to treat depression, because such patients should be depressed. In fact, when cancer patients become depressed, mortality may increase (Brown et al. 2003). With regard to hospitalized elders with cancer, at least one study has shown substantially higher mortality in cancer patients with major depression compared with nondepressed cancer patients (Koenig et al. 1989b). Studies have also shown that "desire for hastened death" among terminally ill cancer patients is significantly increased among those who are depressed or feeling hopeless (Breitbart et al. 2000).

With regard to cardiovascular disease and depression, Schleifer et al. (1989) conducted structured psychiatric interviews of 283 patients (mean age 64 years) admitted to the coronary care unit for myocardial infarction. The interviews were conducted using the Schedule for Affective Disorders and Schizophrenia 8–10 days after infarction and again 3–4 months later. Initially, 45% of the patients met the diagnostic criteria for minor or major depression, including 18% with major depression. Three to 4 months later, 33% of patients continued to meet the criteria for depression, including 77% of those who had initially met the criteria for major depression. In another study, Frasure-Smith et al. (1993) followed 222 patients for 6 months after myocardial infarction; depression was a significant predictor of mortality (hazard ratio, 5.7; $P<0.001$), even after other relevant risk factors were controlled. In an extensive review of this literature, Glassman and Shapiro (1998) reported that 9 of 10 studies found increased cardiovascular mortality in depressed patients; even when community-dwelling populations were examined and prospectively followed, the relationship between depression and cardiovascular mortality persisted (after controlling for smoking and other risk factors).

Diagnostic Workup of the Depressed Older Adult

At its core, the diagnosis of a mood disorder in older adults is made on the basis of a history, augmented with a physical examination and fine-tuned by laboratory studies (Blazer 2003) (see Table 15–3). No biological markers or tests are available to confirm the diagnosis of depression, yet some tests may assist in identifying subtypes of depression; for example, MRI scans for subcortical white matter hyperintensities to confirm the presence of vascular depression (Krishnan et al. 1988) and polysomnography for unexplained sleep distur-

TABLE 15–3. Diagnostic workup of late-life depression

Routine studies
Screening (especially in a primary care setting, use standard symptom checklists such as the Geriatric Depression Scale [Yesavage et al. 1983] or the Center for Epidemiologic Studies Depression Scale [Radloff 1977])
Thorough history and assessment, including present and past history of depressive episodes, family history, medication history, and assessment of psychological functioning and of social stressors; medical history, including assessment of nutritional status, current medications, past and current medical history, and functional status
Screening for cognitive impairment with an instrument such as the Mini-Mental State Examination (Folstein et al. 1975)
Physical examination
Laboratory tests, such as chemistry screen and electrocardiogram if antidepressants are prescribed (previous medical records may provide these data)
Elective studies
Magnetic resonance imaging to establish the diagnosis of vascular depression
Blood screens for evidence of vitamin deficiency such as a deficiency of B_{12} or folate
Polysomnography when sleep abnormalities persist and cannot be explained
Screen for thyroid dysfunction (triiodothyronine, thyroxine, radioactive iodine uptake, thyroid-stimulating hormone levels)

bances. Of special importance in evaluating the depressed elder are the following: the duration of the current depressive episode; the history of previous episodes; the history of drug and alcohol abuse; response to previous therapeutic interventions for the depressive illness; a family history of depression, suicide, and/or alcohol abuse; and the severity of the depressive symptoms. Establishing some indication of the risk of suicide is essential, for suicidal risk may determine where the patient is treated.

Screening for depression is helpful, using standardized scales such as the GDS (Yesavage et al. 1983) and the CES-D (Radloff 1977). In primary care settings, the clinical effectiveness of screening is mixed. One reason is that clinical trials typically exclude the type of patients who are most likely to present to the busy internist, such as the patient with comorbid depression and medical illness. Although internists accept responsibility for treating late-life depression, they frequently perceive their clinical skills to be inadequate and are frustrated with their practice environment (Callahan et al. 1992). Assessment of cognitive status is critical to the evaluation of depressed older patients. Use of a screening scale such as the Mini-Mental State Examination (MMSE) is a good adjunct to the diagnostic workup (Folstein et al. 1975).

The physical examination must include a thorough neurological examination to determine whether soft neurological signs (e.g., frontal release signs) or laterality is present. Weight loss and psychomotor retardation in the depressed older adult may lead to peroneal nerve palsy, documented by electromyography and nerve conduction studies (Massey and Bullock 1978). Because the older adult is less occupied with physical activities and therefore tends to be sedentary, the peroneal nerve is subject to chronic trauma.

The laboratory workup of the depressed older adult is important. It should include a thyroid panel (triiodothyronine, thyroxine, and radioactive iodine uptake) and determination of thyroid-stimulating hormone levels. A blood screen enables the clinician to detect the presence of anemia. However, at least one study has shown that red blood cell enlargement and abnormalities are not good predictors of deficits in vitamin B_{12} or folate (Mischoulon et al. 2000). Because both depressive and cognitive symptoms can result from deficits in vitamin B_{12} or folate, it is important to obtain levels of these vitamins.

Treatment

Treatment of depression in late life is four-pronged, involving psychotherapy, pharmacotherapy, electroconvulsive therapy, and family therapy. These four approaches are discussed in this section.

Psychotherapy

Cognitive-behavioral therapy is the only psychotherapy that was designed specifically to treat depression (Beck 1987). Even the more recently developed technique of interpersonal therapy is primarily a cognitive-behavioral orientation to improving interpersonal relationships (Klerman et al. 1984). The advantage of using cognitive-behavioral therapy in treating the older adult is that the therapy is directive and time limited, usually involving between 10 and 25 sessions. Cognitive-behavioral therapy has been found to be effective in depressed elderly patients (Gallagher and Thompson 1982; Steuer 1984) and in patients with chronic medical illnesses such as type II diabetes (Lustman et al. 1998), heart disease (Kohn et al. 2000), and irritable bowel syndrome (Boyce et al. 2000). It may be particularly useful in patients who show only a partial response to antidepressant drug therapy (Scott et al. 2000).

The goal of behavioral and cognitive therapies is to change behavior and modes of thinking. This change is accomplished through behavioral interventions such as weekly activity schedules, mastery and pleasure logs, and graded task assignments. Cognitive approaches to the restructuring of negative cognitions or automatic thoughts include subjecting these cognitions to empirical reality testing, examining distortions (e.g., overgeneralizations, catastrophizing, dichotomous thinking), and generating new ways of viewing one's life (Steuer 1984). Depressed patients typically regard themselves and their present and future in somewhat idiosyncratic or negative ways. Such patients believe that they are inadequate or defective and think that unpleasant experiences are caused by a problem with themselves and that they are therefore worthless, helpless, and hopeless. This cognitive triad leads the older adult to believe that he or she has a never-ending depression and that nothing pleasant will ever happen again. The cognitive model presupposes that these symptoms of depression are consequences of negative thinking patterns.

Thompson et al. (1987) randomly assigned 91 elders with major depression to cognitive therapy, behavioral therapy, or brief dynamic therapy (the latter stresses the importance of the patient-therapist relationship and emphasizes realistic collaborative aspects of the therapeutic alliance). Patients in each group underwent 16–20 sessions of therapy conducted by expert clinicians; 20 additional patients were assigned to a waiting-list control group. By the end of 6 weeks, 52% of the patients in therapy were in complete remission, and 18% showed significant improvement. All therapies were equally efficacious and superior to waiting for treatment.

Results of empirical studies suggest that compared with control subjects, elders who engage in psychotherapy experience incremental improvement. Not only does the percentage of elders who respond to these treatments compare favorably with the percentage of younger subjects who respond, the degree of improvement appears equal to that obtained with medications, especially for individuals with milder forms of depression. Drug therapy is not appropriate for some elders, and cognitive therapy, behavioral therapy, and brief dynamic psychotherapy are viable alternatives. In addition, evidence has emerged that suggests that the long-term benefit of cognitive-behavioral therapy may be greater than that of pharmacotherapy, especially if the medications are discontinued during the first year of treatment (Reynolds et al. 1999).

Older adults who have minor depression or adjustment disorders, or who experience dysphoria because of losses of various types, often require less intensive forms of psychotherapy. Active listening and simple support may be sufficient to help distressed elders cope with their situation. Because religion is an important factor in the lives of many older adults, referral to a pastoral counselor may be particularly helpful and acceptable (Koenig et al. 2004).

Pharmacotherapy

The use of selective serotonin reuptake inhibitors (SSRIs) has been growing in elderly patients (with or without medical illness). Citalopram (Nyth and Gottfries 1990), escitalopram (Gorwood et al. 2007), fluoxetine (Heiligenstein et al. 1995), paroxetine (Bump et al. 2001), and sertraline (Cohn et al. 1990) have been shown to be effective in geriatric depression. SSRIs have also proved effective in depressed older adults who have had a stroke (Cole et al. 2001) or who have vascular disease in general (Krishnan et al. 2001) or Alzheimer's disease (Lyketsos et al. 2000). These agents have become the drugs of first choice for treating mild to moderate forms of depression. Important advantages of the use of these drugs in treating elderly patients are the lack of anticholinergic, orthostatic, and cardiac side effects; lack of sedation; and safety in overdose. Nevertheless, for a significant number of older adults, these newer antidepressants cause other unacceptable effects, including excessive activation and disturbance of sleep, tremor, headache, significant gastrointestinal side effects, hyponatremia, and weight loss.

Other agents that affect both the serotonergic and noradrenergic systems are often considered the best second-line therapy if the patient's response to an SSRI is not adequate. Duloxetine (Raskin et al. 2008) and venlafaxine (Staab and Evans 2000) have been shown to be effective in geriatric depression.

TCAs are the agents of choice for some patients with more severe forms of major depression who can tolerate the side effects and do not respond to the medications mentioned above. Medications that are effective yet relatively free of side effects (especially cardiovascular effects) are preferred. In recent years, nortriptyline and desipramine have become the more popular medications for treating older adults with endogenous or melancholic major depression. However, doxepin remains a favorite among many practitioners. It is recommended that all elderly patients have an electrocardiogram (ECG) before initiation of treatment and again after therapeutic blood levels have been achieved. If the ECG shows a second-degree (or higher) block, a bifascicular bundle branch block, a left bundle branch block, or a QTc interval greater than 480 milliseconds, treatment with TCAs should not be initiated, or should be stopped in patients already taking these medications.

Antidepressant doses administered to persons in late life should be case specific but are generally lower than those given to persons in midlife (see Table 15–4). Starting therapeutic daily doses of antidepressants are as follows: citalopram, 10–40 mg; fluoxetine, 5–20 mg; paroxetine, 10–30 mg; sertraline, 12.5–50 mg; mirtazapine, 7.5–30 mg; and venlafaxine, 37.5–200 mg (in divided doses). Bupropion therapy should be initiated at 75 mg twice daily, with an increase to 150 mg twice daily (not to exceed 150 mg in a single dose). With regard to tricyclics, 25 mg of desipramine orally twice a day or 25–50 mg of nortriptyline orally at bedtime is frequently adequate for relieving depressive symptoms. Plasma levels of tricyclic medications can be helpful in determining dosing: desipramine levels greater than 125 ng/mL and nortriptyline levels between 50 and 150 ng/mL have been found to be therapeutic.

Trazodone and bupropion (Weihs et al. 2000) are alternatives in patients who cannot tolerate TCAs or one of the newer antidepressants. Trazodone has advantages over TCAs in that it is virtually free of anticholinergic effects, and it has advantages over the newer antidepressants in that it has strong sedative effects. Nevertheless, the drug is not without side effects, including excessive daytime sedation, priapism (occasionally), and significant orthostatic hypotension. The therapeutic daily dose of trazodone is 300 mg or more, an amount that many older patients cannot tolerate because of sedation. Bupropion can be effective in treating depression in the elderly but generally is used once other medications have proved ineffective. Agitation is the most common side effect that troubles older adults.

TABLE 15–4. Pharmacological treatment of late-life depression

Medication	Dosage
Selective serotonin reuptake inhibitors	
Citalopram	10–40 mg daily
Escitalopram	10–20 mg daily
Fluoxetine	5–20 mg daily
Paroxetine	10–30 mg daily
Sertraline	12.5–50 mg daily
Serotonin and norepinephrine reuptake inhibitors	
Duloxetine	20 mg bid
Mirtazapine	7.5–30 mg daily
Venlafaxine	37.5–200 mg tid
Tricyclic antidepressants	
Desipramine	25 mg bid
Doxepin	100 mg daily
Nortriptyline	25–50 mg daily
Other agents	
Bupropion	75–150 mg bid
Trazodone	300 mg daily

Monoamine oxidase inhibitors (MAOIs) are another alternative to TCAs and the newer antidepressants. It should be noted, if MAOIs are being considered because of intolerance of side effects of other antidepressants, that older adults usually do not tolerate MAOIs any better. If treatment with an MAOI is to follow treatment with an SSRI, a minimum of 1–2 weeks (following fluoxetine, 2–4 weeks) must elapse after discontinuation of SSRI therapy before initiation of MAOI therapy, to avoid a serotonergic syndrome. If a patient's depression is severe and ECT is contemplated, use of an MAOI also precludes initiation of ECT until 10–14 days after the drug is discontinued. Such a delay may seriously impede clinical management of the suicidal elder.

Some clinicians prescribe low morning doses of stimulant medications, such as 5 mg of methylphenidate, to improve mood in the apathetic older adult. Although the effectiveness of stimulants has not been conclusively demonstrated, these agents are generally safe at low doses, and rarely does the clinician encounter an elder with a propensity to abuse stimulants or to become addicted when these drugs are given once daily.

For further details regarding psychopharmacological treatment of the older adult, see Chapter 26, "Psychopharmacology."

Electroconvulsive Therapy

ECT continues to be the most effective form of treatment for patients with more severe major depressive episodes (O'Conner et al. 2001). The induction of a seizure via ECT appears to be effective in reversing a major depression. ECT was first established as a treatment in 1938, but it is not used as much as it was immediately after its development. Despite its effectiveness, ECT is not the first-line treatment of choice for a patient with major depression and should be prescribed only because other therapeutic modalities have been ineffective. ECT has been shown to be effective in selected individuals, primarily those who have major depression with melancholia, and especially those who have major depression with psychotic symptoms associated with agitation or withdrawal. Many older adults with such syndromes either fail to respond to antidepressant medications or experience toxicity (usually postural hypotension) when taking antidepressants. The presence of self-destructive behavior, such as a suicide attempt or refusal to eat, increases the necessity for intervening effectively; in such situations, ECT may be the treatment of choice.

If ECT is selected as an intervention, the clinician must first discuss in detail with the patient and the family the nature of the treatment and the reasons for this recommendation. It is important to explain why ECT is necessary; what procedures the patient will undergo during a course of ECT; how many treatments can be expected; how long hospitalization will continue; whether ECT can be performed on an outpatient basis; what the risks and side effects of ECT are; and what results, both immediate and long-term, can be expected. Even when an elderly patient is severely depressed, careful and thoughtful discussion with the patient and family will usually result in a willingness by the patient (often with encouragement from the family) to undergo the course of ECT treatments. Once treatment is begun, fears of ECT usually remit.

The medical workup before ECT includes acquisition of a complete medical history, a physical examination, and consultation with a cardiologist if any cardiac abnormalities are recognized. Knowledge of any family history of psychiatric disorders, suicide, or treatment with ECT is helpful in predicting a patient's response to treatment. Laboratory examination includes a complete blood count, a urinalysis, routine chemistries, chest and spinal X rays (the latter to document previous compression fractures), an ECG, and a computed tomography (CT) scan or MRI (with CT or MRI available, an electroencephalogram and skull X ray are not routinely required). The presence of some abnormalities seen in magnetic resonance images does not militate against the use of ECT, however. For example, a series of older adults with major depression were found to have subcortical arteriosclerotic encephalopathy, as demonstrated by MRI, but promptly improved after undergoing ECT (Coffey et al. 1987).

Before an older adult undergoes ECT, all medications should be withdrawn, if possible. As noted in the pharmacotherapy section earlier in this chapter, any MAOIs must be withdrawn 10–14 days before the procedure to prevent any toxic interactions with the anesthetic used during ECT. Reserpine and anticholinesterase drugs should also be withdrawn for at least 1 week prior to ECT. Lithium carbonate, TCAs, antipsychotics, and antianxiety agents (including sedative-hypnotics) are not absolutely contraindicated in patients who are to undergo ECT; however, benzodiazepines increase the seizure threshold and should be avoided. Generally, a short-acting barbiturate, such as chloral hydrate (500 mg orally at bedtime), is the most appropriate sedative-hypnotic, although chloral hydrate should not be given on the night preceding administration of ECT, if possible. Use of low-dose haloperidol or thiothixene is probably the most appropriate means of controlling severe agitation or psychotic symptoms during the course of ECT treatment.

The basic techniques for ECT are well described. Thirty minutes before treatment, an anticholinergic agent is administered intramuscularly to prevent complications of cardiac arrhythmias and aspiration. Directly before treatment, a short-acting anesthetic, such as thiopental or methohexital, is administered until an eyelash response is no longer present. Then a muscle relaxant, such as succinylcholine, is administered to prevent severe muscle contractions. Investigators are increasingly using unilateral electrode placement to the nondominant cerebral hemisphere, because evidence has accumulated that less confusion occurs after unilateral treatment than after bilateral treatment. Nevertheless, unilateral electrode placement does not preclude development of memory difficulties. (Some investigators question the efficacy of unilateral versus bilateral electrode placement, but bilateral electrode placement has not been clearly established as therapeutically superior to unilateral electrode placement.) The electrical stimulus is applied, and the seizure is monitored either by applying a tourniquet to one arm and observing the tonic and clonic movements in the extremity peripheral to the tourniquet or by using direct electroencephalographic monitoring. Direct electroencephalographic monitoring is preferred, and a seizure lasting 25 seconds or more is required for optimal results.

Seizure duration varies with age. In a study involving 228 patients treated with ECT, Hinkle et al. (1986) found that of patients older than 60 years, a greater percentage were likely to have a seizure of 30 seconds or less. When ECT is repeated, use of caffeine may increase the likelihood of inducing a seizure without the necessity of restimulation using higher electrical parameters (which could lead to increased central nervous system toxicity).

ECT treatments are generally administered three times per week, and usually 6–12 treatments are necessary for adequate therapeutic response. A clear improvement is often noted after one of the treatments, with the patient reporting a remarkable improvement in mood and functioning. Two or three treatments are generally given after the ECT administration that leads to improvement.

The risks and side effects of ECT in elderly patients are similar to those in the general population. Cardiovascular effects are of greatest concern and include premature ventricular contractions, ventricular arrhythmias, and transient systolic hypertension. Multiple monitoring during treatment decreases the (infrequent) risk that one of these side effects will lead to permanent problems. Confusion and amnesia often result after a treatment, but the duration of this confusional episode is brief. Even with the use of unilateral nondominant treatment, however, some patients have prolonged memory difficulties. Headaches are a common symptom with ECT; they usually respond to nonnarcotic analgesics. Status epilepticus and vertebral compression fractures are some of the rare but more serious adverse effects. Compression fractures are a particular risk in older women because of the high incidence of osteoporosis in the postmenopausal population.

The overall success rate of ECT in patients who have not responded to drug therapy is usually 80% or greater, and there is no evidence that effectiveness is lower in older adults (Avery and Lubrano 1979). Wesner and Winokur (1989) examined the influence of age on the natural history of major depressive disorder and found that ECT reduced the rate of chronicity when it was used in patients age 40 or older but, surprisingly, not in those younger than 40 years.

A review of records in Canada from 1992 to 2004 found that rates of ECT use in the elderly increased during the 1990s but then stabilized at approximately 12.5 persons per year per 100,000 in the population (Rapaport et al. 2006). Rosenbach et al. (1997) reported that the number of beneficiaries receiving ECT increased from 12,000 in 1987 to 15,560 in 1992, an increase of more than 20% (after calculations were adjusted for increased numbers of beneficiaries between 1987 and 1992). In a prospective, multisite study, Tew et al. (1999) compared characteristics and treatment outcomes of 133 adult (age 59 or younger), 63 young-old (ages 60–74 years), and 72 old-old (age 75 or older) patients treated with ECT for major depression. They found that patients less than 60 years old had a significantly lower rate of response to ECT (54%) than did young-old patients (73%) or old-old patients (67%). The investigators concluded that despite a higher level of physical illness and cognitive impairment, patients age 75 or older who had severe major depression tolerated ECT in a manner similar to the way in which younger patients tolerated the treatment, and the old-old patients demonstrated a similar or even better response. There is also evidence that ECT may be more effective and have fewer side effects than antidepressants when used to treat depression in old-old patients (Manly et al. 2000).

The relapse rate with no prophylactic intervention may exceed 50% in the year after a course of ECT. This relapse rate can be decreased if antidepressants or lithium carbonate is prescribed after the treatment. Maintenance ECT may be necessary for some patients who exhibit a high likelihood of recurrence despite use of prophylactic medication and/or who experience high toxicity and therefore cannot tolerate prophylactic medications. For such patients, weekly or monthly treatments (usually on an outpatient basis) are prescribed, with careful monitoring of response and side effects. Following an effective course of ECT, the combination of continuation ECT and antidepressant drug therapy has been shown to have greater efficacy than use of medications alone (Gagné et al. 2000).

Despite the effectiveness of ECT, few deny that treatment may lead to memory difficulties. In a study by Frith et al. (1983), 70 severely depressed patients were randomly assigned to eight real or sham ECT treatments and were divided according to the degree of recovery from depression afterward. Compared with nondepressed control subjects, the depressed patients were impaired on a wide range of tests of memory and concentration before treatment, but after treatment, performance on most tests improved. Real ECT induced impairments in concentration, short-term memory, and learning but significantly facilitated access to remote memories. At 6-month follow-up, all differences between real and sham ECT groups had disappeared.

Price and McAllister (1989) examined the efficacy of ECT in elderly depressed patients with dementia. Overall, the patients achieved an 86% response rate, with only 21% experiencing a significant worsening of cognition; the cognition problems were transient in most cases. Of particular importance is that 49% of the patients treated with ECT showed improvement in memory function after treatment. Likewise, Stoudemire et al. (1995) found that over time, ECT may lead to significant improvement in memory of cognitively impaired older adults with depression. Although data on the safety and efficacy of ECT in patients with concurrent medical illness derive primarily from retrospective studies involving psychiatric patients with stable disease, these data do support the use of ECT in patients with cardiovascular, neurological, endocrine, or metabolic conditions, as well as a variety of other conditions (Stoudemire et al. 1998).

Family Therapy

The final component of therapy for the depressed elderly patient is work with the family. Not only may family dysfunction contribute to the depressive symptoms experienced by the older adult, but family support is critical to a successful outcome in the treatment of the depressed elder. A clinician must attend to 1) those members of the family who will be available to the elder; 2) the frequency and quality of interactions between the older adult and family members, as well as among other family members; 3) the overall family atmosphere; 4) family values regarding psychiatric disorders; 5) family support and tolerance of symptoms (such as expressions of wishing not to live); and 6) stressors encountered by the family other than the depression experienced by the elder (Blazer 2002).

Most depressed elders do not resist interaction between the clinician and family members. With the patient's permission, the family should be instructed regarding the nature of the depressive disorder and the potential risks associated with depression in late life, especially suicide. Family members can assist the clinician in observing changes in the patient's behavior, such as an increase in discomfort (either physical or emotional), increased withdrawal and decreased verbalization, and preoccupation with medications or weapons. The family can assist by removing possible implements of suicide from places of easy access. The family can also take responsibility for administering medications to an older adult who is unreliable or whose potential for suicide is high.

Family members can benefit from simple instructions regarding how to communicate with an elderly depressed patient. Methods of responding to expressions of low self-esteem and pessimism, such as paraphrase and expression of understanding without a sense of responsibility to intervene, can be especially effective. Families can be taught, for example, to acknowledge to the patient, "I hear what you are saying, and I understand." Behavioral techniques for dealing with demanding or overly dependent elders can be taught to families as well. A depressed elder's demand for constant attention from a family member may necessitate "weaning" the patient from continued contact.

When the symptoms of depression become so severe that hospitalization is required, family members are valuable in facilitating hospitalization. Without a proper alliance between clinician and family, a family may be resistant to hospitalization and undermine the clinician's attempts to treat the older adult appropriately. It is usually necessary for the clinician to take responsibility for saying that hospitalization is essential—that the situation has reached the point at which the family has no choice. The clinician informs the patient—in the presence of the family—of the necessity of hospitalization, and the family in turn can support the clinician's position. In such a situation, the patient rarely resists hospitalization for long.

Key Points

- Late-life depression overall may not be as frequent as at other stages of the life cycle, yet the frequency is much higher in physically and cognitively impaired older adults than in community-based samples.
- The biopsychosocial model works well in placing the origins of late-life depression in context. Most cases derive from a variety of causes.
- Older adults appear more vulnerable to biological causes of depression, such as depression secondary to vascular lesions in the brain.
- Social causes of depression in older adults do not appear to be more frequent but differ from social causes of depression in young or middle-aged adults.
- Older adults who are cognitively intact may experience a buffering of depression because of a lifetime of cumulative wisdom coupled with a different view of events given their age.
- The diagnostic workup of the depressed older adult is centered on a detailed history, ideally from the patient and family.
- For moderately severe depression, a combination of antidepressant therapy and psychotherapy (e.g., interpersonal therapy) is optimal.
- Electroconvulsive therapy is indicated for more severe and treatment-resistant depressive disorders in late life and is generally well tolerated.

References

Alexopoulos GS, Meyers BS, Young RC, et al: The course of geriatric depression with "reversible dementia": a controlled study. Am J Psychiatry 150:1693–1699, 1993

Alexopoulos GS, Meyers BS, Young RC, et al: Recovery in geriatric depression. Arch Gen Psychiatry 53:305–312, 1996

Ambelas A: Live events and mania. Br J Psychiatry 150:235–240, 1987

American Psychiatric Association: Diagnostic and Statistical Manual of Mental Disorders, 4th Edition, Text Revision. Washington, DC, American Psychiatric Association, 2000

Arborelius L, Owens M, Plotsky P, et al: The role of corticotropin-releasing factor in depression and anxiety disorders. J Endocrinol 160:1–12, 1999

Arfken CL, Lichtenberg PA, Tancer ME: Cognitive impairment and depression predict mortality in medically ill older adults. J Gerontol A Biol Sci Med Sci 54:M152–M156, 1999

Atchley RC: A continuity theory of normal aging. Gerontologist 29:183–190, 1989

Avery D, Lubrano A: Depression treated with imipramine and ECT: the DeCarolis study reconsidered. Am J Psychiatry 136:559–562, 1979

Baldwin RC, Jolley DJ: The prognosis of depression in old age. Br J Psychiatry 149:574–583, 1986

Baltes P, Staudinger U: Wisdom: a metaheuristic (pragmatic) to orchestrate mind and virtue toward excellence. Am Psychol 55:122–136, 2000

Beck A: Cognitive model of depression. Journal of Cognitive Psychotherapy 1:2–27, 1987

Beekman A, Deeg D, van Tilberg T, et al: Major and minor depression in later life: a study of prevalence and risk factors. J Affect Disord 36:65–75, 1995

Beekman AT, Deeg DJ, Geerlings SW, et al: Emergence and persistence of late life depression: a 3-year follow-up of the Longitudinal Aging Study Amsterdam. J Affect Disord 65:131–138, 2001

Beekman A, Geerlings S, Deeg D, et al: The natural history of late-life depression. Arch Gen Psychiatry 59:605–611, 2002

Black S: Increased health burden associated with comorbid depression in older diabetic Mexican Americans: results from the Hispanic Established Population for Epidemiologic Study of the Elderly survey. Diabetes Care 22:56–64, 1999

Black S, Goodwin J, Markides K: The association between chronic diseases and depressive symptomology in older Mexican Americans. J Gerontol A Biol Sci Med Sci 53:M118–M194, 1998

Blazer DG: Social support and mortality in an elderly community population. Am J Epidemiol 115:684–694, 1982

Blazer DG: Impact of late-life depression on the social network. Am J Psychiatry 140:162–166, 1983

Blazer DG: Psychiatry and the oldest old. Am J Psychiatry 157:1915–1924, 2000

Blazer DG: Depression in Late Life, 3rd Edition. New York, Springer, 2002

Blazer DG: Depression in late life: review and commentary. J Gerontol A Biol Sci Med Sci 58:249–265, 2003

Blazer DG 2nd, Hybels CF: Origins of depression in later life. Psychol Med 35:1241–1252, 2005

Blazer D, Bachar JR, Hughes DC: Major depression with melancholia: a comparison of middle-aged and elderly adults. J Am Geriatr Soc 35:927–932, 1987a

Blazer D, Hughes DC, George LK: The epidemiology of depression in an elderly community population. Gerontologist 27:281–287, 1987b

Blazer D, Hughes DC, Fowler N: Anxiety as an outcome symptom of depression in elderly and middle-aged adults. Int J Geriatr Psychiatry 4:273–278, 1989

Blazer D, Burchett B, Service C, et al: The association of age and depression among the elderly: an epidemiologic exploration. J Gerontol 46:M210–M215, 1991

Blazer DG, Hybels CF, Pieper CF: The association of depression and mortality in elderly persons: a case for multiple independent pathways. J Gerontol A Biol Sci Med Sci 56A:M505–M509, 2001

Blazer DG, Burchett B, Fillenbaum G: APOE ε4 and low cholesterol as risks for depression in a biracial elderly community sample. Am J Geriatr Psychiatry 10:515–520, 2002a

Blazer DG, Moody-Ayers S, Craft-Morgan J, et al: Depression in diabetes and obesity: racial/ethnic/gender issues in older adults. J Psychosom Res 53:913–916, 2002b

Boyce P, Gilchrist J, Talley NJ, et al: Cognitive-behaviour therapy as a treatment for irritable bowel syndrome: a pilot study. Aust N Z J Psychiatry 34:300–309, 2000

Braam AW, Beekman AT, Deeg DJ, et al: Religiosity as a protective or prognostic factor of depression in later life: results from a community survey in The Netherlands. Acta Psychiatr Scand 96:199–205, 1997a

Braam AW, Beekman AT, van Tilburg TG, et al: Religious involvement and depression in older Dutch citizens. Soc Psychiatry Psychiatr Epidemiol 32:284–291, 1997b

Breitbart W, Rosenfeld B, Pessin H, et al: Depression, hopelessness, and desire for hastened death in terminally ill patients with cancer. JAMA 284:2907–2911, 2000

Bridges P: The drug treatment of depression in old age, in Affective Disorders in the Elderly. Edited by Murphy E. Edinburgh, Scotland, Churchill Livingstone, 1986, pp 91–149

Brodaty H, Luscombe G, Parker G, et al: Early and late onset depression in old age: different aetiologies, same phenomenology. J Affect Disord 66:225–236, 2001

Brown KW, Levy AR, Rosberger Z, et al: Psychological distress and cancer survival: a follow-up 10 years after diagnosis. Psychosom Med 65:636–643, 2003

Bruce ML: Depression and disability in late life: directions for future research. Am J Geriatr Psychiatry 9:102–112, 2001

Bruce ML: Psychosocial risk factors for depressive disorders in late life. Biol Psychiatry 52:175–184, 2002

Bruce ML, Leaf PJ: Psychiatric disorders and 15-month mortality in a community sample of older adults. Am J Public Health 79:727–730, 1989

Bukberg J, Penman D, Holland JC: Depression in hospitalized cancer patients. Psychosom Med 46:199–212, 1984

Bump GM, Mulsant BH, Pollock BG, et al: Paroxetine versus nortriptyline in the continuation and maintenance treatment of depression in the elderly. Depress Anxiety 13:38–44, 2001

Callahan CM, Nienaber NAS, Hendrie HC, et al: Depression of elderly outpatients: primary care physicians' attitudes and practice patterns. J Gen Intern Med 7:26–31, 1992

Carstensen LL, Pasupathi M, Mayr U, et al: Emotional experience in everyday life across the adult life span. J Pers Soc Psychol 79:644–655, 2000

Chi I, Chou KL: Social support and depression among elderly Chinese people in Hong Kong. Int J Aging Hum Dev 52:231–252, 2001

Clayton PJ: Bereavement and depression. J Clin Psychiatry 51(suppl):34–40, 1990

Coffey CE, Hinkle PE, Weiner RD, et al: Electroconvulsive therapy of depression in patients with white matter hyperintensity. Biol Psychiatry 22:629–636, 1987

Coffey CE, Figiel GS, Djang WT: Subcortical hyperintensity on magnetic resonance imaging: a comparison of normal and depressed elderly subjects. Am J Psychiatry 147:187–189, 1990

Cohn CK, Shrivastava R, Mendels J, et al: Double-blind, multicenter comparison of sertraline and amitriptyline in elderly depressed patients. J Clin Psychiatry 51 (suppl B):28–33, 1990

Cole MG, Bellavance F, Mansour A: Prognosis of depression in elderly community and primary care populations: a systematic review and meta-analysis. Am J Psychiatry 156:1182–1189, 1999

Cole MG, Elie LM, McCusker J, et al: Feasibility and effectiveness of treatments of post-stroke depression in elderly inpatients: systematic review. J Geriatr Psychiatry Neurol 14:37–41, 2001

Cornoni-Huntley J, Blazer D, Lafferty M, et al (eds): Established Populations for Epidemiologic Studies of the Elderly: Resource Data Book, Vol 2. Bethesda, MD, National Institute on Aging, 1990

Covinsky KE, Kahana E, Chin MH, et al: Depressive symptoms and 3-year mortality in older hospitalized medical patients. Ann Intern Med 130:563–569, 1999

Cutler NR, Post RM: Life course of illness in untreated manic-depressive patients. Compr Psychiatry 23:101–115, 1982

Czéh B, Michaelis T, Watanabe T, et al: Stress-induced changes in cerebral metabolites, hippocampal volume, and cell proliferation are prevented by antidepressant treatment with tianeptine. Proc Natl Acad Sci U S A 98:12796–12801, 2001

de Beurs E, Beekman A, Geerlings S, et al: On becoming depressed or anxious in late life: similar vulnerability factors but different effects of stressful life events. Br J Psychiatry 179:426–431, 2001

Devanand DP: Comorbid psychiatric disorders in late life depression. Biol Psychiatry 51:236–242, 2002

Devanand DP, Turret N, Moody BJ, et al: Personality disorders in elderly patients with dysthymic disorder. Am J Geriatr Psychiatry 8:188–195, 2000

Devanand DP, Kim MK, Paykina N, et al: Adverse life events in elderly patients with major depression or dysthymia and in healthy-control subjects. Am J Geriatr Psychiatry 10:265–274, 2002

Dunner DL: Affective disorder: clinical features, in Psychiatry, Vol 1. Edited by Michels R, Cavenar J. Philadelphia, JB Lippincott, 1985, pp 59–60

Eastham JH, Jeste DV, Young RC: Assessment and treatment of bipolar disorder in the elderly. Drugs Aging 12:205–224, 1998

Eisses A, Kluiter H, Jongenelis K, et al: Risk indicators of depression in residential homes. Int J Geriatr Psychiatry 19:634–640, 2004

Fassler LB, Gaviria M: Depression in the elderly. J Am Geriatr Soc 26:471–475, 1978

Fillenbaum G: Multidimensional Functional Assessment of Older Adults: The Duke Older Americans Resources and Services Procedures. Hillsdale, NJ, Erlbaum, 1988

Fiske A, Gatz M, Pedersen NL: Depressive symptoms and aging: the effects of illness and non-health-related events. J Gerontol B Psychol Sci Soc Sci 58:P320–P328, 2003

Folstein M, Folstein S, McHugh P: "Mini-mental state": a practical method for grading the cognitive state of patients for the clinician. J Psychiatr Res 12:189–198, 1975

Frasure-Smith N, Lespérance F, Talajic M: Depression following myocardial infarction: impact on 6-month survival. JAMA 270:1819–1825, 1993 [Erratum in: JAMA 271(14):1082, 1994]

Fried L: Frailty, in Principles of Geriatric Medicine and Gerontology, 3rd Edition. Edited by Hazzard W, Bierman E, Blass J, et al. New York, McGraw-Hill, 1994, pp 1149–1156

Frith CD, Stevens M, Johnstone EC, et al: Effects of ECT and depression on various aspects of memory. Br J Psychiatry 142:610–617, 1983

Gagné GG Jr, Furman MJ, Carpenter LL, et al: Efficacy of continuation ECT and antidepressant drugs compared to long-term antidepressants alone in depressed patients. Am J Psychiatry 157:1960–1965, 2000

Gallagher DE, Thompson LW: Treatment of major depressive disorder in older outpatients with brief psychotherapies. Psychotherapy Theory, Research, Practice, Training 19:482–490, 1982

Gallo JJ, Rabins PV, Lyketsos CG: Depression without sadness: functional outcomes of nondysphoric depression in later life. J Am Geriatr Soc 45:570–578, 1997

Gatz M, Pedersen N, Plomin R, et al: Importance of shared genes and shared environments for symptoms of depression in older adults. J Abnorm Psychol 101:701–708, 1992

Geerlings SW, Beekman AT, Deeg DJ, et al: Duration and severity of depression predict mortality in older adults in the community. Psychol Med 32:609–618, 2002

George LK, Blazer DG, Hughes DC, et al: Social support and the outcome of major depression. Br J Psychiatry 154:478–485, 1989

George MS, Ketter TA, Post RM: Prefrontal cortex dysfunction in clinical depression. Depression 2:59–72, 1994

Glasser M, Rabins P: Mania in the elderly. Age Ageing 13:210–213, 1984

Glassman AH, Shapiro PA: Depression and the course of coronary artery disease. Am J Psychiatry 155:4–11, 1998

Gonzalez-Salvador MT, Arango C, Lyketsos CG, et al: The stress and psychological morbidity of the Alzheimer patient caregiver. Int J Geriatr Psychiatry 14:701–710, 1999

Gorwood P, Weiller E, Lemming O, et al: Escitalopram prevents relapse in older adults with major depressive disorder. Am J Geriatr Psychiatry 15:581–593, 2007

Gottfries CG: Neurochemical aspects on aging and diseases with cognitive impairment. J Neurosci Res 27:541–547, 1990

Guttmann CR, Jolesz F, Kikinis R, et al: White matter changes with normal aging. Neurology 50:972–978, 1998

Hays JC, Saunders WB, Flint EP, et al: Social support and depression as risk factors for loss of physical function in late life. Aging Mental Health 3:209–220, 1997

Hays JC, Steffens DC, Flint EP, et al: Does social support buffer functional decline in elderly patients with unipolar depression? Am J Psychiatry 158:1850–1855, 2001

Heiligenstein JH, Ware JE Jr, Beusterien KM, et al: Acute effects of fluoxetine versus placebo on functional health and well-being in late-life depression. Int Psychogeriatr 7(suppl):125–137, 1995

Henderson AS, Jorm AF, MacKinnon A: The prevalence of depressive disorders and the distribution of depressive symptoms in later life: a survey using draft ICD-10 and DSM-III-R. Psychol Med 23:719–729, 1993

Henderson AS, Korten AE, Jacomb PA, et al: The course of depression in the elderly: a longitudinal community-based study in Australia. Psychol Med 27:119–129, 1997

Hickie I, Scott E, Naismith S, et al: Late-onset depression: genetic, vascular and clinical contributions. Psychol Med 31:1403–1412, 2001

Hinkle P, Coffey CE, Weiner R, et al: ECT seizure duration varies with age. Paper presented at the American Geriatrics Society, Chicago, IL, 1986

Holahan CK, Holahan CJ: Self-efficacy, social support, and depression in aging: a longitudinal analysis. J Gerontol 42:65–68, 1987

Holahan CJ, Moos RH: Social support and psychological distress: a longitudinal analysis. J Abnorm Psychol 90:365–370, 1981

Hughes DC, Blazer DG, George LK: Age differences in life events: a multivariate controlled analysis. Int J Aging Hum Dev 127:207–220, 1988

Husain MM, McDonald WM, Doraiswamy PM, et al: A magnetic resonance imaging study of putamen nuclei in major depression. Psychiatry Res 40:95–99, 1991

Hybels CF, Blazer DG, Pieper CF: Toward a threshold for subthreshold depression: an analysis of correlates of depression by severity of symptoms using data from an elderly community sample. Gerontologist 41:357–365, 2001

Hybels CF, Pieper CF, Blazer DG: Sex differences in the relationship between subthreshold depression and mortality in a community sample of older adults. Am J Geriatr Psychiatry 10:283–291, 2002

Hybels CF, Blazer DG, Steffens DC: Predictors of partial remission in older patients treated for major depression: the role of comorbid dysthymia. Am J Geriatr Psychiatry 13:713–721, 2005

Idler EL: Religious involvement and the health of the elderly: some hypotheses and an initial test. Social Forces 66:226–238, 1987

Jang Y, Haley WE, Small BJ: The role of mastery and social resources in the associations between disability and depression in later life. Gerontologist 42:807–813, 2002

Keller MB, Shapiro RW, Lavori PW, et al: Recovery in major depressive disorder: analyses with the life table and regression models. Arch Gen Psychiatry 39:905–910, 1982a

Keller MB, Shapiro RW, Lavori PW, et al: Relapse in major depressive disorder: analysis with the life table. Arch Gen Psychiatry 39:911–915, 1982b

Kennedy GJ, Kelman HR, Thomas C: The emergence of depressive symptoms in late life: the importance of declining health and increasing disability. J Community Health 15:93–104, 1990

Kessler RC, Chiu WT, Demler O, et al: Prevalence, severity, and comorbidity of 12-month DSM-IV disorders in the National Comorbidity Survey Replication. Arch Gen Psychiatry 62:617–627, 2005 [Erratum in: Arch Gen Psychiatry 62(7):709, 2005]

Klerman GL, Weissman MM, Rounsaville BJ, et al: Interpersonal Psychotherapy of Depression. New York, Basic Books, 1984

Koenig HG: Religion and depression in older medical inpatients. Am J Geriatr Psychiatry 15:282–291, 2007a

Koenig HG: Religion and remission of depression in medical inpatients with heart failure/pulmonary disease. J Nerv Ment Dis 195:389–395, 2007b

Koenig HG, Blazer DG: Epidemiology of geriatric affective disorders. Clin Geriatr Med 8:235–251, 1992

Koenig HG, Meador KG, Cohen HJ, et al: Depression in elderly hospitalized patients with medical illness. Arch Intern Med 148:1929–1936, 1988

Koenig HG, Goli V, Shelp F, et al: Antidepressant use in elderly medical inpatients: lessons from an attempted clinical trial. J Gen Intern Med 4:498–505, 1989a

Koenig HG, Shelp F, Goli V, et al: Survival and health care utilization in elderly medical inpatients with major depression. J Am Geriatr Soc 37:599–606, 1989b

Koenig HG, Cohen HJ, Blazer DG, et al: Religious coping and depression among elderly, hospitalized medically ill men. Am J Psychiatry 149:1693–1700, 1992

Koenig HG, George LK, Peterson BL: Religiosity and remission of depression in medically ill older patients. Am J Psychiatry 155:536–542, 1998

Koenig HG, George LK, Titus P: Religion, spirituality, and health in medically ill hospitalized older patients. J Am Geriatr Soc 52:554–562, 2004

Kohn CS, Petrucci RJ, Baessler C: The effect of psychological intervention on patients' long-term adjustment to the ICD: a prospective study. Pacing Clin Electrophysiol 23:450–456, 2000

Kraaij V, de Wilde EJ: Negative life events and depressive symptoms in the elderly: a life span perspective. Aging Ment Health 5:84–91, 2001

Kraaij V, Arensman E, Spinhoven P: Negative life events and depression in elderly persons: a meta-analysis. J Gerontol B Psychol Sci Soc Sci 57:P87–P94, 2002

Krishnan KR, Goli V, Ellinwood EH, et al: Leukoencephalopathy in patients diagnosed as major depressive. Biol Psychiatry 23:519–522, 1988 [Erratum in: Biol Psychiatry 25(6):822, 1989]

Krishnan KR, McDonald WM, Escalona PR, et al: Magnetic resonance imaging of the caudate nuclei in depression: preliminary observations. Arch Gen Psychiatry 49:553–557, 1992
Krishnan KR, McDonald WM, Doraiswamy PM, et al: Neuroanatomical substrates of depression in the elderly. Eur Arch Psychiatry Clin Neurosci 243:41–46, 1993
Krishnan KR, Hays JC, Blazer DG: MRI-defined vascular depression. Am J Psychiatry 154:497–501, 1997
Krishnan KR, Doraiswamy PM, Clary CM: Clinical and treatment response characteristics of late-life depression associated with vascular disease: a pooled analysis of two multicenter trials with sertraline. Prog Neuropsychopharmacol Biol Psychiatry 25:347–361, 2001
Krishnan KR, Taylor WD, McQuoid DR, et al: Clinical characteristics of magnetic resonance imaging–defined subcortical ischemic depression. Biol Psychiatry 55:390–397, 2004
Kumar A, Mintz J, Bilker W, et al: Autonomous neurobiological pathways to late-life depressive disorders: clinical and pathophysiological implications. Neuropsychopharmacology 26:229–236, 2002
Lenze EJ, Munin MC, Skidmore ER, et al: Onset of depression in elderly persons after hip fracture: implications for prevention and early intervention of late-life depression. J Am Geriatr Soc 55:81–86, 2007
Li YS, Meyer JS, Thornby J: Longitudinal follow-up of depressive symptoms among normal versus cognitively impaired elderly. Int J Geriatr Psychiatry 16:718–727, 2001
Liverman C, Blazer D (eds): Testosterone and Aging: Clinical Research Directions. Washington, DC, National Academies Press, 2004
Livingston G, Manela M, Katona C: Depression and other psychiatric morbidity in carers of elderly people living at home. BMJ 312:153–156, 1996
Luisi S, Tonetti A, Bernardi F, et al: Effect of acute corticotropin releasing factor on pituitary-adrenocortical responsiveness in elderly women and men. J Endocrinol Invest 21:449–453, 1998
Lustman PJ, Griffith LS, Freedland KE, et al: Cognitive behavior therapy for depression in type 2 diabetes mellitus: a randomized, controlled study. Ann Intern Med 129:613–621, 1998
Lyketsos CG, Sheppard JM, Steele CD, et al: Randomized, placebo-controlled, double-blind, clinical trial of sertraline in the treatment of depression complicating Alzheimer's disease: initial results from the Depression in Alzheimer's Disease Study. Am J Psychiatry 157:1686–1689, 2000
Lyles KW: Osteoporosis and depression: shedding more light upon a complex relationship. J Am Geriatr Soc 49:827–828, 2001
Lyness JM, Caine ED, King DA, et al: Depressive disorders and symptoms in older primary care patients. Am J Geriatr Psychiatry 10:275–282, 2002
Magaziner J, Simonsick EM, Kashner TM, et al: Predictors of functional recovery one year following hospital discharge for hip fracture: a prospective study. J Gerontol 45:M101–M107, 1990
Manly DT, Oakley SP Jr, Bloch RM: Electroconvulsive therapy in old-old patients. Am J Geriatr Psychiatry 8:232–236, 2000
Massey EW, Bullock R: Peroneal palsy in depression. J Clin Psychiatry 39:287, 291–292, 1978
Meyers BS, Kalayam B, Mei-Tal V: Late-onset delusional depression: a distinct clinical entity? J Clin Psychiatry 45:347–349, 1984
Mischoulon D, Burger JK, Spillmann MK, et al: Anemia and macrocytosis in the prediction of serum folate and vitamin B_{12} status, and treatment outcome in major depression. J Psychosom Res 49:183–187, 2000
Mojtabai R, Olfson M: Major depression in community-dwelling middle-aged and older adults: prevalence and 2- and 4-year follow-up symptoms. Psychol Med 34:623–634, 2004
Morley J, Kraenzle D: Causes of weight loss in a community nursing home. J Am Geriatr Soc 42:583–585, 1994
Morse JQ, Lynch TR: A preliminary investigation of self-reported personality disorders in late life: prevalence, predictors of depressive severity, and clinical correlates. Aging Ment Health 8:307–315, 2004
Murphy E: Social origins of depression in old age. Br J Psychiatry 141:135–142, 1982
Murphy E: The prognosis of depression in old age. Br J Psychiatry 142:111–119, 1983
Murphy E, Smith R, Lindesay J, et al: Increased mortality rates in late-life depression. Br J Psychiatry 152:347–353, 1988
Musselman DL, Evans DL, Nemeroff CB: The relationship of depression to cardiovascular disease: epidemiology, biology, and treatment. Arch Gen Psychiatry 55:580–592, 1998
Nyth AL, Gottfries CG: The clinical efficacy of citalopram in treatment of emotional disturbances in dementia disorders: a Nordic multicentre study. Br J Psychiatry 157:894–901, 1990
O'Conner M, Knapp R, Husain M, et al: The influence of age on the response of major depression to electroconvulsive therapy: a C.O.R.E. Report. Am J Geriatr Psychiatry 9:382–390, 2001
Olin J, Schneider L, Katz I, et al: Provisional diagnostic criteria for depression of Alzheimer disease. Am J Geriatr Psychiatry 10:125–128, 2002
Parker G, Roy K, Hadzi-Pavlovic D, et al: The differential impact of age on the phenomenology of melancholia. Psychol Med 31:1231–1236, 2001
Parmelee PA, Katz IR, Lawton MP: Depression among institutionalized aged: assessment and prevalence estimation. J Gerontol 44:M22–M29, 1989
Penninx BW, Geerlings SW, Deeg DJ, et al: Minor and major depression and the risk of death in older persons. Arch Gen Psychiatry 56:889–895, 1999a
Penninx BW, Leveille S, Ferrucci L, et al: Exploring the effect of depression on physical disability: longitudinal evidence from the Established Populations for Epidemiologic Studies of the Elderly. Am J Public Health 89:1346–1352, 1999b
Pollock BG: Geriatric psychiatry: psychopharmacology: general principles, in Kaplan and Sadock's Comprehensive Textbook of Psychiatry. Edited by Sadock BJ, Sadock VA. Baltimore, MD, Williams and Wilkins, 2000, pp 3086–3090
Post F: The Significance of Affective Symptoms at Old Age. London, Oxford University Press, 1962
Post F: The management and nature of depressive illnesses in late life: a follow-through study. Br J Psychiatry 121:393–404, 1972
Post F: The functional psychoses, in Geriatric Psychiatry. Edited by Isaacs A, Post F. New York, Wiley, 1978, pp 77–98
Pressman P, Lyons JS, Larson DB, et al: Religious belief, depression, and ambulation status in elderly women with broken hips. Am J Psychiatry 147:758–760, 1990
Price TR, McAllister TW: Safety and efficacy of ECT in depressed patients with dementia: a review of clinical experience. Convuls Ther 5:61–74, 1989
Prigerson H, Reynolds CF 3rd, Frank E, et al: Stressful life events, social rhythms, and depressive symptoms among the elderly: an examination of hypothesized causal linkages. Psychiatry Res 51:33–49, 1994
Prince MJ, Harwood RH, Thomas A, et al: A prospective population-based study of the effects of disablement and social milieu

on the onset and maintenance of late-life depression: the Gospel Oak Project VII. Psychol Med 28:337–350, 1998

Rabkin JG, Charles E, Kass F: Hypertension and DSM-III depression in psychiatric outpatients. Am J Psychiatry 140:1072–1074, 1983

Radloff LS: The CES-D Scale: a self-report depression scale for research in the general population. Applied Psychological Measurement 1:385–401, 1977

Rapaport MJ, Mamdani M, Herrman N: Electroconvulsive therapy in older adults: 13-year trends. Can J Psychiatry 51:616–619, 2006

Raskin J, Xu JY, Kajdasz DK: Time to response for duloxetine 60 mg once daily versus placebo in elderly patients with major depressive disorder. Int Psychogeriatr 20:309–327, 2008

Reynolds CF 3rd, Frank E, Perel JM, et al: Combined pharmacotherapy and psychotherapy in the acute and continuation treatment of elderly patients with recurrent major depression: a preliminary report. Am J Psychiatry 149:1687–1692, 1992

Reynolds CF 3rd, Frank E, Perel JM, et al: Nortriptyline and interpersonal psychotherapy as maintenance therapies for recurrent major depression: a randomized controlled trial in patients older than 59 years. JAMA 281:39–45, 1999

Reynolds CF 3rd, Dew MA, Pollock BG, et al: Maintenance treatment of major depression in old age. N Engl J Med 354:1130–1138, 2006

Roberts RE, Kaplan GA, Shema SJ, et al: Does growing old increase the risk for depression? Am J Psychiatry 154:1384–1390, 1997

Robinson RG, Price TR: Post-stroke depressive disorders: a follow-up study of 103 patients. Stroke 13:635–641, 1982

Rosenbach ML, Hermann RC, Dorwart RA: Use of electroconvulsive therapy in the Medicare population between 1987 and 1992. Psychiatr Serv 48:1537–1542, 1997

Rovner BW, German PS, Brant LJ, et al: Depression and mortality in nursing homes. JAMA 265:993–996, 1991 [Erratum in: JAMA 265(20):2672, 1991]

Sapolsky RM: Why stress is bad for your brain. Science 273:749–750, 1996

Sapolsky RM: Depression, antidepressants, and the shrinking hippocampus. Proc Natl Acad Sci U S A 98:12320–12322, 2001

Schleifer SJ, Macari-Hinson MM, Coyle DA, et al: The nature and course of depression following myocardial infarction. Arch Intern Med 149:1785–1789, 1989

Schulz R, Drayer RA, Rollman BL: Depression as a risk factor for non-suicide mortality in the elderly. Biol Psychiatry 52:205–225, 2002

Scott J, Teasdale JD, Paykel ES, et al: Effects of cognitive therapy on psychological symptoms and social functioning in residual depression. Br J Psychiatry 177:440–446, 2000

Seidman SN, Araujo AB, Roose SP, et al: Low testosterone levels in elderly men with dysthymic disorder. Am J Psychiatry 159:456–459, 2002

Sheline YI: Neuroimaging studies of mood disorder effects on the brain. Biol Psychiatry 54:338–352, 2003

Sheline YI, Wang PW, Gado MH, et al: Hippocampal atrophy in recurrent major depression. Proc Natl Acad Sci U S A 93:3908–3913, 1996

Sheline YI, Mintun MS, Moerlein SM, et al: Greater loss of 5-HT(2A) receptors in midlife than in late life. Am J Psychiatry 159:430–435, 2002

Sherwin B, Gelfand M: Sex steroids and affect in the surgical menopause: a double-blind, cross-over study. Psychoneuroendocrinology 10:325–335, 1985

Shulman KI: Mania in old age, in Affective Disorders in the Elderly. Edited by Murphy E. Edinburgh, Scotland, Churchill Livingstone, 1986, pp 203–216

Shulman KI: The influence of age and aging on manic disorder. Int J Geriatr Psychiatry 4:63–65, 1989

Shulman K, Post F: Bipolar affective disorder in old age. Br J Psychiatry 136:26–32, 1980

Smith GS, Gunning-Dixon FM, Lotrich FE, et al: Translational research in late-life mood disorders: implications for future intervention and prevention research. Neuropsychopharmacology 32:1857–1875, 2007

Spar JE, Ford CV, Liston EH: Bipolar affective disorder in aged patients. J Clin Psychiatry 40:504–507, 1979

Spiegel D: Cancer and depression. Br J Psychiatry 169(suppl):109–116, 1996

Staab JP, Evans DL: Efficacy of venlafaxine in geriatric depression. Depress Anxiety 12 (suppl 1):63–68, 2000

Steffens DC, Payne ME, Greenberg DL, et al: Hippocampal volume and incident dementia in geriatric depression. Am J Geriatr Psychiatry 10:62–71, 2002

Steuer JL, Mintz J, Hammen CL, et al: Cognitive-behavioral and psychodynamic group psychotherapy in treatment of geriatric depression. J Consult Clin Psychol 52:180–189, 1984

Stoudemire A, Hill CD, Morris R, et al: Long-term outcome of treatment-resistant depression in older adults. Am J Psychiatry 150:1539–1540, 1993

Stoudemire A, Hill CD, Morris R, et al: Improvement in depression-related cognitive dysfunction following ECT. J Neuropsychiatry Clin Neurosci 7:31–34, 1995

Stoudemire A, Hill CD, Marquardt M, et al: Recovery and relapse in geriatric depression after treatment with antidepressants and ECT in a medical-psychiatric population. Gen Hosp Psychiatry 20:170–174, 1998

Sullivan MD, LaCroix AZ, Baum C, et al: Functional status in coronary artery disease: a one year prospective study of the role of anxiety and depression. Am J Med 103:348–356, 1997

Takeshita J, Masaki K, Ahmed I, et al: Are depressive symptoms a risk factor for mortality in elderly Japanese American men? The Honolulu Asia Aging Study. Am J Psychiatry 159:1127–1132, 2002

Taylor WS, Steffens DC, MacFall JR, et al: White matter hyperintensity progression and late-life depression outcomes. Arch Gen Psychiatry 60:1090–1096, 2003

Tew JD Jr, Mulsant BH, Haskett RF, et al: Acute efficacy of ECT in the treatment of major depression in the old-old. Am J Psychiatry 156:1865–1870, 1999

Thakur M, Hays J, Ranga K [sic], Krishnan KRR: Clinical, demographic, and social characteristics of psychotic depression. Psychiatry Res 86:99–106, 1999

Thomas C, Kelman HR, Kennedy GJ, et al: Depressive symptoms and mortality in elderly persons. J Gerontol 47:S80–S87, 1992

Thompson LW, Gallagher D, Breckenridge JS: Comparative effectiveness of psychotherapies for depressed elders. J Consult Clin Psychol 55:385–390, 1987

Turner R, Turner J: Social integration and support, in Handbook of Sociology of Mental Health. Edited by Aneshensel C, Phelan J. New York, Kluwer Academic, 1999, pp 301–319

Waite A, Bebbington P, Skelton-Robinson M, et al: Social factors and depression in carers of people with dementia. Int J Geriatr Psychiatry 19:582–587, 2004

Weihs KL, Settle EC Jr, Batey SR, et al: Buproprion sustained release versus paroxetine for the treatment of depression in the elderly. J Clin Psychiatry 61:196–202, 2000

Weissman MM, Prusoff BA, Klerman GL: Personality and the prediction of long-term outcome in depression. Am J Psychiatry 135:797–800, 1978

Weissman MM, Bruce ML, Leaf PJ, et al: Affective disorders, in Psychiatric Disorders in America: The Epidemiologic Catchment Area Study. Edited by Robins LN, Regier DA. New York, Free Press, 1991, pp 53–80

Wesner RB, Winokur G: The influence of age on the natural history of unipolar depression when treated with electroconvulsive therapy. Eur Arch Psychiatry Neurol Sci 238:149–154, 1989

Whooley MA, Browner WS: Association between depressive symptoms and mortality in older women: study of Osteoporotic Fractures Research Group. Arch Intern Med 158:2129–2135, 1998

Whyte EM, Pollock BG, Wagner WR, et al: Influence of serotonin-transporter-linked region polymorphism on platelet activation in geriatric depression. Am J Psychiatry 158:2074–2076, 2001

Williams SA, Kasl SV, Heiat A, et al: Depression and risk of heart failure among the elderly: a prospective community-based study. Psychosom Med 64:6–12, 2002

Winokur G: The Iowa 5000: heterogeneity and course of manic-depressive illness (bipolar). Compr Psychiatry 16:125–131, 1975

Wylie ME, Mulsant BH, Pollock BG, et al: Age of onset in geriatric bipolar disorder: effects on clinical presentation and treatment outcomes in an inpatient sample. Am J Geriatr Psychiatry 7:77–83, 1999

Yassa R, Nair V, Nastase C, et al: Prevalence of bipolar disorder in a psychogeriatric population. J Affect Disord 14:197–201, 1988

Yesavage JA, Brink TL, Rose TL, et al: Development and validation of a geriatric depression screening scale: a preliminary report. J Psychiatr Res 17:37–49, 1983

Young RC, Falk JR: Age, manic psychopathology, and treatment response. Int J Geriatr Psychiatry 4:73–78, 1989

Young RC, Klerman GL: Mania in late life: focus on age at onset. Am J Psychiatry 149:867–876, 1992

Zesiewicz TA, Gold M, Chari G, et al: Current issues in depression in Parkinson's disease. Am J Geriatr Psychiatry 7:110–118, 1999

Suggested Readings

Alexopoulos G, Meyers B, Young RC, et al: The course of geriatric depression with "reversible dementia": a controlled study. Am J Psychiatry 150:1693–1699, 1993

Blazer DG: Psychiatry and the oldest old. Am J Psychiatry 157:1915–1924, 2000

Blazer DG: Depression in Late Life, 3rd Edition. New York, Springer, 2002

Blazer DG: Depression in late life: review and commentary. J Gerontol A Biol Sci Med Sci 58:249–265, 2003

Blazer DG 2nd, Hybels CF: Origins of depression in later life. Psychol Med 35:1241–1252, 2005

Koenig HG, Meador KG, Cohen HJ, et al: Depression in elderly hospitalized patients with medical illness. Arch Intern Med 148:1929–1936, 1988

Krishnan KR, Goli V, Ellinwood EH, et al: Leukoencephalopathy in patients diagnosed as major depressive. Biol Psychiatry 23:519–522, 1988 [Erratum in: Biol Psychiatry 25(6):822, 1989]

Reynolds CF 3rd, Dew MA, Pollock BG, et al: Maintenance treatment of major depression in old age. N Engl J Med 354:1130–1138, 2006

Steffens DC, Payne ME, Greenberg DL, et al: Hippocampal volume and incident dementia in geriatric depression. Am J Geriatr Psychiatry 10:62–71, 2002

Taylor WS, Steffens DC, MacFall JR, et al: White matter hyperintensity progression and late-life depression outcomes. Arch Gen Psychiatry 60:1090–1096, 2003

CHAPTER 16

Bipolar Disorder in Late Life

John L. Beyer, M.D.

Bipolar disorder can be a severe, relapsing mental illness, and it shares characteristics with both major depressive disorder and schizophrenia. Like depressive disorders, bipolar disorder features recurrent episodes of altered mood that interfere with cognition and functioning. Like schizophrenia, it is a chronic disorder that often contains psychotic episodes and similar pathological findings. However, in contrast to late-life depression and schizophrenia, information about late-life bipolar disorder is relatively scarce (Bauer et al. 2002; Charney et al. 2003; Depp et al. 2005; Unutzer and Bruce 2002). Even basic facts, such as how age may affect the development or expression of bipolar disorder, where older adults with bipolar disorder live or access their health care, or how late-life bipolar disorder may affect social support, have been relatively lightly studied. Further, answers to elementary questions regarding such issues as the prevalence of late-life bipolar disorder and the best treatment practices are unclear (Charney et al. 2003; Unutzer and Bruce 2002).

Diagnosis

Bipolar disorder is a cycling illness that affects an individual's ability to regulate moods. Under the rubric of bipolar disorders are four main entities: bipolar I, bipolar II, cyclothymia, and bipolar not otherwise specified (NOS) (American Psychiatric Association 2000).

For a diagnosis of bipolar I disorder, the patient must have experienced at least one manic episode. A manic episode is defined as an alteration in mood that is euphoric, expansive, or irritable; lasts for at least 1 week; and occurs with three other associated symptoms (e.g., decreased need for sleep, increased energy, racing thoughts, pressured speech, increased behaviors that may have high likelihood for bad outcome). It is not necessary for a patient to have experienced a depressive episode to be diagnosed with bipolar disorder, although the vast majority of bipolar patients have experienced depression and many report it to be the most commonly experienced mood problem.

For a diagnosis of bipolar II disorder, the patient must have experienced one or more depressive episodes accompanied by at least one hypomanic episode. A hypomanic episode is defined as at least 4 days of altered mood (expansive, euphoric, irritable) occurring with at least three other associated symptoms (see previous paragraph).

Cyclothymia is defined as cycling moods that do not fully meet the criteria for either depression or mania. Bipolar NOS is defined as disorders with bipolar features that do not meet the criteria for specific bipolar disorders. For the most part, little is known about bipolar II, cyclothymia, or bipolar disorder NOS in late life, and therefore all information presented in this chapter will focus on bipolar I disorder unless noted otherwise.

Epidemiology and Clinical Presentation

Prevalence

The exact prevalence of bipolar disorder in late life is uncertain. Based on four large-scale studies that used very different sampling methods, the prevalence of bipolar disorder in the community has been generally reported to range from 0.08% to 0.5%. The Epidemiologic Catchment Area (ECA) study conducted in the early 1990s sampled 18,263 community-dwelling Americans at five sites to determine the prevalence of mental illnesses for those ages 15 years and older (Weissman et al. 1988). The ECA study found that bipolar disorder for adults ages 65 years and older had a 1-year prevalence range of 0.0%–0.5% with a cross-site mean of 0.1%. This was markedly lower than the prevalence among young (ages 18–44 years; 1.4%) and middle-age (ages 45–64 years; 0.4%) adults. Similarly, a large health maintenance organization (HMO) administrative database review containing almost 300,000 unique individuals found a prevalence of 0.25% for bipolar disorder in persons ages 65 years and older and a prevalence rate of 0.46% in adults ages 40–64 years (Unutzer et al. 1998). Hirschfeld et al. (2003) sent the Mood Disorder Questionnaire (a validated screening instrument for bipolar I and II disorders) to 127,000 people. For the 85,258 responders, the overall screen rate for bipolar disorder was 3.4%, but for adults ages 65 years and older, the screen rate was 0.5%. Finally, Klap et al. (2003) conducted a telephone survey of 9,585 households and found a prevalence rate of 0.08% for adults ages 65 years and older compared with 1.17% for adults ages 30–64 years. Interestingly, each of these surveys suggested that the prevalence of bipolar disorder declines with age or in aging cohorts.

Winokur (1975) was the first to propose the concept that manic patients may "burn out" after a finite number of episodes. In a retrospective study, Angst et al. (1973) described a finite number of episodes in patients with mania, suggesting that the illness may be self-limiting. However, in a later prospective study, Angst and Preisig (1995) followed 209 bipolar patients over a period of 40 years until a median age of 68. They found that manic episodes did not decrease with age and that many patients continued to have episodes into their 60s. It should be noted that the decline in prevalence rates with age in bipolar disorder is consistent with findings for other mental illnesses, such as depression and schizophrenia.

Because most of the large-scale prevalence surveys have excluded patients who were institutionalized in hospitals, nursing homes, or other residential treatment centers, critics have suggested that the prevalence data may underrepresent the true prevalence since older mentally ill patients are more likely to require institutionalized care. Two surveys of mental illness in nursing home patients found a prevalence of bipolar disorder of 3%–10% (Koenig and Blazer 1992; Tariot et al. 1993). Speer (1992) reported that bipolar disorder was present in 17.4% of residential psychiatric programs for older adults.

Chart reviews of inpatient admissions revealed prevalence rates of bipolar disorder among older adults in psychiatric inpatient treatment settings to be 4.7%–18.5% (see Depp and Jeste 2004 for a review of published surveys). The mean prevalence was 8.7%, though Depp et al. (2004) argued that this was likely to be an underestimation, because many of the inpatient surveys did not include bipolar depressed subjects or reported prevalence only for those whose bipolar disorder began after age 60 years. A study of Medicare patients admitted for a primary psychiatric diagnosis in the 1990–1991 calendar year found that of the 240,000 admissions, 6.7% were for bipolar disorder (compared with admission rates of 28.1% for unipolar depression and 5.7% for schizophrenia) (Ettner and Hermann 1998).

Surveys of two outpatient geriatric clinics found the prevalence of bipolar disorder in their outpatient population to be 2%–5% (Holroyd and Duryee 1997; Speer 1992), whereas a bipolar disorder prevalence of 25% was found among older adults treated at a community mental health center (Meeks and Murrell 1997).

In summary, the prevalence of bipolar disorder may depend in part on the diagnostic criteria or measurement used and on the population that is sampled. In general, community surveys show that bipolar disorder appears to decrease with age, a change consistent with the declines seen in other mental disorders. Yet the proportion of patients utilizing services (either inpatient or outpatient) appears to be the same as in younger populations. Further, there may be increasing utilization of institutional care with age.

Gender

Epidemiological studies in the United States have indicated that bipolar disorder is approximately equally common in men and women (American Psychiatric Association 2000). Depp and Jeste (2004) pooled 17 studies reporting various samples of late-life bipolar disorder and found that the weighted mean of elderly women with bipolar disorder was 69% (range 45%–89%). However, they noted that this percentage was similar to the gender ratio among older adults in the general population.

Comorbidity

Psychiatric Comorbidity

Psychiatric comorbidity is frequently seen in bipolar patients and has been a major point of discussion in the literature on bipolar disorder, yet there is very little information about its presence in late-life bipolar disorder. There is only a scattering of studies looking at substance abuse comorbidity, while individual reports (mostly regional or individual hospital-based data) are available for personality disorders, posttraumatic stress disorder (PTSD), and other anxiety disorders. There are no published reports on comorbid eating disorders or attention disorders, which have been found to be significant in surveys of mixed-age bipolar subjects.

Sajatovic et al. (2006) conducted a review of the national Veterans Health Administration database to examine the prevalence of dementia, substance abuse, PTSD, and other anxiety disorders in older bipolar patients. They identified 4,668 subjects with bipolar disorder (mean age 70 years), and of these, 4.5% had comorbid dementia, 5.4% were found to have PTSD, and 9.4% had an anxiety disorder.

The best evidence for the prevalence of comorbid substance abuse and bipolar disorders comes from the National Comorbidity Study, in which 61% of individuals with bipolar disorder also had a substance use disorder (Kessler et al. 1997). Unfortunately, this survey excluded adults older than age 55 years from the data set. Cassidy et al. (2001) reviewed rates of substance abuse in 392 patients who were hospitalized at a state psychiatric facility for bipolar disorder. Nearly 60% had some history of lifetime substance abuse (consistent with the finding of the National Comorbidity Study), but in the 51 patients over the age of 60 years, only 29% had a history of lifetime substance abuse. Supporting this finding of lower-than-expected substance abuse disorders in older bipolar patients are two small inpatient retrospective studies (Ponce et al. 1999; Sajatovic et al. 1996), a review of elderly bipolar utilizers of mental health system outpatient services (Depp et al. 2005), and a large review of the Veterans Health Administration database (Sajatovic et al. 2006). The reason for this unexpected finding is unclear.

Only one study has reviewed the presence of personality disorders together with co-occurring late-life mental disorders. Molinari and Marmion (1995) reviewed 76 geriatric outpatients and inpatients and found that 63% of the patients had one of the personality disorders. Of the 27 subjects with bipolar disorder, 70% were found to have a personality disorder. The authors suggest that the unusually high rate of personality disorders may be in part due to the difficult and chronic patterns of affective disorders.

Medical Comorbidity

Because of the high association that secondary mania has with late-life bipolar disorder, there have been more studies assessing the presence of comorbid medical problems—the most common being neurological illnesses—than studies assessing psychiatric comorbidities. Depp and Jeste (2004) reviewed eight studies that reported the presence of illness and noted that despite a wide variety in reporting strategies, the sample-weighted prevalence was 23.1%. Shulman et al. (1992) compared 50 geriatric patients hospitalized for mania to 50 age-matched patients hospitalized for unipolar depression. They found that the rates of neurological illness in manic patients were significantly higher (36% versus 8%), suggesting that neurological disease is a risk factor for the development of mania in late life.

Other comorbid medical disorders are also common in bipolar disorder and especially in late-life bipolar disorder. Regenold et al. (2002) reviewed the inpatient charts of 243 older (ages 50–74 years) psychiatric inpatients. They found that type II diabetes was present in 26% of those with bipolar disorder, which is a much higher rate than for unipolar depression, schizophrenia, and inpatient bipolar patients in other studies (9.9% in mixed-age inpatient sample; Cassidy et al. 1999).

Dementia

Dementia has become an increasing concern for older adults in general and possibly a special concern for older adults with bipolar disorder. Studies of four inpatient samples found that comorbid dementia was highly variable, ranging from 3% to 25% (Broadhead and Jacoby 1990; Himmelhoch et al. 1980; Ponce et al. 1999; Stone 1989). Sajatovic et al. (2006) reported dementia in 4.5% of veterans treated for bipolar disorder through the Veterans Affairs (VA) system. Comorbidity does not necessarily imply an association, which has been a particular concern for late-life bipolar disorder. Tsai et al. (2003) reported that 30.7% of the early-onset patients in his inpatient sample had Mini-Mental State Examination (MMSE) scores below 24. Furthermore, Dhingra and Rabins (1991) reviewed 25 elderly patients who had been hospitalized 5–7 years previously for manic episodes and found that 32% experienced a significant decline in their MMSE scores. Kocsis et al. (1993) followed 38 elderly bipolar patients treated with lithium and found that rates of cognitive and functional impairment were much higher than in the general population.

Mortality

Individuals with mental illness at all ages have higher mortality rates, from both natural and unnatural causes, than does the general population (Laursen et al. 2007). Dhingra and Rabins (1991) found that mortality rates among 25 elderly patients with bipolar disorder who had been hospitalized 5–7 years previously were higher than expected compared to population norms. However, Shulman et al. (1992) found that the mortality rate over a 10- to 15-year follow-up for elderly hospitalized bipolar patients was significantly higher than that of elderly hospitalized unipolar depressed patients (50% versus 20%), suggesting that mania appears to have a poorer prognosis and to be a more severe form of affective illness than unipolar depression.

In summary, psychiatric comorbidity is frequent in bipolar patients, but the prevalence of the comorbidities in older bipolar patients is relatively unknown. Substance abuse, the most common and best-reported comorbid condition in the literature, appears less commonly in older than younger patients with bipolar disorder. Lifetime history also appears less commonly. Dementia and poorer cognitive performance on neurological testing (see "Neurocognitive Testing" section later in this chapter) are possibly increased, or apparent earlier, in older adults with bipolar disorder. Medical comorbidity is also higher in older adults with bipolar disorder (Beyer et al. 2005), with special concern about neurological illness and diabetes. All of these problems may contribute to higher mortality rates for patients with bipolar disorder than for non–psychiatrically ill individuals and unipolar depressed patients.

Course

After reviewing studies that retrospectively looked at course prior to hospitalization, Goodwin and Jamison (1990) reported that depression was the initial episode more often in older adults than younger patients. Shulman and Post (1980) reviewed the course of 67 elderly bipolar patients whose first manic episode occurred around age 60 years. They described a group of patients who had a depressive episode as their index episode and then experienced a long latency period (mean 15 years) before the onset of mania. They hypothesized that this group may have underlying cerebral changes due to aging that convert them to mania. Other investigators have described a similar latency period of 10–20 years in a subgroup of patients between their first depressed episode and the onset of mania (Broadhead and Jacoby 1990; Shulman et al. 1992; Snowdon 1991; Stone 1989).

The symptom presentation in the elderly may differ somewhat from that of younger patients. Post (1968) and Spar et al. (1979) found that most elderly patients with bipolar disorder exhibited more mixed symptoms than the classic manic presentation. Also, a number of case reports have reported rapid-cycling patterns in older patients, though it is unclear if this is more or less common among geriatric patients (Camus et al. 1997; Conlon 1989; Gnam and Flint 1993; King et al. 1979).

As noted previously, Angst and Preisig (1995) followed 209 psychiatrically hospitalized patients with bipolar disorder over a 40-year period until a median age of 68. Of these patients, only 16% had fully recovered (defined as no episodes in the previous 5 years and a Global Assessment of Functioning [GAF] Scale score above 60) while 26% had no episodes and their GAF scores were below 60. The largest group (36%) had still experienced episodes within the previous 5 years, and another 16% exhibited a chronic course. Seven percent had committed suicide.

Interestingly, despite the high risk of suicide reported with aging and among individuals with bipolar disorder, the risk of suicide in late-life bipolar disorder appears be lower than expected. Tsai et al. (2002) studied suicide rates in Taiwan among patients with bipolar disorder and found that the highest risk was during the first 7–12 years after the onset of the illness and for individuals under age 35 years. Depp and Jeste (2004) suggests that older, early-onset bipolar patients may constitute a "survivor cohort." Young and Falk (1989) found that older patients with mania who need hospitalization tend to have a slower resolution of symptoms and a longer duration of hospitalization than do younger adult patients.

A study comparing health-related quality of life and functioning in elderly adults with bipolar disorder ($n=54$) and a non–psychiatrically ill group ($n=38$) found that even patients in remission from bipolar disorder had quality-of-life scores lower than those of the normal comparison group. Overall, bipolar disorder was associated with substantial disability, comparable to schizophrenia, and incomplete improvement in functioning even among those classified as remitters (Depp et al. 2006).

Similar to younger bipolar patients, older adults with bipolar disorder have a high use rate of mental health services. Sajatovic et al. (1996) found that older bipolar patients were hospitalized at the same rate as older patients with schizophrenia. Bartels et al. (2000) found that older adults with bipolar disorder used outpatient services four times as much as a similarly aged group of patients with unipolar depression. Brennan et al. (2002) found that older veterans with comorbid bipolar disorder and substance use disorders had an increased probability of mental health care services use and readmission. However, Depp et al. (2005) compared 2,903 elderly bipolar patients who received outpatient services with younger bipolar groups and found that elderly bipolar patients were less likely to use inpatient, outpatient, and emergency room psychiatric care, but they were more likely to use case management and conservator services. Overall, the elderly bipolar group had less substance use but more cognitive disorders and a lower global functioning than the younger bipolar groups.

Age at Onset

The mean age at onset for bipolar disorder is in the late teens to early 20s (Weissman et al. 1996). However, some researchers have divided bipolar disorder into early- and late-onset subtypes. The definition of late-onset has ranged from after ages 30–50 years in various studies (Hopkinson 1964; James 1977; Taylor and Abrams 1973). The *Diagnostic and Statistical Manual of Mental Disorders,* Fourth Edition, Text Revision (DSM-IV-TR; APA 2000) does not make such a distinction, and while there is some heuristic evidence supporting this division, there are differences in opinion as to the importance of making such a distinction.

In a study of 87 elderly subjects with late-life bipolar disorder, Depp et al. (2004) found few meaningful differences between early- and late-onset groups (onset after age 40 years), except for lower psychopathology in the late-onset group. However, Sajatovic et al. (2006) reviewed the VA database for 16,330 elderly individuals with bipolar disorder and found that a large majority had an earlier-onset bipolar illness, but age at onset suggested two different subgroups of older adults with bipolar disorder. Differences in populations (inpatient versus outpatient) and cohorts may account for these disparities.

While most studies have found bipolar disorder to be unimodal in distribution, a few studies have noted two peaks at the onset of mania, with the first occurring in the mid 20s and a second, smaller peak occurring closer to middle age, in the late 40s (Angst 1978; Goodwin and Jamison 1984; Petterson 1977). This bimodal distribution is more prominent in women, and the second peak is noted to occur around the time of menopause (Angst 1978; Petterson 1977; Sibisi 1990; Zis et al. 1979). Conversely, males have been noted to have an increased incidence of the onset of mania in old age, with a peak in the person's 70s (Spicer et al. 1973) or 80s (Sibisi 1990). Others have described a decline (D'Elia and Perris 1969; Loranger and Levine 1978; Mendlewicz et al. 1972; Taylor and Abrams 1973) or increase (Eagles and Whalley 1985; Spicer et al. 1973) in the incidence of mania with age and no bimodal distribution.

There are several explanations for possible age-of-onset difference. It has been postulated that this could be a marker for different etiologies of bipolar disorder or even treatment response. Two factors that have been the focus of studies are familial affective illness and neurological illness.

Several studies have suggested that patients with an early-onset illness may have an increased prevalence of close family members with affective disorders compared with subjects who had a later onset of illness (Baron et al. 1981; Hopkinson 1964; James 1977; Mendlewicz et al. 1972; Post 1968; Snowdon 1991; Stenstedt 1952; Taylor and Abrams 1973). It is argued that this would suggest a higher genetic loading for early-onset patients and/or a higher incidence of secondary bipolar disorder for late-onset patients. However, this issue is not clear because six other studies did not show any significant difference between early- and late-onset bipolar patients (Broadhead and Jacoby 1990; Carlson et al. 1977; Depp et al. 2004; Glasser and Rabins 1984; Hays et al. 1998; Tohen et al. 1994). It should be noted that even if the number of affectively ill relatives is higher in the early-onset group, the percentage of affectively ill relatives in the late-onset group is still considerable and corresponds to the 4%–22% generally cited for the relatives of manic patients (James 1977; Mendlewicz et al. 1972; Post 1968; Stenstedt 1952; Taylor and Abrams 1973).

The existence of a relationship between late-onset illness and neurological abnormalities is a much more consistent finding. Though the definition of neurological illness varied, three of the five studies assessing this showed significantly higher rates in the late-onset patients (Almeida and Fenner 2002; Tohen et al. 1994; Wylie et al. 1999), while the other two studies showed trends toward increased levels of neurological illness in late-onset patients (Broadhead and Jacoby 1990; Hays et al. 1998).

Late-onset subjects were also more likely to have a higher risk for mortality. Snowdon (1991) reviewed the admission data of 75 elderly bipolar subjects and found that the 13 patients with a known neurological disease had their first episode of mania after age 50 years. Cook et al. (1987) reported that 39 patients with neurological disease preceding the onset of mania had significantly later onsets, less family history of mood disorder, fewer depressive episodes, and more irritability and assaultive behavior during the manic episode. Himmelhoch et al. (1980) found the rate of concurrent neurological disease among elderly bipolar patients to be 46%.

Carlson et al. (1977) found that an early age at onset is not a factor in the variable course and prognosis of bipolar disorder. However, in a later study, Carlson et al. (2000) found that early-onset bipolar patients (first episode before age 21 years) experienced complete episode remission less frequently during the following 24 months than did later-onset (first episode after age 30 years) bipolar patients. They further found that early-onset bipolar subjects were more likely to be male, to have had childhood behavior disorders, to have substance abuse comorbidity, and to exhibit more paranoia in their psychotic features than late-onset bipolar subjects.

Neurocognitive Testing

There have been a few studies that have evaluated the neuropsychological performance among older bipolar patients. Depp et al. (2007) administered a clinical battery of neuropsychological tests to 67 older bipolar subjects, 150 older subjects with schizophrenia who had mild to moderate clinical symptoms, and 87 control subjects. Among clinically stable, middle-aged, and older outpatients, bipolar disorder was associated with substantial neurocognitive impairment, with a pattern that was somewhat distinct from that found in schizophrenia. Depp and colleagues specifically noted that deficits in the bipolar group were not related to severity or duration of psychiatric symptoms but were related to quality of life, suggesting that bipolar disorder often involves disabling and enduring cognitive impairments in older outpatients. Burt et al. (2000) compared inpatient elderly subjects with unipolar and bipolar depression. They found that older unipolar and bipolar patients did not differ in global measurements; on measures of delayed recall, younger bipolar subjects performed best and older bipolar subjects performed the worst.

Neuroimaging

Stroke

Compared with unipolar depression, mania following a stroke is relatively uncommon. However, a controlled study of patients with secondary mania showed that when manic symptoms are present, the right hemisphere of the brain (both cortical and subcortical areas) is more frequently the site of the lesion (Starkstein et al. 1987, 1991). Further research suggests that development of mania after right-sided lesions occurs more often when the basal region of the right temporal lobe is involved (Starkstein et al. 1990).

Volumetric Neuroimaging

Neuroimaging in mixed-age bipolar subjects is still a rising field, but as the literature has evolved, an emerging hypothesis for understanding bipolar disorder has developed, suggesting that affective instability may be the result of changes or altered processes in certain areas of the brain (Phillips 2006). There appears to be increased activity among the subcortical and limbic regions that make an initial assessment of emotive stimuli (amygdala, anterior insula), resulting in increased activity in regions associated with mood generation and decision processing of the emotional material (ventromedial and ventrolateral prefrontal cortices, ventral anterior cingulate gyrus). Finally, there is reduced activity in regions that regulate these responses and attentional processes (dorsomedial prefrontal cortices), causing the mood lability. Neuroimaging results specific to late-life bipolar disorders have been relatively limited, but the published studies have supported significant volumetric abnormalities in certain areas that are consistent with the overall theory presented above.

Volumetric studies of total brain volumes for patients with bipolar disorder have shown only limited changes. Young et al. (1999) compared 30 geriatric manic patients with control subjects but did not find any difference in the ventricular-brain ratios. They did note that bipolar subjects had greater cortical sulcal widening, which correlated with age at onset and age at first manic episode. Tanaka et al. (1982) suggested that atrophy may occur at an earlier age in bipolar subjects, despite the fact that cortical atrophy in their elderly bipolar subjects was similar to that of normal controls. Beyer et al. (2004a) also did not find any differences in total brain volume or lateral ventricular volumes between elderly bipolar subjects and controls; however, they did find a volume decrease in late-onset (after age 45 years) compared with early-onset bipolar subjects.

Other volumetric findings include smaller caudate (Beyer et al. 2004a) and larger hippocampal (Beyer et al. 2004b) volumes in patients with late-life bipolar disorder compared with controls. The latter finding appeared to be consistent with use of lithium, suggesting a role for neuroprotection.

Magnetic Resonance Imaging Hyperintensities

Possibly related to strokes, "hyperintense" signals viewed on T_2-weighted magnetic resonance imaging have been one of the earliest and most consistent neuroimaging findings in the study of bipolar disorder. Hyperintensities represent areas of neuronal cell death, though the mechanism by which this is done is unclear. Pathological examination has found that hyperintensities could characterize areas of arteriosclerotic disease, demyelination, loss of axons, arteriolar hyalinization, rarefaction, infarctions, and necrosis (Bradley et al. 1984; Braffman et al. 1988; Chimowitz et al. 1992; Fazekas et al. 1993; Fujikawa et al. 1997; George et al. 1986). Fujikawa et al. (1997) coined the term *silent cerebral ischemia* to refer to these hyperintensities. Electroencephalographic studies in patients with dementia suggest that white matter hyperintensities may result in a functional brain disconnection. Thus some researchers have suggested that for patients with mood disorders, hyperintensities may "disconnect" different pathways in the mood regulation circuits.

Dupont et al. (1987) were the first to report the presence of hyperintensities in bipolar patients, and most (Altshuler et al. 1995; Aylward et al. 1994; Botteron et al. 1995; Dupont et al. 1990, 1995; Figiel et al. 1991; Krabbendam et al. 2000; McDonald et al. 1991, 1999; Swayze et al. 1990), but not all (Brown et al. 1992; Strakowski et al. 1993), studies supported this finding. Because of differences in study groups and methodology, there is a wide range in frequency of T_2 hyperintensities found in bipolar subjects (5%–62%) and normal controls (0%–42%). However, in all but one study, the odds ratio was in the same direction and the overall effect size was highly significant (Bearden et al. 2001). Two meta-analyses reported similar findings with common odds ratios of 3.3 (Altshuler et al. 1995) and 3.29 (Videbech 1997), strongly supporting the relationship between hyperintensities and bipolar disorder. One of the researchers who did not find a relationship studied bipolar patients at the time of their first hospitalization, though he did find a trend toward the presence of hyperintensities (1.7 times higher rate) (Strakowski et al. 1993). Interestingly, this finding is not inconsistent with data from Aylward et al. (1994) and Hickie et al. (1995), who noted that the presence of hyperintensities was significant only in an older subgroup of bipolar patients (older than age 39 years), or Dupont et al. (1995), who noted a correlation of hyperintensities only in patients with mania onset after adolescence. Thus, increased age is related to the presence of hyperintensities, a finding not unexpected since this is also seen in normal aging populations as well as with subjects with unipolar depression.

The presence of hyperintensities not only is more common in patients with bipolar disorder compared with control subjects (Dupont et al. 1995) but remains significantly more common when medical risk factors (such as hypertension or vascular disease) are controlled for (Altshuler et al. 1995; Hickie et al. 1995; McDonald et al. 1999). Specific studies of bipolar disorder in late life have consistently found higher presence of hyperintensities in bipolar subjects than in controls. McDonald et al. (1991) examined elderly patients (older than age 50 years) with mania. He found no significant difference with respect to the presence of hyperintensities between the elderly patients with bipolar disorder and the control sample, yet the mean number of larger signal hyperintensities (>2.5 mm) was significantly higher in elderly patients with bipolar disorder. A more recent study by McDonald et al. (1999) in a mixed bipolar sample that included elderly patients found increased hyperintensities in the subependymal region, subcortical gray nuclei, and deep white matter, and de Asis et al. (2006) found increased hyperintensities in the frontal deep white matter in a group of older bipolar patients when compared with controls. This was especially prominent on the right side in the late-onset group.

The presence of hyperintensities may be especially important in late-life bipolar disorder because of their impact on treatment response and severity of illness. Data from studies on bipolar disorder are very limited, but it has been found that magnetic resonance imaging hyperintensities are associated with longer hospital stays

(Dupont et al. 1990) and more frequent rehospitalizations (McDonald et al. 1999). After studying a small sample ($n=9$), Robert Young (personal communication, February 2002) noted that the presence of periventricular hyperintensities is associated with less reduction in manic symptoms than in those without the hyperintensities over 3 weeks in a naturalistic treatment setting. Also, hyperintensities appear to be related to cognitive changes. Following a review of the literature, Bearden et al. (2001) concluded that hyperintensities play an increasing role in bipolar cognitive impairment with increasing age and chronicity of disorder and may be considered a risk modifier for cognitive dysfunction in bipolar disorder.

Differential Diagnosis

There are five potential presentations of patients with late-life bipolar disorder: 1) those who had an early-onset of bipolar disease and have now reached old age; 2) those who previously only experienced episodes of depression but have now switched to a manic episode; 3) those who have never had an affective illness but develop mania because of a specific medical or neurological event (e.g., head trauma, cerebrovascular accident, hyperthyroidism); 4) those who have never been recognized as having bipolar symptoms or who have been misdiagnosed with another disorder; and 5) those who have never had an affective illness but develop mania for unknown reasons. It is unknown how common each presentation may be, though personal experience has shown the most frequently encountered presentation to be of a patient who developed bipolar disorder earlier in life and is now seeking treatment. However, based on findings by Hirschfeld et al. (2003), it is not uncommon for the diagnosis of bipolar illness to have been missed previously.

Since the onset of bipolar disorder in late life is relatively uncommon, every patient who presents with a new onset of mania should have a good medical evaluation, with special emphasis on the neurological examination. Since older adults may be receiving a higher number of medications, these should be reviewed for possible temporal association. A laboratory workup consisting of a thyroid panel and basic tests should also be completed. Finally, consideration should be given to neuroimaging, especially if the presentation is associated with psychosis.

Treatment

Treatment of bipolar disorder is often challenging for many reasons. In addition to the challenge of medication management in older adults, elderly bipolar patients often have incomplete response, recurrent episodes, potentially severe psychopathology, and higher mortality rates. Further, the disease itself tends to cause problems with poor insight and poor compliance with treatment. Finally, there are limited data on use of medications and psychotherapies for older bipolar patients. Many of the treatment practices are based on results from clinical trials in younger populations that have been adapted for geriatric use.

Lithium

Lithium has traditionally been identified as the gold standard for treatment of bipolar disorder and has been widely prescribed to geriatric bipolar patients (Shulman et al. 2003; Umapathy et al. 2000). However, there have been no placebo-controlled efficacy trials in geriatric patients. Studies that have focused on geriatric patients have been primarily retrospective and naturalistic. Young et al. (2004) reviewed four studies (Chen et al. 1999; Himmelhoch et al. 1980; Schaffer and Garvey 1984; van der Velde et al. 1970) that included more than 10 elderly patients in their reports. Overall, 66% of the patients improved with lithium treatment, though concentrations varied widely (0.3–2.0 mEq/L). The recommended lithium level for acute mania in geriatric patients is unclear. Case series have suggested that elderly patients may respond to lower lithium levels (0.5–0.8 mEq/L) than what is recommended for younger adults (Chen et al. 1999; Prien et al. 1972; Roose et al. 1979), while other reports have not found a difference (DeBattista and Schatzberg 2006; Young et al. 1992).

Special care must be taken in dosing geriatric patients with lithium. With aging, the renal clearance of lithium decreases and the elimination half-life increases (Foster 1992; Shulman et al. 1987; Sproule et al. 2000). Further, commonly prescribed medications to the elderly, such as thiazide diuretics, nonsteroidal anti-inflammatory agents, and angiotension-converting enzyme inhibitors, can increase lithium concentrations. Other medications, such as theophylline, can decrease lithium concentrations. Finally, since lithium use can contribute to hypothyroidism and a decline in renal clearance, lithium should be used with caution in patients with kidney problems or thyroid disorders. Because of this, lithium toxicity in elderly patients is not uncommon (Foster 1992). Commonly reported adverse effects of lithium in the elderly include cognitive impairment, ataxia, urinary frequency, weight gain, edema, tremor, and worsening of psoriasis and arthritis. Because of adverse effects (including neurotoxicity) that can occur even at therapeutic levels, appropriate lithium serum levels in the elderly are largely determined by medical status, frailty, and conservative dosing (Sajatovic et al. 2005b; Young et al. 2004).

Anticonvulsants

Physicians have increasingly been prescribing anticonvulsants for the treatment of bipolar disorder. Since 1993, three anticonvulsants have been approved by the U.S. Food and Drug Administration (FDA) to treat bipolar disorder: valproate, carbamazepine, and lamotrigine. For information regarding the anticonvulsants, the literature is limited to case reports and the inclusion of some elderly patients in larger studies.

Valproate

The past decade has seen a marked increase in the prescription of valproate for bipolar disorder, especially for the elderly. In 1999, Oshima and Higuchi proposed that lithium be the first choice in treatment guidelines for geriatric bipolar disorder. However, Shulman et al. (2003) noted that prescriptions of valproate for elderly patients with bipolar disorder increased in the late 1990s while prescriptions of lithium decreased, such that valproate is now the most prescribed medication treatment for elderly persons with bipolar disorder, despite there being no published data comparing valproate with placebo or lithium in the elderly.

Similar to the published research on lithium, only retrospective and open-label studies of valproate in the geriatric population have been published. Young et al. (2004) reviewed the five published studies that each included more than 10 elderly manic subjects (Chen et al. 1999; Kando et al. 1996; Niedermier and Nasrallah 1998; Noaguil et al. 1998; Puryear et al. 1995). They found that 59% of the combined sample met the various improvement criteria. Again, however, the dose concentrations varied widely at 25–120 μg/mL. The recommended blood level concentration for valproate in the general population is 50–120 μg/mL (Bowden 2002), and Chen et al. (1999) found that for manic elderly patients, those who had blood level concentrations from 65–90 μg/mL improved more than patients with lower concentrations.

As patients age, the elimination half-life of valproate may be prolonged and the free fraction of plasma valproate increases. The clinical significance of this is unknown, although it should be noted that usual laboratory tests measure the total valproate level. Thus, the reported level may underrepresent the actual dose available to the brain in geriatric patients (Sajatovic et al. 2005b; Young et al. 2004). Common medications taken concurrently may also influence the level of valproate: aspirin can increase the valproate free fraction, and phenytoin and carbamazepine may decrease the valproate level. In turn, valproate may affect the effects of other medications. It can inhibit the metabolism of lamotrigine so that the dose of lamotrigine may need to be lowered in order to minimize side effects. Valproate also may increase the unbound fraction of warfarin; coagulation parameters should therefore be monitored in patients on anticoagulation therapy (Panjehshahin et al. 1991).

The most common side effects associated with valproate are nausea, somnolence, and weight gain. Less common side effects that may be particularly important to geriatric patients are the possibility of hair thinning, thrombocytopenia, hepatotoxicity, and pancreatitis (the latter two are less likely to occur with age) (Bowden et al. 2002). It also should be noted that valproate is available in sprinkle and liquid formulations for patients who have difficulty swallowing. In addition, Regenold and Prasad (2001) have reported on the intravenous use of valproate in three geriatric patients.

Carbamazepine

Carbamazepine was approved for the treatment of bipolar mania in 1996, and the extended release formulation was approved in 2005. Some researchers have suggested that carbamazepine may be the preferred mood-stabilizing agent (in contrast to lithium) for patients with secondary mania (Evans et al. 1995; Sajatovic 2002); however, there is very little information on the use of carbamazepine (in either preparation) for the elderly bipolar patient. Okuma and colleagues (1990) noted that seven elderly manic patients were included in a larger sample of 50 treated with carbamazepine in a double-blind study that showed good efficacy.

Before initiating carbamazepine, the physician should check liver enzymes, electrolytes, and complete blood cell count. Because carbamazepine can also affect the heart's rhythm, an electrocardiogram should be considered. In elderly patients, carbamazepine may be started at 100 mg either once or twice daily and gradually increased every 3–5 days to 400–800 mg/day (McDonald et al. 2000). Target serum levels are between 6 and12 μg/L.

Carbamazepine is metabolized in the liver by cytochrome P450 (CYP) enzyme 3A4/5. Because carbamazepine can induce its own metabolism, dose increases may need to be adjusted in the first 1–2 months. Further, carbamazepine clearance is decreased in an age-dependent manner, presumably due to a reduction in CYP 3A4/5 metabolism, suggesting (Battino et al. 2003) that elderly patients may require lower doses compared with younger patients to achieve similar blood levels. Notably, carbamazepine may also alter the pharmacokinetics of other medications, including oral hormones, calcium channel blockers, cimetidine, terfenadine, and erythromycin (Sajatovic 2002).

Possible adverse effects associated with carbamazepine include sedation, ataxia, nystagmus/blurred vision, leukopenia, hyponatremia (secondary to the syndrome of inappropriate antidiuretic hormone secretion [SIADH]) and agranulocytosis. The U.S. Food and Drug Administration ([FDA] 2008) has recommended that patients of Asian ancestry have a genetic blood test to identify an inherited variant of the gene *HLA=B*1502* (found almost exclusively in people of Asian ancestry) before starting therapy. Patients testing positive should not be treated with carbamazepine.

Lamotrigine

A recent addition to the treatment of bipolar disorder is the anticonvulsant lamotrigine. It was approved by the FDA in 2003 for the maintenance phase of bipolar disorder. Sajatovic et al. (2005a) conducted a retrospective analysis of two placebo-controlled, double-blind clinical trials for maintenance therapy in bipolar disorder focusing on 98 subjects who were age 55 years or older. They found that, similar to the parent study, lamotrigine significantly delayed the time to intervention for any mood episode, while lithium and placebo did not. In a subanalysis of the type of mood episode that was more likely to recur, the authors found that lamotrigine was significantly more effective than lithium and placebo at increasing time to intervention for depressive recurrences, but lithium performed much better in increasing time to intervention for manic episodes. Overall, the authors found that lamotrigine was well tolerated (compared with lithium) by the older bipolar patients and no increased incidence of rash was noted (Sajatovic et al. 2007). A small case series (Robillard and Conn 2002) of five female geriatric bipolar patients with depressive episodes suggested good efficacy when lamotrigine was used as an augmenting agent as well.

Lamotrigine is metabolized in the liver and eliminated through the hepatic glucuronide conjugation. There are some minor decreases in hepatic glucuronidation with aging, though the impact of this on dosing lamotrigine to the elderly is not thought to be significant (Hussein and Posner 1997; Posner et al. 1991). Overall, lamotrigine is well tolerated, though serious skin rashes (Stevens-Johnson syndrome) have been reported. It has been suggested that lamotrigine may have fewer negative effects on cognition than other anticonvulsant medications, which may be important for some geriatric patients (Aldenkamp et al. 2003).

Antidepressants

Antidepressants are frequently prescribed for the treatment of bipolar depression in the elderly (Beyer et al. 2008), although the use of antidepressants in bipolar disorder is a point of continued concern among psychiatrists (Ghaemi et al. 2003). Three issues highlight the controversy. First, the literature is ambiguous as to the efficacy of antidepressants in bipolar depression. Second, antidepressants have the potential to induce a manic episode. Third, antidepressants may also induce a rapid cycling course. Thase and Denko (2008) have reviewed the general literature, focusing especially on two large clinical trials from the Stanley Foundation and the National Institute of Mental Health (Systematic Treatment Enhancement for Bipolar Disorders [STEP-BD]) that have attempted to clarify the benefits and risks of antidepressant use in bipolar depression. The results of both trials did not show that antidepressant augmentation of mood stabilizers distinguished itself as more effective than placebo or the use of a second mood stabilizer. However, possible benefit was noted for certain subgroups. On the basis of the data, the authors were neither able to recommend the use of antidepressants nor to conclude that antidepressants should be avoided (Thase 2007).

Given these limitations, the American Psychiatric Association (2002) has maintained its recommendations that primary treatment of bipolar depression should be with a mood stabilizer and that antidepressant augmentation of the mood stabilizer may be considered if there is limited or no response.

There are no specific studies of the use of antidepressants in geriatric populations. Young et al. (2003) conducted a retrospective study of elderly inpatients who had antidepressant-induced mania. They found tricyclic antidepressants were more likely than others to induce manias in late life, suggesting the use of selective serotonin reuptake inhibitors may be preferable in the elderly.

Antipsychotic Agents

The atypical antipsychotic agents are increasingly being used for the treatment of various phases of bipolar disorder. Olanzapine, risperidone, quetiapine, ziprasidone, and aripiprazole are currently approved by the FDA for the treatment of acute mania; olanzapine/fluoxetine and quetiapine are approved for the treatment of acute depression; and olanzapine and aripiprazole are approved for the treatment of the maintenance phase. However, there are limited data in the geriatric population for their efficacy.

Beyer et al. (2001) reported on a pooled subanalysis of three double-blind, placebo-controlled acute bipolar mania clinical trials with olanzapine, focusing on subjects older than age 50 years. Compared with placebo, olanzapine was found to be efficacious for the treatment of acute mania without any significant change in the side-effect profile. Information on quetiapine, risperidone, clozapine, ziprasidone, and aripiprazole is much more limited. Case reports and open-label studies in geriatric bipolar patient treatment are published for quetiapine (Madhusoodanan et al. 2000), risperidone (Madhusoodanan et al. 1995, 1999), and clozapine (Frye et al. 1996; Shulman et al. 1997). No published reports are currently available for ziprasidone or aripiprazole.

In general, a lower-dose strategy in the elderly has been recommended for most atypical antipsychotics (Alexopoulos et al. 2004), though this may be less of a concern in the acute state. A major concern of atypical antipsychotic use is the potential risk of metabolic abnormalities such as obesity, diabetes, and dyslipidemia. This may be less of a concern for elderly patients because they have less propensity for weight gain and other metabolic effects associated with atypical antipsychotics (Meyer 2002). In 2006, a black-box warning was added to each of the atypical antipsychotic agents, warning about the use of these agents in the elderly. In studies associated with treatment of psychosis in dementia, these medications carried an increased risk of death. Presumably the risk is for cardiovascular incidents, although no information is available on the incidence of these in late-life bipolar disorder.

Electroconvulsive Therapy

Electroconvulsive therapy (ECT) has long been known to be effective for the treatment of bipolar disorder. However, there are very limited data on the use of ECT in elderly bipolar patients, especially when compared with the literature on ECT for unipolar depression. McDonald and Thompson (2001) reported on a case series of three elderly manic patients who also had some dementia and were resistant to pharmacotherapy but did respond to ECT treatment. Little et al. (2004) reported on a case series of depressed patients that included five elderly bipolar depressed patients treated with bifrontal ECT. They found this method could be effective, although a third experienced cognitive side effects.

Key Points

- As with other mental illnesses, the prevalence of bipolar disorder decreases with age. However, bipolar disorder in late life does continue to be a frequent cause for admission to psychiatric inpatient facilities and disruption of patients' lives.
- The mortality rate for older adults with bipolar disorder is significantly higher than that for the general population and for patients with unipolar depression.
- The onset of bipolar disorder at a later age may be associated with fewer genetic associations and more neurological illnesses.
- Treatment guidelines for late-life bipolar disorder are based primarily on case reports and extrapolation from bipolar treatment in younger adults. As in other geriatric treatment recommendations, the maxim "start low and go slow" is applicable to late-life bipolar treatment.
- Elderly patients may require lower doses of lithium because of decreased renal clearance.

References

Aldenkamp AP, De Krom M, Reijs R: Newer antiepileptic drugs and cognitive issues. Epilepsia 44 (suppl 4):21–29, 2003

Alexopoulos GS, Streim J, Carpenter D, et al: Using antipsychotic agents in older patients. J Clin Psychiatry 65 (suppl 2):5–99, 2004

Almeida OP, Fenner S: Bipolar disorder: similarities and differences between patients with illness onset before and after 65 years of age. Int Psychogeriatr 14:311–322, 2002

Altshuler LL, Curran JG, Hauser P, et al: T2 hyperintensities in bipolar disorder: magnetic resonance imaging comparison and literature meta-analysis. Am J Psychiatry 152:1139–1144, 1995

American Psychiatric Association: Diagnostic and Statistical Manual of Mental Disorders, 4th Edition, Text Revision. Washington, DC, American Psychiatric Association, 2000

American Psychiatric Association: Practice guideline for the treatment of patients with bipolar disorder (revision). Am J Psychiatry 159 (4 suppl):1–50, 2002

Angst J: The course of affective disorders, II: typology of bipolar manic-depressive illness. Arch Psychiatr Nervenkr 226:65–73, 1978

Angst J, Preisig M: Course of a clinical cohort of unipolar, bipolar and schizoaffective patients: results of a prospective study from 1959 to 1985. Schweiz Arch Neurol Psychiatr 146:5–16, 1995

Angst J, Baastrup P, Grof P, et al: The course of monopolar depression and bipolar psychoses. Psychiatr Neurol Neurochir 76:489–500, 1973

Aylward EH, Roberts-Twillie JV, Barta PE, et al: Basal ganglia volumes and white matter hyperintensities in patients with bipolar disorder. Am J Psychiatry 151:687–693, 1994

Baron M, Mendlewicz J, Klotz J: Age-of-onset and genetic transmission in affective disorders. Acta Psychiatr Scand 64:373–380, 1981

Bartels S, Forester B, Miles K, et al: Mental health service use by elderly patients with bipolar disorder and unipolar major depression. Am J Geriatr Psychiatry 8:160–166, 2000

Battino D, Croci D, Rossini A, et al: Serum carbamazepine concentrations in elderly patients: a case-matched pharmacokinetic evaluation based on therapeutic drug monitoring data. Epilepsia 44:923–929, 2003

Bauer M, Unutzer J, Pincus HA, et al: Bipolar disorder. Ment Health Serv Res 4:225–229, 2002

Bearden CE, Hoffman KM, Cannon TD: The neuropsychology and neuroanatomy of bipolar affective disorder: a critical review. Bipolar Disord 3:106–150, 2001

Beyer JL, Siegal A, Kennedy JS, et al: Olanzapine, divalproex, and placebo treatment non-head-to-head comparisons of older adult acute mania. Presented at the annual meeting of the International Psychogeriatric Association, Nice, France, September 2001

Beyer JL, Kuchibhatla M, Payne M, et al: Caudate volume measurement in older adults with bipolar disorder. Int J Ger Psychiatry 19:109–114, 2004a

Beyer JL, Kuchibhatla M, Payne ME, et al: Hippocampal volume measurement in older adults with bipolar disorder. Am J Ger Psychiatry 12:613–620, 2004b

Beyer JL, Kuchibhatla M, Gersing K, et al: Medical comorbidity in an outpatient bipolar clinical population. Neuropsychopharmacology 30:401–404, 2005

Beyer JL, Burchitt B, Gersing K, et al: Patterns of pharmacotherapy and treatment response in elderly adults with bipolar disorder. Psychopharmacol Bull 41:102–114, 2008

Botteron KN, Vannier MW, Geller B, et al: Preliminary study of magnetic resonance imaging characteristics in 8- to 16-year-olds with mania. J Am Acad Child Adolesc Psychiatry 34:742–749, 1995

Bowden CL, Lawson DM, Cunningham M, et al: The role of divalproex in the treatment of bipolar disorder. Psychiatr Ann 32:742–750, 2002

Bradley WG, Waluch V, Brant-Zawadzki M, et al: Patchy, periventricular white matter lesions in the elderly: a common observation during NMR imaging. Noninvasive Medical Imaging 1:35–41, 1984

Braffman BH, Zimmerman RA, Trojanowski JQ, et al: Brain MR: pathologic correlation with grass and histopathology, II: hyperintense white-matter foci in the elderly. AJR Am J Roentgenol 151:559–566, 1988

Brennan P, Nichols K, Moos R: Long-term use of VA mental health services by older patients with substance use disorders. Psychiatr Serv 53:836–841, 2002

Broadhead J, Jacoby R: Mania in old age: a first prospective study. Int J Geriatr Psychiatry 5:215–222, 1990

Brown FW, Lewine RJ, Hudgins PA, et al: White matter hyperintensity signals in psychiatric and nonpsychiatric subjects. Am J Psychiatry 149:620–625, 1992

Burt T, Prudic J, Peyser S, et al: Learning and memory in bipolar and unipolar major depression: effects of aging. Neuropsychiatry Neuropsychol Behav Neurol 13:246–253, 2000

Camus V, de Mendonca Lima CA, Antonioli D, et al: Rapid-cycling affective disorder in the elderly: clinical subtype or specific course of manic-depressive illness? J Geriatr Psychiatry Neurol 10:105–110, 1997

Carlson GA, Davenport YB, Jamison K: A comparison of outcome in adolescent- and later-onset bipolar manic depressive illness. Am J Psychiatry 134:919–922, 1977

Carlson GA, Bromet EJ, Sievers S: Phenomenology and outcome of subjects with early and adult-onset psychotic mania. Am J Psychiatry 157:213–219, 2000

Cassidy F, Ahearn E, Carroll BJ: Elevated frequency of diabetes mellitus in hospitalized manic-depressive patients. Am J Psychiatry 156:1417–1420, 1999

Cassidy F, Ahearn P, Carroll B: Substance abuse in bipolar disorder. Bipolar Disord 3:181–188, 2001

Charney DS, Reynolds CF 3rd, Lewis L, et al: Depression and Bipolar Support Alliance consensus statement on the unmet needs in diagnosis and treatment of mood disorders in late life. Arch Gen Psychiatry 60:664–672, 2003

Chen ST, Altshuler LL, Melnyk KA, et al: Efficacy of lithium vs. valproate in the treatment of mania in the elderly: a retrospective study. J Clin Psychiatry 60:181–185, 1999

Chimowitz MI, Estes ML, Furlan AJ, et al: Further observations on the pathology of subcortical lesions identified on magnetic resonance imaging. Arch Neurol 49:747–752, 1992

Conlon P: Rapid cycling mood disorder in the elderly. J Geriatr Psychiatry Neurol 2:106–108, 1989

Cook BL, Shukla S, Hoff AL, et al: Mania with associated organic factors. Acta Psychiatr Scand 76:674–677, 1987

de Asis JM, Greenwald BS, Alexopoulos GS, et al: Frontal signal hyperintensities in mania in old age. Am J Geriatr Psychiatry 14:598–604, 2006

DeBattista C, Schatzberg AF: Current psychotropic dosing and monitoring guidelines. Primary Psychiatry 13(6):61–81, 2006

D'Elia G, Perris C: Suicide attempts in bipolar and unipolar depressed psychotics. Arch Gen Psychiatry 28:656–658, 1969

Depp CA, Jeste DV: Bipolar disorder in older adults: a critical review. Bipol Disord 6:343–367, 2004

Depp CA, Jin H, Mohamed S, et al: Bipolar disorder in middle-aged and elderly adults: is age of onset important? J Nerv Ment Dis 192:796–799, 2004

Depp CA, Lindamer LA, Folsom DP, et al: Differences in clinical features and mental health service use in bipolar disorder across the lifespan. Am J Geriatr Psychiatry 13:290–298, 2005

Depp CA, Davis CE, Mittal D, et al: Health-related quality of life and functioning of middle-aged and elderly adults with bipolar disorder. J Clin Psychiatry 67:215–221, 2006

Depp CA, Moore DJ, Sitzer D, et al: Neurocognitive impairment in middle-aged and older adults with bipolar disorder: comparison to schizophrenia and normal comparison subjects. J Affect Disord 101:201–209, 2007

Dhingra U, Rabins PV: Mania in the elderly: a 5–7 year follow-up. J Am Geriatr Soc 39:581–583, 1991

Dupont RM, Jernigan TL, Gillin JC, et al: Subcortical signal hyperintensities in bipolar patients detected by MRI. Psychiatry Res 21:357–358, 1987

Dupont RM, Jernigan TL, Butters N, et al: Subcortical abnormalities detected in bipolar affective disorder using magnetic resonance imaging: clinical and neuropsychological significance. Arch Gen Psychiatry 47:55–59, 1990

Dupont RM, Jernigan TL, Heindel W, et al: Magnetic resonance imaging and mood disorders: localization of white matter and other subcortical abnormalities. Arch Gen Psychiatry 52:747–755, 1995

Eagles JM, Whalley LJ: Ageing and affective disorders: the age at first onset of affective disorders in Scotland, 1969–1978. Br J Psychiatry 147:180–187, 1985

Ettner S, Hermann R: Inpatient psychiatric treatment of elderly Medicare beneficiaries. Psychiatr Serv 49:1173–1179, 1998

Evans DL, Byerly MJ, Greer RA: Secondary mania: diagnosis and treatment. J Clin Psychiatry 56 (suppl 3):31–37, 1995

Fazekas R, Kleimert R, Offenbacher H, et al: Pathologic correlates of incidental MRI white matter hyperintensities. Neurology 3:1683–1689, 1993

Figiel GS, Krishnan KR, Rao VP, et al: Subcortical hyperintensities on brain magnetic resonance imaging: a comparison of normal and bipolar subjects. J Neuropsychiatry 3:18–22, 1991

Foster JR: Use of lithium in elderly psychiatric patients: a review of the literature. Lithium 3:77–93, 1992

Frye MA, Altshuler LL, Bitran JA: Clozapine in rapid cycling bipolar disorder. J Clin Psychopharmacol 16:87–90, 1996

Fujikawa T, Yanai I, Yamawaki S: Psychosocial stressors in patients with major depression and silent cerebral infarction. Stroke 28:1123–1125, 1997

George AE, de Leon M, Kalmin A, et al: Lucoencepholopathy in normal and pathologic aging, II: MRI of brain lucencies. Am J Neuroradiology 7:567–570, 1986

Ghaemi SN, Hsu DJ, Soldani F, et al: Antidepressants in bipolar disorder: the case for caution. Bipolar Disord 5:421–433, 2003

Glasser M, Rabins P: Mania in the elderly. Age Ageing 13:210–213, 1984

Gnam W, Flint AJ: New onset rapid cycling bipolar disorder in an 87 year old woman. Can J Psychiatry 38:324–326, 1993

Goodwin FK, Jamison KR: The natural course of manic depressive illness, in Neurobiology of Mood Disorders. Edited by Post RM, Ballenger JC. Baltimore, MD, Williams & Wilkens, 1984, pp 20–37

Goodwin FK, Jamison KR: Manic-Depressive Illness. New York, Oxford University Press, 1990

Hays JC, Krishnan KR, George LK, et al: Age of first onset of bipolar disorder: demographic, family history, and psychosocial correlates. Depress Anxiety 7:76–82, 1998

Hickie I, Scott E, Mitchell P, et al: Subcortical hyperintensities on magnetic resonance imaging: clinical correlates and prognostic significance in patients with severe depression. Biol Psychiatry 37:151–160, 1995

Himmelhoch J, Neil J, May S, et al: Age, dementia, dyskinesias, and lithium response. Am J Psychiatry 137:941–945, 1980

Hirschfeld RM, Lewis L, Vornik LA: Perceptions and impact of bipolar disorder: how far have we really come? Results of the national depressive and manic-depressive association 2000 survey of individuals with bipolar disorder. J Clin Psychiatry 64:161–174, 2003

Holroyd S, Duryee JJ: Characteristics of persons utilizing a geriatric psychiatry outpatient clinic. J Geriatr Psychiatry Neurol 10:136–141, 1997

Hopkinson G: A genetic study of affective illness in patients over 50. Br J Psychiatry 110:244–254, 1964

Hussein Z, Posner J: Population pharmacokinetics of lamotrigine monotherapy in patients with epilepsy: retrospective analysis of routine monitoring data. Br J Clin Pharmacol 43:457–465, 1997

James NM: Early- and late-onset bipolar affective disorder: a genetic study. Arch Gen Psychiatry 34:715–717, 1977

Judd LL, Akiskal HS, Schettler PJ, et al: The long-term natural history of the weekly symptomatic status of bipolar I disorder. Arch Gen Psychiatry 59:530–537, 2002

Judd LL, Akiskal HS, Schettler PJ, et al: A prospective investigation of the natural history of the long-term weekly symptomatic status of bipolar II disorder. Arch Gen Psychiatry 60:261–269, 2003

Kando JC, Tohen M, Castillo J, et al: The use of valproate in an elderly population with affective symptoms. J Clin Psychiatry 57:238–240, 1996

Kessler RC, Rubinow DR, Holmes C, et al: The epidemiology of DSM-III-R bipolar I disorder in a general population survey. Psychol Med 27:1079–1089, 1997

King DJ, Salem SA, Meimary NS: A 48-hour periodic manic-depressive illness presenting in late life. Br J Psychiatry 135:190–191, 1979

Klap R, Unroe KT, Unutzer J: Caring for mental illness in the United States: a focus on older adults. Am J Geriatr Psychiatry 11:517–524, 2003

Kocsis JH, Shaw ED, Stokes PE, et al: Neuropsychologic effects of lithium discontinuation. J Clin Psychopharmacol 13:268–276, 1993

Koenig HG, Blazer DG: Epidemiology of geriatric affective disorders. Clin Geriatr Med 8:235–251, 1992

Krabbendam L, Honig A, Wiersma J, et al: Cognitive dysfunctions and white matter lesions in patients with bipolar disorder in remission. Acta Psychiatr Scand 101:274–280, 2000

Laursen TM, Munk-Olsen T, Nordentoft M, et al: Increased mortality among patients admitted with major psychiatric disorders: a register-based study comparing mortality in unipolar depressive disorder, bipolar affective disorder, schizoaffective disorder, and schizophrenia. J Clin Psychiatry 68:899–907, 2007

Little JD, Atkins MR, Munday J, et al: Bifrontal electroconvulsive therapy in the elderly: a 2-year retrospective. J ECT 20:139–141, 2004

Loranger A, Levine PM: Age at onset of bipolar affective illness. Arch Gen Psychiatry 35:1345–1348, 1978

Madhusoodanan S, Brenner R, Araujo L, et al: Efficacy of risperidone treatment for psychoses associated with schizophrenia, schizoaffective disorder, bipolar disorder, or senile dementia in 11 geriatric patients: a case series. J Clin Psychiatry 56:514–518, 1995

Madhusoodanan S, Brecher M, Brenner R, et al: Risperidone in the treatment of elderly patients with psychotic disorders. Am J Geriatr Psychiatry 7:132–138, 1999

Madhusoodanan S, Brenner R, Alcantra A: Clinical experience with quetiapine in elderly patients with psychotic disorders. J Geriatr Psychiatry Neurol 13:28–32, 2000

McDonald WM: Epidemiology, etiology, and treatment of geriatric mania. J Clin Psychiatry 61 (suppl 13):3–11, 2000

McDonald WM, Thompson TR: Treatment of mania in dementia with electroconvulsive therapy. Psychopharmacol Bull 35:72–82, 2001

McDonald WM, Krishnan KR, Doraiswamy PM, et al: Occurrence of subcortical hyperintensities in elderly subjects with mania. Psychiatric Res 40:211–220, 1991

McDonald WM, Tupler LA, Marsteller FA, et al: Hyperintense lesions on magnetic resonance images in bipolar disorder. Biol Psychiatry 45:965–971, 1999

Meeks S, Murrell SA: Mental illness in late life: socioeconomic conditions, psychiatric symptoms, and adjustment of long-term sufferers. Psychol Aging 12:296–308, 1997

Mendlewicz J, Fieve RR, Rainer JD, et al: Manic-depressive illness: a comparative study of patients with and without a family history. Br J Psychiatry 120:523–530, 1972

Meyer JM: A retrospective comparison of weight, lipid, and glucose changes between risperidone- and olanzapine-treated inpatients: metabolic outcomes after 1 year. J Clin Psychiatry 63:425–433, 2002

Molinari V, Marmion J: Relationship between affective disorders and axis II diagnoses in geropsychiatric patients. J Geriatr Psychiatry Neurol 8:61–64, 1995

Niedermier JA, Nasrallah HA: Clinical correlates of response to valproate in geriatric inpatients. Ann Clin Psychiatry 10:165–168, 1998

Noagiul S, Narayan M, Nelson CJ: Divalproex treatment of mania in elderly patients. Am J Geriatr Psychiatry 6:257–262, 1998

Okuma T, Yamashita I, Takahashi R, et al: Comparison of the antimanic efficacy of carbamazepine and lithium carbonate by double-blind controlled study. Pharmacopsychiatry 23:143–150, 1990

Oshima A, Higuchi T: Treatment guidelines for geriatric mood disorders. Psychiatry Clin Neurosci 53 (suppl 3):26S–31S, 1999

Panjehshahin MR, Bowman CJ, Yates MS: Effect of valproic acid, its unsaturated metabolites and some structurally related fatty acids on the binding of warfarin and dansylsacrosine to human albumin. Biochem Pharmacol 41:1227–1233, 1991

Petterson U: Manic-depressive illness: a clinical, social and genetic study. Acta Psychiatrica Scandinavica 269:1–93, 1977

Phillips ML: The neural basis of mood dysregulation in bipolar disorder. Cognit Neuropsychiatry 11:233–249, 2006

Ponce H, Kunik M, Molinari V, et al: Divalproex sodium treatment in elderly male bipolar patients. J Geriatr Drug Therapy 12:55–63, 1999

Posner J, Holdrich T, Crome P: Comparison of lamotrigine pharmacokinetics in young and elderly healthy volunteers. J Pharm Med 1:121–128, 1991

Post F: The factor of ageing in affective illness, in Recent Developments in Affective Disorders, Special Publication 2. Edited by Coppen A, Walk A. London, Royal Medico-Psychological Association, 1968, pp. 105–116

Prien RF, Caffey EM, Klett CJ: Relationship between serum lithium level and clinical response in acute mania treated with lithium. Br J Psychiatry 120:409–414, 1972

Puryear LJ, Kunik ME, Workman R: Tolerability of divalproex sodium in elderly psychiatric patients with mixed diagnoses. J Geriatr Psychiatry Neurol 8:234–237, 1995

Regenold WT, Prasad M: Uses of intravenous valproate in geriatric psychiatry. Am J Geriatr Psychiatry 9:306–308, 2001

Regenold WT, Thapar RK, Marano C, et al: Increased prevalence of type 2 diabetes mellitus among psychiatric inpatients with bipolar I affective and schizoaffective disorders independent of psychotropic drug use. J Affect Disord 70:19–26, 2002

Robillard M, Conn DK: Lamotrigine use in geriatric patients with bipolar depression. Can J Psychiatry 47:767–770, 2002

Roose SP, Bone S, Haidorfer C, et al: Lithium treatment in older patients. Am J Psychiatry 136:843–844, 1979

Sajatovic M: Treatment of bipolar disorder in older adults. Int J Geriatr Psychiatry 17:865–873, 2002

Sajatovic M, Popli A, Semple W: Health resource utilization over a ten-year period by geriatric veterans with schizophrenia and bipolar disorder. J Geriatr Psychiatry Neurol 15:128–133, 1996

Sajatovic M, Gyulai L, Calabrese JR, et al: Maintenance treatment outcomes in older patients with bipolar I disorder. Am J Geriatr Psychiatry 13:305–311, 2005a

Sajatovic M, Madhusoodanan S, Coconcea N: Managing bipolar disorder in the elderly: defining the role of the newer agents. Drugs Aging 22:39–54, 2005b

Sajatovic M, Blow FC, Ignacio RV: Psychiatric comorbidity in older adults with bipolar disorder. Int J Geriatr Psychiatry 21:582–587, 2006

Sajatovic M, Ramsay E, Nanry K, et al: Lamotrigine therapy in elderly patients with epilepsy, bipolar disorder or dementia. Int J Geriatr Psychiatry 22:945–950, 2007

Schaffer CB, Garvey MJ: Use of lithium in acutely manic elderly patients. Clin Gerontol 3:58–60, 1984

Shulman K, Post F: Bipolar affective disorder in old age. Br J Psychiatry 136:26–32, 1980

Shulman KI, Mackenzie S, Hardy B: The clinical use of lithium carbonate in old age: a review. Prog Neuropsychopharmacol Biol Psychiatry 11:159–164, 1987

Shulman KI, Tohen M, Satlin A, et al: Mania compared with unipolar depression in old age. Am J Psychiatry 149:341–345, 1992

Shulman KI, Rochon P, Sykora K, et al: Changing prescription patterns for lithium and valproic acid in old age: shifting practice without evidence. BMJ 326:960–961, 2003

Shulman RW, Singh A, Shulman KI: Treatment of elderly institutionalized bipolar patients with clozapine. Psychopharmacol Bull 33:113–118, 1997

Sibisi CDT: Sex differences in the age of onset of bipolar affective illness. Br J Psychiatry 156:842–845, 1990

Snowdon J: A retrospective case-note study of bipolar disorder in old age. Br J Psychiatry 158:485–490, 1991

Spar JE, Ford CV, Liston EH: Bipolar affective disorder in aged patients. J Clinical Psychiatry 40:504–507, 1979

Speer DC: Differences in social resources and treatment history among diagnostic groups of older adults. Hosp Community Psychiatry 43:270–274, 1992

Spicer CC, Hare EH, Slater E: Neurotic and psychotic forms of depressive illness: evidence from age-incidence in a national sample. Br J Psychiatry 123:535–541, 1973

Sproule BA, Hardy BG, Shulman KI: Differential pharmacokinetics of lithium in elderly patients. Drugs Aging 16:165–177, 2000

Starkstein SE, Robinson RG, Price TR: Comparison of cortical and subcortical lesions in the production of post-stroke mood disorders. Brain 110:1045–1059, 1987

Starkstein SE, Mayberg HS, Berthier ML, et al: Mania after brain injury: neuroradiological and metabolic findings. Ann Neurol 27:652–659, 1990

Starkstein SE, Fedoroff P, Berthier ML, et al: Manic-depressive and pure manic states after brain lesions. Biol Psychiatry 29:149–158, 1991

Stenstedt A: Study in manic-depressive psychosis: clinical, social, and genetic investigations. Acta Psychiatr Neurol Scand Suppl 79:1–111, 1952

Stone K: Mania in the elderly. Br J Psychiatry 155:220–224, 1989

Strakowski SM, Woods BT, Tohen M, et al: MRI subcortical signal hyperintensities in mania at first hospitalization. Biol Psychiatry 33:204–206, 1993

Swayze VW, Andreasen NC, Alliger RJ, et al: Structural brain abnormalities in bipolar affective disorder. Arch Gen Psychiatry 47:1054–1059, 1990

Tanaka Y, Hazama H, Fukuhara T, et al: Computerized tomography of the brain in manic-depressive patients—a controlled study. Folia Psychiatr Neurol Jpn 36:137–143, 1982

Tariot P, Podgorski C, Blazina L, et al: Mental disorders in the nursing home: another perspective. Am J Psychiatry 150:1063–1069, 1993

Taylor M, Abrams R: Manic states: a genetic study of early and late onset affective disorders. Arch Gen Psychiatry 28:656–658, 1973

Thase ME: Bipolar depression: issues in diagnosis and treatment. Harv Rev Psychiatry 13:257–271, 2005

Thase ME: STEP-BD and bipolar depression: what have we learned. Curr Psychiatry Rep 9:497–503, 2007

Thase ME, Denko T: Pharmacotherapy of mood disorders. Ann Rev Clin Psychol 4:53–91, 2008

Tohen M, Shulman KI, Satlin A: First-episode mania in late life. Am J Psychiatry 151:130–132, 1994

Tsai S, Kuo C, Chen C, et al: Risk factors for completed suicide in bipolar disorder. J Clin Psychiatry 63:469–476, 2002

Tsai S, Lee H, Shang C, et al: The correlates of cognitive dysfunction in early onset elderly bipolar patients. Presented at the international congress of the International Psychogeriatrics Association, Chicago, IL, August 2003

Umapathy C, Mulsant BH, Pollock BG: Bipolar disorder in the elderly. Psychiatr Ann 30:473–480, 2000

Unutzer J, Bruce M: The elderly. National Institute of Mental Health Affective Disorders Workgroup. Mental Health Serv Res 4:245–247, 2002

Unutzer J, Simon G, Pabiniak C, et al: The treated prevalence of bipolar disorder in a large staff-model HMO. Psychiatr Serv 49:1072–1078, 1998

U.S. Food and Drug Administration: Carbamazepine prescribing information to include recommendation of genetic test for patients with Asian ancestry. FDA News, December 12, 2007. Available at http://www.fda.gov/bbs/topics/NEWS/2007/NEW01755.html. Accessed February 17, 2008.

van der Velde CD: Effectiveness of lithium carbonate in the treatment of manic-depressive illness. Am J Psychiatry 123:345–351, 1970

Videbech P: MRI findings in patients with affective disorder: a meta-analysis. Acta Pscyhiatr Scand 96:157–168, 1997

Weissman MM, Leaf PJ, Tischler GL, et al: Affective disorders in five United States communities. Psychol Med 18:141–153, 1988

Weissman MM, Bland RC, Canino GJ, et al: Cross-national epidemiology of major depression and bipolar disorder. JAMA 276:293–299, 1996

Winokur G: The Iowa 500: heterogeneity and course in manic-depressive illness (bipolar). Comp Psychiatry 16:125–131, 1975

Wylie M, Mulsant B, Pollock B, et al: Age at onset in geriatric bipolar disorder. Am J Geriatr Psychiatry 7:77–83, 1999

Young RC, Falk JR: Age, manic psychopathology and treatment response. Int J Geriatr Psychiatry 4:73–78, 1989

Young RC, Kalayam B, Tsuboyama G, et al: Mania: response to lithium across the age spectrum (abstract). Society for Neuroscience 18:669, 1992

Young RC, Nambudiri DE, Jain H, et al: Brain computed tomography in geriatric manic disorder. Biol Psychiatry 45:1063–1065, 1999

Young RC, Jain H, Kiosses DN, et al: Antidepressant-associated mania in late life. Int J Geriatr Psychiatry 18:421–424, 2003

Young RC, Gyulai L, Mulsant BH, et al: Pharmacotherapy of bipolar disorder in old age: review and recommendations. Am J Geriatr Psychiatry 12:342–357, 2004

Zis AP, Grof P, Goodwin FK: The natural course of affective disorders: implications for lithium prophylaxis, in Lithium: Controversies and Unsolved Issues. Edited by Cooper TB, Gershon S, Kline NS, Shou M. Amsterdam, The Netherlands, Excerpta Medica, 1979, pp 381–398

Suggested Readings

Beyer JL, Burchitt B, Gersing K, et al: Patterns of pharmacotherapy and treatment response in elderly adults with bipolar disorder. Psychopharmacol Bull 41:102–114, 2008

Depp CA, Jeste DV: Bipolar disorder in older adults: a critical review. Bipol Disord 6:343–367, 2004

Sajatovic M, Madhusoodanan S, Coconcea N: Managing bipolar disorder in the elderly: defining the role of the newer agents. Drugs Aging 22:39–54, 2005

Young RC, Gyulai L, Mulsant BH, et al: Pharmacotherapy of bipolar disorder in old age: review and recommendations. Am J Geriatr Psychiatry 12:342–357, 2004

CHAPTER 17

Schizophrenia and Paranoid Disorders

Dilip V. Jeste, M.D.
Nicole M. Lanouette, M.D.
Ipsit V. Vahia, M.D.

Delusions, hallucinations, and other psychotic symptoms can accompany a number of conditions in late life. These symptoms may be more common than previously thought; Swedish investigators found that the prevalence of any psychotic symptom in a population-based sample of 95-year-old individuals without dementia was 7.1%, with 6.7% experiencing hallucinations, 10.4% having delusions, and 0.6% experiencing paranoid ideation (Ostling and Skoog 2002; Ostling et al. 2007), and in a sample of 85-year-old people, the prevalence of psychotic symptoms was 10.1%, with 6.9% experiencing hallucinations, 5.5% having delusions, and 6.9% experiencing paranoid ideation (Ostling and Skoog 2002).

Some conditions that cause psychotic symptoms, such as delirium and substance-induced psychosis, are acute, and the psychotic symptoms tend to resolve when the underlying condition is treated. These conditions are discussed elsewhere in this volume. In this chapter, we review the epidemiology, presentation, and treatment of chronic late-life psychotic disorders that are not secondary to a mood disorder or a general medical condition other than dementia. Thus, we discuss early-onset schizophrenia, late-onset schizophrenia, very late-onset schizophrenia-like psychosis (with onset after age 60), delusional disorder, psychosis of Alzheimer's disease, and psychosis associated with other dementias.

Schizophrenia

Early-Onset Schizophrenia

Typically, individuals with schizophrenia develop the disease in the second or third decade of life (American Psychiatric Association 2000). Although mortality rates in general, and suicide and homicide rates in particular, are higher among individuals with schizophrenia than in the general population (Hannerz et al. 2001; Hiroch et al. 2001; Joukamaam et al. 2001), many of these patients with early-onset schizophrenia are now living into older adulthood. Thus, most older adults with schizophrenia typically have had an early onset of the disease and have a chronic course of illness spanning several decades. The prevalence of schizophrenia among adults between ages 45 and 64 is approximately 0.6%, and prevalence estimates for schizophrenia among elderly individuals range from 0.1% to 0.5% (Castle and Murray 1993; Copeland et al. 1998; Keith et al. 1991).

Longitudinal follow-up of patients with schizophrenia indicates considerable heterogeneity of outcome. A minority of patients experience remission of both positive and negative symptoms (Ciompi 1980; Harding et al. 1987; Huber 1997). Auslander and Jeste (2004) reported that nearly 10% of community-dwelling older patients with schizophrenia met strict research criteria for sustained remission. A small proportion of patients experience deterioration of symptoms.

The course in a majority of patients is largely unchanged over time (Belitsky and McGlashan 1993; Cohen 1990; Harvey et al. 1999), although there is generally an improvement in positive symptoms (Jeste et al. 2003).

Factors associated with poor prognosis for early-onset schizophrenia include chronicity, insidious onset, premorbid psychosocial or functional deficits, and prominent negative symptoms (Ram et al. 1992). In a sample of chronically institutionalized patients with schizophrenia, older age was associated with lower levels of positive symptoms and higher levels of negative symptoms (Davidson et al. 1995). However, Harding (2002) noted that the strength of the association between predictors of outcome and actual outcome in patients with schizophrenia weakens over time.

Cognition in Older Patients With Schizophrenia

The pattern of cognitive deficits in schizophrenia differs significantly from that in Alzheimer's disease (AD); patients with AD have less efficient learning and more rapid forgetting than patients with schizophrenia (Heaton et al. 2001). Among community-dwelling older outpatients with schizophrenia, cognitive functioning seems to remain relatively stable, other than the changes expected from normal aging (Heaton et al. 2001). A small proportion of chronically institutionalized older patients with schizophrenia tend to have cognitive decline greater than that expected for their age (Putnam and Harvey 2000).

Depression in Older Patients With Schizophrenia

Depression is a common source of comorbidity in older patients with schizophrenia. Studies have shown depressive symptoms to be distinct from negative symptoms (Baynes et al. 2000). Depression is also a major predictor of suicidality in this population (Montross et al. 2006). Depression may be associated with positive symptoms, and it predicts worse functional outcome as well. An important recent finding in studies of depression in older patients with schizophrenia has been the role of subsyndromal depression in increasing morbidity (Diwan et al. 2007; Zisook et al. 2007). Detection and management of subsyndromal depression may have an important role to play in management of this population.

Functional Capacity

The level of functional impairment varies considerably among older adults with schizophrenia. In a study of a group of middle-aged and older schizophrenia outpatients, Palmer et al. (2002) found that 30% had been employed at least part time since the onset of psychosis, 43% were current drivers, and 73% were living independently. In general, worse neuropsychological test performance, lower educational level, and negative symptoms but not positive symptoms are associated with poorer functional capacity in older outpatients with schizophrenia (Evans et al. 2003).

Quality of Life

Self-appraisal is considered to be essential in studies of quality of life for patients with schizophrenia. Several studies found self-assessed lower quality of life to be associated with depression, positive and negative symptoms, cognitive deficits, financial strain, poor social support, and poor social skills (Vahia et al. 2007). These findings suggest that a multimodal approach to management of these patients is necessary to improve quality of life.

Late-Onset Schizophrenia

Historically, schizophrenia has been considered a disease of younger adulthood. Kraepelin (1971) termed schizophrenia *dementia praecox* to distinguish it from organic disorders arising in late life and to indicate a poor prognosis with a course of progressive deterioration. However, in later years, Kraepelin himself observed that some cases arose for the first time in older age and that progressive decline was not a universal feature of the disease. Bleuler (1943) and Roth (1955) developed this concept further, with studies describing the late-onset phenotype as a distinct entity from the early-onset form. A literature review found that approximately 23% of patients with schizophrenia reportedly had an onset after age 40, with 3% being older than age 60 (Harris and Jeste 1988). An investigation involving first-contact patients found that 29% of patients had an onset after age 44, with 12% reporting onset after age 64 (Howard et al. 1993). Although DSM-III-R labeled schizophrenia with onset after age 45 as a late-onset type (American Psychiatric Association 1987), DSM-IV-TR (American Psychiatric Association 2000) does not specify age at onset. The consensus statement by the International Late-Onset Schizophrenia Group suggested that schizophrenia with an onset after age 40 should be called "late-onset schizophrenia" and should be considered a subtype of schizophrenia rather than a related disorder (Howard et al. 2000).

Risk factors and clinical presentation associated with late-onset schizophrenia are similar to those associated with early-onset schizophrenia (Brodaty et al. 1999; Jeste et al. 1995). Similar proportions of individuals with early-onset or late-onset schizophrenia reported having a family history of schizophrenia (10%–15%), and no consistent relationship has been found between age at onset and genetic risk of schizophrenia (Jeste et al. 1997b; Kendler et al. 1987). Levels of childhood maladjustment, measured retrospectively, were similar in late-onset and early-onset schizophrenia patients and higher in both groups than in healthy subjects (Jeste et al. 1997b). Patients with late-onset schizophrenia show increased rates of minor physical anomalies relative to healthy subjects but similar rates to those of patients with early-onset schizophrenia (Lohr et al. 1997).

Neuroimaging studies show that patients with late-onset schizophrenia, compared with patients with early-onset schizophrenia, have more nonspecific structural abnormalities, such as enlarged ventricles and increased white matter hyperintensities (Sachdev et al. 1999), and a larger volume of thalamus on magnetic resonance imaging (Corey-Bloom et al. 1995). Other imaging studies have ruled out strokes, tumors, or other abnormalities as potential causes of schizophrenia in late life (Rivkin et al. 2000). Finally, long-term neuropsychological follow-up of a group of patients with late-onset schizophrenia revealed no evidence of cognitive decline, suggesting a neurodevelopmental rather than a neurodegenerative process (Palmer et al. 2003).

Women predominate among individuals with onset of schizophrenia in middle to late life (Hafner et al. 1998; Jeste et al. 1997b). It has been speculated that estrogen may serve as an endogenous antipsychotic, masking schizophrenic symptoms in vulnerable women until after menopause (Seeman 1996). However, investigations on efficacy of hormone replacement therapy as an adjunct treatment for postmenopausal women with psychosis (Kulkarni et al. 1996, 2001; Lindamer et al. 2001) have not had promising results.

Data from our center suggest a higher prevalence of the paranoid subtype of schizophrenia among patients with late-onset schizophrenia (approximately 75%) than among patients with early-onset schizophrenia (approximately 50%) (Jeste et al. 1997b). Patients with late-onset schizophrenia tend to have more organized delusions, auditory hallucinations or hallucinations with a running commentary, and persecutory delusions with and without hallucinations (Howard et al. 2000). Patients with late-onset schizophrenia also have lower levels of negative symptoms on average than patients with early-onset schizophrenia; however, they have higher levels of negative symptoms than healthy subjects (Jeste et al. 1988, 1997b; Palmer et al. 2001).

On neuropsychological testing, after correction for age, education, and gender, patients with late-onset schizophrenia tend to have less impairment in learning, abstraction, and flexibility in thinking than patients with early-onset schizophrenia (Jeste et al. 1997b). Compared with patients with early-onset schizophrenia, a greater proportion of patients with late-onset schizophrenia have successful occupational and marital histories and generally higher premorbid functioning.

Sensory deficits, particularly hearing loss, are associated with psychotic symptoms in late life and have been proposed as a risk factor for late-onset schizophrenia (Howard et al. 1994; Raghuram et al. 1980). However, other data suggest that both early- and late-onset schizophrenia patients may be less likely than healthy older adults to receive appropriate correction for vision and hearing impairments (Prager and Jeste 1993). Thus, uncorrected sensory deficits may reflect generally poorer health care utilization by older psychotic patients and may not be a potential cause of psychosis in the elderly population.

In summary, although there are several similarities between early-onset schizophrenia and late-onset schizophrenia, there are also notable differences. Analyses of large data sets should be carried out to find differences between the two groups in epidemiology, symptomatology, etiology, pathophysiology, and treatment so as to determine the optimal age cutoff for defining late-onset schizophrenia (Jeste et al. 2005).

Very-Late-Onset Schizophrenia-Like Psychosis

In its consensus statement, the International Late-Onset Schizophrenia Group proposed the diagnostic term *very-late-onset schizophrenia-like psychosis* (VLOSLP) for patients whose psychosis begins after age 60 (Howard et al. 2000). Table 17–1 compares risk factors for and clinical features of early-onset schizophrenia, late-onset schizophrenia, and VLOSLP. Very late-onset schizophrenia-like psychosis may be difficult to diagnose clinically because its clinical picture can be confused with other conditions (e.g., delirium, psychosis due to underlying medical illness). Nevertheless, new-onset primary psychotic symptoms have been described

TABLE 17–1. Comparison of early-onset schizophrenia, late-onset schizophrenia, and very late-onset schizophrenia-like psychosis

Feature	Early-onset schizophrenia	Late-onset schizophrenia	Very-late-onset schizophrenia-like psychosis
Age at onset	Before 40	Middle age (~40–60)	Late life (60+)
Female preponderance	–	+	++
Negative symptoms	++	+	–
Minor physical anomalies	+	+	–
Neuropsychological impairment			
Learning	++	+	?++
Retention	–	–	?++
Progressive cognitive deterioration	–	–	++
Brain structure abnormalities (e.g., strokes, tumors)	–	–	++
Family history of schizophrenia	+	+	–
Early childhood maladjustment	+	+	–
Daily neuroleptic dose	++	+	+
Risk of tardive dyskinesia	+	+	++

+=mildly present; ++=strongly present; ?++=probably strongly present, but limited data exist; –=absent.

Source. Adapted from Palmer et al. 2001.

in older adults. Indeed, Cervantes et al. (2006) described a clinical case of primary-onset psychosis in a 100-year-old patient.

Factors distinguishing patients with VLOSLP from "true" schizophrenia patients include a lower genetic load, less evidence of early childhood maladjustment, a relative lack of thought disorder and negative symptoms (including blunted affect), a greater risk of tardive dyskinesia, and evidence of a neurodegenerative rather than a neurodevelopmental process (Andreasen 1999; Howard et al. 1997). Although the term was initially considered a catchall phrase for several different entities, recent research suggests that VLOSLP may be a distinct entity. It has been noted to be more common in immigrant populations, suggesting that psychosocial factors might play a role (Mitter et al. 2005). Imaging studies have shown underlying focal white matter abnormalities in cerebral tracts (Jones et al. 2005). One study has suggested that the cognitive biases that are common in younger persons with delusions are absent in patients with VLOSLP (Moore et al. 2006). A study by Mazeh et al. (2005) suggested that patients with VLOSLP may have somewhat more stable cognitive and everyday functioning than do chronically institutionalized elderly patients with schizophrenia. In summary, clinical vigilance must be exercised when treating apparent primary-onset psychotic symptoms in older patients, and "organic" causes should be meticulously ruled out.

Delusional Disorder

At least 6% of older adults have paranoid symptoms such as persecutory delusions, but most of these individuals have dementia (Christenson and Blazer 1984; Forsell and Henderson 1998; Henderson et al. 1998). The essential feature of a delusional disorder is a nonbizarre delusion (e.g., a persecutory, somatic, erotomanic, grandiose, or jealous delusion) without prominent auditory or visual hallucinations. Symptoms must be present for at least 1 month. When delusional disorder arises in late life, basic personality features, intellectual performance, and occupational function are preserved, but social functioning is compromised. To diagnose delusional disorder, the clinician must rule out delirium, dementia, psychotic disorders due to general medical conditions or substance use, schizophrenia, and mood disorders with psychotic features. The course of persecutory delusional disorder is typically chronic, but patients with other types of delusions may have partial remissions and relapses.

According to DSM-IV-TR, the prevalence of delusional disorder is 0.03% and is slightly higher among women than among men. The disorder typically first appears in middle to late adulthood, with an average age at onset of 40–49 years for men and 60–69 years for women.

Risk factors for delusional disorder include a family history of schizophrenia or avoidant, paranoid, or schizoid personality disorder (Kendler and Davis 1981). Evidence supporting hearing loss as a risk factor for paranoia is mixed (Cooper and Curry 1976; Moore 1981). In one neuroimaging study, brain atrophy and white matter hyperintensities did not distinguish older psychotic patients with somatic delusions from those without such delusions (Rockwell et al. 1994). According to Maher (2005), a subset of the population that is prone to primary perceptual abnormalities may be prone to developing delusions as a result. Maher (2005) also pointed out that "normal" persons may demonstrate "delusional" behavior as a result of sensory disturbances. Evans et al. (1996) compared middle-aged and older patients with schizophrenia or delusional disorder and found no differences in neuropsychological impairment but more severe psychopathology associated with delusional disorder. Finally, immigration and low socioeconomic status may be risk factors for delusional disorder (American Psychiatric Association 2000).

Psychosis of Alzheimer's Disease

Based on a review of 55 studies, Ropacki and Jeste (2005) estimated the median prevalence of psychosis in Alzheimer's disease to be about 41% (range 12.2%–74.1%). Psychosis is associated with more rapid cognitive decline. Some studies found a significant association between psychosis and age, age at onset of AD, and illness duration; however, gender, education, and family history of dementia or psychiatric illness showed weak or inconsistent relationships with psychosis. In a large sample of patients with probable AD, Paulsen et al. (2000) found a cumulative incidence of psychotic symptoms of 20% at 1 year, 36% at 2 years, 50% at 3 years, and 51% at 4 years. Delusions, especially of a persecutory nature, tend to be the most common symptom (median prevalence 36%); visual hallucinations (median prevalence 18.7%) and auditory hallucinations (median prevalence 9.2%) are less common (Ropacki and Jeste 2005). These symptoms often need to be inferred from the patient's behavior, because the patient may be unable to verbalize thoughts or perceptions due to cognitive impairment, particularly in the later stages of the disease. In one large naturalistic study of the course of psychotic symptoms in dementia, Devanand et al. (1997) found that hallucinations and paranoid delusions were more persistent than depressive symptoms over time but less prevalent and less persistent than behavioral disturbances, particularly agitation.

In Table 17–2, characteristics associated with psychosis of AD are compared with characteristics of schizophrenia in elderly patients (Jeste and Finkel 2000). Two common psychotic symptoms in AD are misidentification of caregivers and delusions of theft (Jeste et al. 2007). Schneiderian first-rank symptoms, such as hearing multiple voices talking to one another or hearing a running commentary on the patient's actions, are rare (Burns et al. 1990a, 1990b). Disorganization of speech and behavior and negative symptoms are also uncommon (Jeste et al. 2007). Active suicidal ideation and past history of psychosis are rare. Because psychotic symptoms in patients with dementia tend to remit in the late stages of the disease, very long-term maintenance therapy on antipsychotics is typically unnecessary.

AD patients with psychosis and those without psychosis differ in several important ways. Neuropsychologically, AD patients with psychosis have shown greater impairment in executive functioning, more rapid cognitive decline (Jeste et al. 1992; Stern et al. 1994), and greater prevalence of extrapyramidal symptoms (Stern et al. 1994) than have AD patients without psychosis. Delusions in dementia have been associated with dysfunction in paralimbic areas of the frontotemporal cortex (Sultzer 1996). Neuropathologically, dementia patients with psychosis have shown increased neurodegenerative changes in the cortex, increased norepinephrine in subcortical regions, and reduced serotonin levels in both cortical and subcortical areas (Zubenko et al. 1991). In one study, AD patients with psychosis had much higher levels of tau protein in the entorhinal and temporal cortices than did nonpsychotic AD patients (Mukaetova-Ladinska et al. 1995). Furthermore, Wilkosz et al. (2006) have suggested that

TABLE 17–2. Comparison of psychosis of Alzheimer's disease with schizophrenia in older patients

Feature	Psychosis of AD	Schizophrenia
Prevalence	35%–50% of AD patients	Less than 1% of general population
Bizarre or complex delusions	Rare	Frequent
Misidentification of caregivers	Frequent	Rare
Common form of hallucinations	Visual	Auditory
Schneiderian first-rank symptoms	Rare	Frequent
Active suicidal ideation	Rare	Frequent
Past history of psychosis	Rare	Very common
Eventual remission of psychosis	Frequent	Uncommon
Need for years of maintenance on antipsychotic medication	Uncommon	Very common
Usual optimal daily doses of commonly used atypical antipsychotics:		
Risperidone	0.75–1.5 mg	1.5–2.5 mg
Olanzapine	2.5–7.5 mg	7.5–12.5 mg
Recommended adjunctive psychosocial treatment	Sensory enhancement, structured activities, social contact, behavior therapy[a]	Cognitive-behavioral therapy, social skills training[b]

Note. AD=Alzheimer's disease.
[a]Cohen-Mansfield 2001.
[b]Granholm et al. 2002; McQuaid et al. 2000.
Source. Adapted from Jeste DV, Finkel SI: "Psychosis of Alzheimer's Disease and Related Dementias: Diagnostic Criteria for a Distinct Syndrome. *American Journal of Geriatric Psychiatry* 8:29–34, 2000. Used with permission.

the misidentification subtype and the paranoid subtype of psychosis of AD may be distinct.

Jeste and Finkel (2000) recommended specific diagnostic criteria for psychosis of AD to facilitate epidemiological, clinical, and therapeutic research. These criteria include the presence of visual or auditory hallucinations or delusions, a primary diagnosis of AD, a duration of at least 1 month, and a chronology indicating that symptoms of AD preceded those of psychosis. Alternative causes of psychosis must be excluded, and sufficient functional impairment should be present for this diagnosis to be made. There is evidence for good interrater and test-retest reliability of these criteria (Jeste et al. 2007).

Psychosis in Other Dementias

Psychosis is also common in other dementias. Visual hallucinations and secondary delusions are common in Lewy body disease, and vascular dementia may also be accompanied by delusions or hallucinations (Schneider 1999). Naimark et al. (1996) found psychotic symptoms in approximately one-third of a sample of patients with Parkinson's disease, with hallucinations being more common than delusions. Psychosis in frontotemporal dementias is poorly characterized but may be as common as psychosis in AD (Srikanth et al. 2005).

Treatment

The modern era of pharmacological treatment for schizophrenia and related disorders began with the introduction of chlorpromazine in the early 1950s. Although this and other conventional agents substantially improved the positive symptoms of schizophrenia (e.g., hallucinations and delusions), a number of treatment liabilities have been recognized over the years, such as movement disorders, sedation, orthostatic hypotension, and increased prolactin concentrations. In addition, older adults have a significantly higher risk for developing tardive dyskinesia than do younger adults, making use of conventional antipsychotics in this population highly problematic.

Therefore, when atypical antipsychotics—which are associated with significantly lower incidence of tardive dyskinesia—were introduced, they were hailed as the drugs of choice for older adults with psychotic disorders. However, these agents have since been linked to an increased risk of metabolic dysfunction, including diabetes, dyslipidemia, and obesity, thereby leading to a worsened cardiovascular risk profile. In elderly patients with dementia, atypical antipsychotics have been associated with an increased risk of cerebrovascular adverse events and mortality compared to placebo; therefore, leading pharmaceutical regulatory agencies have issued warnings about the use of these agents in patients with dementia. At the same time, because of the paucity of evidence-based pharmacological treatment alternatives to antipsychotics for patients with dementia, clinicians are restricted to off-label treatments, which must be used with caution and close monitoring. Psychosocial treatments for older adults with psychosis have been developed and tested in randomized, controlled trials and show promise as adjunctive treatments.

Treatment of Schizophrenia and Delusional Disorder

Pharmacological Treatments

Pharmacotherapy for older adults with schizophrenia and delusional disorder can be challenging. Although few randomized, placebo-controlled, double-blind clinical trials have been conducted in this population, some information has become available. Maintenance pharmacotherapy is usually required for older patients with schizophrenia due to risk of relapse. Because older patients are at higher risk of adverse antipsychotic effects, due to age-related pharmacokinetic and pharmacodynamic factors (Hammerlein et al. 1998), coexisting medical illnesses, and concomitant medications, the recommended starting and maintenance doses of antipsychotics in older adults are much lower than the usual doses in younger adults (American Psychiatric Association 1997). Patients with late-onset schizophrenia respond well to low-dose antipsychotic medication, requiring about 50% of the dose typically taken by older patients with early-onset schizophrenia and 25%–33% of the dose used in younger patients with schizophrenia.

Use of conventional or typical antipsychotics in older adults with schizophrenia and delusional disorder is problematic because of the higher incidence of tardive dyskinesia in older patients. Aging appears to be the most important risk factor for the development of tardive dyskinesia (American Psychiatric Association 2000; Yassa and Jeste 1992). The cumulative 1-year incidence of tardive dyskinesia is 29% among older patients (mean age 65 years) despite low dosing (Jeste et al. 1999b), whereas the annual cumulative incidence of tardive dyskinesia in young adults is 4%–5% (Kane et al. 1993). The risk of severe tardive dyskinesia is also higher in older patients (Caligiuri et al. 1997). Other side effects of conventional neuroleptics include sedation, anticholinergic effects, cardiovascular effects including orthostatic hypotension, parkinsonian reactions, and neuroleptic malignant syndrome. Despite these side effects, occasionally a conventional antipsychotic may be the most reasonable treatment option for an individual patient, and these agents can be used at flexible, individualized low doses to minimize side effects (Jeste et al. 1999b).

Few efficacy comparisons have been done of conventional antipsychotics versus atypical antipsychotics in patients with schizophrenia over age 65. In a study of 42 elderly inpatients, Howanitz et al. (1999) found that clozapine (≤300 mg/day) and chlorpromazine (≤600 mg/day) had similar efficacy. Kennedy et al. (2003) compared olanzapine (5–20 mg/day) and haloperidol (5–20 mg/day) in a 6-week trial of 117 patients ages 60 years and older who had schizophrenia and related disorders. Olanzapine (mean modal dose 11.9 mg/day) produced significantly greater symptomatic improvement and had fewer motor side effects than did haloperidol (mean modal dose 9.4 mg/day) (Kennedy et al. 2003). The National Institute of Mental Health Clinical Antipsychotic Trials of Intervention Effectiveness (CATIE) study (Lieberman et al. 2005), which included adults ages 18–65, found no significant differences in effectiveness between the conventional antipsychotic perphenazine and the atypical antipsychotics risperidone, olanzapine, quetiapine, or ziprasidone, but it is unknown how these findings would translate to patients older than age 65.

Generally, atypical antipsychotics carry a much lower risk of tardive dyskinesia than conventional neuroleptics, even when taken by very high-risk patients such as middle-aged and older adults with borderline tardive dyskinesia (Dolder and Jeste 2003; Jeste et al. 1999a). Preexisting tardive dyskinesia may improve after switching from a conventional antipsychotic to an atypical antipsychotic. Clozapine has shown efficacy in reducing tardive dyskinesia in patients with existing tardive dyskinesia (Kane et al. 1993; Lieberman et al. 1991; Simpson et al. 1978; Small et al. 1987); however, other side effects limit its use, particularly in elderly patients. A beneficial effect of other atypical agents, specifically risperidone and olanzapine, on preexisting tardive dyskinesia has also been reported (Jeste et al. 1997a; Kinon et al. 2004; Littrell et al. 1998; Street et al. 2000).

Atypical antipsychotics have a less favorable side-effect profile, however, in terms of metabolic function. Common metabolic side effects include excessive weight gain and obesity, glucose intolerance, new-onset type II diabetes mellitus, diabetic ketoacidosis, and dyslipidemia (Allison et al. 1999; Jin et al. 2002, 2004; Wirshing et al. 1998). Although there are no guidelines for management of these side effects specifically in older patients with schizophrenia, the monitoring recommendations developed by the American Diabetes Association et al. (2004) are potentially applicable. Because elderly patients tend to be at higher risk for cardiovascular disease than younger patients, closer monitoring is necessary for older adults.

The only large-scale randomized, double-blind controlled trial comparing two atypical antipsychotics in adults older than age 60 has been Jeste et al.'s (2003) multisite international study of risperidone and olanzapine. In that trial, 175 patients with schizophrenia or schizoaffective disorder ages 60 years and older were randomly assigned to receive risperidone (1–3 mg/day, median dose 2 mg/day) or olanzapine (5–20 mg/day, median dose 10 mg/day). Both groups had significant improvement in symptoms and had lower scores on rating scales of extrapyramidal symptoms (EPS). Clinically relevant weight gain was significantly less frequent in patients treated with risperidone.

To date, quetiapine, ziprasidone, and aripiprazole have been studied in older adults with schizophrenia only in open-label or retrospective studies. Although clozapine has been shown to have superior effectiveness compared to other antipsychotics in younger adults (Jones et al. 2006; Lieberman et al. 2005), the medication is difficult to use in elderly persons due to the risk of leukopenia and agranulocytosis, as well as other side effects such as orthostasis, sedation, and anticholinergic effects. The necessity of weekly blood draws also may pose a problem for older patients. Risperidone in higher doses carries a greater risk of extrapyramidal side effects. Both olanzapine and clozapine appear to carry the greatest liability in terms of metabolic side effects. All of the atypical agents have other possible side effects that are especially relevant for older patients, including orthostatic hypotension and sedation.

Because of the dearth of randomized, controlled data, Alexopoulos et al. (2004) conducted a consensus survey of 48 American experts on the use of antipsychotic drugs in older adults. The experts' first-line recommendation for late-life schizophrenia was risperidone (1.25–3.5 mg/day). The second-line recommendations included quetiapine (100–300 mg/day), olanzapine (7.5–15 mg/day), and aripiprazole (15–30 mg/day). There was limited support for the use of clozapine, ziprasidone, and high-potency conventional antipsychotics. Given the data on the increased risk of strokes and mortality in elderly patients with dementia treated with atypical antipsychotics and the consequent U.S. Food and Drug Administration (FDA) black-box warnings (discussed in "Treatment of Psychosis of Alzheimer's Disease and Other Dementias," later in this chapter), clinicians should exercise caution, clinical judgment, and shared decision making when using these drugs in older patients with schizophrenia, although there are no data to support or refute the applicability of these findings to people with schizophrenia.

Few data are available specifically on the pharmacological treatment of delusional disorder in elderly patients. Alexopoulos et al.'s (2004) survey of 48 experts in geriatric care concluded that antipsychotics are the only recommended treatment, and their first-line recommendation for older adults with delusional disorder was risperidone (0.75–2.5 mg/day), followed by olanzapine (5–10 mg/day) and quetiapine (50–200 mg/day).

Psychosocial Treatments

Recent years have seen the development and testing of psychosocial interventions for older adults with chronic psychotic disorders. Granholm et al. (2005) conducted a randomized, controlled trial in 76 middle-aged and elderly stable outpatients with schizophrenia to examine the effects of adding cognitive-behavioral social skills training to treatment as usual. This training intervention teaches cognitive and behavioral coping techniques, social functioning skills, problem-solving techniques, and compensatory aids for neurocognitive impairments. The investigators found that cognitive-behavioral social skills training led to significantly increased frequency of social functioning activities, greater cognitive insight (more objectivity in reappraising psychotic symptoms), and greater skill mastery. Although cognitive-behavioral social skills training did not show a significant effect on symptoms, this was not surprising because the patients had already been on stable dosages of antipsychotic medications, and these were continued during the study. An increase in cognitive insight was significantly correlated with a greater reduction in positive symptoms. At 12-month follow-up, the cognitive-behavioral social skills training group had maintained their greater skill acquisition and performance of everyday living skills. The greater cognitive insight seen in the cognitive-behavioral social skills training group at the end of the treatment was not maintained at 12-month follow-up, however, suggesting a possible need for booster sessions (Granholm et al. 2007).

Patterson et al. (2006) conducted a randomized, controlled trial to compare a behavioral group intervention called Functional Adaptation Skills Training (FAST) with a time-equivalent attention control condition. FAST is a manualized behavioral intervention designed to improve everyday living skills (including medication management, social skills, communication skills, organization and planning, transportation, and financial management) of middle-aged and older adults with schizophrenia or schizoaffective disorder. Compared with participants randomized to attention control, the FAST group showed significant improvement in daily living skills and social skills but not medication management. The FAST intervention has also been culturally adapted and pilot-tested in middle-aged and older Spanish-speaking Mexican American patients with schizophrenia or schizoaffective disorder. This intervention, called Programa de Entrenamiento para el Desarrollo de Aptitudes para Latinos (PEDAL), was compared in a randomized, controlled pilot study to a time-equivalent friendly support group (Patterson et al. 2005). The PEDAL group demonstrated a significant improvement in everyday living skills that was maintained at 12-month follow-up.

Following an examination of employment outcomes among middle-aged and older adults with schizophrenia who each participated in one of three types of work rehabilitation program, Twamley et al. (2005) reported that the highest rates of volunteer or paid work (81%) and competitive/paid work (69%) occurred for the patients who were placed in a job chosen with a vocational counselor and who then received individualized on-site support. The less successful programs (achieving at best a 44% rate of volunteer or paid work) employed a train-then-place approach.

Treatment of Psychosis of Alzheimer's Disease and Other Dementias

Over the past decade, atypical antipsychotics have for the most part replaced conventional antipsychotics in treating psychosis, aggression, and agitation in patients with dementia because of greater tolerability, lower risk for acute extrapyramidal symptoms, and comparatively lower risk of tardive dyskinesia. Most antipsychotics that are prescribed for older adults are for behavioral disturbances associated with dementia, despite their lacking this FDA-approved indication (Weiss et al. 2000).

Atypical antipsychotics seem to have modest efficacy for treating psychosis of AD (Ballard et al. 2006; Sink et al. 2005); however, studies have not always found a significant advantage over placebo in treating psychotic symptoms (Kindermann et al. 2002; Schneider et al. 2006a). In the CATIE Alzheimer's disease trial—the largest (N=421) non–industry-sponsored trial of atypical antipsychotics for psychosis or agitation/aggression in people with dementia—olanzapine, quetiapine, and risperidone were no better than placebo for the primary outcome (time to discontinuation for any reason) (Schneider et al. 2006b). Time to discontinuation due to lack of efficacy favored olanzapine and risperidone, whereas time to discontinuation due to adverse events favored placebo. In Schneider and colleagues' meta-analysis of randomized, controlled trials of atypical antipsychotics in dementia, the number needed to treat ranged from 5 to 14, depending on the outcome measure, criterion for improvement, and methodology used (Schneider et al. 2006a). The reviewers found that the overall average treatment effect was approximately 18%, which is remarkably similar to that reported in a meta-analysis of conventional antipsychotics in this population (Schneider et al. 1990).

There have been only a few randomized, controlled trials comparing atypical and conventional antipsychotics for treatment of dementia: three trials compared risperidone with haloperidol (Chan et al. 2001; De Deyn et al. 1999; Suh et al. 2004), and one compared quetiapine with haloperidol (Tariot et al. 2006). One of these found superior efficacy of the atypical over the typical agent, and the others reported no significant differences between the two types. In all four studies, haloperidol was associated with more extrapyramidal symptoms.

In addition to the liabilities described above, the use of atypical antipsychotics in elderly patients with dementia has been associated with both cerebrovascular adverse events (CVAEs) and death, leading to black-box warnings by the FDA. Currently, risperidone, olanzapine, and aripiprazole carry black-box warnings for stroke risk in older patients with dementia. The data for quetiapine in this population are more limited than for risperidone, olanzapine, and aripiprazole. The attribution of risk of CVAEs to atypical antipsychotics is limited, however, in that these studies were not designed to determine a cause-and-effect relationship between atypical antipsychotics and CVAEs, and serious CVAEs were not operationally defined in the trials. Additionally, retrospective database reviews (Gill et al. 2005; Herrmann et al. 2004) did not find any difference in incidence of CVAEs for typical versus atypical antipsychotic use, although none of these studies were originally designed to examine CVAE risk.

In May 2004, the FDA issued a black-box warning that elderly patients with dementia treated with atypical antipsychotic drugs are at an increased risk for death compared to those treated with placebo. A 2005 meta-analysis of 15 randomized, controlled trials reported a mortality risk of 3.5% for atypical antipsychotic–treated patients compared with a risk of 2.5% for patients given placebo (odds ratio 1.5, 95%; CI, 1.1–2.2) (Schneider et al. 2005). The causes of death were most commonly cardiac or infectious, the two most common causes of death in patients with dementia (Kammoun et al. 2000; Keene et al. 2001). The data on risk of mortality associated with typical versus atypical antipsychotics have been mixed (Jeste et al. 2008).

Unfortunately, insufficient data are available to support the systematic use of any of the following alternatives to antipsychotics: no active treatment, other psychotropic drugs, or psychosocial interventions. Nonuse of active treatment may be a reasonable option for some mild to moderate cases, but in a majority of clinical scenarios, this would be an unacceptably risky alternative. No other psychotropic medications have been approved by the FDA for the treatment of dementia-associated psychosis or agitation, and few clinical trials of psychotropic drugs have been done with older adults, particularly those with dementia. Jeste et al. (2007a) systematically reviewed the randomized, controlled trials ($n = 17$) of non–antipsychotic medications in this population and found mixed results, at best, in terms of efficacy and tolerability.

Also, few well-designed randomized, controlled trials have been done of behavioral and psychosocial interventions in patients with dementia. Although recent reviews have noted several promising treatments (e.g., behavioral management techniques, caregiver education), when strict inclusion criteria are used, such as those of the American Psychological Association, very few of these studies can be considered evidence based because the results are often inconclusive (Ayalon et al. 2006; Livingston et al. 2005).

Patients with Lewy body dementia and parkinsonian dementia are especially sensitive to side effects such as extrapyramidal symptoms and anticholinergic effects; therefore, very low doses and slow titration schedules should be used to avoid worsening of motor symptoms (Stoppe et al. 1999). Low-dose clozapine has demonstrated efficacy in reducing symptoms of psychosis, and the drug does not worsen and can even improve the parkinsonian tremor (Bonuccelli et al. 1997; Masand 2000; Parkinson Study Group 1999; Pollak et al. 2004). Several trials of olanzapine in patients with Parkinson's disease have found worsened motor function without demonstrable efficacy in treating psychosis (Chou et al. 2007; Miyasaki et al. 2006). Quetiapine does not appear to worsen motor functioning, but data about its efficacy for psychosis in Parkinson's disease are mixed (Chou et al. 2007; Yeung et al. 2000). The limited data (generally from small, open-label studies) on ziprasidone and aripiprazole do not clearly support the use of these drugs in patients with movement disorders; however, no large randomized, controlled trials have been published to date (Chou et al. 2007). One double-blind, placebo-controlled trial that addressed the treatment of psychosis in dementia with Lewy bodies ($N = 120$) found that twice as many patients treated with rivastigmine (up to 12 mg/day) (63%) versus placebo (30%) had at least 30% improvement in delusions and hallucinations without worsening of motor symptoms (McKeith et al. 2000).

Key Points

- Schizophrenia may be classified by age at onset into early-onset schizophrenia (onset before age 40), late-onset schizophrenia (onset between ages 40 and 60), and very late-onset schizophrenia-like psychosis (onset after age 60).
- There is marked heterogeneity of outcome with aging in patients with early-onset schizophrenia, although there is generally an improvement in positive symptoms.

- Patients with late-onset schizophrenia are similar to patients with early-onset schizophrenia in terms of risk factors, clinical presentation, family history of schizophrenia, and response to medications. However, women are overrepresented among the late-onset patients. Late-onset schizophrenia is marked by higher rates of delusional symptoms and lower rates of negative symptoms.
- Very-late-onset schizophrenia-like psychosis is a heterogeneous entity with varied etiology.
- Patients with psychosis of Alzheimer's disease tend to have paranoid delusions and visual or auditory hallucinations, as well as greater risk of agitation, faster cognitive decline, and greater likelihood of being institutionalized than patients with Alzheimer's disease without psychosis.
- Older adults have a much higher risk for developing tardive dyskinesia than younger patients. Although atypical antipsychotics are associated with significantly lower risk of tardive dyskinesia than conventional agents, they have problematic metabolic liabilities.
- Psychosocial treatments have an important place as an adjunctive treatment for older adults with schizophrenia.
- There are currently no FDA-approved treatments for psychosis and agitation in dementia; however, off-label use of medications, as well as certain psychosocial interventions, may be appropriate.
- The use of atypical antipsychotics by elderly patients with dementia has been associated with an increased risk of cerebrovascular adverse events and mortality, leading to FDA black-box warnings for this population.
- Principles of pharmacotherapy for older adults with psychosis include careful consideration of indications, shared decision making, and use of the lowest effective doses for the shortest possible time periods.

References

Alexopoulos GS, Streim J, Carpenter D, et al: Using antipsychotic agents in older patients. J Clin Psychiatry 65:5–99, 2004

Allison DB, Mentore JL, Heo M, et al: Antipsychotic-induced weight gain: a comprehensive research synthesis. Am J Psychiatry 156:1686–1696, 1999

American Diabetes Association, American Psychiatric Association, American Association of Clinical Endocrinologists, et al: Consensus Development Conference on Antipsychotic Drugs and Obesity and Diabetes. J Clin Psychiatry 65:267–272, 2004

American Psychiatric Association: Diagnostic and Statistical Manual of Mental Disorders, 3rd Edition, Revised. Washington, DC, American Psychiatric Press, 1987

American Psychiatric Association: Diagnostic and Statistical Manual of Mental Disorders, 4th Edition, Text Revision. Washington, DC, American Psychiatric Association, 2000

American Psychiatric Association: Practice guidelines for the treatment of patients with schizophrenia. Am J Psychiatry 154:1–63, 1997

American Psychiatric Association: Diagnostic and Statistical Manual of Mental Disorders, 4th Edition, Text Revision. Washington, DC, American Psychiatric Association, 2000

Andreasen NC: I don't believe in late onset schizophrenia, in Late-Onset Schizophrenia. Edited by Howard R, Rabins PV, Castle DJ. Philadelphia, PA, Wrightson Biomedical, 1999, pp 111–123

Auslander LA, Jeste DV: Sustained remission of schizophrenia among community-dwelling older outpatients. Am J Psychiatry 161:1490–1493, 2004

Ayalon L, Gum AM, Feliciano L, et al: Effectiveness of nonpharmacological interventions for the management of neuropsychiatric symptoms in patients with dementia: a systematic review. Arch Intern Med 166:2182–2188, 2006

Ballard C, Waite J, Birks J: Atypical antipsychotics for aggression and psychosis in Alzheimer's disease. Cochrane Database Syst Rev, Issue 1, Art. No.: CD003476, 2006

Baynes D, Mulholland C, Cooper SJ, et al: Depressive symptoms in stable chronic schizophrenia: prevalence and relationship to psychopathology and treatment. Schizophr Res 45:47–56, 2000

Belitsky R, McGlashan TH: The manifestations of schizophrenia in late life: a dearth of data. Schizophr Bull 19:683–685, 1993

Bleuler M: Die spatschizophrenen Krankheitsbilder. Fortschr Neurol Psychiatr Grenzgeb 15:259–290, 1943

Bonuccelli U, Ceravolo R, Salvetti S, et al: Clozapine in Parkinson's disease tremor: effects of acute and chronic administration. Neurology 49:1587–1590, 1997

Brodaty H, Sachdev P, Rose N, et al: Schizophrenia with onset after age 50 years, 1: phenomenology and risk factors. Br J Psychiatry 175, 410–415, 1999

Burns A, Jacoby R, Levy R: Psychiatric phenomena in Alzheimer's disease, I: disorders of thought content. Br J Psychiatry 157:72–76, 1990a

Burns A, Jacoby R, Levy R: Psychiatric phenomena in Alzheimer's disease, II: disorders of perception. Br J Psychiatry 157:76–81, 1990b

Caligiuri MP, Lacro JP, Rockwell E, et al: Incidence and risk factors for severe tardive dyskinesia in older patients. Br J Psychiatry 171:148–153, 1997

Castle DJ, Murray RM: The epidemiology of late-onset schizophrenia. Schizophr Bull 19:691–700, 1993

Cervantes AN, Rabins PV, Slavney PR: Onset of schizophrenia at age 100. Psychosomatics 47:356–359, 2006

Chambless DL, Hollon SD: Defining empirically supported therapies. J Consult Clin Psychol 66:7–18, 1998

Chan WC, Lam LC, Choy CN, et al: A double-blind randomised comparison of risperidone and haloperidol in the treatment of behavioural and psychological symptoms in Chinese dementia patients. Int J Geriatr Psychiatry 16:1156–1162, 2001

Chou KL, Borek LL, Friedman JH: The management of psychosis in movement disorder patients. Expert Opin Pharmacother 8:935–943, 2007

Christenson R, Blazer D: Epidemiology of persecutory ideation in an elderly population in the community. Am J Psychiatry 141:1088–1091, 1984

Ciompi L: Catamnestic long-term study on the course of life and aging of schizophrenics. Schizophr Bull 6:606–618, 1980

Cohen CI: Outcome of schizophrenia into later life: an overview. Gerontologist 30:790–797, 1990

Cohen-Mansfield J: Nonpharmacologic interventions for inappropriate behaviors in dementia: a review and critique. Am J Geriatr Psychiatry 9:361–381, 2001

Cooper AF, Curry AR: The pathology of deafness in the paranoid and affective psychoses of later life. J Psychosom Research 20:97–105, 1976

Copeland JRM, Dewey ME, Scott A, et al: Schizophrenia and delusional disorder in older age: community prevalence, incidence, comorbidity and outcome. Schizophr Bull 19:153–161, 1998

Corey-Bloom J, Jernigan T, Archibald S, et al: Quantitative magnetic resonance imaging of the brain in late-life schizophrenia. Am J Psychiatry 152:447–449, 1995

Davidson M, Harvey PD, Powchik P, et al: Severity of symptoms in chronically institutionalized geriatric schizophrenic patients. Am J Psychiatry 152:197–207, 1995

De Deyn P, Rabheru K, Rasmussen A, et al: A randomized trial of risperidone, placebo, and haloperidol for behavioral symptoms of dementia. Neurology 53:946–955, 1999

Devanand DP, Jacobs DM, Tang MX, et al: The course of psychopathologic features in mild to moderate Alzheimer disease. Arch Gen Psychiatry 54:257–263, 1997

Diwan S, Cohen CI, Bankole AO, et al: Depression in older adults with schizophrenia spectrum disorders: prevalence and associated factors. Am J Geriatr Psychiatry 15:991–998, 2007

Dolder CR, Jeste DV: Incidence of tardive dyskinesia with typical versus atypical antipsychotics in very high risk patients. Biol Psychiatry 53:1142–1145, 2003

Evans JD, Paulsen JS, Harris MJ, et al: A clinical and neuropsychological comparison of delusional disorder and schizophrenia. J Neuropsychiatry Clin Neurosci 8:281–286, 1996

Evans JD, Heaton RK, Paulsen JS, et al: The relationship of neuropsychological abilities to specific domains of functional capacity in older schizophrenia patients. Biol Psychiatry 53:422–430, 2003

Forsell Y, Henderson AS: Epidemiology of paranoid symptoms in an elderly population. Br J Psychiatry 172:429–432, 1998

Gill SS, Rochon PA, Herrmann N, et al: Atypical antipsychotic drugs and risk of ischaemic stroke: population based retrospective cohort study. Br Med J 330:445, 2005

Granholm E, McQuaid JR, McClure FS, et al: A randomized controlled pilot study of cognitive behavioral social skills training for older patients with schizophrenia (letter). Schizophr Res 153:167–169, 2002

Granholm E, McQuaid JR, McClure FS, et al: A randomized, controlled trial of cognitive behavioral social skills training for middle-aged and older outpatients with chronic schizophrenia. Am J Psychiatry 162:520–529, 2005

Granholm E, McQuaid JR, McClure FS, et al: Randomized controlled trial of cognitive behavioral social skills training for older people with schizophrenia: 12-month follow-up. J Clin Psychiatry 68:730–737, 2007

Hafner H, Van Der Heiden W, Behrens S, et al: Causes and consequences of the gender differences in age at onset of schizophrenia. Schizophr Bull 24:99–113, 1998

Hammerlein A, Derendorf H, Lowenthal DT: Pharmacokinetic and pharmacodynamic changes in the elderly: clinical implications. Clin Pharmacokinet 35:49–64, 1998

Hannerz H, Borga P, Borritz M: Life expectancies for individuals with psychiatric diagnoses. Public Health 115:328–337, 2001

Harding C: Changes in schizophrenia across time, in Schizophrenia Into Later Life. Edited by Cohen CI. Washington, DC, American Psychiatric Publishing, 2002, pp 19–42

Harding CM, Brooks GW, Ashikaga T, et al: Aging and social functioning in once-chronic schizophrenic patients 22–62 years after first admission: the Vermont story, in Schizophrenia and Aging. Edited by Miller NE, Cohen GD. New York, Guilford Press, 1987, pp 74–82

Harris MJ, Jeste DV: Late-onset schizophrenia: an overview. Schizophr Bull 14:39–55, 1988

Harvey PD, Silverman JM, Mohs RC, et al: Cognitive decline in late-life schizophrenia: a longitudinal study of geriatric chronically hospitalized patients. Biol Psychiatry 45:32–40, 1999

Heaton RK, Gladsjo JA, Palmer BW, et al: Stability and course of neuropsychological deficits in schizophrenia. Arch Gen Psychiatry 58:24–32, 2001

Henderson AS, Korten AE, Levings C, et al: Psychotic symptoms in the elderly: a prospective study in a population sample. Int J Geriatr Psychiatry 13:484–492, 1998

Herrmann N, Mamdani M, Lanctot KL: Atypical antipsychotics and risk of cerebrovascular accidents. Am J Psychiatry 161:1113–1115, 2004

Hiroch U, Appleby L, Mortensen PB, et al: Death by homicide, suicide, and other unnatural causes by people with mental illness. Lancet 358:2110–2112, 2001

Howanitz E, Pardo M, Smelson DA: The efficacy and safety of clozapine versus chlorpromazine in geriatric schizophrenia. J Clin Psychiatry 60:41–44, 1999

Howard R, Castle D, Wessely S, et al: A comparative study of 470 cases of early and late-onset schizophrenia. Br J Psychiatry 163:352–357, 1993

Howard R, Almeida O, Levy R: Phenomenology, demography and diagnosis in late paraphrenia. Psychol Med 24:397–410, 1994

Howard R, Graham C, Sham P, et al: A controlled family study of late-onset non-affective psychosis (late paraphrenia). Br J Psychiatry 170:511–514, 1997

Howard R, Rabins PV, Seeman MV, et al: Late-onset schizophrenia and very-late-onset schizophrenia-like psychosis: an international consensus. Am J Psychiatry 157:172–178, 2000

Huber G: The heterogeneous course of schizophrenia. Schizophr Res 28:177–185, 1997

Jeste DV, Finkel SI: Psychosis of Alzheimer's disease and related dementias: diagnostic criteria for a distinct syndrome. Am J Geriatr Psychiatry 8:29–34, 2000

Jeste DV, Harris MJ, Pearlson GD, et al: Late-onset schizophrenia: studying clinical validity. Psychiatr Clin North Am 11:1–14, 1988

Jeste DV, Wragg RE, Salmon DP, et al: Cognitive deficits of patients with Alzheimer's disease with and without delusions. Am J Psychiatry 149:184–189, 1992

Jeste DV, Harris MJ, Krull A, et al: Clinical and neuropsychological characteristics of patients with late-onset schizophrenia. Am J Psychiatry 152:722–730, 1995

Jeste DV, Klausner M, Brecher M, et al: A clinical evaluation of risperidone in the treatment of schizophrenia: a 10-week, open-label, multicenter trial involving 945 patients. Psychopharmacology 131:239–247, 1997a

Jeste DV, Symonds LL, Harris MJ, et al: Non-dementia non-praecox dementia praecox? Late-onset schizophrenia. Am J Geriatr Psychiatry 5:302–317, 1997b

Jeste DV, Lacro JP, Bailey A, et al: Lower incidence of tardive dyskinesia with risperidone compared with haloperidol in older patients. J Am Geriatr Soc 47:716–719, 1999a

Jeste DV, Rockwell E, Harris MJ, et al: Conventional versus newer antipsychotics in elderly patients. Am J Geriatr Psychiatry 7:70–76, 1999b

Jeste DV, Barak Y, Madhusoodanan S, et al: An international multisite double-blind trial of the atypical antipsychotic risperidone and olanzapine in 175 elderly patients with chronic schizophrenia. Am J Geriatr Psychiatry 11:638–647, 2003

Jeste DV, Blazer DG, First M: Aging-related diagnostic variations: need for diagnostic criteria appropriate for elderly psychiatric patients. Biol Psychiatry 58:265–271, 2005

Jeste DV, Meeks TW, Kim DS, et al: Diagnostic categories and criteria for neuropsychiatric syndromes in dementia: research agenda for DSM-V, in Diagnostic Issues in Dementia: Advancing the Research Agenda for DSM-V. Edited by Sunderlan T, Jeste DV, Baiyewu O, et al. Washington, DC, American Psychiatric Publishing, 2007, pp 77–98

Jeste DV, Blazer D, Casey D, et al: ACNP White Paper: update on the use of antipsychotic drugs in elderly persons with dementia. Neuropsychopharmacology 33:957–970, 2008

Jin H, Meyer JM, Jeste DV: Phenomenology of and risk factors for new-onset diabetes mellitus and diabetic ketoacidosis associated with atypical antipsychotics: an analysis of 45 published cases. Ann Clin Psychiatry 14:59–64, 2002

Jin H, Meyer JM, Jeste DV: Atypical antipsychotics and glucose dysregulation: a systematic review. Schizophr Res 71:195–212, 2004

Jones DK, Catani M, Pierpaoli C, et al: A diffusion tensor magnetic resonance imaging study of frontal cortex connections in very-late-onset schizophrenia-like psychosis. Am J Geriatr Psychiatry 13:1092–1099, 2005

Jones PB, Barnes TR, Davies L, et al: Randomized controlled trial of the effect on quality of life of second- vs. first-generation antipsychotic drugs in schizophrenia: Cost Utility of the Latest Antipsychotic Drugs in Schizophrenia Study (CUtLASS 1). Arch Gen Psychiatry 63:1079–1087, 2006

Joukamaam M, Heliovaara M, Knekt P, et al: Mental disorders and cause-specific mortality. Br J Psychiatry 147:498–502, 2001

Kammoun S, Gold G, Bouras C, et al: Immediate causes of death of demented and non-demented elderly. Acta Neurol Scand 176:96–99, 2000

Kane JM, Woerner MG, Pollack S, et al: Does clozapine cause tardive dyskinesia? J Clin Psychiatry 54:327–330, 1993

Keene J, Hope T, Fairburn CG, et al: Death and dementia. Int J Geriatr Psychiatry 16:969–974, 2001

Keith SJ, Regier DA, Rae DS: Schizophrenic disorders, in Psychiatric Disorders in America: the Epidemiologic Catchment Area Study. Edited by Robins LN, Regier DA. New York, Free Press, 1991, pp 33–52

Kendler KS, Davis KL: The genetics and biochemistry of paranoid schizophrenia and other paranoid psychoses. Schizophr Bull 7:689–709, 1981

Kendler KS, Tsuang MT, Hays P: Age at onset in schizophrenia: a familial perspective. Arch Gen Psychiatry 44:881–890, 1987

Kennedy JS, Jeste DV, Kaiser CJ, et al: Olanzapine vs. haloperidol in geriatric schizophrenia: analysis of data from a double-blind controlled trial. Int J Geriatr Psychiatry 18:1013–1020, 2003

Kindermann SS, Dolder CR, Bailey A, et al: Pharmacologic treatment of psychosis and agitation in elderly patients with dementia: four decades of experience. Drugs Aging 19:257–276, 2002

Kinon BJ, Jeste DV, Kollack-Walker S, et al: Olanzapine treatment for tardive dyskinesia in schizophrenia patients: a prospective clinical trial with patients randomized to blinded dose reduction periods. Prog Neuropsychopharmacol Biol Psychiatry 28:985–996, 2004

Kraepelin E: Dementia Praecox and Paraphrenia (1919). Translated by Barclay RM. Huntington, NY, Krieger, 1971

Kulkarni J, de Castella A, Smith D, et al: A clinical trial of the effects of estrogen in acutely psychotic women. Schizophr Res 20:247–252, 1996

Kulkarni J, Riedel A, de Castella A, et al: Estrogen: a potential treatment for schizophrenia. Schizophr Res 48:137–144, 2001

Lieberman JA, Saltz BL, Johns CA, et al: The effects of clozapine on tardive dyskinesia. Br J Psychiatry 158:503–510, 1991

Lieberman JA, Stroup TS, McEvoy JP, et al: Effectiveness of antipsychotic drugs in patients with chronic schizophrenia. N Engl J Med 353:1209–1223, 2005

Lindamer LA, Buse DC, Lohr JB, et al: HRT in postmenopausal women with schizophrenia: positive effect on negative symptoms? Biol Psychiatry 49:47–51, 2001

Littrell KH, Johnson CG, Littrell S, et al: Marked reduction of tardive dyskinesia with olanzapine. Arch Gen Psychiatry 55:279–280, 1998

Livingston G, Johnston K, Katona C, et al: Systematic review of psychological approaches to the management of neuropsychiatric symptoms of dementia. Am J Psychiatry 162:1996–2021, 2005

Lohr JB, Alder M, Flynn K, et al: Minor physical anomalies in older patients with late-onset schizophrenia, early-onset schizophrenia, depression, and Alzheimer's disease. Am J Geriatr Psychiatry 5:318–323, 1997

Maher B: Delusional thinking and cognitive disorder. Integr Physiol Behav Sci 40:136–146, 2005

Masand PS: Atypical antipsychotics for elderly patients with neurodegenerative disorders and medical conditions. Psychiatr Ann 30:203–208, 2000

Mazeh D, Zemishlani C, Aizenberg D, et al: Patients with very-late-onset schizophrenia-like psychosis: a follow-up study. Am J Geriatr Psychiatry 13:417–419, 2005

McKeith I, Del Ser T, Spano P, et al: Efficacy of rivastigmine in dementia with Lewy bodies: a randomised, double-blind, placebo-controlled international study. Lancet 356:2031–2036, 2000

McQuaid JR, Granholm E, McClure FS, et al: Development of an integrated cognitive-behavioral and social skills training intervention for older patients with schizophrenia. J Psychother Pract Res 9:149–156, 2000

Mitter P, Reeves S, Romero-Rubiales F, et al: Migrant status, age, gender and social isolation in very late-onset schizophrenia-like psychosis. Int J Geriatr Psychiatry 20:1046–1051, 2005

Miyasaki JM, Shannon K, Voon V, et al: Practice parameter: evaluation and treatment of depression, psychosis, and dementia in Parkinson disease (an evidence-based review): report of the Quality Standards Subcommittee of the American Academy of Neurology. Neurology 66:996–1002, 2006

Montross L, Kasckow J, Golshan S, et al: The continued need for suicide assessments among middle-aged and older patients with schizophrenia. Paper presented at the annual meeting of the American Association for Geriatric Psychiatry, San Juan, Puerto Rico, March 2006

Moore NC: Is paranoid illness associated with sensory defects in the elderly? J Psychosom Res 25:69–74, 1981

Moore R, Blackwood N, Corcoran R, et al: Misunderstanding the intentions of others: an exploratory study of the cognitive etiology of persecutory delusions in very late-onset schizophrenia-like psychosis. Am J Geriatr Psychiatry 14:410–418, 2006

Mukaetova-Ladinska EB, Harrington CR, Xuereb J, et al: Biochemical, neuropathological, and clinical correlations of neurofibrillary degeneration in Alzheimer's disease, in Treating Alzheimer's and Other Dementias. Edited by Bergener M, Finkel SI. New York, Springer, 1995, pp 57–80

Naimark D, Jackson E, Rockwell E, et al: Psychotic symptoms in Parkinson's disease patients with dementia. J Am Geriatr Soc 44:296–299, 1996

Ostling S, Skoog I: Psychotic symptoms and paranoid ideation in a nondemented population-based sample of the very old. Arch Gen Psychiatry 59:53–59, 2002

Ostling S, Borjesson-Hanson A, Skoog I: Psychotic symptoms and paranoid ideation in a population-based sample of 95-year-olds. Am J Geriatr Psychiatry 15:999–1004, 2007

Palmer BW, McClure F, Jeste DV: Schizophrenia in late-life: findings challenge traditional concepts. Harv Rev Psychiatry 9:51–58, 2001

Palmer BW, Nayak G, Jeste DV: A comparison of early and late-onset schizophrenia, in Schizophrenia Into Late Life. Edited by Cohen CI. Washington, DC, American Psychiatric Publishing, 2002, pp 43–55

Palmer BW, Bondi MW, Twamley EW, et al: Are late-onset schizophrenia-spectrum disorders neurodegenerative conditions? Annual rates of change on two dementia measures. J Neuropsychiatry Clin Neurosci 15:45–52, 2003

Parkinson Study Group: Low-dose clozapine for the treatment of drug-induced psychosis in Parkinson's disease. N Engl J Med 340:757–763, 1999

Patterson TL, Bucardo J, McKibbin CL, et al: Development and pilot testing of a new psychosocial intervention for older Latinos with chronic psychosis. Schizophr Bull 31:922–930, 2005

Patterson TL, McKibbin C, Mausbach BT, et al: Functional Adaptation Skills Training (FAST): a randomized trial of a psychosocial intervention for middle-aged and older patients with chronic psychotic disorders. Schizophr Res 86:291–299, 2006

Paulsen JS, Salmon DP, Thal LJ, et al: Incidence of and risk factors for hallucinations and delusions in patients with probable AD. Neurology 54:1965–1971, 2000

Pollak P, Tison F, Rascol O, et al: Clozapine in drug induced psychosis in Parkinson's disease: a randomised, placebo controlled study with open follow up. J Neurol Neurosurg Psychiatry 75:689–695, 2004

Prager S, Jeste DV: Sensory impairment in late-life schizophrenia. Schizophr Bull 19:755–772, 1993

Putnam KM, Harvey PD: Cognitive impairment and enduring negative symptoms: a comparative study of geriatric and nongeriatric schizophrenia patients. Schizophr Bull 26:869–878, 2000

Raghuram R, Keshavan MD, Channabasavanna SM: Musical hallucination in a deaf middle-aged patient. J Clin Psychiatry 41:357, 1980

Ram R, Bromet EJ, Eaton WW, et al: The natural course of schizophrenia: a review of first-admission studies. Schizophr Bull 18:185–207, 1992

Rivkin P, Kraut M, Barta P, et al: White matter hyperintensity volume in late-onset and early-onset schizophrenia. Int J Geriatr Psychiatry 15:1085–1089, 2000

Rockwell E, Krull AJ, Dimsdale J, et al: Late-onset psychosis with somatic delusions. Psychosomatics 35:66–72, 1994

Ropacki SA, Jeste DV: Epidemiology of and risk factors for psychosis of Alzheimer's disease: a review of 55 studies published from 1990 to 2003. Am J Psychiatry 162:2022–2030, 2005

Roth M: The natural history of mental disorder in old age. J Ment Sci 101:281–301, 1955

Sachdev P, Brodaty H, Rose N, et al: Schizophrenia with onset after age 50 years, 2: neurological, neuropsychological and MRI investigation. Br J Psychiatry 175:416–421, 1999

Schneider LS: Pharmacologic management of psychosis in dementia. J Clin Psychiatry 60:54–60, 1999

Schneider LS, Pollock VE, Lyness S.A: A meta-analysis of controlled trials of neuroleptic treatment in dementia. J Am Geriatr Soc 38:553–563, 1990

Schneider LS, Dagerman KS, Insel P: Risk of death with atypical antipsychotic drug treatment for dementia: meta-analysis of randomized placebo-controlled trials. JAMA 294:1934–1943, 2005

Schneider LS, Dagerman K, Insel PS: Efficacy and adverse effects of atypical antipsychotics for dementia: meta-analysis of randomized, placebo-controlled trials. Am J Geriatr Psychiatry 14:191–210, 2006a

Schneider LS, Tariot PN, Dagerman KS, et al: Effectiveness of atypical antipsychotic drugs in patients with Alzheimer's disease. N Engl J Med 355:1525–1538, 2006b

Seeman MV: The role of estrogen in schizophrenia. J Psychiatry Neurosci 21:123–127, 1996

Simpson GM, Lee JM, Shrivastava RK: Clozapine in tardive dyskinesia. Psychopharmacology 56:75–80, 1978

Sink KM, Holden KF, Yaffe K: Pharmacological treatment of neuropsychiatric symptoms of dementia: a review of the evidence. JAMA 293:596–608, 2005

Small JG, Milstein V, Marhenke JD, et al: Treatment outcome with clozapine in tardive dyskinesia, neuroleptic sensitivity, and treatment-resistant psychosis. J Clin Psychiatry 48:263–267, 1987

Srikanth S, Nagaraja AV, Ratnavalli E: Neuropsychiatric symptoms in dementia: frequency, relationship to dementia severity and comparison in Alzheimer's disease, vascular dementia and frontotemporal dementia. J Neurol Sci 236:43–48, 2005

Stern Y, Albert M, Brandt J, et al: Utility of extrapyramidal signs and psychosis as predictors of cognitive and functional decline, nursing home admission, and death in Alzheimer's disease: prospective analyses from the Predictors Study. Neurology 44:2300–2307, 1994

Stoppe G, Brandt CA, Staedt JH: Behavioural problems associated with dementia: the role of newer antipsychotics. Drugs Aging 14:41–54, 1999

Street JS, Tollefson GD, Tohen M, et al: Olanzapine for psychotic conditions in the elderly. Psychiatr Ann 30:191–196, 2000

Suh GH, Son HG, Ju YS, et al: A randomized, double-blind, crossover comparison of risperidone and haloperidol in Korean dementia patients with behavioral disturbances. Am J Geriatr Psychiatry 12:509–516, 2004

Sultzer DL: Neuroimaging and the origin of psychiatric symptoms in dementia. Int Psychogeriatr 8 (suppl 3):239–243, 1996

Tariot PN, Schneider L, Katz IR, et al: Quetiapine treatment of psychosis associated with dementia: a double-blind, randomized, placebo-controlled clinical trial. Am J Geriatr Psychiatry 14:767–776, 2006

Twamley EW, Padin DS, Bayne KS, et al: Work rehabilitation for middle-aged and older people with schizophrenia: a comparison of three approaches. J Nerv Ment Dis 193:596–601, 2005

Vahia I, Bankole AO, Reyes P, et al: Schizophrenia in later life. Aging Health 3:383–396, 2007

Weiss E, Hummer M, Koller D, et al: Off-label use of antipsychotic drugs. J Clin Psychopharmacol 20:695–698, 2000

Wilkosz PA, Miyahara S, Lopez OL, et al: Prediction of psychosis onset in Alzheimer disease: the role of cognitive impairment, depressive symptoms, and further evidence for psychosis subtypes. Am J Geriatr Psychiatry 14:352–360, 2006

Wirshing DA, Spellberg BJ, Erhart SM, et al: Novel antipsychotics and new onset diabetes. Biol Psychiatry 44:778–783, 1998

Yassa R, Jeste DV: Gender differences in tardive dyskinesia: a critical review of the literature. Schizophr Bull 18:701–715, 1992

Yeung PP, Tariot PN, Schneider LS, et al: Quetiapine for elderly patients with psychotic disorders. Psychiatr Ann 30:197–201, 2000

Zisook S, Montross L, Kasckow J, et al: Subsyndromal depressive symptoms in middle-aged and older persons with schizophrenia. Am J Geriatr Psychiatry 15:1005–1014, 2007

Zubenko GS, Moossy J, Martinez AJ, et al: Neuropathologic and neurochemical correlates of psychosis in primary dementia. Arch Neurol 48:619–624, 1991

Suggested Readings

Auslander LA, Jeste DV: Sustained remission of schizophrenia among community-dwelling older outpatients. Am J Psychiatry 161:1490–1493, 2004

Chou KL, Borek LL, Friedman JH: The management of psychosis in movement disorder patients. Expert Opin Pharmacother 8:935–943, 2007

Granholm E, McQuaid JR, McClure FS, et al: A randomized, controlled trial of cognitive behavioral social skills training for middle-aged and older outpatients with chronic schizophrenia. Am J Psychiatry 162:520–529, 2005

Howard R, Rabins PV, Seeman MV, et al: Late-onset schizophrenia and very-late-onset schizophrenia-like psychois: an international consensus. Am J Psychiatry 157:172–178, 2000

Jeste DV, Harris MJ, Krull A, et al: Clinical and neuropsychological characteristics of patients with late-onset schizophrenia. Am J Psychiatry 152:722–730, 1995

Jeste DV, Blazer D, Casey D, et al: ACNP White Paper: update on the use of antipsychotic drugs in elderly persons with dementia. Neuropsychopharmacology 33:957–970, 2008

Kendler KS, Tsuang MT, Hays P: Age at onset in schizophrenia: a familial perspective. Arch Gen Psychiatry 44:881–890, 1987

Ropacki SA, Jeste DV: Epidemiology of and risk factors for psychosis of Alzheimer's disease: a review of 55 studies published from 1990 to 2003. Am J Psychiatry 162:2022–2030, 2005

Vahia I, Bankole AO, Reyes P, et al: Schizophrenia in later life. Aging Health 3:383–396, 2007

CHAPTER 18

Anxiety Disorders

Eric J. Lenze, M.D.
Julie Loebach Wetherell, Ph.D.

This chapter reviews the presentation, epidemiology, correlates, and treatment of late-life anxiety disorders. Because of the similarities in pathogenesis and clinical presentation of anxiety disorders and depression, particularly between generalized anxiety disorder (GAD) and major depressive disorder (MDD), this chapter addresses comparisons between late-life anxiety disorders and late-life depression, particularly in terms of presentation, risk factors, and comorbidity. Much more is known about the pathophysiology and treatment of geriatric depression than of geriatric anxiety disorders. Absent are longitudinal or mechanistic studies that would shed light on aging-related pathophysiology for the anxiety disorders or elucidate treatment outcomes. With respect to treatment, few large-scale National Institutes of Health (NIH)–funded clinical trials have been published, although some are in progress. Thus, there remain many unanswered basic questions about anxiety disorders in late life. Despite this, advances in knowledge about the epidemiology and treatment of these disorders in late life provide us with a growing body of information to guide clinicians and researchers (Lenze and Wetherell 2008).

Shared Versus Distinct Clinical Features of the Anxiety Disorders

Anxiety disorders are marked by elevated fear or worry and behavioral avoidance. As Table 18–1 demonstrates, the anxiety disorders have shared and distinct features.

It should be noted that all of the anxiety disorders are associated with some degree of avoidance (e.g., even in GAD) and arousal (e.g., GAD is associated with sleep disturbance and irritability, similar to posttraumatic stress disorder [PTSD] and MDD). However, Table 18–1 delineates the more overt situational fear response from worry. On the basis of these shared and distinct features, the eight DSM-IV-TR anxiety disorders—GAD, panic disorder, specific phobia, social phobia, agoraphobia, obsessive-compulsive disorder (OCD), PTSD, and acute stress disorder (American Psychiatric Association 2000)—can be divided into three main categories based on the nature of their phenomenology: worry/distress disorders (GAD, PTSD, and acute stress disorder), fear disorders (panic disorder and the phobias), and OCD (Watson 2005). Worry/distress disorders can also include MDD and dysthymia. Research in young and middle-aged adults has demonstrated that these categories have distinct genetic diatheses, neurocircuitry, and neuroendocrine responses, lending some credence to this grouping. It should be emphasized that similar research has not been done in older adults; therefore, we know very little about the appropriate subtyping of anxiety presentations in late life to distinguish or group anxiety disorders based on underlying neurobiology. Nevertheless, the next section describes the various anxiety disorders, subtyped into the three categories just mentioned, and what is known about their presentation in relationship to aging as well as their epidemiology.

TABLE 18–1. Shared and distinct clinical features of anxiety disorders

	Situational fear	Situational avoidance	Autonomic arousal	Anticipatory worry	Obsessions and compulsions	Panic attacks
Panic disorder	x	x	x	x		x
Social and specific phobia and agoraphobia	x	x	x	x		x
Obsessive-compulsive disorder	x	x		x	x	
Generalized anxiety disorder				x		
Posttraumatic stress disorder, acute stress disorder	x	x	x	x		

Epidemiology

Opinions on the prevalence of late-life anxiety disorders vary, from the view that they are relatively uncommon, and, if present, are typically comorbid conditions with depression, to the opinion that anxiety disorders are common and in fact more prevalent than mood disorders in the elderly.

These disparate opinions stem from the wide variability in published prevalence estimates of anxiety disorders in community-dwelling older adults. For example, the Longitudinal Aging Study Amsterdam (LASA) is one of the largest epidemiological studies to focus on psychiatric disorders in elderly persons. It demonstrated that more than 10% of elderly persons had GAD, phobias, panic disorder, and/or OCD, in line with estimates in younger adults. Other studies have found that all of the anxiety disorders are less common in older adults, with many studies finding panic disorder rare or nonexistent (Flint 1994). One study, the Australian National Mental Health and Well-Being Survey (NMHWS), found that the prevalence of anxiety disorders in the elderly varied almost threefold depending on whether DSM-IV-TR or ICD-10 (World Health Organization 1992) criteria were used (Trollor et al. 2007).

Table 18–2 shows several large epidemiological studies that included a large sample of elderly persons, using the National Comorbidity Study Replication (NCS-R) as a mixed-age comparator. As a whole, the studies suggest that GAD is at least as common in late life as in younger adults, whereas other anxiety disorders (particularly OCD, and probably panic disorder) are rarer. Because only one of these studies surveyed PTSD (NMHWS), it is likely that anxiety prevalence rates are underestimated among the other investigations.

Age at Onset and Risk Factors for Anxiety Disorders

Published reviews of the literature have taken two different stances on the question of age at onset of anxiety disorders. One camp describes them as rarely of late onset (Flint 2005a), pointing to studies finding that anxiety disorders usually have onset in childhood or early adulthood (Kessler et al. 2007). Another camp, which unsurprisingly includes most of the NIH-funded researchers in late-life anxiety, has found in clinical samples of elderly persons that many have a later onset of anxiety disorder (Le Roux et al. 2005; Lenze et al. 2005a; Sheikh et al. 2004; van Zelst et al. 2003). For example, in a sample of 103 treatment-seeking elderly GAD patients, the mean age at onset was 49, with 46% being of late onset (Lenze et al. 2005a). Other evidence suggests a bimodal distribution of onset, with approximately two-thirds having onset in childhood or adolescence and one-third developing the disorder for the first time at the age of 50 or later (Blazer et al. 1991; Le Roux et al. 2005).

In a sense both camps may be correct, and aging may either protect from anxiety or cause anxiety, depending on circumstances. Congruent with this assertion, some reports have noted a decline in the propensity for negative affect (which underlies anxiety as well as depression) from adulthood to "early" elderly years, with a subsequent rise in the mid-70s (Charles et

TABLE 18–2. Prevalence estimates of late-life anxiety disorders from epidemiological studies

	Epidemiological studies in the elderly					NCS-R (adults)
	LASA	ECA	AMSTEL	NMHWS	CCHS	
N	3,107		4,051	1,792	12,792	9,282
Age range	55–85	65+	65–84	65+	55+	18+
Prevalence						
Any anxiety disorder	10.2%	5.5%	N/A	4.4%	N/A	18.1%
Generalized anxiety disorder	7.3%	1.9%	3.2%	2.4%	N/A	3.1%
Phobic disorder	3.1%	4.8%	N/A	0.6% (social)	1.3% (social) 0.6% (agoraphobia)	8.7%
Panic disorder	1.0%	0.1%	N/A	0.8%	0.8%	2.7%
Obsessive-compulsive disorder	0.6%	0.8%	N/A	0.1%	N/A	1.0%
Posttraumatic stress disorder	N/A	N/A		1.0%	N/A	3.5%

Note. AMSTEL=Amsterdam Study of the Elderly; CCHS=Canadian Community Health Survey; ECA=Epidemiologic Catchment Area; LASA=Longitudinal Aging Study Amsterdam; NCS-R=National Comorbidity Study Replication; NMHWS=National Mental Health and Well-Being Study. N/A=not applicable.

al. 2001; Teachman 2006). It has been suggested that aging provides the opportunity to inoculate against the anxiety-producing nature of stressors and to practice emotion regulation (Jarvik and Russell 1979). Additionally, aging may reduce the propensity for anxiety because of degeneration in anxiety-producing brain regions such as the locus coeruleus (Flint 1994). On the other hand, aging is associated with a number of new stressors, such as chronic illness and disability (in self or loved ones), that may be particularly anxiogenic. Also, age-related degeneration in brain regions associated with adaptive responses to anxiety (e.g., the dorsolateral prefrontal cortex) may reduce the ability of some to manage anxiogenic situations; findings of poststroke GAD (Aström 1996) and cerebral lesions associated with late-onset OCD (Swoboda and Jenike 1995) are congruent with this assertion. Along these lines, clinicians should be aware that many prescription medications can induce anxiety (e.g., anticholinergics, psychostimulants, or steroids), and this should be a part of any differential diagnosis of new-onset anxiety in an elderly person. However, it is our clinical experience that elderly persons, unless cognitively impaired, are usually quite insightful when a medication they take causes clinically significant anxiety.

Another consideration is that some anxiety disorders presenting in later life may have a different nature (Flint 2005b), owing to a potentially different etiology, much as late-onset depression, often in the context of cerebrovascular illness, has different phenomenology than the early-onset variety. Research has not shown this to be the case in anxiety: early- and late-onset disorders do not appear to be qualitatively different (Sheikh et al. 2004; Wetherell et al. 2003b), yet this in itself may be due to the use of DSM-IV-TR diagnoses created for younger adults. Anxiety conditions germane to elderly persons—such as anxiety in the context of dementia (Starkstein et al. 2007), of anxiogenic medical conditions such as heart disease (Todaro et al. 2007), of fear of falling (Gagnon et al. 2005), or of hoarding syndrome (Saxena 2007)—may not be discerned by standard epidemiological assessments or methodology. Thus, the prevalence and significance of such conditions are unknown. In summary, late-onset anxiety disorders are probably more common than appreciated, but they may present differently than in younger adults.

Risk factors for anxiety disorders have been reported in elderly persons (Vink et al. 2007). They include female gender, neurotic personality, early life stress, and chronic disability in self or spouse. However, research uncovering neurobiological risk factors for late-life, or late-onset, anxiety has not been done. Therefore, the basic question of who develops anxiety in older age is largely unanswered.

Worry/Distress Disorders: Generalized Anxiety Disorder and Posttraumatic Stress Disorder

Generalized Anxiety Disorder

Case Example

Mary M., a 65-year-old woman, was interviewed about anxiety by her family physician after she presented with concerns about her memory and voiced a fear that she had Alzheimer's disease. She admits to being "a worrier" all her life but does not feel that her previous anxiety had been excessive or problematic. In the past 3 years, however, she reports spending more time worrying and finding it more distressing and "difficult to turn my mind off." This has occurred in the context of caring for her husband, who has severe cardiac failure and often gets chest pain, resulting in the need for immediate medical attention at any time of the day.

Mary also worries about her own health, her children's health and their financial issues, and other issues (e.g., crime in the neighborhood). In the past 3 years she has had poor sleep, finding it difficult to stop worrying at night. She feels "tense" as well and has seen an orthopedist about "shoulder pain" that was thought to be muscle tension. Her concentration is poor, although she does well with objective testing of memory and other neuropsychological domains. Finally, she feels fatigued much of the day, resulting in workups for anemia and other medical problems.

The central feature of GAD is worry or anticipation of future negative events. Also known as "anxious apprehension," worry is thought to be a separate form of anxiety from fear or "anxious arousal" as seen in the fear disorders (e.g., panic disorder). Phenomenologically, they are quite different: worry may wax and wane but does not have the intense episodic nature of panic attacks (although worry can itself precipitate panic attacks). As such, GAD has evolved diagnostically to be first considered a residual state of phobic/panic anxiety, then a disorder in its own right, and now, in the looming DSM-V era, as a close relative to MDD. Worry in DSM-IV-TR-diagnosed GAD must be excessive, be difficult to control, and cause distress. The actual content of worry in late-life GAD has been noted to be similar to that in older adults without GAD—that is, concerns about health or disability, family relationships, or finances (Diefenbach et al. 2001).

Associated features of GAD are muscle tension, restlessness (or feeling keyed up or on edge), sleep difficulties, concentration problems (often thought by older adults to be memory problems), fatigue, and irritability. It is our clinical experience that elderly persons with GAD often present (to primary care or specialty medical care) with these associated symptoms, which then become the targets of treatment (e.g., benzodiazepines for sleep, muscle relaxants or even physical therapy referral for muscle tension, cholinesterase inhibitors for cognitive complaints) rather than detection of the underlying anxiety syndrome. GAD may wax and wane but is typically chronic, unlike depressive episodes (Lenze et al. 2005a).

The LASA study found a prevalence of 7.3% in adults ages 55 and older; within this sample there was no reduction in prevalence in older cohorts (i.e., those ages 75 and older compared with those ages 55–64). However, several other studies have found lower prevalence estimates of GAD in the elderly, including the National Epidemiologic Survey on Alcohol and Related Conditions (NESARC; Grant et al. 2005), which found a lower prevalence of GAD in older adults (1%) compared with young and middle-aged adults. The tenfold variation in published estimates of late-life GAD may result from important qualitative differences between the ways in which elderly persons versus younger adults describe anxiety. The objects of worry in elderly persons with GAD are largely the same as those in older adults without GAD: health, disability in self or spouse, and finances (Diefenbach et al. 2001). Because these are often realistic sources of concern in aging, older adults with GAD may be unlikely to feel that their worry is excessive or is about "minor things" as described in the GAD criteria, making its diagnosis difficult in epidemiological research or in clinical practice. Clinicians need to consider that it is the amount of worry, the difficulty the individual has in stopping it, and the degree of distress or functional impairment related to worrying that is critical, not the degree to which the worry is realistic.

In any event, GAD is one of the most common mental disorders in elderly persons. The disorder is even more common in medical settings, as might be expected for any affective or anxiety disorder (Todaro et al. 2007; Tolin et al. 2005). Together with data showing that elderly persons with anxiety disorders rarely present to specialty mental health (Ettner and Hermann 1997), this suggests that primary and specialty medical care, not psychiatric settings, are the places to find late-life GAD that is not comorbid with depression.

The overlap between GAD and MDD is great in terms of symptoms such as impaired sleep and concentration, low energy, and irritability. Additionally, low mood is a frequent feature of GAD, and excessive worry is frequently seen in MDD. The underlying genetic predisposition to both disorders is thought to be similar in older as in younger adults (Kendler et al. 1992, 2007). As a whole, there are several reasons for high comorbidity between GAD and MDD. Yet some studies have found that "pure" GAD (non-comorbid with MDD) is more common than the comorbid condition (Beekman et al. 2000; Schoevers et al. 2003).

As previously noted, GAD tends to be chronic rather than episodic. Studies have found that the mean length of GAD symptoms in elderly persons presenting for treatment was 20 (Lenze et al. 2005a) to more than 30 years (Stanley et al. 2003a; Wetherell et al. 2003a), which compares with an average of 9 years among younger adults (Wang et al. 2005). These data fit with evidence showing GAD to be one of the least likely mental disorders in the anxiety/affective spectrum to remit spontaneously over time (Bruce et al. 2005). Other reports have suggested that in elderly persons chronic GAD tends to develop into a somatization condition (Rubio et al. 2007) or mixed GAD/MDD (Schoevers et al. 2003).

Posttraumatic Stress Disorder and Acute Stress Disorder

Case Example

A 78-year-old World War II veteran presented to the VA hospital for complaints related to a possible diagnosis of PTSD. He described being a land-sea transport captain during the invasion of Normandy in 1941 who brought soldiers to Omaha Beach. Many of these soldiers, especially in the initial waves, were killed by gunfire in front of him. He describes still visualizing bodies lapped against his ship by the waves. He describes several symptoms related to this visualization: elevated anxiety and distress, nightmares, poor concentration, irritability, and feelings of being detached or numb. These symptoms have worsened recently as a number of his friends have passed away from illness.

PTSD is characterized by exposure to a traumatic event (an accident, violence, or natural event) that produced intensive fear, helplessness, or horror. The event must have produced at least 1 month of symptoms (less than 1 month for acute stress disorder) in each of three clusters: reexperiencing of the event (via thoughts, flashbacks, or dreams), avoidance (avoiding thoughts of the event or situations that bring it to mind, feeling detached, having diminished interest in or responsiveness to activities, having a sense of foreshortened future), and distress/arousal (e.g., sleep disturbances, exaggerated startle, irritability).

PTSD has received little study in older adults, despite the association of the disorder with many types of traumatic experiences common in this age group, such as combat experiences for veterans of World War II and the Korean conflict (Frueh et al. 2007) or traumatic medical events (Dew et al. 2001). Also of note is an epidemiological report in older African American patients that found PTSD was the most common anxiety disorder in this population, with the highest 12-month prevalence of any mental disorder (Ford et al. 2007). These findings may have reflected methodological differences from other studies or real differences of minorities from Caucasians in this age group. Overall, the research in late-life PTSD is far behind its overall impact in terms of prevalence and morbidity (van Zelst et al. 2003).

Fear Disorders: Panic Disorder, Agoraphobia, Social Phobia, and Specific Phobia

The fear disorders are marked by anxiety that is discrete (clearly episodic) and confined to a specific situation, although in the case of agoraphobia, behavioral avoidance may be continuous and without reference to specific triggers. The fear disorders are also marked by autonomic arousal and situational avoidance.

Panic Disorder

A *panic attack* is an episode of fear or intense anxiety accompanied by multiple somatic and cognitive symptoms (e.g., feeling that one is losing control). Somatic symptoms tend to be autonomic in nature (palpitations, sweating, chills, tremulousness) and also include gastrointestinal distress, numbness and tingling in extremities, and shortness of breath. Attacks build to peak intensity quickly (within 10 minutes at the most) and last up to 30 minutes, although repeated or "status" panic attacks can occur. Attacks can occur at any time, including nocturnally, causing sudden awakening.

Panic disorder is the syndrome of recurrent panic attacks (at least some out of the blue) associated with concern about having further attacks and, often, avoidance of situations associated in the patient's mind with attacks. This avoidance can often lead to agoraphobia.

Most studies have found a low prevalence of panic disorder in older adults in the community. This has led to a line of thinking that perhaps the aging process reduces panic disorder prevalence or that mortality due to panic disorder reduces the likelihood of its being present in older age groups (Flint 1994). Late-onset panic disorder appears to be rare and may often be a prodrome of a medical or neurological problem. However, this assertion is based on the disorder as defined in young adults and cannot exclude the possibility that panic symptoms that do not meet criteria for panic disorder may be more common in late life.

Case Example

A 72-year-old woman was referred to geriatric psychiatry after she presented with complaints of "passing out" to her primary care doctor. She described how, without warning, she would feel like passing out. The feeling was subjective and not tied to exertion, physical activity, or orthostatic changes. On further interview, she reported that these episodes would last for approximately 15 minutes and would be associated with shortness of breath, palpitations, tingling in her hands, and abdominal distress. She did not have any active cardiac problems. These episodes occurred approximately monthly.

Since the onset of these symptoms, her family describes her as more "needy." She goes out less often, and when she does, it is only with a family member present. She describes this change as related to crime in the neighborhood and realistic worries about falling with no one there to help her in the case of an injury.

When panic disorder does occur in elderly persons, it tends to be associated with less severe or less frequent panic attacks than in young adults, who frequently have daily attacks (Sheikh et al. 2004). The lower severity of attacks may be due to older adults having less ability to mount a strong autonomic response (Flint et al. 2002). Nevertheless, because the disability due to panic disorder tends to be related to the behavioral avoidance rather than the frequency of attacks themselves, panic disorder can still be a highly disabling condition in elderly persons.

Phobias

Phobias are marked by an excessive and unreasonable situational fear that is distressing or impairing. Exposure to the situation is either avoided or endured only with distress, even precipitating a panic attack in some instances.

Phobias may be difficult to detect in older adults—particularly if the phobia has been lifelong—because of lifestyle accommodation around it (e.g., avoiding social situations in the case of social phobia). The available evidence suggests that specific phobias are quite common in the elderly, whereas social phobia is less so.

The difficulty of diagnosing phobias is exemplified by a condition called "fear of falling," a common problem in elderly persons which by its very name might be considered a phobia. However, research into this condition suggests that it is not. In the only published study that examined anxiety diagnoses in fear of falling, in no case was the fear diagnosable as a phobia, in part because subjects did not feel their fear to be excessive or unreasonable (Gagnon et al. 2005). It has been noted that the "excessive/unreasonable" criterion is not required for a diagnosis of specific phobia in children, raising the question of whether this criterion should be dropped for phobia diagnoses in the elderly (Flint 2005b).

Social phobia has received little study in elderly persons. In the largest examination of this condition, Cairney et al. (2007) found that aging was associated with reduced prevalence of social phobia, although the condition still remained fairly common in old age and qualitatively appeared strikingly similar to that in young adults.

Agoraphobia can present within the context of panic attacks but frequently does not do so in elderly persons (McCabe et al. 2006). It can appear *de novo* in the context of a stroke or other medical event, in which case it can be highly disabling, leading to inhibition of activities necessary for restoration after the event (Burvill et al. 1995). The largest study to examine agoraphobia in older adults found it to be rare (0.6% prevalence; McCabe et al. 2006), but the condition itself might lead to decreased ability to detect it.

Obsessive-Compulsive Disorder

Most epidemiological studies have concluded that OCD, marked by obsessions and/or compulsions, is fairly uncommon in elderly persons and is rarely of late onset. However, one report from the Epidemiologic Catchment Area data set found a second peak of OCD incidence in women ages 65 and older (Nestadt et al. 1998). In any event, it has not been the topic of research in this age group (Velayudhan and Katz 2006), beyond a few case reports and case series (e.g., Chacko et al. 2000; Weiss and Jenike 2000). These case reports have often found cerebral lesions, often in the basal ganglia, suggesting neurodegenerative disease as potential pathophysiology for late-onset OCD. The observation of hoarding and similar compulsive behavior in dementia, and the observation of greater neuropsychological impairment in late-onset OCD (Hwang et al. 2007), adds to evidence of a connection between neurodegenerative illness and late-onset OCD.

Genetic predisposition for OCD appears limited to those with early-onset illness (Nestadt et al. 2000). Those with a later onset of illness may be more likely to respond to cognitive-behavioral therapy (CBT) for the disorder (Grant et al. 2007), although it is not clear that this would be the case if there was overlying cognitive impairment (as would be expected for patients with neurodegenerative disease).

Neuropsychology and Neurobiology of Late-Life Anxiety Disorders

Some reports examining neuropsychological features in late-life GAD have drawn on literature that demonstrates a relationship of anxiety symptoms or disorders with cognitive decline in older adults (Sinoff and Werner 2003; Wetherell et al. 2002). A preliminary study comparing GAD patients, MDD patients, and healthy elderly individuals found the GAD patients had impaired short-term and delayed memory, but not executive deficits as seen in MDD (Mantella et al. 2007). These results are consistent with another study in late-life GAD that found increased anxiety severity was associated with memory impairments (Caudle et al. 2007). Similar findings have been reported in late-life PTSD (Yehuda et al. 2007). Another study of late-life GAD found that more severe worry was associated with better executive function, in a measure of inhibitory control (Price and Mohlman 2007). As a whole, these studies suggest both similarities and differences between late-life anxiety and depression, but more definitive research in this area is needed. To date, no longitudinal study of clinical anxiety disorders in late life has been carried out that could examine cognitive decline, and there has been little interest in examining these aspects in disorders other than GAD, in part because of their apparent rarity.

Very little translational research has been carried out in late-life anxiety disorders. Some studies have examined the hypothalamic-pituitary-adrenal axis in late-life GAD because dysfunction in this axis is common in late-life depression and in young adults with anxiety disorders. Late-life GAD is associated with 40%–50% higher diurnal cortisol levels than are seen in healthy elderly persons (Mantella et al. 2007). Elevated cortisol in late-life GAD decreases with pharmacological treatment (Pomara et al. 2005) but does not decrease in younger adults with GAD, suggesting some important age-related differences in this syndrome with respect to neurohormonal stress response. These findings of elevated cortisol in late-life GAD may distinguish the disorder from PTSD, for which a study in a largely elderly population found lower urinary cortisol in veterans with PTSD compared with those without (Yehuda et al. 2007). That same study found no relationship of PTSD with hippocampal volume. To date, no other structural or functional neuroimaging studies have been carried out in late-life anxiety disorders.

Comorbidity With Late-Life Depression

Much attention has been given to the issue of anxiety comorbidity with late-life depression because studies have consistently found that response to antidepressants is delayed or diminished in late-life depression in the context of anxiety.

The term *anxious depression* refers to individuals with MDD and either a comorbid anxiety disorder or significant anxiety symptoms. The LASA study, to our knowledge the largest epidemiological study to examine comorbidity of anxiety disorders and depression in the elderly, found that 48% of elderly persons with MDD also had a current comorbid anxiety disorder, whereas approximately one-fourth of those with anxiety disorders had MDD (Beekman et al. 2000). Likewise, rates of severe anxiety symptoms have been seen in as high as one-half of late-life MDD clinical samples (Lenze et al. 2000; Mulsant et al. 1996). Thus, comorbid anxiety is quite common in late-life depression.

The comorbidity is not surprising given the extensive symptomatic overlap of anxiety disorders (particularly GAD and PTSD) with MDD. In the classification system described earlier, MDD and dysthymia are grouped with PTSD and GAD as distress disorders. Many patients with late-life MDD develop significant anxiety only within the depressive episode, whereas others have a long history of an anxiety disorder with later onset of depression (Lenze et al. 2005a). Symptomatically, anxiety symptoms are more stable than those of depression and more likely to lead to depressive symptoms than vice versa (Wetherell et al. 2001). As a result, anxiety disorders might be a risk factor for late-life depression (Hettema et al. 2006). When depression precedes or coexists with the anxiety disorder, anxiety symptoms often persist after remission of depression and increase risk for depressive relapse (Dombrovski et al. 2007; Flint and Rifat 1997). Unfortunately, translational research that might better clarify the convergence of anxiety and depression in late life (e.g., functional neuroimaging) is lacking, although we are aware of ongoing efforts in this area.

The combination of anxiety and depression in elderly persons is a severe and often treatment-resistant illness. Depressed elderly with comorbid anxiety have greater somatic symptoms, greater suicidal ideation (Jeste et al. 2006; Lenze et al. 2000), and a higher risk of suicide (Allgulander and Lavori 1993). Many studies have demonstrated a longer time to response in depression, and/or a reduced response rate, in association with anxiety symptoms (Alexopoulos et al. 2005; Andreescu et al. 2007; Dew et al. 1997; Lenze et al. 2003; Mulsant et al. 1996) or an anxiety disorder (Flint and Rifat 1997; Steffens et al. 2005). The reason for these findings is unclear; it may simply be that the combination of two disorders results in higher symptom levels, which reduces the chance of remitting to "normal" levels of symptoms. However, one study found that even after elderly patients achieved full remission from late-life depression, they were still more likely to relapse if they had high levels of baseline anxiety symptoms (Andreescu et al. 2007) (see Figure 18–1). Additionally, one study found that comorbid GAD or panic disorder was predictive of greater decline in memory over an average of 4 years' naturalistic follow-up in late-life depression after remission of the acute episode (DeLuca et al. 2005). Thus, it may be that anxious depression is a treatment-relevant neurobiological subtype in elderly persons.

Treatment

As in young adults, anxiety disorders have a waning and waxing course in the elderly but are unlikely to remit completely (Schuurmans et al. 2005); additionally, they produce quality-of-life impairments and disability on par with that of late-life depression (DeBeurs et al. 1999; Wetherell et al. 2004) and may be a risk factor for the development of anxious depression, a severe and treatment-resistant illness. All of these issues suggest the importance of treatment.

The treatment of late-life anxiety disorders has been the subject of many reviews and meta-analyses (e.g., Pinquart and Duberstein 2007; Wetherell et al. 2005b) despite the relative lack of treatment trials. The available evidence suggests that both psychotherapy (primarily CBT) and pharmacotherapy are effective. However, considerable gaps exist in our understanding of these treatments. As a result, authors have concluded alternately that psychotherapy (Mohlman and Price 2006) or pharmacotherapy (Pinquart and Duberstein 2007) should be the first-line treatment. The goal here is not to take a side but to describe relevant treatment research as well as management issues with both modalities.

Psychotherapy

There is evidence that older adults can learn new skills in CBT and use them effectively over time (Wetherell et al. 2005a). In the only study to simultaneously compare CBT with a credible attention control condition and a waiting list for late-life GAD, CBT produced large effects on measures of anxiety, depression, and quality of life relative to the waiting list, whereas the control condition produced small to medium effects (Wetherell et al. 2003a). Other research has found that CBT is effective compared with minimal-contact controls (Stanley et al. 2003a) or usual care (Stanley et al. 2003b). These data, although preliminary, suggest that CBT is an efficacious treatment for GAD in older adults.

CBT for late-life anxiety includes education about anxiety and its symptoms, relaxation skills, cognitive therapy, problem-solving skills training, exposure exercises, and sleep hygiene instructions (Stanley et al. 2004). Adaptations for CBT in elderly persons include increased repetition and increased time reviewing previous sessions (Mohlman and Price 2006).

The evidence is more mixed as to whether CBT is a superior treatment to other psychotherapy for late-life anxiety (Barrowclough et al. 2001; Stanley et al. 1996; Wetherell et al. 2003a). The only study directly comparing CBT and pharmacotherapy for late-life anxiety (mostly GAD and panic disorder) found a greater effect size for pharmacotherapy (sertraline), although the study was preliminary (Schuurmans et al. 2006). This raises the question of whether further enhancements or a sequential approach of using medications and CBT would be more effective in older adults. Study of these alternatives is under way by several groups at the time of this writing.

No controlled research on psychotherapy focused on anxiety conditions other than GAD exists. Several

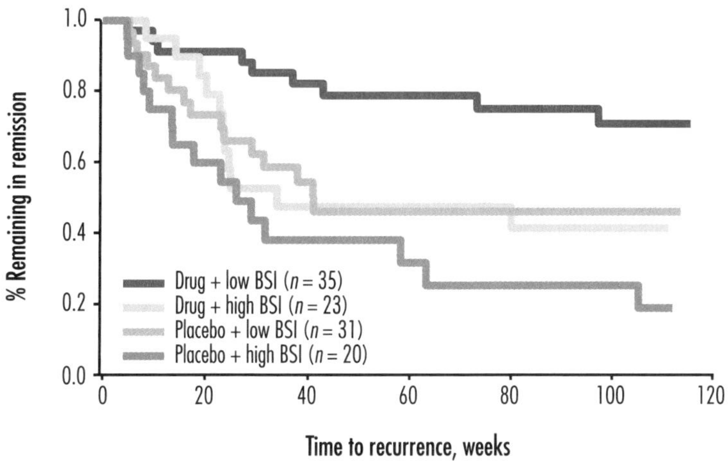

FIGURE 18–1. High pretreatment levels of comorbid anxiety symptoms, as measured by the Brief Symptom Inventory (BSI), predict increased recurrence after remission from major depressive disorder.

Source. Adapted from Andreescu et al. 2007.

studies have included samples with mixed anxiety disorders, including panic disorder and social phobia, but none have published disorder-specific results. Clearly this represents a gap in the research literature.

Pharmacotherapy

Surprisingly little research has been done in late-life anxiety pharmacotherapy. As reviewed elsewhere (Pinquart and Duberstein 2007; Wetherell et al. 2005b), many small clinical trials have been carried out, but they differ to such an extent in terms of the populations studied (e.g. GAD vs. panic vs. anxiety neurosis) and treatments used (benzodiazepine vs. antidepressant vs. other) that it is unhelpful to provide an omnibus summary of the findings.

Some studies have found that benzodiazepines are efficacious in reducing anxiety symptoms in late-life anxiety (Bresolin et al. 1988; Koepke et al. 1982). However, the use of these medications, already common in elderly persons, is concerning given the potential for increased risk of falls (e.g., Landi et al. 2005) and cognitive impairment.

Antidepressants—particularly selective serotonin reuptake inhibitors (SSRIs) such as escitalopram, citalopram, and sertraline, and serotonin-norepinephrine reuptake inhibitors such as duloxetine and venlafaxine—are considered first-line treatment for anxiety disorders in younger adults because of these drugs' lower potential for toxicity or abuse. Some small studies have demonstrated the efficacy of the SSRIs citalopram and sertraline for late-life anxiety disorders (Lenze et al. 2005b; Schuurmans et al. 2006). However, these were small preliminary studies. At the time of this writing, no large-scale prospective clinical trials of pharmacotherapy for late-life anxiety disorders have been published, although we are aware of two studies under way.

No studies have been published examining either second-line strategies (except for a small study of risperidone [Moríñigo et al. 2005]) or maintenance treatment.

No published studies have focused exclusively on late-life PTSD, but a few in mixed-age populations with mean age of 55–60 have suggested that the antidepressants citalopram (English et al. 2006) and mirtazapine (Chung et al. 2004) and the α-adrenergic blocker prazosin (Raskind et al. 2007) are effective. Further research is needed to determine optimal treatment for this illness in elderly persons.

Clinical Management

As we await further research to clarify the extent to which medication, psychotherapy, or their combination is efficacious acutely or long term for late-life anxiety, there are several important management issues for clinicians.

First and foremost, detecting and diagnosing the anxiety (whether primary or comorbid) is of importance. Elderly persons with anxiety disorders may not be insightful or conversant with terms used to define anxiety (e.g., "panic," "social anxiety"). They often feel that anxiety or fear is a realistic response to their environment or current stressors. Yet *undetected* anxiety is likely to persist and have a detrimental effect on treatment of comorbid conditions (such as depression). Anecdotally, we have found that asking about reactions to stress (e.g., "How do you feel in times of stress?") is a useful opener in asking elderly persons about anxiety symptoms. Patients who report anxiety terms (e.g., "anxious," "concerned," "worried") can then be asked additional questions such as "How often does it occur?" and "What do you do to manage these feelings?" In this latter point, asking whether anxiety is "excessive" or "uncontrollable" is unlikely to be fruitful; instead, asking about mechanisms to control anxiety will elicit a more pertinent response. Patients with panic symptoms may not endorse "panic attacks" but may admit to brief periods with multiple physical symptoms (particularly autonomic symptoms such as palpitations).

Second, discuss the management with the patient while keeping in mind how anxiety will affect his or her views about treatment. This is particularly true in the case of medications, especially antidepressants that are well known to have a stimulating or mildly anxiogenic effect initially before an antianxiety effect occurs. Anecdotally, we have noted that most patients with late-life anxiety report being sensitive or intolerant of antidepressant medications if they have tried them. This "intolerance" likely results from anticipatory concern about side effects, vigilance toward interoceptive stimuli, and a tendency to catastrophize about any interoceptive sensations they detect (even if unrelated to the antidepressant). Therefore, management consists of counseling patients in advance about side effects of medication explicitly to reduce the concern that these might somehow be toxic or incapacitating. Additionally, management includes close follow-up after the onset or dosage titration of an antidepressant medication to ensure that the patient did start it and to address the perception of side effects. Clinicians should realize that when these "side effects" occur, the patient is actually most likely to be describing anxiety-related symptoms that preceded the start of the medicine and that are now being attributed to the medicine. It is useful to inform the patient that such symptoms are expected to get better and are not harmful.

The early use of benzodiazepines may produce a fast anxiolytic action that could improve compliance; however, the long-term use of these medications is discouraged in favor of alternative treatments when possible, such as SSRIs, other antidepressants, or psychotherapy. Also it should be noted that benzodiazepines may counteract the effects of psychotherapy, particularly CBT (Westra and Stewart 1998).

In summary, the detection and management of anxiety disorders in elderly persons is challenging, but the high prevalence and significant morbidity associated with these disorders highlight the importance of understanding them. It is expected that as our knowledge base (in diagnosis, etiology, and treatment) of these disorders improves, anxiety disorders will become a core clinical issue in geriatric psychiatry, much like dementia and depression.

Key Points

- Epidemiological studies show wide variation of prevalence and suggest that generalized anxiety disorder (GAD) is the most common anxiety disorder in late life.
- Late-onset anxiety disorders are more common than previously thought but may appear qualitatively different from typical DSM-IV-TR disorders.
- Pharmacological and psychotherapeutic treatments are similar to those in young adults.
- Increased vigilance is required of the clinician to detect and manage anxiety in this age group.
- More research is needed to examine the nature, course, and treatment of these common syndromes.

References

Allgulander C, Lavori PW: Causes of death among 936 elderly patients with "pure" anxiety neurosis in Stockholm County, Sweden, and in patients with depressive neurosis or both diagnoses. Compr Psychiatry 34:299–302, 1993

Alexopoulos GS, Katz IR, Bruce ML, et al: Remission in depressed geriatric primary care patients: a report from the PROSPECT study. The PROSPECT Group. Am J Psychiatry 162:718–724, 2005

American Psychiatric Association: Diagnostic and Statistical Manual of Mental Disorders, 4th Edition, Text Revision. Washington, DC, American Psychiatric Association, 2000

Andreescu C, Lenze EJ, Dew MA, et al: Effect of comorbid anxiety on treatment response and relapse risk in late-life depression: controlled study. Br J Psychiatry 190:344–349, 2007

Aström M: Generalized anxiety disorder in stroke patients: a 3-year longitudinal study. Stroke 27:270–275, 1996

Barrowclough C, King P, Colville J, et al: A randomized trial of the effectiveness of cognitive-behavioral therapy and supportive counseling for anxiety symptoms in older adults. J Consult Clin Psychol 69:756–762, 2001

Beekman ATF, de Beurs E, van Balkom AJLM, et al: Anxiety and depression in later life: co-occurrence and communality of risk factors. Am J Psychiatry 157:89–95, 2000

Blazer D, George KL, Hughes D: The epidemiology of anxiety disorders: an age comparison, in Anxiety in the Elderly: Treatment and Research. Edited by Salzman C, Lebowitz BD. New York, Springer, 1991, pp 17–30

Bresolin N, Monza G, Scarpini E, et al: Treatment of anxiety with ketazolam in elderly patients. Clin Ther 10:536–546, 1988

Bruce SE, Yonkers KA, Otto MW, et al: Influence of psychiatric comorbidity on recovery and recurrence in generalized anxiety disorder, social phobia, and panic disorder: a 12-year prospective study. Am J Psychiatry 162:1179–1187, 2005

Burvill PW, Johnson GA, Jamrozik KD, et al: Anxiety disorders after stroke: results from the Perth Community Stroke Study. Br J Psychiatry 166:328–332, 1995

Cairney J, McCabe L, Veldhuizen S, et al: Epidemiology of social phobia in later life. Am J Geriatr Psychiatry 15:224–233, 2007

Caudle DD, Senior AC, Wetherell JL, et al: Cognitive errors, symptom severity, and response to cognitive behavior therapy in older adults with generalized anxiety disorder. Am J Geriatr Psychiatry 15:680–689, 2007

Chacko RC, Corbin MA, Harper RG: Acquired obsessive compulsive disorder associated with basal ganglia lesions. J Neuropsychiatry Clin Neurosci 12:269–272, 2000

Charles ST, Reynolds CA, Gatz M: Age-related differences and change in positive and negative affect over 23 years. J Pers Soc Psychol 80:136–151, 2001

Chung MY, Min KH, Jun YJ, et al: Efficacy and tolerability of mirtazapine and sertraline in Korean veterans with posttraumatic stress disorder: a randomized open label trial. Hum Psychopharmacol 19:489–494, 2004

DeBeurs E, Beekman ATF, van Balkom AJLM, et al: Consequences of anxiety in older persons: its effect on disability, well-being and use of health services. Psychol Med 29:583–593, 1999

DeLuca AK, Lenze EJ, Mulsant BH, et al: Comorbid anxiety disorder in late-life depression: association with memory decline over four years. Int J Geriatr Psychiatry 20:848–854, 2005

Dew MA, Reynolds CF 3rd, Houck PR, et al: Temporal profiles of the course of depression during treatment: predictors of pathways toward recovery in the elderly. Arch Gen Psychiatry 54:1016–1024, 1997

Dew MA, Kormos RL, DiMartini AF, et al: Prevalence and risk of depression and anxiety-related disorders during the first three years after heart transplantation. Psychosomatics 42:300–313, 2001

Diefenbach GJ, Stanley MA, Beck JG: Worry content reported by older adults with and without generalized anxiety disorder. Aging Ment Health 5:269–274, 2001

Dombrovski AY, Mulsant BH, Houck PR, et al: Residual symptoms and recurrence during maintenance treatment of late-life depression. J Affect Disord 103:77–82, 2007

English BA, Jewell M, Jewell G, et al: Treatment of chronic posttraumatic stress disorder in combat veterans with citalopram: an open trial. J Clin Psychopharmacol 26:84–88, 2006

Ettner SL, Hermann RC: Provider specialty choice among Medicare beneficiaries treated for psychiatric disorders. Health Care Financ Rev 18:43–59, 1997

Flint A: Epidemiology and comorbidity of anxiety disorders in the elderly. Am J Psychiatry 151:640–649, 1994

Flint A: Anxiety and its disorders in late life: moving the field forward. Am J Geriatr Psychiatry 13:3–6, 2005a

Flint A: Generalised anxiety disorder in elderly patients: epidemiology, diagnosis and treatment options. Drugs Aging 22:101–114, 2005b

Flint AJ, Rifat SL: Two-year outcome of elderly patients with anxious depression. Psychiatry Res 66:23–31, 1997

Flint A, Bradwejn J, Vaccarino F, et al: Aging and panicogenic response to cholecystokinin tetrapeptide: an examination of the cholecystokinin system. Neuropsychopharmacology 27:663–671, 2002

Ford BC, Bullard KM, Taylor RJ, et al: Lifetime and 12-month prevalence of DSM–IV disorders among older African Americans: findings from the National Survey of American Life (NSAL). Am J Geriatr Psychiatry 15:652–659, 2007

Frueh BC, Grubaugh AL, Acierno R, et al: Age differences on PTSD, psychiatric disorders, and healthcare service use among veterans in Veterans Affairs primary care clinics. Am J Geriatr Psychiatry 15:660–672, 2007

Gagnon N, Flint AJ, Naglie G, et al: Affective correlates of fear of falling in elderly persons. Am J Geriatr Psychiatry 13:7–14, 2005

Grant BF, Hasin DS, Stinson FS, et al: Prevalence, correlates, comorbidity, and comparative disability of DSM-IV generalized anxiety disorder in the USA: results from the National Epidemiologic Survey on Alcohol and Related Conditions. Psychol Med 35:1747–1759, 2005

Grant JE, Mancebo MC, Pinto A, et al: Late-onset obsessive compulsive disorder: clinical characteristics and psychiatric comorbidity. Psychiatry Res 152:21–27, 2007

Hettema JM, Kuhn JW, Prescott CA, et al: The impact of generalized anxiety disorder and stressful life events on risk for major depressive episodes. Psychol Med 36:789–795, 2006

Hwang SH, Kwon JS, Shin YW, et al: Neuropsychological profiles of patients with obsessive-compulsive disorder: early onset versus late onset. J Int Neuropsychol Soc 13:30–37, 2007

Jarvik LJ, Russell D: Anxiety, aging, and the third emergency response. J Gerontol 37:197–200, 1979

Jeste ND, Hays JC, Steffens DC: Clinical correlates of anxious depression among elderly patients with depression. J Affect Disord 90:37–41, 2006

Kendler KS, Neale MC, Kessler RC, et al: Major depression and generalized anxiety disorder: same genes, (partly) different environments? Arch Gen Psychiatry 49:716–722, 1992

Kendler KS, Gardner CO, Gatz M, et al: The sources of comorbidity between major depression and generalized anxiety disorder in a Swedish national twin sample. Psychol Med 37:453–462, 2007

Kessler RC, Amminger GP, Aguilar-Gaxiola S, et al: Age of onset of mental disorders: a review of recent literature. Curr Opin Psychiatry 20:359–364, 2007

Koepke HH, Gold RL, Linden ME, et al: Multicenter controlled study of oxazepam in anxious elderly outpatients. Psychosomatics 23:641–645, 1982

Landi F, Onder G, Cesari M, et al: Psychotropic medications and risk for falls among community-dwelling frail older people: an observational study. J Gerontol A Biol Sci Med Sci 60:622–626, 2005

Le Roux H, Gatz M, Wetherell JL: Age at onset of generalized anxiety disorder in older adults. Am J Geriatr Psychiatry 13:23–30, 2005

Lenze EJ, Wetherell JL: Bringing the bedside to the bench, and then to the community: a prospectus for intervention research in late-life anxiety disorders. Int J Geriatr Psychiatry, July 9, 2008 [Epub ahead of print]

Lenze EJ, Mulsant BH, Shear MK, et al: Comorbid anxiety disorders in depressed elderly patients. Am J Psychiatry 15:722–728, 2000

Lenze EJ, Mulsant BH, Dew MA, et al: Good treatment outcomes in late-life depression with comorbid anxiety. J Affect Disord 77:247–254, 2003

Lenze EJ, Mulsant BH, Mohlman J, et al: Generalized anxiety disorder in late life: lifetime course and comorbidity with major depressive disorder. Am J Geriatr Psychiatry 13:77–80, 2005a

Lenze EJ, Mulsant BH, Shear MK, et al: Efficacy and tolerability of citalopram in the treatment of late-life anxiety disorders: results from an 8-week randomized, placebo-controlled trial. Am J Psychiatry 162:146–150, 2005b

Mantella RC, Butters MA, Dew MA, et al: Cognitive impairment in late-life generalized anxiety disorder. Am J Geriatr Psychiatry 15:673–679, 2007

McCabe L, Cairney J, Veldhuizen S, et al: Prevalence and correlates of agoraphobia in older adults. Am J Geriatr Psychiatry 14:515–522, 2006

Mohlman J, Price R: Recognizing and treating late-life generalized anxiety disorder: distinguishing features and psychosocial treatment. Expert Rev Neurother 6:1439–1445, 2006

Moríñigo A, Blanco M, Labrador J, et al: Risperidone for resistant anxiety in elderly persons. Am J Geriatr Psychiatry 13:81–82, 2005

Mulsant BH, Reynolds CF, Shear MK, et al: Comorbid anxiety disorders in late-life depression. Anxiety 2:242–247, 1996

Nestadt G, Bienvenu OJ, Cai G, et al: Incidence of obsessive-compulsive disorder in adults. J Nerv Ment Dis 186:401–406, 1998

Nestadt G, Samuels J, Riddle M, et al: A family study of obsessive-compulsive disorder. Arch Gen Psychiatry 57:358–363, 2000

Pinquart M, Duberstein PR: Treatment of anxiety disorders in older adults: a meta-analytic comparison of behavioral and pharmacological interventions. Am J Geriatr Psychiatry 15:639–651, 2007

Pomara N, Willoughby LM, Sidtis JJ, et al: Cortisol response to diazepam: its relationship to age, dose, duration of treatment, and presence of generalized anxiety disorder. Psychopharmacology (Berl) 178:1–8, 2005

Price RB, Mohlman J: Inhibitory control and symptom severity in late life generalized anxiety disorder. Behav Res Ther 45:2628–2639, 2007

Raskind MA, Peskind ER, Hoff DJ, et al: A parallel group placebo controlled study of prazosin for trauma nightmares and sleep disturbance in combat veterans with post-traumatic stress disorder. Biol Psychiatry 61:928–934, 2007

Rubio G, López-Ibor JJ: Generalized anxiety disorder: a 40-year follow-up study. Acta Psychiatr Scand 115:372–379, 2007

Saxena S: Is compulsive hoarding a genetically and neurobiologically discrete syndrome? Implications for diagnostic classification. Am J Psychiatry 164:380–384, 2007

Schoevers RA, Beekman ATF, Deeg DJH, et al: Comorbidity and risk-patterns of depression, generalised anxiety disorder and mixed anxiety-depression in later life: results from the AMSTEL study. Int J Geriatr Psychiatry 18:994–1001, 2003

Schuurmans J, Comijs HC, Beekman ATF, et al: The outcome of anxiety disorders in older people at 6-year follow-up: results from the Longitudinal Aging Study Amsterdam. Acta Psychiatr Scand 111:420–428, 2005

Schuurmans J, Comijs H, Emmelkamp PM, et al: A randomized, controlled trial of the effectiveness of cognitive-behavioral therapy and sertraline versus a waitlist control group for anxiety disorders in older adults. Am J Geriatr Psychiatry 14:255–263, 2006

Sheikh JI, Swales PJ, Carlson EB, et al: Aging and panic disorder: phenomenology, comorbidity, and risk factors. Am J Geriatr Psychiatry 12:102–109, 2004

Sinoff G, Werner P: Anxiety disorder and accompanying subjective memory loss in the elderly as a predictor of future cognitive decline. Int J Geriatr Psychiatry 18:951–959, 2003

Stanley MA, Beck JG, Glassco JD: Treatment of generalized anxiety in older adults: a preliminary comparison of cognitive-behavioral and supportive approaches. Behav Ther 27:565– 581, 1996

Stanley MA, Beck JG, Novy DM, et al: Cognitive-behavioral treatment of late-life generalized anxiety disorder. J Consult Clin Psychol 71:309–319, 2003a

Stanley MA, Hopko DR, Diefenbach GJ, et al: Cognitive-behavior therapy for late-life generalized anxiety disorder in primary care: preliminary findings. Am J Geriatr Psychiatry 11:92–96, 2003b

Stanley MA, Diefenbach GJ, Hopko DR: Cognitive behavioral treatment for older adults with generalized anxiety disorder: a therapist manual for primary care settings. Behav Modif 28:73–117, 2004

Starkstein SE, Jorge R, Petracca G, et al: The construct of generalized anxiety disorder in Alzheimer disease. Am J Geriatr Psychiatry 15:42–49, 2007

Steffens DC, McQuoid DR: Impact of symptoms of generalized anxiety disorder on the course of late-life depression. Am J Geriatr Psychiatry 13:40–47, 2005

Swoboda KJ, Jenike MA: Frontal abnormalities in a patient with obsessive-compulsive disorder: the role of structural lesions in obsessive-compulsive behavior. Neurology 45:2130–2134, 1995

Teachman BA: Aging and negative affect: the rise and fall and rise of anxiety and depression symptoms. Psychol Aging 21:201–207, 2006

Todaro JF, Shen BJ, Raffa SD, et al: Prevalence of anxiety disorders in men and women with established coronary heart disease. J Cardiopulm Rehabil Prev 27:86–91, 2007

Tolin DF, Robison JT, Gaztambide S, et al: Anxiety disorders in older Puerto Rican primary care patients. Am J Geriatr Psychiatry 13:150–156, 2005

Trollor JN, Anderson TM, Sachdev PS, et al: Prevalence of mental disorders in the elderly: the Australian National Mental Health and Well-Being Survey. Am J Geriatr Psychiatry 15:455–466, 2007

van Zelst WH, de Beurs E, Beekman AT, et al: Prevalence and risk factors of posttraumatic stress disorder in older adults. Psychother Psychosom 72:333–342, 2003

Velayudhan L, Katz AW: Late-onset obsessive-compulsive disorder: the role of stressful life events. Int Psychogeriatr 18:341–344, 2006

Vink D, Aartsen MJ, Schoevers RA: Risk factors for anxiety and depression in the elderly: a review. J Affect Disord 106:29–44, 2008

Wang PS, Berglund P, Olfson M, et al: Failure and delay in initial treatment contact after first onset of mental disorders in the National Comorbidity Survey Replication. Arch Gen Psychiatry 62:603–613, 2005

Watson D: Rethinking the mood and anxiety disorders: a quantitative hierarchical model for DSM-V. J Abnorm Psychol 114:522–536, 2005

Weiss AP, Jenike MA: Late-onset obsessive-compulsive disorder: a case series. J Neuropsychiatry Clin Neurosci 12:265–268, 2000

Westra HA, Stewart SH: Cognitive behavioural therapy and pharmacotherapy: complementary or contradictory approaches to the treatment of anxiety? Clin Psychol Rev 18:307–340, 1998

Wetherell JL, Gatz M, Pedersen NL: A longitudinal analysis of anxiety and depressive symptoms. Psychol Aging 16:187–195, 2001

Wetherell JL, Reynolds CA, Gatz M, et al: Anxiety, cognitive performance, and cognitive decline in normal aging. J Gerontol Psychol Sci 57B:P246–P255, 2002

Wetherell JL, Gatz M, Craske MG: Treatment of generalized anxiety disorder in older adults. J Consult Clin Psychol 71:31–40, 2003a

Wetherell JL, Le Roux H, Gatz M: DSM-IV criteria for generalized anxiety disorder in older adults: distinguishing the worried from the well. Psychol Aging 18:622–627, 2003b

Wetherell JL, Thorp SR, Patterson TL, et al: Quality of life in geriatric generalized anxiety disorder: a preliminary investigation. J Psychiatr Res 38:305–312, 2004

Wetherell JL, Hopko DR, Diefenbach GJ, et al: Cognitive-behavioral therapy for late-life generalized anxiety disorder: who gets better? Behav Ther 36:147–156, 2005a

Wetherell JL, Lenze EJ, Stanley MA: Evidence-based treatment of geriatric anxiety disorders. Psychiatr Clin North Am 28:871–896, ix, 2005b

World Health Organization: International Statistical Classification of Diseases and Related Health Problems, 10th Revision. Geneva, Switzerland, World Health Organization, 1992

Yehuda R, Golier JA, Tischler L, et al: Hippocampal volume in aging combat veterans with and without post-traumatic stress disorder: relation to risk and resilience factors. J Psychiatr Res 41:435–445, 2007

Suggested Readings

Beekman ATF, de Beurs E, van Balkom AJLM, et al: Anxiety and depression in later life: co-occurrence and communality of risk factors. Am J Psychiatry 157:89–95, 2000

Charles ST, Reynolds CA, Gatz M: Age-related differences and change in positive and negative affect over 23 years. J Personal Soc Psychol 80:136–151, 2001

Flint A: Epidemiology and comorbidity of anxiety disorders in the elderly. Am J Psychiatry 151:640–649, 1994

Lenze EJ, Wetherell JL: Bringing the bedside to the bench, and then to the community: a prospectus for intervention research in late-life anxiety disorders. Int J Geriatr Psychiatry 2008 Jul 9 [Epub ahead of print] PMID: 18613267

Wetherell JL, Lenze EJ, Stanley MA: Evidence-based treatment of geriatric anxiety disorders. Psychiatr Clin North Am 28:871–896, ix, 2005

CHAPTER 19

SOMATOFORM DISORDERS

MARC E. AGRONIN, M.D.

Somatoform disorders comprise a heterogeneous group of psychiatric illnesses in which physical symptoms or complaints without objective organic causes are present and in which there are strongly associated psychological factors. The seven somatoform disorders listed in DSM-IV-TR (American Psychiatric Association 2000) are 1) somatization disorder, 2) undifferentiated somatoform disorder, 3) hypochondriasis, 4) conversion disorder, 5) pain disorder, 6) body dysmorphic disorder (BDD), and 7) somatoform disorder not otherwise specified. Prevalence rates vary by diagnosis, but in general, across ages, somatoform disorders and their less severe variants have been seen in 16% of primary care outpatients (DeWaal et al. 2004) and in 23% of outpatients with medically unexplained symptoms (Smith et al. 2005).

Older individuals with somatoform disorders are seen in all health care settings, where they frequently overuse medical services (Barsky 1979) and overburden general practitioners (Reid et al. 2001). They often come to the attention of a geriatric psychiatrist after another clinician has attempted unsuccessfully to resolve their physical symptoms. To date, somatoform disorders have not been well studied in late life, in part because many of the disorders tend to begin in early adulthood. In addition, research involving older cohorts has usually focused on reported somatic symptoms rather than on specific diagnoses. A complicating factor is that somatoform symptoms in late life are often obscured by comorbid physical and psychiatric illnesses. In particular, somatoform disorders have been strongly associated with depression, anxiety, psychological trauma, substance abuse, and personality disorders (DeWaal et al. 2004; Hasin and Katz 2007; Otto et al. 2001; Polatin et al. 1993; Sack et al. 2007).

Clinical Features

Medically unexplained symptoms are seen commonly in outpatient settings. When these symptoms shift from transient expressions of somatic concern to more serious bodily preoccupation and impairment, and no organic cause emerges from appropriate workup, a somatoform disorder becomes a more likely diagnosis. Somatoform symptoms are experienced by the affected individual as real physical sensations, pain, or discomfort, usually indistinguishable from symptoms of actual medical disorders and frequently coexisting with them. Despite having no organic basis, these symptoms can lead to significant emotional distress and functional impairment. Associated psychological factors are presumed but not always apparent, and patients vary in their degree of insight into such factors.

Patients with somatoform disorders are often able to accept that their symptoms may be functional and have psychological roots. Unlike malingering, however, somatoform disorders do not represent intentional, conscious attempts by patients to present physical symptoms in order to achieve a specific goal (e.g., to get out of work). They differ from factitious disorders such as Munchausen syndrome in that their etiologies are considered to be wholly unconscious and are not always aimed at achieving the sick role. Neither do they represent delusional thinking as found in psychotic states (although BDD can be associated with beliefs of delusional quality).

Somatoform disorders also differ from psychosomatic disorders, which are characterized by actual disease states with presumed psychological triggers. Instead, somatoform disorders involve a complex interaction between brain and body, in which the affected individual is unknowingly expressing psychological stress or conflict through the body. Not surprisingly, increased somatic symptoms and preoccupation with illness are often associated with anxiety, depression, and psychological trauma.

Somatization Disorder

Somatization disorder is characterized by multiple physical complaints, in excess of what would be expected given the patient's history and examination findings. These complaints cannot be fully explained by medical workup and must include pain at four or more sites, as well as two gastrointestinal symptoms, one sexual symptom, and one pseudoneurological symptom (other than pain). Another term used in the literature for this disorder is *Briquet's syndrome* (Liskow et al. 1986). Symptoms typically appear before age 30 and have usually persisted for years by the time of diagnosis. Cloninger (1986) suggested that symptoms of somatization disorder differ from those of true medical illness in that the former 1) involve multiple body systems simultaneously, 2) have an early onset and a chronic history without later development of pathognomonic symptoms of medical illness, and 3) are not associated with relevant physical or laboratory findings.

Somatization disorder is seen almost exclusively in women and may have a prevalence rate ranging from less than 1%–3% (Faravelli et al. 1997; Rabinowitz et al. 2006). High rates of the disorder have been noted among first-degree female relatives of affected individuals (Cloninger 1986) and in certain medical conditions. For example, definite or probable somatization disorder was diagnosed in 42% of a sample of 50 medical outpatients with irritable bowel disease (Miller et al. 2001). Associated problems include drug abuse and dependence, depression and suicidality, and multiple and unnecessary medical treatments, including surgeries.

The most difficult diagnostic feature to establish in elderly patients is the onset of symptoms before age 30, because such history can rarely be accurately determined. In addition, the presence of multiple physical symptoms in excess of what would be expected is a relative factor in late life, given the high incidence of comorbid illnesses.

Somatization disorder tends to run a chronic course, with the majority of individuals demonstrating consistent symptom patterns as they age, even into later life (Pribor et al. 1994). Rabinowitz et al. (2006) found that older individuals with somatization were more lonely, isolated, and dissatisfied with the support they received from others.

Undifferentiated Somatoform Disorder

In most elderly patients with somatoform symptoms, a diagnosis of undifferentiated somatoform disorder can be more easily made than a diagnosis of somatization disorder. Undifferentiated somatoform disorder is defined by the presence of one of more physical complaints, lasting at least 6 months, that cannot be fully explained by appropriate medical workup and that result in considerable social, occupational, or functional impairment. Again, diagnosis is complicated in late life by the frequency of comorbid medical disorders. Determining whether the impairment is caused by somatoform symptoms rather than comorbid medical disorders is difficult and may be nearly impossible in the case of many debilitated elderly individuals. Prevalence rates for undifferentiated somatoform disorder have not been well established for any age group, although one community study in Italy found a rate of 13.8%—significantly higher than rates for every other somatoform disorder (Faravelli et al. 1997). Patients with chronic pain have been found to have quite high rates of undifferentiated somatoform disorder (Aigner and Bach 1999).

Hypochondriasis

Hypochondriasis is characterized by a preoccupation with fears of having a serious illness. These fears arise from misinterpretation of bodily symptoms, and the individual's preoccupation is resistant to medical evaluation and reassurance. Hypochondriacal symptoms are more common among individuals who are under stress because of medical illness in themselves or a relative or who have a history of serious illness, especially in childhood (Kellner 1987). Physical complaints tend to be based on common but transient symptoms that are viewed as portending a serious illness. In fact, most individuals have one or more somatic symptoms in any given week, and a small but not insignificant percentage of affected individuals and a higher percentage of somewhat neurotic individuals will develop mild anxiety with respect to such symptoms (Kellner 1987).

The line between normal somatic concern and hypochondriasis can be difficult to draw but depends on a pattern of dysfunctional behaviors that ultimately serve to increase anxiety and constrain medical treatment. Barsky (1979) suggested that underlying this pattern is a psychological state that tends to amplify bodily perceptions. Similar psychological states have been described in women who have fibromyalgia (McDermid et al. 1996), although without the behavioral patterns seen in hypochondriasis. In the person with hypochondriasis, it is the resultant conviction of having a disease that leads to a pattern of 1) anxious ruminations that one has a terrible illness and 2) repetitive medical consultations.

Hypochondriasis has been seen in 3% of medical inpatients (Fink et al. 2004) and in around 5% of outpatients (Barsky 2001; Faravelli et al. 1997), and there is some debate regarding whether factors such as low education level, low socioeconomic status, and old age increase these rates (Barsky et al. 1991; Brink et al. 1981; Kellner 1986; Rief et al. 2001). Comorbid psychiatric disorders are common, especially major depression, panic disorder, generalized anxiety disorder, and obsessive-compulsive disorder (Escobar et al. 1998; Fink et al. 2004; Simon et al. 2001).

Conversion Disorder

Conversion disorder is characterized by one or more motor or sensory deficits that cannot be fully explained by appropriate medical workup and that appear to be causally related to psychological factors. The diagnosis should specify whether the symptom or deficit is a motor or sensory one, involves a seizure, or entails a mixed presentation. As with other somatoform symptoms, however, the presence of true medical comorbidity can cloud the picture. The key to the diagnosis of conversion symptoms is identification of the psychological conflict that seems to be prompting the symptom, and this approach often requires in-depth psychotherapeutic investigation. Some researchers have argued that conversion disorder is actually a form of a dissociative disorder (Brown et al. 2007).

Although conversion disorder has been reported in the elderly population (Weddington 1979), it is more common in young women, and the prevalence rate in the community is less than 1% (Cloninger 1986; Faravelli et al. 1997). Dula and DeNaples (1995) reviewed records of 42 patients who were seen in an emergency room and subsequently received a diagnosis of conversion disorder. Of these patients, 24 were women (average age, 33 years) and 18 were men (average age, 34 years). Comorbid diagnoses included substance abuse, chronic illness, head trauma, and previous conversion symptoms. Psychogenic nonepileptic seizures (PNES), sometimes referred to as pseudoseizures, represent one subtype of conversion symptoms. They are characterized by behavioral spells that mimic various forms of seizures but are not associated with electroencephalographic findings and have a presumed psychological etiology (D'Allesio et al. 2006; Mari et al. 2006). PNES are more frequent in young women and are seen in 5%–20% of outpatients with epilepsy, often in combination with an actual seizure disorder (Chabolla et al. 1996). They have been diagnosed in individuals older than 60 years (Behrouz et al. 2006).

Risk factors for conversion disorder include physical and sexual abuse, personality disorder, and other neurological illnesses (O'Sullivan et al. 2007; Roelofs et al. 2002; Sar et al. 2004). Conversion disorder in late life may be even more likely to be associated with an actual comorbid neurological disorder. The prognosis is variable and depends on several factors, including the degree of functional impairment and psychiatric comorbidity and the type of symptoms. In one study, persistent symptoms were present in nearly 40% of subjects at 10-year follow-up (Mace and Trimble 1996). In contrast, a separate small study using physical therapy to treat conversion symptoms noted complete recovery in all affected individuals (Ness 2007). According to a review by Krem (2004), affected individuals with more acute, quickly diagnosed conversion symptoms with minimal comorbidity tend to do better over time compared with individuals who are older or have symptoms of longer duration and more severe disability—especially seizures and paralysis.

Pain Disorder

Pain is the most common medical complaint in elderly persons, with pain caused by musculoskeletal disease (e.g., osteoarthritis, back pain, headache) being the most common type of pain (Leveille et al. 2001). Close to 50% of elderly individuals have chronic pain, and the percentage approaches 70% for those in long-term care

(Otis and McGeeney 2000). Persistent pain is associated with significant functional and social impairment (Scudds and Ostbye 2001) as well as comorbid psychiatric symptoms, including depression, insomnia, and substance abuse. Pain assessment is often limited because of its dependence on subjective patient reports, which can be influenced by numerous confounding factors in late life, including dementia. Dementia may limit an individual's ability to verbalize pain, with the result that caregivers must rely on nonverbal behaviors. It has also been proposed that the pathological process in Alzheimer's disease may alter pain perception, perhaps by increasing the pain threshold (Scherder et al. 2001). Pharmacological treatment of pain, however, can lead to additional problems caused by medication side effects and drug-drug interactions.

In pain disorder, pain is the major focus of the clinical presentation, and psychological factors are believed to play critical roles in the onset, severity, exacerbation, or continuation of the pain. Diagnostic variants of pain disorder in DSM-IV-TR include pain disorder associated with psychological factors, a general medical condition, or both. Even when there are specific causes of pain, diagnosis hinges on identifying an overwhelming preoccupation with pain—a preoccupation sometimes involving a pattern of treatment resistance. The determination of such psychological factors is difficult, especially in late life, and the ensuing divisions between the relative roles of mind and body raise questions about diagnostic validity (Boland 2002).

This dilemma is illustrated by the overwhelming psychiatric comorbidity associated with both chronic pain and somatoform pain disorder. In a study involving individuals with chronic low back pain, 80% of subjects met criteria for at least one lifetime psychiatric disorder—including major depression, substance abuse, anxiety disorders, or personality disorders (Polatin et al. 1993)—usually with onset before the development of chronic pain. In another study involving individuals with chronic pain, 66% of the subjects (ages 18–65 years) met DSM-IV criteria for pain disorder (Aigner and Bach 1999). Of the patients with pain disorder, 22% had depression, 7% had hypochondriasis, 10% had somatization disorder, and more than 90% met criteria for undifferentiated somatoform disorder. Descriptions of pain characteristics did not differ between pain disorder associated with psychological factors and pain disorder caused by both psychological factors and a general medical problem. Similar findings emerged from a study involving individuals with chronic headache (Okasha et al. 1999). In that study, somatoform pain disorder was diagnosed in more than 40% of individuals with no established organic etiology and in 20% of persons with an organic etiology. Personality disorders were diagnosed in 77% of members of the nonorganic etiology group, compared with a rate of 24% in the organic etiology group. Depressive disorders were also relatively common in the nonorganic etiology group.

Body Dysmorphic Disorder

BDD is characterized by a preoccupation with an imagined or small defect in appearance. Common body parts that become the object of focus include facial features (e.g., the nose), breasts, and genitals. If there is an actual physical defect, this preoccupation greatly exceeds what would be expected. Affected individuals often spend considerable time engaging in repetitive behaviors such as looking at the body part in the mirror, touching or picking at it, and seeking reassurance from others regarding their concern. Symptoms tend to be chronic and often lead patients to make extraordinary attempts to deal with the imagined or slight defect, including unnecessary plastic surgery (Grant and Phillips 2005; Phillips and Dufresne 2000). For this reason, BDD often presents to plastic surgeons or dermatologists long before coming to the attention of a psychiatrist. The disorder is commonly diagnosed in young adults and in women around the time of menopause, and it is often associated with comorbid depression, obsessive-compulsive behaviors, personality disorders, and even suicidality (Bellino et al. 2006; Phillips 1998).

The estimated prevalence of BDD in women in the community is 0.7% (Faravelli et al. 1997; Otto et al. 2001). In a study involving 74 individuals with BDD, Phillips and McElroy (2000) found comorbid personality disorders in 57% of the sample; the most common personality disorders were avoidant (43% of patients with a personality disorder), dependent (15%), obsessive-compulsive (14%), and paranoid (14%) personality disorders. In up to 50% of individuals with BDD, the somatic preoccupation may be delusional (Phillips 1998; Phillips et al. 1998). Although no prevalence figures for BDD in late life are available, such specific complaints are less common in older patients.

Somatoform Disorder Not Otherwise Specified

The diagnosis of somatoform disorder not otherwise specified is used when the patient has somatoform symptoms that do not meet the criteria for other somatoform disorders but that result in similar degrees of social, occupational, and functional impairment. Some somatoform presentations that fit this category are hypochondriacal symptoms of less than 6 months' duration, unexplained physical symptoms of less than 6 months' duration, and pseudocyesis, in which the false belief that one is pregnant is associated with objective (albeit false) symptoms of pregnancy.

Etiology

The causes of somatoform disorders are usually multifactorial and are often rooted in early developmental experiences and personality traits. For example, somatization and all somatoform disorders have been associated with the experience of serious illness early in life (Stuart and Noyes 1999), childhood abuse (Roelofs et al. 2002; Samelius et al. 2007; Waldinger et al. 2006), dissociative amnesia (Brown et al. 2005), significant psychological stress (Hollifield et al. 1999; Ritsner et al. 2000), and the personality traits of alexithymia and neuroticism (Bailey and Henry 2007; De Gucht 2003; Phillips and McElroy 2000). As noted throughout the chapter, somatoform disorders are also highly associated with comorbid depression, anxiety and panic disorders, substance abuse, and personality disorders (Noyes et al. 2001; Sar et al. 2004). Somatization may be more common in women and in older individuals, although the prevalence of actual somatoform disorders has not been associated with increased age—with the exception of hypochondriasis. When present in late life, especially with late onset, somatoform disorders may be associated with neuropsychological impairment and/or comorbid neurological illness (Sheehan and Banerjee 1999). Functional magnetic resonance imaging scans have found distinctive patterns of increased cerebral activation in the left inferior frontal lobe and in left limbic structures associated with somatoform symptoms (Stone et al. 2007; Vuilleumier 2005). Specific neuroimaging studies of patients with conversion symptoms have found decreased activity in motor or somatosensory cortex, along with increased activation in orbitofrontal and anterior cingulated cortex (Vuilleumier et al. 2001; Yazící and Kostakoglu 1998). These and other factors associated with somatoform disorders are summarized in Table 19–1.

TABLE 19–1. Factors associated with somatoform disorders

Alexithymia
Childhood physical and/or sexual abuse
Chronic medical illness
Chronic pain
Dissociative amnesia
Female gender
Frontal lobe, anterior cingulate, and limbic dysfunction
Lower educational level
Low socioeconomic status
Neuroticism
Psychiatric illness
Anxiety disorders
Depressive disorders
Other somatoform disorder
Personality disorders
Substance abuse
Severe, persistent psychological stress

Psychodynamic approaches suggest that somatoform disorders result from unconscious conflict in which intolerable impulses or affects are believed to be expressed through more tolerable somatic symptoms or complaints. The classic example of this phenomenon is found in conversion disorder, in which intolerable unconscious impulses are converted into motor or sensory dysfunction. Freud first wrote about such a mechanism based on his studies of young women who had what was then termed *hysteria* (Breuer and Freud 1893–1895/1955). Specifically, psychodynamic theory suggests that excessive and intolerable guilt or hostility are psychological sources of somatization—in particular, hypochondriasis (Barsky and Klerman 1983). In such cases, physical symptoms serve as a means of self-punishment for unacceptable unconscious impulses. Anger directed toward caregivers is indirectly expressed through distrust of and dissatisfaction with multiple physicians. Some researchers have suggested that underlying and complicating this psychodynamic rechannelization of anger or guilt is the trait of alexithymia, in which an individual has a relative inability to identify and express emotional states (Bailey and Henry 2007; Waller and Scheidt 2004). The experiencing and reporting of bodily sensations thus becomes a mode of emotional expression. Although alexithymia has long been postulated to play a role in both somatoform and psychosomatic illnesses, not all empirical research has supported the correlation of alexithymia with somatic complaints (Lundh and Simonsson-Sarnecki 2001).

In late life, somatoform disorders may represent a dysfunctional attempt to cope with accumulating physical and psychosocial losses, especially when these losses are associated with functional disability, anxiety, and depression. These include loss of or isolation from family, friends, and caregivers; loss of beauty and strength; financial setbacks; loss of independence; and loss of social role (e.g., as a result of retirement, loss of a spouse, or occupational disability). The psychological distress and anxiety over such losses may be less threatening and more controllable when they are shifted to somatic complaints or symptoms. In turn, a sick role might be reinforced by increased social contacts and support. The presence of comorbid medical problems and the use of multiple medications may provide somatic symptoms around which psychological conflict can center. In long-term care, older individuals are faced with many additional overwhelming losses, and their own bodies often serve as the last bastion of control. Somatic preoccupation thus serves as a means of coping with stress, even though it is maladaptive and can result in excessive and unnecessary disability. It may also serve to mobilize and control resources and staff attention within the long-term care environment.

Treatment

By definition, somatoform disorders present to clinicians with what appear to be legitimate somatic complaints of unknown organic etiology. It is only after repeated but fruitless workups, multiple and persistent complaints and requests from the patient, and sometimes angry and inappropriate reactions to treatment that clinicians begin to suspect a somatoform disorder. In some cases, the manner of presentation and the symptom complex are more immediately suggestive of a particular somatoform disorder. In any event, it is important for the clinician to remember that the reported symptoms and complaints are quite real and disturbing for the patient. Even after workups have made it obvious that there are psychological factors involved, it is never wise to challenge the patient or suggest that the symptoms are "all in your mind." The typical response to such a suggestion is for the patient to seek additional opinions and medical tests, which in turn can perpetuate a cycle of somatization in which underlying issues are never addressed.

Instead, the role of the physician must be to foster a supportive, consistent, and professional relationship with the affected individual. Such a relationship will provide reassurance as well as protect the patient from excessive and unnecessary medical visits and procedures. The clinician should focus on responding to individual complaints, perhaps with periodic but regularly scheduled appointments, and setting limits on workup and treatment in a firm but empathic manner. This can be difficult to do when patients become demanding and attempt to consume excessive clinic time, but the clinician must endeavor to remain professional and to not personalize the situation or feel as though he or she were failing the patient. The clinician should focus on symptom reduction and rehabilitation and not attempt to force the patient to gain insight into the potential psychological nature of his or her symptoms (Kellner 1987).

It obviously can be hazardous for a clinician to diagnose a somatoform disorder prematurely, because underlying organic pathology might have eluded diagnosis. For example, multiple sclerosis, systemic lupus erythematosus, and acute intermittent porphyria often have complex presentations that elude initial diagnostic workup (Kellner 1987). Somatoform disorders may coexist with actual disease states; for example, many individuals with pseudoseizures also have a seizure disorder (D'Allesio et al. 2006; Mari et al. 2006). Moene et al. (2000) found that slightly more than 10% of patients who received an initial diagnosis of conversion disorder actually had a true neurological disorder. At the same time, it is important for the clinician to set limits on what he or she can offer and to make appropriate referrals to specialists and/or mental health clinicians.

In contrast to a primary care practitioner or a medical specialist, the geriatric psychiatrist will play a more active role in addressing the somatoform disorder itself rather than the actual physical complaints. Because many presentations of somatoform disorders are chronic, the goal of treatment is not always to cure the patient but often to control symptoms. To facilitate this, the clinician must form a therapeutic alliance through empathic listening and acknowledging of physical discomfort, without trivializing the somatic complaints. Sometimes an offer to review all available medical records can be a tangible way of conveying one's seriousness to the patient. Educating the patient about various symptom complexes and involving him or her in part of the decision making can be empowering for the patient, especially a patient with chronic pain.

Individual therapy that takes a psychodynamic approach will focus on helping the patient identify and then discuss psychological conflict and associated emotion. Cognitive-behavioral therapy (CBT) focuses on identifying distorted thought patterns and anxiety triggers and replacing them with more realistic and adaptive strategies, as well as integrating behavioral techniques to desensitize anxious reactions. For example, the somatic preoccupation seen in hypochondriasis and BDD can closely resemble symptoms of obsessive-compulsive disorder and may respond to techniques similar to those used in the latter disorder for extinguishing such thought patterns. There is an impressive body of research supporting the efficacy of psychotherapy—particularly CBT—for treating somatoform disorders (Speed 1996; Thomson and Page 2007; Woolfolk et al. 2007).

Pharmacotherapy is a central component of treatment for somatoform disorders. It can be targeted at a specific disorder or at underlying anxiety, depression, or thought patterns that appear delusional. Somatization disorder has been treated successfully with both antidepressants (Menza et al. 2001) and anticonvulsants or mood stabilizers (Garcia-Campayo and Sanz-Carrillo 2001). Hypochondriacal symptoms have responded to a variety of antidepressant medications—in particular, selective serotonin reuptake inhibitors (SSRIs)—as well as to anxiolytics (Barsky 2001; Fallon et al. 1996; Oosterbaan et al. 2001). A meta-analysis of antidepressant therapy in pain disorder found that pharmacotherapy decreased pain intensity significantly more than placebo (Fishbain et al. 1998). Anticonvulsants have also been found to be useful in treating pain disorder, especially when the disorder is associated with a comorbid mood disorder (Maurer et al. 1999). BDD has responded well to antidepressant treatment, especially high doses (Grant and Phillips 2005; Phillips et al. 2002) and has also been treated with antipsychotics alone or as augmenting agents (Grant 2001; Phillips 1996, 2005). A study by Phillips et al. (2001) demonstrated a 60% response rate with SSRIs, a high relapse rate when medications were discontinued, and increased response with antidepressant augmentation. A double-blind crossover study involving 29 patients with BDD found clomipramine to be superior to desipramine across a variety of symptomatic domains (Hollander et al. 1999). Even the delusional variant of BDD has been shown to respond to antidepressant treatment (Phillips et al. 1998, 2002).

The tendency of many psychiatrists to focus more on pharmacotherapy can become a trap with somatoform disorders, because the therapeutic relationship is such a key element. Given the chronic nature of somatoform symptoms, it is unlikely that pharmacotherapy will be a quick fix. When this narrow focus on treatment with medications fails to result in rapid control of symptoms, the patient may abandon the therapist for alternative treatment. Other patients may welcome such a focus because it keeps them from having to face underlying psychological issues. Instead, clinicians must be in it for the long haul and strike a balance between reasonable pharmacotherapy that targets specific symptoms of anxiety or depression and a supportive alliance in which the most appropriate therapy for the patient is used. If another clinician serves as the therapist, frequent communication between psychiatrist and therapist is necessary to coordinate treatment.

For the older patient with a somatoform disorder, the greatest challenge is always trying to separate out actual medical disease from somatoform symptoms. Sometimes they are so intertwined that the line between where one begins and the other ends cannot be reasonably discerned without successful treatment response of a discrete symptom to either a medical or a psychiatric intervention. Moreover, many patients are quite resistant to psychiatric care because they feel it delegitimates their physical suffering. Teamwork between internist and psychiatrist is key here, allowing both to identify the most important symptoms of concern to the patient, provide appropriate attention and workup, and coordinate medical and psychiatric interventions.

Key Points

- Somatoform disorders represent a heterogeneous group of seven disorders characterized by physical symptoms or complaints without objective organic causes and in which there are strongly associated psychological factors.

- The increased presence of comorbid medical and psychiatric illnesses in late life poses a unique diagnostic challenge for somatoform disorders.
- Somatoform disorders include somatization disorder, undifferentiated somatoform disorder, hypochondriasis, conversion disorder, pain disorder, body dysmorphic disorder, and somatoform disorder not otherwise specified.
- Somatoform disorders are most commonly diagnosed in younger individuals. Major risk factors include childhood abuse, female gender, chronic illness or pain, lower education and socioeconomic status, and comorbid anxiety, depression, personality disorders, and substance abuse.
- There has been little research on somatoform disorders in late life; as a result, assessment and treatment strategies across all age groups are similar.
- Management of somatoform disorders requires a consistent, empathic approach that focuses on symptomatic improvement and rehabilitation, does not challenge the veracity of the patient's reports, and provides efficacious cognitive-behavioral therapy and appropriate pharmacotherapy.

References

Aigner M, Bach M: Clinical utility of DSM-IV pain disorder. Compr Psychiatry 40:353–357, 1999

American Psychiatric Association: Diagnostic and Statistical Manual of Mental Disorders, 4th Edition, Text Revision. Washington, DC, American Psychiatric Association, 2000

Bailey PE, Henry JD: Alexithymia, somatization and negative affect in a community sample. Psychiatry Res 150:13–20, 2007

Barsky AJ: Patients who amplify bodily sensations. Ann Intern Med 91:63–70, 1979

Barsky AJ: The patient with hypochondriasis. N Engl J Med 345:1395–1399, 2001

Barsky AJ, Klerman GL: Overview: hypochondriasis, bodily complaints, and somatic styles. Am J Psychiatry 149:273–283, 1983

Barsky AJ, Frank C, Cleary P, et al: The relation between hypochondriasis and age. Am J Psychiatry 148:923–928, 1991

Behrouz R, Heriaud L, Benbadis SR: Late-onset psychogenic nonepileptic seizures. Epilepsy 8:649–650, 2006

Bellino S, Zizza M, Paradiso E: Dysmorphic concern symptoms and personality disorders: a clinical investigation in patients seeking cosmetic surgery. Psychiatry Res 144:73–78, 2006

Boland RJ: How could the validity of the DSM-IV pain disorder be improved in reference to the concept that it is supposed to identify? Curr Pain Headache Rep 6:23–29, 2002

Breuer J, Freud S: Studies on hysteria (1893–1895), in Standard Edition of the Complete Psychological Works of Sigmund Freud, Vol 2. Translated and edited by Strachey J. London, Hogarth Press, 1955, pp 1–319

Brink T, Janakes C, Martinez N: Geriatric hypochondriasis: situational factors. J Am Geriatr Soc 29:37–39, 1981

Brown RJ, Schrag A, Trimble MR: Dissociation, childhood interpersonal trauma, and family functioning in patients with somatization disorder. Am J Psychiatry 162:899–905, 2005

Brown RJ, Cardena E, Nijenhuis E: Should conversion disorder be reclassified as a dissociative disorder in DSM-V? Psychosomatics 48:369–378, 2007

Chabolla DR, Krahn LE, So EL, et al: Psychogenic nonepileptic seizures. Mayo Clin Proc 71:493–500, 1996

Cloninger CR: Somatoform and dissociative disorders, in The Medical Basis of Psychiatry. Edited by Winokur G, Clayton PJ. Philadelphia, PA, WB Saunders, 1986, pp 123–151

D'Allesio L, Giagante B, Oddo S: Psychiatric disorders in patients with psychogenic non-epileptic seizures, with and without comorbid epilepsy. Seizure 15:333–339, 2006

De Gucht V: Stability of neuroticism and alexithymia in somatization. Compr Psychiatry 44:466–471, 2003

DeWaal MWM, Arnold IA, Eekhof JAH: Somatoform disorders in general practice: prevalence, functional impairment and comorbid anxiety and depressive disorders. Br J Psychiatry 184:470–476, 2004

Dula DJ, DeNaples L: Emergency department presentation of patients with conversion disorder. Acad Emerg Med 2:120–123, 1995

Escobar JI, Gara M, Waitzkin H, et al: DSM-IV hypochondriasis in primary care. Gen Hosp Psychiatry 20:155–159, 1998

Fallon BA, Schneier FR, Marshall R, et al: The pharmacotherapy of hypochondriasis. Psychopharmacol Bull 32:607–611, 1996

Faravelli C, Salvatori S, Galassi F, et al: Epidemiology of somatoform disorders: a community survey in Florence. Soc Psychiatry Psychiatr Epidemiol 32:24–29, 1997

Fink P, Hansen MS, Oxhoj ML: The prevalence of somatoform disorders among medical inpatients. J Psychopharm Res 56:413–418, 2004

Fishbain DA, Cutler RB, Rosomoff HL, et al: Do antidepressants have an analgesic effect in psychogenic pain and somatoform pain disorder? A meta-analysis. Psychosom Med 60:503–509, 1998

Garcia-Campayo J, Sanz-Carrillo C: Gabapentin for the treatment of patients with somatization disorder (letter). J Clin Psychiatry 62:474, 2001

Grant JE: Successful treatment of nondelusional body dysmorphic disorder with olanzapine: a case report. J Clin Psychiatry 62:297–298, 2001

Grant JE, Phillips KA: Recognizing and treating body dysmorphic disorder. Ann Clin Psychiatry 17:205–210, 2005

Hasin D, Katz H: Somatoform and substance use disorders. Psychosom Med 69:870–875, 2007

Hollander E, Allen A, Kwon J, et al: Clomipramine vs. desipramine crossover trial in body dysmorphic disorder: selective efficacy of a serotonin reuptake inhibitor in imagined ugliness. Arch Gen Psychiatry 56:1033–1039, 1999

Hollifield M, Tuttle L, Paine S, et al: Hypochondriasis and somatization related to personality and attitudes towards self. Psychosomatics 40:387–395, 1999

Kellner R: Somatization and Hypochondriasis. New York, Praeger, 1986

Kellner R: Hypochondriasis and somatization. JAMA 258:2718–2722, 1987

Krem MM: Motor conversion disorders reviewed from a neuropsychiatric perspective. J Clin Psychiatry 65:783–790, 2004

Leveille SG, Ling S, Hochberg MC, et al: Widespread musculoskeletal pain and the progression of disability in older disabled women. Ann Intern Med 135:1038–1046, 2001

Liskow B, Othmer E, Penick EC, et al: Is Briquet's syndrome a heterogeneous disorder? Am J Psychiatry 143:626–629, 1986

Lundh LG, Simonsson-Sarnecki M: Alexithymia, emotion, and somatic complaints. J Pers 69:483–510, 2001

Mace CJ, Trimble MR: Ten-year prognosis of conversion disorder. Br J Psychiatry 169:282–288, 1996

Mari F, Bonaventure C, Vanacore N: Video-EEG study of psychogenic nonepileptic seizures: differential characteristics in patients with and without epilepsy. Epilepsia 47 (suppl 5):64–67, 2006

Maurer I, Volz HP, Sauer H: Gabapentin leads to remission of somatoform pain disorder with major depression. Pharmacopsychiatry 32:255–257, 1999

McDermid AJ, Rollman GB, McCain GA: Generalized hypervigilance in fibromyalgia: evidence of perceptual amplification. Pain 66:133–144, 1996

Menza M, Lauritano M, Allen L, et al: Treatment of somatization disorder with nefazodone: a prospective, open-label study. Ann Clin Psychiatry 13:153–158, 2001

Miller AR, North CS, Clouse RE, et al: The association of irritable bowel syndrome and somatization disorder. Ann Clin Psychiatry 13:25–30, 2001

Moene FC, Landberg EH, Hoogduin KA, et al: Organic syndromes diagnosed as conversion disorder: identification and frequency in a study of 85 patients. J Psychosom Res 49:7–12, 2000

Ness D: Physical therapy management for conversion disorder: case series. J Neurol Phys Ther 31:30–39, 2007

Noyes R Jr, Langbehn DR, Happel RL, et al: Personality dysfunction among somatizing patients. Psychosomatics 42:320–329, 2001

Okasha A, Ismail MK, Khalil AH, et al: A psychiatric study of nonorganic chronic headache patients. Psychosomatics 40:233–238, 1999

Oosterbaan DB, van Balkom AJ, van Boeijen CA, et al: An open study of paroxetine in hypochondriasis. Prog Neuropsychopharmacol Biol Psychiatry 25:1023–1033, 2001

O'Sullivan SS, Spillane JE, McMahon EM: Clinical characteristics and outcome of patients diagnosed with psychogenic nonepileptic seizures: a 5-year review. Epilepsy Behav 11:77–84, 2007

Otis JAD, McGeeney B: Managing pain in the elderly. Clin Geriatr 8:48–62, 2000

Otto MW, Cohen WS, Harlow BL: Prevalence of body dysmorphic disorder in a community sample of women. Am J Psychiatry 158:2061–2063, 2001

Phillips KA: Body dysmorphic disorder: diagnosis and treatment of imagined ugliness. J Clin Psychiatry 57 (suppl 8):61–64, 1996

Phillips KA: Body dysmorphic disorder: clinical aspects and treatment strategies. Bull Menninger Clin 62:A33–A48, 1998

Phillips KA: Olanzapine augmentation of fluoxetine in body dysmorphic disorder. Am J Psychiatry 162:1022–1023, 2005

Phillips KA, Dufresne RG: Body dysmorphic disorder: a guide for dermatologists and cosmetic surgeons. Am J Clin Dermatol 1:235–243, 2000

Phillips KA, McElroy SL: Personality disorders and traits in patients with body dysmorphic disorder. Compr Psychiatry 41:229–236, 2000

Phillips KA, Dwight MM, McElroy SL: Efficacy and safety of fluvoxamine in body dysmorphic disorder. J Clin Psychiatry 59:165–171, 1998

Phillips KA, Albertini RS, Siniscalchi JM, et al: Effectiveness of pharmacotherapy for body dysmorphic disorder: a chart-review study. J Clin Psychiatry 62:721–727, 2001

Phillips KA, Albertini RS, Rasmussen SA: A randomized placebo-controlled trial of fluoxetine in body dysmorphic disorder. Arch Gen Psychiatry 59:381–388, 2002

Polatin PB, Kinney RK, Gatchel RJ, et al: Psychiatric illness and chronic low-back pain: the mind and the spine—which goes first? Spine 18:66–71, 1993

Pribor EF, Smith DS, Yutzy SH: Somatization disorder in elderly patients. J Geriatr Psychiatry 2:109–117, 1994

Rabinowitz T, Hirdes JP, Desjardins I: Somatoform disorders in late life, in Principles and Practice of Geriatric Psychiatry. Edited by Agronin ME, Maletta G. Philadelphia, PA, Lippincott Williams & Wilkins, 2006, pp 489–503

Reid S, Whooley D, Crayford T, et al: Medically unexplained symptoms—GPs' attitudes towards their cause and management. Fam Pract 18:519–523, 2001

Rief W, Hessel A, Braehler E: Somatization symptoms and hypochondriacal features in the general population. Psychosom Med 63:595–602, 2001

Ritsner M, Ponizovsky A, Kurs R, et al: Somatization in an immigrant population in Israel: a community survey of prevalence, risk factors, and help-seeking behavior. Am J Psychiatry 157:385–392, 2000

Roelofs K, Keijsers GP, Hoogduin KA, et al: Childhood abuse in patients with conversion disorder. Am J Psychiatry 159:1908–1913, 2002

Sack M, Lahmann C, Jaeger B, et al: Trauma prevalence and somatoform symptoms: are there specific somatoform symptoms related to traumatic experiences? J Nerv Ment Dis 195:928–933, 2007

Samelius L, Wijma B, Wingren G, et al: Somatization in abused women. J Womens Health 6:909–918, 2007

Sar V, Akyüz G, Kundakçi T: Childhood trauma, dissociation, and psychiatric comorbidity in patients with conversion disorder. Am J Psychiatry 161:2271–2276, 2004

Scherder E, Bouma A, Slaets J, et al: Repeated pain assessment in Alzheimer's disease. Dement Geriatr Cogn Disord 12:400–407, 2001

Scudds RJ, Ostbye T: Pain and pain-related interference with function in older Canadians: the Canadian Study of Health and Aging. Disabil Rehabil 23:654–664, 2001

Sheehan B, Banerjee S: Review: somatization in the elderly. Int J Geriatr Psychiatry 14:1044–1049, 1999

Simon GE, Gureje O, Fullerton C: Course of hypochondriasis in an international primary care study. Gen Hosp Psychiatry 23:51–55, 2001

Smith RC, Gardiner JC, Lykes JS, et al: Exploration of DSM-IV criteria in primary care patients with medically unexplained symptoms. Psychosom Med 67:123–129, 2005

Speed J: Behavioral management of conversion disorder: retrospective study. Arch Phys Med Rehabil 77:147–154, 1996

Stone J, Zeman A, Simonotto E, et al: FMRI in patients with motor conversion symptoms and controls with simulated weakness. Psychosom Med 69:961–969, 2007

Stuart S, Noyes R Jr: Attachment and interpersonal communication in somatization. Psychosomatics 40:34–43, 1999

Thomson AB, Page LA: Psychotherapies for hypochondriasis. Cochrane Database Syst Rev CD006520, Oct 17, 2007

Vuilleumier P: Hysterical conversion and brain function. Prog Brain Res 150:309–329, 2005

Vuilleumier P, Chicherio C, Assal F, et al: Functional neuroanatomical correlates of hysterical sensorimotor loss. Brain 124:1077–1090, 2001

Waldinger RJ, Schulz MS, Barsky AJ, et al: Mapping the road from childhood trauma to adult somatization: the role of attachment. Psychosom Med 68:129–135, 2006

Waller E, Scheidt CE: Somatoform disorders as disorders of affect regulation: a study comparing the TAS-20 with non-self-report measures of alexithymia. J Psychosom Res 57:239–247, 2004

Weddington WW: Conversion reaction in an 82 year old man. J Nerv Ment Dis 167:368–369, 1979

Woolfolk RL, Allen LA, Tiu JE: New directions in the treatment of somatization. Psychiatr Clin North Am 30:621–644, 2007

Yazící KM, Kostakoglu L: Cerebral blood flow changes in patients with conversion disorder. Psychiatry Res 83:163–168, 1998

Suggested Readings

Barsky AJ: The patient with hypochondriasis. N Engl J Med 345:1395–1399, 2001

DeWaal MWM, Arnold IA, Eekhof JAH: Somatoform disorders in general practice: prevalence, functional impairment and comorbid anxiety and depressive disorders. Br J Psychiatry 184:470–476, 2004

Grant JE, Phillips KA: Recognizing and treating body dysmorphic disorder. Ann Clin Psychiatry 17:205–210, 2005

Rabinowitz T, Hirdes JP, Desjardins I: Somatoform disorders in late life, in Principles and Practice of Geriatric Psychiatry. Edited by Agronin ME, Maletta G. Philadelphia, PA, Lippincott Williams & Wilkins, 2006, pp 489–503

Sheehan B, Banerjee S: Review: somatization in the elderly. Int J Geriatr Psychiatry 14:1044–1049, 1999

CHAPTER 20

Sexual Disorders

Marc E. Agronin, M.D.

Sexual issues and disorders increasingly have become a part of assessment and treatment by the geriatric psychiatrist, in both outpatient and long-term care settings. One reason for this is that aging individuals are living longer and healthier lives and expect sexuality to continue to play an important role. The renewed interest in sexuality in late life has also been fueled by changing attitudes. On the one hand, the idea of sexuality in late life has often been denied or regarded with humor or even disgust. For many younger individuals, the idea of sexuality clashes with stereotypes of their mom and dad or grandma and grandpa. The denial of sexuality in parents and grandparents then becomes the denial of sexuality in all older individuals. These defensive, distorted, and ageist ways of thinking about sexuality in late life may lead many clinicians to view sexual dysfunction as a normal and untreatable part of aging. However, several factors have led to broadened perspectives on sexuality in late life. Certainly the sexual and feminist revolutions in the 1960s and 1970s shattered many stereotypes. In addition, the widespread use of hormone replacement therapy has allowed many women to maintain more vital and enjoyable sexual function well beyond menopause. For men, the advent of numerous treatments for erectile dysfunction (ED), a relatively common sexual dysfunction in late life, also ensured the persistence of sexual function in later years. In particular, the discovery of oral erectogenic agents has revolutionized the treatment of ED and has made sexuality in late life a more common and comfortable topic of conversation. In turn, the destigmatization of sexual dysfunction has no doubt brought many older couples into treatment who might otherwise have suffered in silence and shame.

Sexual Behaviors in Late Life

Several major studies over the last 20 years have shown that a majority of middle-aged and older individuals continue to be sexually active, although with modest decreases in activity, determined in part by gender and the availability of partners. These studies have indicated that older men are more sexually active than older women and that individuals with steady partners are more active than single individuals. In general, sexual interest and activity in late life depend on the previous level of sexual activity; the availability, health, and sexual interest of the partner; and the individual's overall physical health (Comfort and Dial 1991; Kligman 1991).

One of the more recent series of studies of late-life sexuality was conducted by the American Association of Retired Persons (AARP). In the original 1999 mail survey, researchers gathered responses from 1,384 men and women age 45 years or older (Jacoby 1999). The survey found that three-quarters of both men and women in the sample remained sexually active. Eighty-four percent of men and 78% of women ages 45–59 years had steady sexual partners, compared with 58% of men and 21% of women older than 75 years. In terms of frequency, 50% of individuals ages 45–59 years reported having sex at least once a week, compared with 30% of men and 24% of women ages 60–74 years. Of the respondents, the majority of men without partners said they masturbated, whereas more than 77% of women did not. The study also examined attitudes toward specific aspects of sexuality. Sixty percent of men and 35% of women said that sexual activity was important to their overall quality of life. Two-thirds of all respondents were extremely or somewhat satisfied with sex. Attitudes toward partners were generally favorable, with a majority of both genders describing their partners with terms that included "best friend," "kind and gentle," and "physically attractive." The study also found several generational differences in attitudes toward sex. Individuals older than 60 years were less likely than younger respondents to approve of oral sex, masturbation, and sex between unmarried partners.

A 2004 update of the AARP study surveyed 2,930 men and women age 45 years or older about various sexual issues, and it included samples of Asians, African Americans, and Hispanics (American Association for Retired Persons 2005). Of this group, approximately two-thirds were married or living with a partner, and 5% identified themselves as either homosexual or lesbian. Attitudes toward sexuality were remarkably similar to those seen in the 1999 survey, with only a few new findings. As before, the vast majority of individuals had positive attitudes toward sex, and those with partners described themselves as more satisfied, optimistic, and tolerant than those without partners. African Americans and Hispanics were more likely to be extremely satisfied with their partner. Those who engaged in physical exercise on a regular basis had greater degrees of sexual satisfaction. An increasing number of individuals were seeking information on sex from the Internet and from health care providers. Compared with the 1999 survey, there was less opposition to sex between nonmarried individuals.

The 2004 update of the AARP study found no major changes in sexual behaviors, with 86% of respondents continuing to be sexually active. Men were more active than women, and rates of sexual activity declined with age. The percentage of men seeking potency-enhancing medications doubled from 10% to 22%, with 68% of respondents saying that the treatment helped. The number of women on hormone replacement therapy dropped by 50%, no doubt related to warnings about increased cancer risk. More individuals in 2004 reported engaging in masturbation and oral sex compared with those in 1999. Overall, 60% of men and 50% of women reported engaging in masturbation at least once in the 6 months prior to the survey.

The AARP study findings are consistent with several other surveys. Lindau et al. (2007) interviewed 3,005 adults ages 57–85 years in the United States and found that 73% of those ages 57–64 years were sexually active, declining to 53% of the 65- to 74-year-old group and 26% of those older than 75 years. Rates of having sex at least once a week fell from 40% of men and 34% of women in the youngest cohort to 31% of both men and women in the middle cohort and 23% of men and 24% of women in the oldest cohort. Overall, men were more sexually active than women across all age groups. Older individuals with poorer health rankings were less sexually active and more prone to sexual dysfunction. A large cross-national study of 27,000 older individuals in 29 countries found that men had high levels of sexual satisfaction regardless of the country and that sexual satisfaction decreased with increasing number of partners (Laumann et al. 2006). In an earlier study, Marsiglio and Donnelly (1991) surveyed more than 800 married men and women age 60 years or older and found that more than 50% had sex at least monthly. The mean frequency for respondents between ages 60 and 75 years was 4.26 times per month, which decreased to 2.75 times per month for those age 76 years or older. These figures can be compared with rates of sexual frequency among younger individuals (ages 19–59 years; N=3,432) in an influential University of Chicago study (Michael et al. 1994). In that study, men had sex an average of 6.5 times per month, whereas the average rate for women was 6.2 times per month.

In a mail survey of 1,292 individuals ages 60–90 years, the National Council on the Aging (1998) found that 80% of respondents with sexual partners had sex at least once a month. By gender, 61% of men remained sexually active, compared with 37% of women. Eighty-five percent of women sought partners who were financially secure, whereas 79% of men sought partners who were interested in sex. Compared with women, men were twice as likely to want more sex than they were already having. Satisfaction with sex remained quite high in late life: 61% of respondents with partners indicated that sex was as physically satisfying as it was in their 40s. A sizable number of respondents attributed lower satisfaction to the fact that they or their partners had less physical desire, had a medical condition that interfered with sex, or took medications that reduced desire.

None of the published surveys questioned older individuals about sexually transmitted diseases (STDs), even though they are certainly at risk for contracting them. According to 2006 surveillance data from the Centers for Disease Control, rates of STDs (including chlamydia, gonorrhea, and syphilis) in individuals age 65 years or older were the lowest of any group and had not changed appreciably in the last 5 years (Centers for Disease Control 2006). In a study from Washington State, the most common STDs in older individuals were nongonococcal urethritis in men and genital herpes in women—representing 1.3% of all reported cases of STDs (Xu et al. 2001). With respect to HIV/AIDS, approximately 15% of all cases are in individuals 50 years or older, but not all of these are due to sexual transmission (Centers for Disease Control 2007).

Few studies have examined the sexuality of the estimated 1–3 million gay and lesbian individuals over the age of 60 in the United States. Existing data do, however, consistently support the fact that older gay and lesbian individuals continue to be sexually active and to feel high levels of satisfaction with both their lifestyle and their sex lives (Adelman 1991). In one study of 100 gay men ages 40–77 years, 80% remained sexually active, with 34% reporting having sex more than once a week and 69% reporting the same amount of sexual enjoyment as when they were younger (Pope and Schulz 1990). Kimmel (1977) reported similar findings and suggested a number of age-associated advantages that homosexuals might have, including being less dependent on family and children and having large networks of supportive friends.

The Sexual Response Cycle and Aging

The effects of aging on sexual function must be viewed against the backdrop of normal adult sexual response. A four-stage model of the normal sexual response cycle was developed by sex researchers William Masters and Virginia Johnson (1966) from their pioneering work in human sexuality. The four-stage cycle illustrates the physiological changes that take place in the body during sexual activity. These four stages are *excitement* or *arousal, plateau, orgasm,* and *resolution.* Kaplan (1974) and others (Snarch 1991; Zilbergeld and Ellison 1980) added a fifth stage, *desire,* to account for a psychological and physiological component of sexuality that underlies sexual response. In this later model, sexual response is not a linear process but rather a waxing and waning pattern of sexual arousal that may culminate in orgasm, depending on a host of factors. All of these factors can be influenced by age-related changes in sexual function.

The first stage of the five-stage model, *desire,* involves physical and psychological urges to seek out and respond to sexual interaction. This drive is centered in the limbic system of the brain, particularly in the hypothalamus, and is stimulated in both sexes by testosterone. Desire is intimately linked to the physiological process of sexual *excitement* or *arousal* (the second stage); it is difficult for one to exist without the other. In both men and women, sexual arousal can be triggered by thoughts and fantasies or by direct physical stimulation. Autonomic nervous stimulation leads to predictable physiological responses, including increased muscle tone, increases in heart and respiratory rates, and increased blood flow to the genitals (vasocongestion). In men, these responses result in penile erection, whereas in women, they result in vaginal lubrication and swelling of breast and genital tissues, especially the clitoris. The relatively brief *plateau* stage is characterized by a sense of impending *orgasm* and is followed by orgasm and then a refractory period of relaxation called *resolution.* In both sexes, orgasm is characterized by euphoria associated with rhythmic contractions of genital muscles. In men, orgasm is brief and is accompanied by ejaculation. In women, orgasm tends to last longer and there may be multiple successive occurrences.

Normal aging produces several changes in the sexual response cycle (see Table 20–1). In women, the most significant changes occur during menopause, a 2- to 10-year period that usually ends in the early 50s. The decline and eventual cessation of ovarian estrogen production during menopause leads to important changes in sexual function, including atrophy of urogenital tissue, a decrease in vaginal size, and diminished vaginal lubrication, vasocongestion, and erotic sensitivity of nipple, clitoral, and vulvar tissue. As a result, sexual desire may decrease, sexual arousal may require more time, sexual intercourse may be more uncomfortable because of reduced lubrication of vaginal and clitoral tissue, and orgasms may be felt as less intense. Up to 85% of menopausal women also experience symptoms such as hot flashes, head and neck aches, mood changes, and excess fatigue. During menopause, women also experience decreases in testosterone production that may lead to diminished libido (Nappi et al. 2006).

In most women, hormone replacement therapy largely reverses these menopause-associated changes in sexual function. Estrogen is often prescribed with

TABLE 20–1. Normal age-related changes in sexual function

Men
Testosterone production modestly decreases, with unpredictable effect on sexual function.
Sperm count changes minimally, but amount of functional sperm and rate of conception decrease.
There are no predictable changes in sexual desire (libido).
Increased tactile stimulation is needed for sexual arousal.
Erections take longer to achieve and are more difficult to sustain.
Penile rigidity decreases because of decreases in blood flow and smooth muscle relaxation.
Sensation of urgency during plateau stage is diminished.
Ejaculation is less forceful, with decreased ejaculate volume.
Refractory period increases by hours to days.
Women
During menopause, estrogen production decreases and eventually stops.
Sexual desire (libido) may decrease due in part to decreased testosterone levels.
Blood supply to pelvic region is reduced.
Vagina shortens and narrows. Vaginal mucosa is thinner and less lubricated.
During arousal, vaginal lubrication and swelling occur more slowly and are decreased.
Sexual arousal may take longer and may require increased stimulation.
During orgasm, strength and amount of vaginal contractions decrease.

Source. Goodwin and Agronin 1997; Metz and Miner 1995; Spector et al. 1996.

progesterone to replicate previous hormone levels. It can be administered orally or via a slow-release transdermal patch (Alexander et al. 2004). In addition, estrogen cream can be applied directly to genital tissues to relieve irritation and enhance lubrication (Suckling et al. 2006). Unfortunately, research findings have indicated a small but potentially unacceptable risk of breast and ovarian cancer associated with oral hormone replacement therapy (Lacey et al. 2002; Rossouw et al. 2002).

Compared with women, the sexual changes in aging men occur more gradually, with a less predictable time frame (Metz and Miner 1995; Westheimer and Lopater 2002). As men age, desire may involve less anticipatory physical arousal, and sexual arousal and orgasm may take longer to achieve. Older men require more physical stimulation to achieve erections, and the erections tend to be less frequent, less durable, and less reliable. The volume of ejaculate during orgasm is decreased. In older men, the resolution or refractory stage is much longer, lasting hours to days instead of minutes to hours as in younger men. Testosterone levels in men decline 35% on average by age 80, although some men have more significant declines, with levels dropping below 200 ng/dL, a condition termed *hypogonadism* (Morley 2003). Some researchers have suggested the existence of a male menopause or *andropause* resulting from declining testosterone levels and involving a symptom complex that includes decreased libido and sexual function; diminished bone and muscle mass, muscle power, and body hair; and decreased lean body mass (Heaton and Morales 2001; Morley and Perry 2003; Westheimer and Lopater 2002). Research has suggested, however, that these changes are quite variable and that testosterone replacement therapy has inconsistent results (Harman 2005).

In both sexes, the effects of physiological changes in sexual function are mediated by a number of psychosocial factors. The more an individual knows about what constitutes normal age-associated changes in sexual function, the more easily he or she may be able to accept these changes. For example, a man who does not understand the normal changes in erectile function may misinterpret them and believe that he has a sexual problem. Similarly, a woman may misinterpret vaginal dryness as an indication that she does not want to have sex. Such overreactions to normal changes can lead an individual to engage in less frequent or more limited sexual activity.

In addition, some older individuals may accept ageist stereotypes about sexuality, seeing their behaviors as inappropriate or potentially harmful, despite their relatively normal sexual desire and capacity. Other individuals may lose self-confidence and feel less sexy, especially as they struggle to cope with age-associated changes in physical appearance, strength, and endurance. Such attitudinal barriers may be more damaging to sexuality than actual physiological changes.

The quality of an individual's relationship with a partner is also influential. Couples often have to adapt sexual technique and spend more time on foreplay to preserve previous levels of sexual function and enjoyment. Partners who are not able to work together may experience difficulty with sex and perhaps even sexual dysfunction. On the other hand, aging can bring new possibilities for sexuality in later life. Partners may have more time to spend with each other once children have left home or during retirement. For postmenopausal women, sex may be associated with a reduced level of anxiety because of the impossibility of pregnancy.

Sexuality in Long-Term Care

Sexuality among residents in long-term care settings is stigmatized not only because the residents are elderly but also because they are no longer living independently and often have multiple medical and psychiatric problems, including cognitive impairment. As a result, both residents and staff tend to view sexuality in a negative manner. For example, in one study, even though the majority of long-term care staff acknowledged the sexual needs of residents, most did not think it was necessary for them to be sexually active (Saretsky 1987). Residents often feel sexually unattractive and are pessimistic about whether sex would even be possible or enjoyable (Kaas 1978; Wasow and Loeb 1979). Not surprisingly, the rate of sexual activity is low in most nursing homes (Hajjar and Kamel 2003a; Mulligan and Palguta 1987). For many residents, however, the desire for sexual relationships still exists. In a 1982 study involving 250 nursing home residents, White (1982) found that 91% had not been sexually active in the last month and 17% wanted to be sexually active but lacked privacy or a partner. Other common barriers to sexual activity among long-term care residents include loss of interest, chronic illness, sexual dysfunction, and negative attitudes of staff (Hajjar and Kamel 2003a; Richardson and Lazur 1995; Wasow and Loeb 1979).

When one or both members of a couple are living in a long-term care facility, staff must be aware of residents' rights to sexual expression. Mental health consultants can help remove barriers to sexual activity in long-term care settings in several ways. A key to accomplishing this goal is educating staff about sexuality in late life so that stereotypes are dispelled. Such an education provides staff with an understanding of residents' rights to sexual expression and the role of sexuality in helping residents meet needs for intimacy and physical contact (Spector et al. 1996). Also, residents should be educated about sexuality in late life and about their sexual rights. One way to facilitate these educational goals for residents and staff in long-term care settings is to develop and promote a policy on sexuality.

To carry out such a policy, clinical staff in long-term care facilities should ensure that a sexual history is obtained during intake and as a part of routine nursing, medical, and mental health evaluations. These evaluations can also be used to assess residents' concerns and capacities with respect to sexual function and relationships. Long-term care facilities must ensure adequate privacy for couples wishing to be intimate and must facilitate conjugal or home visits. To this end, facilities might provide private rooms for married couples or individuals with other partners, when this is feasible. Privacy can be increased with "Do Not Disturb" signs, locks on doors, and reminders to staff and residents to knock before entering a resident's room (Spector et al. 1996). Finally, facilities can provide beauty services such as hair styling and manicures (Richardson and Lazur 1995).

Sexual Dysfunction in Late Life

Although the majority of older individuals continue to engage in sexual activity, the prevalence of sexual dysfunction does increase with age (Lindau 2007; Mulligan et al. 2003). The DSM-IV-TR (American Psychiatric Association 2000) classification of sexual disorders is provided in Table 20–2. ED is the most common form of sexual dysfunction in older men, affecting more than 50% of men ages 40–70 years and nearly 70% of men age 70 years or older (Althof and Seftel 1995; Feldman et al. 1994). In older women, the most common forms of sexual dysfunction include hypoactive sexual desire, inhibited orgasm, and dyspareunia (Bachmann and Leiblum 1991; Crenshaw and Goldberg 1996; Lindau et al. 2007). Lindau et al. (2007) found that 43% of women ages 57–85 years reported low desire, 39% had difficulty with lubrication, and 34% had anorgasmia. In the same study, 37% of men reported erectile dysfunction and 14% were taking medications for it.

Unfortunately, physicians often fail to ask older patients about sexual function, perhaps because of their discomfort with the topic or their acceptance of ageist stereotypes. As a result, many older individuals endure treatable forms of sexual dysfunction and are either ignorant about treatment, pessimistic about it, or too ashamed to inquire. The geriatric psychiatrist can play a vital role in providing support, education, and treatment to such individuals.

TABLE 20–2. DSM-IV-TR classification of sexual dysfunction

Sexual desire disorders
Hypoactive sexual desire disorder: persistent or recurrent deficiency of sexual fantasies and desire for sex
Sexual aversion disorder: extreme aversion to and avoidance of genital sexual contact
Sexual arousal disorders
Female sexual arousal disorder: persistent or recurrent difficulty in achieving and/or maintaining vaginal swelling and lubrication during sexual activity
Male erectile disorder (impotence): persistent or recurrent inability to attain and/or maintain an erection adequate for sexual activity
Orgasmic disorders
Female or male orgasmic disorder: persistent or recurrent delay in or absence of orgasm in response to sexual stimulation
Premature ejaculation: persistent or recurrent uncontrollable, rapid ejaculation that occurs just before or shortly after penetration
Sexual pain disorders
Dyspareunia: recurrent or persistent genital pain associated with sexual intercourse
Vaginismus: recurrent or persistent involuntary spasm of vaginal muscles that limits or prohibits vaginal penetration

Although medical and psychiatric problems and medication effects are usually the main causes of sexual dysfunction in late life, numerous psychological factors must be considered, including performance anxiety, the presence of another sexual disorder in one or both partners, fears of self-injury or death caused by medical conditions (e.g., a history of myocardial infarction, shortness of breath), sensitivity to loss of personal appearance or control of bodily functions (e.g., incontinence), relationship problems, and life stress. The first occurrence of psychogenic sexual dysfunction often follows a stressful event such as the loss of a loved one, a divorce, a financial or occupational strain, or a major health scare. Such major stresses may break sexual patterns and lead to uncertainty about how to resume sexual activity. As noted, the availability of partners is an acute issue for women, who outnumber men by more than two to one by age 85 years.

Medical and psychiatric disorders that are the most common causes of sexual dysfunction in geriatric patients are listed in Table 20–3. In both sexes, major risk factors for sexual dysfunction include diabetes mellitus, peripheral vascular disease, cancer, pulmonary disease, depression, stroke, dementia, Parkinson's disease, and substance abuse. These and other medical disorders exert both primary and secondary effects on sexual function. Examples of primary effects include impaired sexual arousal caused by diabetic neuropathy and impaired genital vasocongestion caused by peripheral vascular disease. Secondary effects such as fatigue, pain, and physical disability caused by medical illness can make individuals feel less sexy and less confident in their sexual ability, which in turn can lead to hypoactive desire. Medications can also cause sexual dysfunction and can affect both men and women at any point in the sexual response cycle (Crenshaw and Goldberg 1996; Goodwin and Agronin 1997; Thomas 2003). The most common problematic medications include antihypertensives such as beta-blockers and diuretics, antiandrogens, and many psychotropic medications (Gitlin 1994; Zajecka 2001). Some of the medications most commonly associated with sexual dysfunction in late life are listed in Table 20–4.

TABLE 20–3. Medical and psychiatric conditions commonly associated with sexual dysfunction in late life

Anxiety disorders (generalized anxiety disorder, obsessive-compulsive disorder, panic disorder)
Arthritis and other degenerative joint diseases
Atherosclerosis (peripheral vascular disease, cerebrovascular accident)
Cancer (especially urologic and genital cancers and their treatments)
Cardiac disease (coronary artery disease, congestive heart failure, myocardial infarction)
Chronic obstructive pulmonary disease
Chronic organ failure (renal, hepatic)
Dementia (e.g., Alzheimer's disease, vascular dementia)
Diabetes mellitus
Major depressive disorder and other mood disorders
Multiple sclerosis
Parkinson's disease
Prostate disease and prostate surgery
Schizophrenia and other chronic psychotic disorders
Substance abuse

TABLE 20–4. Medications associated with sexual dysfunction in late life

α-Adrenergic blockers (prazosin, phentolamine)
Antiandrogens (leuprolide, ketoconazole)
Antidepressants (MAOIs, TCAs, SSRIs, venlafaxine)
Antihistamines
Antihypertensives (thiazide diuretics, β-blockers, ACE inhibitors, clonidine, spironolactone, calcium-channel blockers, reserpine)
Antipsychotics (conventional and atypical)
Benzodiazepines
Cancer chemotherapeutic agents
Cardiac medications (e.g., digoxin, amiodarone)
Corticosteroids
Disopyramide
L-Dopa
Histamine subtype 2 (H_2) receptor blockers
Mood stabilizers (lithium, valproic acid, carbamazepine)

Note. ACE=angiotensin-converting enzyme; MAOI=monoamine oxidase inhibitor; SSRI=selective serotonin reuptake inhibitor; TCA=tricyclic antidepressant.
Source. Goodwin and Agronin 1997; Kligman 1991.

Sexual dysfunction in late life is often comorbid with other psychiatric disorders. Symptoms range from transient dysfunction, present only during episodes of illness, to full-blown sexual disorders independent of the primary psychiatric disorder. Major depression often features loss of libido but may also be associated with inhibited arousal and ED. Anxiety disorders and panic disorders, as well as symptomatic anxiety, are frequently associated with sexual dysfunction—in particular, with sexual phobias and sexual aversion (Kaplan 1987). Unfortunately, many of the antidepressants used to treat mood or anxiety disorders can cause or exacerbate sexual dysfunction (see Table 20–4). ED, delayed or inhibited orgasm, and/or a decrease in desire is experienced by 10%–60% of men taking selective serotonin reuptake inhibitors (SSRIs), venlafaxine, or tricyclic antidepressants (Montejo et al. 2001; Segraves 1998). Lower rates of sexual dysfunction have been associated with the antidepressants mirtazapine (25%), bupropion (5%–15%), and nefazodone (8%) (Kavoussi et al. 1997; Montejo et al. 2001).

Schizophrenia and other psychotic disorders often involve sexual problems. Psychotic individuals with negative symptoms—such as social withdrawal or discomfort in the presence of others, apathy, and blunted affect—may have relatively little interest in sexual relationships. Psychotic patients with positive symptoms—such as delusions, hallucinations, and bizarre thought patterns—may have difficulty relating to others and interacting in sexually comfortable or appropriate ways. During periods of symptom remission, however, sexual relationships can be more appropriate. All antipsychotic medications can cause sexual dysfunction, usually in proportion to the dose (Crenshaw and Goldberg 1996; Gitlin 1994). As with antidepressant and anxiolytic medications, antipsychotics can decrease libido, interfere with sexual arousal, and inhibit erections, ejaculation, and orgasm.

Assessment

The assessment of sexual dysfunction in late life involves identifying the specific problem and then obtaining a comprehensive medical, psychiatric, and sexual history in order to determine potential causes. A comprehensive sexual history includes an individual's prior sexual experiences, current sexual functioning, and attitudes toward sexuality and toward any current partner. With older couples, interviewers must be able to identify relevant age-appropriate issues (Sbrocco et al. 1995). It is important to balance the need to gather sexual history with the responsibility to be sensitive to the fact that sexual data may be some of the most personal information that a patient will ever divulge. Finally, accurate assessment of sexual dysfunction in late life depends to a large degree on a comfortable and productive doctor-patient relationship—one in which the patient and his or her partner feel secure enough to disclose adequate history and the physician asks the right questions and has sufficient testing performed. Partner involvement is crucial to a successful outcome.

The medical workup for sexual dysfunction may involve a physical examination, laboratory testing, and specialized diagnostic testing. The focus of the physical examination is on genital and urologic anatomy and function, including underlying vascular and neurological function. Laboratory testing typically involves examination of routine blood chemistry (e.g., blood count, electrolyte levels, glucose levels, lipid profile), testosterone and prolactin levels, thyroid function, and, in men, prostate-specific antigen levels. Specialized diagnostic tests for ED include nocturnal penile tumescence and rigidity testing (to determine whether natural erections occur during sleep) and penile duplex ultrasonography (to assess blood flow in the penis).

Treatment

Preservation and enhancement of sexual activity in geriatric patients requires recognition of and sensitivity to the fact that many of these individuals want and intend to continue with sex, despite changes in physical and sexual function. Once an evaluation is complete, both partners should be educated about normal and dysfunctional sexuality. This information helps to reassure the affected individual that he or she is not the only person with the particular problem, that the problem has specific causes, and that it can be treated. In addition, clinicians can help patients recognize sexuality as a form of physical and psychological intimacy and not solely as sexual intercourse. This discussion will build trust between the patient and the clinician, and it will help the patient feel comfortable about seeking follow-up and being open about emotional reactions to the problem. Many treatments fail at this point, not because the treatments cannot work but because the patient and the clinician never establish a solid working relationship. Treatment can also fail when one partner refuses to cooperate with treatment or when problems within the couple's entire relationship become insurmountable.

Unique challenges are faced by couples in which one or both partners have a chronic medical illness or disability. These couples often need to shift their focus from intercourse to foreplay and to adapt sexual practices to account for physical limitations such as fatigue, loss of muscle strength, and pain (Agronin and Westheimer 2006; Morley and Tariq 2003; Schover and Jensen 1988). Education is key. Organizations such as the American Cancer Society, the United Ostomy Organization, and the National Jewish Center for Immunology and Respiratory Medicine have published helpful guides to maintaining sexual function despite specific medical illnesses. Physicians should work to maximize both rehabilitative and palliative treatments—for example, making use of analgesics for pain, inhalers for shortness of breath, or physical therapy for joint immobility and muscle weakness. In addition, appropriate treatment of depression, anxiety, or psychosis can often lead to significant improvement in sexual function, assuming that the medications used to treat these disorders do not themselves cause problems. Some ways in which an older couple can enhance sexual function and cope with disability are outlined in Table 20–5.

TABLE 20–5. Ten ways to enhance sexual function in late life

1. Cultivate a positive attitude toward sexuality in later life.
2. Maintain optimal health and fitness. Avoid use of tobacco and excessive use of alcohol.
3. Maintain open and honest communication with your partner about how your sexual responsiveness has changed over time.
4. Focus on foreplay as much as on intercourse. Be open-minded about adapting sexual practices to your needs.
5. Maximize treatment of medical problems or disabilities that are interfering with sexual function. Consult a physician about any concerns regarding excess exertion during sex. To achieve adequate stamina, use appropriate exercise to build up strength and self-confidence.
6. *Before* sex, maximize treatment of symptoms that affect sex. For pain, consider taking a warm shower or bath, having a relaxing massage, or taking analgesics before sex. For shortness of breath, adapt sexual activity to minimize exertion and use prescribed inhalers ahead of time. Choose times of day for sex when pain is at a minimum.
7. If you are a woman, consider the use of estrogen cream, which can relieve vaginal dryness and improve vasocongestion in peri- or postmenopausal women. Tender genital or breast tissue may require more gentle stimulation, sometimes along with the use of an external lubricant.
8. Identify problematic medications and investigate alternative agents or strategies.
9. Avoid unrealistic expectations that sex must be the same as when you were younger.
10. Explore sexual positions that decrease exertion or account for equipment such as oxygen tanks or ostomy bags. Suggested positions for intercourse include lying side by side or sitting face-to-face.

Source. Butler and Lewis 1986; Goodwin and Agronin 1997.

When medication side effects impair sexual function, physicians can consider several options (Goodwin and Agronin 1997; Labbate et al. 2003; Zajecka 2001). The first step is to continue administering the medication and wait for tolerance to develop; many side effects diminish or disappear after several weeks. If no change occurs, dose reduction can be tried. Simplifying the overall regimen might also be helpful, given that combinations of medications can cause more sexual side effects than each medication alone. For certain medications, such as antidepressants with short half-lives, a drug holiday in which administration of the medication is temporarily stopped for a day or two (such as for a weekend) can result in transient improvement in sexual function (Rothschild 1995). However, there is a risk of recurrence of psychiatric symptoms during this holiday. Ultimately, the clinician may have to consider replacing the medication with an agent that has less potential for sexual side effects, such as bupropion or mirtazapine (Gelenberg et al. 2000). With regard to antipsychotic medications, more potent agents with less anticholinergic side effects may cause less dysfunction.

When sexual dysfunction is caused by antidepressant medication, the clinician can also consider using antidotes to reverse sexual side effects (Thomas 2003; Zajecka 2001). Several antidotes include yohimbine, amantadine, cyproheptadine (which can also reverse the antidepressant effect of SSRIs), bethanecol, methylphenidate, buspirone, bromocriptine (for antipsychotic-induced sexual dysfunction), and the antidepressants bupropion, nefazodone, mirtazapine, and trazodone. The oral erectogenic agents sildenafil, tadalafil, and vardenafil have also been shown to reverse antidepressant-induced ED (Berigan 2004; Fava et al. 2006; Segraves et al. 2007). Depending on the chosen antidote for sexual side effects, the patient can take a dose anywhere from 30 to 60 minutes before anticipated sex and can take increasing doses until success is achieved. If intermittent use of an antidote does not work, a regularly scheduled daily dose should be considered.

If none of these strategies work, the clinician must consider the trade-off between the benefits of the original medication and the sexual side effects. For some individuals, stopping the medication poses too great a risk of recurrent psychiatric symptoms, and adequate alternatives may not exist. In this frustrating situation, affected individuals must choose between discontinuing a needed medication and coping with persistent sexual dysfunction.

Sex Therapy

In some older couples, sexual dysfunction has clear psychological roots; for example, sexual dysfunction often occurs in the context of a dysfunctional relationship. Sex therapy is always best done conjointly, with both partners participating, because both are integral parts of the problem and solution. Historically, a psychodynamic model was used in sex therapy to uncover underlying unconscious conflicts, but that approach is now viewed as less successful, and cognitive-behavioral techniques are used in current treatment models (Kaplan 1974, 1983; Rosen and Leiblum 1988; Westheimer and Lopater 2002). Brief supportive and educational counseling is a first step in treatment and can help dispel distorted and uninformed attitudes toward sexuality in general and toward a sexual problem in particular. Counseling can also help an individual or couple change sexual practices to resolve a problem. In other cases, more-intensive couples therapy is needed to resolve long-standing relationship issues before work on a sexual problem can begin.

Sex therapy involves both cognitive and behavioral techniques, with an overall goal of building an association between relaxed and sensual physical intimacy and sexual relations. The same principles can be applied across the life span, with several refinements in late life. Using cognitive therapy techniques, the therapist attempts to change distorted cognitive attitudes toward sexual activity into more practical attitudes. For example, many men with ED find it difficult not to assume the role of spectator during sex—that is, not to watch themselves with their partners and be preoccupied with the status of their erections. This spectator role can increase anxiety and distract the man from concentrating on pleasurable sensations, with the result that ED is reinforced (Masters and Johnson 1970). To counter this, the man is taught to shift his mental focus from his erection to pleasurable aspects of the encounter (Kaplan 1974). ED may also be perpetuated by cognitive distortions such as catastrophizing, in which the man thinks that if he does not achieve an erection during sex, he will be rejected not only by his partner but by all women. Another common cognitive distortion is all-or-nothing thinking, in which the man thinks that he must achieve an instant erection during sex or else the whole thing is pointless. The problem with such unrealistic cognitive distortions is that they often become self-fulfilling prophesies. The therapist helps the patient to gain insight into the negative effect of such thoughts and then to practice replacing them with more realistic and hopeful ones, sometimes even with positive assertions or affirmations of success (Goodwin and Agronin 1997).

Behavioral techniques used during sex therapy begin with exercises called *sensate focus,* in which a couple practices physical relaxation techniques during non-pressured sensual touching. Sensate focus helps to reduce performance anxiety and restore the natural flow of the sexual response cycle. Once the partners are able to feel relaxed and physically intimate together without sexual stimulation, they gradually progress to genital stimulation and then intercourse. Several adjustments in these exercises may be required for the older couple. For example, older patients with physical problems that involve some degree of disability may express concerns about being able to exert themselves adequately during sexual activity. The therapist might recommend one of several positions that minimize exertion, such as lying side by side or having one partner kneel on pillows and support him- or herself on a low bed. Other suggestions outlined in Table 20–5 might also apply. Such simple suggestions may remove some of the most anxiety-provoking barriers for an older couple, especially the common but unfounded belief that older persons lack the stamina or dexterity for sexual activity.

During sex therapy, the therapist continues to work with the couple on their relationship and tries to identify and confront resistance that inevitably arises during treatment. Such resistance to these seemingly innocuous exercises often reveals key problems in the relationship that are either causing the sexual dysfunction or impeding its treatment. Regardless of age, many couples find that sexual interest and pleasure reemerge and sexual function improves during sex therapy, allowing them to enjoy once again such a fundamental component of their relationship.

Erectile Dysfunction

ED is the most common sexual dysfunction in men. According to DSM-IV-TR, it is a disorder of sexual arousal characterized by the inability to achieve or sustain an erection that is adequate for sexual function. Historically, ED was seen as a psychological problem; however, current data indicate that in up to 80% of men (and in up to 90% of older men), ED is primarily caused by a problem with erectile physiology (Althof and Seftel 1995; Feldman et al. 1994; Tariq et al. 2003). There are, however, important psychological components of ED in terms of both cause and effect. Many men equate erections with masculinity, potency, and vitality. As a result, ED in late life is often experienced by men as a harbinger of physical and sexual decline. Performance anxiety, stress, depression, and relationship problems can trigger or exacerbate ED. In turn, ED is associated with feelings of anger, anxiety, powerlessness, shame, and humiliation in front of one's partner. Recurrent ED can lead to depression.

The penis contains three cylindrical bodies: two corpora cavernosa lie atop the corpus spongiosum, which contains the urethra. These bodies contain spongy erectile tissue, composed of vascular spaces or sinusoids surrounded by smooth muscle. Erections occur when autonomic innervation leads to relaxation of cavernosal smooth muscle, allowing blood flow into the vascular spaces. This muscle relaxation is mediated by the release of the neurotransmitter nitric oxide, with subsequent activation of cyclic guanosine monophosphate (GMP). As the vascular spaces in the spongy erectile tissue expand, the penile veins that drain them are compressed against the surrounding collagenous sheath or tunica albuginea, preventing outflow. The erection subsides when smooth muscles surrounding the vascular spaces contract, mediated by the breakdown of cyclic GMP to GMP via the key enzyme phosphodiesterase type 5 (PDE5). ED results from one of three physiological problems: 1) failure of erectile initiation because of psychological or neurological inhibition of nervous stimulation, 2) failure to attain penile arterial filling, or 3) failure to maintain penile veno-occlusion. The latter two causes are frequently associated with peripheral vascular disease, which in turn is associated with hypertension, hyperlipidemia, and tobacco use.

Treatment of ED in geriatric patients involves the same approaches as those used in younger men and has been revolutionized with the advent of oral erectogenic agents. Several major causes of ED are reversible and, if present, must be addressed before other treatments are considered. For men with hypogonadism as the likely cause of ED, testosterone replacement therapy in the form of a pill, transdermal gel or patch, intramuscular injection, or subcutaneous implant may be helpful (Howell and Shalit 2001; Morley 2003). This treatment should be avoided in men with a history of prostate or bladder cancer or with bladder outlet obstruction. Some men have ED as a result of vascular damage and may benefit from microsurgical revascularization. Peyronie's disease, characterized by scarring-caused curvature of the penis during erection, can also be treated, with resultant improvement in erectile function.

Penile intracavernosal self-injection was the first pharmacological treatment for ED. Injectable agents work by increasing smooth muscle relaxation and arterial dilatation in the penis. Two of the available agents are preparations of alprostadil, a synthetic form of prostaglandin E_1. Injection of these agents into the base of the penis 10–20 minutes before sex leads to erections in 70%–80% of men (Althof and Seftel 1995). Injection therapy with alprostadil has been associated with local pain, scar tissue formation with chronic use, and, rarely, priapism. Alprostadil is also available as a urethral suppository, the use of which can be associated with some penile discomfort and, rarely, with hypotension (Padma-Nathan et al. 1997).

Sildenafil was the first oral erectogenic agent available for men with ED, followed by tadalafil and vardenafil. All three agents improve erectile function in men with both organic and psychogenic ED by serving as selective inhibitors of PDE5. Sildenafil and vardenafil can be taken 30 minutes to 4 hours before anticipated sexual activity, and tadalafil can be taken up to 30 hours before. Erections do not occur spontaneously on taking these medications but require adequate physical stimulation. The obvious advantages of PDE5 inhibitors are ease of use and high rate of success in up to 70%–80% of affected men (Boolell et al. 1996; Porst et al. 2003a, 2003b). Potential side effects for these medications include headache, skin flushing, dizziness, gastrointestinal discomfort, blurred vision, and the potential for blood pressure decreases when combined with nitrates (e.g., sublingual nitroglycerin, isosorbide). In addition, the PDE5 inhibitors should be used with caution in men with abnormal penile shape, a history of orthostatic hypotension, severe renal or hepatic disease, concomitant use of certain antiviral and antifungal medications, and diseases that increase the risk of priapism, such as sickle cell anemia, multiple myeloma, and leukemia. An extremely rare but potentially devastating side effect of PDE5 inhibitors that has emerged is nonarteritic anterior ischemic optic neuropathy (NOIAN), characterized by the rapid onset of visual loss. Although the exact role of PDE5 inhibitors in the pathogenesis of NOIAN has not been fully established, any changes in visual acuity while taking a PDE5 inhibitor requires immediate assessment (Bella et al. 2006).

Despite the efficacy of all three oral erectogenic agents, it is important for older men to realize that these medications are not substitutes for poor sexual or marital relationships and that these drugs can pose risks for men who have brittle cardiovascular disease and/or men seeking sexual exertion whose bodies are out of condition (Mobley and Baum 1999).

Two other important treatments for ED are the use of vacuum constriction devices and penile implants (Sison et al. 1997). A vacuum constriction device consists of a plastic tube with an attached pump that fits over the penis and creates a vacuum that causes blood flow into the penis. Once an erection is achieved, a ring is placed around the base of the penis to maintain rigidity and the tube is removed. Although vacuum constriction devices are quite effective, their use requires some dexterity and can cause numbing, bruising, and delayed ejaculation (Dutta and Eid 1999). Penile implants are an effective but less frequently used treatment for ED. A number of penile implants are on the market, some of them semirigid and others consisting of inflatable tubes with implantable pumps (Evans 1998). Aside from the risks associated with surgery and the risks of infection, the main problem concerning these implants is mechanical failure, which occurs from 5% to 20% of the time (Lewis 1995). Penile implants can, however, be surgically repaired or reimplanted. Because surgical placement of an implant leads to destruction of erectile tissue, a prosthetic device will always be needed to achieve an erection.

Premature Ejaculation

Premature ejaculation is the most common sexual dysfunction in younger men, reported in 20%–38% of various samples (Porst et al. 2007; Westheimer and Lopater 2002), but its prevalence among older men is unknown (Althof 1995). Premature ejaculation is defined in DSM-IV-TR as persistent or recurrent uncontrollable, rapid ejaculation that occurs just before or shortly after penetration. Such rapid ejaculation usually prohibits adequate sexual intercourse. Historically, treatment involved psychotherapeutic and cognitive-behavioral techniques to slow down perception of sexual stimulation, as well as couples techniques in which the partner gently squeezes on the man's penis before penetration to reduce sensation and stall ejaculation (Kaplan 1989). Treatment has changed significantly since the introduction of antidepressant medications (in particular, SSRIs) that can delay ejaculation without necessarily affecting erectile function (Waldinger 2007). In addition, the PDE5 inhibitor sildenafil has also been found to effectively treat premature ejaculation, both alone and in combination with SSRIs (Wang et al. 2007).

Hypoactive Sexual Desire Disorder in Women

Hypoactive sexual desire is a significant sexual problem for women across the life span and involves multiple psychological and physical factors. In some older women, loss of libido results from a poor self-image—

brought about by age-associated losses of physical strength and beauty—and from changes in sexual function caused by cessation of estrogen production during menopause. An older woman's ability to see herself as a sexual being can be further eroded by exposure to negative societal attitudes and negative images of sexuality in late life. Unfortunately, many women internalize these distorted, ageist beliefs. Treatment of low desire must begin with sex education and counseling to counter those psychological barriers. Estrogen replacement therapy may help improve sexual arousal and comfort, which in turn may lead to increased desire.

The critical physiological cause of low desire in women, however, appears to be menopause-associated reduction in levels of free testosterone. Testosterone replacement therapy has been beneficial in women with hypoactive sexual desire (Basson 1999; Buster et al. 2005; Shifren et al. 2006), although side effects can include weight gain, virilization (e.g., growth of facial and chest hair, lowering of the voice), suppression of clotting factors, and even liver damage (Kingsberg et al. 2007). Sildenafil therapy has also been studied in women with sexual dysfunction (hypoactive desire, orgasmic disorder, or dyspareunia) associated with female sexual arousal disorder, but though well tolerated, it did not lead to improvement (Basson et al. 2002).

Female Orgasmic Disorder

Orgasmic disorder is defined in DSM-IV-TR as persistent or recurrent delay or absence of orgasm after a normal sexual excitement phase. The disorder is common in sexually active women of all ages. Female orgasmic disorder is often comorbid with hypoactive desire and involves many of the same attitudinal barriers to resolution. Many older women who have experienced inhibited orgasm for years resist seeking help, especially if they do not perceive it as a problem for themselves or their relationships. Individual sex therapy involves relaxation techniques that incorporate sensual self-stimulation and masturbation, usually with the aid of a vibrator, to increase clitoral stimulation (Heiman and Lopiccolo 1976). Short-term group therapy can also be helpful, providing education and support (Barbach 1980). When orgasm can be achieved, sensate focus exercises can help to incorporate it into the couple's sexual relations.

Sexual Pain Disorders

The two female sexual pain disorders, dyspareunia and vaginismus, are grouped together in DSM-IV-TR but are very different entities. Dyspareunia is recurrent pain that is associated with sexual intercourse. It is common in late life, especially after menopause. This disorder may be associated with a number of medical conditions that affect the genital region, including vulvitis, vulvodynia, and vulvar vestibulitis (Goodwin and Agronin 1997). Pain can also be associated with many pelvic disorders and can result from surgical or radiation treatment of gynecologic malignancies. Gynecologic examination should always be the first step, because treatment of the underlying condition can help reduce and perhaps resolve discomfort. Estrogen replacement therapy may be helpful for women with atrophic changes and decreased lubrication caused by menopause. However, when dyspareunia is chronic, treatment can be challenging and should incorporate various methods of sex therapy. In older women, dyspareunia can significantly disrupt sexual relations, sometimes leading to abandonment of sex altogether. The goal of therapy may be to introduce the couple to sensual exercises (e.g., massage, foreplay, oral sex) that can substitute for sexual intercourse when pain is prohibitive.

Vaginismus occurs more commonly than suspected and typically presents in a young woman attempting sexual intercourse for the first time. Without treatment, vaginismus can lead to an unconsummated marriage and avoidance of sexual relations throughout life. Treatment is almost always successful and involves both conjoint sex therapy and physical exercises in which the woman uses vaginal dilators in graduated sizes to extinguish the involuntary vaginal muscle contraction (Goodwin and Agronin 1997). It is not known how common vaginismus is in later life.

Sexual Function and Dysfunction in Dementia

Sexuality continues to play an important role in the lives of many individuals with dementia, often by providing a nonverbal means of communication and intimacy. Depending on the degree of dementia, however, the ability to initiate sexual activity and sustain performance may be impaired. Agitation, disinhibition, and psychosis associated with dementia may give rise to sexually aggressive or inappropriate behaviors. Ethical issues also complicate sexuality associated with dementia. For example, one partner may not be fully competent to consent to sex, especially with another individual who has dementia (Haddad and Benbow

1993), or the nonaffected partner may seek to fulfill sexual needs outside the relationship. It is important to understand these issues when assessing and treating dementia patients and their caregivers. Unfortunately, health care professionals often fail to inquire about such issues, despite the frequency with which they affect couples (Duffy 1995).

Dementia affects sexuality in several ways. Sexual desire may remain strong and even increase, especially if inhibitions are reduced by cognitive impairment. As the dementia progresses, the cognitively intact partner may become concerned about whether the affected individual is truly consenting to sexual activity (Hanks 1992). The partner without dementia may also feel frustrated with a partner who does not always recognize him or her or who requests sex repeatedly because he or she cannot remember when they last had sex (Davies et al. 1992; Redinbaugh et al. 1997). The cognitively intact partner's sexual desire may decrease because he or she views the dementia and associated changes in behavior and personality as a sexual turnoff. Partners may be further confused by conflicting feelings of love and fidelity for their spouses with dementia and guilt over their desires for extramarital intimacy.

It is not surprising, then, that there is an overall decrease in sexual activity in affected couples. In one study, only 27% of couples with a partner affected by Alzheimer's disease were sexually active, compared with 82% of couples without dementia (Wright 1991). This decrease may also be attributed in part to sexual dysfunction associated with dementia. For example, cognitive impairment may reduce the capacity for paying attention during sex, as well as the ability to initiate and perform components of lovemaking (Duffy 1995; Redinbaugh et al. 1997). This impairment may explain why men with Alzheimer's disease have high rates of ED (more than 50% in one sample; Zeiss et al. 1990): they are unable to maintain a cognitive focus on physical and mental stimulation during sex. Such reasoning may also explain why inhibited orgasm (or anorgasmia) is common in women with dementia (Wright 1991). Few studies have examined sexual dysfunction in dementia, so the rates of specific sexual disorders in different types of dementia are not known.

Although the percentage of individuals with dementia who demonstrate sexually aggressive or inappropriate behaviors is relatively small, these persons tend to generate a disproportionate amount of anxiety for caregivers and to require a disproportionate amount of clinical attention from long-term care staff. The problematic behaviors associated with dementia include inappropriate sexual comments or demands, hypersexual behaviors (e.g., repeated requests for sexual gratification, compulsive masturbation), disinhibition (e.g., exposing oneself, disrobing, or masturbating in public areas), and sexually aggressive behaviors (e.g., attempts to grope, fondle, or force sex on another person). In various studies, these behaviors were seen in 2%–7% of individuals with Alzheimer's disease (Burns et al. 1990; Kumar et al. 1988; Rabins et al. 1982), although these rates may be higher in institutionalized populations (Mayers 1994). For example, one study found that 25% of residents on a dementia unit engaged in sexually inappropriate behaviors (Hashmi et al. 2000). Because frontal and temporal regions of the brain are involved in behavioral control and inhibition, individuals with dementia affecting these areas of the brain may be particularly vulnerable to developing such inappropriate behaviors (Haddad and Benbow 1993; Raji et al. 2000). Other factors associated with inappropriate or hyperactive sexual behaviors include mania, psychosis, alcohol or drug abuse, stroke, head trauma (Hashmi et al. 2000), and use of levodopa (Bowers et al. 1971).

When assessing an individual who has allegedly demonstrated problematic behaviors, it is critical to identify the context of the behaviors. For example, public disrobing or touching of genitals in public may not be caused by sexual urges but may instead reflect underlying confusion, delirium, motor restlessness, or stereotypy associated with dementia. However, caregivers and long-term care staff sometimes misinterpret innocuous behaviors as evidence of sexual disinhibition (Hajjar and Kamel 2003b; Redinbaugh et al. 1997). A good example would be the aphasic individual with dementia who reaches out or grabs for attention while in his or her wheelchair, inadvertently hitting someone in the waist or chest area. The individual is simply reaching out for help, but the staff member who is touched in the groin or breast area may wrongly view this act as an act of sexual aggression. It is also important to recognize that even individuals with severe dementia have legitimate needs for physical stimulation and intimacy, and these persons may be reacting out of frustration and confusion because they lack the ability to communicate their needs verbally.

The geriatric psychiatrist must be able to address these challenging issues of sexuality in dementia. Regardless of the setting, individuals with dementia have a right to engage in sexual relationships if they still have the capacity to understand the nature of the relationship and provide reasonable consent. If the cognitively intact partner is concerned about the competence of his or her spouse to engage in sexual activity, a psychiatric or psychological consultation may shed light on the affected individual's understanding of the relationship. Lichtenberg and Strzepek (1990) proposed several questions to be answered in any interview to determine an individual's capacity to consent to a sexual relationship: Does the individual know who is initiating sexual contact? Can the individual describe his or her preferred degree of intimacy? Is the sexual activity consistent with the individual's previous beliefs and values? Can he or she say "no" to unwanted activity? Does the individual understand that a sexual relationship with someone other than his or her spouse may be temporary? Can the individual describe how he or she would react if the sexual relationship were to end? Responses to these questions will help determine the affected individual's awareness of the relationship, his or her ability to avoid coercion and exploitation, and his or her awareness of the possible risks.

One main purpose of psychological or psychiatric intervention is to provide education about sexuality to caregivers in the community and to staff in long-term care settings. Such education will improve interpretation of and response to apparent inappropriate sexual behaviors. In addition, educational programs for long-term care staff may foster attitudes that are more open minded (White and Catania 1982).

Behavioral approaches for inappropriate sexual comments include setting verbal limits and directing the individual to a different topic. Staff and caregivers must be careful to avoid reinforcing inappropriate comments, such as by laughing at off-color jokes or teasing patients in a seductive manner in response to sexual comments. In the case of inappropriate or aggressive sexual advances, staff may need to physically remove the individual from the situation or keep him or her away from vulnerable individuals. Sometimes restrictive clothing (e.g., pants without zippers, pants with suspenders) can cut down on public displays of genitals, although caution must be used so that the individual is not inadvertently restrained. Because sexual advances may reflect unmet sexual needs, existing partners can be asked to consider providing more physical and perhaps sexual intimacy, the hope being that doing so will remove the drive to engage in inappropriate behaviors.

When behavioral approaches are insufficient, psychiatric consultation is needed to provide better control through pharmacotherapy. The choice of medication will depend on the nature and severity of the behaviors and on the presence of underlying psychopathology, if any. In general, however, much of sexual aggression can be viewed in the same way as any other form of agitation associated with dementia and can be treated accordingly. Thus, a variety of psychotropic agents—in particular, the atypical antipsychotics—may help treat both agitation and sexual problems associated with dementia. Medications may also be used to treat specific underlying psychopathology. For example, overactive libido can sometimes be reduced through use of an antidepressant with sexual side effects, such as an SSRI or a tricyclic antidepressant (Raji et al. 2000; Segraves 1998), or through use of a beta-blocker. If the inappropriate sexual behaviors are believed to reflect hypersexuality caused by mania, use of an antipsychotic or a mood stabilizer is indicated. Another pharmacological strategy for decreasing libido and sexual aggression is use of hormone therapy. Estrogen has been shown to reduce aggression in men with dementia (Kyomen et al. 1999), a finding that may be applicable to sexually aggressive behaviors. Two steroid hormones with both progesterone and antiandrogen activity are medroxyprogesterone and cyproterone acetate. Medroxyprogesterone works by blocking synthesis of testosterone in the testes. Both agents have been shown to reduce sexually aggressive behaviors in individuals with dementia (Brown 1998; Cooper 1987; Nadal and Allgulander 1992). However, cyproterone acetate is available only in Europe. Side effects of both medroxyprogesterone and cyproterone include weight gain, glucose intolerance, and liver dysfunction.

Key Points

- As individuals are living longer, healthier lives, sexuality continues to play an important role, facilitated by increasingly positive attitudes and newer and more effective treatments for sexual dysfunction.
- Sexual surveys indicate that while a majority of individuals 65 years and older continue to be sexually active, there is a decline in both the rate and the frequency of sexual activity, particularly in older, single women.

- The main predictors of sexual activity in late life include previous sexual behaviors; the availability, health, and interest of a partner; and the individual's overall physical health.
- Rates of sexual dysfunction increase with age, with erectile dysfunction being the most common male disorder and hypoactive sexual desire being the most common female disorder.
- Sexual dysfunction in late life can be treated with a variety of approaches, depending on its form, including treatment of causative medical or medication-related factors, psychoeducation, individual or couples counseling, sex therapy, and the use of disorder-specific medications, such as oral erectogenic agents for erectile dysfunction.

References

Adelman M: Stigma, gay lifestyles, and adjustment to aging: a study of late-life gay men and lesbians. J Homosex 20:7–32, 1991

Agronin ME, Westheimer RK: Sexuality and sexual disorders in late life, in Principles and Practice of Geriatric Psychiatry. Edited by Agronin ME, Maletta G. Philadelphia, PA, Lippincott Williams & Wilkins, 2006, pp 523–546

Alexander JL, Kotz K, Dennerstein L: The effects of postmenopausal hormone therapies on female sexual functioning: a review of double-blind, randomized controlled trials. Menopause 11 (6 part 2):749–765, 2004

Althof SE: Pharmacologic treatment of rapid ejaculation. Psychiatr Clin North Am 18:85–94, 1995

Althof SE, Seftel AD: The evaluation and management of erectile dysfunction. Psychiatr Clin North Am 18:171–192, 1995

American Association for Retired Persons: Sexuality at Midlife and Beyond: 2004 Update of Attitudes and Behaviors. 2005. Available at http://assets.aarp.org/rgcenter/general/2004_sexuality.pdf. Accessed April 8, 2008.

American Psychiatric Association: Diagnostic and Statistical Manual of Mental Disorders, 4th Edition, Text Revision. Washington, DC, American Psychiatric Association, 2000

Bachmann GA, Leiblum SR: Sexuality in sexagenarian women. Maturitas 13:43–50, 1991

Barbach L: Women Discover Orgasm: A Therapist's Guide to a New Treatment Approach. New York, Free Press, 1980

Basson R: Androgen replacement for women. Can Fam Physician 45:2100–2107, 1999

Basson R, McInnes R, Smith MD, et al: Efficacy and safety of sildenafil in estrogenized women with sexual dysfunction associated with female sexual arousal disorder. J Womens Health Gend Based Med 11:367–377, 2002

Bella AJ, Brant WO, Lue TF, et al: Non-arteritic anterior ischemic optic neuropathy (NAION) and phosphodiesterase type-5 inhibitors. Can J Urol 13:3233–3238, 2006

Berigan T: Antidepressant-induced sexual dysfunction treated with vardenafil. Can J Psychiatry 49:643, 2004

Boolell M, Gepi-Attee S, Gingell JC, et al: Sildenafil, a novel effective oral therapy for male erectile dysfunction. Br J Urol 78:257–261, 1996

Bowers MB, Woert MV, Davis L: Sexual behavior during L-dopa treatment for parkinsonism. Am J Psychiatry 127:1691–1693, 1971

Brown FW: Case report: sexual aggression in dementia. Annals of Long-Term Care 6:248–249, 1998

Burns A, Jacoby R, Levy R: Psychiatric phenomena in Alzheimer's disease, IV: disorders of behavior. Br J Psychiatry 157:86–94, 1990

Buster JE, Kingsberg SA, Aguirre O, et al: Testosterone patch for low sexual desire in surgically menopausal women: a randomized trial. Obstet Gynecol 105 (5 part 1):944–952, 2005

Butler RN, Lewis MI: Love and Sex After 40: A Guide for Men and Women for Their Mid and Later Years. New York, Harper & Row, 1986

Centers for Disease Control: Cases of HIV infection and AIDS in the United States and Dependent Areas, 2005. HIV/AIDS Surveillance Report, Volume 17, Revised Edition, June 2007. Available at http://www.cdc.gov/hiv/topics/surveillance/resources/reports/2005report/default.htm. Accessed April 8, 2008.

Centers for Disease Control: STD surveillance report 2006. Available at http://www.cdc.gov/std/stats/default.htm. Accessed April 8, 2008.

Comfort A, Dial LK: Sexuality and aging: an overview. Clin Geriatr Med 7:1–7, 1991

Cooper AJ: Medroxyprogesterone acetate (MPA) treatment of sexual acting out in men suffering from dementia. J Clin Psychiatry 48:368–370, 1987

Crenshaw TL, Goldberg JP: Sexual Pharmacology: Drugs That Affect Sexual Function. New York, WW Norton, 1996

Davies HD, Zeiss A, Tinklenberg JR: 'Til death do us part: intimacy and sexuality in the marriages of Alzheimer's patients. J Psychosoc Nurs Ment Health Serv 30:5–10, 1992

Duffy LM: Sexual behavior and marital intimacy in Alzheimer's couples: a family theory perspective. Sex Disabil 13:239–254, 1995

Dutta TC, Eid JF: Vacuum constriction devices for erectile dysfunction: a long-term, prospective study of patients with mild, moderate, and severe dysfunction. Urology 54:891–893, 1999

Evans C: The use of penile prostheses in the treatment of impotence. Br J Urol 81:591–598, 1998

Fava M, Nurnberg HG, Seidman SN: Efficacy and safety of sildenafil in men with serotonergic antidepressant-associated erectile dysfunction: results from a randomized, double-blind, placebo-controlled trial. J Clin Psychiatry 67:240–246, 2006

Feldman HA, Goldstein I, Hatzichristou DG, et al: Impotence and its medical and psychosocial correlates: results of the Massachusetts Male Aging Study. J Urol 151:54–61, 1994

Gelenberg AJ, McGahuey C, Laukes C, et al: Mirtazapine substitution in SSRI-induced sexual dysfunction. J Clin Psychiatry 61:356–360, 2000

Gitlin MJ: Psychotropic medications and their effects on sexual function: diagnosis, biology, and treatment approaches. J Clin Psychiatry 55:406–413, 1994

Goodwin AJ, Agronin ME: A Women's Guide to Overcoming Sexual Fear and Pain. Oakland, CA, New Harbinger, 1997

Haddad P, Benbow S: Sexual problems associated with dementia, part 2: aetiology, assessment and treatment. Int J Geriatr Psychiatry 8:631–637, 1993

Hajjar RR, Kamel HK: Sexuality in the nursing home, part 1: attitudes and barriers to sexual expression. J Am Med Dir Assoc 5 (suppl 2):152–156, 2003a

Hajjar RR, Kamel HK: Sexuality in the nursing home, part 2: managing abnormal behavior—legal and ethical issues. J Am Med Dir Assoc 5 (suppl 2):203–206, 2003b

Hanks N: The effects of Alzheimer's disease on the sexual attitudes and behaviors of married caregivers and their spouses. Sex Disabil 10:137–151, 1992

Harman SM: Testosterone in older men after the Institute of Medicine Report: where do we go from here? Climacteric 8:124–135, 2005

Hashmi FH, Krady AI, Qayum F, et al: Sexually disinhibited behavior in the cognitively impaired elderly. Clin Geriatr 8:61–68, 2000

Heaton JP, Morales A: Andropause—a multisystem disease. Can J Urol 8:1213–1222, 2001

Heiman L, Lopiccolo J: Becoming Orgasmic: A Sexual and Personal Growth Program for Women, Revised Edition. New York, Prentice-Hall, 1976

Howell S, Shalit S: Testosterone deficiency and replacement. Horm Res 56 (suppl 1):86–92, 2001

Jacoby S: Great sex: what's age got to do with it? Modern Maturity (serial online) September/October 1999. Available at http://www.aarpmagazine.org/lifestyle/relationships/great_sex.html. Accessed July 30, 2008.

Kaas MJ: Sexual expression of the elderly in nursing homes. Gerontologist 18:372–378, 1978

Kaplan HS: The New Sex Therapy. New York, Brunner/Mazel, 1974

Kaplan HS: The Evaluation of Sexual Disorders: Psychological and Medical Aspects. New York, Brunner/Mazel, 1983

Kaplan HS: Sexual Aversion, Sexual Phobias, and Panic Disorder. New York, Brunner/Mazel, 1987

Kaplan HS: Overcoming Premature Ejaculation. New York, Brunner/Mazel, 1989

Kavoussi RJ, Segraves RT, Hughes AR, et al: Double-blind comparison of bupropion sustained release and sertraline in depressed outpatients. J Clin Psychiatry 58:532–537, 1997

Kimmel DC: Patterns of aging among gay men. Psychotherapy Theory, Research, and Practice 14:386–393, 1977

Kingsberg S, Shifren J, Wekselman K, et al: Evaluation of the clinical relevance of benefits associated with transdermal testosterone treatment in postmenopausal women with hypoactive sexual desire disorder. J Sex Med 4 (part 1):1001–1008, 2007

Kligman EW: Office evaluation of sexual function and complaints. Clin Geriatr Med 7:15–39, 1991

Kumar A, Koss E, Metzler D, et al: Behavioral symptomatology in dementia of the Alzheimer type. Alzheimer Dis Assoc Disord 2:363–365, 1988

Kyomen HH, Satlin A, Hennen J, et al: Estrogen therapy and aggressive behavior in elderly patients with moderate-to-severe dementia. Am J Geriatr Psychiatry 7:339–348, 1999

Labbate LA, Croft HA, Oleshansky MA: Antidepressant-related erectile dysfunction: management via avoidance, switching antidepressants, antidotes, and adaptation. J Clin Psychiatry 64 (suppl 10):11–19, 2003

Lacey JV Jr, Mink PJ, Lubin JH, et al: Menopausal hormone replacement therapy and risk of ovarian cancer. JAMA 288:334–341, 2002

Laumann EO, Paik A, Glasser DB, et al: A cross-national study of subjective sexual well-being among older women and men: findings from the Global Study of Sexual Attitudes and Behaviors. Arch Sex Behav 35:145–161, 2006

Lewis RW: Long-term results of penile prosthetic implants. Urol Clin North Am 22:847–856, 1995

Lichtenberg PA, Strzepek DM: Assessments of institutionalized dementia patients' competencies to participate in intimate relationships. Gerontologist 30:117–120, 1990

Lindau ST, Schumm LP, Laumann EO, et al: A study of sexuality and health among older adults in the United States. N Engl J Med 357:762–774, 2007

Marsiglio W, Donnelly D: Sexual relations in later life: a national study of married persons. J Gerontol 46:S338–S344, 1991

Masters WH, Johnson VE: Human Sexual Response. Boston, MA, Little, Brown, 1966

Masters WH, Johnson VE: Human Sexual Inadequacy. Boston, MA, Little, Brown, 1970

Mayers KS: Sexuality and the patient with dementia. Sex Disabil 12:213–219, 1994

Metz ME, Miner MH: Male "menopause," aging, and sexual function: a review. Sex Disabil 13:287–307, 1995

Michael RT, Gagnon JH, Laumann EO, et al: Sex in America: A Definitive Survey. Boston, MA, Little, Brown, 1994

Mobley DF, Baum N: Sildenafil in elderly men: advice and caveats. Clin Geriatr 7:34–41, 1999

Montejo AL, Llorca G, Izquierdo JA.: Incidence of sexual dysfunction associated with antidepressant agents: a prospective multicenter study of 1022 outpatients. Spanish Working Group for the Study of Psychotropic-Related Sexual Dysfunction. J Clin Psychiatry 62 (suppl 3):10–21, 2001

Morley JE: Testosterone and behavior. Clin Geriatric Med 19:605–616, 2003

Morley JE, Perry HM: Andropause: an old concept in new clothing. Clin Geriatric Med 19:507–528, 2003

Morley JE, Tariq SH: Sexuality and disease. Clin Geriatric Med 19:563–574, 2003

Mulligan T, Palguta RF Jr: Sexual interest, activity, and satisfaction among male nursing home residents. Arch Sex Behav 20:199–204, 1987

Mulligan T, Reddy S, Gulur PV, et al: Disorders of male sexual dysfunction. Clin Geriatric Med 19:473–482, 2003

Nadal M, Allgulander S: Normalization of sexual behavior in a female with dementia after treatment with cyproterone. Int J Geriatr Psychiatry 8:265–267, 1992

Nappi RE, Wawra K, Schmitt S: Hypoactive sexual desire disorder in postmenopausal women. Gynecol Endocrinol 22:318–323, 2006

National Council on the Aging: Healthy Sexuality and Vital Aging: Executive Summary. Washington, DC, National Council on the Aging, 1998

Padma-Nathan H, Hellstrom WJG, Kaiser FE, et al: Treatment of men with erectile dysfunction with transurethral alprostadil. Medicated Urethral System for Erection (MUSE) Study Group. N Engl J Med 336:1–7, 1997

Pope M, Schulz R: Sexual attitudes and behavior in midlife and aging homosexual males. J Homosex 20:169–177, 1990

Porst H, Padma-Nathan H, Giuliano F, et al: Efficacy of tadalafil for the treatment of erectile dysfunction at 24 and 36 hours after dosing: a randomized controlled trial. Urology 62:121–125, 2003a

Porst H, Young JM, Schmidt AC, et al: Efficacy and tolerability of vardenafil for treatment of erectile dysfunction in patient subgroups. Urology 62:519–523, 2003b

Porst H, Montorsi F, Rosen RC, et al: The Premature Ejaculation Prevalence and Attitudes (PEPA) survey: prevalence, comorbidities, and professional help-seeking. Eur Urol 51:816–823, 2007

Rabins PV, Mace NL, Lucas MJ: The impact of dementia on the family. JAMA 248:333–335, 1982

Raji M, Liu D, Wallace D: Case report: sexual aggressiveness in a patient with dementia: sustained clinical response to citalopram. Annals of Long-Term Care 8:81–83, 2000

Redinbaugh EM, Zeiss AM, Davies HD, et al: Sexual behavior in men with dementing illnesses. Clin Geriatr 5:45–50, 1997

Richardson JP, Lazur A: Sexuality in the nursing home patient. Am Fam Physician 51:121–124, 1995

Rosen RC, Leiblum SR: Principles and Practice of Sex Therapy: Update for the 1990s. New York, Guilford, 1988

Rossouw JE, Anderson GL, Prentice RL, et al: Writing Group for the Women's Health Initiative Investigators: Risks and benefits of estrogen plus progestin in healthy postmenopausal women: principal results from the Women's Health Initiative randomized controlled trial. JAMA 288:321–333, 2002

Rothschild AJ: Selective serotonin reuptake inhibitor–induced sexual dysfunction: efficacy of a drug holiday. Am J Psychiatry 152:1514–1516, 1995

Saretsky K: The right to be human, how one facility cares. Provider 13:20–23, 1987

Sbrocco T, Weisberg BA, Barlow DH: Sexual dysfunction in the older adult: assessment of psychosocial factors. Sex Disabil 13:201–218, 1995

Schover LR, Jensen SB: Sexuality and Chronic Illness. New York, Guilford, 1988

Segraves RT: Antidepressant-induced sexual dysfunction. J Clin Psychiatry 59 (suppl 4):48–54, 1998

Segraves RT, Lee J, Stevenson R: Tadalafil for treatment of erectile dysfunction in men on antidepressants. J Clin Psychopharmacol 27:62–66, 2007

Shifren JL, Davis SR, Moreau M, et al: Testosterone patch for the treatment of hypoactive sexual desire disorder in naturally menopausal women: results from the INTIMATE NM1 Study. Menopause 13:770–779, 2006

Sison AS, Godschalk MF, Mulligan T: Erectile dysfunction in the elderly: treatment recommendations from the recent American Urological Association guidelines. Clin Geriatr 5:73–76, 1997

Snarch D: Constructing the Sexual Crucible: An Integration of Sexual and Marital Therapy. New York, WW Norton, 1991

Spector IP, Rosen RC, Leiblum SR: Sexuality, in Psychiatric Care in the Nursing Home. Edited by Reichman WE, Katz PR. New York, Oxford University Press, 1996, pp 133–150

Suckling J, Lethaby A, Kennedy R: Local oestrogen for vaginal atrophy in postmenopausal women. Cochrane Database Syst Oct 18:CD001500, 2006

Tariq SH, Haleem U, Omran ML, et al: Erectile dysfunction: etiology and treatment in young and old patients. Clin Geriatric Med 19:539–551, 2003

Thomas DR: Medications and sexual function. Clin Geriatric Med 19:553–562, 2003

Waldinger MD: Premature ejaculation: state of the art. Urol Clin North Am 34:591–599, 2007

Wang WF, Wang Y, Minhas S, et al: Can sildenafil treat primary premature ejaculation? A prospective clinical study. Int J Urol 14:331–335, 2007

Wasow M, Loeb MB: Sexuality in nursing homes. J Am Geriatr Soc 27:73–79, 1979

Westheimer RK, Lopater S: Human Sexuality: A Psychosocial Perspective. Philadelphia, PA, Lippincott Williams & Wilkins, 2002

White CB: Sexual interest, attitudes, knowledge, and sexual history in relation to sexual behavior in the institutionalized aged. Arch Sex Behav 11:11–21, 1982

White CB, Catania JA: Psychoeducational intervention for sexuality with the aged, family members of the aged, and people who work with the aged. Int J Aging Hum Dev 15:121–138, 1982

Wright LK: The impact of Alzheimer's disease on the marital relationship. Gerontologist 31:224–237, 1991

Xu F, Schillinger JA, Aubin MR, et al: Sexually transmitted diseases of older persons in Washington State. Sex Transm Dis 28:287–291, 2001

Zajecka J: Strategies for the treatment of antidepressant-related sexual dysfunction: management via avoidance, switching antidepressants, antidotes, and adaptation. J Clin Psychiatry 64 (suppl 10):11–19, 2001

Zeiss AM, Davies HD, Wood M, et al: The incidence and correlates of erectile problems in patients with Alzheimer's disease. Arch Sex Behav 19:325–332, 1990

Zilbergeld B, Ellison C: Desire discrepancies and arousal problems in sex therapy, in Principles and Practice of Sex Therapy. Edited by Leiblum S, Pervin L. New York, Guilford, 1980, pp 65–101

Suggested Readings

Agronin ME: Geriatric psychiatry: sexuality and aging, in Kaplan and Sadock's Comprehensive Textbook of Psychiatry, 8th Edition. Edited by Sadock BJ, Sadock VA. Philadelphia, PA, Lippincott Williams & Wilkins, 2005, pp 3834–3838

Agronin ME, Westheimer RK: Sexuality and sexual disorders in late life, in Principles and Practice of Geriatric Psychiatry. Edited by Agronin ME, Maletta G. Philadelphia, PA, Lippincott Williams & Wilkins, 2006, pp 523–546

Alexander JL, Kotz K, Dennerstein L: The effects of postmenopausal hormone therapies on female sexual functioning: a review of double-blind, randomized controlled trials. Menopause 11 (6 part 2):749–765, 2004

American Association for Retired Persons: Sexuality at Midlife and Beyond: 2004 Update of Attitudes and Behaviors. 2005. Available at http://assets.aarp.org/rgcenter/general/2004_sexuality.pdf. Accessed April 8, 2008.

Hashmi FH, Krady AI, Qayum F, et al: Sexually disinhibited behavior in the cognitively impaired elderly. Clin Geriatr 8:61–68, 2000

Heaton JP, Morales A: Andropause—a multisystem disease. Can J Urol 8:1213–1222, 2001

Lindau ST, Schumm LP, Laumann EO, et al: A study of sexuality and health among older adults in the United States. N Engl J Med 357:762–774, 2007

Morley JE (ed): Geriatric Sexuality. Clin Geriatr Med 19(3):463–662, 2003

Westheimer RK, Lopater S: Human Sexuality: A Psychosocial Perspective. Philadelphia, PA, Lippincott Williams & Wilkins, 2002

CHAPTER 21

BEREAVEMENT

Moria J. Smoski, Ph.D.
Larry W. Thompson, Ph.D.

Late-life bereavement is an important topic that is affecting a growing number of individuals as the population ages. This chapter begins with a review of the demographics of bereavement, followed by theoretical and empirical perspectives on adjustment to the loss of a loved one. Finally, we review considerations in the diagnosis and treatment of complicated grief.

Late-Life Bereavement

Who Are the Elderly Bereaved?

The terms *bereavement* and *grief reaction* have been used to refer to any number of losses experienced by older adults. These losses include (but are not limited to) the death of a spouse, an adult child, another family member, or a close personal friend; divorce (Cain 1988); prolonged caregiving for a severely impaired relative (Bass et al. 1991); and a significant decline in one's own health, attractiveness, capabilities, opportunities, and so forth (Kalish 1987). When used in its narrowest sense, *bereavement* refers to the reaction or process that results after the death of someone close. Indeed, death of a spouse is generally accepted as the most common and traumatic life event that older people experience (Jacobs and Ostfeld 1977).

In the United States, the mean age at which widowhood or widowerhood takes place is 69 years for men and 66 years for women. Forty-five percent of women and 15% of men over the age of 65 have lost a spouse (Federal Interagency Forum on Aging Related Statistics 2000). The mean duration of widowhood or widowerhood is approximately 14 years for women versus only 7 years for men (U.S. Census Bureau 2001). These data, plus the fact that widowers are more likely to remarry after losing their wives, have often led to the interpretation that widowhood is a women's issue. However, research has shown that after the loss of a spouse, older men are at a higher risk for mortality than are women. For example, in the University of Southern California longitudinal study of spousal bereavement, the first year after bereavement saw a mortality rate of 12% in men but only about 1% in women (Gallagher-Thompson et al. 1993; Thompson et al. 1991).

The rates of widowhood among persons age 65 or older are similar for whites and Hispanics and are slightly higher for African Americans (U.S. Census Bureau 2001). Given the prediction that the elderly population in each of these ethnic groups will increase considerably over the next 20 years (Federal Interagency Forum on Aging Related Statistics 2000), there is a clear need to understand how the processes of bereavement are mediated by cultural factors.

This work was supported in part by grant R01-AG01959 from the National Institute on Aging and grants R01-MH36834 and R01-MH37196 from the National Institute of Mental Health. In addition, author M.J.S. was supported by institutional training grant T32-MH070448 (Principal Investigator: Blazer).

Theories About Adjustment to Permanent Losses

Numerous theoretical perspectives on the function and process of bereavement have been developed over the years. For a more comprehensive review, the interested reader is referred to articles by Osterweis et al. (1984) and, more recently, Stroebe and Schut (1999) and Stroebe et al. (2001a). We begin by presenting a historical perspective on important theoretical perspectives. We then briefly mention major positions that reflect trends in the development of frameworks for describing the symptoms and process of grief.

Early work emphasized that mourning was a process whereby the bereaved gradually "surrendered" their attachment to the lost loved one by engaging in certain specific psychological and behavioral tasks that occurred at appropriate time points during the bereavement (Freud 1917 [1915] /1957; Lindemann 1944). This process was thought to be necessary for the individual to develop new constructive attachments to other people entering their life. Failure to complete these tasks would result in the development of a psychiatric disorder. Bowlby (1961) offered a somewhat different interpretation of grief behaviors. He posited that any involuntary separation, including bereavement, gives rise to many forms of attachment behavior (such as separation anxiety and pining) that reflect the person's desire to reunite with the lost person. Thus the function of bereavement is not a surrendering of attachment but rather an attempt to regain a sense of connection with the lost object of attachment. With time, these behaviors were thought to dissipate through a series of stages, including shock, protest, despair, and finally breakage of the bond and adjustment to a new self.

Although stage theories of adaptation have been widely accepted by health care professionals, little empirical evidence exists to support these theories. For example, although stage theories would predict an eventual end stage in which grieving ceases, grief symptoms often do not abate in elderly widows and widowers (Bierhals et al. 1995). To expect that grief will resolve or end is now considered erroneous by some theorists (Stroebe et al. 2001b). Bereavement, as Rosenblatt (1996) contended, is a dynamic process that may continue for a number of years and even for the remainder of one's life. Also, bereaved individuals do not proceed from one clearly identifiable phase to another in an orderly fashion, a fact particularly true of older adults. From early on, researchers questioned the validity of theories in which most individuals proceed one by one through a specific series of grief stages (Weisman 1974). Many elderly persons experience multiple losses, often without sufficient time in between to complete the grieving for one event before the next one occurs. Kastenbaum (1981) termed this "bereavement overload" and suggested that because of multiple losses, the process of grieving is likely to be significantly different and more complex among older individuals. Again, however, few empirical data exist. Although the specific process of moving through stages has not been supported, the stage models provide a useful descriptive overview of many commonly recognized facets of the bereavement process. Thus, they are described here both for their historical importance and their descriptive value.

Parkes (1972) and Horowitz (1976) proposed models that involve phases or stages of reaction to the death of a loved one (see Wortman and Silver 1987 for a review of stage models). These models are similar to Kübler-Ross's (1969) seminal stage model of the reactions of individuals facing a terminal illness. Parkes' (1972) first phase begins at the time of the death and persists for several weeks. Shock and disbelief, combined with emotional numbness and cognitive confusion, characterize this period, and intense free-floating anxiety and sharp mood fluctuations occur as well. Specific somatic symptoms include sleeplessness, loss of appetite, and vague muscular aches and pains, and these symptoms lead to increased contact with primary care physicians and, commonly, requests for medication.

The second phase generally begins as the numbness and anxiety start to decrease. During this period, family and friends gradually become less available and often convey the message that the bereaved person should be getting on with life and should be getting over his or her grief, although the individual is far from ready to do so. It is only with increased time that the finality of the loss becomes more apparent to the bereaved person and more of the sadness, anger, guilt, relief, and other strong emotions begin to surface, causing emotional lability and confusion. Specific symptoms such as frequent crying, chronic sleep disturbance, blue mood, poor appetite, low energy, feelings of fatigue, loss of interest in daily living, and problems with attention and concentration are common. Nevertheless, most individuals do not develop major depression, despite the fact that certain symptoms of grief and depression overlap.

This second phase is described as a time of "yearning and protest," during which the bereaved may actively search for the deceased (Parkes 1972). They may seek out things that remind them of their loved one or go to places often frequented by the deceased. They may also have a strong sense of the presence of their lost loved one, such as seeing someone that reminds them of the deceased and for a moment feeling certain that it must be them. Vivid experiences of auditory and visual hallucinations of the deceased often occur as a normal part of grieving. Although these experiences may be startling at first glance, they often are reported as positive or comforting (Grimby 1993; Rees 1971).

Other cognitive components of this period include frequent searching for the meaning of the death and for an explanation of why it occurred the way it did. Bereaved persons may frequently relive and recollect memories and scenes associated with the death, as if to confirm that the death has occurred and that it cannot be undone. Continuous emotional and social support are particularly important to continue during this period, although weathering this phase with the bereaved can be difficult for friends and family members (who may feel that they have heard the memories many times before).

The final phase is often referred to as "identity reconstruction" (Lopata 1996). During this period the bereaved person gradually reinvests the psychic energy that has been completely focused on the lost loved one into new relationships and activities. Lopata (1975) estimated that identity reconstruction most often takes a year or more, depending on what she refers to as the "centrality of roles" involved and the complexity of new learning that must occur in developing a new sense of self.

In brief, one might best view these stages or phases of adaptation to loss in descriptive terms without oversimplifying one's understanding of a very complicated phenomenon. Most bereaved individuals will experience some combination of shock and disbelief, yearning for their lost loved one, a search for meaning in the loss, and some attempt to build a life without the deceased. However, these experiences may overlap, abate completely, and return again over the course of the bereaved's lifetime. As Shuchter and Zisook (1993) concluded, "grief's duration may be prolonged, at times even indefinite, and its intensity varies over time, from person to person, and from culture to culture. It cannot be understood from a static or linear perspective" (p. 43).

One item of debate among theories of bereavement is the adaptive or maladaptive nature of sustaining a psychological connection with the deceased. Some theorists have argued that a prolonged connection may reflect psychological problems (Horowitz et al. 1980; Rando 1992–1993). In support of this, Field et al. (2003) found that at 5 years postloss individuals experiencing severe distress were more likely to express a frequent continued connection with the deceased. Yet despite its association with distress, maintaining a strong sense of connection may be both common and adaptive. After reviewing work by Parkes (1972) and Glick et al. (1974), Bowlby (1980) pointed out that more than half of men and women undergoing bereavement still maintained ties to the deceased after 12 months and often had a strong sense of the deceased's presence in any number of situations. That sense of presence was not necessarily aversive or unwelcome, because those situations precipitated a high level of both positive and negative affect. Stroebe and Stroebe (1989) added that bereaved individuals often reflected on past actions of the deceased and used these memories as models for making decisions or solving real-life problems. More recently, these and other arguments have led to a commonly accepted position that bereaved persons maintain and in some instances nourish an active connection with their deceased loved one. Furthermore, the argument has been made that "prolonged grief" as noted by Shuchter and Zisook (1993) does not necessarily reflect psychopathology or poor adaptive functioning (Klass 1996; Reisman 2001; Rosenblatt 1996; Rosenblatt and Elde 1990; Silverman and Klass 1996). Indeed, a feeling of bondedness with a deceased spouse early in the bereavement process is adaptive (Field et al. 1999). Nonetheless, a distinction has been made between adaptive and maladaptive continuing attachment, on the basis of the forms of the attachment. Maintaining abstract rather than concrete ties with the deceased person is suggestive of healthy adaptation (Pincus 1974). In a longitudinal study, Field et al. (1999) found that 7 months after the loss of a spouse, persons who comforted themselves by using special possessions of the deceased spouse experienced more psychological distress and a smaller decrease in grief-specific symptoms over time than did persons who engaged in less searching behavior and were more inclined to maintain a bond with the deceased spouse through positive memories.

Another trend in bereavement theory has been to consider environmental changes and role adaptation along with individual emotional and psychological adjustments. Whereas earlier positions focused solely on intrapsychic processes (e.g., Bowlby 1961, 1980), more recently theorists have incorporated interpersonal and social processes into their models (e.g., Neimeyer 1998). Grieving is not just a process involving preoccupation with the deceased, accepting the loss and trying to make sense of what has happened, and so on; it also involves attempts to construct meaning of the loss and reduce the chaos associated with such traumatic events. As Stroebe and Schut (1999) addressed with their dual-process model, the bereaved oscillate between dealing with *loss-oriented stressors* and *restoration-oriented stressors.* The former focus on the specific components of the loss leading to emotional behavioral and cognitive symptoms and how to deal with these; the latter pertain to how one must interact constructively with social/environmental systems in order to maintain adaptive function in social, vocational, and avocational activities. Grief "tasks" usually have included confronting the loss, restructuring thoughts and memories about the deceased person, and emotionally withdrawing from (but not forgetting) the deceased person. Restoration tasks include accepting the changed world, spending time away from grieving, and developing new relationships and identities. Stroebe and Schut (1999) argued that alternation or "oscillation" in dealing with these two types of stressors is critical in the adjustment process. Psychological mechanisms that help the individual avoid or minimize the massive impact of the loss are helpful in the adjustment process, provided that they are not persistently implemented and are not the only coping efforts employed. Periodically engaging in restoration coping tasks serves to interrupt the process of coping with the loss, and this may in turn facilitate a gradual habituation to the loss. Balance in dealing with the two types of stressors as a result of oscillation thus precludes the preoccupation with one or the other that may lead to prolonged and complicated bereavement.

Cultural Variations in Bereavement Responses

Culture plays an important role in reactions to loss, the course of grieving, and outcomes of bereavement (Brown and Stoudemire 1983; Klass 1996; Wisocki and Skowron 2000). The manifestations, duration, and intensity of grief are likely to be culturally specific, and substantial individual and subcultural variations exist. From the literature describing cross-cultural and ethnic expressions after a death, it is clear that bereavement distress can be communicated and regulated through various pathways. Some theorists challenge the concept that grief is a universal emotional reaction to bereavement; they view death, loss, and grief as social constructs and grief as a cultural artifact that is shaped by the sociocultural environment (Corwin 1995; Neimeyer 1998; Rosenblatt 1993). At present, most of the work on cultural differences in bereavement is descriptive (Wisocki and Skowron 2000). Empirical studies on whether and how older adults in minority groups experience or cope with bereavement differently from European Americans are virtually nonexistent. Most studies of cultural differences appear to focus exclusively on customs, rituals, and perceptions relating to appropriate expressions and behaviors concerning the death of a family member. It is not clear how these customs, rituals, and perceptions, which are considerably different from those in Anglo-Christian traditions, may regulate emotions and facilitate adaptive coping. Nevertheless, Romanoff and Terenzio (1998) suggested that rituals and funerals are a "condensed version of private, emotionally charged material" (p. 698) that enables emotions to be channeled and expressed and bereaved persons to transition from one social role to another.

Older adults living in the pluralistic culture of the United States who have retained at least some aspects of their original culture of heritage are of particular interest. When a cultural or ethnic minority group migrates to a majority culture, some of the group's practices, values, and customs are expected to change, reflecting adaptation to the host culture. In the United States, the proportion of older adults of non-European ancestry is steadily increasing. The Latino population is the fastest-growing ethnic/racial minority and is anticipated to be the largest minority in the 65+ age group by the year 2028 (Administration on Aging 2003). The proportion of Asian Americans in late life is also anticipated to grow in the coming years. Because reactions to death and the perceived meaning of death are likely to be different among different ethnic and cultural groups, cultural influences on bereavement should not be underestimated. Researchers and clinicians alike should familiarize themselves with bereavement practices, common perceptions of death, and what behaviors characterize psychopathology for different cultural groups that they may interact with in their professional work. Braun and Nichols (1997) emphasize that professionals should inquire about 1) cultural traditions for expressing psychological pain resulting from death, 2) rituals and practices associated with mourning, 3) cultural beliefs about the continuing relationship between the deceased and the bereaved, and 4) the potential effects of cultural beliefs and traditions on the eventual outcome of bereavement.

Grief Work Across Cultures

The concept of working through one's grief (Bowlby 1980; Freud 1917 [1915]/1957; Lindemann 1944) or performing grief tasks (Worden 2002) may not be equally applicable to all cultures. The approach also lacks empirical support for its effectiveness in dealing with loss. Euro-American culture has generally conceptualized grief as more loss oriented (Stroebe and Schut's [1999] dual-process model), and the focus has often been on individual manifestations of grief. In contrast, grief in other cultures may be associated with culturally sanctioned rituals, expressions, and meanings that are shared within relationships. Cultural belief systems typically have a major impact on the behavioral and emotional expression of grief as well as customary coping strategies used to cope with the ensuing stressors. For example, in mainstream America, death often signifies a time to terminate the relationship with the deceased, and culturally appropriate ways of expressing this loss occur both publicly and privately (Shuchter and Zisook 1988). However, in other cultures, the norm may be to engage in rituals that signify a continuation of the relationship with the deceased family member, such as ancestor rituals like *sosen suhai* that are practiced in Japan (Goss and Klass 1997). Outward emotional expressions of grief have been shown to be effective in helping bereaved individuals adjust in the mainstream culture (Mawson et al. 1981), but other cultures may view such expressions differently. For example, Tibetans believe that crying for the deceased person hinders that person's liberation or rebirth, and they believe that emotions should be channeled into spiritual practices for the deceased individual. Similarly, Buddhists often discourage open and intense statement of emotions (Goss and Klass 1997). Among the Navajo, excessive expression of emotions is not permitted (Miller and Schoenfeld 1973), and crying is considered inappropriate by some Indonesian Muslims (Wikan 1988). Sometimes denial of death is culturally appropriate (al-Adawi et al. 1997). Moreover, denial may lessen the anxiety associated with the enormous task of accepting the reality of loss and may be beneficial to the bereaved person (Janof-Bulman and Timko 1987; Stroebe 1992–1993). In fact, the concept of working through grief is foreign in many non-Western cultures, such as the Samoan culture (Ablon 1971), and a continuous relationship and continuous communication with the deceased individual are encouraged (al-Issa 1995).

Social Support

Research has shown that perceived social support is vital to maintaining life satisfaction and reducing the risk of depression among elderly persons (Kogan et al. 1995; Newsom and Schulz 1996). Cultures with extensive familial networking and familial support often have well-established mourning practices that involve the entire extended family rather than just the individual most directly affected by the loss. In some cultural traditions this shared grief response can even extend to the community, as for example in recent Mexican immigrants (Block 1998) and in the Rauto culture in Australia (Wisocki and Skowron 2000). In situations in which it appears that this tradition may have been dropped, possibly as a result of acculturation after immigration, interventions to increase familial involvement so that grieving becomes more of a collaborative process for all family members may minimize the onset of a complicated bereavement process (Nadeau 2001).

In one of the early multicultural studies done in the United States, Kalish and Reynolds (1981) found that African Americans had more exposure to persons who died violently (e.g., in accidents, homicides, or wars) than did Caucasian, Hispanic, and Japanese adults. Eisenbruch (1984) surmised that because blacks were less likely to die of old age than through violence, their belief systems, attachment patterns, and grief reactions might change so that the pain of separation through death could be better managed. As a consequence, African Americans may not seek help from health professionals to deal with their grief but may instead rely more on informal supports, such as their religion and church-based relationships. For example, being able to summon emotional support from church members has been regarded as particularly helpful to African Americans during grieving (Rosenblatt 1993).

Japanese ancestor rituals, through which living persons are thought to be able to interact continually with the spirit of the deceased person (Klass 1996), are perhaps the most frequently documented culture-specific bereavement response among Asian groups. Similarly, for Chinese who follow the Taoist tradition, the deceased elderly individual is regarded as an ancestor who can bestow blessings on the surviving spouse and on younger generations. The deceased person's ashes (which are kept in an urn) and a photo of him or her are often placed on an altar at home. Incense is burned twice a day as a symbol of reverence, and food is offered on the altar to the deceased person. Among Chinese who ascribe to more traditional values, it is generally not acceptable to openly discuss either death or plans for death (Bowman and Singer 2001; Crain 1996), and grief is shared only within the family (Braun and Nichols 1997). This value appears to be played out in the effects of social support on bereavement. A study of elders residing in Wuhan, China, found that support by friends had little impact on depressive symptoms following the death of a spouse, whereas family support had a buffering effect (Li et al. 2005). It may therefore be difficult for health professionals to detect bereavement-related psychological problems in elderly Chinese persons, who may seem avoidant and appear to be somatizing. However, other groups may express bereavement-related emotions more freely and explicitly. Younoszai (1993) observed that most Mexicans perceive death as part of life, and the funeral, which everyone connected with the deceased is expected to attend and which is typically organized according to orthodox Catholic practices, is a social event that brings the extended family together. Similarly, Block (1998) noted as a physician that Latinos, particularly first and second generations, value familial input when making treatment decisions, possess extensive social networks, place family interests before interests of the self, more readily accept death as unavoidable, and prefer a caring, personal approach to a scientific, matter-of-fact approach in the treatment process.

In summary, grief clearly is expressed in a variety of ways in different ethnic and cultural groups, and bereavement distress can be communicated and regulated through various pathways. A clear understanding of culturally specific traditions for expressing grief and for successfully coping with the stressors associated with bereavement is an important component of providing helpful assistance to individuals from other cultures. Indeed, successful interventions with culturally diverse individuals require a knowledge of the nuances of each individual's unique history as well as consideration of the larger contexts of both the individual's culture of origin and of the mainstream to which the individual is acculturating.

Operational Definitions of "Normal" and "Abnormal" Grief

Given the wide variability in how people proceed through the grief process, how can one determine what is "normal" and what is not? The lines between abnormal or complicated grief, major depression, and a healthy grief process are not always clear (Shear and Shair 2005; Shuchter and Zisook 1993; Silverman et al. 2000).

DSM-IV-TR Definitions

In DSM-IV-TR (American Psychiatric Association 2000a), bereavement is in the V Code section, meaning it is a condition that may be the focus of attention or treatment but is not directly attributable to a psychiatric disorder. *Uncomplicated bereavement* is defined in DSM-IV-TR as follows:

> This category can be used when the focus of clinical attention is a reaction to the death of a loved one. As part of their reaction to the loss, some grieving individuals present with symptoms characteristic of a Major Depressive Episode (e.g., feelings of sadness and associated symptoms such as insomnia, poor appetite, and weight loss). The bereaved individual typically regards the depressed mood as "normal," although the person may seek professional help for relief of associated symptoms such as insomnia or anorexia. The duration and expression of "normal" bereavement vary considerably among different cultural groups. (American Psychiatric Association 2000a, pp. 740–741)

Differentiating between normal and complicated bereavement has not always been easy. DSM-IV-TR identifies several atypical symptoms that are not associated with a normal course of bereavement:

> 1) guilt about things other than actions taken or not taken by the survivor at the time of the death; 2) thoughts of death other than the survivor feeling that he or she would be better off dead or should have died with the deceased person; 3) morbid preoccupation with worthlessness; 4) marked psychomotor retardation; 5) prolonged and marked functional impairment; and 6) hallucinatory experiences other than thinking that he or she hears the voice of, or

transiently sees the image of, the deceased person. (American Psychiatric Association 2000a, p. 741)

These symptoms may be indicative of a *complicated bereavement,* as discussed in the following section.

Definitional Problems and Issues

Differential diagnostic criteria for normal and abnormal grief, depression, and other stress disorders remain controversial at the present time. For abnormal grief, Horowitz et al. (1997) emphasized the importance of both *intrusive symptoms* and signs of *avoidance and failure to adapt.* Intrusive symptoms include unbidden memories, strong spells of severe emotion related to the lost relationship, and distressingly strong yearnings for the deceased. Signs of avoidance and poor adjustment are characterized by feelings of emptiness or of being very much alone; avoidance of people, places, or activities that remind one of the deceased person; unusual levels of sleep disturbance; and loss of interest and decreased engagement in social, occupational, or recreational activities. Evidence of these signs and symptoms must be present for 14 months after the loss. Similarly, Prigerson and colleagues (Jacobs et al. 2000; Prigerson et al. 1999) have defined a category of "traumatic grief." Primary symptoms include yearning and searching for the deceased person, loneliness, and intrusive thoughts about the deceased person. These are accompanied by traumatic distress that includes purposelessness; numbness or detachment; disbelief; feelings of meaninglessness; loss of a sense of trust, security, or control; and excessive irritability, bitterness, or anger related to the death. Prigerson et al. (1999) do not include symptoms of avoidance and require that the symptoms only need to be present for a period of 2 months.

Although no consensus is yet apparent, the groundwork is being laid for specific criteria to distinguish normal and abnormal (i.e., complicated or traumatic) grief reactions. Continued research is indicated to help refine and solidify what cognitive, affective, and behavioral features characterize these two forms. As data are accumulated, theories and therapies will continue to be modified. For example, as noted earlier, it is becoming increasingly apparent that continued attachment often can be comforting (Field et al. 1999; Wortman and Silver 1987). Variations in grief practices across cultures have also emphasized the impact that cultural traditions and beliefs can have on bereavement practices and have widened the scope of what can be termed as "normal" grief reactions. Thus, one might wonder if it is necessary to minimize one's attachment to a deceased individual in order to resolve one's grief, or if grief resolution itself should be the goal. Other issues include what constitutes a reasonable time period for a "normal" grief reaction and what constitute the indisputable signs of abnormal bereavement patterns predictive of poor adjustment. Until such time as these issues are resolved, the best the clinician can do is to use currently available guidelines, as noted in this chapter, to help evaluate the individual patient.

There is consensus that normal grief is not equivalent to the clinical syndrome of major depression, which should be considered as a possible sequelae of major loss. Results of our own psychometric work in this regard—in which common self-report questionnaires were used to assess both depression and level of grief—generally support this position (Breckenridge et al. 1986; Gallagher-Thompson et al. 1982).

Adaptation to Late-Life Bereavement

Results from several longitudinal studies are consistent in their descriptions of the course of depressed mood, anxiety, well-being, and level of grief following a loss. Generally significant differences between bereaved and nonbereaved individuals are readily apparent during the first 6 months after the loss. However, at approximately 12 months postloss, levels of reported distress in the bereaved are substantially reduced, and often the difference between bereaved and nonbereaved control subjects may be difficult to detect (Harlow et al. 1991; Lund et al. 1989; Thompson et al. 1991). Although considerable recovery has occurred, however, many symptoms are still present (Harlow et al. 1991; Thompson et al. 1984).

A study by Bonnano et al. (2002) examined patterns of depression and recovery after loss based on data collected as a part of the Changing Lives of Older Couples study. Prospective data reflecting level of depression, grief, and psychosocial functioning were obtained from 205 older adults several years prior to the death of their spouse and again at 6 and 18 months after the loss. Five patterns of adjustment were identified based on pre- and postloss levels of adjustment. Those patterns included chronic grief (good adjustment preloss followed by chronic poor adjustment), chronic depression (poor adjustment at all three time points), depression followed by improvement (poor adjustment preloss, with improvement at either 6 or 18 months), common/normal grief (good preloss functioning with a decline at 6 months and subsequent improvement at 18 months), and resilience (good adjustment at all three time points).

The unique inclusion of preloss data enabled Bonanno and colleagues to distinguish postloss chronic grief reactions from chronic depression. Chronic grievers could be distinguished from others by elevated depression and grief symptoms at 6 months after the loss, suggesting that assessment at this point may be especially useful in identifying individuals at high risk for chronic grief. Despite the label of "common/normal" grief for a pattern of lowered adjustment at 6 months postloss followed by recovery, the most frequent pattern of bereavement in their sample (45%) was of stable, low-level depression over time, which they characterized as a *resilient* pattern. Contrary to theoretical perspectives associating "inhibited" grief with poor attachment to the spouse or to a cold or distant interpersonal style, the resilient group was found not to differ from common or chronic grief groups in either relationship quality or interviewer ratings of interpersonal skill or warmth. Follow-up analyses demonstrated that the resilient group reported the most comfort from positive memories of their spouse and the least search for meaning in the death (Bonanno et al. 2004). Little evidence for a delayed grief reaction was found. These results have been pivotal in recommending that initiating "grief work" with those who experience the resilient pattern may not be necessary and may even be counterproductive. These data offer strong support to earlier descriptive work emphasizing that most older individuals who lose their spouse are able to make a satisfactory adjustment over time without the need for professional intervention (Bonnano and Kaltman 2001; Thompson et al. 1991).

One notable exception to these results regarding psychological distress concerns the level of grief reported by the bereaved individual over time. Thompson et al. (1991) reported that elderly men and women had higher mean scores for experienced grief than the normative scores on the Texas Inventory of Grief—Revised (Faschingbauer 1981). These scores were elevated throughout the 30-month period of the study. Furthermore, there were no gender differences on this measure at any time point postloss, which is contrary to the results on other measures of psychological distress. These findings suggest that grief can be distinguished from depression and related symptoms using brief self-report questionnaires and that the latter will abate considerably over time, particularly by 6 months postloss, whereas the former may remain higher than in individuals who are not currently undergoing bereavement, even though they are not reporting other symptoms of distress. The data suggest that prolonged elevated grief may be considered normal for older bereaved adults. This observation is in agreement with earlier work by Zisook and Shuchter (1985, 1986), who reported that a continuing sense of attachment was still quite strong even 4 years after the loss.

Risk Factors for Intensification of Grief

Grief has been characterized by many as not only a highly charged emotional state but also a significant risk factor for a wide range of negative outcomes, including mortality and major physical and mental health disturbances. On the other hand, some clinicians and researchers have been struck by the ability of many older adults to survive and cope quite well overall with the profound losses of old age. Zisook et al. (1993) found that their oldest subjects showed the most consistent improvement in distress levels over time. In contrast, Sable (1991), among others, found that older widows were more distressed throughout the first 3 years of bereavement than were their younger counterparts. In their 10-year follow-up study of a national sample of bereaved men and women, McÇrae and Costa (1993) found that the great majority of individuals showed considerable ability to adapt to this major life stress (although length of recovery seemed to vary considerably). Nevertheless, an attempt to identify elders at risk for negative outcomes after spousal loss is an important mental health objective (for a thorough review, see Sanders 1993 and Stroebe et al. 2001a). Variables often associated with prolonged or complicated bereavement include 1) age and gender of the survivor, 2) the mode of death, 3) presence of significant depression shortly after the death, 4) self-esteem and perceived coping, 5) prior relationship satisfaction, and 6) social support. Strength of religious commitment and involvement, participation in culturally appropriate mourning rituals, and redistribution of roles within the family after the death may also affect the grief process, although these findings are not as robust.

Gender differences in bereavement are complex. Stroebe et al. (2001b) concluded that "widowers are indeed at relatively higher risk [of death] than widows, and, given that death is the most extreme consequence of bereavement, much weight may be attached to this finding" (p. 69). Bowling (1988–1989) followed up with 500 elderly widows and widowers for 6 years after their loss and found that men age 75 or older had excessive mortality compared with men of the same age in the general population. Bowling also found that low social contact predicted mortality. Gallagher-Thompson et al. (1993) found that widowers who died within the first year of spousal bereavement had reported more often than survivors that their wives were their main confidants and that they had minimal involvement in activities with other persons after their wives' deaths. The differential psychological impact of bereavement on men and women also appears unbalanced. Several studies have found a greater impact of bereavement on depression scores in men than women (van Grootheest et al. 1999; Williams 2003) or that men may begin to experience greater depression before the loss of their wives, which is maintained in bereavement (Lee and DeMaris 2007). Women have been found to have less life satisfaction than men following the loss of a spouse (Lichtenstein et al. 1996; Williams 2003) but may also experience more personal growth after the loss (Carr 2004). Referring to their "dual process" model, Stroebe et al. (2001b) hypothesized that women are more focused on psychological aspects of coping with the loss, whereas men are more focused on restoring their life pattern without the loved one. However, societal and structural demands prompt flexible coping in women (e.g., in addition to loss-focused coping, women must adjust to new financial and domestic circumstances), whereas less pressure exists for men to engage with their nonpreferred coping focus. Further research is needed to determine whether less flexibility in coping focus mediates the relationship between gender and psychological outcomes.

Violent, stigmatized (as in the case of AIDS), or unexpected deaths generally are associated with poorer adaptation (O'Neil 1989; Osterweis et al. 1984; Parkes and Weiss 1983; Worden 2002). Farberow et al. (1987) compared older adults whose spouses had died of natural causes with older adults whose spouses had committed suicide and found that the effect of the suicide on the survivor was not notably different from the effects of other modes of death during the early period of bereavement. However, the expected decline in level of depression and other symptoms by the end of 1 year did not occur in those grieving the loss of a loved one by suicide. Both types of survivors seemed to manage their new roles and responsibilities adequately by 30 months postloss. Individuals in the suicide group who had high initial levels of depression were more likely to maintain their depression, whereas this pattern, although evident, was not as severe in the nonsuicide bereaved group.

Similar studies involving elders whose spouses (or other family members) were homicide victims are rare, nor has much research been done on the effect of stigmatized deaths and/or very sudden deaths. In a study examining 552 widows ages 18–74, Kitson (2000) found that, similar to the findings of Farberow et al. (1987), violent deaths (including homicide and suicide) were not associated with greater distress than natural death early in bereavement (5–6 months postloss). Within the oldest third of the sample (ages 51–74), she did find limited evidence for greater distress after homicide than suicide, which she attributed to the relative rarity of homicide in this age range. Across the age range, Kitson found greater distress in women whose husbands died of long-term illness as opposed to unexpected causes. This result contrasts that of Burton et al. (2006), who found an association between unexpected death and depression in older adults both 6 and 18 months postloss. Further research is necessary to determine the long-term course of symptoms after the violent or unexpected death of a loved one.

One potentially important factor in successful coping with a loss, especially a traumatic one, is one's ability to find meaning in the experience. Indeed, 70%–80% of bereaved individuals report seeking sense or meaning in their loss (Neimeyer 2000). Neimeyer (2000) emphasized the importance of how a bereaved person interprets and integrates the loss into his or her personal narrative. Frequent interactions with significant others help to refine and reinforce one's sense of self, and the loss of that feedback due to the death of a loved one can leave the bereaved individual feeling as though the "plot" of their daily lives is disorganized and undefined (Neimeyer et al. 2002). Bereaved individuals who report that they are able to make sense of a loss report better adjustment in the first year after the loss, and the ability to see the benefit in a loss (e.g., through making them a stronger person or through a greater valuing of friends and family) is associated with better adjustment later in the bereavement process (Davis et al. 1998). Although a search for meaning is not a necessary factor for good adjustment following a loss (Davis et al. 2000), the inability to resolve meaning can be a risk factor for poor outcome.

Clinically significant symptoms of depression within the first 2 months postloss is a significant risk factor for poor outcome over time. Lund et al. (1993) found that intense negative emotions at 2 months postloss—such as a desire to die and frequent crying—were associated with poor coping 2 years later. Wortman and Silver (1989) reviewed a number of studies indicating that depression confounds successful resolution of grief. In studies where participants are initially identified by the loss of a spouse with only retrospective information on preloss functioning, it is difficult to determine whether early symptoms of depression were specifically caused by the loss or are the continuation/augmentation of a preloss depression. Both early loss and preloss depression may play a significant role in adjustment. The prospective study by Bonanno et al. (2002) discussed earlier in the chapter found that individuals in the depressed-improved group still showed higher levels of depression than the resilient group at 18 months postloss. In addition, it appears that a higher proportion of individuals with preloss depression remained depressed at 18 months postloss (43%) than those without depression preloss (21%, based on Bonanno et al. 2002). In our own work investigating the relationship between depression and later bereavement outcome (Gilewski et al. 1991), we found that individuals with self-reported depression in the moderate to severe range were at greatest risk for all other psychopathological symptoms, such as increased anxiety, hostility, interpersonal sensitivity, and other indices of global psychiatric distress. This result occurred whether their spouses had committed suicide or died of natural causes. However, subjects whose spouses had committed suicide and who were moderately to severely depressed at the outset had the highest mean score of any subgroup on the depression measure that was used, maintained higher mean levels of depression over time, and were more likely to score high on other distress measures. These data suggest that, again, the interaction of one or more risk factors may contribute to the greatest distress.

Several articles have suggested that bereaved elderly individuals with poor self-esteem and/or inadequate coping skills are at a greater risk for difficult bereavement. Johnson et al. (1986) conducted one of the few studies that directly addressed these variables in elders. As expected, individuals who, early in bereavement, reported themselves to be high in self-esteem and to be effective copers maintained a high self-esteem and remained effective copers throughout the first year of bereavement, whereas those who initially reported high stress levels generally had high levels of stress at subsequent times of measurement. Likewise, Bonanno et al. (2002) found that among those with preloss depression, greater perceived coping skills predicted remittance of depression 18 months postloss. However, perceived coping skills did not appear to affect later depression in those who were not already distressed at the time of loss.

Although often discussed, the effects of preloss relationship satisfaction as a risk factor remain unclear (Parkes and Weiss 1983; Worden 2002). Futterman et al. (1990) found that more positive ratings of marital satisfaction were made by bereaved subjects than by nonbereaved, currently married control subjects. More positive ratings of satisfaction were associated with more severe depression initially, but this relationship was lower at 30 months postloss. The nature of this relationship was not influenced by gender but clearly was affected by level of neuroticism in the bereaved (Itzhar-Nabarro 2004). Older individuals who scored high on the Neuroticism scale of the 16PF (Cattell et al. 1969) reported high levels of depressive symptoms that remained elevated over a 2-year period regardless of marital satisfaction. Individuals who scored low on the scale and also reported high marital satisfaction were high on depression initially but then declined over time, whereas those who were low on the Neuroticism scale and low on marital satisfaction had fewer depressive symptoms initially. These data emphasize that personality factors interact with other risk factors in predicting both short- and long-range adjustment patterns. Bonanno et al. (2002) found that poor relationship quality rated preloss was most strongly associated with either a pattern of preloss depression followed by an improvement in symptoms postloss or chronic depression beginning preloss and continuing throughout bereavement. Follow-up analyses did find increased idealization of the relationship in bereaved individuals, but the degree of idealization did not differ based on level of adjustment (Bonanno et al. 2004). Thus, relationship satisfaction may interact with several other variables, including general psychological health and a change in perspective on the relationship over the course of the bereavement process. Clearly, more research is needed in this area.

The role of social support is less ambiguous overall. Since the publication of Cobb's (1976) seminal paper on the stress-buffering effects of social support, it has been widely recognized as a moderator of many kinds of life stress. In a comprehensive review of the role of social support in mitigating the effects of bereavement, Stylianos and Vachon (1993) made the point that social support should be viewed as a multidimensional process, including such aspects as the size, structure, and quality of the network; types of support provided (and by whom); and the appraisal of the support. Most studies have focused on only one aspect of support, although there is no single aspect that has been most frequently selected for study. With regard to late-life spousal bereavement, Dimond et al. (1987) found in their longitudinal study that the total size of the reported support network at baseline was positively correlated with perceived coping skills and life satisfaction at later times of measurement. They also found that the quality of the network was inversely related to later depression and was positively correlated with later measures of life satisfaction. Finally, through a series of multiple regression analyses, they found that several baseline social network factors made independent contributions to the variance accounted for in predicting depression at later times of measurement. This finding suggests that social support mitigates severe negative reactions to the loss of a spouse in older individuals.

Our own research involving individuals whose spouses had died of natural causes and those whose spouses had committed suicide also confirms and supports this position. In a series of analyses directly comparing these two groups, Farberow et al. (1992a, 1992b) found that persons whose spouses committed suicide received significantly less emotional and practical support for their feelings of depression and grief than did persons whose spouses died of natural causes. This was particularly true about 6 months postloss. Also, individuals whose spouses committed suicide did not feel that they could confide in members of their network any more than did the nonbereaved comparison group. Gender differences were also noted: the bereaved women in both groups reported that they received more support overall compared with either group of bereaved men. The most common sources of support were other family members (particularly adult children), followed by friends and then siblings. Another significant difference concerned how social supports changed over time. The survivors of spouses who had natural deaths reported keeping roughly the same levels of feelings for the people in their network, whereas the feelings of the persons (especially men) whose spouses committed suicide fluctuated considerably over the 30 months. However, by the end point, both practical and emotional supports had increased among individuals whose spouses committed suicide and were more comparable with the levels reported by individuals whose spouses died of natural causes.

On the basis of these data it is apparent that several risk factors are associated with a more difficult subsequent grief process in elderly individuals. It is noteworthy, however, that the available research was conducted using volunteer subjects typically with higher educational levels and often from higher socioeconomic levels. Furthermore, the response rate from this segment of our population tends to be extremely low (around 30%–40%), which clearly limits the generality of these findings. Greater efforts should be made to engage elderly persons who are economically disadvantaged, in poor health, with low social support systems and low community involvement. In addition, more studies are needed on the interactive effect of several of these risk factors (particularly because they may change over time in relative intensity or salience to the individual) as well as on whether the same risk factors apply to bereavement due to other causes, such as divorce and death of a parent or an adult child. Clearly, more research is needed on risk factors among ethnically and culturally diverse elders as well.

Interventions for Late-Life Bereavement

To our knowledge, formal guidelines for interventions in patients with late-life bereavement have not yet been established. However, there is an abundance of clinical comments throughout the bereavement literature indicating that treatment can be immensely helpful to some individuals. The extent to which a treatment might be effective depends in large measure on the intensity and pattern of symptoms present. In some situations it appears that intervention above the usual family and community support is not called for and indeed may even be counterproductive. In others, medication, psychotherapy, or a combination of the two would be advised. Decisions regarding treatment strategy are facilitated by knowing whether the symptom pattern is consistent with what would be termed a "normal grief reaction" for the particular cultural group with which the person is identified, or if it appears that the severity, type of symptoms present, and/or risk factor profile suggests a complicated course. In particular, it is important to determine whether the symptom picture is consistent with the diagnostic criteria for some other psychiatric disorder, such as depression. This distinction is critical for making appropriate intervention choices (Raphael et al. 2001). Although the literature is not conclusive on diagnostic issues, the distinction between complicated and normal bereavement is often made, and given this, it seems reasonable to review treatments that have been used for individuals in one or the other of these categories.

Treatment of Complicated Bereavement

A thorough assessment of any comorbid psychological conditions should be conducted before beginning treatment for bereavement. This is especially important for conditions with similar symptoms to bereavement, such as depression. Clinical levels of depression should be treated with medication and/or psychotherapy before the focus of treatment can effectively shift to bereavement (National Institutes of Health Consensus Conference 1992; Parkes and Weiss 1983; Raphael et al. 2001; Reynolds 1992). Reynolds (1992) stated, "Our clinical practice has been to intervene as early as 2 months, and certainly by 4 months, in the presence of clear syndromal major depression" (p. 50). Remission will enable the focus of treatment to return to the bereavement. Careful attention to the grief process can often then determine whether additional interventions are required. In particular, risk factors may become an important focus for remediation. For example, there is considerable evidence now to indicate that older widowers may not thrive if they do not have a constructive support system. Isolation is a documented risk factor, and men undergoing stress may not have the requisite skills to build or implement a nourishing social network. It may become necessary to provide specific assistance with this problem. Once accomplished, other interventions may not be necessary.

Other common complications that are particularly significant in older bereaved persons (Rosenzweig et al. 1997) and that require treatment include posttraumatic stress disorder, anxiety disorders (that may or may not be related to the bereavement), and subsyndromal depression (Reynolds et al. 1999; Schut et al. 1997). A combination of medication and psychotherapy appears to be more effective than either alone when attempting to reduce psychiatric symptoms that occur with bereavement. For example, the late-life depression research group at the Western Psychiatric Institute tested the efficacy of nortriptyline therapy, interpersonal psychotherapy, and combined treatment in elderly patients with bereavement-related major depression and reported that combined treatment was superior to either intervention alone, particularly among patients age 70 or older (Miller et al. 1997; Reynolds et al. 1999).

In some instances older persons either cannot or refuse to use psychotropic medications. Although recent data have suggested that "counseling" of various kinds may not be all that helpful with individuals undergoing a normal grief reaction, there is evidence that various psychological treatments can have a positive effect in treating complicated bereavement (Neimeyer 2000). Both individual and group psychotherapies reflecting different theoretical perspectives have been used in treating complicated bereavement with mixed results (Raphael et al. 1993; Schut et al. 2001).

One of the more common psychodynamic therapies used with complicated bereavement is Horowitz's (1976) time-limited psychodynamic therapy. This 12-session phase-oriented strategy is designed to help individuals work through emotional reactions to traumatic life events. Careful attention is also paid to tailor treatment to the patient's particular personality type. Abreaction, clarification, and interpretation of defenses and affects are used to facilitate realistic appraisals of the implications of a death and to explore the effect of the loss of a relationship on the bereaved person's self-concept. Empirical data demonstrating its effectiveness are available (Horowitz et al. 1981, 1984; Marmar et al. 1988; Windholz et al. 1985).

Guided mourning is a brief, intensive, structured behavioral program that is helpful in the resolution of chronic grief (Mawson et al. 1981). The effectiveness of this approach has been replicated by Sireling et al. (1988). Ninety-minute sessions are held three times weekly for 2 weeks, with subsequent less intense follow-up for 28 weeks. The treatment is designed to help bereaved individuals repeatedly confront aspects of their loss in order to eventually diminish their negative effects through habituation.

Cognitive and cognitive-behavioral therapies of various forms have been used to treat patients with complex bereavement reactions. One such strategy focuses on core constructs known to be disrupted during intense grief (Viney 1990). As these disrupted constructs are identified through self-monitoring and Socratic questioning during treatment sessions, the client learns methods of reconstructing shattered beliefs about the self, the present surroundings, and future events. A blend of cognitive and behavioral techniques (such as challenging dysfunctional thoughts and teaching specific behavioral skills for use in resolving interpersonal problems) has been applied successfully with individual patients (see Florsheim and Gallagher-Thompson [1990] for an example). Abrahms (1981) developed a conceptual model for illustrating cognitive and behavioral strategies with this population. Detailed case studies can be helpful in understanding and applying this model with bereaved clients (Gantz et al. 1992; Kaplan and Gallagher-Thompson 1995).

Researchers at the Western Psychiatric Institute in Pittsburgh, Pennsylvania (Frank et al. 1997; Shear et al. 2001, 2005), developed a treatment for complicated grief that involves principles similar to those featured in the treatment of posttraumatic stress disorder. The treatment for complicated grief included a series of cognitive-behavioral techniques such as imaginal exposure to the death scene; in vivo, graded exposure to avoided death-related circumstances; mindful breathing; reminiscence of positive and negative memories of the loved one; and writing goodbye letters to the deceased person. Also integral to the treatment were homework assignments involving listening to tapes of imaginal exposure. Following the dual-process model, the treatment also involved motivational enhancement and goal setting to facilitate restorative goals. The results of this treatment were encouraging: complicated grief, anxiety, and depressive symptoms were significantly reduced. In a randomized, controlled trial, individuals undergoing complicated grief treatment showed a greater response than those undergoing interpersonal psychotherapy (Shear et al. 2005).

In a recent revision, Worden (2002) outlined various approaches that he developed for the treatment of normal grief and inhibited or unresolved grief. His methods focus on reviving memories of the deceased person, followed by generating a broad range of emotions possibly associated with these memories. He argued that this helps the person acknowledge and deal with ambivalent feelings, leading to an eventual emotional balance. He also engages patients in an exploration of the meaning of objects that link and maintain a relationship with the deceased. The intent is to help the bereaved individual acknowledge the finality of the loss and say a final goodbye. He also uses psychodrama and role playing at times to intensify the emotional experience. These methods can work within a variety of theoretical frameworks. However, there is little empirical evidence documenting efficacy of these techniques beyond clinical observations.

Prigerson and Jacobs (2001) suggested that for bereavement-related major depression, interventions should follow the practice guideline for depression (American Psychiatric Association 2000b), whereas for bereavement complications, use of selective serotonin reuptake inhibitors combined with cognitive-behavioral interventions is probably most effective. However, few empirical studies have focused on the efficacy of specific treatment programs. Open-label trials of bupropion (Zisook et al. 2001), nortriptyline (Pasternak et al. 1991), antidepressant treatment with either nortriptyline or sertraline (Oakley et al. 2002), and paroxetine (Zygmont et al. 1998) for bereavement-related major depression in older adults have shown promise. As Hensley (2006) noted in her review of medication treatments for bereavement-related depression, antidepressant medications appear to have a larger impact on depressive symptoms than on grief-specific symptoms.

Treatment of Normal Grief Reactions

There is a long history of formal and informal interventions for normal grief reactions, including self-help groups and individual and group counseling. Most bereaved persons (particularly elders) do not seek professional assistance for their grief. Self-help support groups for bereaved persons are often used by those who find the experience too painful and the loneliness overwhelming. Lieberman (1993) argued that the important restorative features in these groups are 1) a family-like atmosphere, 2) encouragement of intense emotional expression, and 3) encouragement in adopting an identity of as single person rather than a couple. Self-help groups specifically for bereaved individuals often are long term, and membership can persist long after the painful grief experiences are no longer evident. Careful review of the few available reports led Lieberman (1993) to the conclusion that such groups are widely used and often may be sufficient for meeting the psychosocial issues confronting persons working through uncomplicated bereavement. Despite conceptual and anecdotal support for the effectiveness of these programs, relatively little empirical support has been found. Several reviews have examined the literature on counseling for normal grief reactions and have concluded that these interventions by and large do not reduce grief or depressive symptoms above and beyond the effects of time, nor do they facilitate better adjustment postintervention (Genevro 2004; Jordan and Neimeyer 2003; Schut et al. 2001). In fact, individuals experiencing uncomplicated bereavement may experience an iatrogenic effect of treatment, appearing worse off at the end of the treatment than if they had not participated (Neimeyer 2000).

Furthermore, the use of medication for the treatment of uncomplicated grief (other than for specific symptoms such as insomnia) has been questioned. Many clinicians feel that medication, if used at all, should be minimal and brief. For example, Raphael et al. (2001) argued that if depression is not evident, then antidepressants should not be prescribed to reduce symptoms of grief. There are concerns that medication may impede recovery by masking the full experience of bereavement (Parkes 1972; Worden 2002) and that prescribing medication pathologizes a natural human process. Others believe that the provider should intervene sooner rather than later, given the tendency of depressive symptoms to persist throughout the first year of spousal bereavement (Reynolds 1992). It has been noted that there is limited empirical evidence that one must go through a difficult grieving process in order to resume one's life effectively (Bonanno et al. 2002; Regehr and Sussman 2004); therefore, it is argued that pharmacological (and other) treatments for pain and suffering should be available to those who request them (Wortman and Silver 1987). Further research is necessary to determine the optimum level of pharmacological intervention to both ease suffering and allow the natural process of bereavement to take its course.

Anticipatory Bereavement: Hospice and Palliative Care

Over the past decade, increasing research has been done on palliative care at the end of life and on hospice treatment approaches in the care of patients with terminal illnesses. Hospice and other end-of-life settings are becoming increasingly common in the care of many elderly patients facing terminal illnesses. In 1998, approximately 3,100 hospice programs in the United States provided care for close to 540,000 people (Hospice Foundation of America 2003). The level of satisfaction with the overall care received in hospice or other palliative care settings is generally high (Medigovich et al. 1999; Ng and von Gunten 1998; Nolen-Hoeksema et al. 2000; Voltz et al. 1997; Wilkinson et al. 1999), and continued proliferation of these settings is likely, given the aging of the population.

Because of the particular focus of hospice on the emotional, interpersonal, and spiritual effects of terminal illness on patients and their loved ones, psychosocial factors implicated in bereavement and anticipatory bereavement understandably are integrated into the counseling component of usual hospice care. Bereavement counseling in the hospice setting is recommended by leading hospice organizations, and it has become a standard component of the Medicare hospice benefit (Hospice Care 42 CFR § 418.88 [2001]). A recent survey of patients, family members, and physicians supports this action. Ninety percent or more of respondents believed that being free from anxiety, having someone who will listen, and saying goodbye to important people are critical to pre- and postloss adjustment and that the counseling component of hospice care should facilitate this process (Steinhauser et al. 2000). Although few empirical studies have been conducted on the effects of hospice or palliative care on bereavement outcomes when compared with more traditional types of care (Berch 1999; Clukey 1997; Franco 1996; Gilbar 1998; Kramer 1997; Quigley and Schatz 1999; Ragow-O'Brien et al. 2000; Seale and Kelly 1997; Thornton 1998), findings suggest that enrollment in hospice, particularly in cases of painful illness and death, has a positive effect on bereavement adjustment (Bradley et al. 2004; Ragow-O'Brien et al. 2000).

The increase in hospice and palliative care treatment settings has increased the interest in anticipatory grief experienced by family members of dying patients. Some studies have found that encouraging forewarning has a positive effect on the bereavement outcome (Kramer 1997; O'Bryant 1990–1991). Additionally, caregivers who feel they are unprepared for the loss are at increased risk for postloss complications (Herbert et al. 2006). Other studies, however, have suggested that anticipatory work focusing on the impending death of a loved one might have negative or no effect on outcome after bereavement (Clayton et al. 1973; Lindemann 1944; Ortiz et al. 1999). Reviews of this literature have led some authors to argue that contradictory findings are a result of different conceptual perspectives and consequent strategies for measuring anticipatory grief (Evans 1994; Fulton et al. 1996; Rando 2000; Siegel and Weinstein 1983; Sweeting and Gilhooly 1990). Rando (2000) coined the phrase "anticipatory mourning" in an attempt to reconcile differences, but agreement on the effects of anticipatory work is still lacking. Clearly, available findings and increased interest indicate that continued research in this area is welcomed and should lead to improved models for interventions during this critical time prior to the loved one's death (Chapman and Pepler 1998; Gilliland and Fleming 1998; Sanders et al. 1979, 1985).

Key Points

- *Bereavement* can refer to a person's reactions to any set of significant losses but typically refers to the loss of a loved one such as a spouse.
- Among persons age 65 and over, 45% of women and 15% of men have experienced the loss of a spouse.
- The *dual-process model* of bereavement outlined by Strobe and Schut focuses on the interplay of loss-oriented stressors and restoration-oriented stressors. These are stressors related to the loss of the presence of the loved one in a person's life (e.g., loneliness, loss of support) as well as stressors related to building a new life without the presence of the loved one (e.g., taking on roles previously performed by the spouse, changing one's identity from one of wife to widow). Bereaved persons oscillate in their focus on these two stressors, and this is thought to promote more healthy adjustment.
- Culture can play a key role in the expected course of grief and should be taken into account when assessing or designing interventions for complicated grief.
- Research by Bonnano and colleagues highlights different potential patterns of adaptation after the loss of a spouse. It is notable that the majority of individuals show resilience to or recovery from depressive symptoms within 18 months after the loss of a spouse. However, symptoms of grief such as missing the deceased person and engaging in fond remembrances of the lost loved one may continue indefinitely, even in individuals who show minimal depressive symptoms.
- Postloss adjustment among bereaved individuals can vary widely. Several risk factors are predictive of poor adjustment. These include male gender; loss through a violent, stigmatized, or unexpected death; the presence of significant depressive symptoms early in the loss; poor coping skills and low self-esteem; and poor breadth and quality of social support.
- Bereavement reactions can be categorized as "normal" or "complicated" grief. Most people experience "normal" grief, which can include the experience of sadness, loneliness, or longing for the deceased; experiencing the "presence" of the deceased; and/or disruptions in sleep and appetite. Although there is no single standard set of criteria for a diagnosis of complicated grief, typical definitions include an element of prolonged duration of symptoms, marked distress, and avoidance of or failure to adapt to new life roles.
- Several empirically validated treatments are available for complicated bereavement, including cognitive-behavioral therapy and a complicated-grief treatment based on the principles of treating posttraumatic stress disorder.
- Normal bereavement typically resolves without the need for treatment beyond targeted interventions for specific symptoms (e.g., disturbed sleep). In fact, some common interventions for normal bereavement have been found to lead to a worsening of symptoms and are not recommended.

References

Ablon J: Bereavement in a Samoan community. Br J Med Psychol 44:329–337, 1971

Abrahms JL: Depression versus normal grief following the death of a significant other, in New Directions in Cognitive Therapy. Edited by Emery G, Hollon S, Bedrosian RC. New York, Guilford, 1981, pp 255–270

Administration on Aging: Snapshot: a statistical profile of Hispanic older Americans aged 65+. 2003. Available at http://www.aoa.gov/press/prodsmats/fact/fact.aspx. Accessed July 18, 2008.

al-Adawi S, Burjorjee R, al-Issa I: Mu-Ghayeb: a culture-specific response to bereavement in Oman. Int J Soc Psychiatry 43:144–151, 1997

al-Issa I: The illusion of reality or the reality of illusion: hallucinations and culture. Br J Psychiatry 166:368–373, 1995

American Psychiatric Association: Diagnostic and Statistical Manual of Mental Disorders, 4th Edition, Text Revision. Washington, DC, American Psychiatric Association, 2000a

American Psychiatric Association: Practice Guideline for the Treatment of Patients With Major Depressive Disorder, 2nd Edition. Washington, DC, American Psychiatric Association, 2000b

Bass DM, Bowman K, Noelker LS: The influence of caregiving and bereavement support on adjusting to an older relative's death. Gerontologist 31:32–42, 1991

Berch DG: Group treatment in a hospice bereavement program (abstract). Dissertation Abstracts International. Section B, The Sciences and Engineering 60:1289, 1999

Bierhals AJ, Prigerson HG, Fasiczka A, et al: Gender differences in complicated grief among the elderly. Omega (Westport) 32:303–317, 1995

Block JB: The meaning of death, in Healing Latinos: The Art of Cultural Competence in Medicine. Edited by Hayes-Bautista D, Chiprut R. Los Angeles, CA, Cedars-Sinai Health System, 1998, pp 79–85

Bonanno GA, Kaltman S: The varieties of grief experiences. Clin Psychol Rev 21:705–734, 2001

Bonanno GA, Wortman CB, Lehman DR, et al: Resilience to loss and chronic grief: a prospective study from pre-loss to 18 months post-loss. J Pers Soc Psychol 83:1150–1164, 2002

Bonanno GA, Wortman CB, Nesse RM: Prospective patterns of resilience and maladjustment during widowhood. Psychol Aging 19:260–271, 2004

Bowlby J: Processes of mourning. Int J Psychoanal 42:317–340, 1961

Bowlby J: Attachment and Loss, Vol 3: Loss: Sadness and Depression. London, England, Hogarth, 1980

Bowling A: Who dies after widow(er)hood? a discriminant analysis. Omega (Westport) 19:135–153, 1988–1989

Bowman KW, Singer PA: Chinese seniors' perspectives on end-of-life decisions. Soc Sci Med 53:455–464, 2001

Bradley EH, Prigerson HG, Carlson MD: Depression among surviving caregivers: does length of hospice enrollment matter? Am J Psychiatry 161:2257–2262, 2004

Braun KL, Nichols R: Death and dying in four Asian American cultures: a descriptive study. Death Stud 21:327–359, 1997

Breckenridge J, Gallagher D, Thompson LW, et al: Characteristic depressive symptoms of bereaved elders. J Gerontol 41:163–168, 1986

Brown JT, Stoudemire GA: Normal and pathological grief. JAMA 250:378–383, 1983

Burton AM, Haley WE, Small BJ: Bereavement after caregiving or unexpected death: effects on elderly spouses. Aging Ment Health 10:319–326, 2006

Cain BS: Divorce among elderly women: a growing social phenomenon. Soc Casework 69:563–568, 1988

Carr D: Gender, preloss marital dependence, and older adults' adjustment to widowhood. J Marriage Fam 66:220–235, 2004

Cattell RB, Eber HW, Delhees KH: A large sample cross validation of the personality trait structure of the 16-PF with some clinical implications. Multivariate Behav Res 4 (special issue):107–131, 1969

Chapman KJ, Pepler C: Coping, hope, and anticipatory grief in family members in palliative home care. Cancer Nurs 21:226–234, 1998

Clayton P, Halikas J, Maurice W, et al: Anticipatory grief and widowhood. Br J Psychiatry 122:47–51, 1973

Clukey L: "Just be there!": the experience of anticipatory grief (abstract). Dissertation Abstracts International. Section B, The Sciences and Engineering 58:1208, 1997

Cobb S: Presidential Address—1996: Social support as a moderator of life stress. Psychosom Med 3:300–314, 1976

Corwin MD: Cultural issues in bereavement therapy: the social construction of mourning. In Session: Psychotherapy in Practice 1:23–41, 1995

Crain M: A cross-cultural study of beliefs, attitudes and values in Chinese-born American and non-Chinese frail homebound elderly. J Long Term Home Health Care 15:9–18, 1996

Davis CG, Nolen-Hoeksema S, Larson J: Making sense of loss and benefiting from the experience. J Pers Soc Psychol 75:561–574, 1998

Davis CG, Wortman CB, Lehman DR, et al: Searching for meaning in loss: are clinical assumptions correct? Death Stud 24:497–540, 2000

Dimond M, Lund DA, Caserta MS: The role of social support in the first two years of bereavement in an elderly sample. Gerontologist 27:599–604, 1987

Eisenbruch M: Cross-cultural aspects of bereavement, II: ethnic and cultural variations in the development of bereavement practices. Cult Med Psychiatry 8:315–347, 1984

Evans AJ: Anticipatory grief: a theoretical challenge. Palliat Med 8:159–165, 1994

Farberow NL, Gallagher DE, Gilewski MJ, et al: An examination of the early impact of bereavement on psychological distress in survivors of suicide. Gerontologist 27:592–598, 1987

Farberow NL, Gallagher-Thompson D, Gilewski M, et al: Changes in grief and mental health of bereaved spouses of older suicides. J Gerontol 47:P357–P366, 1992a

Farberow NL, Gallagher-Thompson D, Gilewski M, et al: The role of social supports in the bereavement process of surviving spouses of suicide and natural deaths. Suicide Life Threat Behav 22:107–124, 1992b

Faschingbauer TR: Texas Inventory of Grief—Revised Manual. Houston, TX, Honeycomb Publishing, 1981

Federal Interagency Forum on Aging Related Statistics: Older Americans 2000: Key Indicators of Well-Being. Washington, DC, Federal Interagency Forum on Aging Related Statistics, 2000

Field NP, Nichols C, Holen A, et al: The relation of continuing attachment to adjustment in conjugal bereavement. J Consult Clin Psychol 67:212–218, 1999

Field NP, Gal-Oz B, Bonanno GA: Continuing bonds and adjustment at 5 years after the death of a spouse. J Consult Clin Psychol 67:212–218, 2003

Florsheim M, Gallagher-Thompson D: Cognitive/behavioral treatment of atypical bereavement: a case study. Clin Gerontologist 10:73–76, 1990

Franco PC: The effect of caregiving during terminal illness on subsequent bereavement (abstract). Dissertation Abstracts International. Section B, The Sciences and Engineering 57:2219, 1996

Frank E, Prigerson HG, Shear MK, et al: Phenomenology and treatment of bereavement related distress in the elderly. Int Clin Psychopharmacol 12(suppl):S25–S29, 1997

Freud S: Mourning and melancholia (1917[1915]), in The Standard Edition of the Complete Psychological Works of Sigmund Freud, Vol 14. Translated and edited by Strachey J. London, Hogarth, 1957, pp 237–260

Fulton G, Madden C, Minichiello V: The social construction of anticipatory grief. Soc Sci Med 43:1349–1358, 1996

Futterman A, Gallagher D, Thompson LW, et al: Retrospective assessment of marital adjustment and depression during the first 2 years of spousal bereavement. Psychol Aging 5:277–283, 1990

Gallagher D, Breckenridge J, Dessonville C, et al: Similarities and differences between normal grief and depression in the elderly. Essence 5:127–140, 1982

Gallagher-Thompson D, Futterman A, Farberow N, et al: The impact of spousal bereavement on older widows and widowers, in Handbook of Bereavement. Edited by Stroebe MS, Stroebe W, Hansson R. Cambridge, United Kingdom, Cambridge University Press, 1993, pp 227–239

Gallagher-Thompson D, Dupart T, Liu W, et al: Assessment and treatment issues in bereavement in later life, in Handbook of Emotional Disorders in Later Life. Edited by Laidlaw K, Knight BG. New York, Oxford University Press, 2008, pp 287–307

Gantz F, Gallagher D, Rodman J: Cognitive/behavioral facilitation of inhibited grief, in Comprehensive Casebook of Cognitive Therapy. Edited by Freeman A, Dattilio F. New York, Plenum, 1992, pp 201–207

Genevro JL: Report on bereavement and grief research. Death Stud 28:491–575, 2004

Gilbar O: Length of cancer patients' stay at a hospice: does it affect psychological adjustment to the loss of the spouse? J Palliat Care 14:16–20, 1998

Gilewski MJ, Farberow NL, Gallagher DE, et al: Interaction of depression and bereavement on mental health in the elderly. Psychol Aging 6:67–75, 1991

Gilliland G, Fleming S: A comparison of spousal anticipatory grief and conventional grief. Death Stud 22:541–569, 1998

Glick IO, Weiss, RS, Parkes CM: The First Year of Bereavement. New York, Wiley, 1974

Goss RE, Klass D: Tibetan Buddhism and the resolution of grief: the Bardo-thodol for the dying and the grieving. Death Stud 21:377–395, 1997

Grimby A: Bereavement among elderly people: grief reactions, post-bereavement hallucinations, and quality of life. Acta Psychiatr Scand 87:72–80, 1993

Harlow SD, Goldberg EL, Comstock GW: A longitudinal study of the prevalence of depressive symptomatology in elderly widowed and married women. Arch Gen Psychiatry 48:1065–1068, 1991

Hensley PL: Treatment of bereavement-related depression and traumatic grief. J Affect Disord 92:117–124, 2006

Herbert RS, Dang Q, Schultz R: Preparedness for the death of a loved one and mental health in bereaved caregivers of dementia patients: findings from the REACH study. J Palliat Med 9:683–693, 2006

Horowitz MJ: Stress Response Syndromes. New York, Jason Aronson, 1976

Horowitz MJ, Wilner N, Marmar C, et al: Pathological grief and the activation of latent self-images. Am J Psychiatry 137:1157–1162, 1980

Horowitz MJ, Krupnick J, Kaltreider N, et al: Initial response to parental death. Arch Gen Psychiatry 38:316–323, 1981

Horowitz MJ, Weiss DS, Kaltreider N, et al: Reactions to the death of a parent: results from patients and field subjects. J Nerv Ment Dis 172:383–392, 1984

Horowitz MJ, Siegel B, Holen A, et al: Diagnostic criteria for complicated grief disorder. Am J Psychiatry 154:904–910, 1997

Hospice Care, 42 CFR § 418.88 (2001)

Hospice Foundation of America: What is hospice? Available at http://www.hospicefoundation.org/hospiceinfo. Accessed August 12, 2008.

Itzhar-Nabarro Z: The relationship between marital satisfaction and bereavement over 30-months period. Doctoral dissertation. Ann Arbor, MI, Proquest, 2004

Jacobs SC, Ostfeld AM: An epidemiological review of the mortality of bereavement. Psychosom Med 39:344–357, 1977

Jacobs SC, Mazure C, Prigerson H: Diagnostic criteria for traumatic grief. Death Stud 24:185–199, 2000

Janof-Bulman R, Timko C: Coping with traumatic life events: the role of denial in light of people's assumptive worlds, in Coping With Negative Life Events: Clinical and Social Psychological Perspectives. Edited by Snyder CR, Ford CE. New York, Plenum, 1987, pp 135–159

Johnson RJ, Lund DA, Dimond M: Stress, self-esteem, and coping during bereavement among the elderly. Soc Psychol Q 49:273–279, 1986

Jordan JR, Niemeyer RA: Does grief counseling work? Death Stud 27:765–786, 2003

Kalish RA: Older people and grief. Generations 11:33–38, 1987

Kalish RA, Reynolds DK: Death and Ethnicity: A Psychocultural Study. New York, Baywood Publishing, 1981

Kaplan C, Gallagher-Thompson D: The treatment of clinical depression in caregivers of spouses with dementia. Journal of Cognitive Psychotherapy 9:35–44, 1995

Kastenbaum RJ: Death, Society, and Human Experience, 2nd Edition. St. Louis, MO, CV Mosby, 1981

Kitson GC: Adjustment to violent and natural deaths in later and earlier life for black and white widows. J Gerontol B Psychol Sci Soc Sci 55:S341–S351, 2000

Klass D: Grief as an Eastern culture: Japanese ancestor worship, in Continuing Bonds: New Understandings of Grief (Series in Death Education, Aging, and Health Care, 0275–3510). Edited by Klass D, Silverman PR, Nickman SL. Washington, DC, Taylor and Francis, 1996, pp 59–70

Kogan ES, Van-Hasselt VB, Hersen M, et al: Relationship of depression, assertiveness, and social support in community-dwelling older adults. Journal of Clinical Geropsychology 1:157–163, 1995

Kramer D: How women relate to terminally ill husbands and their subsequent adjustment to bereavement. Omega (Westport) 34:93–106, 1997

Kübler-Ross E: On Death and Dying. New York, Simon & Schuster, 1969

Lee GR, DeMaris A: Widowhood, gender, and depression: a longitudinal analysis. Res Aging 29:56–72, 2007

Li L, Liang J, Toler A, et al: Widowhood and depressive symptoms among older Chinese: do gender and source of support make a difference? Soc Sci Med 60:637–647, 2005

Lichtenstein P, Gatz M, Pedersen NL, et al: A co-twin-control study of response to widowhood. J Gerontol B Psychol Sci Soc Sci 51B:P279–P289, 1996

Lieberman MA: Bereavement self-help groups: a review of conceptual and methodological issues, in Handbook of Bereavement. Edited by Stroebe MS, Stroebe W, Hansson R. Cambridge, United Kingdom, Cambridge University Press, 1993, pp 411–426

Lindemann E: Symptomatology and management of acute grief. Am J Psychiatry 101:141–148, 1944

Lopata HZ: On widowhood: grief work and identity reconstruction. J Geriatr Psychiatry 8:41–55, 1975

Lopata HZ: Current Widowhood: Myths and Realities. Thousand Oaks, CA, Sage, 1996

Lund DA, Caserta M, Dimond M: Impact of spousal bereavement on the subjective well-being of older adults, in Older Bereaved Spouses. Edited by Lund DA. New York, Hemisphere, 1989, pp 3–15

Lund DA, Caserta M, Dimond M: The course of spousal bereavement in later life, in Handbook of Bereavement. Edited by Stroebe MS, Stroebe W, Hansson R. Cambridge, United Kingdom, Cambridge University Press, 1993, pp 240–254

Marmar C, Horowitz MJ, Weiss DS, et al: A controlled trial of brief psychotherapy and mutual-help group treatment of conjugal bereavement. Am J Psychiatry 145:203–212, 1988

Mawson D, Marks IM, Ramm L, et al: Guided mourning for morbid grief: a controlled study. Br J Psychiatry 138:185–193, 1981

McCrae RR, Costa PT: Psychological resilience among widowed men and women: a 10-year follow-up of a national sample, in Handbook of Bereavement. Edited by Stroebe MS, Stroebe W, Hansson R. Cambridge, United Kingdom, Cambridge University Press, 1993, pp 196–207

Medigovich K, Porock D, Kristjanson LJ, et al: Predictors of family satisfaction with an Australian palliative home care service: a test of discrepancy theory. J Palliat Care 15:48–56, 1999

Miller MD, Wolfson L, Frank E, et al: Using interpersonal psychotherapy (IPT) in a combined psychotherapy/medication research protocol with depressed elders: a descriptive report with case vignettes. J Psychother Pract Res 7:47–55, 1997

Miller SI, Schoenfeld L: Grief in the Navajo: psychodynamics and culture. Int J Soc Psychiatry 19:187–191, 1973

Nadeau JW: Meaning making in family bereavement: a family systems approach, in Handbook of Bereavement Research: Consequences, Coping, and Care. Edited by Stroebe MS, Hansson RO, Stroebe W, et al. Washington, DC, American Psychological Association, 2001, pp 329–347

National Institutes of Health Consensus Conference: Diagnosis and treatment of depression in late life. JAMA 268:1018–1024, 1992

Neimeyer RA: The Lessons of Loss: A Guide to Coping. Raleigh, NC, McGraw-Hill, 1998

Neimeyer RA: Searching for the meaning of meaning: grief therapy and the process of reconstruction. Death Stud 24:531–558, 2000

Neimeyer RA, Prigerson HG, Davies B: Mourning and meaning. Am Behav Sci 46:235–251, 2002

Newsom JT, Schulz R: Social support as a mediator in the relation between functional status and quality of life in older adults. Psychol Aging 11:34–44, 1996

Ng K, von Gunten CF: Symptoms and attitudes of 100 consecutive patients admitted to an acute hospice/palliative care unit. J Pain Symptom Manage 16:307–316, 1998

Nolen-Hoeksema S, Larson J, Bishop M: Predictors of family members' satisfaction with hospice. Hosp J 15:29–48, 2000

Oakley F, Khin NA, Parks L, et al: Improvement in activities of daily living in elderly following treatment for post-bereavement depression. Acta Psychiatr Scand 105:231–234, 2002

O'Bryant SL: Forewarning of a husband's death: does it make a difference for older widows? Omega (Westport) 22:227–239, 1990–1991

O'Neil M: Grief and bereavement in AIDS and aging. Generations 13:80–82, 1989

Ortiz A, Simmons J, Hinton WL: Locations of remorse and homelands of resilience: notes on grief and sense of loss of place of Latino and Irish-American caregivers of demented elders. Cult Med Psychiatry 23:477–500, 1999

Osterweis M, Solomon F, Green M (eds): Bereavement: Reactions, Consequences, and Care. Washington, DC, National Academy Press, 1984

Parkes CM: Bereavement: Studies of Grief in Adult Life. New York, International Universities Press, 1972

Parkes CM, Weiss RS: Recovery From Bereavement. New York, Basic Books, 1983

Pasternak RE, Reynolds CF 3rd, Schlernitzauer M, et al: Acute open-label trial of nortriptyline therapy of bereavement-related depression in late life. J Clin Psychiatry 52:307–310, 1991

Pincus L: Death and the Family. New York, Pantheon, 1974

Prigerson HG, Jacobs SC: Perspectives on care at the close of life: caring for bereaved patients: "all the doctors just suddenly go." JAMA 286:1369–1376, 2001

Prigerson HG, Shear MK, Jacobs SC, et al: Consensus criteria for traumatic grief: a preliminary empirical test. Br J Psychiatry 174:67–73, 1999

Quigley DG, Schatz MS: Men and women and their responses in spousal bereavement. Hosp J 14:65–78, 1999

Ragow-O'Brien D, Hayslip B, Guarnaccia CA: The impact of hospice on attitudes toward funerals and subsequent bereavement adjustment. Omega (Westport) 41:291–305, 2000

Rando TA: The increasing prevalence of complicated mourning: the onslaught is just beginning. Omega (Westport) 26:43–59, 1992–1993

Rando TA: Anticipatory mourning: a review and critique of the literature, in Clinical Dimensions of Anticipatory Mourning. Edited by Rando TA. Champaign, IL, Research Press, 2000, pp 17–49

Raphael B, Middleton W, Martinek N, et al: Counseling and therapy of the bereaved, in Handbook of Bereavement. Edited by Stroebe MS, Stroebe W, Hansson R. Cambridge, United Kingdom, Cambridge University Press, 1993, pp 427–453

Raphael B, Minkov C, Dobson M: Psychotherapeutic and pharmacological intervention for bereaved persons, in Handbook of Bereavement Research: Consequences, Coping, and Care. Edited by Stroebe MS, Hansson RO, Stroebe W, et al. Washington, DC, American Psychological Association, 2001, pp 587–612

Rees WD: The hallucinations of widowhood. Br Med J 4:37–41, 1971

Regehr C, Sussman T: Intersections between grief and trauma: toward an empirically based model for treating traumatic grief. Brief Treatment and Crisis Intervention 4:289–309, 2004

Reisman AS: Death of a spouse: illusory basic assumptions and continuation of bonds. Death Stud 25:445–460, 2001

Reynolds CF 3rd: Treatment of depression in special populations. J Clin Psychiatry 53(suppl):45–53, 1992

Reynolds CF 3rd, Miller MD, Pasternak RE, et al: Treatment of bereavement-related major depressive episodes in later life: a controlled study of acute and continuation treatment with nortriptyline and interpersonal psychotherapy. Am J Psychiatry 156:202–208, 1999

Romanoff BD, Terenzio M: Rituals and the grieving process. Death Stud 22:697–711, 1998

Rosenblatt PC: Cross-cultural variation in the experience, statement, and understanding of grief, in Ethnic Variations in Dying, Death, and Grief: Diversity in Universality. Edited by Irish DP, Lundquist KF, Nelsen VJ. Washington, DC, Taylor and Francis, 1993, pp 13–19

Rosenblatt PC: Grief that does not end, in Continuing Bonds: New Understandings of Grief (Series in Death Education, Aging, and Health Care, 0275-3510). Edited by Klass D, Silverman PR, Nickman SL. Washington, DC, Taylor and Francis, 1996, pp 45–58

Rosenblatt PC, Elde C: Shared reminiscence about a deceased parent: implications for grief education and grief counseling. Fam Relat 39:206–210, 1990

Rosenzweig A, Prigerson H, Miller MD, et al: Bereavement and late-life depression: grief and its complications in the elderly. Annu Rev Med 48:421–428, 1997

Sable P: Attachment, loss of spouse, and grief in elderly adults. Omega (Westport) 23:129–142, 1991

Sanders CM: Risk factors in bereavement outcome, in Handbook of Bereavement. Edited by Stroebe MS, Stroebe W, Hansson R. Cambridge, United Kingdom, Cambridge University Press, 1993, pp 255–267

Sanders CM, Mauger PA, Strong PN Jr: A Manual for the Grief Experience Inventory. Tampa, FL, University of South Florida, 1979

Sanders CM, Mauger PA, Strong PN Jr: A Manual for the Grief Experience Inventory. Palo Alto, CA, Consulting Psychologists Press, 1985

Schut HA, Stroebe MS, van den Bout J: Intervention for the bereaved: gender differences in the efficacy of two counselling programmes. Br J Clin Psychol 36:63–72, 1997

Schut H, Stroebe MS, van den Bout J, et al: The efficacy of bereavement interventions: determining who benefits, in Handbook of Bereavement Research: Consequences, Coping, and Care. Edited by Stroebe MS, Hansson RO, Stroebe W, et al. Washington, DC, American Psychological Association, 2001, pp 705–737

Seale C, Kelly M: A comparison of hospice and hospital care for the spouses of people who die. Palliat Med 11:101–106, 1997

Shear [M]K, Shair H: Attachment, loss, and complicated grief. Dev Psychobiol 47:253–267, 2005

Shear MK, Frank E, Foa E, et al: Traumatic grief treatment: a pilot study. Am J Psychiatry 158:1506–1508, 2001

Shear [M]K, Frank E, Houck PR, et al: Treatment of complicated grief: a randomized controlled trial. JAMA 293:2601–2608, 2005

Shuchter SR, Zisook S: Widowhood: the continuing relationship with the dead spouse. Bull Menninger Clin 52:269–279, 1988

Shuchter SR, Zisook S: The course of normal grief, in Handbook of Bereavement. Edited by Stroebe MS, Stroebe W, Hansson R. Cambridge, United Kingdom, Cambridge University Press, 1993, pp 23–43

Siegel K, Weinstein L: Anticipatory grief reconsidered. J Psychosoc Oncol 1:61–72, 1983

Silverman GK, Jacobs SC, Kasl SV, et al: Quality of life impairments associated with diagnostic criteria for traumatic grief. Psychol Med 30:857–862, 2000

Silverman PR, Klass D: Introduction: what's the problem? in Continuing Bonds: New Understandings of Grief (Series in Death Education, Aging, and Health Care, 0275-3510). Edited by Klass D, Silverman PR, Nickman SL. Washington, DC, Taylor and Francis, 1996, pp 3–27

Sireling L, Cohen D, Marks I: Guided mourning for morbid grief: a controlled replication. Behav Ther 19:121–132, 1988

Steinhauser KE, Christakis NA, Clipp EC, et al: Factors considered important at the end of life by patients, family, physicians, and other care providers. JAMA 284:2476–2482, 2000

Stroebe MS: Coping with bereavement: a review of the grief work hypothesis. Omega (Westport) 26:19–42, 1992–1993

Stroebe M, Stroebe W: Who participates in bereavement research? A review and empirical study. Omega (Westport) 20:1–29, 1989

Stroebe M, Schut H: The dual process model of coping with bereavement: rationale and description. Death Stud 23:197–224, 1999

Stroebe MS, Hansson RO, Stroebe W, et al: Introduction: concepts and issues in contemporary research on bereavement, in Handbook of Bereavement Research: Consequences, Coping, and Care. Edited by Stroebe MS, Hansson RO, Stroebe W, et al. Washington, DC, American Psychological Association, 2001a, pp 3–22

Stroebe MS, Stroebe W, Schut H: Gender differences in adjustment to bereavement: an empirical and theoretical review. Rev Gen Psychol 5:62–83, 2001b

Stylianos S, Vachon M: The role of social support in bereavement, in Handbook of Bereavement. Edited by Stroebe MS, Stroebe W, Hansson R. Cambridge, United Kingdom, Cambridge University Press, 1993, pp 397–410

Sweeting HN, Gilhooly ML: Anticipatory grief: a review. Soc Sci Med 30:1073–1080, 1990

Thompson LW, Breckenridge JN, Gallagher D, et al: Effects of bereavement on self-perceptions of physical health in elderly widows and widowers. J Gerontol 39:309–314, 1984

Thompson LW, Gallagher-Thompson D, Futterman A, et al: The effects of late-life spousal bereavement over a 30-month interval. Psychol Aging 6:434–441, 1991

Thornton JCB: The hospice widow and grief resolution: perceived marital satisfaction and social support as factors influencing bereavement (abstract). Dissertation Abstracts International. Section B, The Sciences and Engineering 59:1337, 1998

U.S. Census Bureau: Marital status of people 15 years and over, by age, sex, personal earnings, race, and Hispanic origin, March 2000. Released June 29, 2001. Available at http://www.census.gov/population/www/socdemo/hh-fam/cps2001.html. Accessed August 12, 2008.

van Grootheest DS, Beekman ATF, Broese van Groenou MI, et al: Sex differences in depression after widowhood: do men suffer more? Soc Psychiatry Psychiatr Epidemiol 34:391–398, 1999

Viney L: The construing widow: dislocation and adaptation in bereavement. Psychotherapy Patient 6:207–222, 1990

Voltz R, Akabayashi A, Reese C, et al: Organization and patients' perception of palliative care: a cross-cultural comparison. Palliat Med 11:351–357, 1997

Weisman A: The Realization of Death: A Guide for the Psychological Autopsy. Northvale, NJ, Jason Aronson, 1974

Wikan U: Bereavement and loss in two Muslim communities: Egypt and Bali compared. Soc Sci Med 27:451–460, 1988

Wilkinson EK, Salisbury C, Bosanquet N, et al: Patient and carer preference for, and satisfaction with, specialist models of palliative care: a systematic literature review. Palliat Med 13:197–216, 1999

Williams K: Has the future of marriage arrived? A contemporary examination of gender, marriage, and psychological well-being. J Health Soc Behav 44:470–487, 2003

Windholz MJ, Weiss DS, Horowitz MJ: An empirical study of the natural history of time-limited psychotherapy for stress response syndromes. Psychotherapy: Theory, Research, Practice, Training 22:547–554, 1985

Wisocki PA, Skowron J: The effects of gender and culture on adjustment to widowhood, in Handbook of Gender, Culture, and Health. Edited by Eisler RM, Hersen M. Mahwah, NJ, Erlbaum, 2000, pp 429–448

Worden JW: Grief Counseling and Grief Therapy, 3rd Edition. New York, Springer, 2002

Wortman C, Silver RC: Coping with irrevocable loss, in Cataclysms, Crises, and Catastrophes: Psychology in Action (The Master Lectures). Edited by VandenBos G, Bryant BK. Washington, DC, American Psychological Association, 1987, pp 185–235

Wortman C, Silver RC: The myths of coping with loss. J Consult Clin Psychol 57:349–357, 1989

Younoszai B: Mexican American perspectives related to death, in Ethnic Variations in Dying, Death, and Grief: Diversity in Universality. Edited by Irish DP, Lundquist KF, Nelsen VJ. Washington, DC, Taylor and Francis, 1993, pp 67–78

Zisook S, Shuchter SR: Time course of spousal bereavement. Gen Hosp Psychiatry 7:95–100, 1985

Zisook S, Shuchter SR: The first four years of widowhood. Psychiatr Ann 15:288–294, 1986

Zisook S, Shuchter SR, Sledge P, et al: Aging and bereavement. J Geriatr Psychiatry Neurol 6:137–143, 1993

Zisook S, Shuchter SR, Pedrelli P, et al: Bupropion sustained release for bereavement: results of an open trial. J Clin Psychiatry 62:227–230, 2001

Zygmont M, Prigerson HG, Houck PR, et al: A post hoc comparison of paroxetine and nortriptyline for symptoms of traumatic grief. J Clin Psychiatry 59:241–245, 1998

Suggested Readings

Bonanno GA, Wortman CB, Lehman DR, et al: Resilience to loss and chronic grief: a prospective study from pre-loss to 18 months post-loss. J Pers Soc Psychol 83:1150–1164, 2002

Breckenridge J, Gallagher D, Thompson LW, et al: Characteristic depressive symptoms of bereaved elders. J Gerontol 41:163–168, 1986

Horowitz MJ, Siegel B, Holen A, et al: Diagnostic criteria for complicated grief disorder. Am J Psychiatry 154:904–910, 1997

Neimeyer R: Searching for the meaning of meaning: grief therapy and the process of reconstruction. Death Stud 24:531–558, 2000

Parkes CM: Bereavement: Studies of Grief in Adult Life. New York, International Universities Press, 1972

Prigerson HG, Shear MK, Jacobs SC, et al: Consensus criteria for traumatic grief: a preliminary empirical test. Br J Psychiatry 174:67–73, 1999

Stroebe M, Schut H: The dual process model of coping with bereavement: rationale and description. Death Stud 23:197–224, 1999

Stroebe MS, Hansson RO, Stroebe W, et al: Handbook of Bereavement Research: Consequences, Coping, and Care. Washington, DC, American Psychological Association, 2001

Worden JW: Grief Counseling and Grief Therapy, 3rd Edition. New York, Springer, 2002

Wortman C, Silver RC: Coping with irrevocable loss, in Cataclysms, Crises, and Catastrophes: Psychology in Action (The Master Lectures). Edited by VandenBos G, Bryant BK. Washington, DC, American Psychological Association, 1987, pp 185–235

CHAPTER 22

SLEEP AND CIRCADIAN RHYTHM DISORDERS

Andrew D. Krystal, M.D., M.S.
Jack D. Edinger, Ph.D.
William K. Wohlgemuth, Ph.D.

Sleep disorders are an important aspect of geriatric psychiatry. In the United States, more than half of noninstitutionalized individuals older than 65 years report chronic sleep difficulties (Foley et al. 1995; National Institutes of Health Consensus Development Conference Statement 1991; Prinz et al. 1990). Sleep disturbances affect quality of life, increase the risk of accidents and falls, and, perhaps most importantly, are among the leading reasons for long-term care placement (Pollak and Perlick 1991; Pollak et al. 1990; Sanford 1975). Working effectively with elderly individuals requires expertise in the diagnosis and treatment of sleep disorders.

Reviewing the basic nomenclature used to describe sleep disorders provides a first step in understanding sleep disorders in the elderly. The major disorders of sleep are typically divided into three groups: 1) difficulties in initiating and maintaining sleep (insomnias), 2) disorders involving excessive daytime sleepiness, and 3) disorders of circadian rhythm. Insomnias are characterized by complaints of sustained difficulty in initiating or maintaining sleep and/or complaints of nonrestorative sleep, along with significant distress or impairment in daytime function (American Psychiatric Association 2000; American Sleep Disorders Association 1997). These disorders frequently are classified as either primary insomnia (in which no psychiatric or medical disorder is associated with the condition) or comorbid insomnia (in which a psychiatric or medical disorder occurs along with the sleep disturbance) (American Psychiatric Association 2000).

Disorders of excessive daytime sleepiness are characterized by persistent daytime sleepiness that causes significant distress or impairment in function (American Psychiatric Association 2000; American Sleep Disorders Association 1997). The most important disorders of excessive sleepiness are sleep apnea, periodic limb movement disorder (PLMD), and narcolepsy.

Circadian rhythm disorders manifest as a misalignment between an individual's sleep-wake cycle and the pattern that is desired or required (American Psychiatric Association 2000; American Sleep Disorders Association 1997). Affected individuals report that they cannot sleep at the times when sleep is desired, needed, or expected and that they fall asleep at times when wakefulness is desired, needed, or expected. The circadian rhythm is important for function because it is a cycle not only of sleep and wakefulness but also of many physiological processes and phenomena, including body temperature, alertness, cognitive performance, and hormone release (Czeisler et al. 1990; Folkard and Totterdell 1994; Minors et al. 1994).

Despite the variety and differing pathophysiologies of sleep disorders, the incidence of nearly all these disorders increases with age. The majority of age-related changes in sleep appear to stem from an increased incidence of sleep disturbances that lead to secondary sleep-related symptoms such as sleep apnea, PLMD, and medical and psychiatric disorders (Bliwise 1993; Foley et al. 1995; Gislason and Almqvist 1987; Prinz 1995; Prinz et al. 1990). However, evidence shows that changes in sleep and the circadian rhythm occur even in healthy elderly individuals without such disorders (Bliwise 1993; Foley et al. 1995; Gislason and Almqvist 1987; Prinz 1995; Prinz et al. 1990). Given that these changes are not necessarily associated with complaints of sleep disturbance or diminished daytime function, sleep and circadian rhythm disturbances may not be an inevitable consequence of aging. These factors provide some challenges for clinical care. One of these challenges is the need to use a different threshold for normality in elderly patients. Sleep attributes that are considered abnormal in a younger individual may not be associated with symptoms in an elderly person. Furthermore, clinical care of the elderly population requires a heightened awareness of and expertise in identifying underlying medical and psychiatric disorders.

Although these challenges can be formidable, they are not insurmountable. In this chapter, we first review the changes in sleep and circadian rhythm that occur in individuals without medical and psychiatric disorders. We then review the disorders that can cause disturbances of sleep and chronobiology and whose likelihood increases with age. Finally, we discuss evaluation and treatment of elderly individuals with a sleep complaint or suspected sleep-related dysfunction.

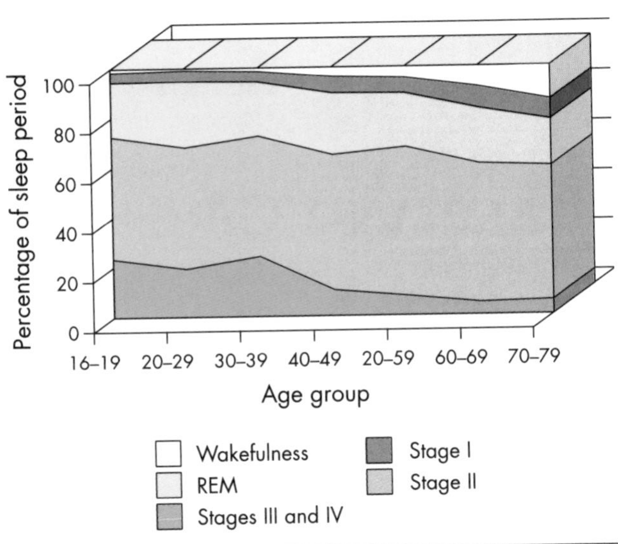

FIGURE 22–1. Sleep-stage distributions across age groups.

REM=rapid-eye movement.

Influence of Aging on Sleep and Circadian Functions

Since the 1970s, extensive research has shown that marked changes in sleep and circadian rhythm accompany aging. Normative data derived from adults without complaints of sleep disturbance have implied that marked changes in the duration, continuity, and depth of nocturnal sleep accompany normal aging (Hirshkowitz et al. 1992). As shown in Figure 22–1, nocturnal sleep time steadily decreases across the life span, and nocturnal wake time increases because of an increase in arousals. Accompanying these changes are marked reductions in stages III and IV sleep (these stages are the deeper stages of non–rapid eye movement [NREM] sleep). Although the clinical significance of these changes is unknown, they may relate to the reported reduction in subjective sleep quality and lowering of the arousal threshold with age (Riedel and Lichstein 1998; Zepelin et al. 1984).

The sleep-wake cycle appears to change significantly with age as well. The amplitudes of both the sleep-wake cycle and the 24-hour body temperature rhythm appear to decrease with aging (Bliwise 2000; Czeisler et al. 1999). Additionally, compared with younger age groups, older adults tend to awaken at an earlier phase (i.e., closer to the nadir of their 24-hour temperature rhythms), and they show a greater propensity to awaken during the later portions of their sleep episodes (Dijk et al. 1997; Duffy et al. 1998). Furthermore, multiple psychosocial changes that accompany aging may alter or eliminate important *zeitgebers* ("time markers") for the circadian system and promote the onset of sleep difficulties among older adults.

Disorders Associated With Sleep and Circadian Rhythm Disturbances

A number of medical and psychiatric conditions are associated with sleep difficulties, and these conditions occur more frequently with increasing age. The longstanding view was that such medical and psychiatric conditions caused disorders of sleep and circadian rhythm, which were best viewed as symptoms (National Institutes of Health Consensus Conference 1984). This point of view discouraged targeting treatment specifically to address the associated sleep disorders. More recent data suggest that in a number of situations (the best examples are insomnia occurring with major depression, generalized anxiety disorders, and chronic pain), the relationship is more complex than previously believed, and in some cases the causality appears to be bidirectional (Krystal 2006; National Institutes of Health 2005). The emerging view is that sleep disorders occurring with medical and psychiatric disorders have been undertreated, and the term *comorbid* has been proposed to replace *secondary* as a means of describing conditions where sleep disorders occur with medical and psychiatric conditions (National Institutes of Health 2005).

Primary Sleep Disorders

Sleep Apnea

In patients with sleep apnea, breathing ceases for periods of 10 seconds or more (Aldrich 2000), either because no effort is made to breathe (central sleep apnea) or because the oropharynx collapses during attempts to breathe (obstructive sleep apnea). The predominant type of sleep apnea seen in elderly individuals is obstructive sleep apnea (Ancoli-Israel et al. 1987). A number of studies suggest that the frequency of obstructive sleep apnea increases with age (Ancoli-Israel 1989; Ancoli-Israel et al. 1991; Dickel and Mosko 1990; Roehrs et al. 1983). Apnea generally causes excessive sleepiness, although mild to moderate apnea can be associated with insomnia. Referral to a sleep disorders specialist is required for diagnosis and treatment. The treatment of choice for obstructive sleep apnea is continuous positive airway pressure (CPAP). This treatment involves blowing air through the nose at night to increase pressure within the upper airway, thereby preventing the collapse that leads to apnea. Some individuals (particularly those with anatomical anomalies predisposing them to apnea) are treated with upper airway surgery. Central sleep apnea is relatively rare, constituting 4%–10% of patients with apnea (White 2000). This disorder can be caused by a number of different pathophysiologies, including any cause of waking alveolar hypoventilation, congestive heart failure, neurological disorders, and nasal and upper airway obstruction. Therapy should be targeted to the particular underlying process, although in many cases no such problem can be identified, and CPAP is usually the first treatment attempted (White 2000).

Periodic Limb Movement Disorder and Restless Legs Syndrome

In PLMD, repetitive muscular contractions occur during sleep; these contractions most commonly involve the legs and often cause sleep disturbances. When these events occur infrequently, they are not considered pathological, because they tend not to be associated with any symptoms (Roehrs et al. 1983). The frequency of these events is characterized in terms of the number of movements associated with arousal that occur per hour of sleep (the movement-arousal index). There is some debate about what movement-arousal index is abnormal. Thresholds ranging from 5 to 15 movements per hour have been suggested (Ancoli-Israel et al. 1991; Dickel and Mosko 1990). Some authors have suggested that a higher threshold for abnormality should be applied to elderly patients, who tend to be symptom free at movement-arousal indices typically associated with significant symptoms in younger individuals (Ancoli-Israel 1989). Perhaps even more relevant for those working with elderly patients is that PLMD, as with sleep apnea, is more prevalent in the elderly (Roehrs et al. 1983). Several studies indicate that clinically significant PLMD is seen in 30%–45% of adults age 60 years or older, compared with 5%–6% of all adults (Ancoli-Israel et al. 1991).

Individuals with PLMD may complain of leg kicks (most commonly noticed by the bed partner), cold feet, excessive daytime sleepiness, and insomnia (Ancoli-Israel 1989; Ancoli-Israel et al. 1991; Roehrs et al. 1983). The insomnia may be characterized by difficulty in falling asleep or staying asleep (Ancoli-Israel 1989). Unfortunately, the presence of this disease is difficult to predict reliably on the basis of the patient's history (Ancoli-Israel 1989; Dickel and Mosko 1990). Furthermore, a high level of confidence in the diagnosis is needed before institution of treatment, because treatment typically involves long-term use of medications that can have significant side effects (see "Pharmacological Treatment" later in this chapter). Therefore, when a history is suggestive of PLMD, standard practice is to make a referral for a polysomnogram for definitive diagnosis (Ancoli-Israel 1989). Polysomnography is also indicated when an individual has significant insomnia or hypersomnia that does not respond to usual treatment. Such a patient may have significant PLMD that was undetected when the patient's history was obtained.

Restless legs syndrome (RLS) is often associated with PLMD and is described as an uncomfortable feeling in the lower extremities that creates an irresistible urge to move. RLS occurs in 6% of the adult population and is present in up to 28% of patients older than 65 years (Clark 2001). Polysomnography is not needed for a diagnosis of RLS, which is made through history taking.

When compared in the general population, RLS is almost twice as prevalent in elderly women as in elderly men. RLS, as well as PLMD, has been associated with anemia (O'Keeffe et al. 1994). In elderly patients, ferritin levels less than 45 μg/L have a positive correlation with an increased risk of RLS, and such patients often benefit from administration of supplemental iron (O'Keeffe et al. 1994). Also associated with PLMD and RLS are diabetes mellitus, pregnancy, iron deficiency anemia, and use of certain medications, including antidepressants (Bliwise et al. 1985). Workup to exclude these conditions is typically carried out before initiating medication treatment.

The same medications are effective for both RLS and PLMD. The primary treatment for these conditions is dopaminergic agonists (Bliwise et al. 2005; Montplaisir et al. 1999). Second-line treatment options include anticonvulsants (gabapentin) and benzodiazepines (clonazepam). Opiates are typically reserved for patients who do not respond to these other drugs. Because of the high prevalence of PLMD and RLS in the elderly population, the geriatric psychiatrist should be acquainted with the symptoms of these disorders. Effective treatment often significantly improves the quality of life of affected individuals.

Neuropsychiatric Disorders

Bereavement

Psychological factors that most commonly affect sleep in elderly persons are reactions to loss, such as loss of health or functional capacity, and reactions to the death of a friend or loved one. Although bereavement is normal, it is often associated with substantial sleep disturbance (American Psychiatric Association 2000). When bereavement is associated with more frequent intrusive thoughts and avoidance behaviors, there appears to be more sleep disturbance, predominantly in the form of difficulty in falling asleep (Hall et al. 1997). Bereavement and depression are closely linked, however. Depression is usually diagnosed only when symptoms have persisted for more than 2 months after a loss or when symptoms are severe, such as suicidal ideation, psychotic symptoms, malnutrition, or dehydration (American Psychiatric Association 2000). Antidepressant medication may be helpful. A short course of sedative-hypnotic therapy may provide substantial symptomatic relief. If this approach is taken, the medication should be tapered off when the other symptoms of bereavement diminish. Because the clinician will not know at the outset how long treatment will be needed, considerations related to longer-term treatment pertain (see "Pharmacological Treatment" later in this chapter). Although unlikely, it is possible for rebound insomnia to occur after a relatively short course (3–4 weeks) of treatment. As a result, clinicians should warn patients of this possibility and wait at least several days after discontinuing the medication to determine whether there is persistent insomnia. If all symptoms of bereavement have resolved except insomnia, cognitive-behavioral therapy for insomnia should be considered (see "Cognitive-Behavioral Treatment" later in this chapter). Grief counseling should also be considered.

Major Depression

Depression is frequently associated with sleep disruption in individuals older than 60 years. Roughly 10%–15% of individuals older than 65 years experience clinically significant depressive symptoms (Hoch et al. 1989). The most frequent complaints in affected individuals are 1) experiencing a decrease in total sleep time and 2) waking earlier than desired. Daytime sleepiness may occur but is less common.

Major depression is the condition in which there is the strongest evidence for a complex bidirectional relationship with sleep disturbance (Krystal 2006). Although insomnia has long been viewed as a secondary symptom of underlying depression, the results of a series of relatively recent studies are inconsistent with this point of view (National Institutes of Health Consensus Conference 1984). The findings include evidence that those with insomnia have an increased future risk of major depression, that insomnia is an independent risk factor for suicide in depressed individuals, that antidepressant treatment frequently does not result in resolution of insomnia, and that this residual insomnia is associated with an increased risk of depression relapse (Breslau et al. 1996; Fawcett et al. 1990; Livingston et al. 1994; Reynolds et al. 1997).

The strongest evidence of the importance of depression is a study that examined the administration of the insomnia agent eszopiclone along with the antidepressant fluoxetine for initial therapy of depression (N=545) (Fava et al. 2006; Krystal et al. 2007). Compared with subjects treated with fluoxetine and placebo, those receiving fluoxetine and eszopiclone not only slept significantly better but also experienced more rapid and greater improvement in nonsleep aspects of depression. Although studies of this type have not been carried out in older adults, these data nonetheless make a strong case for the importance of treating insomnia in those with depression. The available research literature provides little guidance on the optimal management of insomnia occurring in this setting. The relative utility of sedating antidepressants versus the combination of nonsedating antidepressants (such as selective serotonin reuptake inhibitors) and insomnia agents has not been evaluated. Data also are lacking on the treatment of insomnia that is comorbid with depression by using insomnia agents other than eszopiclone or by using cognitive-behavioral therapy for the insomnia (see "Pharmacological Treatment" later in this chapter).

Alzheimer's Disease

Individuals with Alzheimer's disease have been found to experience an increased number of arousals and awakenings, to take more daytime naps, and to have a diminished amount of REM sleep and slow-wave sleep (Prinz et al. 1982). Individuals with dementia often experience evening or nocturnal agitation and confusion. This phenomenon, called *sundowning,* is among the leading reasons that individuals with dementia become institutionalized (Pollak and Perlick 1991; Pollak et al. 1990; Sanford 1975). The pathophysiology of sundowning is poorly understood. A number of features appear to increase the risk of sundowning, including greater dementia severity, pain, fecal impaction, malnutrition, polypharmacy, infections, rapid eye movement (REM) sleep behavior disorder, PLMD, and environmental sleep disruptions (Bliwise 2000).

Treatment of sundowning should begin with an assessment for such conditions. If no causative condition can be found, or if attempts to eliminate the cause are unsuccessful, treatment should be instituted. Nonmedication management includes light therapy, elimination of daytime napping, and a structured activity program (Bliwise 2000). More research is needed to determine the efficacy of these interventions.

Medication management of sundowning is also an area in which more research is needed. Several studies have examined the use of benzodiazepines for the treatment of sleep problems in patients with Alzheimer's disease and sundowning, and these studies suggest that benzodiazepines are ineffective (Bliwise 2000).

Nonbenzodiazepines (agents chemically unrelated to benzodiazepines that have a related mechanism of action) have been prescribed to treat insomnia (see "Pharmacological Treatment" later in this chapter). Of the nonbenzodiazepines currently available in the United States to treat insomnia (zaleplon, zolpidem, and eszopiclone), only a preliminary study of zolpidem has been carried out, and the study findings suggest that it may have some efficacy (Shaw et al. 1992). Of all medications prescribed for sundowning, antipsychotic medications have the most evidence supporting efficacy (Bliwise 2000). Most studies involved older agents. The newer antipsychotics, such as risperidone, olanzapine, and quetiapine, have fewer side effects (Bliwise 2000). However, these newer agents have relatively recently been linked to an increased risk of mortality in this population, the mechanism of which remains to be determined (Kales et al. 2007). Preliminary data suggest that melatonin may also have some utility. Clearly, more research is needed to address the highly important and difficult-to-treat problem of sleep disorders in patients with Alzheimer's disease.

Parkinson's Disease

Sleep complaints are noted in 60%–90% of individuals with Parkinson's disease (Trenkwalder 1998). The majority of Parkinson's disease patients with affected sleep experience difficulty in initiating and maintaining sleep, daytime fatigue, RLS, and an inability to turn over in bed. The last of these features was rated as the most troublesome symptom of sleep disturbance in a study by Lees et al. (1988). Another sleep problem seen in patients with Parkinson's disease is REM sleep behavior disorder, in which the patient acts out dreams because the paralysis that usually occurs during REM sleep is absent (Clarenbach 2000). Dopaminergic medications used to treat Parkinson's disease, such as carbidopa/levodopa, may contribute to sleep initiation problems and sleep difficulties in the first half of the night and may cause nightmares (Trenkwalder 1998). No study findings indicate how to manage sleep difficulties in patients with Parkinson's disease. The use of sedative-hypnotics and the use of tricyclic antidepressants have been described.

Medical Conditions

Pain

Pain is a central feature of many medical conditions that occur with increased frequency in elderly individuals; these conditions include arthritis, neuropathies, angina, reflux esophagitis, and peptic ulcer disease (Aldrich 2000). Disruption of sleep is frequently noted in persons with significant pain (Pilowsky et al. 1985). Attempts to ameliorate the condition causing the pain should be the first step. When these attempts fail, treatment for the pain should be instituted. Often, combined behavioral and pharmacological treatment is needed. There is some evidence that, as with depression, pain may have a bidirectional relationship with sleep disturbance. Two studies suggest that the treatment of insomnia leads to improvement in pain. These studies involved the treatment of individuals with fibromyalgia with cognitive-behavioral therapy for insomnia and treatment of individuals with rheumatoid arthritis with the benzodiazepine triazolam (Edinger et al. 2005; Walsh et al. 1996). These data speak to the importance of treating insomnia in those with chronic pain (see "Treatment of Insomnia" later in this chapter).

Chronic Obstructive Pulmonary Disease

Individuals with chronic obstructive pulmonary disease (COPD) have been found to have both subjective and objective evidence of disturbed sleep, but the degree of sleep disruption is unrelated to hypoxemia (Douglas 2000). Also, daytime sleepiness, which is seen in patients with sleep apnea, does not appear to occur. Polysomnography is not routinely indicated for individuals with COPD who have sleep difficulties (Connaughton et al. 1988), and the need for polysomnography in COPD patients should be determined in the same way that the need in other patients is determined. Sleep apnea appears to be no more common in persons with COPD than in the general population. Nocturnal oxygen may be needed in some patients; however, patients who tend to become most hypoxemic at night are patients who are most hypoxemic during the day (Connaughton et al. 1988). Oral theophyllines, which are frequently used in COPD treatment, are adenosine-receptor antagonists and may have a sleep-disruptive effect (Douglas 2000). Also, patients with COPD should be instructed to avoid alcohol, which can exacerbate hypoxemia and promote other complications. Benzodiazepines should be used with caution because they may increase inhibition of ventilatory or arousal responses and may worsen nocturnal hypoxemia (Douglas 2000). In severe COPD the benzodiazepines triazolam and flunitrazepam but not the nonbenzodiazepine zolpidem adversely affected oxygenation (Murciano et al. 1993). However, in patients with mild to moderate COPD, both zolpidem and triazolam improved awakenings compared with placebo, and neither had an adverse effect on respiration versus placebo (Steens et al. 1993). The melatonin receptor agonist ramelteon has also been found to improve sleep without adversely affecting respiration in patients with mild to moderate COPD (Kryger et al. 2007).

Cerebrovascular Disease

The sleep pathology associated with cerebrovascular disease depends on which areas of the brain are affected by the condition. Hypersomnia has been associated with lesions of the cephalad portions of the ascending reticular activating system, which includes the midbrain and paramedian region of the thalamus (the thalamic lesions most commonly occur in the dorsomedial nucleus, intralaminar nuclei, and centromedian nucleus) (Bassetti and Chervin 2000). Large lesions of the cerebral hemispheres and lesions of other regions such as the caudate and striatum have been less commonly associated with hypersomnia. Insomnia directly related to damage of specific areas of the brain is much less common than insomnia caused by multifactorial complications of strokes or other medical or psychiatric conditions associated with an individual's cerebrovascular disease (Bassetti and Chervin 2000). Therefore, treatment should be directed toward these associated conditions.

Nocturia

The urge to urinate is an often-overlooked cause of awakenings in the elderly population (Bliwise 2000). Surprisingly, it has been reported that nocturia (excessive urination at night) is the most common explanation given by elderly individuals for difficulty in maintaining sleep; 63%–72% of elderly persons cite nocturia as a reason for sleep maintenance problems (Middelkoop et al. 1996). Furthermore, several studies have documented the sleep disturbance caused by and daytime adverse effects of nocturia (Bliwise 2000). The most common causes of nocturia are conditions that increase in frequency with age: benign prostatic hypertrophy in men and decreased urethral resistance due to decreased estrogen levels in women (Bliwise 2000). Sleep apnea, which increases in prevalence in the elderly population, can also lead to nocturia (Bliwise 2000). Thus, when evaluating elderly individuals with complaints of sleep maintenance, the clinician should assess for nocturia and the associated conditions that increase the risk of nocturia. If detected, this disorder can generally be treated effectively by addressing the underlying condition.

Menopause

Despite the enormous number of individuals with menopause-related sleep difficulties, there is a striking lack of research in this area (Krystal et al. 1998). Although little is known, there appears to be clear evidence that many women experience sleep disruption in association with vasomotor symptoms (night sweats, hot flashes, decreased urethral resistance often leading to nocturia) that are caused by decreased levels of circulating estrogen and progesterone (Bliwise 2000; Krystal et al. 1998). Several factors hinder elucidation of menopausal sleep disturbance. One is that many disorders that cause insomnia increase in frequency with age and are highly prevalent during the period in which women experience menopausal changes. Another factor is that although hormone replacement therapy is highly effective in ameliorating the vasomotor symptoms of menopause, the subjective reports of sleep disturbance often do not change (Krystal et al. 1998). Although menopausal sleep disturbance is poorly understood, it has been suggested that behavioral conditioning occurs, just as is often the case with individuals who, having experienced insomnia during a period of high stress, continue to have insomnia after the stress has resolved (Krystal et al. 1998).

Given these considerations, elderly women with insomnia should be evaluated for underlying causes of sleep disturbance (e.g., medical and psychiatric conditions, primary sleep disorders), and it should be determined whether there is an association between changes in menstrual periods, vasomotor symptoms, and insomnia symptoms. If an association between insomnia and menopausal changes appears to exist, a trial of hormone replacement therapy could be considered. If hormone replacement therapy ameliorates vasomotor symptoms but insomnia complaints persist, behavioral therapy should be considered. If hormone replacement therapy is contraindicated or if use of this treatment is not preferred, other treatments such as pharmacological management of insomnia or cognitive-behavioral sleep therapy should be considered (see discussions in "Pharmacological Treatment" and "Cognitive-Behavioral Treatment" later in this chapter). Two studies have been carried out in women with insomnia occurring in association with menopause (Dorsey et al. 2004; Soares et al. 2006). These studies document the efficacy of zolpidem 10 mg and eszopiclone 3 mg for improving sleep difficulties that occur in association with hot flashes. Further studies are needed to determine the efficacy of cognitive-behavioral therapy for insomnia and of other insomnia agents.

Loss of Hearing, Vision, and Mobility

Many elderly individuals experience decrements in hearing, vision, and mobility (e.g., walking, driving). These changes are caused by a variety of medical conditions that increase in frequency with age. Changes in these vital functions can have a profound effect on sleep. Most frequently, this effect stems from a loss of activities in which the affected individual can engage. The person then takes unplanned naps or tries to sleep more than he or she is physiologically able to, in order to pass the time. The result is fragmentation of sleep and loss of circadian rhythmicity. Affected individuals report spending many frustrating hours awake in bed at night. Although this problem should be easily solved by increasing activity and developing new activity options, in practice, making these changes is difficult to achieve.

Evaluation of Individuals With Sleep-Related Complaints

The first step in evaluating a patient with sleep-related complaints is a comprehensive clinical evaluation. The patient should be carefully assessed for sleep disorders and for underlying medical, psychiatric, and environmental conditions. A physical examination should be performed if the history suggests a need for it. Several laboratory tests are available to the clinician, including overnight polysomnography and the Multiple Sleep Latency Test (MSLT; Buysse et al. 2006). Subjective sleep logs and actigraphy can also be used. Each of these methods of assessment may be useful, depending on the nature of the complaint.

Polysomnography is the primary laboratory test in sleep medicine. It allows the determination of stages of sleep (wakefulness; stage I, II, III, and IV sleep; and REM sleep) throughout the night as well as the monitoring of nocturnal breathing, movements, cardiac function, and brain function. Polysomnography is primarily used to evaluate for sleep apnea, PLMD, nocturnal seizures, and nocturnal medical or psychiatric events.

The MSLT is a daytime test in which the patient takes a series of four or five naps spaced 2 hours apart throughout the day. This test provides a physiological assessment of daytime sleepiness and is part of the assessment of narcolepsy.

A subjective sleep log can be useful, particularly in the assessment of complaints of insomnia and circadian rhythm disturbances (Buysse et al. 2006). Each morning on awakening, for at least a week, the patient records information about the previous night's sleep. This information typically includes the time to bed, time to onset of sleep, number of awakenings during the night, length of awakenings, time of final awakening, rise time, quality of the night's sleep, and level of restedness. In addition, naps during the previous day and the use of sleep aids are recorded.

Actigraphy is an objective assessment of activity throughout the day and night (American Academy of Sleep Medicine 2007). Patients wear an actigraph, which is much like a wristwatch, 24 hours a day for several days. Data are typically recorded in 1-minute epochs and stored in the actigraph's memory. The information is used to characterize the typical sleep-wake patterns and to determine the amount of wakefulness during the sleep period.

Choice of these methods is determined by the presenting complaint. For example, an individual complaining of excessive daytime sleepiness and snoring at night usually requires overnight polysomnography. Someone complaining of difficulty in staying asleep at night requires a sleep log assessment. An individual suspected of having narcolepsy requires polysomnography followed by an MSLT the next day. A person who complains of an inability to fall asleep until 3 A.M. and difficulty in awakening before noon may need actigraphy and a sleep log assessment.

To develop a diagnosis and a treatment plan, the clinician must combine the results of laboratory tests with the information obtained during the comprehensive evaluation. The treatment plan may include further testing, consultation, or institution of a treatment regimen.

Treatment of Insomnia

Although changes in sleep appear to be a part of aging, insomnia is not an inevitable consequence of aging. No treatment is needed to address the changes in sleep that normally occur. However, when individuals experience insomnia as defined in the chapter introduction, treatment should be instituted, because untreated insomnia is associated with significant morbidity and decreased quality of life (Breslau et al. 1996; National Institutes of Health 2005; Ohayon 2002; Ozminkowski et al. 2007; Weissman et al. 1997; Zammit et al. 1999). Treatment of insomnia in elderly patients poses some particular challenges. We now discuss the two major types of treatment for insomnia: cognitive-behavioral therapy and pharmacological treatment. In this discussion, we focus on issues relevant to elderly patients.

Cognitive-Behavioral Treatment

Myriad lifestyle changes that accompany aging increase risks of insomnia among older adults (Morgan 2000). With aging comes the increased incidence of infirmities that lead to reduced activity levels and a general flattening of the sleep-wake activity rhythm. Retirement leads to increased vacant time and a loss of both routine and zeitgebers that regulate and stabilize the sleep-wake cycle. Retirement coupled with loss of a spouse may lead to dramatically reduced social contacts and increased boredom. Many individuals attempt to reduce hours of daytime boredom by daytime napping and by staying in bed longer during their nighttime sleep period. Such practices often lead to increased nocturnal wake time. Dysfunctional beliefs about sleep, such as "Everyone should try to get 8 hours a night" and "Older adults can do little to improve their sleep," may actually perpetuate sleep difficulties over time (Means and Edinger 2002; Morin et al. 1993). Nonpharmacological interventions that address these misconceptions and the sleep-disruptive habits they sustain are often useful for combating insomnia in older patients.

Currently, a range of behavioral interventions are available for treating these patients, including relaxation therapies, cognitive therapies, and treatments that target disruptive sleep habits. Among the more effective of these interventions is stimulus control therapy, developed by Bootzin (1972). This treatment is particularly useful for older adults who have fallen out of a normal sleep-wake routine and for those who compromise their nighttime sleep by excessive daytime napping. Stimulus control therapy addresses such problems by curtailing daytime napping and by enforcing a consistent sleep-wake schedule. In addition, this treatment enhances sleep-inducing qualities of the bedroom by eliminating sleep-incompatible behaviors in bed. The patient with insomnia is instructed to go to bed only when sleepy; establish a standard wake-up time; get out of bed whenever he or she is awake for more than 15–20 minutes; avoid reading, watching TV, eating, worrying, and engaging in other sleep-incompatible behaviors in the bed and bedroom; and refrain from daytime napping. This treatment has appeal because it is easily understood and usually can be outlined in one visit. However, follow-up visits are usually needed to ensure compliance and achieve optimal success.

Because older adults appear to have a reduced homeostatic sleep drive (Dijk et al. 1997) as well as a propensity to spend excessive time in bed (Carskadon et al. 1982), measures are often needed to reduce the amount of time older patients with insomnia routinely allot for nocturnal sleep. Such a reduction is the aim of sleep restriction therapy (Spielman et al. 1987; Wohlgemuth and Edinger 2000). Typically this treatment begins with the patient maintaining a sleep log. After 2–3 weeks, the average total sleep time (TST) is calculated. Subsequently, an initial time-in-bed (TIB) prescription may be set either at the average TST or at a value equal to the average TST plus an amount of time that is deemed to represent normal nocturnal wakefulness (e.g., 30 minutes). However, unless evidence suggests that the individual has an unusually low sleep requirement, the initial TIB prescription is seldom set at less than 5 hours per night. The TIB prescription is increased by 15- to 20-minute increments after weeks in which the person with insomnia sleeps more than 85%–90% of the TIB, on average, and continues to report daytime sleepiness. Conversely, TIB is usually reduced by similar increments after weeks in which the individual sleeps less than 80% of the time spent in bed, on average. Because TIB adjustments are usually necessary, sleep restriction therapy typically entails an initial visit, when treatment instructions are given, and follow-up visits, when TIB prescriptions are altered.

Research suggests that stimulus-control and sleep-restriction therapies are more effective than most other nonpharmacological interventions (Morin et al. 1999, 2006; Murtagh and Greenwood 1995). Moreover, a meta-analytic comparison suggests that behavioral therapies compare favorably with hypnotic pharmacotherapies in terms of short-term treatment effects and, unlike hypnotics, have enduring benefits and few side effects (Smith et al. 2002). Clinical trials have also generally suggested that therapies combining stimulus control, sleep restriction, and cognitive strategies to alter dysfunctional sleep-related beliefs hold particular promise for treatment of the sleep maintenance difficulties so common in older age groups (Edinger et al. 2001, 2007; Morin et al. 1999). Given such findings, behavioral interventions should be included in treatment plans for older patients with insomnia, particularly when improper sleep scheduling and other lifestyle factors contribute to sleep complaints.

Pharmacological Treatment

It is well established that untreated insomnia is associated with significant adverse effects (Gislason and Almqvist 1987; Krystal 2007; Zammit et al. 1999). Although a number of medications have been demonstrated to have potent therapeutic effects on this condition (see Table 22–1), the utility of insomnia pharmacotherapy has remained controversial primarily because of concerns about the risks of long-term treatment.

The long-standing view of the medication management of insomnia has been that tolerance and withdrawal are inevitable with use for longer than several weeks (National Institutes of Health Consensus Conference 1984). As a result, treatment for longer periods was discouraged (National Institutes of Health Consensus Conference 1984). It is important to note that this view was not empirically based. It is only more recently that data from placebo-controlled studies of the treatment of insomnia with these agents for periods longer than 3 weeks have been available (Nowell et al. 1997). These studies examining periods up to 1 year of nightly treatment demonstrate that tolerance and withdrawal are not inevitably associated with longer therapy duration (Ancoli-Israel et al. 2005; Krystal et al. 2003, 2008; Walsh et al. 2007). They established the efficacy and safety of the nonbenzodiazepine eszopiclone 3 mg in adults less than age 65 in two 6-month placebo-controlled studies, one of which had a subsequent 6-month open-label extension phase (Krystal et al. 2003; Walsh et al. 2007). Another nonbenzodiazepine, zolpidem 10 mg, was dosed 3–7 nights per week for 6 months in younger adults and was found to improve sleep without evidence of significant adverse effects related to the duration of therapy (Krystal et al. 2008). The only study to examine long-term treatment in older adults identified that in up to 1 year of nightly treatment with the nonbenzodiazepine zaleplon 5–10 mg in an open-label study, there were no significant risks associated with long-term therapy or significant discontinuation effects (Ancoli-Israel et al. 2005). The

TABLE 22–1. Attributes of medications used to treat insomnia

	Half-life (hours)	Principal side effects
Benzodiazepines	2.9–74[a]	Motor and cognitive impairment
Zolpidem	2.6±1	Motor and cognitive impairment
Zaleplon	1	Motor and cognitive impairment
Eszopiclone	6	Motor and cognitive impairment
Ramelteon	1	Dizziness, myalgia
Tricyclic antidepressants	12–43	Anticholinergic effects, weight gain, orthostatic hypotension, sexual dysfunction
Trazodone	11±5	Orthostatic hypotension, priapism (rare)
Mirtazapine	20–40	Dry mouth, weight gain
Diphenhydramine	4±2	Anticholinergic effects, motor impairment
Chloral hydrate	7±3	Alcohol interaction, gastric irritation, motor and cognitive impairment, respiratory depression at high doses

[a]Benzodiazepine half-lives: flurazepam=74±24; diazepam=43±13; quazepam=39; lorazepam=14±5; estazolam=12±12; temazepam=11±6; triazolam=2.9±1.

Source. Golden et al. 1998; Hobbs et al. 1996; Krystal (in press); *Physicians' Desk Reference* 2002; Potter et al. 1998.

long-term efficacy and safety of eszopiclone and zolpidem in older adults remain to be established, as do the efficacy and safety of other agents.

Studies of treatment for up to 2 weeks have established the risk-benefit profile for seven agents available in the United States for the treatment of insomnia. These are the benzodiazepines flurazepam, triazolam, and temazepam; the nonbenzodiazepines eszopiclone, zaleplon, and zolpidem; and the melatonin agonist ramelteon (Krystal, in press). The half-lives and principal side effects of these agents appear in Table 22–1. A number of the benzodiazepines have half-lives that are so long that they are unsuitable insomnia agents because of inevitable daytime impairment. Only triazolam and temazepam have half-lives in a range that makes them reasonable to use in the treatment of insomnia. Of the medications most frequently used to treat insomnia, the nonbenzodiazepine hypnotic zaleplon and the melatonin receptor agonist ramelteon have the shortest half-lives (approximately 1 hour), making them well suited for treating problems falling asleep. Because of its short half-life, zaleplon may also be useful in the middle of the night for individuals who sometimes wake up at that time (Stone et al. 2002). Zolpidem, with a half-life of approximately 2.5 hours, is another agent approved for the treatment of difficulties falling asleep. Although the agent with the shortest half-life that effectively treats the sleep difficulty should always be used in order to minimize risks, individuals with difficulty staying asleep generally need longer-acting agents. Of the agents available in the United States, eszopiclone is the only one demonstrated to improve the ability to stay asleep in older adults with insomnia (McCall et al. 2006). Although antidepressants are widely used to treat insomnia in the United States (most notably trazodone, mirtazapine, doxepin, and amitriptyline), there has yet to be a study of any of these agents in older adults with insomnia (Walsh 2004).

The primary adverse effects of the benzodiazepines and nonbenzodiazepines are motor and cognitive impairment. Many older adults may be particularly vulnerable to adverse outcomes because of these effects. In terms of motor impairment, these agents might be expected to increase the risks for falls in older adults. Although there is evidence for an association of falls with benzodiazepines, nonbenzodiazepines, and medications with anticholinergic and antiadrenergic effects (includes antihistamines and antidepressants), there are also studies suggesting that untreated insomnia increases the risks for falls (Allain et al. 2005; Avidan et al. 2005; Brassington et al. 2000; Koski et al. 1998; Nebes et al. 2007; Neutel et al. 2002; Suzuki et al. 1992). Further research will be needed to provide guidance, when managing insomnia in clinical practice, as to how to take into account the risks of falls caused by being awake at night versus the risks of falls caused by medications.

In this regard, as with the treatment of any condition, decisions regarding the treatment of insomnia should involve weighing the risks and benefits associated with each of the available treatment options (each of the insomnia medications versus cognitive-behavioral therapy for insomnia versus no treatment). The available studies of the pharmacological treatment represent the empirical basis for making such decisions. Although these studies establish a favorable risk-benefit profile for a number of agents over periods of treatment up to 2 weeks, clearly more studies are needed to provide a more effective guide for the treatment of insomnia in older adults. Given the limited number of studies in older adults, it is tempting to apply the results of studies carried out in younger adults to the treatment of older insomnia patients. However, this should be done with great caution given the greater vulnerability to adverse effects of older adults and the likelihood that medication blood levels will be higher and the effects will be longer lasting because of slower drug metabolism in this population (Krystal, in press).

In summary, although cognitive-behavioral therapy should always be considered for the treatment of insomnia, medications may be needed in some cases. In general, it is best to use agents with relatively short half-lives to minimize risks of daytime impairment. However, some older adults require an agent that addresses difficulty staying asleep. A number of medications have been demonstrated to have a favorable risk-benefit profile for the treatment of insomnia in older individuals and can be used in such cases. However, it is important to be cognizant of the risks of treatment in this highly vulnerable population. More studies of insomnia therapies in older adults and, in particular, of longer-term trials of treatment are needed.

Conclusion

Management of sleep disorders in elderly patients is challenging. Although sleep disorders are not an inevitable consequence of aging, elderly persons are more prone to primary sleep disorders and medical and psychiatric conditions that cause sleep difficulties. Therefore, evaluation of a sleep complaint in an elderly individual should include a thorough workup to determine whether primary sleep pathology and associated psychiatric and medical disorders are present. Effective behavioral and medication treatments exist for treating sleep and circadian rhythm disorders in elderly patients, but these treatments have significant limitations. More research is needed to develop and assess nonmedication therapies that are effective in treating insomnia and normalizing the circadian rhythm. Particularly promising areas include cognitive-behavioral sleep therapy, and exercise programs.

In addition, research to improve medication treatment is needed. More medications are needed that can help elderly individuals stay asleep without causing next-day sedation. Furthermore, medications are needed that do not cause motor or cognitive impairment or anticholinergic side effects and that have been evaluated in trials of long-term treatment in older adults. Studies of the efficacy and safety of antidepressants in the treatment of insomnia in older adults are also needed.

Finally, a better understanding of sundowning is needed, as are more effective treatments for this common condition.

Key Points

- More than one-half of noninstitutionalized individuals older than 65 years report chronic sleep difficulties.
- Although disturbed sleep is not an inevitable consequence of aging, the elderly are at increased risk of experiencing a number of sleep disorders and are uniquely vulnerable to the consequences of these disorders, which include insomnia, restless legs syndrome, sleep apnea, and disorders of circadian rhythm.
- Effective behavioral and medication treatments exist for treating sleep and circadian rhythm disorders in elderly patients, but more research is needed to develop improved treatments and to establish the risk-benefit profiles of some of the most commonly administered therapies.

References

Aldrich MS: Cardinal manifestations of sleep disorders, in Principles and Practice of Sleep Medicine, 3rd Edition. Edited by Kryger MH, Roth T, Dement WC. Philadelphia, PA, WB Saunders, 2000, pp 526–534

Allain H, Bentué-Ferrer D, Polard E, et al: Postural instability and consequent falls and hip fractures associated with use of hypnotics in the elderly: a comparative review. Drugs Aging 22:749–765, 2005

American Academy of Sleep Medicine: Practice parameters for the use of actigraphy in the assessment of sleep and sleep disorders: an update for 2007. Sleep 30:519–529, 2007

American Psychiatric Association: Diagnostic and Statistical Manual of Mental Disorders, 4th Edition, Text Revision. Washington, DC, American Psychiatric Association, 2000

American Sleep Disorders Association: The International Classification of Sleep Disorders: Diagnostic and Coding Manual, Revised Edition. Rochester, MN, American Sleep Disorders Association, 1997

Ancoli-Israel S: Epidemiology of sleep disorders. Clin Geriatr Med 5:347–362, 1989

Ancoli-Israel S, Kripke DF, Mason W: Characteristics of obstructive and central sleep apnea in the elderly: an interim report. Biol Psychiatry 22:741–750, 1987

Ancoli-Israel S, Kripke DF, Klauber MR, et al: Periodic limb movements in sleep in community-dwelling elderly. Sleep 14:496–500, 1991

Ancoli-Israel S, Richardson GS, Mangano RM, et al: Long-term use of sedative hypnotics in older patients with insomnia. Sleep Med 6:107–113, 2005

Avidan AY, Fries BE, James ML, et al: Insomnia and hypnotic use, recorded in the minimum data set, as predictors of falls and hip fractures in Michigan nursing homes. J Am Geriatr Soc 53:955–962, 2005

Bassetti C, Chervin R: Cerebrovascular diseases, in Principles and Practice of Sleep Medicine, 3rd Edition. Edited by Kryger MH, Roth T, Dement WC. Philadelphia, PA, WB Saunders, 2000, pp 1072–1086

Bliwise DL: Sleep in normal aging and dementia. Sleep 16:40–81, 1993

Bliwise DL: Normal aging, in Principles and Practice of Sleep Medicine, 3rd Edition. Edited by Kryger MH, Roth T, Dement WC. Philadelphia, PA, WB Saunders, 2000, pp 26–42

Bliwise DL, Petta D, Seidel W, et al: Periodic leg movements during sleep in the elderly. Arch Gerontol Geriatr 4:273–281, 1985

Bliwise DL, Freeman A, Ingram CD, et al: Randomized, double-blind, placebo-controlled, short-term trial of ropinirole in restless legs syndrome. Sleep Med 6:141–147, 2005

Bootzin RR: A stimulus control treatment for insomnia. Proc Am Psychol Assoc 7:395–396, 1972

Brassington GS, King AC, Bliwise DL: Sleep problems as a risk factor for falls in a sample of community-dwelling adults aged 64–99 years. J Am Geriatr Soc 48:1234–1240, 2000

Breslau N, Roth T, Rosenthal L, et al: Sleep disturbance and psychiatric disorders: a longitudinal epidemiological study of young adults. Biol Psychiatry 39:411–418, 1996

Buysse DJ, Ancoli-Israel S, Edinger JD, et al: Recommendations for a standard research assessment of insomnia. Sleep 29:1155–1173, 2006

Carskadon MA, Brown ED, Dement WC: Sleep fragmentation in the elderly: relationship to daytime sleep tendency. Neurobiol Aging 3:321–327, 1982

Clarenbach P: Parkinson's disease and sleep. J Neurol 247 (suppl 4): IV20–IV23, 2000

Clark MM: Restless legs syndrome. J Am Board Fam Pract 14:368–374, 2001

Connaughton JJ, Catterall JR, Elton RA, et al: Do sleep studies contribute to the management of patients with severe chronic obstructive pulmonary disease? Am Rev Respir Dis 138:341–344, 1988

Czeisler CA, Johnson MP, Duffy JF, et al: Exposure to bright light and darkness to treat physiologic maladaptation to night work. N Engl J Med 322:1253–1259, 1990

Czeisler CA, Duffy JF, Shanahan TL, et al: Stability, precision, and near-24-hour period of the human circadian pacemaker. Science 284:2177–2181, 1999

Dickel MJ, Mosko SS: Morbidity cut-offs for sleep apnea and periodic leg movements in predicting subjective complaints in seniors. Sleep 13:155–166, 1990

Dijk DJ, Duffy JF, Riel E, et al: Altered interaction of circadian and homeostatic aspects of sleep propensity results in awakening at an earlier circadian phase in older people. Sleep Research 26:710, 1997

Dorsey CM, Lee KA, Scharf MB. Effect of zolpidem on sleep in women with perimenopausal and postmenopausal insomnia: a 4-week, randomized, multicenter, double-blind, placebo-controlled study. Clin Ther 26:1578–1586, 2004

Douglas NJ: Chronic obstructive pulmonary disease, in Principles and Practice of Sleep Medicine, 3rd Edition. Edited by Kryger MH, Roth T, Dement WC. Philadelphia, PA, WB Saunders, 2000, pp 965–975

Duffy JF, Dijk DJ, Klerman EB, et al: Later endogenous circadian temperature nadir relative to an earlier wake time in older people. Am J Physiol 275:R1478–R1487, 1998

Edinger JD, Wohlgemuth WK, Radtke RA, et al: Cognitive behavioral therapy for treatment of chronic primary insomnia: a randomized controlled trial. JAMA 285:1856–1864, 2001

Edinger JD, Wohlgemuth WK, Krystal AD, et al: Behavioral insomnia therapy for fibromyalgia patients: a randomized clinical trial. Arch Intern Med 165:2527–2535, 2005

Edinger JD, Wohlgemuth WK, Radtke RA, et al: Dose response effects of cognitive-behavioral insomnia therapy: a randomized clinical trial. Sleep 30:203–212, 2007

Fava M, McCall WV, Krystal A, et al: Eszopiclone co-administered with fluoxetine in patients with insomnia co-existing with major depressive disorder. Biol Psychiatry 59:1052–1060, 2006

Fawcett J, Scheftner WA, Fogg L, et al: Time-related predictors of suicide in major affective disorder. Am J Psychiatry 147:1189–1894, 1990

Foley DJ, Monjan AA, Brown SL, et al: Sleep complaints among elderly persons: an epidemiologic study of three communities. Sleep 18:425–432, 1995

Folkard S, Totterdell P: "Time since sleep" and "body clock" components of alertness and cognition. Acta Psychiatr Belg 94:73–74, 1994

Gislason T, Almqvist M: Somatic diseases and sleep complaints: an epidemiological study of 3,201 Swedish men. Acta Med Scand 221:475–481, 1987

Golden RN, Dawkins K, Nicholas L, et al: Trazodone, nefazodone, bupropion, and mirtazapine, in Textbook of Psychopharmacology, 2nd Edition. Edited by Schatzberg AF, Nemeroff CB. Washington, DC, American Psychiatric Press, 1998, pp 251–269

Hall M, Buysse DJ, Dew MA, et al: Intrusive thoughts and avoidance behaviors are associated with sleep disturbances in bereavement-related depression. Depress Anxiety 6:106–112, 1997

Hirshkowitz M, Moore CA, Hamilton CR, et al: Polysomnography of adults and elderly: sleep architecture, respiration, and leg movement. J Clin Neurophysiol 9:56–62, 1992

Hobbs WR, Rall TW, Verdoorn TA: Hypnotics and sedatives: ethanol, in Goodman and Gilman's The Pharmacological Basis of Therapeutics, 9th Edition. Edited by Hardman JG, Limbird LE. New York, McGraw-Hill, 1996, pp 361–398

Hoch CC, Buysse DJ, Reynolds CF: Sleep and depression in late life. Clin Geriatr Med 5:259–272, 1989

Kales HC, Valenstein M, Kim HM, et al: Mortality risk in patients with dementia treated with antipsychotics versus other psychiatric medications. Am J Psychiatry 164:1568–1576, 2007

Koski K, Luukinen H, Laippala P, et al: Risk factors for major injurious falls among the home-dwelling elderly by functional abilities: a prospective population-based study. Gerontology 44:232–238, 1998

Kryger M, Wang-Weigand S, Zhang J, et al: Effect of Ramelteon, a selective MT(1)/MT (2)-receptor agonist, on respiration during sleep in mild to moderate COPD. Sleep Breath Dec 1, 2007 [Epub ahead of print]

Krystal AD: Sleep and psychiatry: future directions. Psychiatr Clin North Am 29:1115–1130, 2006

Krystal AD: Treating the health, quality of life, and functional impairments in insomnia. J Clin Sleep Med 3:63–72, 2007

Krystal AD: A compendium of placebo-controlled trials of the risks/benefits of pharmacologic treatments for insomnia: the empirical basis for clinical practice. Sleep Med Rev (in press)

Krystal AD, Edinger J, Wohlgemuth W, et al: Sleep in peri-menopausal and post-menopausal women. Sleep Med Rev 2:243–253, 1998

Krystal AD, Walsh JK, Laska E, et al: Sustained efficacy of eszopiclone over six months of nightly treatment: results of a randomized, double-blind, placebo controlled study in adults with chronic insomnia. Sleep 26:793–799, 2003

Krystal AD, Fava M, Rubens R, et al: Evaluation of eszopiclone discontinuation after co-therapy with fluoxetine for insomnia with co-existing depression. J Clin Sleep Med 3:48–55, 2007

Krystal AD, Erman M, Zammit GK, et al: Long-term efficacy and safety of zolpidem extended-release 12.5 mg, administered 3 to 7 nights per week for 24 weeks, in patients with chronic primary insomnia: a 6-month, randomized, double-blind, placebo-controlled, parallel-group, multicenter study. Sleep 31:79–90, 2008

Lees AJ, Blackburn NA, Campbell VL: The nighttime problems of Parkinson's disease. Clin Neuropharmacol 11:512–519, 1988

Livingston G, Blizard B, Mann A: Does sleep disturbance predict depression in elderly people? A study in inner London. Br J Gen Pract 44:445–448, 1994

McCall WV, Erman M, Krystal AD, et al: A polysomnography study of eszopiclone in elderly patients with insomnia. Curr Med Res Opin 22:1633–1642, 2006

Means MK, Edinger JD: Behavioral treatment of insomnia. Expert Review of Neurotherapeutics 2:127–137, 2002

Middelkoop HA, Smilde-van den Doel DA, Neven AK, et al: Subjective sleep characteristics of 1,485 males and females aged 50–93: effects of sex and age and factors related to self-evaluated quality of sleep. J Gerontol A Biol Sci Med Sci 51:M108–M115, 1996

Minors DS, Waterhouse JM, Akerstedt T: The effect of the timing, quality, and quantity of sleep upon the depression (masking) of body temperature on an irregular sleep/wake schedule. J Sleep Res 3:45–51, 1994

Montplaisir J, Nicolas A, Denesle R, et al: Restless legs syndrome improved by pramipexole: a double-blind randomized trial. Neurology 52:938–943, 1999

Morgan K: Sleep and aging, in Treatment of Late-Life Insomnia. Edited by Lichstein KL, Morin CM. Thousand Oaks, CA, Sage, 2000, pp 3–36

Morin CM, Stone J, Trinkle D, et al: Dysfunctional beliefs and attitudes about sleep among older adults with and without insomnia complaints. Psychol Aging 8:463–467, 1993

Morin CM, Colecchi C, Stone J, et al: Behavioral and pharmacological therapies for late-life insomnia: a randomized controlled trial. JAMA 281:991–1035, 1999

Morin CM, Bootzin R, Buysse DJ, et al: Psychological and behavioral treatment for insomnia. Sleep 29:1398–1414, 2006

Murciano D, Armengaud MH, Cramer PH, et al: Acute effects of zolpidem, triazolam and flunitrazepam on arterial blood gases and control of breathing in severe COPD. Eur Respir J 6:625–629, 1993

Murtagh DR, Greenwood KM: Identifying effective psychological treatments for insomnia: a meta-analysis. J Consult Clin Psychol 63:79–89, 1995

National Institutes of Health: National Institutes of Health State of the Science Conference statement on manifestations and management of chronic insomnia in adults, June 13–15, 2005. Sleep 28:1049–1057, 2005

National Institutes of Health Consensus Conference: Drugs and insomnia: the use of medications to promote sleep. JAMA 251:2410–2414, 1984

National Institutes of Health Consensus Development Conference Statement: The treatment of sleep disorders in older people, March 26–28, 1990. Sleep 14:169–177, 1991

Nebes RD, Pollock BG, Halligan EM, et al: Serum anticholinergic activity and motor performance in elderly persons. J Gerontol A Biol Sci Med Sci 62:83–85, 2007

Neutel CI, Perry S, Maxwell C: Medication use and risk of falls. Pharmacoepidemiol Drug Saf 11:97–104, 2002

Nowell PD, Mazumdar S, Buysse DJ, et al: Benzodiazepines and zolpidem for chronic insomnia: a meta-analysis of treatment efficacy. JAMA 278:2170–2177, 1997

Ohayon MM: Epidemiology of insomnia: what we know and what we still need to learn. Sleep Med Rev 6:97–111, 2002

O'Keeffe ST, Gavin K, Lavan JN: Iron status and restless legs syndrome in the elderly. Age Ageing 23:200–203, 1994

Ozminkowski RJ, Wang S, Walsh JK: The direct and indirect costs of untreated insomnia in adults in the United States. Sleep 30:263–273, 2007

Physicians' Desk Reference, 56th Edition. Montvale, NJ, Medical Economics, 2002

Pilowsky I, Crettenden I, Townley M: Sleep disturbance in pain clinic patients. Pain 23:27–33, 1985

Pollak CP, Perlick D: Sleep problems and institutionalization of the elderly. J Geriatr Psychiatry Neurol 4:204–210, 1991

Pollak CP, Perlick D, Linsner JP, et al: Sleep problems in the community elderly as predictors of death and nursing home placement. J Community Health 15:123–135, 1990

Potter WZ, Manji HK, Rudorfer MV: Tricyclics and tetracyclics, in Textbook of Psychopharmacology, 2nd Edition. Edited by Schatzberg AF, Nemeroff CB. Washington, DC, American Psychiatric Press, 1998, pp 239–250

Prinz PN: Sleep and sleep disorders in older adults. J Clin Neurophysiol 12:139–146, 1995

Prinz PN, Peskind ER, Vitaliano PP, et al: Changes in the sleep and waking EEGs of nondemented and demented elderly subjects. J Am Geriatr Soc 30:86–93, 1982

Prinz PN, Vitiello MV, Raskind MA, et al: Geriatrics: sleep disorders and aging. N Engl J Med 323:520–526, 1990

Reynolds CF 3rd, Frank E, Houck PR, et al: Which elderly patients with remitted depression remain well with continued interpersonal psychotherapy after discontinuation of antidepressant medication? Am J Psychiatry 154:958–962, 1997

Riedel BW, Lichstein KL: Objective sleep measures and subjective sleep satisfaction: how do older adults with insomnia define a good night's sleep? Psychol Aging 13:159–163, 1998

Roehrs T, Zorick F, Sicklesteel J, et al: Age-related sleep-wake disorders at a sleep disorder center. J Am Geriatr Soc 31:364–370, 1983

Sanford JRA: Tolerance of debility in elderly dependants by supporters at home: its significance for hospital practice. Br Med J 3:471–473, 1975

Shaw SH, Curson H, Coquelin JP: A double-blind comparative study of zolpidem and placebo in the treatment of insomnia in elderly psychiatric inpatients. J Int Med Res 20:150–161, 1992

Smith MT, Perlis ML, Park A, et al: Comparative meta-analysis of pharmacotherapy and behavior therapy for persistent insomnia. Am J Psychiatry 159:5–11, 2002

Soares CN, Joffe H, Rubens R, et al: Eszopiclone in patients with insomnia during perimenopause and early postmenopause: a randomized controlled trial. Obstet Gynecol 108:1402–1410, 2006

Spielman AJ, Saskin P, Thorpy MJ: Treatment of chronic insomnia by restriction of time in bed. Sleep 10:45–55, 1987

Steens RD, Pouliot Z, Millar TW, et al: Effects of zolpidem and triazolam on sleep and respiration in mild to moderate chronic obstructive pulmonary disease. Sleep 16:318–326, 1993

Stone BM, Turner C, Mills SL, et al: Noise-induced sleep maintenance insomnia: hypnotic and residual effects of zaleplon. Br J Clin Pharmacol 53:196–202, 2002

Suzuki M, Okamura T, Shimazu Y, et al: A study of falls experienced by institutionalized elderly. Nippon Koshu Eisei Zasshi 39:927–940, 1992

Trenkwalder C: Sleep dysfunction in Parkinson's disease. Clin Neurosci 5:107–114, 1998

Walsh JK: Drugs used to treat insomnia in 2002: regulatory-based rather than evidence-based medicine. Sleep 27:14441–14442, 2004

Walsh JK, Muehlbach MJ, Lauter SA, et al: Effects of triazolam on sleep, daytime sleepiness, and morning stiffness in patients with rheumatoid arthritis. J Rheumatol 23:245–252, 1996

Walsh JK, Krystal AD, Amata DA, et al: Nightly treatment of primary insomnia with eszopiclone for six months: effect on sleep, quality of life, and work limitations. Sleep 30:959–968, 2007

Weissman MM, Greenwald S, Niño-Murcia G, et al: The morbidity of insomnia uncomplicated by psychiatric disorders. Gen Hosp Psychiatry 19:245–250, 1997

White DP: Central sleep apnea, in Principles and Practice of Sleep Medicine, 3rd Edition. Edited by Kryger MH, Roth T, Dement WC. Philadelphia, WB Saunders, 2000, pp 827–839

Wohlgemuth WK, Edinger JD: Sleep restriction therapy, in Treatment of Late-Life Insomnia. Edited by Lichstein KL, Morin CM. Thousand Oaks, CA, Sage, 2000, pp 147–184

Zammit GK, Weiner J, Damato N, et al: Quality of life in people with insomnia. Sleep 22 (suppl 2):S379–S385, 1999

Zepelin H, McDonald CS, Zammit GK: Effects of age on auditory awakening thresholds. J Gerontol 39:294–300, 1984

Suggested Readings

Ancoli-Israel S, Richardson GS, Mangano RM, et al: Long-term use of sedative hypnotics in older patients with insomnia. Sleep Med 6:107–113, 2005

Bliwise DL: Sleep in normal aging and dementia. Sleep 16:40–81, 1993

National Institutes of Health Consensus Development Conference Statement: The treatment of sleep disorders in older people, March 26–28, 1990. Sleep 14:169–177, 1991

Pollak CP, Perlick D: Sleep problems and institutionalization of the elderly. J Geriatr Psychiatry Neurol 4:204–210, 1991

Pollak CP, Perlick D, Linsner JP, et al: Sleep problems in the community elderly as predictors of death and nursing home placement. J Community Health 15:123–135, 1990

CHAPTER 23

Alcohol and Drug Problems

David W. Oslin, M.D.
Shahrzad Mavandadi, Ph.D.

Alcohol and drug misuse are associated with a wide array of negative physical and mental health outcomes that are exacerbated with advancing age, such as functional and cognitive decline, compromised immune function, and depression. Yet relatively little work has examined the correlates and consequences of substance use among older adults. Accordingly, substance misuse in later life, which encompasses alcohol and illicit, prescription, and over-the-counter drugs, has been called an "invisible epidemic" (Widlitz and Marin 2002). Epidemiological work, which has focused on younger populations, demonstrates that beginning in the mid to late 20s, overall rates of alcohol and illicit drug use begin to decline, with the majority of older adults reporting no substance use. Nevertheless, changes in demographic and cohort trends suggest that substance misuse in later life is a pressing public health matter and that older adults represent a group in growing need of specialized substance treatment programs and services (Gfroerer et al. 2003).

With the aging of the U.S. population and the resultant increase in the proportion of adults living to advanced ages, recent years have seen a concomitant increase in the number of older adults who misuse alcohol and drugs. Not only are older adults the fastest-growing segment of the U.S. population, but in the next several decades the aging population will be composed primarily of "baby boomers," individuals born between the years 1946 and 1964. The aging of the baby boom cohort poses unique challenges to providers; in addition to reporting higher rates of illicit drug and alcohol use and addiction than earlier cohorts, the baby boom cohort also is significantly larger than previous cohorts (Koenig et al. 1994).

The potential public health impact of these demographic trends is highlighted by examining changes in rates of substance use and misuse in the last several decades. For example, it has been estimated that from the early 1990s until 2002, the prevalence of alcohol abuse or dependence tripled to 3.1% among adults ages 65 and older (Grant et al. 2004). Heavy and binge drinking among adults over age 65 also has increased, with recent reports citing rates near 7.6% (Office of Applied Studies 2007) (Figure 23–1). Reports of substance use among the baby boomers are notably higher; 22% of adults ages 50–54 were heavy or binge drinkers in 2006 (Figure 23–1), and rates of illicit drug use among those in this age group increased from 3.4% to 6.0% from 2002 to 2006 (Office of Applied Studies 2007) (Figure 23–2).

In light of these epidemiological changes, it is projected that by the year 2020, the number of older adults requiring substance abuse treatment will increase to 4.4 million, a significant departure from the estimated 1.7 million in need of treatment in 2000 and 2001 (Gfroerer et al. 2003). Hence, in order to meet the special needs of older adults experiencing problems with alcohol and drugs, it is imperative that social services professionals and providers within primary and specialty care settings, particularly specialty mental health care, learn to recognize signs and symptoms of substance misuse and gain a firm understanding of

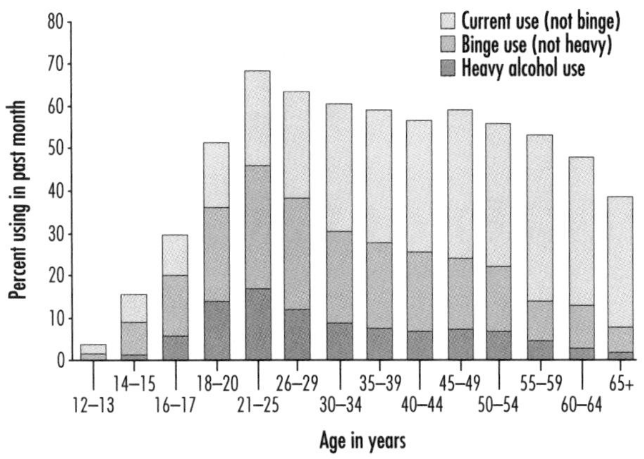

FIGURE 23–1. Current, binge, and heavy alcohol use across the life span in 2006.

Source. Reprinted from Office of Applied Studies: *Results From the 2006 National Survey on Drug Use and Health: National Findings* (DHHS Publ No SMA 07-4293, NSDUH Series H-32). Rockville, MD, Substance Abuse and Mental Health Services Administration, 2007. Available at http://www.oas.samhsa.gov/NSDUH/2k6NSDUH/2k6results.cfm#Ch3. Accessed February 5, 2008.

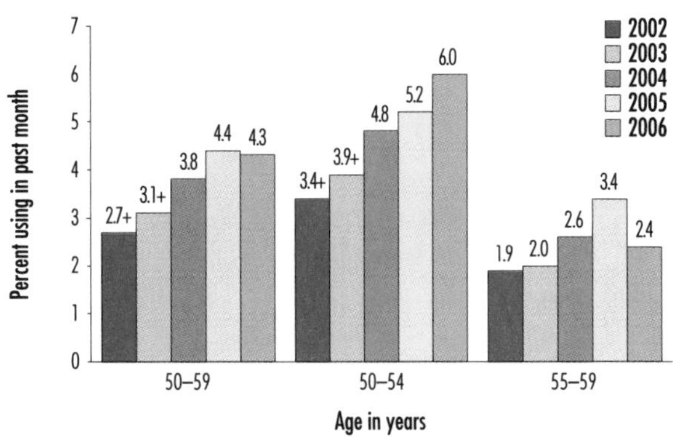

FIGURE 23–2. Rise in the prevalence of illicit drug use among late-middle-aged adults over the last 5 years.

Source. Reprinted from Office of Applied Studies: *Results From the 2006 National Survey on Drug Use and Health: National Findings* (DHHS Publ No SMA 07-4293, NSDUH Series H-32). Rockville, MD, Substance Abuse and Mental Health Services Administration, 2007. Available at http://www.oas.samhsa.gov/NSDUH/2k6NSDUH/2k6Results.cfm#2.1. Accessed February 5, 2008.

available treatment options. Doing so will enhance efforts directed toward reducing problematic use and foster improvements in overall quality of life among older adults with substance use problems.

Guidelines and Classification: A Spectrum of Use

Proper screening, diagnosis, and treatment of individuals with drug and/or alcohol problems requires an understanding of both drinking guidelines and the full range of substance use behavior seen among older adults. Because physiological factors render older adults more sensitive not only to alcohol and illicit drugs but also to over-the-counter and prescription medications, guidelines and recommendations for use of these substances by older adults differ from those applied to younger adults. For example, lean body mass and total water volume decrease relative to total fat volume in later life. As a result, total body volume decreases, thereby increasing the serum concentration, absorption, and distribution of alcohol and drugs in the body (Moore et al. 2007). Age-related declines in the efficiency of metabolic enzymes that target these substances as well as increases in central nervous system sensitivity also contribute to an amplified response to drug and alcohol use among older adults. Furthermore, interactions between alcohol and over-the-counter or prescription medications, which are commonly used by older adults for a variety of acute and chronic medical and psychiatric conditions, may be especially harmful. Consuming alcohol in combination with prescription or over-the-counter drugs may lead to exaggerated or adverse therapeutic effects or, conversely, a blunting of the effectiveness of some medications (Moore et al. 2007).

Taking these age-related factors into account, guidelines for alcohol use are lower for older relative to younger adults. Recommendations set forth by the National Institute on Alcohol Abuse and Alcoholism and the Center for Substance Abuse Treatment's Treatment Improvement Protocol on older adults state that adults ages 65 and older should consume no more than one standard drink per day (Table 23–1) (Blow 1998; National Institute on Alcohol Abuse and Alcoholism 1995). Moreover, older adults should not consume more than two standard drinks on any one occasion (binge drinking). These drinking-limit recommendations are in accord with data concerning the relationship between heavy consumption and alcohol-related problems (Chermack et al. 1996) as well as evidence for the beneficial health effects of low-risk drinking among older adults (Klatsky and Armstrong 1993; Poikolainen 1991).

Recommendations regarding the appropriate prescription and use of over-the-counter and prescription

TABLE 23–1. Alcohol conversion chart

"1 standard drink"	
Beverage type	*Quantity*
Beer	12 oz.
Wine	5 oz.
Fortified wine	3 oz.
Hard liquor (80-proof distilled spirits)	1½ oz. (i.e., "a shot")
Malt liquor	8 oz.
Liqueur or aperitif	4 oz.
Additional conversions	
Beverage type/quantity	*No. of standard drinks*
Beer	
1 6-pack of 16-oz. cans/bottles	8
1 quart	3
1 liter (33.8 oz.)	2.8
Wine (e.g., red, white, Chianti)	
1 bottle (25 oz.)	5
1 bottle (40 oz.)	8
Fifth	6
1 magnum	12
½ gallon	16
Fortified wine (e.g., sherry, port; low-end wines [e.g., Thunderbird, "bum wine"])	
Pint	7
Fifth	12
Hard liquor (e.g., bourbon, rum, gin, tequila, vodka)	
Fifth	18
Pint	11
Quart	20
½ gallon	40
1 bottle (25 oz.)	17
1 bottle (40 oz.)	27
Malt liquor (e.g., Old English)	
12 oz.	1½
Forty (40 oz.)	5

drugs must be considered on a case-by-case basis, with special consideration given to the potential benefits relative to the potential risks of medication use for each patient. There are no accepted safe limits for tobacco, marijuana, or other illicit drug use.

Although the guidelines and recommendations for substance use outlined above address acceptable limits, it is important to recognize that there is still a great deal of variability in the degree to which older adults use alcohol and drugs. Understanding patterns of use can help inform the treatment and counseling of older adults in numerous settings. Thus, in order to capture this variability, or "spectrum of use," a number of categories have been created. The following categories and their definitions, which primarily focus on patterns of alcohol use, reflect both the clinical experience and research findings of addiction specialists (Blow 1998).

Abstainers is the term used to describe individuals who report drinking less than 1–2 drinks in the previous year. This is the most common drinking pattern in later life, with approximately 50%–70% of older adults reporting abstinence (Blow 1998; Kirchner et al. 2007). Nevertheless, determining the reasons for abstinence has important implications for subsequent treatment and counseling of older adults who do not drink. For example, although some individuals may have had lifelong patterns of abstinence, others may not drink because of the onset or presence of acute or chronic illness. Furthermore, some individuals may abstain from alcohol use because of a previous history of alcohol problems or abuse. This latter group, in particular, deserves special consideration and would benefit from preventive monitoring and screening. Not only could new stressors cause relapse among those with a history of problematic drinking or abuse, but past use may make older adults more vulnerable to other mental health problems such as psychiatric disorders or cognitive declines.

Low-risk, social, or moderate drinkers include individuals who drink within the recommended guidelines (i.e., drink no more than one drink per day) and do not exhibit any alcohol-related problems. Older adults in this group also observe caution and do not drink when driving a motor vehicle or boat, nor do they drink when using contraindicated medications.

Low-risk medication/drug use involves adhering to physicians' prescriptions. Nevertheless, it is important to evaluate the number and types of medications being used by low-risk users, because harmful medication interactions may still occur among this group.

At-risk or excessive substance users among older adults are those who consume substances above recommended levels yet experience minimal or no substance-related health, social, or emotional problems. At-risk substance use in older adults generally applies to the consumption of alcohol or prescription and over-the-counter medications rather than illicit drugs. Given the guidelines outlined above, excessive alcohol use readily can be defined as drinking more than one drink per day. On the other hand, determining a prespecified threshold beyond which drug use poses a risk is more challenging. This is because of the high variability in appropriate pharmacological treatment regimens and recommendations that result from individuals having different medical circumstances and needs. However, identification of older adults who are taking high doses of medication and have also been on medications for a period of time exceeding what would be reasonable clinical practice would help target individuals who may be at risk. For example, the prolonged or improper use of psychoactive medications, such as benzodiazepines, presents a particularly high risk of negative health outcomes and adverse drug reactions (Simon et al. 1996). Targeting and identifying older adults in this category is important; although they currently may not be experiencing any substance use–related problems, these individuals may have a high risk of developing alcohol- or medication-related health problems should their substance use remain consistent or increase over time. Preventive brief interventions for at-risk users are valuable and effective, and abstinence or reductions in substance use have been shown to improve quality of life for this group.

Problem use or abuse describes a pattern in older adults in which alcohol or drug consumption is at a level whereby adverse medical, psychological, or social consequences have occurred or are significantly likely to occur. Thus, this category of use is not dependent on the quantity or frequency of use but rather the extent to which substance use impairs physical and/or psychosocial functioning. As seen in Table 23–2, problems reported by problem users fall short of meeting diagnostic criteria for substance dependence (described later in this chapter). It is important to note, however, that some of the standardized symptoms of abuse listed in DSM-IV-TR (American Psychiatric Association 2000), such as employment problems or interpersonal difficulties, may not be as readily applied to older adults, given age-related factors such as retirement, widowhood, and resultant changes in occupational and social roles and network composition. As a result, the risks associated with this pattern of substance use may be underestimated. Nevertheless, because older adults in this group are at a greater risk of negative consequences such as falls, liver disease, pancreatitis, and harmful alcohol-medication interactions (Moore et al. 2000), they represent a group that would greatly benefit from screening, identification, and intervention.

Alcohol or drug dependence is defined, according to DSM-IV-TR criteria, as a medical disorder marked by clinically significant distress or impairment coupled with preoccupation with alcohol or drugs, loss of control, continued substance use despite adverse consequences, and/or physiological symptoms such as tolerance and withdrawal (American Psychiatric Association 2000) (Table 23–2). As is the case for substance use, DSM-IV-TR criteria are based mostly on research with young to middle-aged adults and have not been sufficiently validated among older populations; therefore, the symptoms and consequences set forth in DSM may not be sensitive enough to capture dependence in later life. Moreover, determining whether individuals meet diagnostic criteria relies heavily on self-reported behavioral symptoms. This is potentially problematic because self-report is susceptible to bias because of memory impairments, lack of insight or knowledge regarding the adverse effects of substance use, or unwillingness to admit symptoms. For example, benzodiazepine abuse and dependence may go unnoticed or unreported because of older adults not linking the consequences of medication use to health or social problems. Notwithstanding these limitations in diagnostic criteria, identifying older adults with alcohol or drug dependence is essential because this represents a group in need of specialized treatment and services.

Epidemiology of Late-Life Substance Use

Alcohol

Even though alcohol misuse is often underreported and thus underestimated in later life, epidemiological work suggests that alcohol problems are common among older adults. For instance, the most recent National Survey on Drug Use and Health reported that 48.0% of adults ages 60 to 64 had consumed alcohol in the past month, with 35.2% currently reporting nonbinge or nonheavy use, 10.1% reporting bingeing behavior, and 2.7% reporting

TABLE 23–2. DSM-IV-TR criteria for substance abuse and dependence

Criteria for Substance Abuse

A. A maladaptive pattern of substance use leading to clinically significant impairment or distress, as manifested by one (or more) of the following, occurring within a 12-month period:

(1) recurrent substance use resulting in a failure to fulfill major role obligations at work, school, or home (e.g., repeated absences or poor work performance related to substance use; substance-related absences, suspensions, or expulsions from school; neglect of children or household)

(2) recurrent substance use in situations in which it is physically hazardous (e.g., driving an automobile or operating a machine when impaired by substance use)

(3) recurrent substance-related legal problems (e.g., arrests for substance-related disorderly conduct)

(4) continued substance use despite having persistent or recurrent social or interpersonal problems caused or exacerbated by the effects of the substance (e.g., arguments with spouse about consequences of intoxication, physical fights)

B. The symptoms have never met the criteria for substance dependence for this class of substance.

Criteria for Substance Dependence

A maladaptive pattern of substance use, leading to clinically significant impairment or distress, as manifested by three (or more) of the following, occurring at any time in the same 12-month period:

(1) tolerance, as defined by either of the following:

(a) a need for markedly increased amounts of the substance to achieve intoxication or desired effect

(b) markedly diminished effect with continued use of the same amount of the substance

(2) withdrawal, as manifested by either of the following:

(a) the characteristic withdrawal syndrome for the substance (refer to Criteria A and B of the criteria sets for withdrawal from the specific substances)

(b) the same (or a closely related) substance is taken to relieve or avoid withdrawal symptoms

(3) the substance is often taken in larger amounts or over a longer period than was intended

(4) there is a persistent desire or unsuccessful efforts to cut down or control substance use

(5) a great deal of time is spent in activities necessary to obtain the substance (e.g., visiting multiple doctors or driving long distances), use the substance (e.g., chain-smoking), or recover from its effects

(6) important social, occupational, or recreational activities are given up or reduced because of substance use

(7) the substance use is continued despite knowledge of having a persistent or recurrent physical or psychological problem that is likely to have been caused or exacerbated by the substance (e.g., current cocaine use despite recognition of cocaine-induced depression, or continued drinking despite recognition that an ulcer was made worse by alcohol consumption)

Specify if:

With Physiological Dependence: evidence of tolerance or withdrawal (i.e., either Item 1 or 2 is present)
Without Physiological Dependence: no evidence of tolerance or withdrawal (i.e., neither Item 1 nor 2 is present)

Course specifiers (see text for definitions):

Early Full Remission
Early Partial Remission
Sustained Full Remission
Sustained Partial Remission
On Agonist Therapy
In a Controlled Environment

Source. Reprinted from *Diagnostic and Statistical Manual of Mental Disorders,* 4th Edition, Text Revision. Washington, DC, American Psychiatric Association, 2000. Copyright 2000, American Psychiatric Association. Used with permission.

heavy use (Office of Applied Studies 2007). Although rates of use were lower for those age 65 or older, they were nonetheless significant: 38.4% of respondents reported past-month alcohol use (30.8% nonbinge or nonheavy use, 6.0% bingeing, 1.6% heavy use). With respect to alcohol abuse or dependence, epidemiological census-based work estimates that 2.4% of older men and 0.4% of older women meet diagnostic criteria for alcohol abuse, whereas an additional 0.4% and 0.13% of older men and older women, respectively, meet criteria for alcohol dependence (Grant et al. 2004).

Because substance misuse is more likely to be presented in health care settings, rates of alcohol problems and dependence are higher among clinical than among community-based samples. For example, in their screening program of over 12,000 primary care patients, Barry et al. (1998) found that 5% of patients screened positive for at-risk or problem drinking, as measured by alcohol consumption, binge drinking, or the presence of alcohol-related problems. Similarly, Callahan and Tierney (1995) found that 10.6% of their sample of 3,954 primary care patients ages 60 and older met criteria for problem drinking. In a more recent study of older adults in primary care settings, Kirchner et al. (2007) reported that of the 24,863 individuals screened, 21.5% drank within the recommended levels (1–7 drinks per week), while 4.1% were at-risk drinkers (8–14 drinks per week), and 4.5% were heavy (>14 drinks per week) or binge drinkers. Rates of abuse and dependence appear to be particularly high among patients in mental health clinics and nursing homes. In their study of 140 patients enrolled in a geriatric mental health outpatient clinic, Holroyd and Duryee (1997) found that 8.6% of patients met DSM-IV criteria for alcohol dependence. Furthermore, results from a study of mostly male nursing home residents in a short-term rehabilitation facility revealed that 49% of residents had a lifetime diagnosis of alcohol dependence, with 18% reporting active symptoms of dependence within 1 year of admission (Joseph et al. 1995). Likewise, Oslin et al. (1997b) found that 29% of male nursing home residents had a lifetime diagnosis of alcohol abuse or dependence, with 10% of residents meeting criteria for abuse or dependence within 1 year of admission to the home.

Prescription and Over-the-Counter Medications

The use of pharmaceutical drugs is prevalent in older adulthood, and the risk of misusing prescription and over-the-counter medications, which include substances such as sedatives/hypnotics, narcotic and nonnarcotic analgesics, diet aids, and decongestants, also increases with age. According to a review of the scant literature on this topic, up to 11% of older women misuse prescription drugs, and it is projected that by the year 2020, 2.7 million adults will be using prescription drugs for nonmedical purposes (Simoni-Wastila and Yang 2006). A large proportion of medications prescribed to older adults include psychoactive, mood-altering drugs. Psychotherapeutic medications, in particular, are subject to improper use and can lead to negative health consequences, both when used alone and in combination with other drugs and alcohol. This is troubling when considering that the use of benzodiazepines, which are one of the most commonly prescribed medications in the United States, increases with age and tends to be chronic in later life (Simon et al. 1996).

Examination of pharmaceutical data supports the notion that older adults are more likely than younger people to take multiple medications (Golden et al. 1999; Lassila et al. 1996). For instance, in one study of rural, community-dwelling older adults, 71% of the 1,360 participants sampled reported regularly taking at least 1 prescription medication, and 10% reported taking 5 or more medications (Lassila et al. 1996). In fact, it has been estimated that the average older patient takes 5.3 prescription medications each day (Golden et al. 1999). Over-the-counter drug use also is quite common; in one study, 87% of older adults reported regular use of over-the-counter medications, and 5.7% were taking 5 or more over-the-counter medications concurrently (Stoehr et al. 1997). Polypharmacy, or the concomitant use of multiple drugs, may have negative consequences in cases in which complex medication regimens are not carefully and appropriately adhered to by patients or monitored by physicians (Montamat and Cusack 1992). Thus, clinicians should be cautious when prescribing or recommending a treatment, take both risks and benefits into account when determining a treatment plan, and clearly communicate guidelines for appropriate use to patients. Clinicians also should carefully consider discontinuing medications that do not prove effective. For example, medications often are continued from one care setting to another without clear justification for use as older adults are navigated through the health care system.

Illicit Drugs

Unlike alcohol and prescription/over-the-counter medication use, illicit drug use among older adults is rare. Based on data from the Epidemiologic Catchment Area study, analyses in the early 1990s estimated that the lifetime prevalence rate of drug abuse and dependence was 0.12% for older men and 0.06% for older women, whereas the lifetime history of illicit drug use was 2.88% and 0.66% for men and women, respectively (Anthony and Helzer 1991). However, other work suggests that illicit substance use is more common among older adults than previous estimates suggest. For example, results from a study of 684 adults age 50 or older who had a lifetime history of intravenous cocaine and heroin use revealed that 13% were actively using cocaine more than once per day (McBride et al. 1992). An even higher rate of illicit substance use—38%—was reported among older veterans in a Veterans Affairs addiction treatment program (Schonfeld and Dupree 2000). Finally, according to the most recent National Household Survey on Drug Use and Health, the percentage of adults ages 55–59 using illicit drugs in the past month increased from 1.9% in 2002 to 2.4% in 2006 (Office of Applied Studies 2007). Although this increase in drug use may not seem significant, it is important to keep in mind that the baby boomers represent the only age group that showed notable increases in illicit substance use during the designated time period. Thus, rates of illicit substance use and abuse will likely continue to rise in the next several decades because of the aging of the baby boom cohort.

Correlates and Consequences of Substance Use Problems

Correlates and Risk Factors of Substance Abuse

Several studies have sought to identify factors that are related to increased vulnerability to substance misuse and the maintenance of problematic substance use patterns in later life. Factors such as gender, medical comorbidity, history of past use, and social and family environment are all correlated with problematic substance use. Longitudinal work, for instance, suggests that older men tend to drink greater quantities of alcohol than women and are more likely to have alcohol-related problems (Moore et al. 2005). Older men also are more likely to have had a longer history of problem drinking (D'Archangelo 1993). The relationship between certain factors and alcohol abuse also may vary across genders; among alcohol abusers, women are more likely to have been married to a problem drinker, to report negative life events and ongoing difficulties with spouses and other family members, and to have had a history of depression than their male counterparts (Brennan and Moos 1990; Gomberg 2003). Furthermore, increases in free time coupled with a reduction in role obligations may have a large impact on problem drinking in older women (Wilsnack and Wilsnack 1995). Indeed, age-related losses in social, physical, and occupational/role domains, such as widowhood, the death of family and friends, reduced physical function, and retirement, help contribute to the adoption or maintenance of abusive drinking patterns in later life among men and women (Blow 1998).

Finally, longitudinal work has demonstrated that additional social context and life history factors, such as friends' approval of drinking and a history of heavy drinking or alcohol problems, also are related to a higher likelihood of late-life drinking problems (Moos et al. 2004).

With respect to prescription and over-the-counter drugs, factors such as declining physical health and physiological changes that accompany the aging process increase exposure and reactivity to medications and, thus, the potential for misuse of these substances in later life. Women, though less likely than men to use and abuse alcohol, are more likely than men to use and misuse psychoactive medications (Simoni-Wastila and Yang 2006), particularly if they are divorced or widowed, have lower socioeconomic status (e.g., education and income), or have been diagnosed with a mood disorder such as depression or anxiety (Closser and Blow 1993). Comorbid psychiatric diagnoses, in general, increase the risk for prescription drug abuse and dependence, regardless of gender (Simoni-Wastila and Yang 2006). When considering the full range of factors associated with drug misuse, it also is important to recognize factors such as inappropriate prescribing practices and insufficient monitoring of drug reactions and patient adherence by health care providers (Montamat and Cusack 1992).

Consequences of Substance Use

Although the literature presented thus far has alluded to the adverse effects of problematic substance use and dependence, there is some evidence to suggest that low-risk or moderate alcohol consumption may have a positive impact on physical health and mental well-being. For example, low-risk or moderate alcohol consumption is associated with a reduced risk of cardiovascular disease in both men and women and a reduced risk of cardiovascular disease–related disability (Rimm et al. 1991; Stampfer et al. 1988). Furthermore, researchers in one study of older adults without cardiovascular disease found that moderate alcohol consumption was related to lipoprotein subclass distribution (Mukamal et al. 2007a). Specifically, results indicated that moderate alcohol use was associated with fewer small low-density lipoprotein particles (LDL) and a greater number of large- and medium-sized high-density lipoprotein (HDL) particles.

Studies also have demonstrated that moderate use may protect against type 2 diabetes mellitus and functional decline and may also affect additional indicators of well-being. In their prospective study of 4,655 older adults with no diabetes at baseline, Djousse et al. (2007) found that regardless of the type of beverage consumed, light to moderate alcohol consumption was associated with a lower incidence of diabetes approximately 6.3 years later. With respect to functional decline, findings from cross-sectional work suggest that among older men, low to moderate alcohol consumption is associated with lower odds of reporting physical limitations when compared with abstinence or heavy use (Cawthon et al. 2007). Finally, light to moderate alcohol use has beneficial effects on subjective well-being for both men and women (Lang et al. 2007) and improves self-esteem, reduces stress, and provides relaxation, particularly in social situations (Dufour et al. 1992).

Although the literature cited previously does suggest that low to moderate use of alcohol can lead to various health benefits among older adults, it is important to recognize that there is no evidence to support the notion that recommending that nondrinkers initiate drinking will translate into reduced health risks. Moreover, there is no evidence to suggest that an individual with a medical condition, such as cardiovascular disease, will benefit from continued drinking or the initiation of drinking. In fact, abstinence should still be recommended for individuals who are taking certain medications, those who have been diagnosed with certain acute or chronic conditions (e.g., diabetes and cardiovascular disease), and those who present with a history of alcohol or drug abuse, because substance use is detrimental in these cases.

Drinking that exceeds levels of low risk or moderate use should be carefully monitored and targeted for intervention, given the mounting evidence of the risks of drinking above these recommendations (Oslin 2000). Even moderate use can lead to adverse health outcomes. For example, although moderate alcohol consumption decreases the risk of strokes caused by blocked blood vessels, it increases the risk of having a stroke caused by bleeding or hemorrhaging. Similarly, although there is a graded positive correlation between moderate alcohol use and bone mineral density at the hip, moderate use has a U-shaped relationship with risk of hip fracture (Mukamal et al. 2007b). Low to moderate consumption of alcohol also has been demonstrated to impair one's ability to drive and may increase the risk of accidents and fatal injuries due to falls, motor vehicle crashes, and suicides (Sorock et al. 2006). Depression, memory problems, liver disease, cardiovascular disease, cognitive changes, and sleep problems also have been linked to moderate alcohol use (Gambert and Katsoyannis 1995; Liberto et al. 1992), whereas alcohol dependence is associated with an increased probability of morbidity and mortality from disease-specific disorders such as acute pancreatitis, alcohol-induced cirrhosis, or alcohol-related cardiomyopathy.

When assessing and treating older adults, it is pertinent not only that clinicians take the above factors into account but that they also consider the potential interaction between alcohol and both prescribed and over-the-counter medications, especially psychoactive medications such as benzodiazepines, barbiturates, and antidepressants. As mentioned previously, alcohol use represents one of the leading risk factors for the occurrence of adverse drug reactions and is known to interfere with the metabolism of medications such as digoxin and warfarin (Fraser 1997; Hylek et al. 1998; Onder et al. 2002). Certain medications may themselves have a wide array of negative consequences on health if not used and prescribed carefully. For example, benzodiazepines are associated with an increased risk of falls and fractures, impaired driving, disruptions in sleep cycles, and, among the frail elderly, excessive disability (Hemmelgarn et al. 1997; Herings et al. 1995; Newman et al. 1997). Likewise, diphenhydramine has been linked to cognitive deficits in healthy older adults, which may translate into excessive cognitive deficits in patients with dementing illnesses (Katz et al. 1998). Vulnerability to these adverse consequences is increased when the medication is used for a longer duration than intended or warranted, or when the medication is improperly prescribed by giving an excessive dose or prescribing the medication for the wrong indication.

Finally, mental health providers should be well versed in the impact of moderate alcohol consumption on other mental health disorders. In a study of over 2,000 elderly patients, Oslin et al. (2000) demonstrated that reducing moderate alcohol use (defined as 1–7 drinks per week) while treating a depressive disorder enhanced treatment outcomes. Results further indicated that the greater the alcohol consumption, the larger the negative effect on the treatment of depression. Although data are sparse, there is speculation that moderate alcohol use also may have a negative impact on the prognosis and course of dementing illnesses such as Alzheimer's disease. Moreover, alcohol use may elicit the onset of, or exacerbate preexisting, personality changes or behavioral disturbances in patients with dementia.

Screening and Diagnosis of Substance Use Problems

Potential Barriers to Screening and Diagnosis

As outlined previously, alcohol and drug problems are common in later life. However, substance misuse remains largely underrecognized and undertreated among older adults. It has been suggested that adults over the age of 60 be screened for alcohol and prescription drug use as part of their routine mental and physical health care (Blow 1998). Routine screening would enable the identification of not only those older adults who have problematic substance use, but also those who are at risk of misusing drugs and alcohol. Further, proper screening helps determine if additional assessment is needed. Nonetheless, various factors may interfere with screening and diagnostic processes.

At the provider level, the common misconception that older substance users have a lifelong history of problem use may make it difficult for clinicians to identify individuals who either have or are at high risk for late-onset conditions. Although this assumption is more likely to hold for patterns of illicit drug use, as many as one-third of older adults seeking treatment for alcohol problems have developed these problems in later life. Furthermore, insufficient knowledge regarding symptoms or the potential health impact of at-risk or problematic drinking may inhibit screening efforts.

TABLE 23–3. Common signs and symptoms of potential substance misuse and abuse in older adults

Anxiety
Blackouts, dizziness
Depression, mood swings
Disorientation
Falls, bruises, and burns
Family problems
Financial problems
Headaches
Idiopathic seizures
Incontinence
Increased tolerance to alcohol or medications
Legal difficulties
Memory loss
New difficulties in decision making
Poor hygiene
Poor nutrition
Sleep problems
Social isolation

Source. Adapted from Barry KL, Blow FC, Oslin DW: "Substance Abuse in Older Adults: Review and Recommendations for Education and Practice in Medical Settings. *Substance Abuse* 23:105–131, 2002.

As discussed previously, diagnostic criteria and symptoms for alcohol and prescription drug misuse are not easily applied to older adults and are often confounded with symptoms of comorbid medical illnesses, further complicating the screening and diagnostic process for providers (see Table 23–3). Additionally, the use of multiple diagnostic terms can lead to confusion as to who should be screened, how screening should proceed, and which problems or patterns of use should be treated. A general lack of appreciation of the benefits of reduced substance use in the absence of abuse or dependence, and the belief that there are few accessible and effective treatments for substance use, can also significantly lower a clinician's motivation to screen for or to recognize at-risk or problem drinking. Assuming a clinician does have a desire to assess patients for at-risk or problematic use, the self-report nature of screening instruments may interfere with accurate and appropriate decision making because of various biases related to self-report measures. The dilemma inherent in these issues is consistent with results from studies that have demonstrated lower rates of detection and treatment of alcohol problems among older adults compared with younger adults (Curtis et al. 1986).

At the patient level, confusion as to what constitutes a substance use problem and who might benefit from an intervention also affects patients' behavior with regard to seeking assessment. Like providers, older adults may perceive physical symptoms (e.g., fatigue, sleep problems, anxiety, and confusion) as normative or attribute them to other medical illnesses. Older adults and their families also may not feel that their substance use is problematic, either due to denial or to lack of knowledge regarding recommendations and guidelines for acceptable drinking and prescription/over-the-counter drug use levels. In addition to these factors, age- and substance-related declines in memory may contribute to underreporting of past and current alcohol or drug use. Despite these potential issues, research suggests that retrospective self-report is as reliable as a prospective diet record in identifying patterns of alcohol use (Werch 1989).

Assessing the Frequency and Quantity of Use

Notwithstanding the barriers mentioned above, successful screening techniques have been designed and implemented. Techniques used to assess the quantity and frequency of alcohol and drug use fall into one of three categories: questions regarding average consumption practices, retrospective accounts of daily use over some defined period of time (i.e., the timeline follow-back method (TLFB), and prospective monitoring and recording of alcohol and drug use. The prospective diary method is considered to be the gold standard because it elicits the greatest number of reports of consumption and is highly associated with sales data for alcoholic beverages among younger adults (Lemmens et al. 1992). However, proper completion of this type of measure is time-consuming and requires multiple visits, and therefore this method is impractical for screenings or brief assessments.

The TLFB method represents the most commonly used technique in treatment studies for addiction and has become the method of choice for such studies. Among older adults, 7-day TLFB assessments are highly correlated with reports from prospective diaries. Nevertheless, certain difficulties arise when using this method. First, the specific week of measurement under assessment may not be representative of the individual's usual drinking behavior. Second, although the TLFB closely matches prospective diary reports for nondrinkers or daily drinkers, it underestimates use for less frequent users of alcohol (Lemmens et al. 1992). The TLFB also takes longer to administer than assessments assessing average frequency and, because of the varying individual definitions of a "standard" drink, is more effective and accurate when administered by an interviewer as opposed to self-administration.

Finally, although general questions about the average, rather than daily, quantity and frequency of use over a specified time period are least likely to match prospective diary reports and may underestimate the frequency of moderate drinking, it is the method of choice among many clinicians because of its ease of administration. Likewise, the "brown bag" approach, in which patients are asked to bring in all prescribed and over-the-counter medications they are currently taking, is a useful and convenient aid for determining medication use and misuse. Although reports of the quantity and frequency of use can be independently used to screen and identify at-risk patients, this information must be combined with other measures when the clinician is attempting to recognize problem drinking or a diagnosis of substance abuse or dependence.

Standardized Screening Instruments

Brief, low-cost, convenient, standardized assessments that can be used to screen not only for frequency and quantity of alcohol use but also for drinking consequences and alcohol/medication interactions are essential in the success of efforts targeted toward prevention and early intervention for older adults at risk. As described earlier, screening should be a component of routine mental and physical health care and should be updated annually, before the older adult begins taking any new medications, or in response to problems that may be alcohol- or medication-related. Standardized screening questions can be administered by various methods, including verbal interview and paper-and-pencil or computerized questionnaire. All three methods have demonstrated equivalent reliability and validity (Barry and Fleming 1990; Greist et al. 1987).

To complement questions assessing the quantity and frequency of use discussed in the previous section, the Short Michigan Alcoholism Screening Test–Geriatric Version (SMAST-G), the Alcohol Use Disorders Iden-

In the past year:	Yes	No
1. When talking with others, do you ever underestimate how much you actually drink?	____ (1)	____ (0)
2. After a few drinks, have you sometimes not eaten or been able to skip a meal because you didn't feel hungry?	____ (1)	____ (0)
3. Does having a few drinks help decrease your shakiness or tremors?	____ (1)	____ (0)
4. Does alcohol sometimes make it hard for you to remember parts of the day or night?	____ (1)	____ (0)
In the past year:		
5. Do you usually take a drink to relax or calm your nerves?	____ (1)	____ (0)
6. Do you drink to take your mind off your problems?	____ (1)	____ (0)
7. Have you ever increased your drinking after experiencing a loss in your life?	____ (1)	____ (0)
8. Has a doctor or nurse ever said they were worried or concerned about your drinking?	____ (1)	____ (0)
9. Have you ever made rules to manage your drinking?	____ (1)	____ (0)
10. When you feel lonely, does having a drink help?	____ (1)	____ (0)
TOTAL SMAST-G SCORE (0–10)		____

FIGURE 23–3. Short Michigan Alcohol Screening Test–Geriatric Version (SMAST-G).

Three or more positive responses is indicative of an alcohol abuse problem.

Source. Reprinted from the University of Michigan Alcohol Research Center. Copyright 1991 The Regents of the University of Michigan. Used with permission.

How often did you have a drink containing alcohol in the past year?

____	Never	(0 points)
____	Monthly or less	(1 point)
____	Two to four times a month	(2 points)
____	Two to three times per week	(3 points)
____	Four or more times a week	(4 points)

If you answered "never," score questions 2 and 3 as zero.

How many drinks did you have on a typical day when you were drinking in the past year?

____	1 or 2	(0 points)
____	3 or 4	(1 point)
____	5 or 6	(2 points)
____	7 to 9	(3 points)
____	10 or more	(4 points)

How often did you have six or more drinks on one occasion in the past year?

____	Never	(0 points)
____	Less than monthly	(1 point)
____	Monthly	(2 points)
____	Weekly	(3 points)
____	Daily or almost daily	(4 points)

Possible range=0–12. For older adults, a score of 3 or more is considered positive.

FIGURE 23–4. Alcohol Use Disorders Identification Test–C (AUDIT-C) alcohol screening.

Possible range 0–12. For older adults, a score of 3 or more is considered positive.

Source. Adapted from Bush K, Kivlahan DR, McDonell MB, et al.: "The AUDIT Alcohol Consumption Questions (AUDIT-C): An Effective Brief Screening Test for Problem Drinking." *Archives of Internal Medicine* 158:1789–1795, 1998. Copyright © 1998, American Medical Association. All rights reserved. Adapted with permission.

tification Test (AUDIT), and the CAGE often are used to screen for at-risk substance use or misuse among older adults. Of these three screening tools, the SMAST-G was developed specifically for older adults (Figure 23–3). The SMAST-G (Barry and Blow 1999) was developed at the University of Michigan as a screening instrument for elderly alcohol abuse or dependence in a variety of settings. Psychometric properties of this instrument exceed those of other screening tests for the identification of older adults with alcohol abuse/dependence. The AUDIT and its abbreviated version, the AUDIT-C (Figure 23–4), are simple screening measures that capture the frequency of drinking and bingeing in the past year (Bush et al. 1998; Dawson et al. 2005). The AUDIT-C is scored on a scale of 0–12, with a score of 0 indicating no alcohol use during the preceding year. For older adults, a score of 3 or more reflects a positive screen and suggests the need for further evaluation. Generally, the higher the AUDIT-C score, the more likely it is that the individual's drinking is affecting his or her health and safety (Bush et al. 1998; Dawson et al. 2005).

The CAGE questionnaire (Mayfield et al. 1974), however, is the most widely used alcohol screening test in clinical practice. Four items regarding alcohol use are designed to assess whether patients have 1) felt that they should **C**ut down, 2) felt **A**nnoyed that people criticized their drinking, 3) felt **G**uilty about their drinking, and 4) had a drink upon waking in the morning to get rid of a hangover—an **E**ye-opener. A modified version of the

CAGE questionnaire only asks about recent problems, and the threshold is often reduced to one positive response as an indicator of problems in older adults. This modified version of the CAGE has demonstrated high specificity for detecting alcohol abuse but relatively low sensitivity for alcohol dependence or problem drinking (Buchsbaum et al. 1992; Moore et al. 2002).

As this last point suggests, it important to recognize that the utility of the questionnaires described above may vary as a function of the category of drinking (e.g., at-risk drinking, alcohol abuse, or dependence) that is being assessed. In one comparison of the relative sensitivity and specificity of self-administered versions of the CAGE and AUDIT, Bradley et al. (1998) demonstrated that an augmented version of the CAGE (i.e., a measure including the CAGE items, the first two items of the AUDIT, and the question "Have you ever had a drinking problem?") performed better than the traditional CAGE and AUDIT when screening for active alcohol abuse or dependence. However, the AUDIT was superior to both versions of the CAGE in identifying heavy drinkers. Finally, although both the augmented CAGE and the AUDIT were effective in identifying both heavy drinkers and those actively abusing or dependent on alcohol, the AUDIT performed better. In sum, these results suggest that the selection of screening instruments used in clinical practice should be driven by the goals of screening (Bradley et al. 1998). For example, when screening for both heavy drinking and alcohol abuse or dependence, clinicians might consider using the AUDIT or AUDIT-C as opposed to the CAGE.

Following administration of a screening instrument such as the SMAST-G, AUDIT, or CAGE, clinicians can ask follow-up questions about consequences, health risks, and social/family issues related to substance use. In accordance with DSM-IV-TR criteria, in order to assess dependence, questions should be asked about alcohol-related problems, a history of failed attempts to stop or to cut back, or withdrawal symptoms (e.g., anxiety, tremors, sleep disturbance). The use of a substance abuse assessment instrument such as DSM-IV-TR criteria can assist clinicians and researchers by providing a structured approach to assessment as well as a checklist of items that can be evaluated across older adults. Further, such assessments can inform clinicians' decision making and help determine whether specialized alcohol treatment might be needed.

Use of Biological Markers for Screening

Lastly, it should be noted that biological markers of alcohol and drug use have proved to be less accepted in clinical practice but can be useful. Several laboratory values indicate recent use or abuse, including blood alcohol or acetate level, which is a metabolite of alcohol (Salaspuro 1994). Long-term markers of alcohol use include γ-glutamyl transferase (GGT), mean corpuscular volume, HDL level, and carbohydrate-deficient transferrin (Oslin et al. 1998b). Finally, urine drug screens are useful as both screening tools and confirmation of self-report when assessing prescription/over-the-counter medication and illicit drug abuse. The majority of drugs of abuse will remain detectable in a urine drug screen for 4 or more days, with some still detectable after several weeks.

Treatments for Substance Use Problems

Although there are numerous treatment options for substance use in later life, little formal research has been conducted to compare the relative efficacy of these various approaches among older adults. Nevertheless, results from naturalistic studies are promising: older adults who engage in treatment not only have comparable or significantly better outcomes than their younger counterparts (Lemke and Moos 2003b; Oslin et al. 2002; Satre et al. 2003, 2004a), they also are more likely to complete treatment than are younger patients (Schuckit and Pastor 1978; Wiens et al. 1982). Moreover, brief interventions and therapies have been shown to reduce drinking levels among older at-risk drinkers (F. Blow, "Brief Interventions in the Treatment of At-Risk Drinking in Older Adults," personal communication, 2003). Therefore, despite popular belief, older adults are quite receptive and responsive to treatment, especially in programs that offer age-appropriate care and have providers who are knowledgeable about aging issues. These various treatments are described in more detail in the following sections of this chapter.

Brief Interventions and Therapies

Low-intensity brief interventions or brief therapies are cost-effective and practical techniques that can be used in the initial treatment of at-risk and problem drinkers in a variety of clinical settings (Barry 1999). Brief interventions are time-limited and nonconfrontational in their approach. Given that these interventions are based on concepts and techniques from the behavioral self-control literature, one of the hallmarks of brief interventions is to encourage individuals to change their behavior through motivational interviewing (Miller and Rollnick 1991).

Randomized clinical trials of brief interventions for alcohol problems among older populations reveal that older adults can be engaged in brief intervention protocols and find the protocols acceptable. Results also point to a greater reduction in alcohol consumption among at-risk drinkers receiving interventions as compared with control groups. For example, in one randomized clinical study, older primary care patients randomly assigned to a brief intervention arm received two 10- to 15-minute physician counseling visits and two follow-up telephone calls from clinic staff that involved advice, education, and the creation of contracts (Fleming et al. 1999). Results from this study demonstrated that rates of alcohol use at 12-month follow-up were significantly lower for patients randomized to the brief intervention arm relative to those in the control group. Likewise, older primary care patients randomized to a single brief intervention session have been shown to have significantly greater reductions in alcohol consumption compared with usual care 1 year later (F. Blow, "Brief Interventions in the Treatment of At-Risk Drinking in Older Adults," personal communication, 2003). Although these trials were conducted in primary care settings, brief interventions for older adults are likely to be effective in mental health care settings as well. Thus, geriatric mental health providers are encouraged to gain familiarity with brief intervention therapy both as a primary treatment tool and, if needed, as a way to motivate patients for more formal addiction treatment.

Psychosocial Treatments

The literature regarding the efficacy of psychological therapies specifically for the treatment of substance abuse and dependence in older adulthood is sparse. In one study of older veterans with substance abuse problems, Schonfeld and Dupree (2000) showed that individuals who completed 16 weeks of a group intervention for relapse prevention were more likely to abstain at 6-month follow-up than noncompleters. Using cognitive-behavioral and self-management approaches, the group sessions included modules on coping with factors such as social problems, loneliness, depression, and anxiety and on dealing with high-risk situations for relapse. In yet another treatment study, three different manual-guided, individually delivered psychosocial treatments (cognitive-behavioral therapy, motivational enhancement therapy, and 12-Step facilitation) that spanned 12 weeks were found to be effective in reducing alcohol consumption among adults (7% of whom were age 60 or over) with alcohol dependence 1 year posttreatment (Cooney et al. 1997).

Twelve-Step Programs

A large proportion of community-based and residential treatment programs incorporate the traditional 12-Step peer support model of recovery and rehabilitation. Originally developed by Alcoholics Anonymous (AA) and later adapted by groups such as Narcotics Anonymous (NA), the 12-Step model involves group support and encouragement to help members achieve and maintain sobriety. Participants share their experiences with one another and follow the 12 steps, which include admitting to one's addiction, recognizing the influence of a greater power as a source of strength, and acknowledging and atoning for past mistakes (Alcoholics Anonymous 2004).

Although self-help groups have been associated with positive outcomes for many individuals, findings regarding rates of group engagement and outcomes among older adults remain mixed. In their matched comparison of older versus younger and middle-aged adults who participated in age-integrated residential treatment, Lemke and Moos (2003a) found that older patients engaged in 12-Step programs as frequently as their younger and middle-aged counterparts when assessed at follow-up. Results also indicated that more involvement in self-help groups posttreatment was associated with better outcomes across all three age groups.

Similarly, an investigation of patients who had completed an outpatient treatment program for chemical dependency yielded no age group differences in AA affiliation 5 years posttreatment (Satre et al. 2004a). Upon examination of a subset of participants in the sample who reported attending 12-Step meetings in the prior year, no age group differences in the actual number of meetings attended emerged as significant. However, despite the fact that rates of attendance appeared to be comparable across age groups, the depth of involvement differed; older adults were less likely than middle-aged adults to self-identify as being a 12-Step group member and were less likely than younger and middle-aged adults to report calling a fellow group member for help. Comparable results were observed in examining 1-month postdischarge outcomes among alcohol-dependent patients admitted to a 12-Step residential rehabilitation program (Oslin et al. 2005). Although rates of postdischarge abstinence and AA attendance did not differ across middle-aged and older adults, older adults were significantly less likely to contact a sponsor. Furthermore, older adults were less likely than middle-aged adults to engage in formal aftercare (31.2% vs. 56.4%).

Taken together, these findings highlight the importance of more careful examination of factors that may be related to 12-Step program attendance, degree of engagement, and outcomes among older adults. These include but are not limited to perceived stigma, level of comfort regarding disclosure of personal information in group settings, degree to which age-relevant issues are addressed during group meetings, and logistic barriers such as lack of transportation and health problems that may preclude older adults from attending group sessions and engaging with sponsors (Oslin et al. 2005; Satre et al. 2004a).

Pharmacotherapy

Until recently, the long-term treatment of older alcohol-dependent adults did not involve the use of pharmacological agents. Although disulfiram was originally the only medication approved for the treatment of alcohol dependence, it was seldom used in older patients because of the potential for adverse effects. In 1995, the opioid antagonist naltrexone became the first pharmacological agent approved by the U.S. Food and Drug Administration in over 50 years for use in the treatment of alcohol dependence. Approval of the drug was based on findings from clinical trials that showed that naltrexone was safe and effective in preventing relapse and reducing alcohol cravings (O'Malley et al. 1992; Volpicelli et al. 1992). Although these original clinical trials used samples of middle-aged adults, naltrexone also has been shown to be effective among older adults. For example, results from a double-blind, placebo-controlled, randomized trial demonstrated that among older veterans ages 50–70, half as many naltrexone-treated subjects relapsed to significant drinking when compared with those treated with placebo (Oslin et al. 1997a).

Acamprosate has emerged as another promising agent in the treatment of alcohol dependence. Although the exact action of acamprosate is still unclear, it is believed to reduce glutamate response (Pelc et al. 1997). The clinical evidence favoring acamprosate is impressive. Sass et al. (1996), for example, found that 43% of alcohol-dependent subjects treated with acamprosate were abstinent at the conclusion of their 48-week randomized, placebo-controlled trial compared with 21% in the placebo group. Unfortunately, no studies of the efficacy or safety of acamprosate among older patients have been conducted to date.

Detoxification and Withdrawal

In situations where patients stop consuming substances or drastically cut down their consumption after heavy use, withdrawal symptoms are likely to occur. During hospitalizations, patients may be particularly vulnerable to alcohol or benzodiazepine withdrawal if the clinical team is unaware of problems with these substances. In light of the potential for life-threatening complications, clinicians caring for patients who abuse substances, particularly in settings in which withdrawal management or treatment is available, need to have a fundamental understanding of withdrawal symptoms and be able to provide detoxification management. Clinicians also should be aware of the anticipated time course of various symptoms.

Alcohol withdrawal symptoms can range from unnoticeable and mild to severe and life-threatening. The classic set of symptoms associated with alcohol withdrawal includes autonomic hyperactivity (increased pulse rate, increased blood pressure, and increased temperature), restlessness, disturbed sleep, anxiety, nausea, and tremor. Severe withdrawal is marked by auditory, visual, or tactile hallucinations; delirium; seizures; and coma. Commonly abused prescription and illicit drugs such as benzodiazepines, opioids, and cocaine cause distinct withdrawal symptoms that are also potentially life-threatening. It is important to recognize that among older patients the duration of withdrawal symptoms is longer, and withdrawal has the potential to complicate other medical and psychiatric illnesses. Nonetheless, there is no evidence to suggest that older patients are more prone to alcohol withdrawal or require longer treatment for withdrawal symptoms (Brower et al. 1994).

Moderators and Correlates of Treatment Response and Adherence

There is some evidence that certain factors may have an impact on the degree of treatment response and adherence among older adults receiving treatment. For example, age-specific treatment, or age matching, has been shown to improve treatment completion and to result in higher rates of attendance at group meetings when compared with mixed-age treatments. In one study of male veterans with alcohol problems who were randomly assigned after detoxification to either age-specific or standard mixed-age treatment, outcomes at 6 months and 1 year showed that elder-specific program patients were 2.9 times more likely at 6 months and 2.1 times more likely at 1 year to report abstinence compared with mixed-age group patients (Kashner et al. 1992).

The type of treatment setting also may affect rates of adherence. In a study comparing engagement outcomes among older primary care patients referred to specialty mental health providers versus those referred to an integrated care model using a brief intervention, 60.4% of at-risk drinkers attended at least one visit in the integrated care model (Bartels et al. 2004). In contrast, only 33% of patients attended at least one visit to a specialty provider. It is important to note that these differences emerged in spite of efforts to address barriers to specialty care, such as copayments and insurance claims, and to assure appointments within 2 weeks of patients being identified with at-risk drinking.

Finally, certain patient-level characteristics may differentially predict treatment outcomes. For example, women may have more favorable treatment outcomes than men. Satre et al. (2004b) demonstrated that 6 months after treatment at a private outpatient chemical dependency program, older alcohol-dependent women were significantly more likely to report abstinence from alcohol and drugs during the prior 30 days than men (79.3% vs. 54.0%, P=0.02). Similarly, among patients who were not abstinent, whereas men reported a mean of 4 heavy drinking days over the prior 30 days, none of the women reported heavy drinking. In addition to gender, variables associated with older age that may be related to more favorable treatment outcomes include longer retention in treatment and not having close social network members (e.g., family and friends) who encourage alcohol or drug use (Satre et al. 2004b).

Medical and Psychiatric Comorbidity

The co-occurrence of problematic substance use and other medical and psychiatric conditions deserves special attention because such comorbidity may affect the course, treatment, and prognosis of both conditions. Although epidemiological studies have clearly demonstrated that comorbidity between alcohol use and other psychiatric symptoms is common in younger age groups, less is known about comorbidity between alcohol use and psychiatric illness in late life. Nevertheless, a few studies have demonstrated that concurrent alcohol dependence is common among older adults who have mental health problems. For example, in a review of 3,986 Veterans Affairs hospital patients between the ages of 60–69 presenting for alcohol treatment, the most common comorbid psychiatric disorder was an affective disorder (present in 21% of the patients) (Blow et al. 1992). Of these patients, 43% had major depression. Similarly, in a study of community-dwelling elderly, of the 4.5% of older adults who had a history of alcohol abuse, almost half had a comorbid diagnosis of depression or dysthymia (Blazer et al. 1987).

Comorbid depressive and alcohol symptoms are not only common in late life but also may have a reciprocal effect upon one another. Depressed individuals with alcoholism may have a more complicated clinical course of depression, marked by an increased risk of suicide and more social dysfunction, than nondepressed alcoholic individuals (Conwell 1991; Cook et al. 1991; Waern 2003). In the same vein, alcohol use prior to late life has been shown to influence treatment of late life depression; for example, a prior history of alcohol abuse is associated with a more severe and chronic course of depression (Cook et al. 1991).

Co-occurrence of alcohol use and dementing illnesses such as Alzheimer's disease is also a complex issue. Although Wernicke-Korsakoff syndrome is well defined and often caused by alcohol dependence, alcohol-related dementia (ARD) may be difficult to differentiate from Alzheimer's disease because of a lack of well-specified diagnostic criteria. As a result, clinical diagnostic criteria for ARD have been proposed and validated in at least one trial examining a method for distinguishing ARD, including Wernicke-Korsakoff syndrome, from other types of dementia (Oslin and Cary 2003; Oslin et al. 1998a). Despite these diagnostic issues, it is generally agreed that alcohol abuse contributes to cognitive deficits in later life. In one of the few community-based studies to include alcohol survey data, the Epidemiologic Catchment Area study found the prevalence of a lifetime history of alcohol abuse or dependence was 1.5 times greater among persons with mild and severe cognitive impairment than those with no cognitive impairment (George et al. 1991). Similarly, among older adults seeking alcohol treatment, 23% had dementia associated with alcohol dependence (Finlayson et al. 1988). Finally, patients with ARD who become abstinent do not show a progression in cognitive impairment comparable to that found in Alzheimer's disease (Oslin and Cary 2003).

Sleep disorders and disturbances also frequently co-occur with excessive alcohol use. It is well established that alcohol causes changes in sleep patterns, such as decreased sleep latency, decreased stage 4 sleep, and precipitation or aggravation of sleep apnea (Wagman et al. 1977). Age-related changes in sleep patterns also occur with advancing age and include increased rapid eye movement (REM) episodes, a decrease in REM length and stage 3 and 4 sleep, and increased awakenings. Age-associated changes in sleep can be exacerbated by factors such as alcohol use and depression. For instance, in their study of younger subjects, Moeller et al. (1993) demonstrated that alcohol and depression had additive effects on sleep disturbances when occurring together. Furthermore, Wagman et al. (1977) demonstrated that abstinent alcoholics had poor sleep due to insomnia, frequent awakenings, and REM fragmentation. Nevertheless, upon drinking alcohol, sleep periodicity normalized and REM sleep was temporarily suppressed, suggesting that alcohol use could be used to self-medicate for sleep disturbances.

Future Directions

Substance misuse among older adults represents a pressing public health issue, both now and for years to come. In light of changes in demographic and cohort trends, recent years have seen an increase in the number of older adults who misuse or abuse alcohol and drugs. Moreover, there is a growing awareness that older adults often engage in at-risk or problem substance use. Nevertheless, individuals in need of treatment or at risk for future problems often go unidentified and untreated. Thus, research and clinical efforts aimed at improving screening efforts and identifying system, provider, and patient-level factors that may interfere with screening and referral processes for older adults at risk are warranted. In this vein, a better understanding among clinicians and patients of recommended drinking levels and the risks associated with moderate to heavy alcohol consumption is needed, particularly in light of the high prevalence of co-occurring medical and psychiatric problems in this age group. Clinicians also should ensure that screening becomes a part of routine practice when caring for their older patients.

Furthermore, because both provider recommendations and patient engagement are influenced, in part, by the availability of effective treatment, better dissemination of information regarding currently available and efficacious treatments for at-risk use and substance dependence is needed. It is important to note, however, that treatment studies in addiction have traditionally excluded patients over the age of 65, resulting in a gap in knowledge regarding treatment outcomes and an understanding of the neurobiology of addiction in older adults. Thus, research endeavors should continue to focus on developing more effective treatments for substance misuse in later life, taking into consideration and empirically assessing the various factors (e.g., patient-, treatment-, and system-related) that may moderate treatment engagement and outcomes. Along these lines, more formal research that focuses on the relative efficacy of various treatment modalities, specifically among older adults, is needed. Finally, given that these issues are particularly relevant to older adults, future work may benefit from examining nutrition, vitamin supplementation, and comorbid medical and psychiatric illness, both as foci for treatment and as aspects of health that may be complicated by substance use.

Key Points

- Despite demographic and cohort trends that suggest rates of substance misuse among older adults are increasing, the misuse of alcohol and/or drugs among this group remains largely underrecognized and undertreated. Accordingly, substance misuse in later life has been referred to as an "invisible epidemic."
- Proper screening, diagnosis, and treatment of older adults with drug and/or alcohol problems require an understanding of both age-specific guidelines and the full range of substance use behavior seen among older adults.
- In light of physiological changes that accompany aging, it is recommended that adults ages 65 and older should consume no more than 1 standard drink per day.
- The use of multiple pharmaceutical drugs is prevalent in older adulthood, and thus the risk of misusing prescription and over-the-counter medications

increases with age. Psychotherapeutic medications, in particular, should be closely monitored, as they are subject to improper use and can lead to negative health outcomes and interactions, both used alone and in combination with other drugs and alcohol.

- Factors such as medical comorbidity, history of past use, gender, and social and family environment are related to increased late-life vulnerability to substance misuse and the maintenance of problematic substance use patterns.
- Diagnostic criteria and symptoms for alcohol and drug misuse are not easily applied to older adults, as they are often confounded with symptoms of comorbid medical illnesses. Thus, when diagnosing and treating older adults, it is important that providers be able to distinguish between symptoms of substance misuse and those stemming from comorbid conditions.
- Routine screening allows for the identification of not only problematic and dependent drinkers, but also older adults who are at risk of misusing drugs and alcohol. Proper screening also helps determine needs for additional assessment and/or intervention. Standardized brief, low-cost assessments exist that can be used to assess the quantity and frequency of alcohol and drug use in clinical practice.
- A variety of treatments for substance misuse, such as brief interventions, psychotherapy, 12-step programs, and pharmacotherapy, have been shown to be effective among older adults.
- Special attention should be paid to co-occurrence of problematic substance use and other medical and psychiatric conditions (e.g., depression, dementia, sleep disturbance) because such comorbidity may affect the course, treatment, and prognosis of both conditions.

References

Alcoholics Anonymous Services: Twelve Steps and Twelve Traditions. New York, Alcoholics Anonymous, 2004

American Psychiatric Association: Diagnostic and Statistical Manual of Mental Disorders, 4th Edition, Text Revision. Washington, DC, American Psychiatric Association, 2000

Anthony JC, Helzer JE: Syndromes of drug abuse and dependence, in Psychiatric Disorders in America: The Epidemiologic Catchment Area Study. Edited by Robins LN, Regier DA. New York, Free Press, 1991, pp 116–154

Barry KL (Consensus Panel Chair): Brief Interventions and Brief Therapies for Substance Abuse. Treatment Improvement Protocol (TIP) Series 34 (DHHS SAMHSA Publ No SMA-99-3353). Rockville, MD, Center for Substance Abuse Treatment, 1999

Barry KL, Blow FC: Screening and assessment of alcohol problems in older adults, in Handbook of Assessment in Clinical Gerontology. Edited by Lichtenburg PA. New York, Wiley, 1999, pp 243–269

Barry KL, Fleming M: Computerized administration of alcoholism screening tests in a primary care setting. J Am Board Fam Pract 3:93–98, 1990

Barry KL, Blow FC, Walton MA, et al: Elder-specific brief alcohol intervention: 3-month outcomes. Alcohol Clin Exp Res 22:30A, 1998

Bartels S, Coakley E, Zubritsky C, et al: Improving access to geriatric mental health services: a randomized trial comparing treatment engagement with integrated versus enhanced referral care for depression, anxiety, and at-risk alcohol use. Am J Psychiatry 16:1455–1462, 2004

Blazer DG, Hughes DC, George LK: The epidemiology of depression in an elderly community population. Gerontologist 27:281–287, 1987

Blow FC (Consensus Panel Chair): Substance Abuse Among Older Adults. Treatment Improvement Series Protocol (TIP) Series No. 26. Center for Substance Abuse Treatment. Rockville, MD, U.S. Department of Health and Human Services, 1998

Blow F, Cook CL, Booth B, et al: Age-related psychiatric comorbidities and level of functioning in alcoholic veterans seeking outpatient treatment. Hosp Community Psychiatry 43:990–995, 1992

Bradley KA, Bush KR, McDonell MB, et al: Screening for problem drinking: comparison of CAGE and AUDIT. J Gen Intern Med 13:379–388, 1998

Brennan PL, Moos RH: Life stressors, social resources, and late-life problem drinking. Psychol Aging 5:491–501, 1990

Brower KJ, Mudd S, Blow FC, et al: Severity and treatment of alcohol withdrawal in elderly versus younger patients. Alcohol Clin Exp Res 18:196–201, 1994

Buchsbaum DG, Buchanan R, Welsh J, et al: Screening for drinking disorders in the elderly using the CAGE questionnaire. J Am Geriatr Soc 40:662–665, 1992

Bush K, Kivlahan DR, McDonell MB, et al: The AUDIT alcohol consumption questions (AUDIT-C): an effective brief screening test for problem drinking. Ambulatory Care Quality Improvement Project (ACQUIP). Alcohol Use Disorders Identification Test. Arch Intern Med 158:1789–1795, 1998

Callahan CM, Tierney WM: Health services use and mortality among older primary care patients with alcoholism. J Am Geriatr Soc 43:1378–1383, 1995

Cawthon PM, Fink HA, Barrett-Connor E, et al: Alcohol use, physical performance, and functional limitations in older men. J Am Geriatr Soc 55:212–220, 2007

Chermack ST, Blow FC, Hill EM, et al: The relationship between alcohol symptoms and consumption among older drinkers. Alcohol Clin Exp Res 20:1153–1158, 1996

Closser MH, Blow FC: Special populations: women, ethnic minorities, and the elderly. Psychiatr Clin North Am 16:199–209, 1993

Conwell Y: Suicide in elderly patients, in Diagnosis and Treatment of Depression in Late Life. Edited by Schneider LS, Reynolds CF, Lebowitz BD, et al. Washington, DC, American Psychiatric Press, 1991, pp 397–418

Cook B, Winokur G, Garvey M, et al: Depression and previous alcoholism in the elderly. Br J Psychiatry 158:72–75, 1991

Cooney NL, DiClemente CC, Carbonari J, et al: Matching alcoholism treatments to client heterogeneity–Project Match posttreatment drinking outcomes. J Stud Alcohol 58:7–29, 1997

Curtis J, Millman E, Joseph M, et al: Prevalence rates for alcoholism, associated depression and dementia on the Harlem hospital medicine and surgery services. Adv Alcohol Subst Abuse 6:45–65, 1986

D'Archangelo E: Substance abuse in later life. Can Fam Physician 39:1986–1993, 1993

Dawson DA, Grant BF, Stinson FS, et al: Effectiveness of the derived Alcohol Use Disorders Identification Test (AUDIT-C) in screening for alcohol use disorders and risk drinking in the U.S. general population. Alcohol Clin Exp Res 29:844–854, 2005

Djousse L, Biggs ML, Mukamal KJ, et al: Alcohol consumption and type 2 diabetes among older adults: the cardiovascular health study. Obesity 15:1758–1765, 2007

Dufour MC, Archer L, Gordis E: Alcohol and the elderly. Clin Geriatr Med 8:127–141, 1992

Finlayson R, Hurt R, Davis L, et al: Alcoholism in elderly persons: a study of the psychiatric and psychosocial features of 216 inpatients. Mayo Clin Proc 63:761–768, 1988

Fleming MF, Manwell LB, Barry KL, et al: Brief physician advice for alcohol problems in older adults: a randomized community-based trial. J Fam Pract 48:378–384, 1999

Fraser AG: Pharmacokinetic interactions between alcohol and other drugs. Clin Pharmacokinet 33:79–90, 1997

Gambert S, Katsoyannis K: Alcohol-related medical disorders of older heavy drinkers, in Alcohol and Aging. Edited by Beresford T, Gomberg E. New York, Oxford University Press, 1995, pp 70–81

George LK, Landerman R, Blazer DG, et al: Cognitive impairment, in Psychiatric Disorders in America: The Epidemiologic Catchment Area Study. Edited by Robins LN, Regier DA. New York, Free Press, 1991, pp 291–327

Gfroerer J, Penne M, Pemberton M, et al: Substance abuse treatment need among older adults in 2020: the impact of the aging baby-boom cohort. Drug Alcohol Depend 69:127–135, 2003

Golden AG, Preston RA, Barnett SD, et al: Inappropriate medication prescribing in homebound older adults. J Am Geriatr Soc 47:948–953, 1999

Gomberg ES: Treatment for alcohol-related problems: special populations: research opportunities. Recent Dev Alcohol 16:313–333, 2003

Grant BF, Dawson DA, Stinson FS, et al: The 12-month prevalence and trends in DSM-IV alcohol abuse and dependence: United States, 1991–1992 and 2001–2002. Drug Alcohol Depend 74:223–234, 2004

Greist J, Klein M, Erdman H, et al: Comparison of computer- and interviewer-administered versions of the Diagnostic Interview Schedule. Hosp Community Psychiatry 38:1304–1311, 1987

Hemmelgarn B, Suissa S, Huang A, et al: Benzodiazepine use and the risk of motor vehicle crash in the elderly. JAMA 278:27–31, 1997

Herings RMC, Stricker BHC, deBoer A, et al: Benzodiazepines and the risk of falling leading to femur fractures. Arch Intern Med 155:1801–1807, 1995

Holroyd S, Duryee J: Substance use disorders in a geriatric psychiatry outpatient clinic: prevalence and epidemiologic characteristics. J Nerv Ment Dis 185:627–632, 1997

Hylek EM, Heiman H, Skates SJ, et al: Acetaminophen and other risk factors for excessive warfarin anticoagulation. JAMA 279: 657–662, 1998

Joseph CL, Ganzini L, Atkinson R: Screening for alcohol use disorders in the nursing home. J Am Geriatr Soc 43:368–373, 1995

Kashner TM, Rodell DI, Ogden SR, et al: Outcomes and costs of two VA inpatient treatment programs for older alcoholic patients. Hosp Community Psychiatry 43:985–989, 1992

Katz IR, Sands LP, Bilker W, et al: Identification of medications that cause cognitive impairment in older people: the role of oxybutynin chloride. J Am Geriatr Soc 46:8–13, 1998

Kirchner JE, Zubritsky C, Cody M, et al: Alcohol consumption among older adults in primary care. J Gen Intern Med 22:92–97, 2007

Klatsky AL, Armstrong A: Alcohol use, other traits and risk of unnatural death: a prospective study. Alcohol Clin Exp Res 17:1156–1162, 1993

Koenig HG, George LK, Schneider R: Mental health care for older adults in the year 2020: a dangerous and avoided topic. Gerontologist 34:674–679, 1994

Lang I, Wallace RB, Huppert FA, et al: Moderate alcohol consumption in older adults is associated with better cognition and well-being than abstinence. Age Ageing 36:256–261, 2007

Lassila HC, Stoehr GP, Ganguli M, et al: Use of prescription medications in an elderly rural population: the MoVIES project. Ann Pharmacother 30:589–595, 1996

Lemke S, Moos RH: Outcomes at 1 and 5 years for older patients with alcohol disorders. J Subst Abuse Treat 24:43–50, 2003a

Lemke S, Moos RH: Treatment and outcomes of older patients with alcohol use disorders in community residential programs. J Stud Alcohol 64:219–226, 2003b

Lemmens P, Tan ES, Knibbe RA: Measuring quantity and frequency of drinking in a general population survey: a comparison of five indices. J Stud Alcohol 53:476–486, 1992

Liberto JG, Oslin DW, Ruskin PE: Alcoholism in older persons: a review of the literature. Hosp Community Psychiatry 43:975–984, 1992

Mayfield D, McLeod G, Hall P: The CAGE questionnaire: validation of a new alcoholism instrument. Am J Psychiatry 131: 1121–1123, 1974

McBride DC, Inciardi JA, Chitwood DD, et al: Crack use and correlates of use in a national population of stress heroin users. J Psychoactive Drugs 24:411–416, 1992

Miller W, Rollnick S: Motivational Interviewing: Preparing People to Change Addictive Behavior. New York, Guilford, 1991

Moeller FG, Gillin JC, Irwin M, et al: A Comparison of sleep EEGs in patients with primary major depression and major depression secondary to alcoholism. J Affective Disord 27:39–42, 1993

Montamat SC, Cusack B: Overcoming problems with polypharmacy and drug misuse in the elderly. Clin Geriatr Med 8:143–158, 1992

Moore AA, Hays RD, Reuben DB, et al: Using a criterion standard to validate the Alcohol-Related Problems Survey (ARPS): a screening measure to identify harmful and hazardous drinking in older persons. Aging (Milano) 12:221–227, 2000

Moore AA, Beck JC, Babor TF, et al: Beyond alcoholism: identifying older, at-risk drinkers in primary care. J Stud Alcohol 63:316–324, 2002

Moore AA, Gould R, Reuben DB, et al: Longitudinal patterns and predictors of alcohol consumption in the United States. Am J Public Health 95:458–465, 2005

Moore AA, Whiteman EJ, Ward KT: Risks of combined alcohol/medication use in older adults. Am J Geriatr Pharmacother 5:64–74, 2007

Moos RH, Schutte K, Brennan P, et al: Ten-year patterns of alcohol consumption and drinking problems among older women and men. Addiction 99:829–838, 2004

Mukamal KJ, Mackey RH, Kuller LH, et al: Alcohol consumption and lipoprotein subclasses in older adults. J Clin Endocrinol Metab 92:2559–2566, 2007a

Mukamal KJ, Robbins JA, Cauley JA, et al: Alcohol consumption, bone density, and hip fracture among older adults: The Cardiovascular Health Study. Osteoporos Int 18:593–602, 2007b

National Institute on Alcohol Abuse and Alcoholism: Diagnostic criteria for alcohol abuse. Alcohol Alert No. 30 (October) PH 359, 1995. Bethesda, MD, U.S. Department of Health and Human Services, Public Health Services, National Institutes of Health, 1995, pp 1–6

Newman A, Enright P, Manolio T, et al: Sleep disturbances, psychosocial correlates, and cardiovascular disease in 5201 older adults: the cardiovascular health study. J Am Geriatr Soc 45:1–7, 1997

O'Malley SS, Jaffe AJ, Chang G, et al: Naltrexone and coping skills therapy for alcohol dependence: a controlled study. Arch Gen Psychiatry 49:881–887, 1992

Office of Applied Studies: Results from the 2006 National Survey on Drug Use and Health: National Findings (DHHS Publ No SMA 07-4293, NSDUH Series H-32). Rockville, MD, Substance Abuse and Mental Health Services Administration, 2007

Onder G, Pedone C, Landi F, et al: Adverse drug reactions as cause of hospital admissions: results from the Italian Group of Pharmacoepidemiology in the Elderly (GIFA). J Am Geriatr Soc 50:1962–1968, 2002

Oslin DW: Alcohol use in late life: disability and comorbidity. J Geriatr Psychiatry Neurol 13:134–140, 2000

Oslin DW, Cary MS: Alcohol-related dementia: validation of diagnostic criteria. Am J Geriatr Psychiatry 11:441–447, 2003

Oslin D, Liberto JG, O'Brien J, et al: Naltrexone as an adjunctive treatment for older patients with alcohol dependence. Am J Geriatr Psychiatry 5:324–332, 1997a

Oslin D, Streim JE, Parmelee P, et al: Alcohol abuse: a source of reversible functional disability among residents of a VA nursing home. Int J Geriatr Psychiatry 12:825–832, 1997b

Oslin D, Atkinson RM, Smith DM, et al: Alcohol related dementia: proposed clinical criteria. Int J Geriatr Psychiatry 13:203–212, 1998a

Oslin DW, Pettinati HM, Luck G, et al: Clinical correlations with carbohydrate-deficient transferrin levels in women with alcoholism. Alcohol Clin Exp Res 22:1981–1985, 1998b

Oslin DW, Katz IR, Edell WS, et al: Effects of alcohol consumption on the treatment of depression among elderly patients. Am J Geriatr Psychiatry 8:215–220, 2000

Oslin DW, Pettinati HM, Volpicelli JR: Alcoholism treatment adherence: older age predicts better adherence and drinking outcomes. Am J Geriatr Psychiatry 10:740–747, 2002

Oslin DW, Slaymaker VJ, Blow FC, et al: Treatment outcomes for alcohol dependence among middle-aged and older adults. Addict Behav 30:1431–1436, 2005

Pelc I, Verbanck P, Le Bon O, et al: Efficacy and safety of acamprosate in the treatment of detoxified alcohol-dependent patients: a 90-day placebo-controlled dose-finding study. Br J Psychiatry 171:73–77, 1997

Poikolainen K: Epidemiologic assessment of population risks and benefits of alcohol use. Alcohol Alcohol Suppl 1:27–34, 1991

Rimm EB, Giovannucci EL, Willett WC, et al: Prospective study of alcohol consumption and risk of coronary disease in men. Lancet 338:464–468, 1991

Salaspuro M: Biological state markers of alcohol abuse. Alcohol Health Res World 18:131–135, 1994

Sass H, Soyka M, Mann K, et al: Relapse prevention by acamprosate: results from a placebo-controlled study in alcohol dependence. Arch General Psychiatry 53:673–680, 1996

Satre DD, Mertens JR, Arean PA, et al: Contrasting outcomes of older versus middle-aged and younger adult chemical dependency patients in a managed care program. J Stud Alcohol 64:520–530, 2003

Satre DD, Mertens JR, Arean PA, et al: Five-year alcohol and drug treatment outcomes of older adults versus middle-aged and younger adults in a managed care program. Addiction 99:1286–1297, 2004a

Satre DD, Mertens JR, Weisner C: Gender difference in treatment outcomes for alcohol dependence among older adults. J Stud Alcohol 65:638–642, 2004b

Schonfeld L, Dupree LW: Antecedents of drinking for early- and late-onset elderly alcohol abusers. J Stud Alcohol 52:587–592, 1991

Schonfeld L, Dupree LW: Cognitive-behavioral treatment of older veterans with substance abuse problems. J Geriatr Psychiatry Neurol 13:124–129, 2000

Schuckit M, Pastor P: The elderly as a unique population. Alcohol Clin Exp Res 2:31–38, 1978

Simon G, VonKorff M, Barlow W, et al: Predictors of chronic benzodiazepine use in a health maintenance organization sample. J Clin Epidemiol 49:1067–1073, 1996

Simoni-Wastila L, Yang HK: Psychoactive drug abuse in older adults. Am J Geriatr Pharmacother 4:380–394, 2006

Sorock GS, Chen LH, Gonzalgo SR, et al: Alcohol-drinking history and fatal injury in older adults. Alcohol 40:193–199, 2006

Stampfer MJ, Colditz GA, Willett WC, et al: A prospective study of moderate alcohol consumption and the risk of coronary disease and stroke in women. N Engl J Med 319:267–273, 1988

Stoehr GP, Ganguli M, Seaberg EC, et al: Over-the-counter medication use in an older rural community: the MoVIES project. J Am Geriatr Soc 45:158–165, 1997

Volpicelli JR, Alterman AI, Hayashida M, et al: Naltrexone in the treatment of alcohol dependence. Arch Gen Psychiatry 49:876–880, 1992

Waern M: Alcohol dependence and misuse in elderly suicides. Alcohol Alcohol 38:249–254, 2003

Wagman AM, Allen RP, Upright D: Effects of alcohol consumption upon parameters of ultradian sleep rhythms in alcoholics. Adv Exp Med Biol 85A:601–616, 1977

Werch C: Quantity-frequency and diary measures of alcohol consumption for elderly drinkers. Int J Addict 24:859–865, 1989

Widlitz M, Marin D: Substance abuse in older adults: an overview. Geriatrics 57:29–34, 2002

Wiens AN, Menustik CE, Miller SI, et al: Medical-behavioral treatment for the older alcoholic patient. Am J Drug Alcohol Abuse 9:461–475, 1982

Wilsnack SC, Wilsnack RW: Drinking and problem drinking in U.S. women: patterns and recent trends. Recent Dev Alcohol 12:29–60, 1995

Suggested Readings

Blow FC (Consensus Panel Chair): Substance Abuse Among Older Adults. Treatment Improvement Series Protocol (TIP) Series No. 26. Center for Substance Abuse Treatment. Rockville, MD, U.S. Department of Health and Human Services, 1998

Fleming MF, Manwell LB, Barry KL, et al: Brief physician advice for alcohol problems in older adults: a randomized community-based trial. J Fam Pract 48:378–384, 1999

Gfroerer J, Penne M, Pemberton M, et al: Substance abuse treatment need among older adults in 2020: the impact of the aging baby-boom cohort. Drug Alcohol Depend 69:127–135, 2003

Grant BF, Dawson DA, Stinson FS, et al: The 12-month prevalence and trends in DSM-IV alcohol abuse and dependence: United States, 1991-1992 and 2001-2002. Drug Alcohol Depend 74:223–234, 2004

Kirchner JE, Zubritsky C, Cody M, et al: Alcohol consumption among older adults in primary care. J Gen Intern Med 22:92–97, 2007

Oslin D, Liberto JG, O'Brien J, et al: Naltrexone as an adjunctive treatment for older patients with alcohol dependence. Am J Geriatr Psychiatry 5:324-332, 1997

Satre DD, Mertens JR, Arean PA, et al: Five-year alcohol and drug treatment outcomes of older adults versus middle-aged and younger adults in a managed care program. Addiction 99:1286–1297, 2004

Schonfeld L, Dupree LW: Cognitive-behavioral treatment of older veterans with substance abuse problems. J Geriatr Psychiatry Neurol 13:124–129, 2000

Simoni-Wastila L, Yang HK: Psychoactive drug abuse in older adults. Am J Geriatr Pharmacother 4:380–394, 2006

Widlitz M, Marin D: Substance abuse in older adults. an overview. Geriatrics 57:29–34, 2002

CHAPTER 24

Personality Disorders

Thomas E. Oxman, M.D.

The diagnosis and treatment of personality disorders are relatively difficult and time-intensive in comparison with those of many other psychiatric disorders. In elderly persons, these problems are confounded by a variety of additional issues, both negative and positive. The natural history of personality in later life is affected by the combination of increasing medical-neuropsychiatric comorbidity with ongoing normal psychosocial development.

With aging, the likelihood of multiple chronic diseases increases. The existence of comorbidity results in more functional impairment and requires adaptation (Besdine 1988; Blazer 2000). It can become more difficult to ascertain the primary cause of increased impairment and where best to focus therapeutic interventions. The risk of dementing disorders also increases dramatically in later life. A common feature of dementias is a change in personality or an exacerbation of preexisting characteristics. Without longitudinal history it can be difficult to know whether such presentations are manifestations of a personality disorder, a dementing disorder, or both.

In contrast with these difficulties, it is not uncommon for geriatric psychiatrists to comment that they do not have to deal with problems of patients with personality disorders as much as do their general psychiatry colleagues. Prevalence studies tend to support this observation. If these prevalence studies are valid, there are several explanations for why personality disorders might fade with age. One that deserves attention is that of maturation, described in adult development theory and research.

Although general research in personality disorders has increased, there is a relative dearth of such studies with respect to elderly persons (Agronin and Maletta 2000). This lack is particularly clear in the area of treatment. Substantial evidence shows the negative effect of personality disorders on the outcome of depressive disorders in elderly persons. Other than explaining poor outcomes, however, evidence on the methods and benefits of psychotherapy or pharmacotherapy for personality disorders in elderly persons remains limited. There is even less evidence on treatment and outcomes in nursing homes and general hospitals, the settings in which the geriatric psychiatrist is most likely to be called on to diagnose and treat personality disorders.

Definitions

Personality refers to an individual's habitual ways of relating to other people, interacting with the environment, and thinking about him- or herself (American Psychiatric Association 2000). Personality consists of both temperament (i.e., genetic dispositions) and character (i.e., qualities developed through interaction with the environment) (Robinson 2005). To classify a problem as a personality disorder, DSM-IV (American Psychiatric Association 1994) and its text revision, DSM-IV-TR (American Psychiatric Association 2000), posit several necessary elements: a personality disorder is a pattern of experience and behavior that is noticeably different from cultural expectations. The pattern develops by early adulthood and is intractable and relatively stable across the life span. A personality disorder influences a wide range of both social and personal situations. As is the case with all DSM-IV-TR disorders, a personality disorder results in significant distress or functional impairment. Finally, the enduring pattern must not be a manifestation of another mental disorder, a medical disorder, or use of a substance.

In treating elderly persons, ruling out manifestations of other disorders is particularly important because of the high prevalence of chronic medical disorders. When a change in personality occurs because of the comorbidity of another mental disorder, a medical disorder, or use of a substance, the DSM-IV-TR diagnosis of *personality change due to a general medical condition* is the appropriate diagnostic term. However, dementias are also increasingly prevalent with age and are often associated with changes in personality. A change in personality is often the chief complaint when an older person is brought in by caregivers for a specialist evaluation (Streams et al. 2003). These changes may be totally unrelated to premorbid personality, as occurs in frontal lobe dementias (Lebert et al. 1995), or may be marked exaggerations of preexisting traits, as occurs in Alzheimer's disease (Archer et al. 2007; Holst et al. 1997; Niederehe and Oxman 1994). Because of the progressive pervasiveness of a dementing disorder, the DSM-IV-TR diagnosis of personality change due to a general medical condition does not apply. Although these issues are important in differential diagnosis, for the purposes of this chapter the discussion of personality disorder is focused more closely on conditions that meet DSM-IV-TR personality disorder criteria.

After making a global assessment of the presence or absence of a personality disorder based on the key features listed previously, the next step is to identify a specific personality disorder or a personality cluster. Since 1980, DSM has categorized three different personality disorder clusters: A—odd, eccentric (including paranoid, schizoid, and schizotypal personality disorders); B—dramatic, erratic (including borderline, histrionic, narcissistic, and antisocial personality disorders); and C—anxious, fearful (including obsessive-compulsive, avoidant, and dependent personality disorders; see Table 24–1). The number of specific disorders has varied slightly over the past 20 years. Likewise, over the length of a life span often reaching 75–85 years, both personality and a personality disorder are likely to change somewhat; thus, attention to the identification of a cluster is particularly helpful. Because older patients with personality disorders commonly show symptoms of more than one personality disorder, diagnosis of a specific disorder is likely to be more difficult than in younger adults; thus, *personality disorder not otherwise specified* is a more common descriptive diagnosis for older patients.

Prevalence

The prevalence of personality disorders in the general population is less accurately known than that of Axis I disorders but is estimated at 10%–15% for all ages (Agronin and Maletta 2000; Grant et al. 2004; Lenzenweger et al. 1997; Weissman 1990), a relatively high rate compared with many Axis I disorders. The prevalence of personality disorders in psychiatric settings is usually three to four times higher than that in the community, with frequent comorbidity of Axis I and Axis II disorders (Kunik et al. 1994; Zweig and Hillman 1999).

The prevalence of personality disorders in older persons generally is lower by about half than that in younger persons in the general population (i.e., 5%–10%). The prevalence in selected outpatient or inpatient samples of older persons can be as high as 25%–65% (Agbayewa 1996; Agronin and Maletta 2000; Ames and Molinari 1994; Camus et al. 1997; Cohen et al. 1994; Fogel and Westlake 1990; Kenan et al. 2000). In part, this lower prevalence appears to be due to a decline in severity over the years, especially of Cluster B disorders (Black et al. 1995; Engels et al. 2003; Kenan et al. 2000; McGlashan 1986; Molinari et al. 1994; Robins et al. 1984; Snyder et al. 1985; Tyrer and Seiverwright 1988). Zanarini et al. (2007) recently reported the results of a 10-year follow-up study of 362 patients with personality disorders diagnosed at an inpatient admission. Twelve of 24 symptoms followed showed patterns of sharp decline, reported by less than 15% of patients who reported them at baseline. Symptoms related to impulsivity (such as self-mutilation and suicide attempts) and entitlement resolved relatively quickly. Mood symptoms such as anger, loneliness, and emptiness were more stable.

The association of personality disorders with depressive disorders in the elderly population is probably the single most reported comorbidity—especially Cluster C avoidant and dependent personality disorders (Abrams et al. 1994; Agbayewa 1996; Camus et al. 1997; Devanand et al. 2000; Fogel and Westlake 1990; Kunik et al. 1993; Morse and Lynch 2004; Nubukpo et

TABLE 24–1. Personality disorders and related aspects of aging

Cluster and types	Characteristics	Developmental needs	Related aspects of aging
A. Odd, eccentric			
Paranoid	Perception that people are dangerous, vigilance, suspiciousness	Trust, acceptance	Forced intimate contact from physical dependence highlights the disorder.
Schizoid	Isolation, autonomy	Reciprocity, intimacy	The disorder is relatively persistent.
Schizotypal	Bizarre behavior	Trust, social skills, abstract thinking	Individuals who do not have the disorder are subject to theft and ageism, leading to suspiciousness.
B. Dramatic, erratic			
Borderline	Sensitivity to rejection, feelings of abandonment	Reflection, systematization	Prevalence and/or severity of the disorder declines.
Histrionic	Expressiveness, exhibitionism	Self-esteem beyond attractiveness, reflection	With older age there is less energy and less opportunity for promiscuity, shoplifting, impulse expression.
Narcissistic	Self-aggrandizement, perceived specialness, competitiveness	Group identification, ability to share	
Antisocial	Exploitiveness, taking advantage of others	Empathy	
C. Anxious, fearful			
Obsessive-compulsive	Perfectionism, responsibility, systematization	Playfulness, spontaneity	The disorder is relatively persistent.
Avoidant	Vulnerability, inhibition	Self-assertion, expressiveness	This disorder is associated with poor outcome in major depression.
Dependent	Helplessness, attachment	Mobility, self-reliance	Individuals who do not have the disorder but have fewer social opportunities and more medical illness may be subject to overdiagnosis.

al. 2005), Cluster B personality disorders (Abrams et al. 2001; Sato et al. 1999; Vine and Steingart 1994), and personality disorder not otherwise specified (Kunik et al. 1993). The association is higher for early-onset than for late-onset depressive disorders (Abrams et al. 1994; Camus et al. 1997; Devanand et al. 2000; Fava et al. 1996; Nubukpo et al. 2005). This association of personality disorders and depressive disorders is an important relationship because the presence of a personality disorder in the context of a depressive disorder complicates differential diagnosis and treatment planning. For depressive disorders, the worst outcomes occur among patients with comorbid personality disorders (Abrams et al. 2001; Brodaty et al. 1995; Morse and Lynch 2004; Papakostas et al. 2003; Stek et al. 2002; Thompson et al. 1988; Vine and Steingart 1994). This comorbidity is associated with a longer time to response and more nonresponse to treatment. Expectations about treatment outcomes with antidepressants, electroconvulsive therapy, or hospitalization are thus lowered, and decisions about the need for psychotherapy are increased. The relationship between personality disorder and depression may be etiological. That is, personality disorders predispose to the occurrence of affective dysregulation and depressive disorders (Abrams et al. 1994; Sato et al. 1999). Alternatively, some chronic depression is the equivalent of a depressive disorder (Akiskal 1994, 2001).

The reports of lower prevalence of personality disorders in older persons have raised substantial controversy. There is some concern that the criteria for personality disorders used in earlier life may not adequately apply in later life (Abrams 1990; Kroessler 1990; Rosowsky and Gurian 1991; van Alphen et al.

2006), thus falsely lowering the prevalence in the elderly population. One suggested response is to modify the criteria for personality disorders in later life (Agronin and Maletta 2000; van Alphen et al. 2006). These arguments have some parallel to those positing that many DSM-IV-TR diagnostic criteria are age inappropriate for the elderly (Jeste et al. 1999).

Another suggested response is to adopt a dimensional approach. Personality researchers frequently use dimensional concepts, relating to personality traits, rather than the categorical language of disorders (American Psychiatric Association 2000; Costa and McCrae 1990; Eysenck 1998; Widiger et al. 2006). From this perspective, the categorical diagnostic approach is problematic because of co-occurring disorders, heterogeneity within diagnoses, and the limited evidence base. With respect to age, in nonclinical samples younger persons are somewhat higher on traits of extraversion, neuroticism, and openness, whereas older persons are higher on agreeableness and conscientiousness, with most of the change occurring in young adulthood rather than later life (Roberts et al. 2006). Longitudinal studies of personality traits show relative stability even over 30-year periods (Bengston et al. 1985; Costa and McCrae 1988; Costa et al. 1987; Duggan et al. 1991; Schaie and Willis 1986; Steunenberg et al. 2007). Perhaps most important with respect to geriatrics is that longitudinal studies of twins show that childhood personality change is primarily genetic, whereas in adulthood the majority is environmental, including change caused by experience and by disease (Roberts et al. 2006).

DSM-V, targeted for 2011, has the opportunity to revisit a dimensional versus a categorical approach. More than 18 proposals have been submitted for a dimensional approach to personality disorders (not confining this approach to normal traits as previously) in DSM-V (Widiger et al. 2006). It should be noted that although a dimensional approach may improve description and identification, it is less clear how the approach would be used in treatment, other than to revert to a categorical approach that uses cutoff scores on the dimensional scales. One current dimensional approach included in an appendix in DSM-IV-TR involves levels of defense mechanisms (the Defensive Functioning Scale in Appendix B). It addresses one of the important goals of a dimensional approach—that is, identifying a hierarchy (Widiger et al. 2006). The clinical relevance of defense mechanisms is due to their being reversible and adaptive as well as potentially pathological (Vaillant 1994). In this approach, defense mechanisms thus become categorized as immature, intermediate, or mature.

Rather than different criteria being needed for the elderly population, it is possible that the criteria are relevant but that at least some disorders, particularly those in Cluster B, do improve with age (Kernberg 1984; Sadavoy and Fogel 1992; Solomon 1981; Tyrer and Seivewright 1988; Zanarini et al. 2007). For example, older substance abusers showed lower levels of crime and drug use compared with when they were younger (Hanlon et al. 1990), and in general the elderly are more law abiding, with far fewer arrests (Harlow 1998). Thus, it is not inconsistent for older patients with personality disorders to exhibit fewer "high-energy" diagnostic criteria (e.g., lawbreaking, identity disturbance, promiscuity). Do these research results mean that a maturational change has occurred—or merely that the symptom displays are more subtle because of physical and institutional restrictions (Abrams 1990; Hillman et al. 1997; Rosowsky and Gurian 1991)? Although arguments for modified criteria may ultimately be valid, equal theory and evidence from adult development research at least support the current criteria and the resulting epidemiological findings.

Adult Development

Erikson's concept of epigenesis is important in understanding how personality disorders might improve with age. Erikson was a strong proponent of the interaction of the psychosocial environment with development across the life span. Erikson's stage theory of late-life development (Erikson et al. 1986) proposed that the major developmental task of older age is to look back and seek meaning across the life span, rather than looking forward as in previous developmental modes that are now in decline. The goal of this task as discussed by Erikson is to maintain more integrity than despair about one's life. In this process, as at previous life stages, each earlier life stage conflict must be reconciled and integrated with the current stage, allowing resolution of earlier conflicts. Persons with personality disorders might be expected to have greater difficulty in accomplishing this resolution than other individuals. However, this resolution is not an all-or-nothing phenomenon. The achievement of even some resolution may contribute to the mellowing of a personality disorder.

Vaillant and others (e.g., Diehl et al. 1996) have provided empirical verification for Erikson's life-stage concepts through longitudinal study of the maturation of defenses across the life span (Vaillant 2000, 2002; Vaillant and Milofsky 1980). Defenses are involuntary mental mechanisms for regulating the realities that persons are powerless to change. Vaillant and others (Haan 1977) have described a hierarchy of defenses from immature and maladaptive to mature and adaptive. Mature defenses include humor, altruism, sublimation, anticipation, and suppression. Mature and adaptive defenses synthesize and attenuate conflicts rather than distorting or denying them. Across several longitudinal studies that included privileged persons (Heath 1945), gifted persons (Terman 1925), and persons from the core inner cities (Glueck and Glueck 1968), Vaillant established that mature defenses were more consistently identified primarily in Erikson's later developmental stages (Vaillant 1993; Vaillant and Drake 1985) and that the development of these defenses was independent of education and social privilege (Vaillant 1993). Similarly, others have identified a socioemotional selectiveness for optimizing positive emotional meaningfulness with age (Charles et al. 2003) and improved coping skills with aging (Ryff 1999).

Events with psychological and social impact can reveal previously submerged difficulty. For example, the death of a spouse may unmask dependency problems. Retirement or bereavement may lead to narcissistic problems such as poor regulation of self-esteem and faulty adaptation to loss. However, experience—something that the elderly have more of than any other age group—may attenuate the impact of such later-life events, even for older persons with personality disorders (Birditt and Fingerman 2005; Ryff 1999). For example, in order to cope effectively with stress, persons must learn to recognize the difference between situations that can and cannot be changed and then must match the right coping skill with the right situation. Emotion-focused coping is used when a situation cannot be changed; problem-focused coping is used when a situation can be changed. It is only through repeated experience that these skills develop (Ryff 1999). Although stressful situations certainly exacerbate the symptoms of personality disorders, Neugarten (1970) pointed out how the meaning of stressful situations changes over time. We expect to experience the death of loved ones and our own declining health when we are older and have time to mentally rehearse how we will respond to these "on-time" losses. When these losses occur "off time"—at earlier stages of life—the stress is usually experienced as much greater.

Consideration of this line of evidence should not minimize the impact of personality disorders or the need for some management of them in later life. Even if the prevalence of personality disorders truly does decline, there are still some elderly persons with continuing disorders that cause impairment to themselves and their environment. Consideration of adult development helps us understand how some persons with personality disorders may improve and to understand that this improvement is consistent with the epidemiological findings of reduced psychopathology in later life. Equally important, adult developmental theory helps the clinician consider the positive aspects of development, even in persons with severe psychopathology (Erikson et al. 1986; Ryff 1999). Until the debate on the validity of the epidemiological findings versus the criteria used to make those findings is more definitively settled, perhaps designations of personality disorder "in remission" or "in partial remission" would be a more appropriate and parsimonious way of addressing diagnoses of personality disorder in the elderly population.

Evaluation

Because personality disorders typically have a lifelong pattern, diagnosis generally requires greater historical and collateral information than for Axis I disorders. Complete understanding of the causes of signs and symptoms in geriatric psychiatry is a difficult accomplishment. The interplay of multiple etiologic factors is the rule, not the exception. The Structured Clinical Interview for DSM-IV Axis II Personality Disorders (SCID-II; First et al. 1997) and the Personality Disorders Examination (PDE; Loranger 1988) are semistructured interviews for personality disorders that can be used to guide a diagnostic interview and increase reliability. Historical information, from medical records and from persons who have known a patient over a long period, is still an essential component of an accurate and valid diagnosis. The interview requires a longitudinal inquiry about various life stages to establish the historical presence of a personality disorder, even if not all current criteria are met. Several ancillary self-report instruments are available for initial screening purposes—for example, the Millon Clinical Multiaxial Inventory—III (MCMI-III; Millon 1994), the Personality

Diagnostic Questionnaire (PDQ-IV; Hyler et al. 1988), the Schedule for Nonadaptive and Adaptive Personality (Clark 1993), and the Wisconsin Personality Disorders Inventory (Klein et al. 1993). However, the results of these self-reports have a low concordance with the results of interview methods (Perry 1992), and their use is best established and tolerated in younger populations, not among elderly persons, in whom acquired brain disease is an increasing issue. The Neuroticism, Extraversion, Openness Five-Factor Model (NEO-FFM; Costa and McCrae 1985, 1997) is a reliable and valid dimensional assessment tool for personality traits that has been used with the elderly. This tool has also proved useful as a screening tool for personality disorders (Miller et al. 2005).

Geriatric psychiatrists are familiar with the phenomenon that acquired brain disease in later life appears to strengthen undesirable personality traits that were present, but less intense and conspicuous, in earlier adult life. However, if signs and symptoms of personality disorder were not present before the onset of dementing illness or brain injury, it is rational to assume that such illnesses play a causative role in the personality change. A reasonable approach to a diagnosis in geriatrics, as always, includes these elements: 1) careful and detailed review of the medical and psychosocial history, 2) mental status and physical examinations, with special attention to the neurological examination, and 3) a screening laboratory examination—including, in some cases, brain imaging, an electroencephalogram, and neuropsychological tests.

In many instances, those most able to provide the historical information providing the best clues are family members. Whenever possible, their help should be sought concerning the older patient in whom personality disorder is suspected. Viewing the patient within the family context usually gives added depth of understanding to the clinical perspective.

Syndromes based on frontal lobe pathology that result in loss of normal executive function present some of the most difficult diagnostic challenges—especially if the onset of symptoms is subtle, the rate of progression is slow, and the main attributes of the premorbid personality are obscure. Patients with frontal or frontotemporal lobe disease may show good preservation of memory function. They are, however, prone to trouble with "mechanistic planning, verbal reasoning, or problem solving" and "obeying the rules of interpersonal social behaviour, the experience of reward and punishment, and the interpretation of complex emotions" (Grafman and Litvan 1999, p. 1921; Passant et al. 2005).

These difficulties are similar to some of the problems experienced by many people with borderline, narcissistic, histrionic, paranoid, and antisocial personality disorders. Could one develop a later-life personality disorder de novo, without the presence of underlying brain disease or substance abuse? The answer is not definitively known, but the occurrence is probably rare. It is also possible that signs and symptoms of personality disorders can be quite evident in early adult life, then be diminished or quiescent in mid-adult life, and then reemerge under the stress of social losses or physical illness in later life (Rosowsky and Gurian 1992). The manifestations of personality disorders may vary in different parts of the life cycle. For example, in persons with borderline personality disorder, phenomena such as splitting, intense and unstable interpersonal relationships, impaired affective regulation, and extreme difficulty with control and regulation of anger often persist throughout the life cycle. Problems such as severe impulsivity, risky behavior, and self-mutilation tend to diminish with advancing age (Zanarini et al. 2007). However, other self-injurious behaviors may take their place. These include self-starvation, abuse of medicines, and noncompliance with medical treatment (Rosowsky and Gurian 1992). These behaviors may occur for other reasons, but their presence should at least alert the clinician to the possibility of borderline personality disorder. Late-onset obsessive-compulsive symptoms or traits are particularly likely to have a basis in brain disease.

Treatment Issues

The broad focus of treatment is on reducing symptoms, improving social functioning, and changing responses to the environment (Robinson 2005). Off-label use of psychotropic agents is sometimes valuable for symptom reduction, whereas psychotherapy and caregiver education are helpful for addressing environmental response. All should be considered for their contribution to improved function of older persons.

Psychotherapy

In contrast to the unconscious maturation of defenses, the conscious alteration of personality is unusual. Although people are sometimes able to change patterns of behavior, attitudes, ways of thinking, and ways of feeling, changing the fundamental personality structure is extremely difficult. At the same time, it is possible and important to try to help patients avoid behavior that significantly harms them or others. Helping patients recognize and alter erroneous or distorted thinking is thus also important and possible. Cognitive-behavioral or insight-oriented psychotherapy may significantly help older individuals who are functioning at higher levels and who are not otherwise seriously ill or incapacitated (Beck et al. 2004; Clarkin et al. 2007). For patients in psychiatric hospitals and for residents of group homes or nursing homes, intensive psychotherapy with a goal of changing lifelong maladaptive personality features is neither an available nor an indicated treatment modality. However, for such individuals, supportive and consistent psychotherapeutic contact can be of great benefit (Bienenfeld 1990).

As noted, psychotherapy of any type, either by itself or in combination with pharmacotherapy, with a goal of a global revision of maladaptive aspects of personality in later life, is unlikely to succeed. Individualized treatment targeting specific symptoms that discomfort, threaten, or endanger patients or their family or caregivers—for example, behavioral management to minimize harm from impaired social judgment—is far more realistic and more likely to realize success. However, it is still important not to be rigid or negative about the psychotherapeutic potential of older patients. It is illness, not merely age, that limits or impairs the plasticity of the personality and the potential for self-change. Older patients are often impressive in their resilience, courage, open-mindedness, and willingness to try new ways of thinking and behaving—and those showing these characteristics include some individuals whose adaptation to life in earlier years was far from optimal. This observation is in keeping with Erikson's view of progressive development throughout life. Psychoanalytically oriented psychotherapy, cognitive-behavioral therapy, interpersonal therapy, dialectical behavior therapy, and other forms of psychotherapy all have their adherents and proponents (De Leo et al. 1999). All are probably helpful to certain individuals. The principal features of successful psychotherapy for geriatric patients are a structure with consistency, availability, empathic and respectful listening, flexibility, and open-mindedness on the part of the psychotherapist. These features are probably more important than a particular theoretical orientation (Clarkin et al. 2007).

Therapists who are not yet old themselves have a difficult challenge. They have no direct experience with or memory of being old (Rosowsky 1999). Some geriatric psychiatrists may be two full generations younger than their patients. Extraordinary empathy is required of these clinicians, but also of most practicing geriatric psychiatrists, who are usually caring for persons older than themselves.

Pharmacotherapy

A diagnosis of personality disorder should not preclude pharmacological treatment of concomitant psychiatric disorders such as affective illness or psychosis as well as specific symptoms that may respond to psychotropic medications (Kunik et al. 1993). Successful treatment of affective or psychotic symptoms may show that the symptoms were the result of these eminently treatable diseases, not entrenched maladaptive personality traits. Personality disorder, depressive illness, and acquired brain disease share overlapping symptom constellations: symptoms such as irritability, hostility, and uncooperativeness can derive from all three. Even the most perspicacious diagnostician may not be able to tease out a clear etiological diagnosis for these difficult behavioral symptoms. In such cases, an empirical treatment trial with antidepressant medicine is indicated.

Patients with other symptoms—such as anger outbursts, apathy, and impaired social judgment—may also benefit from pharmacotherapy (Hollander et al. 2003). Pharmacological treatment should be guided by systematic trials of pharmacotherapy for identified target symptom areas (affect, impulsivity/aggression, anxiety, thinking/psychosis) (see Table 24–2), an assessment strategy (global rating, self-reports, or caregiver reports targeted to the symptom area), and a specified duration. Selective serotonin reuptake inhibitors and other newer antidepressant drugs, anticonvulsants, and atypical antipsychotic drugs, used alone or in combinations, may be useful in systematic trials for specified symptoms.

Caregiver Education

Education of caregivers is an important function of geriatric psychiatrists. Family members may be having great difficulty in dealing with unfamiliar negative, disinhibited, or inappropriate behavior. If an underlying medical or neurological etiology can be discerned, caregivers can be reassured about the cause of the otherwise inexplicable changes in their relationship with their loved one. This reassurance helps reduce guilt, anxiety, and uncertainty in the family of the afflicted person.

TABLE 24–2. Symptom areas and pharmacotherapy classes in personality disorders

Symptom area and types	Principal neurotransmitter	Pharmacotherapy class
Cognition/Perception		
Loose associations, thought blocking	Dopamine	Antipsychotics
Overvalued ideas, delusions		
Hallucinations, depersonalization		
Affect/Mood		
Harm/Avoidance	Serotonin	SSRIs
Depression, lability	GABA	Mood stabilizers
Anger		Benzodiazepines
Anxiety		
Behavior		
Impulsivity	Norepinephrine	Mood stabilizers
Aggression	Dopamine	TCAs, MAOIs
Novelty seeking		Antipsychotics
Reward/Dependence		

Note. GABA=γ-aminobutyric acid; MAOIs-monoamine oxidase inhibitors; SSRIs=selective serotonin reuptake inhibitors; TCAs=tricyclic antidepressants.

Primary caregivers in nursing homes, who are usually overworked and underpaid, may not realize that much of the unpleasant behavior of patients that they encounter in their work is not under full volitional control. Uncooperativeness or angry outbursts may have the appearance of simple willfulness or intentionally oppositional behavior. Patients with long-standing personality disorders (as well as those with dementia, stroke, or other types of brain injury) typically have significant deficits in volitional capacity. Understanding this point does not necessarily make the care of these patients easier, but it does provide a perspective on behavior that is otherwise difficult to comprehend and tolerate.

Conclusion

Understanding of the causes of disordered personality development is far from adequate. Diagnosis, and especially treatment, of personality disorders in elderly patients is difficult. Understanding the differentiation between lifelong development and acquired neuropsychiatric illness is an important diagnostic challenge. Geriatric psychiatrists usually try to manage personality disorder symptoms and ameliorate their harmful effects rather than attempt to cure the underlying disorder. Behavioral management, psychotherapy, pharmacotherapy, and caregiver support are the tools that must be judiciously used.

Key Points

- The natural history of personality in later life is influenced by the combination of increasing medical-neuropsychiatric comorbidity and ongoing normal psychosocial maturation.
- Without longitudinal history, it can be difficult to know whether presumed personality problems in later life are a manifestation of a personality disorder, a dementing disorder, or both.
- The prevalence of personality disorders in older persons is generally lower than in younger persons in the general population.
- Positive adaptation in late-life development can mediate the severity and presentation of personality disorders.
- Substantial evidence shows the negative effect of personality disorders on the outcome of depressive disorders in elderly persons.
- It is possible and important to use psychotherapeutic and caregiver interventions to try to help older

patients with personality disorders avoid behavior that significantly harms themselves or others.

- Pharmacological treatment should be guided by systematic trials of pharmacotherapy for identified target symptom areas, an assessment strategy, and a specified duration.

References

Abrams RC: Personality disorders in the elderly, in Verwoerdt's Clinical Geropsychiatry, 3rd Edition. Edited by Bienenfeld D. Baltimore, MD, Williams & Wilkins, 1990, pp 151–163

Abrams RC, Rosendahl E, Card C, et al: Personality disorder correlates of late and early onset depression. J Am Geriatr Soc 42:727–731, 1994

Abrams RC, Alexopoulos GS, Spielman LA, et al: Personality disorder symptoms predict declines in global functioning and quality of life in elderly depressed patients. Am J Geriatr Psychiatry 9:67–71, 2001

Agbayewa MO: Occurrence and effects of personality disorders in depression: are they the same in the old and young? Can J Psychiatry 41:223–226, 1996

Agronin ME, Maletta G: Personality disorders in late life: understanding and overcoming the gap in research. Am J Geriatr Psychiatry 8:4–18, 2000

Akiskal HS: Dysthymia: clinical and external validity. Acta Psychiatr Scand 383(suppl):19–23, 1994

Akiskal HS: Dysthymia and cyclothymia in psychiatric practice a century after Kraepelin. J Affect Disord 62:17–31, 2001

Ames A, Molinari V: Prevalence of personality disorders in community-living elderly. J Geriatr Psychiatry Neurol 7:189–194, 1994

American Psychiatric Association: Diagnostic and Statistical Manual of Mental Disorders, 4th Edition. Washington, DC, American Psychiatric Association, 1994

American Psychiatric Association: Diagnostic and Statistical Manual of Mental Disorders, 4th Edition, Text Revision. Washington, DC, American Psychiatric Association, 2000

Archer N, Brown RG, Reeves SJ, et al: Premorbid personality and behavioral and psychological symptoms in probable Alzheimer disease. Am J Geriatr Psychiatry 15:202–213, 2007

Beck AT, Freeman A, Davis DD: Cognitive Therapy of Personality Disorders, 2nd Edition. New York, Guilford, 2004

Bengston V, Reedy M, Gordon C: Aging and self-conceptions: personality processes and social contexts, in Handbook of the Psychology of Aging. Edited by Birren JE, Schaie KW. New York, Van Nostrand Reinhold, 1985, pp 544–593

Besdine RW: Functional assessment in the elderly, in Geriatric Medicine, 2nd Edition. Edited by Rowe JW, Besdine RW. Boston, MA, Little, Brown, 1988, pp 37–51

Bienenfeld D: Verwoerdt's Clinical Geropsychiatry, 3rd Edition. Baltimore, MD, Williams & Wilkins, 1990

Birditt KS, Fingerman KL: Do we get better at picking our battles? Age group differences in descriptions of behavioral reactions to interpersonal tensions. J Gerontol B Psychol Sci Soc Sci 60B:P121–P12, 2005

Black DW, Baumgard CH, Bell SE: The long-term outcome of antisocial personality disorder compared with depression, schizophrenia, and surgical conditions. Bull Am Acad Psychiatry Law 23:43–52, 1995

Blazer D: Psychiatry and the oldest old. Am J Psychiatry 157:1915–1924, 2000

Brodaty H, Harris L, Peters K: A 16- to 45-year follow-up of 71 men with antisocial personality disorder. Compr Psychiatry 36:130–140, 1995

Camus V, De Mendonca Lima CA, Gaillard M, et al: Are personality disorders more frequent in early onset geriatric depression? J Affect Disord 46:297–302, 1997

Charles ST, Mather M, Carstensen LL: Aging and emotional memory: the forgettable nature of negative images for older adults. J Exp Psychol Gen 132:310–324, 2003

Clark LA: Manual for the Schedule for Nonadaptive and Adaptive Personality (SNAP). Minneapolis University of Minnesota Press, 1993

Clarkin JF, Levy KN, Lenzenweger MF, et al: Evaluating three treatments for borderline personality disorder: a multiwave study. Am J Psychiatry 164:922–928, 2007

Cohen BJ, Nestadt G, Samuels JF, et al: Personality disorder in later life: a community study. Br J Psychiatry 165:493–499, 1994

Costa PT, McCrae RR: The NEO Personality Inventory Manual. Odessa, FL, Psychological Assessment Resources, 1985

Costa PT Jr, McCrae RR: Personality in adulthood: a six-year longitudinal study of self-reports and spouse ratings on the NEO Personality Inventory. J Pers Soc Psychol 54:853–863, 1988

Costa PT Jr, McCrae RR: Personality disorders and the five-factor model of personality. J Personal Disord 4:362–371, 1990

Costa PT Jr, McCrae RR: Stability and change in personality assessment: the revised NEO Personality Inventory in the year 2000. J Pers Assess 68:86–94, 1997

Costa PT Jr, Zonderman AB, McCrae RR, et al: Longitudinal analyses of psychological well-being in a national sample: stability of mean levels. J Gerontol 42:50–55, 1987

De Leo D, Scocco P, Meneghel G: Pharmacological and psychotherapeutic treatment of personality disorders in the elderly. Int Psychogeriatr 11:191–206, 1999

Devanand DP, Turret N, Moody BJ, et al: Personality disorders in elderly patients with dysthymic disorder. Am J Geriatr Psychiatry 8:188–195, 2000

Diehl M, Coyle N, Labouvie-Vief G: Age and sex differences in strategies of coping and defense across the life span. Psychol Aging 11:127–136, 1996

Duggan CF, Shap P, Lee AS, et al: Does recurrent depression lead to a change in neuroticism? Psychol Med 21:985–990, 1991

Engels GI, Duijsens IJ, Haringsma R, et al: Personality disorders in the elderly compared to four younger age groups: a cross-sectional study of community residents and mental health patients. J Personal Disord 17:447–459, 2003

Erikson EH, Erikson JM, Kivnick HQ: Vital Involvement in Old Age. New York, WW Norton, 1986

Eysenck HJ: Dimensions of Personality. New Brunswick, NJ, Transaction Publishers, 1998

Fava M, Alpert JE, Borus JS, et al: Patterns of personality disorder comorbidity in early onset versus late-onset major depression. Am J Psychiatry 153:1308–1312, 1996

First MB, Gibbon M, Spitzer RL, et al: Structured Clinical Interview for DSM-IV Axis II Personality Disorders (SCID-II). Washington, DC, American Psychiatric Press, 1997

Fogel BS, Westlake R: Personality disorder diagnoses and age in inpatients with major depression. J Clin Psychiatry 51:232–235, 1990

Glueck S, Glueck E: Delinquents and Non-Delinquents in Perspective. Cambridge, MA, Harvard University Press, 1968

Grafman J, Litvan I: Importance of deficits in executive function. Lancet 354:1921–1922, 1999

Grant BF, Hasin DS, Stinson FS, et al: Prevalence, correlates, and disability of personality disorders in the United States: results from the national epidemiologic survey on alcohol and related conditions. J Clin Psychiatry 65:948–958, 2004

Haan NA: Coping and Defending. San Francisco, CA, Jossey-Bass, 1977

Hanlon TE, Nurco DN, Kinlock TW, et al: Trends in criminal activity and drug use over an addiction career. Am J Drug Alcohol Abuse 16:223–238, 1990

Harlow CW: Special Report: Profile of Jail Inmates 1996 (Publ No NCJ 164620). Washington, DC, U.S. Department of Justice, 1998

Heath C: What People Are. Cambridge, MA, Harvard University Press, 1945

Hillman J, Stricker G, Zweig R: Clinical psychologists' judgment of older adult patients with character pathology: implications for practice. Prof Psychol Res Pr 28:179–183, 1997

Hollander E, Tracy KA, Swann AC, et al: Divalproex in the treatment of impulsive aggression: efficacy in cluster B personality disorders. Neuropsychopharmacology 28:1186–1197, 2003

Holst G, Hallberg IR, Gustafson L: The relationship of vocally disruptive behavior and previous personality in severely demented institutionalized patients. Arch Psychiatr Nurs 11:147–154, 1997

Hyler SE, Rieder RO, Williams JBW, et al: The Personality Diagnostic Questionnaire: development and preliminary results. J Personal Disord 2:229–237, 1988

Jeste DV, Alexopoulos GS, Bartels SJ, et al: Consensus statement on the upcoming crisis in geriatric mental health: research agenda for the next two decades. Arch Gen Psychiatry 56:848–853, 1999

Kenan MM, Kendjelic EM, Molinari VA, et al: Age-related differences in the frequency of personality disorders among inpatient veterans. Int J Geriatr Psychiatry 15:831–837, 2000

Kernberg O: Severe Personality Disorders: Psychotherapeutic Strategies. New Haven, CT, Yale University Press, 1984

Klein MH, Benjamin L, Rosenfelt R: The Wisconsin Personality Disorders Inventory. J Personal Disord 7:285–303, 1993

Kroessler D: Personality disorder in the elderly. Hosp Community Psychiatry 41:1325–1329, 1990

Kunik ME, Mulsant B, Rifai AH, et al: Personality disorders in elderly inpatients with major depression. Am J Geriatr Psychiatry 1:38–45, 1993

Kunik ME, Mulsant B, Rifai AH, et al: Diagnostic rate of comorbid personality disorder in elderly psychiatric inpatients. Am J Psychiatry 151:603–605, 1994

Lebert F, Pasquier F, Petit H: Personality traits and frontal lobe dementia. Int J Geriatr Psychiatry 10:1047–1049, 1995

Lenzenweger MF, Loranger AW, Korfine L, et al: Detecting personality disorders in a nonclinical population: application for a two-stage procedure for case identification. Arch Gen Psychiatry 54:345–351, 1997

Loranger AW: Personality Disorders Examination (PDE) Manual. Yonkers, NY, DV Communications, 1988

McGlashan TH: The Chestnut Lodge follow-up study, III: long-term outcome of borderline personalities. Arch Gen Psychiatry 43:20–30, 1986

Miller JD, Bagby RM, Pilkonis PA, et al: A simplified technique for scoring DSM-IV personality disorders with the Five-Factor Model. Assessment 12:404–415, 2005

Millon T: Clinical Multiaxial Inventory—III (MCMI-III). Minneapolis, MN, National Computer Systems, 1994

Molinari V, Ames A, Essa M: Prevalence of personality disorders in two geropsychiatric inpatient units. J Geriatr Psychiatry Neurol 7:209–215, 1994

Morse JQ, Lynch TR: A preliminary investigation of self-reported personality disorders in late life: prevalence, predictors of depressive severity, and clinical correlates. Aging Ment Health 8:307–315, 2004

Neugarten BL: Adaptation and the life cycle. J Geriatr Psychol 4:71–87, 1970

Niederehe GT, Oxman TE: The spectrum of dementias: construct and nosologic validity, in Dementia Presentations, Differential Diagnosis, and Nosology. Edited by Emery O, Oxman TE. Baltimore, MD, Johns Hopkins University Press, 1994, pp 19–45

Nubukpo P, Hartmann J, Clement JP: [Role of personality in depression of the elderly: difference between early and late life depression (in French)]. Psychol Neuropsychiatr Vieil 3:63–69, 2005

Papakostas GI, Petersen TJ, Farabaugh AH, et al: Psychiatric comorbidity as a predictor of clinical response to nortriptyline in treatment-resistant major depressive disorder. J Clin Psychiatry 64:1357–1361, 2003

Passant U, Elfgren C, Englund E, et al: Psychiatric symptoms and their psychosocial consequences in frontotemporal dementia. Alzheimer Dis Assoc Disord 19 (suppl 1):S15–S18, 2005

Perry JC: Problems and considerations in the valid assessment of personality disorders. Am J Psychiatry 149:1645–1653, 1992

Roberts BW, Walton KE, Viechtbauer W: Patterns of mean-level change in personality traits across the life course: a meta-analysis of longitudinal studies. Psychol Bull 132:1–25, 2006

Robins LN, Helzer JE, Weissman MM, et al: Lifetime prevalence of specific psychiatric disorders in three sites. Arch Gen Psychiatry 41:949–958, 1984

Robinson DJ: Field Guide to Personality Disorders, 2nd Edition. Port Huron, MI, Rapid Psychler Press, 2005

Rosowsky E: Personality disorders and the difficult nursing home resident, in Personality Disorders in Older Adults: Emerging Issues in Diagnosis and Treatment. Edited by Rosowsky E, Abrams RC. Mahwah, NJ, Erlbaum, 1999, pp 257–274

Rosowsky E, Gurian B: Borderline personality disorder in late life. Int Psychogeriatr 3:39–52, 1991

Rosowsky E, Gurian B: Impact of borderline personality disorder in late life on systems of care. Hosp Community Psychiatry 43:386–389, 1992

Ryff CD: Psychology and aging, in Principles of Geriatric Medicine and Gerontology, 4th Edition. Edited by Hazzard WR, Blass JP, Ettinger WH, et al. New York, McGraw-Hill, 1999, pp 159–169

Sadavoy J, Fogel BS: Personality disorders in old age, in Handbook of Mental Health and Aging. Edited by Birren J, Sloane R, Cohen G. San Diego, CA, Academic Press, 1992, pp 433–462

Sato T, Sakado K, Uehara T, et al: Personality disorder comorbidity in early onset versus late-onset major depression in Japan. J Nerv Ment Dis 187:237–242, 1999

Schaie KW, Willis S: Adult Development and Aging, 2nd Edition. Boston, MA, Little, Brown, 1986

Snyder S, Goodpaster WA, Pitts WM, et al: Demography of psychiatric patients with borderline traits. Psychopathology 18:38–49, 1985

Solomon K: Personality disorder in the elderly, in Personality Disorders: Diagnosis and Management, 2nd Edition. Edited by

Lion JR. Baltimore, MD, Williams & Wilkins, 1981, pp 310–338

Stek ML, Van Exel E, Van Tilburg W, et al: The prognosis of depression in old age: outcome six to eight years after clinical treatment. Aging Ment Health 6:282–285, 2002

Steunenberg B, Beekman AT, Deeg DJ, et al: Mastery and neuroticism predict recovery of depression in later life. Am J Geriatr Psychiatry 15:234–242, 2007

Streams ME, Wackerbarth SB, Maxwell A: Diagnosis-seeking at subspecialty memory clinics: trigger events. Int J Geriatr Psychiatry 18:915–924, 2003

Terman LM: Genetic Studies of Genius, Vol 1: Mental and Physical Traits of a Thousand Gifted Children. Palo Alto, CA, Stanford University Press, 1925

Thompson LW, Gallagher D, Czirr R: Personality disorder and outcome in the treatment of late-life depression. J Geriatr Psychiatry 21:133–153, 1988

Tyrer P, Seiverwright H: Studies of outcome, in Personality Disorders: Diagnosis, Management and Course. Edited by Tyrer P. London, Wright, 1988, pp 119–136

Vaillant GE: The Wisdom of the Ego. Cambridge, MA, Harvard University Press, 1993

Vaillant GE: Ego mechanisms of defense and personality psychopathology. J Abnorm Psychol 130:44–50, 1994

Vaillant GE: Adaptive mental mechanisms: their role in a positive psychology. Am Psychol 55:89–98, 2000

Vaillant GE: Aging Well. Boston, MA, Little, Brown, 2002

Vaillant GE, Drake RE: Maturity of ego defenses in relation to DSM-III axis II personality disorder. Arch Gen Psychiatry 42:597–601, 1985

Vaillant GE, Milofsky E: Natural history of male psychological health, IX: empirical evidence for Erikson's model of the life cycle. Am J Psychiatry 137:1348–1359, 1980

van Alphen SP, Engelen GJ, Kuin R, et al: The relevance of a geriatric sub-classification of personality disorders in the DSM-V. Int J Geriatr Psychiatry 21:205–209, 2006

Vine RG, Steingart AB: Personality disorder in the elderly depressed. Can J Psychiatry 39:392–398, 1994

Weissman M: The epidemiology of personality disorders: a 1990 update. J Personal Disord 7 (suppl):44–62, 1990

Widiger TA, Simonsen E, Sirovatka PJ, et al (eds): Dimensional Models of Personality Disorders: Refining the Research Agenda for DSM-V. Washington, DC, American Psychiatric Association, 2006

Zanarini MC, Frankenburg FR, Reich DB, et al: The subsyndromal phenomenology of borderline personality disorder: a 10-year follow-up study. Am J Psychiatry 164:929–935, 2007

Zweig R, Hillman J: Personality disorders in adults: a review, in Emerging Issues in Diagnosis and Treatment: LEA Series in Personality and Clinical Psychology. Edited by Rosowsky E, Abrams RC. Mahwah, NJ, Erlbaum, 1999, pp 31–53

Suggested Readings

Agronin ME, Maletta G: Personality disorders in late life: understanding and overcoming the gap in research. Am J Geriatr Psychiatry 8:4–18, 2000

Beck AT, Freeman A, Davis DD: Cognitive Therapy of Personality Disorders, 2nd Edition. New York, Guilford, 2004

Clarkin JF, Levy KN, Lenzenweger MF, et al: Evaluating three treatments for borderline personality disorder: a multiwave study. Am J Psychiatry 164:922–928, 2007

Costa PT Jr, McCrae RR: Changes in personality and their origins: comment on Roberts, Walton, and Viechtbauer (2006). Psychol Bull 132:26–28, 2006

Roberts BW, Walton KE, Viechtbauer W: Patterns of mean-level change in personality traits across the life course: a meta-analysis of longitudinal studies. Psychol Bull 132:1–25, 2006

Widiger TA, Simonsen E, Sirovatka PJ, et al (eds): Dimensional Models of Personality Disorders: Refining the Research Agenda for DSM-V. Washington, DC, American Psychiatric Association, 2006

Zanarini MC, Frankenburg FR, Reich DB, et al: The subsyndromal phenomenology of borderline personality disorder: a 10-year follow-up study. Am J Psychiatry 164:929–935, 2007

CHAPTER 25

Agitation and Suspiciousness

Harold W. Goforth, M.D.
Lisa P. Gwyther, M.S.W.

Suspiciousness and Paranoia

Psychiatrists working with older adults frequently encounter suspicious or paranoid behaviors, especially in patients with agitation. In fact, such ideation is not very uncommon in community populations of elderly adults. In a community study of elderly persons in San Francisco, 17% of the subjects reported that they were highly suspicious, and 13% reported delusions (Lowenthal and Berkman 1967). Another study that included elderly persons in both urban and rural areas of North Carolina found that 4% of older adults experienced a sense of persecution by those around them (Christenson and Blazer 1984). Perceptions of a hostile social environment or ideas of persecution lead to greater stress, vigilance, and agitation among elderly persons, resulting in alienation from families and friends. Such individuals represent a challenge for clinicians who care for them.

Among suspicious or paranoid elderly persons, one group has long been recognized, particularly in Europe. The term *late-life paraphrenia* has been used to identify psychosis that has a late age at onset and to distinguish the condition from both chronic schizophrenia and dementia. Kraepelin used *paraphrenia* to classify a small group of patients who exhibited paranoid delusions and yet were able to maintain functioning in their social milieu for months or years. He observed that persons with paraphrenia were typically women, usually living alone. Although current DSM diagnostic nomenclature would classify many of those individuals as having delusional disorder, this late-life syndrome may be more complex. Sometimes paranoid ideation is accompanied by hallucinations. In addition, patients with this condition may have comorbid sensory deficits, especially visual or hearing loss. Thus, although the condition may have features of delusional disorder, it may also have features and comorbidities that point to its being a different entity, perhaps along a continuum with schizophrenia. When the condition is accompanied by agitation, neuroleptics are usually the first-line treatment, although information is lacking on the effectiveness of this class of medications in delusional disorder. Caution with these medications is also warranted, given the increased sensitivity of elderly persons to neuroleptics (Soares and Gershon 1997).

Clearly, chronic paranoid schizophrenia persisting into late life is a major cause of suspiciousness and agitation in elderly persons. With accompanying functional decline and problematic behaviors occurring earlier in life in patients with schizophrenia, it is unusual for new cases of chronic schizophrenia to be diagnosed in elderly patients. Multimodal treatment—including neuroleptic medication, case management, and family education and involvement—is essential for ensuring adequate care. The occurrence of agitation in chronic paranoid schizophrenia patients is common and may indicate a need for an adjustment in neuroleptic dosing.

Lisa Gwyther gratefully acknowledges support from the Joseph and Kathleen Bryan Alzheimer's Disease Research Center at Duke University Medical Center, grant P30 AGO28377 from the National Institute on Aging.

However, new agitation arising in a previously stable older patient with schizophrenia may also indicate another problem, and clinicians need to be particularly attuned to the possibility of an acute medical problem. The medical causes of agitation discussed below for patients with dementia may also affect older patients with schizophrenia, who may require the same level of medical scrutiny.

Classic delusional disorder may occur at any age and is usually characterized by delusions centered on a single theme or a series of connected themes. In elderly patients, delusions tend to be nonbizarre—for example, paranoid jealousy may be seen in individuals with a relatively intact premorbid personality (Yassa and Suranyi-Cadotte 1993). Agitation may become an issue when such individuals are confronted by family or clinicians about their delusion. Data are lacking on treatment for this disorder. Neuroleptics, particularly pimozide, have been reported to be helpful for the delusion (Opler and Feinberg 1991), but behavioral intervention and non-neuroleptic medication may be better choices for sporadic agitation that may arise.

Diagnostic Approach to Patients With New Onset of Suspiciousness and Paranoia

As with most mental disorders, a careful psychiatric evaluation and history are key components of the initial approach to the suspicious or paranoid patient. Interviews of family members may be necessary for establishing a diagnosis, particularly if delusions and agitation are present. Part of the task of the clinician is to determine whether suspicious behavior is warranted. Older adults are occasionally abused or neglected; therefore, confronting family members about a patient's accusations of harm or neglect is often part of the assessment. If after such a confrontation the clinician is not convinced that the accusations are totally explained by the delusion, a social services agency or department should be requested to investigate further.

On the other hand, challenging the delusional patient is usually not recommended. It is important to seek an understanding of the patient's thought processes, so providing an atmosphere of acceptance (although not necessarily agreement) will allow the patient to express his or her beliefs and feelings. Reassurance should be provided in a manner conveying that although the clinician may not fully understand the whole situation, the goal is for the patient to feel better and more secure.

A laboratory workup is usually needed in new cases of paranoia to rule out an organic delusional syndrome. Blood chemistry, a complete blood count, and a thyroid profile should be obtained. If respiratory symptoms are present, a chest X ray may be needed. A computed tomography or magnetic resonance imaging brain scan may be indicated, especially if cognitive impairment or focal neurological findings are present. Because suspiciousness is often associated with sensory impairment, particularly visual and auditory deficits, audiometric and visual testing may identify potential areas for further intervention.

Treatment of paranoia may include neuroleptic medication, depending on the diagnosis, as discussed earlier in this chapter. (For a complete discussion of neuroleptics, please see Chapter 26, "Psychopharmacology.") Regardless of whether neuroleptics are prescribed, key components of management of paranoia include reassurance for the patient, education for the family, and careful monitoring for development of agitation.

Agitation in Elderly Persons

Behavioral manifestations of dementia are common (Lyketsos et al. 2000) and represent major predictors of caregiver depression, burden, and stress across cultures (Chen et al. 2000; Gallicchio et al. 2002; Teri 1997). Anxiety and agitation, the most commonly cited psychiatric manifestations of dementia, can be as disruptive and painful for the person with dementia as they are for family caregivers. Disruptive or resistive behaviors resulting from anxiety and agitation increase the risk of harm to the affected individual and others (Chow and MacLean 2001; Tractenberg et al. 2001), and caregivers frequently become frightened, upset, or simply exhausted by the demands of caring for a family member with agitation.

Nonpharmacological Approaches

Nonpharmacological strategies are recommended as first-line approaches for the noncognitive manifestations of dementia. These approaches can be taught effectively to family and nonprofessional caregivers (Belle et al. 2006; Cohen-Mansfield et al. 2007; Doody et al. 2001; Hepburn et al. 2007; Logsdon et al. 2007; Teri et al. 2005). Nonpharmacological approaches are most effective as adjuncts to pharmacotherapy, when pharmacotherapy is contraindicated, and when behaviors are manifested in response to unmet needs and environmental or interpersonal triggers.

These strategies focus on changing the patient's activities, routines, and/or human, physical, and social environments to provide reassurance, appropriate stimulation, and security. As the person with dementia becomes less adaptable to change, the human and physical environment must adapt to him or her. Behavioral approaches generally include person-specific problem solving, enriched cues, adapted work or expressive activities, exercise, communication strategies, and caregiver skills training.

Key Messages for Families About Agitation in Dementia

Families of persons with dementia should be told directly that anxiety, suspiciousness, and restless agitation are common symptoms of brain disorders, even in the context of excellent, well-intentioned family care. At the same time, it is helpful to suggest that disruptive behaviors do not occur in a vacuum. Agitation has a person-specific situational context and meaning that may often, but not always, be understood. Agitated or even aggressive behavior is often beyond a dementia patient's control or intentionality. In fact, he or she may not be aware of agitation or a change in behavior.

Frequent or escalating agitation requires a prompt and multimodal response. Ignoring agitated or disruptive behaviors will not make them go away. Persons with dementia are most likely to be angry at what they perceive as an intolerable situation that no longer makes sense. For this reason it is wise for families not to take attacks or accusations personally. Families should also be reminded that persons with dementia are more likely to take out their frustration on those closest to them while appearing gracious and appropriate with strangers.

Families should be told that people with dementia generally cannot "try harder." A corollary is that reasoning, arguing, coaxing, pleading, confronting, or punishing agitated persons may only escalate the distressing behavior. Families respond effectively if they understand that agitated people with dementia are likely to be scared and overwhelmed by disorientation and that they may forget appropriate public or private behavior. Agitation is frequently accompanied by a loss of impulse control that can result in uncharacteristic cursing, insensitivity, tactlessness, or sexually inappropriate behavior. Although people with dementia may seem insensitive to others' feelings, they are extremely sensitive to and will respond negatively to patronizing, angry, tense, rushed, or demanding nonverbal communication from family members.

Agitated persons with dementia generally respond well to calm, familiar settings with predictable routines and to requests tailored to their capacities, remaining strengths, and energy levels. Although Alzheimer's disease patients may appear to do less as a result of apathy, they can become fatigued from just trying to make sense of what is going on around them. Late-day fatigue or wearing out may explain some agitated behavior associated with "sundowning" (patients' becoming more confused, agitated, or psychotic in the late afternoon or early evening) and extremely exaggerated reactions to minor incidents. Furthermore, patients with mild to moderate Alzheimer's disease may resist activities they perceive as too difficult or too demeaning in order to limit embarrassment or failure.

Questions to Guide Problem Solving for Agitation in Dementia

Consideration of the following nine questions can help pinpoint and resolve caregivers' problems with a patient's agitated behavior:

1. Which agitated, anxious, or resistive behaviors are most disruptive to family life at this point?
2. Describe the behavior. Is it harmful or does it cause distress to the person with dementia or to others? Can the family change expectations or increase tolerance for this change in the person as they knew him or her?
3. Is there any pattern, trigger, or time of day that sets off the behavior (e.g., a move, travel, hospitalization, or a request to do a complex task)?
4. Does anything happen afterwards that makes it worse (e.g., caregiver anger or abandonment or patient failure)?
5. Is the person uncomfortable (e.g., pain, hunger, thirst, constipation, full bladder, fatigue, infection, cold, fear, misperceived threats, difficult communication)?
6. Is the person looking for something familiar from the past (e.g., rummaging in drawers, searching for an outhouse or an old employer)?
7. Will a change in environment help (e.g., reduce number of people, confusion, stimuli, noise)?
8. Can the caregiver use familiar phrases to calm or reassure the person (e.g., "I'll get right on it"; "Ain't that the truth?"; "Even the Lord rested on Sundays")?

9. Can routines be changed or adapted to prevent future occurrences of the behavior (e.g., exercising early in the day, bathing less frequently, avoiding rush-hour shopping)?

Common Strategies to Reduce Agitation

Nonpharmacological strategies for reducing agitation usually involve redirection of the person's attention away from triggering events or contexts or distraction with offers of pleasant events specific to the person (going out for ice cream or a ride, listening to favorite music, or watching old videotapes). Other strategies include breaking down complex tasks into one-step guided directions, simplifying instructions, and allowing adequate rest or passive observation between stimulating activities. Environmental strategies include using labels, cues, or pictures; hazard-proofing the environment to reduce dangers of exploration or egress; removing guns or hazardous equipment; and using lighting or security objects to reduce nighttime confusion or daytime fear or uncertainty.

Communication Begins With Understanding

Families begin to communicate effectively when they can understand the experience and perspectives of people with dementia. With the current focus on early diagnosis and treatment of Alzheimer's disease, more individuals with insight who have new diagnoses of Alzheimer's disease are willing to provide direction. The following excerpts from a Canadian support group of patients with early-stage Alzheimer's disease can offer guidance to family caregivers:

> Please don't correct me. Remember, my feelings are intact and I get hurt easily. Try to ignore offhand remarks that I wouldn't have made in the past. If you focus on my mistakes, it just makes me feel worse. I may say something that is real to me but not factual to you. It is not a lie. Don't argue—it won't solve anything. (Snyder 2001, p. 2)

When a person with dementia is agitated, he or she may be thinking along the following lines (Gwyther 2000, p. 998):

> How dare you question me? I have always taken care of myself.
>
> I make sense—you and events don't.
>
> Your reality and reasoning wear me out.
>
> I am only protecting what is mine from those people—things keep disappearing.
>
> Can't you see this is not a good time? I'm overwhelmed and scared.

Communication Strategies to Reduce Agitation

First it is necessary to get the person's attention. Make sure vision and hearing are adequate or "tuned up." Use eye contact, call the person by name in a clear adult tone, approach slowly from the side or front or crouch down at his or her level, and offer your hand, palm up. Listen, but do not feel compelled to talk constantly. Words are not as important as a calm tone, pleasant expression, and nondistracting environment (turn off the TV or turn down the radio). Use familiar words and speak in a normal tone and tempo, but give the person time to process and respond. Repeat your words exactly, if necessary. Ask questions if you are unsure of his or her meaning ("Am I getting closer to what you want?"). Be patient—you may need to repeat to reassure him or her.

If frustration mounts, take a deep breath and suggest a better time to talk or another topic. Avoid popular expressions that may be ambiguous or vague, such as "Don't go there," "NOT," or "bottom line." Use concrete subjects, names, and references. Avoid pronouns. Do not test or ask the person if he or she remembers you. Use positive statements such as "Let's go" rather than "Do you want to go now?" Explain what happens next, but wait until just before it will happen. Demonstrate or model so he or she can follow your lead. Use appropriate, respectful humor or his or her favorite phrases ("See ya later, alligator"). It is always appropriate to make fun of yourself, especially if you forget. Smile, nod, gesture, or use photos when words fail.

Summary of Nonpharmacological Approaches

Families often want brief, concrete suggestions for dealing with agitation. The following format may be helpful (Alzheimer's Association 2001; Gwyther 2001):

DO—slow down, soothe the person, or structure the situation. Encourage and reinforce positive adaptations that work for the person ("I depend on my husband for brute strength in carrying those grocery bags"). Be extra gracious and polite. Back off and ask permission. Repeatedly reassure. Use visual and verbal cues and add light. Offer guided choices between two options. Avoid complex multistep directions or ambiguity. Distract with a favorite snack, or ask for help with raking or another adult repetitive task. Increase time spent in pleasant activities like sitting in a porch glider at sunset. Offer a security object, rest, or privacy after an upset. Limit caffeine and alcohol. Use comforting rituals like holding hands during grace, an afternoon tea break, checking the bird feeder, or a hand massage or manicure. Do for the person what she can no longer comfortably do on her own. Join her in modified favorite activities—social, creative, or sports. Remove her from confusing, frustrating, or scary experiences like TV shows that she believes are happening to her.

DO NOT—raise your voice, take offense, corner, crowd, restrain, rush, criticize, ignore, confront, argue, reason, shame, blame, demand, lecture, condescend, moralize, force, explain, teach, show alarm, or make a sudden move out of the person's view.

SAY—May I help you? Do you have time to help me? Let's take a break now—we have earned it. You're safe here. I will get right on it. Everything is under control. I apologize (even if you didn't do it!). I'm sorry you are upset. I know it's hard. We're in this together. I will make sure those men can't get in here. Do what you can and I'll finish up. We're doing fine now.

Pharmacological/Medical Approaches

There are times when agitation warrants pharmacological intervention, and the risks of persistent agitation versus the risks and benefits of treating the agitation must be weighed carefully. This is especially true given the emergence of recent data suggesting an increased risk of stroke or death in agitated patients with dementia who are treated chronically with atypical antipsychotic agents. An accurate risk estimation of using these agents in patients with dementia remains unclear, with some studies estimating up to a 3% risk, whereas other large population-based studies suggesting no increased risk at all (Herrmann and Lanctôt 2005; Kales et al. 2007; Layton et al. 2005; Raivio et al. 2007). At present, all atypical antipsychotic agents carry a black-box warning regarding these risks in patients with dementia, so documentation of a risk assessment in the medical record is prudent.

Most clinicians view agitation as a condition manifested by excessive verbal and/or motor behavior. It is distinguished from aggression, which can also be verbal (e.g., cursing or threats) or physical (e.g., hitting, kicking, shoving objects or people). Agitation can escalate to aggression, so it is vital for the clinician to intervene early in approaching agitated patients. However, it remains essential to determine the cause of agitation so that interventions can then be directed at both treating the underlying cause and managing the agitation itself, given that uncontrolled agitation has been demonstrated to have multiple deleterious effects on patient safety and welfare. Potential medical causes of agitation are shown in Table 25–1.

Agitation most commonly occurs in the context of delirium or dementia, and often these conditions coexist in frail elderly patients. These conditions are discussed in depth later in this section of the chapter. Agitation can also be a feature of late-life depression, and although treatment of the underlying depression should also treat the agitation, the full effect of antidepressant medications may not be apparent for several weeks. However, acute, severe, or escalating agitation may require medication such as the newer atypical neuroleptics for adequate control. Benzodiazepines should generally be avoided in an agitated population because of their high potential for worsening delirium as well as potentially disinhibiting the patient further. They may be appropriately used in cases of alcohol or benzodiazepine (GABAergic) withdrawal, or when the agitation

TABLE 25–1. Common medical causes of agitation in elderly persons

Medication
Drug-drug interaction
Accidental misuse
Central nervous system toxic side effect
Systemic disturbance (e.g., medication-induced electrolyte imbalance)
Urinary tract infection
Poor nutrition, decreased oral intake of food and fluid
Respiratory infection
Recent stroke
Occult head trauma if patient fell recently
Pain
Constipation
Alcohol/substance withdrawal
Chronic obstructive pulmonary disease

can be assumed to be the result of severe anxiety rather than delirium or the nonspecific agitation that can accompany dementia. Chronic treatment of agitation may require the clinician to consider other medications, including antidepressants and mood stabilizers. Choice of medication will depend on the setting and on the severity and chronicity of symptoms, as discussed below.

Agitation in the Context of Delirium

Delirium is a common disorder, with an estimated prevalence of 15%–50% among hospitalized elderly patients (Inouye et al. 2007; Levkoff et al. 1991). Characterized by a disturbance of consciousness and a change in cognition, delirium typically has a rapid onset and runs a short course. More recent data, however, reflect the clinical observation that delirium may independently advance cognitive decline such that patients may not fully recover their predelirium baseline level of cognitive function (Bellelli et al. 2007; McCusker et al. 2001). The principal elements of the DSM-IV-TR diagnosis of delirium are 1) a disturbance of consciousness indicated by reduced awareness of the environment, along with diminished ability to focus, sustain, or shift attention; 2) a change in cognition (which may include deficits of memory, language, or orientation) or onset of a perceptual disturbance not better accounted for by a dementia; and 3) development of the condition over a short period, with a tendency to fluctuate during the course of the day (American Psychiatric Association 2000). DSM-IV-TR categorizes delirium by presumed etiology (including delirium secondary to a medical condition, substance intoxication, and substance withdrawal), mixed or multiple etiologies, and uncertain etiology.

Delirium typically develops over hours to days and is provoked by certain medical illnesses, metabolic derangements, intoxications, and withdrawal states (Lipowski 1989). A prodromal period of subtle confusion, irritability, or psychomotor behavior change may precede the advent of the full syndrome. Confusion, clouding of sensorium or consciousness, and alterations in perception commonly occur, as do frankly psychotic symptoms such as paranoia. Marked disturbances of the sleep cycle contribute to delirium and are highly present (if not ever-present) in these patients. Autonomic changes such as tachycardia and hypertension can also occur, particularly in the hyperactive form of delirium or in delirium secondary to substance withdrawal. Patients with hyperactive delirium often have increased irritability and startle responses and may be acutely sensitive to stimuli. In addition, delirious patients may experience profound shifts in mood and use rambling, illogical language while still having lucid intervals of relatively normal mental functioning. Although short-term memory may be disturbed, long-term memory is typically preserved. The syndrome usually runs a course of several days; however, the duration of illness is largely controlled by the course of the underlying condition that provoked the delirious episode, and in susceptible individuals the episode may portend a permanent decline in mental functioning (Bellelli et al. 2007; McCusker et al. 2001). Hypoactive delirium is not generally accompanied by agitation and may mimic a depressive syndrome with accompanying extreme fear. The need for treatment for hypoactive delirium with neuroleptics remains controversial, but identification of hypoactive delirium is important in that it is generally associated with higher mortality rates compared with nondelirious or hyperactive delirium (Kiely et al. 2007).

Management of delirium is focused primarily on identifying and treating the underlying cause, which will have profound implications for appropriate treatment of the agitation. However, the agitated delirious patient often requires immediate attention prior to completion of the workup, because agitated behavior can impede ongoing medical care and can place the patient and others at physical risk.

Acute treatment of agitation generally requires the administration of intramuscular or intravenous (IV) neuroleptics, with the exception of delirium secondary to GABAergic withdrawal (alcohol or benzodiazepine withdrawal delirium), in which case benzodiazepines become the treatment of choice. If no intravenous access exists, initial treatment with intramuscular haloperidol or lorazepam, alone or in combination, may be required for adequate control. Once intravenous access is present, IV haloperidol remains the standard of care for agitated delirium due to general medical conditions, and IV use of haloperidol is associated with markedly fewer extrapyramidal side effects than the oral formulation.

Oral administration of atypical neuroleptics is frequent in practice, and data regarding effective use in delirium are available for risperidone, quetiapine, and olanzapine (Breitbart et al. 2002; Han and Kim 2004; Pae et al. 2004; Rea et al. 2007; Sasaki et al. 2003). The use of ziprasidone or aripiprazole in delirium currently is limited to case reports (Alao et al. 2005; Leso and Schwartz 2002).

Treatment of alcohol or benzodiazepine withdrawal delirium depends primarily on administration of sufficient doses of benzodiazepines to arrest the withdrawal process; identification of this form of delirium is important because of the high morbidity and mortality associated with it if it is not treated appropriately. Similarly, delirium secondary to hepatic encephalopathy has its own treatment pathway and relies primarily on the administration of either lactulose or antibiotics designed to reduce bowel flora (neomycin or rifaximin).

Agitation in the Context of Dementia

Agitation is a frequent behavioral symptom in dementia, with 24% of caregivers in one survey reporting agitation and/or aggression (Lyketsos et al. 2000). It occurs at some time in about half of all patients with dementia (Small et al. 1997). A person with dementia may become agitated throughout the day, intermittently through the day, or at specific times of day. For example, sundowning commonly occurs in dementia, although this is a nonspecific term that refers to nonspecific agitation. One-fourth of inpatients with Alzheimer's disease were found on nursing evaluation to exhibit sundowning behavior (Little et al. 1995). Behaviors associated with agitation in patients who have dementia include aggression, combativeness, disinhibition, wandering, and hyperactivity. As with all behavioral problems, the first step in treatment is to identify potential precipitants. Evaluation should include assessment for common systemic causes (e.g., infection, dehydration, constipation, and other illnesses) as well as changes in medication.

Pharmacological Treatment

If environmental measures are insufficient to control agitated or aggressive behavior, medication is usually needed. Guidelines for pharmacological treatment of agitation in elderly patients with dementia have been developed (Alexopoulos et al. 1998). High-potency neuroleptics (e.g., haloperidol) are effective for controlling acute agitation, especially when psychotic features are present (Small et al. 1997), but care needs to be taken with these agents given the increased risk of extrapyramidal side effects in elderly patients. Although there is no evidence to suggest that one neuroleptic agent is more effective than another, the atypical antipsychotics—clozapine, risperidone, olanzapine, quetiapine, and ziprasidone—have a lesser frequency of extrapyramidal side effects (e.g., parkinsonism, tardive dyskinesia) than high-potency typical neuroleptic agents. These medications (especially quetiapine) are particularly useful in patients with Parkinson's disease who become agitated or psychotic because the selective dopaminergic blockade is less likely to interfere with dopamine's therapeutic effect on the basal ganglia. However, atypical antipsychotics are expensive, and recent data suggest increased cerebrovascular disease and mortality risks when used chronically in populations with dementia. Benzodiazepines can also be used to treat anxiety or infrequent agitation, but they are less effective than other agents for long-term treatment because of already noted limitations.

In general, when agitation is a consistent problem and neuroleptic treatment is required, we recommend starting with a low-dose agent (e.g., 0.5 mg of haloperidol or 0.25–0.5 mg of risperidone) and administering it on a regular basis rather than attempting to treat specific episodes of agitation. Treating frequently occurring agitation on an as-needed basis makes administering medication difficult, requires larger doses of medication for adequate control, and is likely to cause sedation and further clouding of thought.

The anticonvulsants carbamazepine and divalproex sodium (Depakote) have also been noted to be effective in treating behavioral disturbances in dementia and have a side-effect profile distinct from that of neuroleptics (Lemke 1995). In a double-blind study, Tariot et al. (1998) found that compared with the placebo group, patients taking carbamazepine showed significant improvement in agitation and aggression. The drug was well tolerated. The modal daily dose of carbamazepine was 300 mg, achieving a mean serum level of 5.3 μg/mL. Divalproex has also been shown to be an effective treatment for agitation in dementia (Narayan and Nelson 1997). In this study, the mean final divalproex dose was 1,650 mg/day, with a mean blood level of 64 mg/mL. Divalproex was well tolerated in this population except for reversible sedation in eight patients and transient worsening gait and confusion in one patient. However, both carbamazepine and divalproex have the ability to suppress blood cell lines; therefore, periodic blood monitoring is required. Similarly, divalproex has the capacity to induce liver dysfunction and pancreatitis, and thus periodic liver function testing should be performed for this agent as well—especially during initial dosing.

Other classes of drugs can be useful for treating agitation in particular circumstances. Antidepressants, especially selective serotonin reuptake inhibitors (SSRIs) and trazodone, are effective even in the absence of clear depressive symptoms. There is no established dose range for treatment of agitation with SSRIs, and in our experience the final doses used to achieve successful treatment of agitation have ranged widely. The acetylcholinesterase inhibitors donepezil, rivastigmine, and galantamine have been shown to decrease agitation, possibly by stimulating attention and concentration (Levy et al. 1999). Similarly, the newer *N*-methyl-D-aspartate antagonist memantine has been shown to have some degree of favorable outcome on functional measures and agitation at doses of 10–20 mg daily (Gauthier et al. 2008). The β-blocker propranolol hydrochloride inhibits impulsive behavior after frontal lobe injury and can be used to decrease agitation and aggressive behavior in dementia, but it may cause bradycardia and hypotension so should be used cautiously (Shankle et al. 1995).

The need for continued pharmacological treatment of agitation should be regularly reassessed. Generally, medication for agitation should not be viewed as long-term therapy because of the inherent risks involved with these agents. In one study, neuroleptic treatment was discontinued after agitation was successfully treated in nine patients with dementia (Borson and Raskind 1997). A placebo was then administered, and behavior was monitored for the next 6 weeks. Of the nine patients, eight did not need additional pharmacological treatment. Interestingly, five of the patients were less agitated after drug treatment was stopped. Thus, after agitation is sufficiently controlled, trial reductions in the required dose of medication should be periodically attempted to minimize the need for polypharmacy and the incidence of adverse events.

However, some patients may require chronic medication treatment for agitation. In such cases, antidepressants (especially SSRIs) or anticonvulsants are emerging as the preferred treatments. Benzodiazepines and neuroleptics have obvious inherent risks when used chronically in elderly patients with dementia, and close monitoring for side effects (e.g., sedation and extrapyramidal symptoms) is required. In the case of neuroleptics, agitated patients without an established psychotic illness should have clear documentation of previous failed trials of other medications or the presence of markedly agitated behavior that appears to pose a significant risk to the patient or others.

Key Points

- Agitation is a common and disabling nonspecific condition in the elderly.
- The causes of agitation include a wide differential that must be evaluated prior to treatment.
- A nonpharmacological approach should be a core component to address agitation.
- When the patient does not respond to nonpharmacological approaches, there is a wide range of pharmacological strategies that can be attempted to provide effective intervention.
- If pharmacological means are used, they should not be continued indefinitely; rather, they should be reevaluated periodically and dosages tapered or eliminated if possible.

References

Alao AO, Soderberg M, Pohl EL, et al: Aripiprazole in the treatment of delirium. Int J Psychiatry Med 35:429–433, 2005

Alexopoulos GS, Silver JM, Kahn DA, et al (eds): Agitation in Older Persons With Dementia: A Postgraduate Medicine Special Report (The Expert Consensus Guideline Series). New York, McGraw-Hill, 1998

Alzheimer's Association: Fact Sheet: About Agitation and Alzheimer's Disease. Chicago, IL, Alzheimer's Association, 2001. Available at http://www.nia.nih.gov/Alzheimers/Publications/adfact.htm. Accessed July 18, 2008.

American Psychiatric Association: Diagnostic and Statistical Manual of Mental Disorders, 4th Edition, Text Revision. Washington, DC, American Psychiatric Association, 2000

Belle SH, Burgio L, Burns R, et al: Enhancing the quality of life of dementia caregivers from different ethnic and racial groups: a randomized, controlled trial. Ann Intern Med 145:727–738, 2006

Bellelli G, Frisoni GB, Turco R, et al: Delirium superimposed on dementia predicts 12-month survival in elderly patients discharged from a postacute rehabilitation facility. J Gerontol A Biol Sci Med Sci 62:1306–1309, 2007

Borson S, Raskind MA: Clinical features and pharmacologic treatment of behavioral symptoms of Alzheimer's disease. Neurology 48 (suppl 6):S17–S24, 1997

Breitbart W, Tremblay A, Gibson C: An open trial of olanzapine for the treatment of delirium in hospitalized cancer patients. Psychosomatics 43:175–182, 2002

Chen JC, Borson S, Scanlan JM: Stage-specific prevalence of behavioral symptoms in Alzheimer's disease in a multi-ethnic community sample. Am J Geriatr Psychiatry 8:123–133, 2000

Chow TW, MacLean CH: Quality indicators for dementia in vulnerable community-dwelling and hospitalized elders. Ann Intern Med 135:668–676, 2001

Christenson R, Blazer D: Epidemiology of persecutory ideation in an elderly population in the community. Am J Psychiatry 141:1088–1091, 1984

Cohen-Mansfield J, Libin A, Marx MS: Nonpharmacological treatment of agitation: a controlled trial of systematic individualized intervention. J Gerontol A Biol Sci Med Sci 62:908–916, 2007

Doody RS, Stevens JC, Beck C, et al: Practice parameter: management of dementia (an evidence-based review): Report of the Quality Standards Subcommittee of the American Academy of Neurology. Neurology 56:1154–1166, 2001

Gallicchio L, Siddiqui N, Langenberg P, et al: Gender differences in burden and depression among informal caregivers of demented elders in the community. Int J Geriatr Psychiatry 17:154–163, 2002

Gauthier S, Loft H, Cummings J: Improvement in behavioural symptoms in patients with moderate to severe Alzheimer's disease by memantine: a pooled data analysis. Int J Geriatr Psychiatry 23:537–545, 2008

Gwyther L: Family issues in dementia: finding a new normal. Neurol Clin 18:993–1010, 2000

Gwyther L: Caring for People With Alzheimer's Disease: A Manual for Facility Staff. Washington, DC, American Health Care Association and Alzheimer's Association, 2001

Han CS, Kim YK: A double-blind trial of risperidone and haloperidol for the treatment of delirium. Psychosomatics 45:297–301, 2004

Hepburn K, Lewis M, Tomatore J, et al: The Savvy Caregiver Program: the effectiveness of a transportable dementia caregiver psychoeducational program. J Gerontol Nurs 33:30–36, 2007

Herrmann N, Lanctôt KL: Do atypical antipsychotics cause stroke? CNS Drugs 19:91–103, 2005

Inouye SK, Zhang Y, Jones RN, et al: Risk factors for delirium at discharge: development and validation of a predictive model. Arch Intern Med 167:1406–1413, 2007

Kales HC, Valenstein M, Kim HM, et al: Mortality risk in patients with dementia treated with antipsychotics versus other psychiatric medications. Am J Psychiatry 164:1568–1576, 2007

Kiely DK, Jones RN, Bergmann MA, et al: Association between psychomotor activity delirium subtypes and mortality among newly admitted post-acute facility patients. J Gerontol A Biol Sci Med Sci 62:174–179, 2007

Layton D, Harris S, Wilton LV, et al: Comparison of incidence rates of cerebrovascular accidents and transient ischaemic attacks in observational cohort studies of patients prescribed risperidone, quetiapine or olanzapine in general practice in England including patients with dementia. J Psychopharmacol 19:473–482, 2005

Lemke MR: Effect of carbamazepine on agitation in Alzheimer's inpatients refractory to neuroleptics. J Clin Psychiatry 56:354–357, 1995

Leso L, Schwartz TL: Ziprasidone treatment of delirium. Psychosomatics 43:61–62, 2002

Levkoff S, Cleary P, Liptzin B, et al: Epidemiology of delirium: an overview of research issues and findings. Int Psychogeriatr 3:149–167, 1991

Levy ML, Cummings JL, Kahn-Rose R: Neuropsychiatric symptoms and cholinergic therapy for Alzheimer's disease. Gerontology 45 (suppl 1):15–22, 1999

Lipowski ZJ: Delirium in the elderly patient. N Engl J Med 320:578–582, 1989

Little JT, Satlin A, Sunderland T, et al: Sundown syndrome in severely demented patients with probable Alzheimer's disease. J Geriatr Psychiatry Neurol 8:103–106, 1995

Logsdon RG, McCurry SM, Teri L: Evidence-based psychological treatments for disruptive behaviors in individuals with dementia. Psychol Aging 22:28–36, 2007

Lowenthal MF, Berkman PL: Aging and Mental Disorders in San Francisco: A Social Psychiatry Study. San Francisco, CA, Jossey-Bass, 1967

Lyketsos CG, Steinberg M, Tschanz JT, et al: Mental and behavioral disturbances in dementia: findings from the Cache County Study on Memory in Aging. Am J Psychiatry 157:708–714, 2000

McCusker J, Cole M, Dendukuri N, et al: Delirium in older medical inpatients and subsequent cognitive and functional status: a prospective study. CMAJ 165:575–583, 2001

Narayan M, Nelson JC: Treatment of dementia with behavioral disturbance using divalproex or a combination of divalproex and a neuroleptic. J Clin Psychiatry 58:351–354, 1997

Opler LA, Feinberg SS: The role of pimozide in clinical psychiatry: a review. J Clin Psychiatry 52:221–233, 1991

Pae CU, Lee SJ, Lee CU, et al: A pilot trial of quetiapine for the treatment of patients with delirium. Hum Psychopharmacol 19:125–127, 2004

Raivio MM, Laurila JV, Strandberg TE, et al: Neither atypical nor conventional antipsychotics increase mortality or hospital admissions among elderly patients with dementia: a two-year prospective study. Am J Geriatr Psychiatry 15:416–424, 2007

Rea RS, Battistone S, Fong JJ, et al: Atypical antipsychotics versus haloperidol for treatment of delirium in acutely ill patients. Pharmacotherapy 27:588–594, 2007

Sasaki Y, Matsuyama T, Inoue S, et al: A prospective, open-label, flexible-dose study of quetiapine in the treatment of delirium. J Clin Psychiatry 64:1316–1321, 2003

Shankle WR, Nielson KA, Cotman CW: Low-dose propranolol reduces aggression and agitation resembling that associated with orbitofrontal dysfunction in elderly demented patients. Alzheimer Dis Assoc Disord 9:233–237, 1995

Small GW, Rabins PV, Barry PP, et al: Diagnosis and treatment of Alzheimer disease and related disorders: consensus statement of the American Association for Geriatric Psychiatry, the Alzheimer's Association, and the American Geriatrics Society. JAMA 278:1363–1371, 1997

Snyder L: Perspectives: A Newsletter for Individuals Diagnosed With Alzheimer's Disease. Alzheimer's Disease Research Center, University of California, San Diego, 2001, p 2

Soares JC, Gershon S: Therapeutic targets in late-life psychoses: review of concepts and critical issues. Schizophr Res 27:227–239, 1997

Tariot PN, Erb R, Podgorski CA, et al: Efficacy and tolerability of carbamazepine for agitation and aggression in dementia. Am J Psychiatry 155:54–61, 1998

Teri L: Behavior and caregiver burden: behavioral problems in patients with Alzheimer disease and its association with caregiver burden. Alzheimer Dis Assoc Disord 11 (suppl 4):S35–S38, 1997

Teri L, Huda P, Gibbons L, et al: STAR: a dementia-specific training program for staff in assisted living residences. Gerontologist 45:686–693, 2005

Tractenberg RE, Garmst A, Weiner MF, et al: Frequency of behavioral symptoms characterizes agitation in Alzheimer's disease. Int J Geriatr Psychiatry 16:886–891, 2001

Yassa R, Suranyi-Cadotte B: Clinical characteristics of late-onset schizophrenia and delusional disorder. Schizophr Bull 19:701–707, 1993

Suggested Readings

Caine ED: Clinical perspectives on atypical antipsychotics for treatment of agitation. J Clin Psychiatry 67 (suppl 10):22–31, 2006

Nassisi D, Korc B, Hahn S, et al: The evaluation and management of the acutely agitated elderly patient. Mt Sinai J Med 73:976–984, 2006

Roger KS: A literature review of palliative care, end of life, and dementia. Palliat Support Care 4:295–303, 2006

Spira AP, Edelstein BA: Behavioral interventions for agitation in older adults with dementia: an evaluative review. Int Psychogeriatr 18:195–225, 2006

Zuidema S, Koopmans R, Verhey F: Prevalence and predictors of neuropsychiatric symptoms in cognitively impaired nursing home patients. J Geriatr Psychiatry Neurol 20:41–49, 2007

PART IV

Treatment of Psychiatric Disorders in Late Life

CHAPTER 26

Psychopharmacology

Benoit H. Mulsant, M.D.
Bruce G. Pollock, M.D., Ph.D.

Pharmacological intervention in late life requires special care. Elderly patients are more susceptible to drug-induced adverse events. Particularly troublesome among older persons are peripheral and central anticholinergic effects such as constipation, urinary retention, delirium, and cognitive dysfunction; antihistaminergic effects such as sedation; and antiadrenergic effects such as postural hypotension. Sedation and orthostatic hypotension not only interfere with basic activities but also pose a significant safety risk to elderly patients because they can lead to falls and fractures. Increased susceptibility to adverse effects in elders may be a result of the pharmacokinetic and pharmacodynamic changes associated with aging, such as diminished glomerular filtration, changes in the density and activity of target receptors, reduced liver size and hepatic blood flow, and decreased cardiac output (Lotrich and Pollock 2005) (Table 26–1).

Illnesses that affect many elderly persons (e.g., diabetes) further diminish the processing and removal of medications from the body. In addition, polypharmacy and the associated risk of drug interactions add another level of complexity to pharmacological treatment in older patients. Poor adherence to treatment regimens—which can be a result of impaired cognitive function, confusing drug regimens, or lack of motivation or insight associated with the psychiatric disorder being treated—is a significant obstacle to effective and safe pharmacological treatment. Finally, it should be appreciated that psychotropic medications are not as extensively studied in elders as in younger subjects or those without comorbid medical illness with respect to pharmacokinetic and dosing information (Pollock 2005). For example, only 28% of the package inserts for the drugs most commonly prescribed in the elderly have specific dosing recommendations (Steinmetz et al. 2005). New methodologies such as population pharmacokinetics can help to address this lack of information regarding dosage and drug-drug interactions (Bigos et al. 2006). Nonetheless, even with currently available knowledge, medications cause considerable morbidity in elders. In a 2007 study by Laroche et al., 66% of the admissions to an acute geriatric medical unit were preceded by the prescription of at least one inappropriate medication; among patients taking appropriate medications, the prevalence of adverse drug reactions was 16%.

Despite these challenges, psychiatric disorders can be treated successfully in late life with psychotropic drugs. In this chapter, we summarize relevant data published in scientific journals as of mid-2008 on the efficacy, tolerability, and safety of the major psychotropic drugs.

Antidepressant Medications

Selective Serotonin Reuptake Inhibitors

Selective serotonin reuptake inhibitors (SSRIs) remain first-line drugs for treating late-life depression (Alexopoulos et al. 2001; Pinquart et al. 2006) because of their efficacy for both depressive and anxiety syndromes, their ease of use, and their safety and good tolerability. As with most drugs, few clinical trials of

TABLE 26–1. Physiological changes in elderly persons associated with altered pharmacokinetics

Organ system	Change	Pharmacokinetic consequence
Circulatory system	Decreased concentration of plasma albumin and increased α_1-acid glycoprotein	Increased or decreased free concentration of drugs in plasma
Gastrointestinal tract	Decreased intestinal and splanchnic blood flow	Decreased rate of drug absorption
Kidney	Decreased glomerular filtration rate	Decreased renal clearance of active metabolites
Liver	Decreased liver size; decreased hepatic blood flow; variable effects on cytochrome P450 isozyme activity	Decreased hepatic clearance
Muscle	Decreased lean body mass and increased adipose tissue	Altered volume of distribution of lipid-soluble drugs, leading to increased elimination half-life

Source. Adapted from Pollock BG: "Psychotropic Drugs and the Aging Patient." *Geriatrics* 53 (suppl 1):S20–S24, 1998. Used with permission.

SSRIs have been conducted under "real-life" geriatric situations (e.g., in long-term care facilities) or in very old patients. However, as of June 2007, more than 30 randomized, controlled trials of SSRIs involving more than 5,000 geriatric patients with depression had been published (Table 26–2). Those age 70 and older who have experienced major depression are at high risk for relapse. Maintenance SSRI therapy has been shown to be an effective treatment (Gorwood et al. 2007; Reynolds et al. 2006). Several controlled and open studies also have been conducted in special populations (Solai et al. 2001); reviews of many of these trials concluded that SSRIs are efficacious, safe, and well tolerated in older patients, including those with mild cognitive impairment (Devanand et al. 2003), dementia (Katona et al. 1998; Lyketsos et al. 2003; Nyth and Gottfries 1990; Nyth et al. 1992; Olafsson et al. 1992; Petracca et al. 2001; Taragano et al. 1997), minor depression (Rocca et al. 2005), schizophrenia (Kasckow et al. 2001), cardiovascular disease (Glassman et al. 2002; Serebruany et al. 2003), cerebrovascular disease (Y. Chen et al. 2007; Rasmussen et al. 2003; Robinson et al. 2000), or other medical conditions (Arranz and Ros 1997; Evans et al. 1997; Goodnick and Hernandez 2000; Karp et al. 2005; Lotrich et al. 2007; Trappler and Cohen 1998).

Data show that all available SSRIs have similar efficacy and tolerability in the treatment of depression in younger adults (Kroenke et al. 2001) and older adults (Schneider and Olin 1995; Solai et al. 2001). However, experts favor the use of citalopram, escitalopram, or sertraline over fluvoxamine, fluoxetine, or paroxetine (Alexopoulos et al. 2001; Mulsant et al. 2001a). This preference is in large part because of their favorable pharmacokinetic profiles (Table 26–3), their lower potential for clinically significant drug interactions (Table 26–4), and data suggesting their superiority in terms of cognitive improvement (Burrows et al. 2002; Doraiswamy et al. 2003; Furlan et al. 2001; Newhouse et al. 2000; Nyth and Gottfries 1990; Nyth et al. 1992).

SSRIs have well-established efficacy for anxiety disorders in younger adults (Nemeroff 2002). However, to date, only one published placebo-controlled trial (Lenze et al. 2005) and two small open studies (Sheikh et al. 2004b; Wylie et al. 2000) support their efficacy in older patients with anxiety disorders. In the absence of such data, the use of SSRIs to treat geriatric anxiety disorders is mostly based on extrapolation from studies in younger adults and expert opinion (Flint 2005; Lenze et al. 2002). By contrast, some published studies—including three randomized, placebo-controlled trials—suggest that SSRIs may be efficacious in the treatment of behavioral disturbances associated with dementia, including not only agitation and disinhibition but also delusions and hallucinations (Nyth and Gottfries 1990; Nyth et al. 1992; Pollock et al. 1997, 2002, 2007).

In older patients, SSRI starting dosages are typically half the minimal efficacious dosage (see Table 26–3), and the dosage is usually doubled after 1 week. All the SSRIs can be administered in a single daily dose except for fluvoxamine, which should be given in two divided doses. Although even the frailest older patients typically tolerate these drugs relatively well (Oslin et al. 2000), some patients experience some gastrointestinal distress (e.g., nausea) during the first few days of treatment.

TABLE 26–2. Summary of published randomized, controlled trials of selective serotonin reuptake inhibitors for acute treatment of geriatric depression

	Number of published trials (cumulative number of older participants)	Dosages studied (mg/day)	Comments
Citalopram	7[a] (*N*=1,343)	10–40	Citalopram was more efficacious than placebo in one of two trials and as efficacious as amitriptyline and venlafaxine. It was better tolerated than nortriptyline but associated with a lower remission rate. Several trials included patients with stroke and dementia.
Escitalopram	1[b] (*N*=517)	10	In this failed study, escitalopram and fluoxetine were well tolerated but not superior to placebo on primary end point.
Fluoxetine	13[c] (*N*=2,092)	10–80	Fluoxetine was more efficacious than placebo in two of five trials and as efficacious as amitriptyline, doxepin, escitalopram, paroxetine, sertraline, trimipramine, and venlafaxine. In patients with dysthymic disorder, fluoxetine was marginally superior to placebo. In patients with dementia of the Alzheimer's type, fluoxetine did not differ from placebo.
Fluvoxamine	4[d] (*N*=278)	50–200	Fluvoxamine was more efficacious than placebo and as efficacious as dothiepin, imipramine, mianserin, and sertraline.
Paroxetine	8[e] (*N*=1,444)	10–40	Paroxetine was more efficacious than placebo and as efficacious as amitriptyline, bupropion, clomipramine, doxepin, fluoxetine, and imipramine. Mirtazapine was marginally superior to paroxetine. In very old long-term care patients with minor depression, paroxetine was not more efficacious but was more cognitively toxic than placebo. One trial included patients with dementia.
Sertraline	10[f] (*N*=1,817)	50–200	Sertraline was more efficacious than placebo and as efficacious as amitriptyline, fluoxetine, fluvoxamine, imipramine, nortriptyline, and venlafaxine. Sertraline was better tolerated than imipramine and venlafaxine. Greater cognitive improvement occurred with sertraline than with nortriptyline or fluoxetine. Some trials included long-term care patients and patients with dementia of the Alzheimer's type.

[a]Allard et al. 2004; Andersen et al. 1994; Kyle et al. 1998; Navarro et al. 2001; Nyth and Gottfries 1990; Nyth et al. 1992; Roose et al. 2004b; Rosenberg et al. 2007.
[b]Kasper et al. 2005.
[c]Altamura et al. 1989; Devanand et al. 2005; Doraiswamy et al. 2001; Evans et al. 1997; Feighner and Cohn 1985; Finkel et al. 1999; Kasper et al. 2005; Petracca et al. 2001; Schatzberg and Roose 2006; Schone and Ludwig 1993; Taragano et al. 1997; Tollefson et al. 1995; Wehmeier et al. 2005.
[d]Phanjoo et al. 1991; Rahman et al. 1991; Rossini et al. 2005; Wakelin 1986.
[e]Burrows et al. 2002; Dunner et al. 1992; Geretsegger et al. 1995; Guillibert et al. 1989; Katona et al. 1998; Mulsant et al. 1999, 2001b; Rapaport et al. 2003; Schatzberg et al. 2002; Schone and Ludwig 1993.
[f]Bondareff et al. 2000; Cohn et al. 1990; Doraiswamy et al. 2003; Finkel et al. 1999; Forlenza et al. 2001; Lyketsos et al. 2003; Newhouse et al. 2000; Oslin et al. 2000, 2003; Rossini et al. 2005; Schneider et al. 2003; Sheikh et al. 2004a.

Significant hyponatremia resulting from the syndrome of inappropriate secretion of antidiuretic hormone (SIADH) is a rare but potentially dangerous adverse effect that is observed almost exclusively in the elderly (Fabian et al. 2004).

In contrast to tricyclic antidepressants (TCAs), SSRIs may directly affect platelet activation (Pollock et al. 2000), and data have shown that use of SSRIs is associated with a small but significant increase in the risk of gastrointestinal or postsurgical bleeding (Dalton et al.

TABLE 26–3. Pharmacokinetic properties of selective serotonin reuptake inhibitors

	Half-life (days), including active metabolite(s)	Proportionality of dosage to plasma concentration	Risk of uncomfortable withdrawal symptoms	Age-related pharmacokinetic changes?	Efficacious dosage range in elderly (mg/day)[a]
Citalopram	1–3	Linear across therapeutic range	Low	Yes	20–40
Escitalopram	1–3	Linear across therapeutic range	Low	Yes	10–20
Fluoxetine	7–10	Nonlinear at higher dosages	Very low	Yes	20–40
Fluvoxamine	0.5–1	Nonlinear at higher dosages	Moderate	Yes	50–300
Paroxetine	1	Nonlinear at higher dosages	Moderate	Yes	20–40
Sertraline	1–3	Linear across therapeutic range	Low	No	50–200

[a]Starting dosage is typically half of the lowest efficacious dosage; all the selective serotonin reuptake inhibitors can be administered in single daily doses except for fluvoxamine, which should be given in two divided doses.

2006; Looper 2007). Because SSRIs may act synergistically with other medications that increase the risk of gastrointestinal bleeding, such as nonsteroidal anti-inflammatory drugs (NSAIDs) and low-dose aspirin, SSRIs should be used cautiously in older patients taking these medications.

SSRIs also can be associated with bradycardia and should be started with caution in patients with low heart rates (e.g., patients taking β-blockers). They also may cause extrapyramidal symptoms in older patients, although this is not common (Mamo et al. 2000), and they are well tolerated by most patients with Parkinson's disease (P. Chen et al. 2007). The risk of falls and hip fracture unfortunately has not been shown to differ among different classes of antidepressants (Liu et al. 1998). There is also concern that chronic use of SSRIs may contribute to the risk of fractures through direct effects on bone metabolism (Richards et al. 2007).

A large pharmacoepidemiological study found that SSRIs in elders, compared with non-SSRI antidepressants, are associated with a greater risk for suicide during the first month of therapy (Juurlink et al. 2006). However, the absolute risk is low, which suggests that there may be a vulnerable subgroup at risk for an idiosyncratic response. Controlled data available to the U.S. Food and Drug Administration (FDA) indicated a substantial reduction in the risk for suicidal ideation in older patients taking SSRIs compared with those taking placebo (Friedman and Leon 2007; Nelson et al. 2007).

Other Newer Antidepressants

Only limited controlled data support the efficacy and safety of bupropion, duloxetine, mirtazapine, nefazodone, and venlafaxine in older patients (Table 26–5). Nevertheless, because of their usually favorable side-effect profiles in younger patients and their various mechanisms of action, these drugs are the preferred alternatives in older patients who do not respond to or who cannot tolerate SSRIs (Alexopoulos et al. 2001). Still, controlled data suggest that venlafaxine may be less safe than sertraline in a frail elderly population, without evidence for an increase in efficacy (Oslin et al. 2003). Thus, in the absence of systematic research in older patients, newer agents should be used cautiously (Oslin et al. 2003; Rabins and Lyketsos 2005).

Bupropion

Published data supporting the safety and efficacy of bupropion in geriatric depression are limited to two small controlled trials (see Table 26–5) and one small open study (Steffens et al. 2001). Expert consensus favors the use of bupropion—alone or as an augmentation agent—in older depressed patients who have not responded to SSRIs or who cannot tolerate them (Alexopoulos et al. 2001). In particular, bupropion can be helpful for patients who complain of nausea, diarrhea, unbearable fatigue, or sexual dysfunction during SSRI treatment (Nieuwstraten and Dolovich 2001; Thase et al. 2005b). Although augmentation with bupropion has been reported to be helpful in younger and older patients who were partial responders to SSRIs or ven-

TABLE 26–4. Newer antidepressants' inhibition of cytochrome P450 (CYP) and potential for clinically significant drug-drug interactions

	CYP1A2	CYP2C9/2C19	CYP2D6	CYP3A4	Potential for clinically significant drug-drug interaction
Bupropion	0	0	++	0	Moderate
Citalopram	+	0	+	0	Low
Duloxetine	0	0	+	+	Low
Escitalopram	+	0	+	0	Low
Fluoxetine	+	++	+++	++	High
Fluvoxamine	+++	+++	+	++	High
Mirtazapine	0	0	0	+	Low
Nefazodone	0	+	0	+++	High
Paroxetine	+	+	+++	+	Moderate
Sertraline	+	+	+	+	Low
Venlafaxine	0	0	0	0	Low

Note. 0=minimal or no inhibition; +=mild inhibition; ++=moderate inhibition; +++=strong inhibition.

Source. Belpaire et al. 1998; Brosen et al. 1993; Crewe et al. 1992; Ereshefsky and Dugan 2000; Gram et al. 1993; Greenblatt et al. 1998, 1999; Greene and Barbhaiya 1997; Hua et al. 2004; Iribarne et al. 1998; Jeppesen et al. 1996; Kashuba et al. 1998; Kobayashi et al. 1995; Kotlyar et al. 2005; Pollock 1999; Preskorn and Magnus 1994; Preskorn et al. 1997; B.B. Rasmussen et al. 1998; Rickels et al. 1998; Solai et al. 1997, 2002; Spina and Scordo 2002; von Moltke et al. 1995, 2001; Weigmann et al. 2001.

lafaxine (Bodkin et al. 1997; Spier 1998), the safety of this combination has not been established (Joo et al. 2002).

In addition to the three small geriatric trials supporting its safety, controlled data on the use of bupropion in patients with heart disease (Kiev et al. 1994; Roose et al. 1991), in smokers (Tashkin et al. 2001), and in patients with neuropathic pain (Semenchuk et al. 2001) confirm clinical experience that bupropion is relatively well tolerated by medically ill patients. Bupropion is contraindicated in patients who have or are at risk for seizure disorders (e.g., poststroke patients). However, the sustained-release preparation of bupropion appears to be associated with a very low incidence of seizure, comparable to that of other antidepressants (Dunner et al. 1998). Bupropion also has been associated with the onset of psychosis in case reports (Howard and Warnock 1999), and it is prudent to avoid this medication in psychotic patients or in agitated patients at risk for the development of psychotic symptoms. The propensity of bupropion to induce psychosis in patients at risk has been attributed to its action on dopaminergic neurotransmission (Howard and Warnock 1999). The same mechanism has been hypothesized to underlie the association of bupropion with gait disturbance and falls in some patients (Joo et al. 2002; Szuba and Leuchter 1992).

Bupropion is a moderate inhibitor of cytochrome P450 (CYP) 2D6 (Kotlyar et al. 2005). It appears to be metabolized by the CYP2B6 isoform (Hesse et al. 2000, 2004), and adverse effects of bupropion such as seizures or gait disturbance may be more likely in patients who take drugs that can inhibit CYP2B6, such as fluoxetine or paroxetine (Joo et al. 2002).

Duloxetine

Duloxetine is the newest antidepressant approved in the United States. Like venlafaxine, duloxetine is a dual serotonin-norepinephrine reuptake inhibitor (SNRI) (Chalon et al. 2003). Randomized, controlled trials in younger patients support its efficacy and tolerability in the treatment of major depression (Hudson et al. 2005; Kirwin and Goren 2005). It is also approved for the treatment of pain associated with diabetic neuropathy (Goldstein et al. 2005), and some data support its efficacy in the treatment of stress urinary incontinence (Mariappan et al. 2005). Published placebo-controlled data on duloxetine in the elderly have also found it to

TABLE 26–5. Summary of published randomized, controlled trials of bupropion, duloxetine, mirtazapine, nefazodone, and venlafaxine for acute treatment of geriatric depression

	Number of published trials (cumulative number of older participants)	Dosages studied (mg/day)	Comments
Bupropion	2[a] (*N*=163)	100–450	Bupropion was as efficacious as imipramine and paroxetine.
Duloxetine	2[b] (*N*=610)	20–60	Duloxetine also showed efficacy on pain measures.
Mirtazapine	2[c] (*N*=370)	15–45	Mirtazapine was as efficacious as low-dose (total daily dose=30–90 mg) amitriptyline and marginally superior to paroxetine.
Nefazodone	0	NA	NA
Venlafaxine	7[d] (*N*=921)	50–150	Venlafaxine was as efficacious as citalopram, clomipramine, dothiepin, fluoxetine, nortriptyline, and sertraline and was more efficacious than trazodone. It was less well tolerated than fluoxetine and sertraline, tolerated as well as citalopram and dothiepin, and better tolerated than clomipramine, nortriptyline, and trazodone.

Note. NA=not applicable.
[a]Branconnier et al. 1983; Doraiswamy et al. 2001; Weihs et al. 2000.
[b]Nelson et al. 2005; Raskin et al. 2007.
[c]Hoyberg et al. 1996; Schatzberg et al. 2002.
[d]Allard et al. 2004; Gasto et al. 2003; Mahapatra and Hackett 1997; Oslin et al. 2003; Schatzberg and Roose 2006; Smeraldi et al. 1998; Trick et al. 2004.

be efficacious in the treatment of depression and to alleviate associated pain symptoms (Nelson et al. 2005; Raskin et al. 2007). A small pharmacokinetic study in 12 older and 12 younger healthy volunteers suggested that age has a minimal effect on duloxetine pharmacokinetics and that specific dose recommendations for the elderly are not warranted (Skinner et al. 2004). Similarly, on the basis of currently available data, duloxetine appears to have a low likelihood to be involved in clinically significant drug-drug interactions (Hua et al. 2004) (see Table 26–4).

The effect of duloxetine on the reuptake of norepinephrine raises some concerns about its use in older patients with heart disease (Davidson et al. 2005; Johnson et al. 2006; Oslin et al. 2003). In healthy younger patients, duloxetine has only a modest effect on heart rate and blood pressure and no clinically meaningful effect on electrocardiographic parameters (Thase et al. 2005c). However, it often takes many years before specific drug toxicity is recognized in older patients. See the related discussions later in this chapter on venlafaxine (another SNRI) and atypical antipsychotics. Thus, in the absence of evidence suggesting any clear advantage over other antidepressants (Hansen et al. 2005; Vis et al. 2005), it is prudent not to use duloxetine as a first-line agent until its safety has been established in numerous older patients with a variety of physical illnesses (Oslin et al. 2003; Rabins and Lyketsos 2005).

Mirtazapine

The antidepressant activity of mirtazapine has been attributed to its blockade of α_2 autoreceptors, resulting in a direct enhancement of noradrenergic neurotransmission and an increase in the synaptic levels of serotonin (5-hydroxytryptamine [5-HT]), indirectly enhancing neurotransmission mediated by serotonin type 1A (5-HT_{1A}) receptors. In addition, like the antinausea drugs granisetron and ondansetron, mirtazapine inhibits the 5-HT_2 and 5-HT_3 receptors. Thus, mirtazapine could be particularly helpful for patients who do not tolerate SSRIs because of sexual dysfunction (Gelenberg et al. 2000; Montejo et al. 2001), tremor

(Pact and Giduz 1999), or severe nausea (Pedersen and Klysner 1997). In one case series, mirtazapine was successfully used to treat depression in 19 mixed-age oncology patients who were receiving chemotherapy (Thompson 2000). In some cases, it has been combined with SSRIs (Pedersen and Klysner 1997). However, such a combination should be used very cautiously because its safety has not been established, and it has been associated with a serotonin syndrome in an older patient (Benazzi 1998). Similarly, the Sequenced Treatment Alternatives to Relieve Depression study (STAR*D) found that a combination of mirtazapine and venlafaxine extended-release (XR) had modest efficacy in patients with treatment-resistant depression, comparable to the efficacy of the monoamine oxidase inhibitor (MAOI) tranylcypromine (Rush et al. 2006). However, only a few STAR*D participants were elderly, and the safety of this combination has not been established in older patients.

No published placebo-controlled trials and only two comparator-controlled trials of mirtazapine in geriatric depression have been done (Hoyberg et al. 1996; Schatzberg et al. 2002) (Table 26–5). Consistent with this paucity of controlled data, experts favor the use of mirtazapine as a third-line drug in older depressed patients who cannot tolerate or whose symptoms have not responded to SSRIs or venlafaxine (Alexopoulos et al. 2001). Mirtazapine also has been used to treat depression in frail nursing home patients (Roose et al. 2003) and in older patients with dementia (Raji and Brady 2001), but there are concerns about its effect on cognition. It has been shown to impair driving performance in two placebo- and active comparator–controlled trials in healthy volunteers (Ridout et al. 2003; Wingen et al. 2005) and to cause delirium in older patients with organic brain syndromes (Bailer et al. 2000). This deleterious effect on cognition is possibly a result of mirtazapine's antihistaminergic and sedative effect. Other adverse effects of mirtazapine include weight gain with lipid increase (Nicholas et al. 2003) and neutropenia or even agranulocytosis (Hutchison 2001; Stimmel et al. 1997). Although these hematological adverse effects are very rare, they may occur more frequently in patients with compromised immune function (Stimmel et al. 1997).

Nefazodone

Given the absence of any controlled trials in geriatric depression, mediocre outcomes in an open study (Saiz-Ruiz et al. 2002), and reports that the incidence of hepatic toxicity or even liver failure is 10- to 30-fold higher with nefazodone than with other antidepressants (Carvajal García-Pando et al. 2002; Lucena et al. 1999), nefazodone is very rarely used in older patients. When it is prescribed, one needs to be mindful of potentially problematic drug-drug interactions caused by its strong inhibition of CYP3A4, an isozyme responsible for the metabolism of most drugs, including alprazolam, triazolam, carbamazepine, and cyclosporine (Rickels et al. 1998; Spina and Scordo 2002) (see Table 26–4). Also, because older persons metabolize nefazodone more slowly than do younger patients, geriatric doses should be about 50% of the doses used in younger adults (Barbhaiya et al. 1996). Finally, a cognitive study in a small group of healthy volunteers found that a higher dosage of nefazodone (i.e., 200 mg twice daily) was associated with impairment of cognitive functions (van Laar et al. 1995).

Venlafaxine

Like duloxetine, venlafaxine is an SNRI: it inhibits the reuptake of both serotonin and norepinephrine (Harvey et al. 2000). Published geriatric data comprise seven randomized, controlled trials (see Table 26–5) and several case series or open trials (Amore et al. 1997; Dahmen et al. 1999; Dierick 1996; Khan et al. 1995), including those in older patients with atypical depression (Roose et al. 2004a), dysthymic disorder (Devanand et al. 2004), and poststroke depression (Dahmen et al. 1999).

In younger depressed patients, several meta-analyses suggested that venlafaxine produces a similar rate of response but a higher rate of remission than do SSRIs (Shelton et al. 2005; Smith et al. 2002; Stahl et al. 2002; Thase et al. 2001). This difference in remission rates seems to be most marked in women ages 50 and older (Thase et al. 2005a). Also, some open data support the use of venlafaxine in geriatric patients whose symptoms have not responded to SSRIs (Whyte et al. 2004).

However, venlafaxine shows a clear dose-response relation (Kelsey 1996), and younger patients require higher dosages (i.e., 225 mg/day or more) to obtain the benefits of its dual action (Harvey et al. 2000). Because venlafaxine pharmacokinetics are similar in younger and older patients (Klamerus et al. 1996), geriatric patients also may require high dosages, which are associated with some safety concerns (see the following paragraphs). Venlafaxine also can be useful in the treatment of generalized anxiety disorder (Katz et al. 2002) or chronic pain syndromes (Grothe et al. 2004) in older patients. For the treatment of pain syndromes, higher dosages (i.e., 225 mg/day or more) are usually needed because venlafaxine's antinociceptive effect seems to be mediated through its adrenergic action (Harvey et al. 2000; Schreiber et al. 1999).

Venlafaxine does not inhibit any of the major cytochrome P450 isoenzymes, and thus it is unlikely to cause clinically significant drug-drug interactions (Table 26–4). However, venlafaxine is metabolized by CYP2D6, and its concentration can increase markedly in genetically poor metabolizers or in patients who are taking drugs that inhibit this isozyme (Whyte et al. 2006). Even at low doses, venlafaxine inhibits the reuptake of serotonin. Thus, it shares the side-effect profile of SSRIs, including not only nausea, diarrhea, headaches, and excessive sweating but also SIADH and hyponatremia (Kirby et al. 2002), sexual dysfunction (Montejo et al. 2001), serotonin syndrome (McCue and Joseph 2001; Perry 2000), and discontinuation symptoms (even with venlafaxine XR) (Fava et al. 1997).

Venlafaxine is also associated with adverse effects that can be linked to its action on the adrenergic system. Adverse effects usually seen with TCAs that also affect the adrenergic system have been described, including dry mouth, constipation, urinary retention, increased ocular pressure, cardiovascular problems, and transient agitation (Aragona and Inghilleri 1998; Benazzi 1997). These effects are usually benign, but cardiovascular adverse effects are of concern in the elderly. Most clinicians are aware that venlafaxine can cause hypertension, generally in a dose-dependent fashion (Thase 1998; Zimmer et al. 1997). It also has been associated with clinically significant hypotension, electrocardiographic changes, arrhythmia, and acute ischemia (Davidson et al. 2005; Johnson et al. 2006; Lessard et al. 1999; Reznik et al. 1999). In Great Britain, the National Institute for Clinical Excellence has recommended that venlafaxine should not be prescribed to patients with preexisting heart disease, that an electrocardiogram should be obtained at baseline, and that blood pressure and cardiac functions should be monitored in those patients taking higher doses (National Collaborating Centre for Mental Health 2004). In a randomized trial conducted under double-blind conditions in older nursing home residents, venlafaxine was found to be less well tolerated and less safe than sertraline without evidence for an increase in efficacy (Oslin et al. 2003). Therefore, at present, it seems prudent not to use venlafaxine as a first-line agent in older patients but to reserve it for those whose symptoms do not respond to SSRIs (Alexopoulos et al. 2001; Mulsant et al. 2001a; Whyte et al. 2004). This recommendation is congruent with the results from STAR*D (Rush et al. 2006). In this study, patients who had failed a first-line SSRI had similar outcomes when the next treatment step was augmenting the SSRI with sustained-release bupropion or buspirone, switching to another SSRI, or switching to an agent from another class (i.e., bupropion or venlafaxine XR). The following steps included using a combination of venlafaxine XR and mirtazapine, with outcomes similar to those associated with switching to the MAOI tranylcypromine (Rush et al. 2006).

Tricyclic Antidepressants and Monoamine Oxidase Inhibitors

As is the case in younger patients (Rush et al. 2006), TCAs and MAOIs have become third- and fourth-line drugs in the treatment of late-life depression because of their adverse effects and the special precautions that their use in older patients entail (Mottram et al. 2006; Mulsant et al. 2001a; Wilson and Mottram 2004). The tertiary-amine TCAs—amitriptyline, clomipramine, doxepin, and imipramine—can cause significant orthostatic hypotension and anticholinergic effects, including cognitive impairment, and they should be avoided in the elderly (Beers 1997). MAOIs, now rarely used in older depressed patients, are discussed later in this section.

When one needs to use a TCA in an older patient, the secondary amines desipramine and nortriptyline are preferred because of their lower propensity to cause orthostasis and falls, their linear pharmacokinetics, and their more modest anticholinergic effects (Chew et al. 2008). Typically, the entire dose of desipramine or nortriptyline can be given at bedtime. The relatively narrow therapeutic index (i.e., the plasma level range separating efficacy and toxicity) of the secondary amines necessitates monitoring of plasma levels and electrocardiograms in older patients. After initiation of desipramine at 50 mg and nortriptyline at 25 mg, plasma levels can be measured after 5–7 days and dosages adjusted linearly, targeting plasma levels of 200–400 ng/mL for desipramine and 50–150 ng/mL for nortriptyline. These narrow ranges may ensure efficacy while decreasing risks of cognitive toxicity and other side effects. Like the tertiary-amine TCAs, desipramine and nortriptyline are type 1 antiarrhythmics: they have quinidine-like effects on cardiac conduction and should not be used in patients who have or are at risk for cardiac conduction defects (Roose et al. 1991).

Most anticholinergic side effects of desipramine or nortriptyline (e.g., dry mouth, constipation) resolve with time or usually can be mitigated with symptomatic treatment (Mulsant et al. 1999; Rosen et al. 1993). However, TCAs have been associated with cognitive worsening (Reifler et al. 1989) and with less cognitive improvement than sertraline (Bondareff et al. 2000; Doraiswamy et al. 2003) or other SSRIs.

Even though they have been found to be efficacious in older depressed patients (Georgotas et al. 1986), MAOIs are now rarely used because of the significant hypotension that can be associated with their use and the risk of life-threatening hypertensive or serotonergic crises that is associated with dietary noncompliance or drug interactions. When MAOIs are used in older patients whose symptoms have typically failed to respond to SSRIs, SNRIs, and TCAs, phenelzine is preferred to tranylcypromine because it has been more extensively studied in older patients (Georgotas et al. 1983, 1986). A typical starting dosage would be 15 mg/day, with a target dosage of 45–90 mg/day in three divided doses. Patients need to be advised about dietary restrictions and should be instructed to inform any health care providers (including pharmacists) that they are taking an MAOI.

Psychostimulants

Even though psychostimulants are widely used in the treatment of late-life mood disorders by some clinicians, this practice has very little empirical support. A few small double-blind trials suggested that methylphenidate is generally well tolerated and modestly efficacious for medically burdened depressed elders (Satel and Nelson 1989; Wallace et al. 1995). Methylphenidate also has been used for the treatment of apathy and anergia accompanying late-life depression or dementia (Herrmann et al. 2008). Nonetheless, caution is advised regarding the possible exacerbation by methylphenidate and other psychostimulants of anxiety, psychosis, anorexia, and hypertension and potential interactions with warfarin. The results of a recent study suggested that methylphenidate also can be used to augment SSRIs in older depressed patients (Lavretsky et al. 2006). Given that SSRIs may inhibit dopamine release, contributing to apathy in this population with diminished dopaminergic function, further exploration of methylphenidate as an augmenting agent is warranted.

Experience with other dopaminergic medications—such as pemoline, piribedil, pramipexole, and ropinirole—in the elderly has been more limited than experience with methylphenidate, but there have been encouraging reports in cognitively impaired elders (Eisdorfer et al. 1968; Nagaraja and Jayashree 2001; Ostow 2002). Paradoxically, sleepiness has been reported as a side effect in patients with Parkinson's disease taking pramipexole and ropinirole (Etminan et al. 2001). The wakefulness-promoting agent modafinil, which appears to induce a calm alertness through nondopaminergic mechanisms, also may have utility in treating residual apathy and fatigue, but systematic geriatric data are currently nonexistent.

Antipsychotic Medications

As in other age groups, atypical antipsychotics are being prescribed in late life as first-line drugs for the treatment of psychotic symptoms of any etiology (Rapoport et al. 2005). An increasing number of studies support the efficacy of these agents in the treatment of schizophrenia, behavioral and psychological symptoms of dementia, or delirium in older patients. At the same time, a series of reports are raising questions about their tolerability and safety in older patients (discussed later in this section). In the face of the rapidly changing knowledge base, we summarize the data relevant to the use of antipsychotics in older patients circa September 2007.

Comparisons of Conventional and Atypical Antipsychotics

As in other age groups, atypical antipsychotics have become first-line drugs in late life for the treatment of psychotic symptoms of any etiology (Rapoport et al. 2005). Despite this major shift in prescribing practice, only seven published randomized, controlled trials have compared atypical and conventional antipsychotics in older patients: 1) olanzapine, risperidone, and promazine were compared in patients with behavioral and psychological symptoms of dementia (Gareri et al. 2004); 2) olanzapine and haloperidol were compared in two trials involving older patients with schizophrenia (Barak et al. 2002; Kennedy et al. 2003) and one trial involving patients with behavioral and psychological symptoms of dementia (Verhey et al. 2006); and 3) risperidone and haloperidol were compared in three trials in patients with behavioral and psychological symptoms of dementia (Chan et al. 2001; De Deyn et al. 1999; Suh et al. 2004). In addition, two randomized, controlled trials of relevance to geriatric patients compared oral haloperidol with olanzapine or risperidone (Han and Kim 2004; Skrobik et al. 2004). Overall, in these nine trials, olanzapine and risperidone showed similar or superior efficacy and tolerability to promazine or haloperidol. In particular, they were associated with fewer and less severe extrapyramidal symptoms. In addition to these controlled data, several large case series (e.g., Curran et al. 2005; Frenchman and Prince 1997) and expert opinion (Alexopoulos et al. 2004) support that a shift away from conventional antipsychotics may benefit the elderly who are particularly prone to develop extrapyramidal symptoms or tardive dyskinesia (Caligiuri et al. 2000; Dolder and Jeste 2003; Jeste 2004; Jeste et al. 1995; Miller et al. 2005; Pollock and Mulsant 1995).

A highly publicized report and an FDA warning have indicated a nearly twofold increase in the rate of deaths in older patients with behavioral and psychological symptoms of dementia treated with atypical antipsychotics when compared with patients randomly assigned to receive placebo (Kuehn 2005; Schneider et al. 2005). Other reports have questioned the notion that atypical antipsychotics cause fewer falls (Hien et al. 2005; Landi et al. 2005) or fewer extrapyramidal symptoms (Lee et al. 2004; Rochon et al. 2005; van Iersel et al. 2005), than do conventional antipsychotics, particularly when doses of atypical antipsychotics are increased. Some studies suggest that conventional antipsychotics have a lower risk of cerebrovascular events (Percudani et al. 2005), venous thromboembolism (Liperoti et al. 2005b), and pancreatitis (Koller et al. 2003). By contrast, a series of meta-analyses and large pharmacoepidemiological studies have found that conventional antipsychotics have comparable (or even higher) risks for diabetes mellitus (Feldman et al. 2004), cerebrovascular events (Finkel et al. 2005; Liperoti et al. 2005a; Moretti et al. 2005), stroke (Gill et al. 2005; Herrmann et al. 2004), or death (Ray et al. 2001; Wang et al. 2005). Given the current uncertainty regarding the safety of both conventional and atypical antipsychotics—and the absence of consistent evidence supporting the efficacy or safety of drugs from alternative classes (Sink et al. 2005)—clinicians need to consider the risk-benefit ratio for each individual patient (Rabins and Lyketsos 2005). The National Institute of Mental Health Clinical Antipsychotic Trials of Intervention Effectiveness (CATIE) Alzheimer disease trial (Schneider et al. 2006b) showed modest treatment benefit compared with placebo for olanzapine and risperidone that was mitigated by greater extrapyramidal symptoms, sedation, and confusion. In this trial, relatively low doses of quetiapine did not appear to be efficacious compared with placebo but caused greater sedation. Therefore, the selection of a specific drug to treat a specific patient should be guided by the strength of the available evidence relevant to the disorder being treated and, in the absence of such evidence, by the differing side-effect profiles of the drugs currently available (Schneider et al. 2006a).

Risperidone

Of the atypical antipsychotics currently available in the United States, risperidone has the most published geriatric data for a variety of conditions (Alexopoulos et al. 2004; Schneider et al. 2005, 2006a; Sink et al. 2005). The efficacy and safety of risperidone in the treatment of behavioral and psychological symptoms of dementia have been reported in several randomized, placebo-controlled trials (e.g., Brodaty et al. 2003; De Deyn et al. 1999, 2005b; Katz et al. 1999; Schneider et al. 2006a, 2006b; Sink et al. 2005); randomized comparisons with haloperidol (Chan et al. 2001; De Deyn et al. 1999; Suh et al. 2004), promazine, and olanzapine (Gareri et al. 2004) or olanzapine (Fontaine et al. 2003; Mulsant et al. 2004); and uncontrolled studies or large case series (e.g., Herrmann et al. 1998; Irizarry et al. 1999; Lane et al. 2002; Lavretsky and Sultzer 1998; Rainer et al. 2001; Zarate et al. 1997).

The efficacy and tolerability of risperidone in the treatment of late-life schizophrenia are supported by one randomized comparison with olanzapine (Harvey et al. 2003; Jeste et al. 2003) and one randomized open-label study of crossover from conventional antipsychotics to risperidone or olanzapine (Ritchie et al. 2003, 2006). The parallel study showed similar efficacy between olanzapine and risperidone but more weight gain and less cognitive improvement with olanzapine. In the crossover study, patients switched to olanzapine were more likely to complete the switching process and to show an improvement in psychological quality of life. The results from these two controlled trials are supported by a large body of uncontrolled data in older patients with schizophrenia and other psychotic disorders (e.g., Davidson et al. 2000; Madhusoodanan et al. 1999a, 1999b; Sajatovic et al. 1996; Zarate et al. 1997). In addition, an analysis of the patients with schizophrenia ages 65 and older (*N*=57) who participated in randomized studies of the long-acting injectable ("depot" or Risperdal Consta) risperidone found that it was well tolerated and produced significant symptomatic improvements (Lasser et al. 2004).

One randomized comparison with haloperidol (Han and Kim 2004) and some uncontrolled data (e.g., Horikawa et al. 2003; Liu et al. 2004; Mittal et al. 2004; Parellada et al. 2004) support the efficacy and tolerability of risperidone in the treatment of delirium. However, there have been several case reports of delirium induced by risperidone (e.g., Kato et al. 2005; Ravona-Springer et al. 1998; Tavcar and Dernovsek 1998). One small randomized comparison with clozapine (*N*=10) (Ellis et al. 2000) and several open trials of low-dose risperidone in the treatment of patients with Parkinson's disease and drug-induced psychosis or with Lewy body dementia have had inconsistent results, with clear worsening of parkinsonian symptoms in some studies (e.g., Leopold 2000; Meco et al. 1997; Mohr et al. 2000; Rich et al. 1995; Workman et al. 1997). Thus, risperidone should be used with great caution in the treatment of these disorders (Parkinson Study Group 1999).

As with other atypical antipsychotics, the efficacy and tolerability of risperidone in younger patients with bipolar disorder (and possibly other mood disorders) (Andreescu et al. 2006) are well established. However, no efficacy data in older patients with bipolar disorder would favor the selection of a specific atypical antipsychotic for these patients. As a result, experts favor the use of mood stabilizers as first-line agents except in the presence of severe mania or mania with psychosis, in which case they favor combining risperidone, olanzapine, or quetiapine with a mood stabilizer (Alexopoulos et al. 2004; Sajatovic et al. 2005b; Young et al. 2004).

Commonly reported side effects of risperidone include orthostatic hypotension (on initiation of treatment) and extrapyramidal symptoms that are dose-dependent (Katz et al. 1999). At a given dosage, concentrations of risperidone (and possibly of its active metabolite paliperidone or 9-hydroxyrisperidone) seem to increase with age (Aichhorn et al. 2005; Feng et al. 2006). Therefore, typical dosages should be between 0.5 and 2 mg/day for older patients with dementia and lower than 4 mg/day for older patients without dementia. Of all the atypical antipsychotics, risperidone appears to be the most likely to be associated with hyperprolactinemia (Kinon et al. 2003). Risperidone causes only moderate electroencephalographic abnormalities (Centorrino et al. 2002), and it is rarely associated with cognitive impairment, probably because of its low affinity for muscarinic receptors (Chew et al. 2006; Harvey et al. 2003; Mulsant et al. 2004). Like other antipsychotics, risperidone can cause weight gain, diabetes, or dyslipidemia. It is more likely to do so than are aripiprazole and ziprasidone but less likely than are clozapine and olanzapine (Alexopoulos et al. 2004; American Diabetes Association et al. 2004; Feldman et al. 2004).

Olanzapine

Next to risperidone, olanzapine has the most published geriatric data. Its efficacy and tolerability in the treatment of behavioral and psychological symptoms of dementia have been reported in several randomized, placebo-controlled trials (e.g., Clark et al. 2001; De Deyn et al. 2004; Street et al. 2000) and in randomized comparisons with haloperidol (Verhey et al. 2006), promazine and risperidone (Gareri et al. 2004), and risperidone (Fontaine et al. 2003; Mulsant et al. 2004). However, a recent meta-analysis of all published and nonpublished placebo-controlled trials of olanzapine in the treatment of behavioral and psychological symptoms of dementia concluded that "olanzapine was not associated with efficacy overall" (Schneider et al. 2006a, p. 205). Also, the study by Street and colleagues (2000) found an inverted dose-response relation (i.e., patients receiving 15 mg/day had worse outcomes than did patients receiving 5 mg/day), suggesting that higher doses may be toxic in these patients (see discussion later in this subsection). As discussed earlier in this section, the efficacy and tolerability of olanzapine in the treatment of late-life schizophrenia have been confirmed in two randomized comparisons with haloperidol (Barak et al. 2002; Kennedy et al. 2003) and two randomized comparisons with risperidone (Harvey et al. 2003; Jeste et al. 2003; Ritchie et al. 2003, 2006).

In one of only three published randomized, controlled trials of pharmacotherapy for delirium, and the largest to date, olanzapine and haloperidol were found to have comparable efficacy (Skrobik et al. 2004).

However, caution is needed when using olanzapine in patients with delirium because some controlled trials have reported some cognitive worsening in patients with dementia treated with olanzapine (Kennedy et al. 2005; Mulsant et al. 2004), and several case reports of delirium induced by olanzapine have been published (Lim et al. 2006; Morita et al. 2004; Samuels and Fang 2004). Similarly, two controlled trials suggested that olanzapine may not be a drug of choice for treating drug-induced psychosis in patients with Parkinson's disease. In one placebo-controlled study, olanzapine was not significantly different from placebo in terms of reduction of psychotic symptoms but was significantly worse in terms of parkinsonian symptoms and activities of daily living (Breier et al. 2002). In another small randomized study (N=15), olanzapine was not as efficacious as clozapine and was more toxic (Goetz et al. 2000). The need for caution when olanzapine is used to treat psychosis in patients with Parkinson's disease or Lewy body dementia is reinforced by several open trials or case series: although a few have shown positive results (e.g., Cummings et al. 2002; Sa and Lang 2001), most have reported a significant worsening of motor symptoms in these patients (e.g., Marsh et al. 2001; Molho and Factor 1999; Onofrj et al. 2000; Parkinson Study Group 1999; Walker et al. 1999; Wolters et al. 1996).

The evidence supporting the efficacy and safety of olanzapine in younger patients with bipolar disorder and other mood disorders (Andreescu et al. 2006; Shelton et al. 2001; Thase 2002) is particularly strong. However, as discussed earlier, no relevant data in older patients with mood disorders are available (Alexopoulos et al. 2004; Sajatovic et al. 2005a, 2005b; Young et al. 2004). Similarly, no relevant geriatric data are available on the rapidly dissolving or the intramuscular preparations of olanzapine (Belgamwar and Fenton 2005).

On review of all evidence available in 2004, a consensus conference concluded that among the atypical antipsychotics, clozapine and olanzapine were associated with the highest risk for diabetes and caused the greatest weight gain and dyslipidemia (American Diabetes Association et al. 2004). However, this consensus was based on data in younger patients with psychotic and mood disorders. Relevant geriatric data are very limited, and the risks for metabolic problems may be different in older patients (Etminan et al. 2003; Feldman et al. 2004; Hwang et al. 2003; Lipkovich et al. 2007; Micca et al. 2006). Other common side effects include sedation and gait disturbance. Extrapyramidal symptoms appear to be dose-dependent and are rare at the lower dosages typically used in older patients (5–10 mg/day). Olanzapine also has been associated with electroencephalographic abnormalities (Centorrino et al. 2002), and its strong blocking of the muscarinic receptor (Chew et al. 2005, 2006; Mulsant et al. 2003) (Table 26–6) may explain why it has been associated with constipation in a large series of long-term care patients (Martin et al. 2003); decreased efficacy at higher doses in a randomized trial in older agitated or psychotic patients with dementia (Street et al. 2000); a differential cognitive effect from risperidone in randomized trials involving older patients with schizophrenia (Harvey et al. 2003) or dementia (Mulsant et al. 2004); worsening of cognition in a large placebo-controlled trial in older nonagitated, nonpsychotic patients with Alzheimer's disease (Kennedy et al. 2005); and frank delirium in some clinical cases (Lim et al. 2006; Morita et al. 2004; Samuels and Fang 2004). Patients who are older, female, or nonsmokers, or who are taking a drug that inhibits CYP1A2 (e.g., fluvoxamine or ciprofloxacin) have higher concentrations of olanzapine and may be at higher risk for adverse effects (Gex-Fabry et al. 2003). Because of its adverse-effect profile, experts do not recommend olanzapine as a first-line antipsychotic in older patients with cognitive impairment, constipation, diabetes, diabetic neuropathy, dyslipidemia, obesity, xerophthalmia, or xerostomia (Alexopoulos et al. 2004).

Quetiapine

Results of randomized, placebo-controlled trials in older patients with behavioral and psychological symptoms of dementia—both published and unpublished—are inconclusive (Schneider et al. 2006a). For instance, in a large trial of 333 institutionalized participants, quetiapine, 200 mg/day (but not 100 mg/day) differed from placebo on global impressions and positive symptom ratings but not on the important primary outcome measures of agitation and psychosis (Zhong et al. 2007). By contrast, published but uncontrolled or unblinded studies in older patients with primary psychotic disorders, dementia, or delirium suggest that quetiapine is effective for these disorders (Kim et al. 2003; Madhusoodanan et al. 2000; McManus et al. 1999; Mintzer et al. 2004; Pae et al. 2004; Sasaki et al. 2003; Tariot et al. 2000; Yang et al. 2005). The good tolera-

TABLE 26–6. Receptor blockade of atypical antipsychotics

	D_2	5-HT_2	M_1	α_2
Aripiprazole	*	++	0	+
Clozapine	+	++	+++	+
Olanzapine	++	++	+++	+
Quetiapine	+	++	+	++
Risperidone	+++	+++	0	++
Ziprasidone	++	++	0	+

Note. Receptor types: α_2=alpha-adrenergic type 2; D_2=dopamine type 2; 5-HT_2=5-hydroxytryptamine (serotonin) type 2; M_1=muscarinic type 1.
0=none; +=minimal; ++=intermediate; +++=high.
*High-affinity partial agonist.

bility of quetiapine observed clinically in patients at high risk for extrapyramidal symptoms suggests that quetiapine should be the first-line antipsychotic for older patients with Parkinson's disease, dementia with Lewy body, or tardive dyskinesia (Alexopoulos et al. 2004; Poewe 2005). Indeed, the use of quetiapine in older patients with Parkinson's disease and drug-induced psychosis has been encouraged (Fernandez et al. 1999, 2002; Menza et al. 1999; Targum and Abbott 2000). However, quetiapine was not found to be efficacious in a double-blind trial that had a high dropout rate in quetiapine-treated patients (Rabey et al. 2007). Similarly, in a double-blind trial in patients with dementia and parkinsonism, quetiapine did not show efficacy for agitation or psychosis compared with placebo (Kurlan et al. 2007). Like other antipsychotics, quetiapine can cause somnolence or dizziness (Jaskiw et al. 2004; Yang et al. 2005), but the incidence of these adverse effects can be minimized by a slower dose titration. The risk for weight gain, diabetes, or dyslipidemia associated with the use of quetiapine appears similar to the risk associated with the use of risperidone but lower than the risk associated with the use of clozapine or olanzapine (American Diabetes Association et al. 2004; Feldman et al. 2004).

Clozapine

Clozapine is still considered the drug of choice for younger patients with treatment-refractory schizophrenia (Meltzer 1998), and one small case series suggested that it can be similarly helpful for the treatment of primary psychotic disorders that are refractory to other treatments in older patients (Sajatovic et al. 1997). A randomized, controlled trial comparing clozapine and chlorpromazine in older patients with schizophrenia (Howanitz et al. 1999) and one large case series (Barak et al. 1999) also supported the use of clozapine in moderate dosages (i.e., approximately 50–200 mg/day) in older patients with primary psychotic disorders. The strongest published geriatric studies of clozapine are focused on the treatment of drug-induced psychosis in patients with Parkinson's disease (Ellis et al. 2000; Goetz et al. 2000; Parkinson Study Group 1999). The results of these studies suggest that clozapine at low dosages (12.5–50 mg/day) is the preferred treatment for this condition (Parkinson Study Group 1999). However, the use of clozapine in older patients is severely limited because of its significant hematological, neurological, cognitive, metabolic, and cardiac adverse effects (Alvir et al. 1993; Centorrino et al. 2002, 2003; Chew et al. 2006; Koller et al. 2001; Melkersson and Hulting 2001; Modai et al. 2000; Sernyak et al. 2002).

Aripiprazole

Aripiprazole has a high dopamine type 2 (D_2) receptor affinity and, as a partial agonist, a higher affinity for the G protein–coupled state of the D_2 receptor (i.e., its active state) (Burris et al. 2002). With partial D_2 agonist properties, aripiprazole is conceived as a dopamine system stabilizer: in high dopaminergic states, it acts as an antagonist, and in low dopaminergic states, it acts as an agonist (Coward et al. 1989). This may explain why it is unlikely to cause extrapyramidal side effects or prolactin elevation (associated with osteoporosis), even at high D_2 receptor occupancy (Kane et al. 2002; Mamo et al. 2007; Yokoi et al. 2002). It has only moderate affinity to the adrenergic α_1 receptor and histamine H_1 receptor and negligible affinity to the muscarinic receptor (Chew et al. 2006). As a result, orthostatic hypotension and antihistaminergic and anticholinergic adverse effects are less likely to occur than with other atypical agents. Also, it has not been associated with increases in mean QTc interval. These pharmacodynamic features make aripiprazole attractive for use in older patients. However, lack of published geriatric data had limited its use in older patients to second-line treatments (Alexopoulos et al. 2004). More recently, three randomized, placebo-controlled trial of aripiprazole in older patients with behavioral and psychological symptoms of dementia have been published (De Deyn et al. 2005a; Mintzer et al. 2007; Streim et al. 2008). A meta-analysis of these placebo-controlled trials concluded that "efficacy on rating scales was observed by meta-analysis for aripiprazole" (Schneider et al. 2006a, p. 191). Additional data relevant to older patients with bipolar disorder have been published (Sajatovic et al. 2008; Suppes et al. 2008).

Ziprasidone and Paliperidone

Ziprasidone and paliperidone are two atypical antipsychotics available in the United States for which very limited geriatric data are available. On the basis of ziprasidone's lower effect on glucose, lipids, and weight (American Diabetes Association et al. 2004) and its lack of affinity for the muscarinic receptor (Table 26–6) (Chew et al. 2006) and thus its low potential to cause cognitive impairment, ziprasidone is an attractive medication for older patients with psychosis. One published case series (Berkowitz 2003) and one pharmacokinetic study (Wilner et al. 2000) have reported on oral ziprasidone in the elderly. In addition, two published studies on the use of intramuscular ziprasidone found no adverse cardiovascular or electrocardiographic changes in a total of 38 older patients (Greco et al. 2005; Kohen et al. 2005). However, in the absence of systematic study, there is lingering concern regarding the potential effects of ziprasidone on cardiac conduction, and ziprasidone should not be used in older patients with QTc prolongation or congestive heart failure (Alexopoulos et al. 2004).

Paliperidone is the newest atypical antipsychotic in the United States, and at this time, it is only FDA-approved for the treatment of schizophrenia. It is the active 9-OH-metabolite of risperidone, and therefore its pharmacological action, efficacy, and side effects should be very similar to those of risperidone. It is being marketed as a once-daily XR formulation that takes 24 hours to reach a maximum concentration. As a hydroxylated metabolite, paliperidone clearance is not affected by hepatic impairment or CYP2D6 metabolism, but it is affected by renal function. FDA approval was based on three 6-week trials that included a total of only 125 subjects age 65 years or older (e.g., Davidson et al. 2007; Kane et al. 2007). However, paliperidone has not yet been studied in patients with dementia, and doses remain speculative for this population.

Mood Stabilizers

As a class, mood stabilizers are high-risk medications for elderly patients. There is a paucity of controlled studies and an abundance of concerns regarding their potential toxicity, problematic side effects, and drug interactions. Beyond their approved indications, anticonvulsants are often used in the management of agitation accompanying dementia. Despite the age-linked risks associated with lithium, it continues to be used commonly in elderly patients with bipolar disorder (Umapathy et al. 2000) and, less commonly, for antidepressant augmentation. Currently, no consensus exists as to whether it is still appropriate to prescribe lithium as a first-line mood stabilizer for elders, nor is there agreement on the management of secondary mania (Sajatovic et al. 2005b; Young et al. 2004).

Lithium

Open and naturalistic trials suggest that lithium is efficacious in the acute treatment and prophylaxis of mania in older patients (Eastham et al. 1998; Wylie et al. 1999). However, reductions in renal clearance and decreased total body water significantly affect the pharmacokinetics of lithium in older patients, increasing the risk of toxicity. Moreover, specific psychiatric and medical comorbidities common in late life—such as renal dysfunction, hyponatremia, dehydration, and heart failure—also exacerbate the risk of toxicity (Sajatovic et al. 2006). Thiazide diuretics, angiotensin-converting enzyme inhibitors, and NSAIDs may precipitate toxicity by further diminishing the renal clearance of lithium. For all these reasons, older patients require lower dosages than do younger patients to produce similar serum lithium levels.

Elderly persons are more sensitive to neurological side effects at lower lithium levels. This sensitivity may be a consequence of increased permeability of the blood-brain barrier and subtle changes in sodium-lithium countertransport. Neurotoxicity may manifest as coarse tremor, slurred speech, ataxia, hyperreflexia, and muscle fasciculations. In vitro, lithium has moderate anticholinergic activity (Chew et al. 2008). This may explain why cognitive impairment has been observed with levels well below 1 mEq/L, and frank delirium has been reported with serum levels as low as 1.5 mEq/L (Sproule et al. 2000). Consequently, treatment of older patients may require lithium levels to be kept as low as 0.4–0.8 mEq/L.

In addition to lithium levels, electrolytes and the electrocardiogram should be monitored regularly. Older patients are at higher risk for lithium-induced hypothyroidism and should have thyroid-stimulating hormone concentration monitored at 6-month intervals. Lithium toxicity can produce persistent central nervous system impairment or can be fatal. Thus, it is a medical emergency that requires careful correction of fluid and electrolyte imbalances and that may require administration of aminophylline and mannitol (or even hemodialysis) to increase lithium excretion.

Anticonvulsants

Anticonvulsants are used as alternatives to lithium in the treatment of bipolar disorder and as alternatives to antipsychotics for the symptomatic management of agitation accompanying dementia. In general, side effects are better tolerated and less severe than those of lithium. Furthermore, there may be a subgroup of bipolar patients with dysphoria or rapid cycling who respond poorly to lithium but do well with anticonvulsants (Post et al. 1998). Similarly, given its putative etiology, mania associated with dementia and other neurological illnesses ("secondary mania") may respond preferentially to anticonvulsants (Shulman 1997).

Valproate

Valproate is a broad-spectrum anticonvulsant that has been approved in the United States for the treatment of mania. Small case series have suggested that valproic acid is relatively well tolerated by older patients with bipolar disorder (Kando et al. 1996; Noaghiul et al. 1998) and those with agitation in the context of dementia (Kunik et al. 1998). Nonetheless, in four negative placebo-controlled trials, valproate was not more effective than placebo in treating agitation of dementia (Tariot et al. 2005).

Sedation, nausea, weight gain, and hand tremors are common dose-related side effects. Mild stomach upset may be decreased by use of the enteric-coated divalproex salt. Thrombocytopenia can occur in as many as half of the elderly patients taking valproate and may ensue at lower total drug levels than in younger patients (Conley et al. 2001). Other dose-related adverse effects include reversible elevations in liver enzymes and transient elevations in blood ammonia levels (Davis et al. 1994). Liver failure and pancreatitis are rare. Valproate has other metabolic effects of concern to aging patients, such as increases in bone turnover and reductions of serum folate, with concomitant elevations in plasma homocysteine concentrations (Sato et al. 2001; Schwaninger et al. 1999).

The pharmacokinetics of valproate vary according to formulation, and valproic acid, divalproex sodium, and its extended-release preparation are not interchangeable. Valproate is metabolized principally by mitochondrial β-oxidation and secondarily by the cytochrome P450 system; typical half-lives are in the range of 5–16 hours and are not affected by aging alone. Concomitant administration of valproate will increase concentrations of phenobarbital, primidone, carbamazepine, diazepam, and lamotrigine. Conversely, concurrent administration of carbamazepine, lamotrigine, topiramate, and phenytoin may decrease levels of valproate. Fluoxetine and erythromycin may potentiate the effects of valproate. Changes in protein binding as a result of drug interactions are no longer considered clinically important beyond causing the misinterpretation of total (i.e., free and bound) drug levels (Benet and Hoener 2002). Valproate binding to plasma proteins is generally reduced in the elderly, suggesting that use of free drug levels may be preferable (Kodama et al. 2001).

Carbamazepine and Oxcarbazepine

Carbamazepine is effective for the acute treatment and prophylaxis of mania in younger patients (Post et al. 1998), and it is FDA-approved for the acute treatment of mania. In a placebo-controlled trial in 51 nursing home patients, carbamazepine also has been shown to be efficacious in treating agitation and aggression associated with dementia (Tariot et al. 1998). Side effects of carbamazepine include nausea, dizziness, ataxia, and neutropenia. Older patients are at higher risk for drug-induced leukopenia and agranulocytosis, ataxia, and, of course, drug interactions (Cates and Powers 1998). Carbamazepine is primarily eliminated by CYP3A4, and its clearance is reduced with aging (Bernus et al. 1997). Its interactions with other drugs are protean and complex. Carbamazepine concentrations are increased to potential toxicity by CYP3A4 inhibitors such as macrolide antibiotics, antifungals, and some antidepressants (see Table 26–4). CYP3A4 inducers—such as phenobarbital, phenytoin, and carbamazepine itself—

will lower the concentration of carbamazepine and the concentrations of many drugs metabolized by this isoenzyme (Spina et al. 1996). Oxcarbazepine, the 10-keto analog of carbamazepine, is a less potent CYP3A4 inducer, and although it has been studied in some small trials in bipolar patients, it has not been studied in dementia (Lima 2000).

Gabapentin and Pregabalin

Although gabapentin has been used in bipolar disorder, trials have not borne out its effectiveness, and only anecdotal reports of its use in dementia are available (Pande et al. 2000). Nonetheless, it has a generally favorable side-effect profile and modest anxiolytic and analgesic effects, particularly for neuropathic pain. Gabapentin does not bind to plasma proteins and is not metabolized, being eliminated by renal excretion. In patients with renal impairment, neurological adverse effects such as ataxia, involuntary movements, disorganized thinking, excitation, and extreme sedation have been noted. Even in the absence of renal dysfunction, elderly patients may be prone to excessive sedation. Therefore, in the elderly, initial dosages of 100 mg twice a day are more prudent than the 900 mg/day recommended as a starting dosage for younger patients with epilepsy.

Pregabalin is a structural congener of gabapentin. It has an improved pharmacokinetic profile and may be helpful for neuropathic pain in the elderly. Nonetheless, it is a controlled substance, and no data pertaining to it are available in the geriatric population (Guay 2005).

Lamotrigine

Lamotrigine is approved in the United States for the maintenance treatment of bipolar disorder to prevent mood episodes (depressive, manic, or mixed episodes). Data from a randomized, controlled trial support that lamotrigine is more effective than placebo in treating bipolar disorder in older patients (Sajatovic et al. 2005a). In contrast with many other mood stabilizers and antidepressants, lamotrigine does not seem to be associated with weight gain (Morrell et al. 2003). Somnolence, rashes, and headaches have been observed in a significant number of older patients. In geriatric patients, rashes were the most common reason for study withdrawal, but they were less frequent with lamotrigine (3%) than with carbamazepine (19%) (Brodie et al. 1999). Severe rashes, including Stevens-Johnson syndrome or toxic epidermal necrolysis, have been observed in about 0.3% of adult patients (Messenheimer 1998). At the first sign of rash or other evidence of hypersensitivity (e.g., fever, lymphadenopathy), unless the signs are clearly not drug-related, lamotrigine should be discontinued, and the patient should be evaluated. The incidence of rashes can be reduced by using a slower dose titration. Also, because valproate increases lamotrigine plasma concentration, the titration of lamotrigine needs to be slowed down, and its target dosage needs to be halved in patients who are receiving valproate.

Anxiolytics and Hypnotics

Social isolation, financial concerns, and declining intellectual and physical function may predispose elderly patients to anxiety. New-onset anxiety is a frequent accompaniment of physical illness, depression, or medication side effects. The SSRIs and venlafaxine have displaced the long-acting benzodiazepines (e.g., diazepam) and medications with very short half-lives (e.g., alprazolam) as initial treatments for anxiety in late life, whereas the intermediate half-life benzodiazepine lorazepam and the nonbenzodiazepines (e.g., eszopiclone, zaleplon, zolpidem) have become the most commonly used hypnotics.

Benzodiazepines and Nonbenzodiazepine Hypnotics

Detrimental effects of benzodiazepines in elderly patients frequently outweigh any short-term symptomatic relief that they may provide. Continuous benzodiazepine use increases the risk of falls, hip fractures, and cognitive impairment in elderly patients (Sorock and Shimkin 1988). The popular nonbenzodiazepine zolpidem was found in a very large case-control study to double the risk of hip fracture, after age, gender, and medical conditions were controlled (Wang et al. 2001). Even single small doses of diazepam, nitrazepam, and temazepam have been shown to cause significant impairment in memory and psychomotor performance in elderly subjects (Nikaido et al. 1990; Pomara et al. 1989).

Nevertheless, treatment with benzodiazepines may be indicated for a few weeks in the acute treatment of depression-related sleep disturbance when the primary pharmacotherapy is an antidepressant. Relative contraindications include heavy snoring (because it suggests sleep apnea), dementia (because such patients are at increased risk for daytime confusion, impairment in activities of daily living, and daytime sleepiness), and the use of other sedating medications or alcohol.

In the elderly, compounds with long half-lives (clonazepam, diazepam, and flurazepam) should be avoided. Also, several drugs with shorter half-lives (i.e., alprazolam, triazolam, midazolam, and the nonbenzodiazepines eszopiclone, zaleplon, and zolpidem) undergo phase 1 hepatic metabolism by CYP3A4 that is subject to specific interactions and age-associated decline (Freudenreich and Menza 2000; Greenblatt et al. 1991). Sedatives with very short half-lives also may increase the likelihood that confused elders will awake in the middle of the night to stagger off to the bathroom. Oxazepam and lorazepam do not undergo phase 1 hepatic metabolism, have no active metabolites, have acceptable half-lives that do not increase with age, and are not subject to drug interactions. Lorazepam is preferred for inducing sleep because oxazepam has a relatively slow and erratic absorption. Lorazepam is available in appropriately small doses (0.5-mg pills) and is well absorbed intramuscularly.

Buspirone

The anxiolytic buspirone, a partial 5-HT_{1A} agonist, may be beneficial for some anxious patients and appears to be well tolerated by the elderly without the sedation or addiction liability of the benzodiazepines (Steinberg 1994). Thus, it may be helpful for elderly patients with generalized anxiety disorder who are prone to falls, confusion, or chronic lung disease. Nonetheless, buspirone may take several weeks to exert an anxiolytic effect, has no cross-tolerance with benzodiazepines, and may cause side effects such as dizziness, headache, and nervousness (Strand et al. 1990). Unlike the SSRIs, buspirone is of limited use for panic or obsessive-compulsive disorders. The pharmacokinetics of buspirone are not affected by age or gender, but coadministration with verapamil, diltiazem, erythromycin, or itraconazole will substantially increase buspirone concentrations, and overenthusiastic combinations with serotonergic medications may result in the serotonin syndrome (Mahmood and Sahajwalla 1999). Buspirone should be started at 5 mg three times a day and gradually increased by 5-mg increments every week to a maximum dosage of 60 mg/day.

Cognitive Enhancers

Cholinesterase Inhibitors

Four of the five currently approved drugs available in the United States for the symptomatic improvement of Alzheimer's disease—tacrine, donepezil, galantamine, and rivastigmine—are cholinesterase inhibitors (Table 26–7). The use of tacrine is no longer recommended because of its potential hepatotoxic effects. The principal side effects of these medications are concentration dependent and result from their peripheral cholinergic actions. With these side effects in mind, clinicians should be aware of the drugs' specific pathways of elimination and potential pharmacokinetic drug interactions with CYP2D6 or CYP3A4 inhibitors and CYP3A4 inducers when prescribing donepezil and galantamine (Carrier 1999; Crismon 1998). Rivastigmine is affected by renal function, and FDA warnings have emphasized the need for careful dose titration (and retitration if restarting) to prevent severe vomiting. Drugs with potent anticholinergic effects directly antagonize cholinesterase inhibitors (Chew et al. 2005, 2008; Lu and Tune 2003; Mulsant et al. 2003).

The currently available cognitive enhancers have been found in controlled trials to result in modest improvements in cognition and function (Cummings 2000). A rapid symptomatic deterioration may occur when these drugs are discontinued, and no evidence suggests that they alter the underlying neuropathology of Alzheimer's disease or its eventual progression. Before initiating anticholinesterase therapy, it is imperative that unnecessary anticholinergic medications be discontinued (Lu and Tune 2003). In patients with diminished cognitive reserve, even small anticholinergic effects can substantially impair cognition (Chew et al. 2005; Mulsant et al. 2003; Nebes et al. 1997, 2005). Cholinesterase inhibitors may have a role to play in the prevention and treatment of behavioral and psychological symptoms of dementia (Cummings et al. 2006; Sink et al. 2005), but more research is needed in this area.

NMDA Receptor Antagonist

Memantine, the first drug in the *N*-methyl-D-aspartate (NMDA) receptor antagonist class, is FDA-approved for the treatment of moderate to severe Alzheimer's disease. Glutamatergic overstimulation may cause excitotoxic neuronal damage. As an uncompetitive antagonist with moderate affinity for NMDA receptors, meman-

TABLE 26–7. Cholinesterase inhibitors

	Clearance	Dosing	Significant side effects	Pharmacodynamics
Donepezil	Half-life=70–80 hr CYP 3A4, 2D6	5–10 mg/day in one dose per day; start at 5 mg at bedtime	Mild nausea, diarrhea, agitation	Reversible acetylcholinesterase inhibition
Galantamine, Galantamine ER	Half-life=7 hr CYP 2D6, 3A4	8–24 mg/day divided into two doses; start at 8 mg/day twice daily	Moderate nausea, vomiting, diarrhea, anorexia, tremor, insomnia	Reversible acetylcholinesterase inhibition; nicotinic modulation may increase acetylcholine release
Rivastigmine	Half-life=1.25 hr Renal	6–12 mg/day divided into two doses; start at 1.5 mg twice daily, and retitrate if drug is stopped	Severe nausea, vomiting, anorexia, weight loss, sweating, dizziness	Pseudoirreversible acetylcholinesterase inhibition; also butylcholinesterase inhibition

Note. CYP=cytochrome P450; ER=extended release.

tine may attenuate neurotoxicity without interfering with glutamate's normal physiological actions. In patients with moderate to severe Alzheimer's disease, a daily dosage of 20 mg of memantine was well tolerated and significantly slowed the rate of deterioration compared with placebo in a 28-week U.S. multicenter trial (Reisberg et al. 2003). A 6-month placebo-controlled study in 401 donepezil-treated patients showed benefits of the combination therapy on cognition and activities of daily living relative to baseline (Tariot et al. 2004). In both studies, memantine was well tolerated, although it may cause confusion in some patients. It does not appear to be implicated in drug-drug interactions, but it is excreted by the kidneys, and its dosage needs to be reduced in patients with significant impairment in renal function.

Key Points

- Psychiatric disorders can be successfully treated in late life with psychotropic drugs, but pharmacological intervention requires special care because the elderly are more susceptible to drug-induced adverse events.

Antidepressants

- Selective serotonin reuptake inhibitors (SSRIs) remain first-line drugs for treating late-life depression because of their efficacy for both depressive and anxiety syndromes, ease of use, and safety and good tolerability. All available SSRIs have similar efficacy and tolerability; however, in late life, experts favor the use of citalopram, escitalopram, or sertraline because of their favorable pharmacokinetic profiles. In older patients, SSRI starting dosages are typically half the minimal efficacious dosage. They can cause SIADH; act synergistically with other medications that increase the risk of gastrointestinal bleeding, such as NSAIDs; and be associated with bradycardia.
- Even though only limited controlled data support the efficacy and safety of bupropion, duloxetine, mirtazapine, nefazodone, or venlafaxine in older patients, these drugs are the preferred alternatives in older patients who do not respond to or who cannot tolerate SSRIs.
- When one needs to use a tricyclic antidepressant in treating late-life depression in an older patient, the secondary amines desipramine and nortriptyline are preferred because of their lower propensity to cause orthostasis and falls, their linear pharmacokinetics, and their more modest anticholinergic effects. Because of their relatively narrow therapeutic index, monitoring of plasma levels and electrocardiograms in older patients is required.

Antipsychotics

- For the treatment of psychotic symptoms of any etiology in late life, atypical antipsychotics are first-line drugs. Evidence supports their efficacy in the treatment of schizophrenia, behavioral and psychological symptoms of dementia, or delirium in older patients.

However, significant questions remain regarding their tolerability and safety in older patients. They have been associated with a nearly twofold increase in the rate of deaths in older patients with behavioral and psychological symptoms of dementia. The selection of a specific drug to treat a specific patient should be guided by the strength of the available evidence relevant to the disorder being treated and, in the absence of such evidence, by the differing side-effect profiles of the drugs currently available.

Cognitive enhancers

- The cognitive enhancers that are currently available have been shown in controlled trials to result in modest improvements in cognition and function. Before initiating anticholinesterase therapy, it is imperative that unnecessary anticholinergic medications be discontinued.

Other psychotropic medications

- The efficacy and safety of lithium and divalproex are supported only by open and naturalistic data at present. Both can cause significant adverse effects and require close monitoring. Minimal geriatric data are available for carbamazepine or lamotrigine.
- Detrimental effects of the benzodiazepines in elderly patients frequently outweigh any short-term symptomatic relief that they may provide.

References

Aichhorn W, Weiss U, Marksteiner J, et al: Influence of age and gender on risperidone plasma concentrations. J Psychopharmacol 19:395–401, 2005

Alexopoulos GS, Katz IR, Reynolds CF 3rd, et al: Pharmacotherapy of depression in older patients: a summary of the expert consensus guidelines. J Psychiatr Pract 7:361–376, 2001

Alexopoulos GS, Streim J, Carpenter D, et al: Using antipsychotic agents in older patients. J Clin Psychiatry 65 (suppl 2):5–104, 2004

Allard P, Gram L, Timdahl K, et al: Efficacy and tolerability of venlafaxine in geriatric outpatients with major depression: a double-blind, randomised 6-month comparative study. Int J Geriatr Psychiatry 19:1123–1130, 2004

Altamura AC, De Novellis F, Guercetti G, et al: Fluoxetine compared with amitriptyline in elderly depression: a controlled clinical trial. Int J Clin Pharmacol Res 9:391–396, 1989

Alvir JJ, Lieberman JA, Safferman AZ, et al: Clozapine-induced agranulocytosis: incidence and risk factors in the United States. N Engl J Med 329:162–167, 1993

American Diabetes Association, American Psychiatric Association, American Association of Clinical Endocrinologists, et al: Consensus development conference on antipsychotic drugs and obesity and diabetes. Diabetes Care 27:596–601, 2004

Amore M, Ricci M, Zanardi R, et al: Long-term treatment of geropsychiatric depressed patients with venlafaxine. J Affect Disord 46:293–296, 1997

Andersen G, Vestergaard K, Lauritzen L: Effective treatment of poststroke depression with the selective serotonin reuptake inhibitor citalopram. Stroke 25:1099–1104, 1994

Andreescu C, Mulsant BH, Rothschild AJ, et al: Pharmacotherapy of major depression with psychotic features: what is the evidence? Psychiatr Ann 35:31–38, 2006

Aragona M, Inghilleri M: Increased ocular pressure in two patients with narrow angle glaucoma treated with venlafaxine. Clin Neuropharmacol 21:130–131, 1998

Arranz FJ, Ros S: Effects of comorbidity and polypharmacy on the clinical usefulness of sertraline in elderly depressed patients: an open multicentre study. J Affect Disord 46:285–291, 1997

Bailer U, Fischer P, Kufferle B, et al: Occurrence of mirtazapine-induced delirium in organic brain disorder. Int Clin Psychopharmacol 15:239–243, 2000

Barak Y, Wittenberg N, Naor S, et al: Clozapine in elderly psychiatric patients: tolerability, safety, and efficacy. Compr Psychiatry 40:320–325, 1999

Barak Y, Shamir E, Zemishlani H, et al: Olanzapine vs. haloperidol in the treatment of elderly chronic schizophrenia patients. Prog Neuropsychopharmacol Biol Psychiatry 26:1199–1202, 2002

Barbhaiya RH, Buch AB, Greene DS: A study of the effect of age and gender on the pharmacokinetics of nefazodone after single and multiple doses. J Clin Psychopharmacol 16:19–25, 1996

Beers MH: Explicit criteria for determining potentially inappropriate medication use by the elderly. Arch Intern Med 157:1531–1536, 1997

Belgamwar RB, Fenton M: Olanzapine IM or velotab for acutely disturbed/agitated people with suspected serious mental illnesses. Cochrane Database Syst Rev (2):CD003729, 2005

Belpaire FM, Wijnant P, Temmerman A, et al: The oxidative metabolism of metoprolol in human liver microsomes: inhibition by the selective serotonin reuptake inhibitors. Eur J Clin Pharmacol 54:261–264, 1998

Benazzi F: Urinary retention with venlafaxine-haloperidol combination. Pharmacopsychiatry 30:27, 1997

Benazzi F: Serotonin syndrome with mirtazapine-fluoxetine combination. Int J Geriatr Psychiatry 13:495–496, 1998

Benet LZ, Hoener B: Changes in plasma protein binding have little clinical relevance. Clin Pharmacol Ther 71:115–121, 2002

Berkowitz A: Ziprasidone for dementia in elderly patients: case review. J Psychiatr Pract 9:469–473, 2003

Bernus I, Dickinson RG, Hooper WD: Anticonvulsant therapy in aged patients: clinical pharmacokinetic considerations. Drugs Aging 10:278–289, 1997

Bigos KL, Bies RR, Pollock BG: Population pharmacokinetics in geriatric psychiatry. Am J Geriatr Psychiatry 14:993–1003, 2006

Bodkin JA, Lasser RA, Wines JD Jr, et al: Combining serotonin reuptake inhibitors and bupropion in partial responders to antidepressant monotherapy. J Clin Psychiatry 58:137–145, 1997

Bondareff W, Alpert M, Friedhoff AJ, et al: Comparison of sertraline and nortriptyline in the treatment of major depressive disorder in late life. Am J Psychiatry 157:729–736, 2000

Branconnier RJ, Cole JO, Ghazvinian S, et al: Clinical pharmacology of bupropion and imipramine in elderly depressives. J Clin Psychiatry 44 (5 pt 2):130–133, 1983

Breier A, Sutton VK, Feldman PD, et al: Olanzapine in the treatment of dopamimetic-induced psychosis in patients with Parkinson's disease. Biol Psychiatry 52:438–445, 2002

Brodaty H, Ames D, Snowdon J, et al: A randomized placebo-controlled trial of risperidone for the treatment of aggression, agitation, and psychosis of dementia. J Clin Psychiatry 64:134–143, 2003

Brodie MJ, Overstall PW, Giorgi L: Multicentre, double-blind, randomised comparison between lamotrigine and carbamazepine in elderly patients with newly diagnosed epilepsy. The UK Lamotrigine Elderly Study Group. Epilepsy Res 37:81–87, 1999

Brosen K, Skjelbo E, Rasmussen BB, et al: Fluvoxamine is a potent inhibitor of cytochrome P4501A2. Biochem Pharmacol 45:1211–1214, 1993

Burris KD, Molski TF, Xu C, et al: Aripiprazole, a novel antipsychotic, is a high-affinity partial agonist at human dopamine D2 receptors. J Pharmacol Exp Ther 302:381–389, 2002

Burrows AB, Salzman C, Satlin A, et al: A randomized, placebo-controlled trial of paroxetine in nursing home residents with non-major depression. Depress Anxiety 15:102–110, 2002

Caligiuri MR, Jeste DV, Lacro JP: Antipsychotic-induced movement disorders in the elderly: epidemiology and treatment recommendations. Drugs Aging 17:363–384, 2000

Carrier L: Donepezil and paroxetine: possible drug interaction. J Am Geriatr Soc 47:1037, 1999

Carvajal García-Pando A, García del Pozo J, Sánchez AS, et al: Hepatotoxicity associated with the new antidepressants. J Clin Psychiatry 63:135–137, 2002

Cates M, Powers R: Concomitant rash and blood dyscrasias in geriatric psychiatry patients treated with carbamazepine. Ann Pharmacother 32:884–887, 1998

Centorrino F, Price BH, Tuttle M, et al: EEG abnormalities during treatment with typical and atypical antipsychotics. Am J Psychiatry 159:109–115, 2002

Centorrino F, Albert MJ, Drago-Ferrante G, et al: Delirium during clozapine treatment: incidence and associated risk factors. Pharmacopsychiatry 36:156–160, 2003

Chalon SA, Granier LA, Vandenhende FR, et al: Duloxetine increases serotonin and norepinephrine availability in healthy subjects: a double-blind, controlled study. Neuropsychopharmacology 28:1685–1693, 2003

Chan WC, Lam LC, Choy CN, et al: A double-blind randomised comparison of risperidone and haloperidol in the treatment of behavioural and psychological symptoms in Chinese dementia patients. Int J Geriatr Psychiatry 16:1156–1162, 2001

Chen P, Kales HC, Weintraub D, et al: Antidepressant treatment of veterans with Parkinson's disease and depression: analysis of a national sample. J Geriatr Psychiatry Neurol 20:161–165, 2007

Chen Y, Patel NC, Guo JJ, et al: Antidepressant prophylaxis for poststroke depression: a meta-analysis. Int Clin Psychopharmacol 22:159–166, 2007

Chew ML, Mulsant BH, Rosen J, et al: Serum anticholinergic activity and cognition in patients with moderate to severe dementia. Am J Geriatr Psychiatry 13:535–538, 2005

Chew ML, Mulsant BH, Pollock BG, et al: A model of anticholinergic activity of atypical antipsychotic medications. Schizophr Res 88:63–72, 2006

Chew ML, Mulsant BH, Pollock BG, et al: Anticholinergic activity of 107 medications commonly used by older adults. J Am Geriatr Soc 56:1333–1341, 2008

Clark WS, Street JS, Feldman PD, et al: The effects of olanzapine in reducing the emergence of psychosis among nursing home patients with Alzheimer's disease. J Clin Psychiatry 62:34–40, 2001

Cohn CK, Shrivastava R, Mendels J, et al: Double-blind, multicenter comparison of sertraline and amitriptyline in elderly depressed patients. J Clin Psychiatry 51 (suppl B):28–33, 1990

Conley EL, Coley KC, Pollock BG, et al: Prevalence and risk of thrombocytopenia with valproic acid: experience at a psychiatric teaching hospital. Pharmacotherapy 21:1325–1330, 2001

Coward D, Dixon K, Enz A, et al: Partial brain dopamine D2 receptor agonists in the treatment of schizophrenia. Psychopharmacol Bull 25:393–397, 1989

Crewe HK, Lennard MS, Tucker GT, et al: The effect of selective serotonin re-uptake inhibitors on cytochrome P4502D6 (CYP2D6) activity in human liver microsomes. Br J Clin Pharmacol 34:262–265, 1992

Crismon ML: Pharmacokinetics and drug interactions of cholinesterase inhibitors administered in Alzheimer's disease. Pharmacotherapy 18:47–54, 1998

Cummings JL: Cholinesterase inhibitors: a new class of psychotropic compounds. Am J Psychiatry 157:4–15, 2000

Cummings JL, Street J, Masterman D, et al: Efficacy of olanzapine in the treatment of psychosis in dementia with Lewy bodies. Dement Geriatr Cogn Disord 13:67–73, 2002

Cummings JL, McRae T, Zhang R, et al: Effects of donepezil on neuropsychiatric symptoms in patients with dementia and severe behavioral disorders. Am J Geriatr Psychiatry 14:605–612, 2006

Curran S, Turner D, Musa S, et al: Psychotropic drug use in older people with mental illness with particular reference to antipsychotics: a systematic study of tolerability and use in different diagnostic groups. Int J Geriatr Psychiatry 20:842–847, 2005

Dahmen N, Marx J, Hopf HC, et al: Therapy of early poststroke depression with venlafaxine: safety, tolerability, and efficacy as determined in an open, uncontrolled clinical trial. Stroke 30:691–692, 1999

Dalton SO, Sorensen HT, Johansen C: SSRIs and upper gastrointestinal bleeding: what is known and how should it influence prescribing? CNS Drugs 20:143–151, 2006

Davidson J, Watkins L, Owens M, et al: Effects of paroxetine and venlafaxine XR on heart rate variability in depression. J Clin Psychopharmacol 25:480–484, 2005

Davidson M, Harvey PD, Vervarcke J, et al: A long-term, multicenter, open-label study of risperidone in elderly patients with psychosis. On behalf of the Risperidone Working Group. Int J Geriatr Psychiatry 15:506–514, 2000

Davidson M, Emsley R, Kramer M, et al: Efficacy, safety and early response of paliperidone extended-release tablets (paliperidone ER): results of a 6-week, randomized, placebo-controlled study. Schizophr Res 93:117–130, 2007

Davis R, Peters DH, McTavish D: Valproic acid: a reappraisal of its pharmacological properties and clinical efficacy in epilepsy. Drugs 47:332–372, 1994

De Deyn PP, Rabheru K, Rasmussen A, et al: A randomized trial of risperidone, placebo, and haloperidol for behavioral symptoms of dementia. Neurology 53:946–955, 1999

De Deyn PP, Carrasco MM, Deberdt W, et al: Olanzapine versus placebo in the treatment of psychosis with or without associated behavioral disturbances in patients with Alzheimer's disease. Int J Geriatr Psychiatry 19:115–126, 2004

De Deyn PP, Jeste DV, Swanik R, et al: Aripiprazole for the treatment of psychosis in patients with Alzheimer's disease: a randomized placebo-controlled study. J Clin Psychopharmacol 25:463–467, 2005a

De Deyn PP, Katz IR, Brodaty H, et al: Management of agitation, aggression, and psychosis associated with dementia: a pooled analysis including three randomized, placebo-controlled double-blind trials in nursing home residents treated with risperidone. Clin Neurol Neurosurg 107:497–508, 2005b

Devanand DP, Pelton GH, Marston K, et al: Sertraline treatment of elderly patients with depression and cognitive impairment. Int J Geriatr Psychiatry 18:123–130, 2003

Devanand DP, Juszczak N, Nobler MS, et al: An open treatment trial of venlafaxine for elderly patients with dysthymic disorder. J Geriatr Psychiatry Neurol 17:219–224, 2004

Devanand DP, Nobler MS, Cheng J, et al: Randomized, double-blind, placebo-controlled trial of fluoxetine treatment for elderly patients with dysthymic disorder. Am J Geriatr Psychiatry 13:59–68, 2005

Dierick M: An open-label evaluation of the long-term safety of oral venlafaxine in depressed elderly patients. Ann Clin Psychiatry 8:169–178, 1996

Dolder CR, Jeste DV: Incidence of tardive dyskinesia with typical versus atypical antipsychotics in very high risk patients. Biol Psychiatry 53:1142–1145, 2003

Doraiswamy PM, Khan ZM, Donahue RM, et al: Quality of life in geriatric depression: a comparison of remitters, partial responders, and nonresponders. Am J Geriatr Psychiatry 9:423–428, 2001

Doraiswamy PM, Krishnan KR, Oxman T, et al: Does antidepressant therapy improve cognition in elderly depressed patients? J Gerontol A Biol Sci Med Sci 58:M1137–M1144, 2003

Dunner DL, Cohn JB, Walshe TD, et al: Two combined, multicenter double-blind studies of paroxetine and doxepin in geriatric patients with major depression. J Clin Psychiatry 53 (suppl):57–60, 1992

Dunner DL, Zisook S, Billow AA, et al: A prospective safety surveillance study for bupropion sustained-release in the treatment of depression. J Clin Psychiatry 59:366–373, 1998

Eastham JH, Jeste DV, Young RC: Assessment and treatment of bipolar disorder in the elderly. Drugs Aging 12:205–224, 1998

Eisdorfer C, Conner JF, Wilkie FL: The effect of magnesium pemoline on cognition and behavior. J Gerontol 23:283–288, 1968

Ellis T, Cudkowicz ME, Sexton PM, et al: Clozapine and risperidone treatment of psychosis in Parkinson's disease. J Neuropsychiatry Clin Neurosci 12:364–369, 2000

Ereshefsky L, Dugan D: Review of the pharmacokinetics, pharmacogenetics, and drug interaction potential of antidepressants: focus on venlafaxine. Depress Anxiety 12 (suppl 1):30–44, 2000

Etminan M, Samii A, Takkouche B, et al: Increased risk of somnolence with the new dopamine agonists in patients with Parkinson's disease: a meta-analysis of randomised controlled trials. Drug Saf 24:863–868, 2001

Etminan M, Streiner DL, Rochon PA: Exploring the association between atypical neuroleptic agents and diabetes mellitus in older adults. Pharmacotherapy 23:1411–1415, 2003

Evans M, Hammond M, Wilson K, et al: Treatment of depression in the elderly: effect of physical illness on response. Int J Geriatr Psychiatry 12:1189–1194, 1997

Fabian TJ, Amico JA, Kroboth PD, et al: Paroxetine-induced hyponatremia in older adults: a 12-week prospective study. Arch Intern Med 164:327–332, 2004

Fava M, Mulroy R, Alpert J, et al: Emergence of adverse events following discontinuation of treatment with extended-release venlafaxine. Am J Psychiatry 154:1760–1762, 1997

Feighner JP, Cohn JB: Double-blind comparative trials of fluoxetine and doxepin in geriatric patients with major depressive disorder. J Clin Psychiatry 46 (3 pt 2):20–25, 1985

Feldman PD, Hay LK, Deberdt W, et al: Retrospective cohort study of diabetes mellitus and antipsychotic treatment in a geriatric population in the United States. J Am Med Dir Assoc 5:38–46, 2004

Feng Y, Pollock BG, Coley KC, et al: Assessing sources of variability in risperidone pharmacokinetics: a population analysis of risperidone using highly sparse sampling measurements from the CATIE Study. Society of Biological Psychiatry's 61st Annual Scientific Program. Biol Psychiatry 59:230S, 2006

Fernandez HH, Friedman JH, Jacques C, et al: Quetiapine for the treatment of drug-induced psychosis in Parkinson's disease. Mov Disord 14:484–487, 1999

Fernandez HH, Trieschmann ME, Burke MA, et al: Quetiapine for psychosis in Parkinson's disease versus dementia with Lewy bodies. J Clin Psychiatry 63:513–515, 2002

Finkel SI, Richter EM, Clary CM, et al: Comparative efficacy of sertraline vs. fluoxetine in patients age 70 or over with major depression. Am J Geriatr Psychiatry 7:221–227, 1999

Finkel S, Kozma C, Long S, et al: Risperidone treatment in elderly patients with dementia: relative risk of cerebrovascular events versus other antipsychotics. Int Psychogeriatr 17:617–629, 2005

Flint AJ: Generalised anxiety disorder in elderly patients: epidemiology, diagnosis and treatment options. Drugs Aging 22:101–114, 2005

Fontaine CS, Hynan LS, Koch K, et al: A double-blind comparison of olanzapine versus risperidone in the acute treatment of dementia-related behavioral disturbances in extended care facilities. J Clin Psychiatry 64:726–730, 2003

Forlenza OV, Almeida OP, Stoppe A Jr, et al: Antidepressant efficacy and safety of low-dose sertraline and standard-dose imipramine for the treatment of depression in older adults: results from a double-blind, randomized, controlled clinical trial. Int Psychogeriatr 13:75–84, 2001

Frenchman IB, Prince T: Clinical experience with risperidone, haloperidol, and thioridazine for dementia-associated behavioral disturbances. Int Psychogeriatr 9:431–435, 1997

Freudenreich O, Menza M: Zolpidem-related delirium: a case report. J Clin Psychiatry 61:449–450, 2000

Friedman RA, Leon AC: Expanding the black box: depression, antidepressants, and the risk of suicide. N Engl J Med 356:2343–2346, 2007

Furlan PM, Kallan MJ, Ten Have T, et al: Cognitive and psychomotor effects of paroxetine and sertraline on healthy elderly volunteers. Am J Geriatr Psychiatry 9:429–438, 2001

Gareri P, Cotroneo A, Lacava R, et al: Comparison of the efficacy of new and conventional antipsychotic drugs in the treatment of behavioral and psychological symptoms of dementia (BPSD). Arch Gerontol Geriatr Suppl 9:207–215, 2004

Gasto C, Navarro V, Marcos T, et al: Single-blind comparison of venlafaxine and nortriptyline in elderly major depression. J Clin Psychopharmacol 23:21–26, 2003

Gelenberg AJ, Laukes C, McGahuey C, et al: Mirtazapine substitution in SSRI-induced sexual dysfunction. J Clin Psychiatry 61:356–360, 2000

Georgotas A, Friedman E, McCarthy M, et al: Resistant geriatric depressions and therapeutic response to monoamine oxidase inhibitors. Biol Psychiatry 18:195–205, 1983

Georgotas A, McCue RE, Hapworth W, et al: Comparative efficacy and safety of MAOIs versus TCAs in treating depression in the elderly. Biol Psychiatry 21:1155–1166, 1986

Geretsegger C, Stuppaeck CH, Mair M, et al: Multicenter double blind study of paroxetine and amitriptyline in elderly depressed inpatients. Psychopharmacology (Berl) 119:277–281, 1995

Gex-Fabry M, Balant-Gorgia AE, Balant LP: Therapeutic drug monitoring of olanzapine: the combined effect of age, gender, smoking, and comedication. Ther Drug Monit 25:46–53, 2003

Gill SS, Rochon PA, Herrmann N, et al: Atypical antipsychotic drugs and risk of ischaemic stroke: population based retrospective cohort study. BMJ 330:445, 2005

Glassman AH, O'Connor CM, Califf RM, et al: Sertraline treatment of major depression in patients with acute MI or unstable angina [published erratum appears in JAMA 288:1720, 2002]. JAMA 288:701–709, 2002

Goetz CG, Blasucci LM, Leurgans S, et al: Olanzapine and clozapine: comparative effects on motor function in hallucinating PD patients. Neurology 55:789–794, 2000

Goldstein DJ, Lu Y, Detke MJ, et al: Duloxetine vs. placebo in patients with painful diabetic neuropathy. Pain 116:109–118, 2005

Goodnick PJ, Hernandez M: Treatment of depression in comorbid medical illness. Expert Opin Pharmacother 1:1367–1384, 2000

Gorwood P, Weiller E, Lemming O, et al: Escitalopram prevents relapse in older patients with major depressive disorder. Am J Geriatr Psychiatry 15:581–593, 2007

Gram LF, Hansen MG, Sindrup SH, et al: Citalopram: interaction studies with levomepromazine, imipramine, and lithium. Ther Drug Monit 15:18–24, 1993

Greco KE, Tune LE, Brown FW, et al: A retrospective study of the safety of intramuscular ziprasidone in agitated elderly patients. J Clin Psychiatry 66:928–929, 2005

Greenblatt DJ, Harmatz JS, Shapiro L, et al: Sensitivity to triazolam in the elderly. N Engl J Med 324:1691–1698, 1991

Greenblatt DJ, von Moltke LL, Harmatz JS, et al: Drug interactions with newer antidepressants: role of human cytochromes P450. J Clin Psychiatry 59 (suppl 15):19–27, 1998

Greenblatt DJ, von Moltke LL, Harmatz JS, et al: Human cytochromes and some newer antidepressants: kinetics, metabolism, and drug interactions. J Clin Psychiatry 19 (suppl 1):23S–35S, 1999

Greene DS, Barbhaiya RH: Clinical pharmacokinetics of nefazodone. Clin Pharmacokinet 33:260–275, 1997

Grothe DR, Scheckner B, Albano D: Treatment of pain syndromes with venlafaxine. Pharmacotherapy 24:621–629, 2004

Guay DR: Pregabalin in neuropathic pain: a more "pharmaceutically elegant" gabapentin? Am J Geriatr Pharmacother 3:274–287, 2005

Guillibert E, Pelicier Y, Archambault JC, et al: A double-blind, multicentre study of paroxetine versus clomipramine in depressed elderly patients. Acta Psychiatr Scand Suppl 350:132–134, 1989

Han CS, Kim YK: A double-blind trial of risperidone and haloperidol for the treatment of delirium. Psychosomatics 45:297–301, 2004

Hansen RA, Gartlehner G, Lohr KN, et al: Efficacy and safety of second-generation antidepressants in the treatment of major depressive disorder. Ann Intern Med 143:415–426, 2005

Harvey AT, Rudolph RL, Preskorn SH: Evidence of the dual mechanisms of action of venlafaxine. Arch Gen Psychiatry 57:503–509, 2000

Harvey PD, Napolitano JA, Mao L, et al: Comparative effects of risperidone and olanzapine on cognition in elderly patients with schizophrenia or schizoaffective disorder. Int J Geriatr Psychiatry 18:820–829, 2003

Herrmann N, Rivard MF, Flynn M, et al: Risperidone for the treatment of behavioral disturbances in dementia: a case series. J Neuropsychiatry Clin Neurosci 10:220–223, 1998

Herrmann N, Mamdani M, Lanctot KL: Atypical antipsychotics and risk of cerebrovascular accidents. Am J Psychiatry 161:1113–1115, 2004

Herrmann N, Rothenburg LS, Black SE, et al: Methylphenidate for the treatment of apathy in Alzheimer disease: prediction of response using dextroamphetamine challenge. J Clin Psychopharmacol 28:296–301, 2008

Hesse LM, Venkatakrishnan K, Court MH, et al: CYP2B6 mediates the in vitro hydroxylation of bupropion: potential drug interactions with other antidepressants. Drug Metab Dispos 28:1176–1183, 2000

Hesse LM, He P, Krishnaswamy S, et al: Pharmacogenetic determinants of interindividual variability in bupropion hydroxylation by cytochrome P450 2B6 in human liver microsomes. Pharmacogenetics 14:225–238, 2004

Hien le TT, Cumming RG, Cameron ID, et al: Atypical antipsychotic medications and risk of falls in residents of aged care facilities. J Am Geriatr Soc 53:1290–1295, 2005

Horikawa N, Yamazaki T, Miyamoto K, et al: Treatment for delirium with risperidone: results of a prospective open trial with 10 patients. Gen Hosp Psychiatry 25:289–292, 2003

Howanitz E, Pardo M, Smelson DA, et al: The efficacy and safety of clozapine versus chlorpromazine in geriatric schizophrenia. J Clin Psychiatry 60:41–44, 1999

Howard WT, Warnock JK: Bupropion-induced psychosis. Am J Psychiatry 156:2017–2018, 1999

Hoyberg OJ, Maragakis B, Mullin J, et al: A double-blind multicentre comparison of mirtazapine and amitriptyline in elderly depressed patients. Acta Psychiatr Scand 93:184–190, 1996

Hua TC, Pan A, Chan C, et al: Effect of duloxetine on tolterodine pharmacokinetics in healthy volunteers. Br J Clin Pharmacol 57:652–656, 2004

Hudson JI, Wohlreich MM, Kajdasz DK, et al: Safety and tolerability of duloxetine in the treatment of major depressive disorder: analysis of pooled data from eight placebo-controlled clinical trials. Hum Psychopharmacol 20:327–341, 2005

Hutchison LC: Mirtazapine and bone marrow suppression: a case report. J Am Geriatr Soc 49:1129–1130, 2001

Hwang JP, Yang CH, Lee TW, et al: The efficacy and safety of olanzapine for the treatment of geriatric psychosis. J Clin Psychopharmacol 23:113–118, 2003

Iribarne C, Picart D, Dreano Y, et al: In vitro interactions between fluoxetine or fluvoxamine and methadone or buprenorphine. Fundam Clin Pharmacol 12:194–199, 1998

Irizarry MC, Ghaemi SN, Lee-Cherry ER, et al: Risperidone treatment of behavioral disturbances in outpatients with dementia. J Neuropsychiatry Clin Neurosci 11:336–342, 1999

Jaskiw GE, Thyrum PT, Fuller MA, et al: Pharmacokinetics of quetiapine in elderly patients with selected psychotic disorders. Clin Pharmacokinet 43:1025–1035, 2004

Jeppesen U, Gram L, Vistisen K: Dose-dependent inhibition of CYP1A2, CYP2C19, and CYP2D6 by citalopram, fluoxetine, fluvoxamine, and paroxetine. Eur J Clin Pharmacol 51:73–78, 1996

Jeste DV: Tardive dyskinesia rates with atypical antipsychotics in older adults. J Clin Psychiatry 65 (suppl 9):21–24, 2004

Jeste DV, Caligiuri MP, Paulsen JS, et al: Risk of tardive dyskinesia in older patients: a prospective longitudinal study of 266 outpatients. Arch Gen Psychiatry 52:756–765, 1995

Jeste DV, Barak Y, Madhusoodanan S, et al: International multisite double-blind trial of the atypical antipsychotics risperidone and olanzapine in 175 elderly patients with chronic schizophrenia. Am J Geriatr Psychiatry 11:638–647, 2003

Johnson EM, Whyte E, Mulsant BH, et al: Cardiovascular changes associated with venlafaxine in the treatment of late life depression. Am J Geriatr Psychiatry 14:796–802, 2006

Joo JH, Lenze EJ, Mulsant BH, et al: Risk factors for falls during treatment of late-life depression. J Clin Psychiatry 63:936–941, 2002

Juurlink DN, Mamdani MM, Kopp A, et al: The risk of suicide with selective serotonin reuptake inhibitors in the elderly. Am J Psychiatry 163:813–821, 2006

Kando JC, Tohen M, Castillo J, et al: The use of valproate in an elderly population with affective symptoms. J Clin Psychiatry 57:238–240, 1996

Kane JM, Carson WH, Saha AR, et al: Efficacy and safety of aripiprazole and haloperidol versus placebo in patients with schizophrenia and schizoaffective disorder. J Clin Psychiatry 63:763–771, 2002

Kane J, Canas F, Kramer M, et al: Treatment of schizophrenia with paliperidone extended-release tablets: a 6-week placebo-controlled trial. Schizophr Res 90:147–161, 2007

Karp JF, Weiner D, Seligman K, et al: Body pain and treatment response in late-life depression. Am J Geriatr Psychiatry 13:188–194, 2005

Kasckow JW, Mohamed S, Thallasinos A, et al: Citalopram augmentation of antipsychotic treatment in older schizophrenia patients. Int J Geriatr Psychiatry 16:1163–1167, 2001

Kashuba AD, Nafziger AN, Kearns GL, et al: Effect of fluvoxamine therapy on the activities of CYP1A2, CYP2D6, and CYP3A as determined by phenotyping. Clin Pharmacol Ther 64:257–268, 1998

Kasper S, de Swart H, Andersen HF: Escitalopram in the treatment of depressed elderly patients. Am J Geriatr Psychiatry 13:884–891, 2005

Kato D, Kawanishi C, Kishida I, et al: Delirium resolving upon switching from risperidone to quetiapine: implication of CYP2D6 genotype. Psychosomatics 46:374–375, 2005

Katona CLE, Hunter BN, Bray J: A double-blind comparison of the efficacy and safety of paroxetine and imipramine in the treatment of depression with dementia. Int J Geriatr Psychiatry 13:100–108, 1998

Katz IR, Jeste DV, Mintzer JE, et al: Comparison of risperidone and placebo for psychosis and behavioral disturbances associated with dementia: a randomized, double-blind trial. Risperidone Study Group. J Clin Psychiatry 60:107–115, 1999

Katz IR, Reynolds CF 3rd, Alexopoulos GS, et al: Venlafaxine ER as a treatment for generalized anxiety disorder in older adults: pooled analysis of five randomized placebo-controlled clinical trials. J Am Geriatr Soc 50:18–25, 2002

Kelsey JE: Dose-response relationship with venlafaxine. J Clin Psychopharmacol 16 (3 suppl 2):21S–26S; discussion, 26S–28S, 1996

Kennedy JS, Jeste D, Kaiser CJ, et al: Olanzapine vs. haloperidol in geriatric schizophrenia: analysis of data from a double-blind controlled trial. Int J Geriatr Psychiatry 18:1013–1020, 2003

Kennedy J, Deberdt W, Siegal A, et al: Olanzapine does not enhance cognition in non-agitated and non-psychotic patients with mild to moderate Alzheimer's dementia. Int J Geriatr Psychiatry 20:1020–1027, 2005

Khan A, Rudolph R, Baumel B, et al: Venlafaxine in depressed geriatric outpatients: an open-label clinical study. Psychopharmacol Bull 31:753–758, 1995

Kiev A, Masco HL, Wenger TL, et al: The cardiovascular effects of bupropion and nortriptyline in depressed outpatients. Ann Clin Psychiatry 6:107–115, 1994

Kim KY, Bader GM, Kotlyar V, et al: Treatment of delirium in older adults with quetiapine. J Geriatr Psychiatry Neurol 16:29–31, 2003

Kinon BJ, Stauffer VL, McGuire HC, et al: The effects of antipsychotic drug treatment on prolactin concentrations in elderly patients. J Am Med Dir Assoc 4:189–194, 2003

Kirby D, Harrigan S, Ames D: Hyponatraemia in elderly psychiatric patients treated with selective serotonin reuptake inhibitors and venlafaxine: a retrospective controlled study in an inpatient unit. Int J Geriatr Psychiatry 17:231–237, 2002

Kirwin JL, Goren JL: Duloxetine: a dual serotonin-norepinephrine reuptake inhibitor for treatment of major depressive disorder. Pharmacotherapy 25:396–410, 2005

Klamerus KJ, Parker VD, Rudolph RL, et al: Effects of age and gender on venlafaxine and O-desmethylvenlafaxine pharmacokinetics. Pharmacotherapy 16:915–923, 1996

Kobayashi K, Yamamoto T, Chiba K, et al: The effects of selective serotonin reuptake inhibitors and their metabolites on S-mephenytoin 4′-hydroxylase activity in human liver microsomes. Br J Clin Pharmacol 40:481–485, 1995

Kodama Y, Kodama H, Kuranari M, et al: Gender- or age-related binding characteristics of valproic acid to serum proteins in adult patients with epilepsy. Eur J Pharm Biopharm 52:57–63, 2001

Kohen I, Preval H, Southard R, et al: Naturalistic study of intramuscular ziprasidone versus conventional agents in agitated elderly patients: retrospective findings from a psychiatric emergency service. Am J Geriatr Pharmacother 3:240–245, 2005

Koller E, Schneider B, Bennett K, et al: Clozapine-associated diabetes. Am J Med 111:716–723, 2001

Koller EA, Cross JT, Doraiswamy PM, et al: Pancreatitis associated with atypical antipsychotics: from the Food and Drug Administration's MedWatch surveillance system and published reports. Pharmacotherapy 23:1123–1130, 2003

Kotlyar M, Brauer LH, Tracy TS, et al: Inhibition of CYP2D6 activity by bupropion. J Clin Psychopharmacol 25:226–229, 2005

Kroenke K, West SL, Swindle R, et al: Similar effectiveness of paroxetine, fluoxetine, and sertraline in primary care: a randomized trial. JAMA 286:2947–2955, 2001

Kuehn BM: FDA warns antipsychotic drugs may be risky for elderly. JAMA 293:2462, 2005

Kunik ME, Puryear L, Orengo CA, et al: The efficacy and tolerability of divalproex sodium in elderly demented patients with behavioral disturbances. Int J Geriatr Psychiatry 13:29–34, 1998

Kurlan R, Cummings J, Raman R, et al: Quetiapine for agitation or psychosis in patients with dementia and parkinsonism. Neurology 68:1356–1363, 2007

Kyle CJ, Petersen HE, Overo KF: Comparison of the tolerability and efficacy of citalopram and amitriptyline in elderly depressed patients treated in general practice. Depress Anxiety 8:147–153, 1998

Landi F, Onder G, Cesari M, et al: Psychotropic medications and risk for falls among community-dwelling frail older people: an observational study. J Gerontol A Biol Sci Med Sci 60:622–626, 2005

Lane HY, Chang YC, Su MH, et al: Shifting from haloperidol to risperidone for behavioral disturbances in dementia: safety, response predictors, and mood effects. J Clin Psychopharmacol 22:4–10, 2002

Laroche ML, Charmes JP, Nouaille Y, et al: Is inappropriate medication use a major cause of adverse drug reactions in the elderly? Br J Clin Pharmacol 63:177–186, 2007

Lasser RA, Bossie CA, Zhu Y, et al: Efficacy and safety of long-acting risperidone in elderly patients with schizophrenia and schizoaffective disorder. Int J Geriatr Psychiatry 19:898–905, 2004

Lavretsky H, Sultzer D: A structured trial of risperidone for the treatment of agitation in dementia. Am J Geriatr Psychiatry 6:127–135, 1998

Lavretsky H, Park S, Siddarth P, et al: Methylphenidate-enhanced antidepressant response to citalopram in the elderly: a double-blind, placebo-controlled pilot trial. Am J Geriatr Psychiatry 142:181–185, 2006

Lee PE, Gill SS, Freedman M, et al: Atypical antipsychotic drugs in the treatment of behavioural and psychological symptoms of dementia: systematic review. BMJ 329:75, 2004

Lenze EJ, Mulsant BH, Shear MK, et al: Anxiety symptoms in elderly patients with depression: what is the best approach to treatment? Drugs Aging 19:753–760, 2002

Lenze EJ, Mulsant BH, Shear MK, et al: Efficacy and tolerability of citalopram in the treatment of late-life anxiety disorders: results from an 8-week randomized, placebo-controlled trial. Am J Psychiatry 162:146–150, 2005

Leopold NA: Risperidone treatment of drug-related psychosis in patients with parkinsonism. Mov Disord 15:301–304, 2000

Lessard E, Yessine MA, Hamelin BA, et al: Influence of CYP2D6 activity on the disposition and cardiovascular toxicity of the antidepressant agent venlafaxine in humans. Pharmacogenetics 9:435–443, 1999

Lim CJ, Trevino C, Tampi RR: Can olanzapine cause delirium in the elderly? Ann Pharmacother 40:135–138, 2006

Lima JM: The new drugs and the strategies to manage epilepsy. Curr Pharm Des 6:873–878, 2000

Liperoti R, Gambassi G, Lapane KL, et al: Cerebrovascular events among elderly nursing home patients treated with conventional or atypical antipsychotics. J Clin Psychiatry 66:1090–1096, 2005a

Liperoti R, Pedone C, Lapane KL, et al: Venous thromboembolism among elderly patients treated with atypical and conventional antipsychotic agents. Arch Intern Med 165:2677–2682, 2005b

Lipkovich I, Ahl J, Nichols R, et al: Weight changes during treatment with olanzapine in older adult patients with dementia and behavioral disturbances. J Geriatr Psychiatry Neurol 20:107–114, 2007

Liu B, Anderson G, Mittmann N, et al: Use of selective serotonin reuptake inhibitors or tricyclic antidepressants and risk of hip fractures in elderly people. Lancet 351:1303–1307, 1998

Liu CY, Juang YY, Liang HY, et al: Efficacy of risperidone in treating the hyperactive symptoms of delirium. Int Clin Psychopharmacol 19:165–168, 2004

Looper KJ: Potential medical and surgical complications of serotonergic antidepressants. Psychosomatics 48:1–9, 2007

Lotrich FE, Pollock BG: Aging and clinical pharmacology: implications for antidepressants. J Clin Pharmacol 45:1106–1122, 2005

Lotrich FE, Rabinovitz F, Gironda P, et al: Depression following pegylated interferon-alpha: characteristics and vulnerability. J Psychosom Res 63:131–135, 2007

Lu CJ, Tune LE: Chronic exposure to anticholinergic medications adversely affects the course of Alzheimer disease. Am J Geriatr Psychiatry 14:458–461, 2003

Lucena MI, Andrade RJ, Gomez-Outes A, et al: Acute liver failure after treatment with nefazodone. Dig Dis Sci 44:2577–2579, 1999

Lyketsos CG, DelCampo L, Steinberg M, et al: Treating depression in Alzheimer disease: efficacy and safety of sertraline therapy, and the benefits of depression reduction: the DIADS. Arch Gen Psychiatry 60:737–746, 2003

Madhusoodanan S, Brecher M, Brenner R, et al: Risperidone in the treatment of elderly patients with psychotic disorders. Am J Geriatr Psychiatry 7:132–138, 1999a

Madhusoodanan S, Suresh P, Brenner R, et al: Experience with the atypical antipsychotics—risperidone and olanzapine in the elderly. Ann Clin Psychiatry 11:113–118, 1999b

Madhusoodanan S, Brenner R, Alcantra A: Clinical experience with quetiapine in elderly patients with psychotic disorders. J Geriatr Psychiatry Neurol 13:28–32, 2000

Mahapatra SN, Hackett D: A randomised, double-blind, parallel-group comparison of venlafaxine and dothiepin in geriatric patients with major depression. Int J Clin Pract 51:209–213, 1997

Mahmood I, Sahajwalla C: Clinical pharmacokinetics and pharmacodynamics of buspirone, an anxiolytic drug. Clin Pharmacokinet 36:277–287, 1999

Mamo DC, Sweet RA, Mulsant BH, et al: The effect of nortriptyline and paroxetine on extrapyramidal signs and symptoms: a prospective double-blind study in depressed elderly patients. Am J Geriatr Psychiatry 8:226–231, 2000

Mamo D, Graff A, Mizrahi R, et al: Differential effects of aripiprazole on D2, 5-HT2, and 5-HT1A receptor occupancy in patients with schizophrenia: a triple tracer PET study. Am J Psychiatry 164:1411–1417, 2007

Mariappan P, Ballantyne Z, N'Dow JMO, et al: Serotonin and noradrenaline reuptake inhibitors (SNRI) for stress urinary incontinence in adults. Cochrane Database Syst Rev (3):CD004742, 2005

Marsh L, Lyketsos C, Reich SG: Olanzapine for the treatment of psychosis in patients with Parkinson's disease and dementia. Psychosomatics 42:477–481, 2001

Martin H, Slyk MP, Deymann S, et al: Safety profile assessment of risperidone and olanzapine in long-term care patients with dementia. J Am Med Dir Assoc 4:183–188, 2003

McCue RE, Joseph M: Venlafaxine- and trazodone-induced serotonin syndrome. Am J Psychiatry 158:2088–2089, 2001

McManus DQ, Arvanitis LA, Kowalcyk BB: Quetiapine, a novel antipsychotic: experience in elderly patients with psychotic disorders. Seroquel Trial 48 Study Group. J Clin Psychiatry 60:292–298, 1999

Meco G, Alessandri A, Giustini P, et al: Risperidone in levodopa-induced psychosis in advanced Parkinson's disease: an open-label, long-term study. Mov Disord 12:610–612, 1997

Melkersson KI, Hulting AL: Insulin and leptin levels in patients with schizophrenia or related psychoses—a comparison between different antipsychotic agents. Psychopharmacology 154:205–212, 2001

Meltzer HY: Suicide in schizophrenia: risk factors and clozapine treatment. J Clin Psychiatry 59 (suppl 3):15–20, 1998

Menza MM, Palermo B, Mark M: Quetiapine as an alternative to clozapine in the treatment of dopamimetic psychosis in patients with Parkinson's disease. Ann Clin Psychiatry 11:141–144, 1999

Messenheimer JA: Rash in adult and pediatric patients treated with lamotrigine. Can J Neurol Sci 25:S14–S18, 1998

Micca JL, Hoffmann VP, Lipkovich I, et al: Retrospective analysis of diabetes risk in elderly patients with dementia in olanzapine clinical trials. Am J Geriatr Psychiatry 14:62–70, 2006

Miller DD, McEvoy JP, Davis SM, et al: Clinical correlates of tardive dyskinesia in schizophrenia: baseline data from the CATIE schizophrenia trial. Schizophr Res 80:33–43, 2005

Mintzer JE, Mullen JA, Sweitzer DE: A comparison of extrapyramidal symptoms in older outpatients treated with quetiapine or risperidone. Curr Med Res Opin 20:1483–1491, 2004

Mintzer JE, Tune LE, Breder CD, et al: Aripiprazole for the treatment of psychoses in institutionalized patients with Alzheimer dementia: a multicenter, randomized, double-blind, placebo-controlled assessment of three fixed doses. Am J Geriatr Psychiatry 15:918–931, 2007

Mittal D, Jimerson NA, Neely EP, et al: Risperidone in the treatment of delirium: results from a prospective open-label trial. J Clin Psychiatry 65:662–667, 2004

Modai I, Hirschmann S, Rava A, et al: Sudden death in patients receiving clozapine treatment: a preliminary investigation. J Clin Psychopharmacol 20:325–327, 2000

Mohr E, Mendis T, Hildebrand K, et al: Risperidone in the treatment of dopamine-induced psychosis in Parkinson's disease: an open pilot trial. Mov Disord 15:1230–1237, 2000

Molho ES, Factor SA: Worsening of motor features of parkinsonism with olanzapine. Mov Disord 14:1014–1016, 1999

Montejo AL, Llorca G, Izquierdo JA, et al: Incidence of sexual dysfunction associated with antidepressant agents: a prospective multicenter study of 1022 outpatients. Spanish Working Group for the Study of Psychotropic-Related Sexual Dysfunction. J Clin Psychiatry 62 (suppl 3):10–21, 2001

Moretti R, Torre P, Antonello RM, et al: Olanzapine as a possible treatment of behavioral symptoms in vascular dementia: risks of cerebrovascular events: a controlled, open-label study. J Neurol 252:1186–1193, 2005

Morita T, Tei Y, Shishido H, et al: Olanzapine-induced delirium in a terminally ill cancer patient. J Pain Symptom Manage 28:102–103, 2004

Morrell MJ, Isojärvi J, Taylor AE, et al: Higher androgens and weight gain with valproate compared with lamotrigine for epilepsy. Epilepsy Res 54:189–199, 2003

Mottram P, Wilson K, Strobl J: Antidepressants for depressed elderly. Cochrane Database Syst Rev (1):CD003491, 2006

Mulsant BH, Pollock BG, Nebes RD, et al: A double-blind randomized comparison of nortriptyline and paroxetine in the treatment of late-life depression: 6-week outcome. J Clin Psychiatry 60 (suppl 20):16–20, 1999

Mulsant BH, Alexopoulos GS, Reynolds CF 3rd, et al: Pharmacological treatment of depression in older primary care patients: the PROSPECT algorithm. Int J Geriatr Psychiatry 16:585–592, 2001a

Mulsant BH, Pollock BG, Nebes R, et al: A twelve-week, double-blind, randomized comparison of nortriptyline and paroxetine in older depressed inpatients and outpatients. Am J Geriatr Psychiatry 9:406–414, 2001b

Mulsant BH, Pollock BG, Kirshner M, et al: Serum anticholinergic activity in a community-based sample of older adults: relationship with cognitive performance. Arch Gen Psychiatry 60:198–203, 2003

Mulsant BH, Gharabawi GM, Bossie CA, et al: Correlates of anticholinergic activity in patients with dementia and psychosis treated with risperidone or olanzapine. J Clin Psychiatry 65:1708–1714, 2004

Murray V, von Arbin M, Bartfai A, et al: Double-blind comparison of sertraline and placebo in stroke patients with minor depression and less severe major depression. J Clin Psychiatry 66:708–716, 2005

Nagaraja D, Jayashree S: Randomized study of the dopamine receptor agonist piribedil in the treatment of mild cognitive impairment. Am J Psychiatry 158:1517–1519, 2001

National Collaborating Centre for Mental Health: Management of Depression in Primary and Secondary Care (Clinical Guideline 23). London, England, National Institute for Clinical Excellence, 2004

Navarro V, Gasto C, Torres X, et al: Citalopram versus nortriptyline in late-life depression: a 12-week randomized single-blind study. Acta Psychiatr Scand 103:435–440, 2001

Nebes RD, Pollock BG, Mulsant BH, et al: Low-level serum anticholinergicity as a source of baseline cognitive heterogeneity in geriatric depressed patients. Psychopharmacol Bull 33:715–719, 1997

Nebes RD, Pollock BG, Meltzer CC, et al: Cognitive effects of serum anticholinergic activity and white matter hyperintensities. Neurology 65:1487–1489, 2005

Nelson JC, Wohlreich MM, Mallinckrodt CH, et al: Duloxetine for the treatment of major depressive disorder in older patients. Am J Geriatr Psychiatry 13:227–235, 2005

Nelson JC, Delucchi K, Schneider L: Suicidal thinking and behavior during treatment with sertraline in late-life depression. Am J Geriatr Psychiatry 15:573–580, 2007

Nemeroff CB: Comorbidity of mood and anxiety disorders: the rule, not the exception? Am J Psychiatry 159:3–4, 2002

Newhouse PA, Krishnan KR, Doraiswamy PM, et al: A double-blind comparison of sertraline and fluoxetine in depressed elderly outpatients. J Clin Psychiatry 61:559–568, 2000

Nicholas LM, Ford AL, Esposito SM, et al: The effects of mirtazapine on plasma lipid profiles in healthy subjects. J Clin Psychiatry 64:883–889, 2003

Nieuwstraten CE, Dolovich LR: Bupropion versus selective serotonin-reuptake inhibitors for treatment of depression. Ann Pharmacother 35:1608–1613, 2001

Nikaido AM, Ellinwood EH Jr, Heatherly DG, et al: Age-related increase in CNS sensitivity to benzodiazepines as assessed by task difficulty. Psychopharmacology 100:90–97, 1990

Noaghiul S, Narayan M, Nelson JC: Divalproex treatment of mania in elderly patients. Am J Geriatr Psychiatry 6:257–262, 1998

Nyth AL, Gottfries CG: The clinical efficacy of citalopram in treatment of emotional disturbances in dementia disorders: a Nordic multicentre study. Br J Psychiatry 157:894–901, 1990

Nyth AL, Gottfries CG, Lyby K, et al: A controlled multicenter clinical study of citalopram and placebo in elderly depressed patients with and without concomitant dementia. Acta Psychiatr Scand 86:138–145, 1992

Olafsson K, Jorgensen S, Jensen HV, et al: Fluvoxamine in the treatment of demented elderly patients: a double-blind, placebo-controlled study. Acta Psychiatr Scand 85:453–456, 1992

Onofrj M, Thomas A, Bonanni L, et al: Leucopenia induced by low dose clozapine in Parkinson's disease recedes shortly after drug withdrawal: clinical case descriptions with commentary on switch-over to olanzapine. Neurol Sci 21:209–215, 2000

Oslin DW, Streim JE, Katz IR, et al: Heuristic comparison of sertraline with nortriptyline for the treatment of depression in frail elderly patients. Am J Geriatr Psychiatry 8:141–149, 2000

Oslin DW, Ten Have TR, Streim JE, et al: Probing the safety of medications in the frail elderly: evidence from a randomized clinical trial of sertraline and venlafaxine in depressed nursing home residents. J Clin Psychiatry 64:875–882, 2003

Ostow M: Pramipexole for depression. Am J Psychiatry 159:320–321, 2002

Pact V, Giduz T: Mirtazapine treats resting tremor, essential tremor, and levodopa-induced dyskinesias. Neurology 53:1154, 1999

Pae CU, Lee SJ, Lee CU, et al: A pilot trial of quetiapine for the treatment of patients with delirium. Hum Psychopharmacol 19:125–127, 2004

Pande AC, Crockatt JG, Janney C, et al: Gabapentin in bipolar disorder: a placebo-controlled trial of adjunctive therapy. Bipolar Disord 2 (3 pt 2):249–255, 2000

Parellada E, Baeza I, de Pablo J, et al: Risperidone in the treatment of patients with delirium. J Clin Psychiatry 65:348–353, 2004

Parkinson Study Group: Low-dose clozapine for the treatment of drug-induced psychosis in Parkinson's disease. N Engl J Med 340:757–763, 1999

Pedersen L, Klysner R: Antagonism of selective serotonin reuptake inhibitor-induced nausea by mirtazapine. Int Clin Psychopharmacol 12:59–60, 1997

Percudani M, Barbui C, Fortino I, et al: Second-generation antipsychotics and risk of cerebrovascular accidents in the elderly. J Clin Psychopharmacol 25:468–470, 2005

Perry NK: Venlafaxine-induced serotonin syndrome with relapse following amitriptyline. Postgrad Med J 76:254–256, 2000

Petracca GM, Chemerinski E, Starkstein SE: A double-blind, placebo-controlled study of fluoxetine in depressed patients with Alzheimer's disease. Int Psychogeriatr 13:233–240, 2001

Phanjoo AL, Wonnacott S, Hodgson A: Double-blind comparative multicentre study of fluvoxamine and mianserin in the treatment of major depressive episode in elderly people. Acta Psychiatr Scand 83:476–479, 1991

Pinquart M, Duberstein PR, Lyness JM: Treatments for later-life depressive conditions: a meta-analytic comparison of pharmacotherapy and psychotherapy. Am J Psychiatry 163:1493–1501, 2006

Poewe W: Treatment of dementia with Lewy bodies and Parkinson's disease dementia. Mov Disord 20 (suppl 12):S77–S82, 2005

Pollock BG: Psychotropic drugs and the aging patient. Geriatrics 53 (suppl 1):S20–S24, 1998

Pollock BG: Adverse reactions of antidepressants in elderly patients. J Clin Psychiatry 60 (suppl 20):4–8, 1999

Pollock BG: The pharmacokinetic imperative in late-life depression. J Clin Psychopharmacol 25 (suppl 1):S19–S23, 2005

Pollock BG, Mulsant BH: Antipsychotics in older patients: a safety perspective. Drugs Aging 6:312–323, 1995

Pollock BG, Mulsant BH, Sweet R, et al: An open pilot study of citalopram for behavioral disturbances of dementia. Am J Geriatr Psychiatry 5:70–78, 1997

Pollock BG, Laghrissi-Thode F, Wagner WR: Evaluation of platelet activation in depressed patients with ischemic heart disease after paroxetine or nortriptyline treatment. J Clin Psychopharmacol 20:137–140, 2000

Pollock BG, Mulsant BH, Rosen J, et al: Comparison of citalopram, perphenazine, and placebo for the acute treatment of psychosis and behavioral disturbances in hospitalized, demented patients. Am J Psychiatry 159:460–465, 2002

Pollock BG, Mulsant BH, Rosen J, et al: A double-blind comparison of citalopram and risperidone for the treatment of behavioral and psychotic symptoms associated with dementia. Am J Geriatr Psychiatry 15:942–952, 2007

Pomara N, Deptula D, Medel M, et al: Effects of diazepam on recall memory: relationship to aging, dose, and duration of treatment. Psychopharmacol Bull 25:144–148, 1989

Post RM, Frye MA, Denicoff KD, et al: Beyond lithium in the treatment of bipolar illness. Neuropsychopharmacology 19:206–219, 1998

Preskorn SH, Magnus RD: Inhibition of hepatic P-450 isoenzymes by serotonin selective reuptake inhibitors: in vitro and in vivo findings and their implications for patient care. Psychopharmocol Bull 30:251–259, 1994

Preskorn SH, Alderman J, Greenblatt DJ, et al: Sertraline does not inhibit cytochrome P450 3A-mediated drug metabolism in vivo. Psychopharmocol Bull 33:659–665, 1997

Rabey JM, Prokhorov T, Miniovitz A, et al: Effect of quetiapine in psychotic Parkinson's disease patients: a double-blind labeled study of 3 months' duration. Mov Disord 22:313–318, 2007

Rabins PV, Lyketsos CG: Antipsychotic drugs in dementia: what should be made of the risks? JAMA 294:1963–1965, 2005

Rahman MK, Akhtar MJ, Savla NC, et al: A double-blind, randomised comparison of fluvoxamine with dothiepin in the treatment of depression in elderly patients. Br J Clin Pract 45:255–258, 1991

Rainer MK, Masching AJ, Ertl MG, et al: Effect of risperidone on behavioral and psychological symptoms and cognitive function in dementia. J Clin Psychiatry 62:894–900, 2001

Raji MA, Brady SR: Mirtazapine for treatment of depression and comorbidities in Alzheimer disease. Ann Pharmacother 35:1024–1027, 2001

Rampello L, Chiechio S, Nicoletti G, et al: Prediction of the response to citalopram and reboxetine in post-stroke depressed patients. Psychopharmacology (Berl) 173:73–78, 2004

Rapaport MH, Schneider LS, Dunner DL, et al: Efficacy of controlled-release paroxetine in the treatment of late-life depression. J Clin Psychiatry 64:1065–1074, 2003

Rapoport M, Mamdani M, Shulman KI, et al: Antipsychotic use in the elderly: shifting trends and increasing costs. Int J Geriatr Psychiatry 20:749–753, 2005

Raskin J, Wiltse CG, Siegal A, et al: Efficacy of duloxetine on cognition, depression, and pain in elderly patients with major depressive disorder: an 8-week, double-blind, placebo-controlled trial. Am J Psychiatry 164:900–909, 2007

Rasmussen A, Lunde M, Poulsen DL, et al: A double-blind, placebo-controlled study of sertraline in the prevention of depression in stroke patients. Psychosomatics 44:216–221, 2003

Rasmussen BB, Nielsen TL, Brosen K: Fluvoxamine is a potent inhibitor of the metabolism of caffeine in vitro. Pharmacol Toxicol 83:240–245, 1998

Ravona-Springer R, Dolberg OT, Hirschmann S, et al: Delirium in elderly patients treated with risperidone: a report of three cases. J Clin Psychopharmacol 18:171–172, 1998

Ray WA, Meredith S, Thapa PB, et al: Antipsychotics and the risk of sudden cardiac death. Arch Gen Psychiatry 58:1161–1167, 2001

Reifler BV, Teri L, Raskind M: Double-blind trial of imipramine in Alzheimer's disease in patients with and without depression. Am J Psychiatry 146:45–49, 1989

Reisberg B, Doody R, Stöffler A, et al: Memantine in moderate-to-severe Alzheimer's disease. N Engl J Med 348:1333–1341, 2003

Reynolds CF, Dew MA, Pollock BG, et al: Maintenance treatment of major depression in old age. N Engl J Med 354:1130–1138, 2006

Reznik I, Rosen Y, Rosen B: An acute ischaemic event associated with the use of venlafaxine: a case report and proposed pathophysiological mechanisms. J Psychopharmacol 13:193–195, 1999

Rich SS, Friedman JH, Ott BR: Risperidone versus clozapine in the treatment of psychosis in six patients with Parkinson's disease and other akinetic-rigid syndromes. J Clin Psychiatry 56:556–559, 1995

Richards JB, Papaioannou A, Adachi JD for the Canadian Multicentre Osteoporosis Study Research Group: Effect of selective serotonin reuptake inhibitors on the risk of fracture. Arch Intern Med 167:188–194, 2007

Rickels K, Schweizer E, Case WG, et al: Nefazodone in major depression: adjunctive benzodiazepine therapy and tolerability. J Clin Psychopharmacol 18:145–153, 1998

Ridout F, Meadows R, Johnsen S, et al: A placebo controlled investigation into the effects of paroxetine and mirtazapine on measures related to car driving performance. Hum Psychopharmacol 18:261–269, 2003

Ritchie CW, Chiu E, Harrigan S, et al: The impact upon extrapyramidal side effects, clinical symptoms and quality of life of a switch from conventional to atypical antipsychotics (risperidone or olanzapine) in elderly patients with schizophrenia. Int J Geriatr Psychiatry 18:432–440, 2003

Ritchie CW, Chiu E, Harrigan S, et al: A comparison of the efficacy and safety of olanzapine and risperidone in the treatment of elderly patients with schizophrenia: an open study of six months duration. Int J Geriatr Psychiatry 21:171–179, 2006

Robinson R, Schultz S, Castillo C, et al: Nortriptyline versus fluoxetine in the treatment of depression and in short-term recovery after stroke: a placebo-controlled, double-blind study. Am J Psychiatry 157:351–359, 2000

Rocca P, Calvarese P, Faggiano F, et al: Citalopram versus sertraline in late-life nonmajor clinically significant depression: a 1-year follow-up clinical trial. J Clin Psychiatry 66:360–369, 2005

Rochon PA, Stukel TA, Sykora K, et al: Atypical antipsychotics and parkinsonism. Arch Intern Med 165:1882–1888, 2005

Roose SP, Dalack GW, Glassman AH, et al: Cardiovascular effects of bupropion in depressed patients with heart disease. Am J Psychiatry 148:512–516, 1991

Roose SP, Nelson JC, Salzman C, et al: Open-label study of mirtazapine orally disintegrating tablets in depressed patients in the nursing home. Mirtazapine in the Nursing Home Study Group. Curr Med Res Opin 19:737–746, 2003

Roose SP, Miyazaki M, Devanand D, et al: An open trial of venlafaxine for the treatment of late-life atypical depression. Int J Geriatr Psychiatry 19:989–994, 2004a

Roose SP, Sackeim HA, Krishnan KR, et al: Antidepressant pharmacotherapy in the treatment of depression in the very old: a randomized, placebo-controlled trial. Am J Psychiatry 161:2050–2059, 2004b

Rosen J, Sweet R, Pollock BG, et al: Nortriptyline in the hospitalized elderly: tolerance and side effect reduction. Psychopharmacol Bull 29:327–331, 1993

Rosenberg C, Lauritzen L, Brix J, et al: Citalopram versus amitriptyline in elderly depressed patients with or without mild cognitive dysfunction: a Danish multicentre trial in general practice. Psychopharmacol Bull 40:63–73, 2007

Rossini D, Serretti A, Franchini L, et al: Sertraline versus fluvoxamine in the treatment of elderly patients with major depression: a double-blind, randomized trial. J Clin Psychopharmacol 25:471–475, 2005

Rush AJ, Trivedi MH, Wisniewski SR, et al: Acute and longer-term outcomes in depressed outpatients requiring one or several treatment steps: a STAR*D report. Am J Psychiatry 163:1905–1917, 2006

Sa DS, Lang AE: Olanzapine and clozapine: comparative effects on motor function in hallucinating PD patients. Neurology 57:747, 2001

Saiz-Ruiz J, Ibanez A, Diaz-Marsa M, et al: Nefazodone in the treatment of elderly patients with depressive disorders: a prospective, observational study. CNS Drugs 16:635–643, 2002

Sajatovic M, Ramirez LF, Vernon L, et al: Outcome of risperidone therapy in elderly patients with chronic psychosis. Int J Psychiatry Med 26:309–317, 1996

Sajatovic M, Jaskiw G, Konicki PE, et al: Outcome of clozapine therapy for elderly patients with refractory primary psychosis. Int J Geriatr Psychiatry 12:553–558, 1997

Sajatovic M, Gyulai L, Calabrese JR, et al: Maintenance treatment outcomes in older patients with bipolar I disorder. Am J Geriatr Psychiatry 13:305–311, 2005a

Sajatovic M, Madhusoodanan S, Coconcea N: Managing bipolar disorder in the elderly: defining the role of the newer agents. Drugs Aging 22:39–54, 2005b

Sajatovic M, Blow FC, Ignacio RV: Psychiatric comorbidity in older adults with bipolar disorder. Int J Geriatr Psychiatry 21:582–587, 2006

Sajatovic M, Coconcea N, Ignacio RV, et al: Aripiprazole therapy in 20 older adults with bipolar disorder: a 12-week, open-label trial. J Clin Psychiatry 69:41–46, 2008

Samuels S, Fang M: Olanzapine may cause delirium in geriatric patients. J Clin Psychiatry 65:582–583, 2004

Sasaki Y, Matsuyama T, Inoue S, et al: A prospective, open-label, flexible-dose study of quetiapine in the treatment of delirium. J Clin Psychiatry 64:1316–1321, 2003

Satel SL, Nelson JC: Stimulants in the treatment of depression: a critical overview. J Clin Psychiatry 50:241–249, 1989

Sato Y, Kondo I, Ishida S, et al: Decreased bone mass and increased bone turnover with valproate therapy in adults with epilepsy. Neurology 57:445–449, 2001

Schatzberg A, Roose S: A double-blind, placebo-controlled study of venlafaxine and fluoxetine in geriatric outpatients with major depression. Am J Geriatr Psychiatry 14:361–370, 2006

Schatzberg AF, Kremer C, Rodrigues HE, et al: Double-blind, randomized comparison of mirtazapine and paroxetine in elderly depressed patients. Am J Geriatr Psychiatry 10:541–550, 2002

Schneider LS, Olin JT: Efficacy of acute treatment for geriatric depression. Int Psychogeriatr 7(suppl):7–25, 1995

Schneider LS, Nelson JC, Clary CM, et al: An 8-week multicenter, parallel-group, double-blind, placebo-controlled study of sertraline in elderly outpatients with major depression. Am J Psychiatry 160:1277–1285, 2003

Schneider LS, Dagerman KS, Insel P: Risk of death with atypical antipsychotic drug treatment for dementia: meta-analysis of randomized placebo-controlled trials. JAMA 294:1934–1943, 2005

Schneider LS, Dagerman K, Insel PS: Efficacy and adverse effects of atypical antipsychotics for dementia: meta-analysis of randomized placebo-controlled trials. Am J Geriatr Psychiatry 14:191–210, 2006a

Schneider LS, Tariot PN, Dagerman KS, et al: Effectiveness of atypical antipsychotic drugs in patients with Alzheimer's disease. N Engl J Med 355:1525–1538, 2006b

Schone W, Ludwig M: A double-blind study of paroxetine compared with fluoxetine in geriatric patients with major depression. J Clin Psychopharmacol 13 (6 suppl 2):34S–39S, 1993

Schreiber S, Backer MM, Pick CG: The anti-nociceptive effect of venlafaxine in mice is mediated through opioid and adrenergic mechanisms. Neurosci Lett 273:85–88, 1999

Schwaninger M, Ringleb P, Winter R, et al: Elevated plasma concentrations of homocysteine in antiepileptic drug treatment. Epilepsia 40:345–350, 1999

Semenchuk MR, Sherman S, Davis B: Double-blind, randomized trial of bupropion SR for the treatment of neuropathic pain. Neurology 57:1583–1588, 2001

Serebruany VL, Glassman AH, Malinin AI, et al: Platelet/endothelial biomarkers in depressed patients treated with the selective serotonin reuptake inhibitor sertraline after acute coronary events: the Sertraline AntiDepressant Heart Attack Randomized Trial (SADHART) Platelet Substudy. Circulation 108:939–944, 2003

Sernyak MJ, Leslie DL, Alarcon RD, et al: Association of diabetes mellitus with use of atypical neuroleptics in the treatment of schizophrenia. Am J Psychiatry 159:561–566, 2002

Sheikh JI, Cassidy EL, Doraiswamy PM, et al: Efficacy, safety, and tolerability of sertraline in patients with late-life depression and comorbid medical illness. J Am Geriatr Soc 52:86–92, 2004a

Sheikh JI, Lauderdale SA, Cassidy EL: Efficacy of sertraline for panic disorder in older adults: a preliminary open-label trial. Am J Geriatr Psychiatry 12:230, 2004b

Shelton C, Entsuah R, Padmanabhan SK, et al: Venlafaxine XR demonstrates higher rates of sustained remission compared to fluoxetine, paroxetine or placebo. Int Clin Psychopharmacol 20:233–238, 2005

Shelton RC, Tollefson GD, Tohen M, et al: A novel augmentation strategy for treating resistant major depression. Am J Psychiatry 158:131–134, 2001

Shulman KI: Disinhibition syndromes, secondary mania and bipolar disorder in old age. J Affect Disord 46:175–182, 1997

Sink KM, Holden KF, Yaffe K: Pharmacological treatment of neuropsychiatric symptoms of dementia: a review of the evidence. JAMA 293:596–608, 2005

Skinner MH, Kuan HY, Skerjanec A, et al: Effect of age on the pharmacokinetics of duloxetine in women. Br J Clin Pharmacol 57:54–61, 2004

Skrobik YK, Bergeron N, Dumont M, et al: Olanzapine vs. haloperidol: treating delirium in a critical care setting. Intensive Care Med 30:444–449, 2004

Smeraldi E, Rizzo F, Crespi G: Double-blind, randomized study of venlafaxine, clomipramine and trazodone in geriatric patients with major depression. Primary Care Psychiatry 4:189–195, 1998

Smith D, Dempster C, Glanville J, et al: Efficacy and tolerability of venlafaxine compared with selective serotonin reuptake inhibitors and other antidepressants: a meta-analysis. Br J Psychiatry 180:396–404, 2002

Solai LK, Mulsant BH, Pollock BG, et al: Effect of sertraline on plasma nortriptyline levels in depressed elderly. J Clin Psychiatry 58:440–443, 1997

Solai LK, Mulsant BH, Pollock BG: Selective serotonin reuptake inhibitors for late-life depression: a comparative review. Drugs Aging 18:355–368, 2001

Solai LK, Pollock BG, Mulsant BH, et al: Effect of nortriptyline and paroxetine on CYP2D6 activity in depressed elderly patients. J Clin Psychopharmacol 22:481–486, 2002

Sorock GS, Shimkin EE: Benzodiazepine sedatives and the risk of falling in a community-dwelling elderly cohort. Arch Intern Med 148:2441–2444, 1988

Spier SA: Use of bupropion with SRIs and venlafaxine. Depress Anxiety 7:73–75, 1998

Spina E, Scordo MG: Clinically significant drug interactions with antidepressants in the elderly. Drugs Aging 19:299–320, 2002

Spina E, Pisani F, Perucca E: Clinically significant pharmacokinetic drug interactions with carbamazepine: an update. Clin Pharmacokinet 31:198–214, 1996

Sproule BA, Hardy BG, Shulman KI: Differential pharmacokinetics of lithium in elderly patients. Drugs Aging 16:165–177, 2000

Stahl SM, Entsuah R, Rudolph RL: Comparative efficacy between venlafaxine and SSRIs: a pooled analysis of patients with depression. Biol Psychiatry 52:1166–1174, 2002

Steffens DC, Doraiswamy PM, McQuoid DR: Bupropion SR in the naturalistic treatment of elderly patients with major depression. Int J Geriatr Psychiatry 16:862–865, 2001

Steinberg JR: Anxiety in elderly patients: a comparison of azapirones and benzodiazepines. Drugs Aging 5:335–345, 1994

Steinmetz K, Coley K, Pollock BG: Assessment of the quantity and quality of geriatric information in the drug label for commonly prescribed drugs in the elderly. J Am Geriatr Soc 53:891–894, 2005

Stimmel GL, Dopheide JA, Stahl SM: Mirtazapine: an antidepressant with noradrenergic and specific serotonergic effects. Pharmacotherapy 17:10–21, 1997

Strand M, Hetta J, Rosen A, et al: A double-blind controlled trial in primary care patients with generalized anxiety: a comparison between buspirone and oxazepam. J Clin Psychiatry 51(suppl):40–45, 1990

Street JS, Clark WS, Gannon KS, et al: Olanzapine treatment of psychotic and behavioral symptoms in patients with Alzheimer disease in nursing care facilities: a double-blind, randomized, placebo-controlled trial. The HGEU Study Group. Arch Gen Psychiatry 57:968–976, 2000

Streim JE, Porsteinsson AP, Breder CD, et al: A randomized, double-blind, placebo-controlled study of aripiprazole for the treatment of psychosis in nursing home patients with Alzheimer disease. Am J Geriatr Psychiatry 16:537–550, 2008

Suh GH, Son HG, Ju YS, et al: A randomized, double-blind, crossover comparison of risperidone and haloperidol in Korean dementia patients with behavioral disturbances. Am J Geriatr Psychiatry 12:509–516, 2004

Suppes T, Eudicone J, McQuade R, et al: Efficacy and safety of aripiprazole in subpopulations with acute manic or mixed episodes of bipolar I disorder. J Affect Disord 107:145–154, 2008

Szuba MP, Leuchter AF: Falling backward in two elderly patients taking bupropion. J Clin Psychiatry 53:157–159, 1992

Taragano FE, Lyketsos CG, Mangone CA, et al: A double-blind, randomized, fixed-dose trial of fluoxetine vs. amitriptyline in the treatment of major depression complicating Alzheimer's disease. Psychosomatics 38:246–252, 1997

Targum SD, Abbott JL: Efficacy of quetiapine in Parkinson's patients with psychosis. J Clin Psychopharmacol 20:54–60, 2000

Tariot PN, Erb R, Podgorski CA, et al: Efficacy and tolerability of carbamazepine for agitation and aggression in dementia. Am J Psychiatry 155:54–61, 1998

Tariot PN, Salzman C, Yeung PP, et al: Long-term use of quetiapine in elderly patients with psychotic disorders. Clin Ther 22:1068–1084, 2000

Tariot PN, Farlow MR, Grossberg GT, et al: Memantine treatment in patients with moderate to severe Alzheimer disease already receiving donepezil: a randomized controlled trial. JAMA 291:317–324, 2004

Tariot PN, Raman R, Jakimovich L, et al: Divalproex sodium in nursing home residents with possible or probable Alzheimer disease complicated by agitation: a randomized, controlled trial. Am J Geriatr Psychiatry 13:942–949, 2005

Tashkin D, Kanner R, Bailey W, et al: Smoking cessation in patients with chronic obstructive pulmonary disease: a double-blind, placebo-controlled, randomised trial. Lancet 357:1571–1575, 2001

Tavcar R, Dernovsek MZ: Risperidone-induced delirium. Can J Psychiatry 43:194, 1998

Thase ME: Effects of venlafaxine on blood pressure: a meta-analysis of original data from 3744 depressed patients. J Clin Psychiatry 59:502–508, 1998

Thase ME: What role do atypical antipsychotic drugs have in treatment-resistant depression? J Clin Psychiatry 63:95–103, 2002

Thase ME, Entsuah AR, Rudolph RL: Remission rates during treatment with venlafaxine or selective serotonin reuptake inhibitors. Br J Psychiatry 178:234–241, 2001

Thase ME, Entsuah R, Cantillon M, et al: Relative antidepressant efficacy of venlafaxine and SSRIs: sex-age interactions. J Womens Health 14:609–616, 2005a

Thase ME, Haight BR, Richard N, et al: Remission rates following antidepressant therapy with bupropion or selective serotonin reuptake inhibitors: a meta-analysis of original data from 7 randomized controlled trials. J Clin Psychiatry 66:974–981, 2005b

Thase ME, Tran PV, Wiltse C, et al: Cardiovascular profile of duloxetine, a dual re-uptake inhibitor of serotonin and norepinephrine. J Clin Psychopharmacol 25:132–140, 2005c

Thompson DS: Mirtazapine for the treatment of depression and nausea in breast and gynecological oncology. Psychosomatics 41:356–359, 2000

Tollefson GD, Bosomworth JC, Heiligenstein JH, et al: A double-blind, placebo-controlled clinical trial of fluoxetine in geriatric patients with major depression. The Fluoxetine Collaborative Study Group. Int Psychogeriatr 7:89–104, 1995

Trappler B, Cohen CI: Use of SSRIs in "very old" depressed nursing home residents. Am J Geriatr Psychiatry 6:83–89, 1998

Trick L, Stanley N, Rigney U, et al: A double-blind, randomized, 26-week study comparing the cognitive and psychomotor effects and efficacy of 75 mg (37.5 mg b.i.d.) venlafaxine and 75 mg (25 mg mane, 50 mg nocte) dothiepin in elderly patients with moderate major depression being treated in general practice. J Psychopharmacol 18:205–214, 2004

Umapathy C, Mulsant BH, Pollock BG: Bipolar disorder in the elderly. Psychiatr Ann 30:473–480, 2000

van Iersel MB, Zuidema SU, Koopmans RT, et al: Antipsychotics for behavioral and psychological problems in elderly people with dementia: a systematic review of adverse events. Drugs Aging 22:845–858, 2005

van Laar MW, van Willigenburg AP, Volkerts ER: Acute and subchronic effects of nefazodone and imipramine on highway driving, cognitive functions, and daytime sleepiness in healthy adult and elderly subjects. J Clin Psychopharmacol 15:30–40, 1995

Verhey FR, Verkaaik M, Lousberg R: Olanzapine versus haloperidol in the treatment of agitation in elderly patients with dementia: results of a randomized controlled double-blind trial. Dement Geriatr Cogn Disord 21:1–8, 2006

Vis PM, van Baardewijk M, Einarson TR: Duloxetine and venlafaxine-XR in the treatment of major depressive disorder: a meta-analysis of randomized clinical trials. Ann Pharmacother 39:1798–1807, 2005

von Moltke LL, Greenblatt DJ, Court MH, et al: Inhibition of alprazolam and desipramine hydroxylation in vitro by paroxetine and fluvoxamine: comparison with other selective serotonin reuptake inhibitor antidepressants. J Clin Psychopharmacol 15:125–131, 1995

von Moltke LL, Greenblatt DJ, Giancarlo GM, et al: Escitalopram (S-citalopram) and its metabolites in vitro: cytochromes mediating biotransformation, inhibitory effects, and comparison to R-citalopram. Drug Metab Dispos 29:1102–1109, 2001

Wakelin JS: Fluvoxamine in the treatment of the older depressed patient: double-blind, placebo-controlled data. Int Clin Psychopharmacol 1:221–230, 1986

Walker Z, Grace J, Overshot R, et al: Olanzapine in dementia with Lewy bodies: a clinical study. Int J Geriatr Psychiatry 14:459–466, 1999

Wallace AE, Kofoed LL, West AN: Double-blind placebo-controlled trial of methylphenidate in older, depressed, medically ill patients. Am J Psychiatry 152:929–931, 1995

Wang PS, Bohn RL, Glynn RJ, et al: Zolpidem use and hip fractures in older people. J Am Geriatr Soc 49:1685–1690, 2001

Wang PS, Schneeweiss S, Avorn J, et al: Risk of death in elderly users of conventional vs. atypical antipsychotic medications. N Engl J Med 353:2335–2341, 2005

Wehmeier PM, Kluge M, Maras A, et al: Fluoxetine versus trimipramine in the treatment of depression in geriatric patients. Pharmacopsychiatry 38:13–16, 2005

Weigmann H, Gerek S, Zeisig A, et al: Fluvoxamine but not sertraline inhibits the metabolism of olanzapine: evidence from a therapeutic drug monitoring service. Ther Drug Monit 23:410–413, 2001

Weihs KL, Settle EC Jr, Batey SR, et al: Bupropion sustained release versus paroxetine for the treatment of depression in the elderly. J Clin Psychiatry 61:196–202, 2000

Whyte EM, Basinski J, Farhi P, et al: Geriatric depression treatment in nonresponders to selective serotonin reuptake inhibitors. J Clin Psychiatry 65:1634–1641, 2004

Whyte E, Romkes M, Mulsant BH, et al: CYP2D6 genotype and venlafaxine-XR concentrations in depressed elderly. Int J Geriatr Psychiatry 21:1–8, 2006

Wilner KD, Tensfeldt TG, Baris B, et al: Single- and multiple-dose pharmacokinetics of ziprasidone in healthy young and elderly volunteers. Br J Clin Pharmacol 49 (suppl 1):15S–20S, 2000

Wingen M, Bothmer J, Langer S, et al: Actual driving performance and psychomotor function in healthy subjects after acute and subchronic treatment with escitalopram, mirtazapine, and placebo: a crossover trial. J Clin Psychiatry 66:436–443, 2005

Wilson K, Mottram P: A comparison of side effects of selective serotonin reuptake inhibitors and tricyclic antidepressants in older depressed patients: a meta-analysis. Int J Geriatr Psychiatry 19:754–762, 2004

Wolters EC, Jansen EN, Tuynman-Qua HG, et al: Olanzapine in the treatment of dopaminomimetic psychosis in patients with Parkinson's disease. Neurology 47:1085–1087, 1996

Workman RH Jr, Orengo CA, Bakey AA, et al: The use of risperidone for psychosis and agitation in demented patients with Parkinson's disease. J Neuropsychiatry Clin Neurosci 9:594–597, 1997

Wylie ME, Mulsant BH, Pollock BG, et al: Age of onset in geriatric bipolar disorder: effects on clinical presentation and treatment outcomes in an inpatient sample. Am J Geriatr Psychiatry 7:77–83, 1999

Wylie ME, Miller MD, Shear MK, et al: Fluvoxamine pharmacotherapy of anxiety disorders in late life: preliminary open-trial data. J Geriatr Psychiatry Neurol 13:43–48, 2000

Yang CH, Tsai SJ, Hwang JP: The efficacy and safety of quetiapine for treatment of geriatric psychosis. J Psychopharmacol 19:661–666, 2005

Yokoi F, Gründer G, Biziere K, et al: Dopamine D2 and D3 receptor occupancy in normal humans treated with the antipsychotic drug aripiprazole (OPC 14597): a study using positron emission tomography and [11C]raclopride. Neuropsychopharmacology 27:248–259, 2002

Young RC, Gyulai L, Mulsant BH, et al: Pharmacotherapy of bipolar disorder in old age: review and recommendations. Am J Geriatr Psychiatry 12:342–357, 2004

Zarate CA Jr, Baldessarini RJ, Siegel AJ, et al: Risperidone in the elderly: a pharmacoepidemiologic study. J Clin Psychiatry 58:311–317, 1997

Zhong KX, Tariot PN, Mintzer J, et al: Quetiapine to treat agitation in dementia: a randomized, double-blind, placebo-controlled study. Curr Alzheimer Res 4:81–93, 2007

Zimmer B, Kant R, Zeiler D, et al: Antidepressant efficacy and cardiovascular safety of venlafaxine in young vs. old patients with comorbid medical disorders. Int J Psychiatry Med 27:353–364, 1997

Suggested Readings

- **Key readings are bulleted.**

• Alexopoulos GS, Katz IR, Reynolds CF 3rd, et al: Pharmacotherapy of depression in older patients: a summary of the expert consensus guidelines. J Psychiatr Pract 7:361–376, 2001

• Alexopoulos GS, Streim J, Carpenter D, et al: Using antipsychotic agents in older patients. J Clin Psychiatry 65 (suppl 2):5–104, 2004

Chew ML, Mulsant BH, Pollock BG, et al: Anticholinergic activity of 107 medications commonly used by older adults. J Am Geriatr Soc 56:1333–1341, 2008

Cummings JL, McRae T, Zhang R, et al: Effects of donepezil on neuropsychiatric symptoms in patients with dementia and severe behavioral disorders. Am J Geriatr Psychiatry 14:605–612, 2006

Jeste DV: Tardive dyskinesia rates with atypical antipsychotics in older adults. J Clin Psychiatry 65 (suppl 9):21–24, 2004

Jeste DV, Barak Y, Madhusoodanan S, et al: International multisite double-blind trial of the atypical antipsychotics risperidone and olanzapine in 175 elderly patients with chronic schizophrenia. Am J Geriatr Psychiatry 11:638–647, 2003

Lenze EJ, Mulsant BH, Shear MK, et al: Efficacy and tolerability of citalopram in the treatment of late-life anxiety disorders: results from an 8-week randomized, placebo-controlled trial. Am J Psychiatry 162:146–150, 2005

Oslin DW, Ten Have TR, Streim JE, et al: Probing the safety of medications in the frail elderly: evidence from a randomized clinical trial of sertraline and venlafaxine in depressed nursing home residents. J Clin Psychiatry 64:875–882, 2003

• Pinquart M, Duberstein PR, Lyness JM: Treatments for later-life depressive conditions: a meta-analytic comparison of pharmacotherapy and psychotherapy. Am J Psychiatry 163:1493–1501, 2006

Pollock BG, Mulsant BH, Rosen J, et al: A double-blind comparison of citalopram and risperidone for the treatment of behavioral and psychotic symptoms associated with dementia. Am J Geriatr Psychiatry 15:942–952, 2007

• Rabins PV, Lyketsos CG: Antipsychotic drugs in dementia: what should be made of the risks? JAMA 294:1963–1965, 2005

Reisberg B, Doody R, Stöffler A, et al: Memantine in moderate-to-severe Alzheimer's disease. N Engl J Med 348:1333–1341, 2003

Reynolds CF, Dew MA, Pollock BG, et al: Maintenance treatment of major depression in old age. N Engl J Med 354:1130–1138, 2006

Roose SP, Sackeim HA, Krishnan KR, et al: Antidepressant pharmacotherapy in the treatment of depression in the very old: a randomized, placebo-controlled trial. Am J Psychiatry 161: 2050–2059, 2004

Schatzberg A, Roose S: A double-blind, placebo-controlled study of venlafaxine and fluoxetine in geriatric outpatients with major depression. Am J Geriatr Psychiatry 14:361–370, 2006

Schneider LS, Nelson JC, Clary CM, et al: An 8-week multicenter, parallel-group, double-blind, placebo-controlled study of sertraline in elderly outpatients with major depression. Am J Psychiatry 160:1277–1285, 2003

Schneider LS, Dagerman KS, Insel P: Risk of death with atypical antipsychotic drug treatment for dementia: meta-analysis of randomized placebo-controlled trials. JAMA 294:1934–1943, 2005

• Schneider LS, Dagerman KS, Insel P: Efficacy and adverse effects of atypical antipsychotics for dementia: meta-analysis of randomized placebo-controlled trials. Am J Geriatr Psychiatry 14:191–210, 2006a

Schneider LS, Tariot PN, Dagerman KS, et al: Effectiveness of atypical antipsychotic drugs in patients with Alzheimer's disease. N Engl J Med 355:1525–1538, 2006b

Sheikh JI, Lauderdale SA, Cassidy EL: Efficacy of sertraline for panic disorder in older adults: a preliminary open-label trial. Am J Geriatr Psychiatry 12:230, 2004

• Sink KM, Holden KF, Yaffe K: Pharmacological treatment of neuropsychiatric symptoms of dementia: a review of the evidence. JAMA 293:596–608, 2005

Tariot PN, Farlow MR, Grossberg GT, et al: Memantine treatment in patients with moderate to severe Alzheimer disease already receiving donepezil: a randomized controlled trial. JAMA 291:317–324, 2004

Wang PS, Schneeweiss S, Avorn J, et al: Risk of death in elderly users of conventional vs. atypical antipsychotic medications. N Engl J Med 353:2335–2341, 2005

Whyte EM, Basinski J, Farhi P, et al: Geriatric depression treatment in nonresponders to selective serotonin reuptake inhibitors. J Clin Psychiatry 65:1634–1641, 2004

• Young RC, Gyulai L, Mulsant BH, et al: Pharmacotherapy of bipolar disorder in old age: review and recommendations. Am J Geriatr Psychiatry 12:342–357, 2004

CHAPTER 27

Electroconvulsive Therapy

Richard D. Weiner, M.D., Ph.D.
Andrew D. Krystal, M.D., M.S.

Electroconvulsive therapy (ECT) involves the electrical induction of a series of seizures as a treatment for mental disorders, most notably major depression. This chapter covers the history of ECT; the extent to which it is used; indications; risks; the evaluation of patients for ECT; ECT technique; the use of ECT to alleviate episodes of illness (index ECT); management of patients after completion of the ECT course, including the use of ECT to prevent relapse (maintenance ECT); and a brief discussion of what can be expected in the future of this treatment modality. Throughout the chapter, a particular focus is placed on the use of ECT in the elderly. With the mean age of individuals referred for ECT increasing, the importance of ECT in geriatric psychiatry continues to grow.

History

In 1935, the Hungarian neuropsychiatrist Ladislas von Meduna chemically induced seizures in a small series of patients with schizophrenia (Fink 1984). His rationale for doing so was based on the hypothesis (later shown to be incorrect) that individuals with epilepsy had a reduced incidence of schizophrenia. Having achieved some partial success in therapeutic outcome, von Meduna's new convulsive therapy was greeted with great acclaim as a means to manage what had been an otherwise untreatable illness. When the use of pharmacoconvulsive therapy spread to Italy shortly thereafter, another neuropsychiatrist, Ugo Cerletti, was impressed not only by the efficacy of this new treatment but also by its technical difficulty (Endler 1988; Shorter and Healey 2007). From his work as an experimental epileptologist, Cerletti was aware of an electrical model of seizure induction that had been tried in animals. After further experimentation, Cerletti and his assistant Lucio Bini were successful in using electrical seizure induction to treat one of their patients with schizophrenia. After more trials, electroconvulsive therapy rapidly replaced pharmacoconvulsive therapy throughout the world.

Although ECT was first used in the treatment of schizophrenia, clinicians soon realized that its highest therapeutic potency was in treating mood disorders. The peak in ECT utilization was from the early 1940s through the mid-1950s, at which point the first effective antipsychotic and antidepressant medications came into clinical use. Although these new psychopharmacological agents obviated the need for ECT in many individuals with applicable disorders, trials comparing the antidepressant efficacy of ECT and these medications indicate that ECT remains the most rapid and effective means to induce remission (Husain et al. 2004; UK ECT Review Group 2003; Weiner and Coffey 1988).

In the early days of ECT, there was considerable fear concerning the use of ECT in older adults, largely because of the medical comorbidity that is common in this age group. The cardiovascular physiology of ECT was not well understood at the time, and more recent procedural innovations—such as oxygenation, muscular relaxation, general anesthesia, and physiological monitoring—had not yet been instituted. Instead, ECT during that early period was accomplished in a distinctly nonmedical setting, often in psychiatrists' offices, without the presence of other medical staff or medical support resources.

As ECT methodology became more refined, practitioners became more willing to utilize it with previously underserved populations, including older adults, for whom ECT treatment has steadily grown in recent decades (Glen and Scott 1999; Thompson et al. 1994). Thompson et al. (1994) reported that in 1986 approximately one-third of people receiving ECT were age 65 years or older. Since that time, the relative use of ECT in the elderly appears to have risen further. Rosenbach et al. (1997) observed a nationwide rise in ECT use from 4.2/10,000 to 5.1/10,000 among Medicare recipients between 1987 and 1992. In Texas, 48% of those treated with ECT during a 19-month period from 1993 to 1995 were at least age 65 years (Reid et al. 1998). Similarly, using California data, Kramer (1999) reported an ECT treatment rate of 3.82/10,000 for individuals ages 65 and older versus rates of 1.21/10,000 for those ages 45–64 and 0.48/10,000 for those ages 25–44.

There has been considerable speculation about the reasons for the growing use of ECT among older adults. Some evidence shows that depressive episodes in this age group tend to be relatively more severe and also more resistant to medication, yet current data are not conclusive in this regard. In addition, older adults are more likely to be intolerant of medications. Although the lay press has sometimes asserted that increased use of ECT in older adults may reflect a desire on the part of ECT practitioners to obtain Medicare reimbursement funding, low reimbursement rates have made that argument less than credible. Instead, the available evidence indicates that ECT is used because it is safe, it works well, and it works rapidly (Kamat et al. 2003; van der Wurff et al. 2003).

Indications for ECT

Diagnostic Indications

The most common diagnostic indication for ECT is major depression (American Psychiatric Association 2001; Thompson et al. 1994). A significant body of literature not only supports the efficacy of ECT for major depression but suggests that it is the most rapid and effective treatment for this condition (Husain et al. 2004; Weiner and Krystal 2001). This literature includes a series of randomized, double-blind, placebo-controlled studies in which the placebo control was "sham ECT," whereby subjects received all aspects of a usual clinical ECT treatment except the electrical stimulus (Brandon 1986). Evidence from meta-analytical studies also suggests greater efficacy with ECT than with antidepressant medication (Janicak et al. 1985; UK ECT Review Group 2003); however, it should be noted that this type of analysis has not been carried out comparing ECT with newer antidepressant medications.

Regarding subtypes of depression, ECT appears to be effective in treating both melancholic and severe nonmelancholic depression (Sackeim and Rush 1995), as well as bipolar and unipolar major depression (Weiner and Krystal 2001). In addition, it may be particularly effective in treating psychotic major depression (Petrides et al. 2001; Sobin et al. 1996).

Although ECT is used more frequently for major depression than for other illnesses and the vast majority of ECT research studies have been carried out on this condition, evidence suggests that ECT has efficacy in a number of other mental disorders. A series of reports suggest that ECT has efficacy in the treatment of acute mania (Mukherjee et al. 1994; Small et al. 1988). In this regard, ECT has been reported to achieve a response rate as high as 80%, to have efficacy equal to that of lithium, and to have a significant advantage over lithium in patients who have not responded to lithium or antipsychotic medication. The relative efficacy of ECT compared with anticonvulsant, antimanic agents has not yet been studied, and no systematic studies exist to indicate the utility of ECT in individuals with rapid-cycling bipolar disorder (Weiner and Krystal 2001).

Another disorder for which ECT appears to have efficacy is schizophrenia. Although ECT was first employed as a treatment for this condition, the superior response to ECT of patients with mood disorders was soon evident (Weiner and Krystal 2001). Following the development of antipsychotic medications in the late 1950s, the use of ECT as a treatment for schizophrenia gradually declined. Regardless, a number of studies have suggested that antipsychotic medications and ECT have comparable efficacy (Fink and Sackeim 1996; Krueger and Sackeim 1995). In addition, evidence suggests that for treatment of acute psychotic episodes, the combination of antipsychotic medications and ECT may have greater efficacy than either ECT or medications alone (Klapheke 1993; Sajatovic and Meltzer 1993). However, no evidence indicates that ECT has efficacy for the treatment of deficit or "negative" symptoms of schizophrenia (Weiner and Krystal 2001).

The presence of affective symptoms appears to increase the likelihood of response to ECT in individuals with schizophrenia. In this regard, case reports and case series suggest that individuals with schizoaffective disorder may respond better to ECT than those with schizophrenia (Fink and Sackeim 1996; Krueger and Sackeim 1995). Catatonia, which can be associated with both schizophrenia and mood disorders, is highly responsive to ECT (Krystal and Coffey 1997), even when this condition is associated with medical conditions such as systemic lupus erythematosus, uremia, hepatic encephalopathy, porphyria, and hyperparathyroidism (Fricchione et al. 1990; Rummans and Bassingthwaighte 1991).

Some evidence suggests that ECT may also be a useful treatment for Parkinson's disease when medication management fails or is not tolerated (Andersen et al. 1987; Kellner and Bernstein 1993; Krystal and Coffey 1997; Pritchett et al. 1994; Rasmussen and Abrams 1991). However, it should also be noted that patients with Parkinson's disease may be at increased risk for developing cognitive side effects and delirium with ECT (Figiel et al. 1991).

Response to ECT in Older Adults

Several prospective studies suggest that ECT is a highly effective acute treatment for major depression in elderly individuals (Kamat et al. 2003; O'Connor et al. 2001; Tew et al. 1999; van der Wurff et al. 2003; Wesson et al. 1997). Furthermore, one study indicates that ECT has a significant impact on the course of major depression in older adults, in terms of both efficacy and morbidity and mortality rates (Philibert et al. 1995). Also, evidence based on data from 584 subjects suggests that, if anything, the response to ECT increases with advancing age (Sackeim 1998). These data provide support for a role for ECT in the practice of geriatric psychiatry.

Continuation or Maintenance ECT

Although ECT is a highly effective treatment for a number of neuropsychiatric conditions, it is not a cure in the sense that it does not ensure that future episodes will not occur (Weiner and Krystal 2001; Weiner et al. 2000). Also, evidence indicates that the relapse rate of major depressive disorder may be particularly high for older adults (Huuhka et al. 2004). As a result, it is important to institute some form of continuation or maintenance therapy (American Psychiatric Association 2001). This point is underscored by the findings from a study by Sackeim et al. (2001), in which roughly 80% of patients successfully treated with ECT for major depression relapsed within 6 months. Most commonly, continuation or maintenance pharmacotherapy is instituted after a successful course of ECT. Nevertheless, prophylactic pharmacotherapy is not universally effective, and roughly 50%–60% of depressed patients will relapse within a year of the end of the ECT course when treated with typical continuation or maintenance pharmacotherapy (Sackeim et al. 1990, 2001). The relapse rate appears to be even higher among those whose depression was resistant to medication before the ECT course (Sackeim et al. 1990). One study suggests that rather than single-agent therapy, more aggressive pharmacotherapy—specifically the combination of nortriptyline and lithium—is associated with a decrease in the relapse rate to roughly 40% 6 months after ECT (Sackeim et al. 2001).

An alternative to continuation or maintenance pharmacotherapy is continuation or maintenance ECT. Although a number of case series and retrospective reports have suggested the efficacy of continuation or maintenance ECT, not until recently has a randomized, controlled trial of maintenance ECT versus maintenance pharmacotherapy been carried out; Kellner et al. (2006) reported similar 6-month outcomes for patients treated with maintenance bilateral ECT and for patients treated with a combination of lithium and nortriptyline maintenance pharmacotherapy. At the present time, pharmacotherapy is usually instituted after a successful course of ECT unless at least one of the following conditions exists: 1) prophylactic pharmacotherapy has failed in the past, 2) the patient is intolerant of medications, 3) the patient has a medical illness that contraindicates medication management, or 4) the patient has a preference for prophylactic ECT (American Psychiatric Association 2001; Weiner and Krystal 2001).

When to Recommend an Index ECT Course

In general, the decision about whether to recommend ECT for a given patient should rest on a careful assessment of risks and benefits (American Psychiatric Association 2001). Even though ample evidence suggests that ECT is a highly effective treatment for a number of neuropsychiatric disorders, it is generally not used as a first-line treatment. However, first-line treatment with ECT should be considered when there is an urgent need for response in a patient with major depression or mania (American Psychiatric Association 2001; Quitkin et al. 1996). This situation typically occurs when the presenting condition threatens the patient's life because of suicidality, malnutrition, dehydration, or inability to comply with treatment of a critical medical problem. In addition, the first-line use of ECT should be considered when, because of circumstances such as medical illness, ECT is deemed to be safer than pharmacotherapy (American Psychiatric Association 2001; Weiner et al. 2000). ECT should also be considered on a primary basis when a patient has an informed preference for ECT or when there has been a preferential response to ECT in prior episodes (American Psychiatric Association 2001).

The secondary use of ECT is generally undertaken because of either medication intolerance or a lack of response to pharmacotherapy (American Psychiatric Association 2001). Unfortunately, there is no currently accepted definition for medication failure. Operationally, when making this decision, practitioners generally take into account the number of medications tried, the duration of treatment, the dosage administered, symptom severity, tolerance of pharmacotherapy, the expected risks associated with ECT, and patient preference (American Psychiatric Association 2001). In support of the use of ECT following medication failure are several studies indicating that a significant number of individuals respond to ECT after one or more failed trials of medication (Avery and Lubrano 1979; Paul et al. 1981; Prudic et al. 1996).

Risks of ECT and Its Use in Patients With Neurological and Medical Disorders

Because the decision about whether to pursue a course of ECT should involve an evaluation of both the expected risks and benefits of ECT, it is important to be able to carry out an assessment of the likelihood of potential adverse sequelae for each patient.

Mortality

Although it is difficult to establish an accurate mortality rate associated with any medical procedure, it has been estimated that the overall mortality rate for ECT is roughly 1 death per 80,000 treatments (American Psychiatric Association 2001). This relatively low mortality rate appears to be comparable to the rate associated with minor surgery and has been considered to be less than that associated with pharmacotherapy with tricyclic antidepressants (Sackeim 1998). Furthermore, some studies have suggested that depressed inpatients who receive ECT have a lower mortality rate after discharge than individuals who receive other types of treatment (Avery and Winokur 1976; Philibert et al. 1995). It is important to understand, however, that the likelihood of ECT-related death in high-risk populations—most commonly in older adults (see below)—can be substantially higher than that mentioned above. Still, even in such situations, the risk of undertaking ECT may be lower than the risk of not doing it.

Cognitive Side Effects

The most important side effect with ECT is cognitive dysfunction, which appears to be a key factor limiting the use of this treatment modality (American Psychiatric Association 2001). The most common cognitive side effects are anterograde amnesia (difficulty retaining new information) and retrograde amnesia (difficulty recalling information learned in the past). Both anterograde and retrograde memory side effects tend to most strongly affect information encountered during the period of time closest to the ECT treatment course. Anterograde amnesia typically resolves within a few weeks after the treatment course, whereas retrograde amnesia tends to resolve more slowly (American Psychiatric Association 2001; Weiner et al. 1986). Despite objective evidence that memory performance transiently decreases after ECT, some patients indicate that their memory function improves, likely a result of the lifting of depressive symptoms (American Psychiatric Association 2001; Weiner et al. 1986). This finding appears to be present in older adults as well as in younger individuals (Bosboom and Deijen 2006).

Both the degree and the duration of objective and subjective memory side effects of ECT vary substantially among individuals who receive ECT. A number of research studies have identified factors that can affect objective memory side effects of ECT (American Psychiatric Association 2001). Compared with unilateral placement of stimulus electrodes, bilateral placement has repeatedly been shown to increase the risk of amnesia, including in elderly populations (Stoppe et al. 2006). In addition, greater risk is associated with higher stimulus intensity (compared with the seizure threshold), larger numbers of ECT treatments, higher dosages of barbiturate anesthetic, and less time between treatments. Furthermore, some patients—including those taking lithium and medications with anticholinergic properties, as well as those having preexisting cerebral disease—appear to be at increased risk of cognitive side effects (American Psychiatric Association 2001). Individuals with diseases affecting the basal ganglia and subcortical white matter may be at particular risk (Figiel et al. 1990).

Other Risks With ECT

It is important to identify individuals at risk for medical complications with ECT and to be aware of the modifications in ECT technique that may minimize risks. Elderly patients referred for ECT frequently have preexisting medical illnesses (Christopher 2003; Weiner and Krystal 2001). Although some illnesses appear to increase the risks of ECT (Weiner and Coffey 1988; Zielinski et al. 1993), none should be considered "absolute" contraindications to its use, given, as noted earlier, that risk is relative rather than absolute (Weiner and Krystal 2001; Weiner et al. 2000). The decision about whether to pursue a course of ECT should always involve a careful weighing of the risks and benefits of carrying out ECT versus those of not using it. Conditions for which evidence suggests increased risks with ECT are discussed in the following subsections, as are modifications in ECT technique that may decrease these risks, as well as the specific issue of adverse effects of ECT in older adults.

Central Nervous System Disorders

The primary central nervous system (CNS) risks of ECT stem from the increase in intracranial and intravascular pressure that can occur with ECT seizures (Krystal and Coffey 1997). Despite these increases in pressure, the CNS complication rate is generally quite low. A number of CNS disorders leave individuals more vulnerable to increases in pressure than the general ECT population. These include the presence of any space-occupying CNS lesions such as tumors, subdural hematomas, intracranial arachnoid cysts, or normal pressure hydrocephalus (Krystal and Coffey 1997). Patients with these conditions have been considered to be at increased risk for noncardiogenic pulmonary edema, cerebral edema, brain hemorrhage, and cerebral herniation (Krystal and Coffey 1997). Although space-occupying cerebral lesions were once considered an absolute contraindication to ECT, a number of reports describe successful ECT in individuals with these lesions. Patients with small lesions but no edema or pretreatment elevation of intracranial pressure can usually be safely treated with ECT (Krystal and Coffey 1997). For the remainder of patients with space-occupying CNS lesions, the risks may be diminished (although not removed) by pretreating with an antihypertensive agent, osmotic diuretics, and steroids and by employing hyperventilation during treatment.

The increase in intravascular pressure that occurs with ECT theoretically might be expected to lead to an increased risk of intracranial hemorrhage; however, such events are extremely rare (Krystal and Coffey 1997). Nonetheless, individuals with recent strokes, arteriovenous malformations, and aneurysms are considered to be at increased risk (Krystal and Coffey 1997). In two case series involving a total of 34 patients who received ECT while recovering from strokes, no occurrences of hemorrhages or worsening of any stroke-associated deficits were reported (Currier et al. 1992; Murray et al. 1986). Nevertheless, the American Psychiatric Association (2001) recommends waiting as long as possible after a stroke before administering ECT. The use of antihypertensive agents should be considered to diminish the rise in intravascular pressure in patients with a history of hemorrhagic stroke; however, such prophylaxis may be counterproductive in individuals who have suffered cerebral ischemic events (American Psychiatric Association 2001).

Other adverse CNS conditions that can be associated with ECT include prolonged seizures (lasting longer than 3 minutes) and status epilepticus (a single seizure lasting at least 30 minutes, or more than one seizure in which consciousness is not regained during the interictal period) (American Psychiatric Association 2001). Prolonged seizures can lead to increased cognitive side effects, which can be minimized by rapidly administering antiepileptic drugs to terminate such events. It appears that the risk of both prolonged seizures and status epilepticus may be increased by some medications (including theophylline and lithium), as well as by medical conditions that lower the seizure threshold (such as hyponatremia), and also by the induction of multiple seizures in the same treatment session (American Psychiatric Association 2001).

As noted above, patients with preexisting cerebral disease may be particularly likely to experience problems with ECT-related amnesia. At times, even frank delirium may occur. These risks, which appear to be most prominent in individuals with dementia or with basal ganglia disease, can be minimized by decreasing the frequency of treatments and using unilateral electrode placement.

Cardiovascular Disorders

Fluctuations in pulse and blood pressure that occur during ECT treatments may be associated with cardiovascular complications (Weiner et al. 2000). Immediately after the stimulus, there is an increase in parasympathetic tone, which can lead to a sudden but transient decrease in heart rate, not uncommonly presenting as a brief period of asystole. The subsequent induced seizure, however, is associated with a sympathetic surge that markedly increases both blood pressure and heart rate. This sympathetic surge is then followed by a relative increase in parasympathetic tone as the induced seizure ends.

Despite these autonomic fluctuations, cardiovascular complications from ECT rarely occur in individuals without preexisting cardiovascular risk factors (Takada et al. 2005; Weiner et al. 2000). The risk is increased in those with recent myocardial infarction, uncompensated congestive heart failure, severe valvular disease, unstable aneurysm, unstable angina or active cardiac ischemia, uncontrolled hypertension, high-grade atrioventricular block, symptomatic ventricular arrhythmia, and supraventricular arrhythmia with uncontrolled ventricular rate (American Psychiatric Association 2001; Applegate 1997). For patients with these conditions, a consultation with a cardiologist is recommended to help with the risk-benefit analysis and to suggest treatment modifications that may decrease risks. It has been proposed that an assessment of functional cardiac status (such as a stress test) should be considered in 1) men younger than 60 and women under 70 with definite angina, 2) men older than 60 and women over 70 with probable angina, 3) all patients with angina and two risk factors for myocardial infarction, and 4) those with clinically significant extracardiac vascular disease (Applegate 1997). A finding of good functional status indicates that the risk is low; otherwise, further cardiac evaluation is indicated.

Individuals with coronary artery disease are at risk for ischemia during both the periods of relative parasympathetic tone and the periods of increased sympathetic system tone (Christopher 2003; Weiner et al. 2000). When parasympathetic tone is increased, there is a risk of ischemia due to hypoperfusion, whereas when sympathetic activity rises, the increased cardiac workload can lead to complications. The risks of complications due to these factors can be decreased pharmacologically. Anticholinergic medications such as atropine can be used to decrease the occurrence and severity of bradycardia, β-adrenergic blockers can be used to decrease cardiac workload, and nitrates or calcium channel blockers may be used to decrease the risks of ischemia (Weiner et al. 2000). Typically, patients who are receiving medications for the treatment of coronary artery disease at the time of referral for ECT are maintained on those medications throughout the ECT course, including administration before ECT on treatment days (Applegate 1997). Changes to the medication regimen or the addition of other medications to decrease the risks of complications should generally be considered in conjunction with a cardiologic consultant.

Patients with pathologies associated with low cardiac output such as heart failure or those with severe valvular disease are at particular risk during the sympathetic surge because of the increase in afterload and decreased diastolic filling time (Stern et al. 1997). Such patients should not be administered large volumes of fluid (Rayburn 1997). A number of medications have been suggested as means to decrease risks in these situations, including β-adrenergic blockers, α-adrenergic blockers, nitrites, digitalis, and anticholinergic agents; however, all these agents remain controversial (Weiner et al. 2000). There does not appear to be a single regimen that is optimal for all patients with these diseases, and the treatment plan should be individualized on the basis of risk-benefit considerations.

Arrhythmias may increase the risks of ECT (Takada et al. 2005). Bradyarrhythmias are typically best managed with atropine to prevent exacerbation during increases in parasympathetic tone. Because of the anticonvulsant effects of lidocaine, ventricular ectopy should be treated with other agents before the ECT treatment (Hood and Mecca 1983). There is a risk that individuals with atrial fibrillation may experience spontaneous cardioversion with ECT that can lead to an embolic event (Petrides and Fink 1996). As a result, consideration should be given to echocardiography (to rule out a mural thrombus) and the use of anticoagulants (Weiner et al. 2000).

Endocrinological Disorders

Several endocrinological disorders require special consideration before ECT. The most commonly encountered is diabetes mellitus. Patients with diabetes are more likely than other ECT patients to have problems stemming from the need to fast from midnight until the time of the ECT treatment. Insulin doses may need to be adjusted, and pretreatment intravenous glucose administration can be considered if indicated (Weiner et al. 2000).

In patients with hyperthyroidism and pheochromocytoma, β-adrenergic blockers are typically administered to prevent evoking a thyroid storm or hypertensive crisis, which can be elicited by the sympathetic surge (Weiner et al. 2000). In cases of pheochromocytoma, α-adrenergic and tyrosine hydroxylase blockers may be needed.

Metabolic Disorders

The metabolic problems that are of primary concern are hyperkalemia and hypokalemia, both of which may lead to cardiac arrhythmias. The former is of particular concern because of the transient rise in serum potassium caused by succinylcholine and the muscle activity that may occur during the induced seizures (Christopher 2003; Weiner et al. 2000). In individuals with hyperkalemia, prolonged paralysis and associated apnea induced by succinylcholine may be seen. Although it is best to correct these conditions before administering ECT, in cases where correction is not possible, the use of paralytic agents other than succinylcholine should be considered.

Hematological Disorders

Thrombophlebitis carries with it the risk of embolism with ECT, a risk that is generally easily avoided with the use of anticoagulant medications. The use of warfarin has been recommended, with a goal of achieving an International Normalized Ratio (prothrombin time normalized to the laboratory control value) between 1.5 and 2.5 (Petrides and Fink 1996).

Pulmonary Disorders

Patients with asthma or chronic obstructive pulmonary disease have an increased risk of posttreatment bronchospasm, which should be mitigated by the use of bronchodilators (Weiner et al. 2000). Theophylline should be avoided if possible, or the dose should be kept to a minimum because of an increased risk of prolonged seizures.

Gastrointestinal Disorders

Patients with gastroesophageal reflux are commonly encountered in the practice of ECT. Complications of aspiration may be diminished with the use of a pretreatment histamine-2 antagonist the night before and the morning of treatment (Weiner et al. 2000). To increase gastric emptying, pretreatment metoclopramide may be considered, and sodium citrate may also be used to neutralize the acidity of stomach contents. Although it has not been reported, fecal impaction has been mentioned as a risk factor for intestinal rupture with ECT (Weiner et al. 2000). Consequently, in patients referred for ECT, it is important to address constipation, which is particularly common in the elderly population.

Genitourinary Disorders

Urinary retention could, in theory, lead to bladder rupture with ECT. As a result, it has been recommended that patients void before ECT, and urinary catheterization should be considered in those with significant obstruction or difficulty urinating (Weiner et al. 2000).

Musculoskeletal Disorders

Musculoskeletal conditions—such as osteoporosis, unstable fractures, and loose or damaged teeth—are common in older adults and carry an increased risk of complications with ECT. Patients with osteoporosis or with recent or unstable fractures are at risk for bone damage during the induced convulsion. This risk can be addressed by using an increased dose of succinylcholine to ensure good neuromuscular relaxation. In extremely fragile individuals, even the muscle fasciculations that accompany the action of succinylcholine may be of concern, and therefore pretreatment with a short-acting nondepolarizing muscle relaxant, such as mivacurium or rocuronium, should be considered. The contraction of the jaw muscles that leads to teeth clenching cannot be diminished with the use of paralytic agents because it occurs by direct electrical stimulation of the muscle tissue and not via neuromuscular transmission. Therefore, the use of a mouth guard is always necessary. However, those with loose or damaged teeth may require customized devices, dental treatment, or tooth extraction before ECT.

Adverse Effects in Older Adults

Advanced age itself does not appear to increase the medical risks of ECT. As a group, however, older adults have a higher frequency of comorbid medical and neurological conditions that increase the risks of treatment, as outlined above (Kujala et al. 2002; Nuttall et al. 2004; Takada et al. 2005; Tomac et al. 1997). In addition, several studies have reported that older adults tend to have greater and more prolonged cognitive impairment with ECT (see American Psychiatric Association 2001; Sackeim et al. 2007). As a result, in elderly patients, particularly those with preexisting cognitive impairment, modifications of treatment technique should be considered to minimize cognitive side effects.

The greater frequency of comorbid medical and neurological disease in elderly persons also increases the risks associated with pharmacological management of their neuropsychiatric conditions. In some cases, these risks can make pharmacological management extremely difficult and may lead to a referral for ECT. In this regard, Manly et al. (2000) compared the frequency of side effects associated with ECT and pharmacotherapy in a group of depressed patients older than 75 years who were matched for age, sex, and diagnosis. These researchers reported that ECT resulted in fewer side effects (particularly cardiovascular and gastrointestinal) and greater efficacy than pharmacological management. This study underscores that ECT is a relatively safe treatment for older adults and that in many cases it may be both the safest and most effective option.

Pre-ECT Evaluation

Basic Components of the Evaluation

Each pre-ECT evaluation should be carried out by an individual clinically privileged to administer ECT in conjunction with an anesthesia provider. This evaluation should include 1) a thorough psychiatric history and examination, including history of response to ECT and other treatments; 2) a medical history and examination, with special attention paid to cardiovascular, respiratory, neurological, and musculoskeletal systems; 3) a history of dental problems and examination for loose or missing teeth; and 4) a history of personal and family experiences with anesthesia (American Psychiatric Association 2001). Laboratory tests are generally performed, although there is no agreed-on routine set of tests to carry out in each case. The most commonly administered pre-ECT screening battery of tests includes a complete blood count, serum chemistry (including sodium and potassium), and electrocardiogram (American Psychiatric Association 2001). A chest radiograph is indicated in the setting of cardiovascular or pulmonary disease or where there is a history of smoking (American Psychiatric Association 2001; Weiner et al. 2000).

The decision about whether to pursue testing of cerebral function and structure (e.g., electroencephalographic, neuroradiological, and/or neuropsychological assessment) should be made on an individual basis, guided by the history and examination. In addition, spinal radiographs should be considered in individuals with known or suspected spinal disease. Further testing or consultation should be considered when the nature or extent of a problem is uncertain, when the risks of ECT in the setting of the existing medical disease are unclear, or when there is uncertainty about how to modify ECT technique to decrease risks. In every case, the pre-ECT assessment should include an evaluation of the risks of cognitive impairment based on the considerations described above and the information obtained by history, examination, and testing. This evaluation should play a key role in recommendations about treatment technique in terms of electrode placement, treatment frequency, dosing, and medications to be avoided.

Decision About Whether to Administer ECT

The decision about whether to recommend ECT should be based on a careful assessment of risks and benefits of ECT versus alternative treatments, the data obtained in the evaluation, and information presented in the available literature. The starting point for this decision should be the psychiatric diagnosis. ECT should be seriously considered only when the patient has a condition for which there is evidence of ECT efficacy. For individuals with an ECT-responsive disease, a number of factors should be considered in developing a recommendation about ECT. These factors include the severity of the illness, the degree of refractoriness to other treatments, an assessment of the risks of ECT, and the patient's preference.

In conditions such as major depression, for which ECT is the most effective treatment known, the greater the severity of illness, the stronger the indication for ECT (Weiner and Krystal 2001). When psychosis is present or when there is a high degree of lethality because of suicidality, dehydration or malnutrition, or the patient's inability to cooperate with necessary medical treatment, ECT is frequently the treatment of choice. Unfortunately, no proven guidelines exist for how to define treatment refractoriness in terms of medication dosage or duration or number of failed trials. Consequently, the choice of when to refer a patient for ECT on the basis of medication resistance or intolerance is generally based on factors such as symptom severity, morbidity of the episode, and patient preference as much as it is on the characteristics of prior medication trials.

The assessment of risks based on the evaluation described above is an important part of deciding whether to pursue ECT. The greater the perceived risk, the stronger the indication for ECT must be for a recommendation to be made. When the risks of ECT are assessed to be significantly life-threatening, ECT should be pursued only if the illness is so lethal that the risks of not pursuing ECT are determined to be greater. As noted earlier, however, risk is a relative index.

Informed Consent

The collaborative aspect of decision making has been formalized as the legal doctrine of informed consent (American Psychiatric Association 2001). No patient with the capacity to give voluntary consent should be treated with ECT without his or her written, informed consent. Although there is no clear consensus about how to determine capacity to give consent, this capacity has generally been interpreted as evidence that the patient can understand information about the procedure and can act responsibly on the basis of this information (American Psychiatric Association 2001). The process of determining competency, the process for giving ECT involuntarily in cases of emergency, and the specific procedures regarding informed consent should be carried out as specified by applicable state statutes. Because of the increased likelihood of cognitive dysfunction in older adults, capacity to consent is of particular concern (Rabheru 2001).

At a minimum, written consent should be obtained before a course of ECT, if an unusually large number of treatments become necessary, and before initiating continuation or maintenance ECT (American Psychiatric Association 2001). To adequately convey the risks and benefits, the consent form should include the following information: 1) a description of treatment alternatives; 2) a detailed description of how, when, and where ECT will be carried out; 3) a discussion of options regarding electrode placement; 4) the typical range of number of treatments; 5) a statement that there is no guarantee that the treatment will be successful; 6) a statement that continuation or maintenance treatment of some kind will be necessary; 7) a discussion of the possible risks, including death, cardiac dysfunction, confusion, and memory impairment; 8) a statement that the consent also applies to emergency treatment that may be clinically necessary at times when the patient is unconscious; 9) a listing of patient requirements during the ECT course, such as taking nothing by mouth after midnight before treatment; 10) a statement that there has been an opportunity to ask questions and an indication of who can be contacted with further questions; and 11) a statement that consent is voluntary and can be withdrawn at any time (American Psychiatric Association 2001).

Informed consent involves more than just signing a consent form; it requires a consent discussion with the patient or surrogate (and, if possible, a significant other). The consent discussion should include any significant differences in likelihood of benefit or extent of risk from that depicted in the consent form, and mention of such discussion should be briefly documented in the patient's medical record.

Management of Medications

Each pre-ECT assessment should include an evaluation of the patient's medications and recommendations about how medications should be taken before and during the ECT course. Medications that are needed to decrease medical risks should be continued, but their dosing and timing of administration may need to be changed (American Psychiatric Association 2001). Similarly, orders should be written specifying dosage and timing of any medications that are to be added to decrease risks based on the pre-ECT evaluation. Other nonpsychotropic medications should be withheld until after the treatment on ECT days or—in the case of those that interfere with or increase the risks of ECT—should be discontinued.

Regarding the use of psychotropic medications during the ECT course, there are considerable differences of opinion and great variation in practice. The only situation in which compelling evidence exists for a potentiating effect of psychotropic medication on ECT is the use of antipsychotic agents in schizophrenic individuals (and inferentially in those with psychotic depression) (American Psychiatric Association 2001). The literature regarding the benefits of antidepressant medication as a means to augment the ECT response is unclear, although it does not appear that such a combination is associated with significantly increased risk. The primary reasons that have been given for the use of antidepressant medication augmentation are that it is difficult at times to accomplish drug withdrawal before instituting ECT, that there is a desire to decrease the risk of early relapse after ECT, and that "there is nothing to lose."

When possible, antidepressant medications should be chosen that have relatively fewer effects on cardiac function. The following psychotropic medications are among those that are best avoided or maintained at the lowest possible levels: 1) lithium—it may increase the risks for delirium or prolonged seizures; 2) benzodiazepines—their anticonvulsant properties may decrease efficacy (but can be reversed with flumazenil at the time of ECT) (Krystal et al. 1998); 3) antiepileptic drugs—their anticonvulsant properties may decrease efficacy, but they may be needed in those with epilepsy or with very brittle bipolar disorder (in which case they should be withheld the night before and the morning of treatment if possible); 4) bupropion and clozapine—they may increase the risk of prolonged seizures (the dosage should be kept at low to moderate levels).

ECT Technique

Inpatient Versus Outpatient Administration

Although ECT has traditionally been an inpatient treatment modality, a shift has occurred in recent years—much like the one that has occurred in the realm of surgical procedures—to offer it on an outpatient basis (American Psychiatric Association 2001). At present, inpatient ECT is reserved for situations in which 1) the patient's psychiatric illness itself requires an inpatient level of care or 2) such a level is required to ensure that ECT can be safely administered (e.g., for patients with high medical risk factors and no support system). These situations are particularly likely to occur with older adults. Even when inpatient treatments are initially required, consideration should be given to switching to an outpatient mode when it is clinically feasible.

Anesthetic Considerations

ECT is a procedure involving general anesthesia. Airway management, the administration of medications necessary for anesthesia, and the handling of medical emergencies during and immediately following the ECT procedure are the responsibility of the anesthesia provider (American Psychiatric Association 2001). Appropriate medical backup should be present, particularly for high-risk cases.

The patient is ventilated by mask with 100% oxygen throughout the procedure, beginning at least a few minutes before anesthesia induction and lasting until a satisfactory level of spontaneous respiration is maintained during the postictal period. General anesthesia is usually provided by intravenous methohexital, typically 1 mg/kg (American Psychiatric Association 2001; Ding and White 2002; Saito 2005). Because seizure threshold (the amount of electricity necessary to induce a seizure) appears to increase with age, and stimulus output of ECT devices is limited by the U.S. Food and Drug Administration, difficulties in seizure induction can be experienced with older adults, particularly late in an index ECT course. In such situations, methohexital dosage can be slightly diminished by concurrent usage of a short-acting sedative narcotic such as remifentanyl, or the anesthetic itself can be switched to one with less anticonvulsant properties (e.g., etomidate or ketamine).

After loss of consciousness, the muscle relaxant succinylcholine is administered intravenously, again with a typical dosage of 1 mg/kg (American Psychiatric Association 2001). When the patient's muscles are relaxed (ascertainable by disappearance of relaxant-induced fasciculations and loss of deep tendon reflexes or twitch response to a peripheral nerve stimulator), the electrical stimulus can be delivered.

An anticholinergic medication, such as glycopyrrolate or atropine, may be administered before anesthesia to minimize the risk of stimulus-related asystole and the occurrence of postictal oral secretions. However, most practitioners use such agents selectively because they potentiate seizure-related tachycardia. When seizure-related hypertension and tachycardia are severe or when prophylaxis is indicated on the basis of preexisting cardiovascular disease, β-blocking medications (e.g., labetalol) are often used to minimize these effects. Again, it is best to use such agents selectively. When necessary, postictal agitation or delirium can be managed with the use of intravenous midazolam (1 mg) or haloperidol (2–5 mg), as well as by providing reassurance and maintaining a quiet, low-light environment for the postictal recovery process.

With older adults, it is important to recognize that lower dosages of medications may be indicated because of altered metabolism or tolerance. In addition, time to effect may be longer in older adults. On the other hand, under some circumstances, higher doses may be necessary (e.g., more relaxant agent may be needed for an individual with osteoporosis).

Physiological Monitoring

During ECT, as with any procedure utilizing general anesthesia, vital signs and pulse oximetry are monitored throughout the procedure and during the immediate postictal period until stabilization occurs. After spontaneous respiration resumes and vital signs and oxygen saturation are trending toward baseline, the patient is moved to a postanesthesia care unit or area (previously referred to as a recovery room), where monitoring of vital signs and oxygenation continues.

Both the motor and electroencephalographic representations of seizure activity are monitored during ECT. To allow monitoring of the motor response in a patient whose muscles are relaxed, a blood pressure cuff is placed around the ankle and inflated to approximately 200 mm Hg just before administration of the muscle relaxant. This action prevents muscle activity distal to the cuff from being suppressed during the seizure. Ictal electroencephalographic recordings are made, using recording leads placed on the head, in conjunction with amplification and display instrumentation built into the ECT device. It is recommended that two electroencephalographic channels be recorded so that seizure activity from both the left and the right cerebral hemispheres can be monitored. Such recording can be accomplished by placing one pair of recording electrodes over the left prefrontal and left mastoid areas and the other pair over the homologous areas on the right.

Stimulus Electrode Placement

There are three major types of stimulus electrode placement: bitemporal, bifrontal, and unilateral nondominant (the right side for the great majority of individuals). Bitemporal ECT involves placement of both stimulus electrodes over the frontotemporal regions, with the center of the electrode approximately 1 inch above the midpoint of a line transecting the external canthus of the eye and the tragus of the ear. Bifrontal electrode placement involves locating the center of the stimulus electrodes approximately 5 cm superior to each external canthus. The preferred type of unilateral nondominant placement involves location of one electrode over the right frontotemporal area (as above) and the other over the right centroparietal area, just to the right of the vertex of the scalp, a point defined by the intersection of lines between the inion and nasion and between the tragi of both ears.

There is significant controversy over the choice of stimulus electrode placement (American Psychiatric Association 2001). Although unilateral ECT appears to be effective in many patients as long as stimulus intensity is sufficient (see "Stimulus Dosing" below), some patients may preferentially respond to bitemporal ECT. On the other hand, ECT-associated amnesia is greater with bitemporal ECT. A reasonable trade-off is to use unilateral ECT initially, unless an urgent response is necessary or the patient has indicated a preference for or has shown a past preferential response to bitemporal ECT. With bifrontal electrode placement, the newest of the three techniques (Bailine et al. 2000), data are mixed, with some studies suggesting that both efficacy and cognitive effects of bifrontal ECT may be less than with bitemporal ECT and perhaps slightly greater than with unilateral ECT (Bakewell et al. 2004; Heikman et al. 2002).

The choice of stimulus electrode placement is particularly challenging in older adults, for whom an urgent need for a rapid response is often present, yet in whom adverse cognitive effects are of concern, especially in those who have preexisting cerebral impairment. One recent study reported that high-dosage unilateral ECT was as effective in older adults as bitemporal ECT (Stoppe et al. 2006), although the placement controversy is still not resolved.

Stimulus Dosing

All contemporary ECT devices used in the United States utilize a bidirectional, constant-current, brief-pulse stimulus waveform. This waveform is more efficient than the older sine wave stimulus for inducing seizures and allows ECT to be administered with fewer adverse cognitive effects (Weiner et al. 1986). Recently, these devices have also incorporated the use of the ultrabrief pulse stimulus, defined as a pulse duration of less than 0.5 milliseconds, which is considered a more efficient way to induce seizures (Loo et al. 2007). The paradigm for the choice of stimulus dose intensity, however, appears to be as controversial as the choice of electrode placement. The disagreement centers on whether to dose with respect to an empirically determined seizure threshold estimate obtained at the first treatment (dose-titration technique) or to use a formula based on factors such as age, gender, and electrode placement to make this decision (formula-based technique) (American Psychiatric Association 2001).

We have found that the dose-titration technique is better in that it offers a more precise means to determine the patient's seizure threshold (which can vary manyfold) and thereby allows the practitioner to more effectively control stimulus intensity (Coffey et al. 1995). In practice, seizure threshold is estimated at the first treatment by incrementally increasing the dose from a low level until a seizure is induced.

Regardless of the dosing paradigm, compelling evidence suggests that stimulus intensity for unilateral ECT should be somewhere between 2.5 and 8 times seizure threshold (in terms of electrical charge), with the range reflecting current uncertainty as to the minimum dose necessary to optimize therapeutic outcome (McCall et al. 2000). In this regard, it is important to note that increasing stimulus intensity also increases the severity of ECT-associated memory impairment, although to a lesser degree than a switch to bilateral ECT. Stimulus intensity is less of an issue with bilateral ECT, in which a stimulus 1.5 times seizure threshold appears to be sufficient. However, at least theoretically, stimulus intensity may be of most concern with ultrabrief pulse ECT, certainly for unilateral electrode placement but likely also for bitemporal and bifrontal placement.

As alluded to above, seizure threshold is a function of age, with substantially higher thresholds being present in older adults. This higher threshold leaves older adults at greater risk for being unable to receive a stimulus of sufficient intensity, because the maximum output of ECT devices used in the United States is limited by U.S. Food and Drug Administration regulations (Krystal et al. 2000a). The risk that the threshold will exceed the maximum available stimulus intensity is even greater late in the treatment course, because seizure threshold rises to a varying extent with the number of treatments.

Determination of Seizure Adequacy

ECT-induced seizures are identical to spontaneous grand mal seizures except that with ECT the motor response is attenuated pharmacologically. The electroencephalographic recording during ECT (ictal electroencephalogram) manifests the typical electroencephalographic features of a grand mal seizure, with chaotic polyspike activity marking the tonic portion of the seizure and repetitive polyspike and slow-wave discharges during the clonic component. During the immediate postictal period, a relative suppression (i.e., flattening) of electroencephalographic activity can typically be seen (Weiner et al. 1991).

Compelling evidence indicates that not all seizures are equally potent from a therapeutic perspective. With unilateral ECT, barely suprathreshold seizures—despite having identical durations as seizures from more moderately suprathreshold stimuli—are only minimally therapeutic (Sackeim et al. 1993). Based on findings that seizures with higher stimulus intensity exhibit attributes such as higher amplitude, greater regularity in shape, and greater postictal electroencephalographic suppression (Krystal et al. 1995) and that such features are associated with the therapeutic response to ECT, a growing interest has developed in the possibility that electroencephalographically based stimulus dosing may one day be feasible. This type of innovation would be particularly attractive because it would allow practitioners a means to tailor the stimulus intensity to the minimum therapeutic dose for each individual and control for the variable rise in seizure threshold that occurs over the ECT course (Krystal et al. 2000b). Already, ECT device manufacturers in the United States have incorporated "seizure quality" features into their devices, although their utility for routine clinical usage remains to be established (see American Psychiatric Association 2001; Rasmussen et al. 2007).

Frequency and Number of ECT Treatments

In the United States, ECT is typically administered three times a week, with an index course usually lasting between 6 and 12 treatments, although more or fewer are sometimes necessary. The frequency of ECT may be reduced to twice a week or even once a week if amnesia or confusion becomes a major problem (American Psychiatric Association 2001). The decision about when to end the index ECT course depends on treatment outcome as well as the wishes of the consenter. In general, the treatments are stopped when a therapeutic plateau has occurred—that is, when the patient has reached a maximum level of response. If no substantial improvement occurs by the sixth treatment, consideration should be given to making changes in the ECT technique, such as switching stimulus electrode placement, increasing stimulus intensity, or discontinuing medications with anticonvulsant properties. If no response occurs after 8–10 treatments, alternative treatment modalities should be considered. At the present time, these modalities would generally involve combination pharmacotherapy utilizing multiple agents of different classes.

Maintenance Therapy

The conditions for which ECT is used are typically recurrent. The risk of relapse, particularly during the first 2–3 months, is extremely high, necessitating an aggressive program of maintenance treatment to minimize the likelihood of relapse. This maintenance treatment may be pharmacological or in the form of continued ECT (at a greatly lowered frequency).

Pharmacological Maintenance Therapy

Pharmacological maintenance treatment is usually attempted after the initial index ECT course unless the patient indicates a strong preference for maintenance ECT. With major depression, evidence suggests that a combination of antidepressant and mood stabilizer may be more effective in maintaining remission than an antidepressant drug alone (Sackeim et al. 2001). Unfortunately, evidence shows that medication resistance during the index episode diminishes the likelihood of a sustained prophylactic effect (Sackeim et al. 1990). Maintenance pharmacotherapy following ECT treatment of mania or schizophrenia has not been well studied. In the absence of applicable data, an aggressive regimen of different drug classes should be considered.

Maintenance ECT

The high relapse rate following ECT, even with pharmacological maintenance therapy, has created renewed interest in the practice of maintenance ECT. After a flurry of largely positive case-series reports (Rabheru and Persad 1997), a randomized trial of maintenance ECT versus pharmacotherapy in patients treated for major depression was carried out, with results indicating that the efficacy of maintenance ECT over a 6-month period was comparable to that obtained by combination pharmacotherapy with both lithium and nortriptyline (Kellner et al. 2006).

Although there are no established guidelines for a maintenance ECT regimen, practitioners typically start with weekly treatments for 2–4 weeks, followed by another 1–2 months of biweekly treatments, followed by 3-week and then 4-week intervals. After 12 months, treatments are either stopped or continued at an even lower frequency. Although many maintenance ECT patients do well with such a regimen, others appear to require more frequent treatments or even supplementation with psychotropic medications. Others eventually relapse, leading to another index ECT course or a switch to alternative treatment modalities.

In terms of cognitive effects, maintenance ECT is significantly better tolerated than index ECT treatments, particularly if the interval between treatments is kept large. Still, some patients do have cumulative difficulties with amnesia, and these should be taken into account in treatment planning. Given the general good tolerance of maintenance ECT, there is no maximum lifetime number of ECT treatments.

Future of ECT

The use of ECT has persisted for 70 years, despite the development of many alternative treatment options. Its continued viability, however, depends not only on innovations in alternative treatments but also on the continued optimization of ECT in terms of both efficacy and adverse effects. As noted above, research is under way to improve on the available options for both stimulus electrode placement and electrical stimulus parameters. Other work is being done to enable practitioners to better predict which patients might be ECT responders.

Future alternatives to ECT include not only new psychopharmacological agents but also new electromagnetic therapies such as transcranial magnetic stimulation, vagal nerve stimulation, and deep brain stimulation (Wyche et al. 2007). Whether or not any of these new experimental techniques will partially or even fully replace ECT remains to be established. In the meantime, a clear role remains for ECT in the treatment of a variety of disorders, most notably major depression, for which older adults are at a particularly high risk.

Key Points

- ECT is the most rapid and effective treatment for major depressive episodes in older adults.
- Major risks of ECT are largely a function of medical comorbidity.
- An index ECT treatment course can be ended once a therapeutic plateau has been reached.
- The risk for relapse after an acute course of ECT is high, and aggressive continuation treatment is needed.

References

American Psychiatric Association: The Practice of ECT: Recommendations for Treatment, Training, and Privileging. Washington, DC, American Psychiatric Press, 2001

Andersen K, Balldin J, Gottfries CG, et al: A double-blind evaluation of electroconvulsive therapy in Parkinson's disease with "on-off" phenomena. Acta Neurol Scand 76:191–199, 1987

Applegate RJ: Diagnosis and management of ischemic heart disease in the patient scheduled to undergo electroconvulsive therapy. Convuls Ther 13:128–144, 1997

Avery D, Lubrano A: Depression treated with imipramine and ECT: the DeCarolis study reconsidered. Am J Psychiatry 136:549–562, 1979

Avery D, Winokur G: Mortality in depressed patients treated with ECT and antidepressants. Arch Gen Psychiatry 33:1029–1037, 1976

Bailine SH, Rifkin A, Kayne E, et al: Comparison of bifrontal and bitemporal ECT for major depression. Am J Psychiatry 157:121–123, 2000

Bakewell CJ, Russo J, Tanner C, et al: Comparison of clinical efficacy and side effects for bitemporal and bifrontal electrode placement in electroconvulsive therapy. J ECT 20:145–153, 2004

Bosboom PR, Deijen JB: Age-related cognitive effects of ECT and ECT-induced mood improvement in depressive patients. Depress Anxiety 23:93–101, 2006

Brandon S: Efficacy in depression: controlled trials. Psychopharmacol Bull 22:465–468, 1986

Christopher EJ: Electroconvulsive therapy in the medically ill. Curr Psychiatry Rep 5:225–230, 2003

Coffey CE, Lucke J, Weiner RD, et al: Seizure threshold in electroconvulsive therapy, I: initial seizure threshold. Biol Psychiatry 37:713–720, 1995

Currier MB, Murray GB, Welch CC: ECT for post-stroke depression. J Neuropsychiatry Clin Neurosci 4:140–144, 1992

Ding Z, White PF: Anesthesia for electroconvulsive therapy. Anesth Analg 94:1351–1364, 2002

Endler NS: The origins of electroconvulsive therapy. Convuls Ther 4:5–23, 1988

Figiel GS, Coffey CE, Djang WT, et al: Brain magnetic resonance imaging findings in ECT-induced delirium. J Neuropsychiatry Clin Neurosci 2:53–58, 1990

Figiel GS, Hassen MA, Zorumski C, et al: ECT-induced delirium in depressed patients with Parkinson's disease. J Neuropsychiatry Clin Neurosci 3:405–411, 1991

Fink M: Meduna and the origins of convulsive therapy. Am J Psychiatry 141:1034–1041, 1984

Fink M, Sackeim HA: Convulsive therapy in schizophrenia? Schizophr Bull 22:27–39, 1996

Fricchione GL, Kaufman LD, Gruber BL, et al: Electroconvulsive therapy and cyclophosphamide in combination for severe neuropsychiatric lupus with catatonia. Am J Med 88:442–443, 1990

Glen T, Scott AI: Rates of electroconvulsive therapy use in Edinburgh (1992–1997). J Affect Disord 54:81–85, 1999

Heikman P, Kalska H, Katila H, et al: Right unilateral and bifrontal electroconvulsive therapy in the treatment of depression: a preliminary study. J ECT 18:26–30, 2002

Hood DA, Mecca RS: Failure to initiate electroconvulsive seizures in a patient pretreated with lidocaine. Anesthesiology 58:379–381, 1983

Husain MM, Rush AJ, Fink M, et al: Speed of response and remission in major depressive disorder with acute electroconvulsive therapy (ECT): a Consortium for Research in ECT (CORE) report. J Clin Psychiatry 65:485–491, 2004

Huuhka M, Korpisammal L, Haataja R, et al: One-year outcome of elderly inpatients with major depressive disorder treated with ECT and antidepressants. J ECT 20:179–185, 2004

Janicak PG, Davis JM, Gibbons RD, et al: Efficacy of ECT: a meta-analysis. Am J Psychiatry 142:297–302, 1985

Kamat SM, Lefevre PJ, Grossberg GT: Electroconvulsive therapy in the elderly. Clin Geriatr Med 19:825–839, 2003

Kellner CH, Bernstein JH: ECT as a treatment for neurologic illness, in The Clinical Science of Electroconvulsive Therapy. Edited by Coffey CE. Washington, DC, American Psychiatric Press, 1993, pp 183–210

Kellner CH, Knapp RG, Petrides G, et al: Continuation electroconvulsive therapy vs pharmacotherapy for relapse prevention in major depression: a multisite study from the Consortium for Research in Electroconvulsive Therapy (CORE). Arch Gen Psychiatry 63:1337–1344, 2006

Klapheke MM: Combining ECT and antipsychotic agents: benefits and risks. Convuls Ther 9:241–255, 1993

Kramer BA: Use of ECT in California, revisited: 1984–1994. J ECT 15:245–251, 1999

Krueger RB, Sackeim HA: Electroconvulsive therapy and schizophrenia, in Schizophrenia. Edited by Hirsch SR, Weinberger D. Oxford, UK, Blackwell, 1995, pp 503–545

Krystal AD, Coffey CE: Neuropsychiatric considerations in the use of electroconvulsive therapy. J Neuropsychiatry Clin Neurosci 9:283–292, 1997

Krystal AD, Weiner RD, Coffey CE: The ictal EEG as a marker of adequate stimulus intensity with unilateral ECT. J Neuropsychiatry Clin Neurosci 7:295–303, 1995

Krystal AD, Watts BV, Weiner RD, et al: The use of flumazenil in the anxious and benzodiazepine-dependent ECT patient. J ECT 14:5–14, 1998

Krystal AD, Dean MD, Weiner RD, et al: ECT stimulus intensity: are present ECT devices too limited? Am J Psychiatry 157:963–967, 2000a

Krystal AD, Weiner RD, Lindahl V, et al: The development and retrospective testing of an electroencephalographic seizure quality-based stimulus dosing paradigm with ECT. J ECT 16:338–349, 2000b

Kujala I, Rosenvinge B, Bekkelund SI: Clinical outcome and adverse effects of electroconvulsive therapy in elderly psychiatric patients. J Geriatr Psychiatry Neurol 15:73–76, 2002

Loo C, Sheehan P, Pigot M, et al: A report on mood and cognitive outcomes with right unilateral ultrabrief pulsewidth (0.3 ms) ECT and retrospective comparison with standard pulsewidth right unilateral ECT. J Affect Disord 103:277–281, 2007

Manly DT, Oakley SP Jr, Bloch RM: Electroconvulsive therapy in old-old patients. Am J Geriatr Psychiatry 8:232–236, 2000

McCall WV, Reboussin DM, Weiner RD, et al: Titrated moderately suprathreshold vs fixed high-dose right unilateral electroconvulsive therapy: acute antidepressant and cognitive effects. Arch Gen Psychiatry 57:438–444, 2000

Mukherjee S, Sackeim HA, Schnur DB: Electroconvulsive therapy of acute mania episodes: a review of 50 years' experience. Am J Psychiatry 151:169–176, 1994

Murray GB, Shea V, Conn DK: ECT for post-stroke depression. J Clin Psychiatry 47:258–260, 1986

Nuttall GA, Bowersox MR, Douglass SB, et al: Morbidity and mortality in the use of electroconvulsive therapy. J ECT 20:237–241, 2004

O'Connor MK, Knapp R, Husain M, et al: The influence of age on the response of major depression to electroconvulsive therapy: a C.O.R.E. report. Am J Geriatr Psychiatry 9:382–390, 2001

Paul SM, Extein I, Calil HM, et al: Use of ECT with treatment-resistant depressed patients at the National Institute of Mental Health. Am J Psychiatry 138:486–489, 1981

Petrides G, Fink M: Atrial fibrillation, anticoagulation, and ECT. Convuls Ther 12:91–98, 1996

Petrides G, Fink M, Husain MM, et al: ECT remission rates in psychotic versus nonpsychotic depressed patients: a report from CORE. J ECT 17:244–253, 2001

Philibert RA, Richards L, Lynch CF, et al: Effect of ECT on mortality and clinical outcome in geriatric unipolar depression. J Clin Psychiatry 56:390–394, 1995

Pritchett JT, Kellner CH, Coffey CE: Electroconvulsive therapy in geriatric neuropsychiatry, in Textbook of Geriatric Neuropsychiatry. Edited by Coffey CE, Cummings JL. Washington, DC, American Psychiatric Press, 1994, pp 633–659

Prudic J, Haskett RF, Mulsant B, et al: Resistance to antidepressant medications and short-term clinical response to ECT. Am J Psychiatry 153:985–992, 1996

Quitkin FM, McGrath PJ, Stewart JW, et al: Can the effects of antidepressants be observed in the first two weeks of treatment? Neuropsychopharmacology 15:390–394, 1996

Rabheru K: The use of electroconvulsive therapy in special patient populations. Can J Psychiatry 46:710–719, 2001

Rabheru K, Persad E: A review of continuation and maintenance electroconvulsive therapy. Can J Psychiatry 42:476–484, 1997

Rasmussen K, Abrams R: Treatment of Parkinson's disease with electroconvulsive therapy. Psychiatr Clin North Am 14:925–933, 1991

Rasmussen KG, Varghese R, Stevens SR, et al: Electrode placement and ictal EEG indices in electroconvulsive therapy. J Neuropsychiatry Clin Neurosci 19:453–457, 2007

Rayburn BK: ECT in patients with heart failure or valvular heart disease. Convuls Ther 13:145–156, 1997

Reid WH, Keller S, Leatherman M, et al: ECT in Texas: 19 months of mandatory reporting. J Clin Psychiatry 59:8–13, 1998

Rosenbach ML, Hermann RC, Dorwart RA: Use of electroconvulsive therapy in the Medicare population between 1987 and 1992. Psychiatr Serv 48:1537–1542, 1997

Rummans TA, Bassingthwaighte ME: Severe medical and neurologic complications associated with near-lethal catatonia treated with electroconvulsive therapy. Convuls Ther 7:121–124, 1991

Sackeim HA: The use of electroconvulsive therapy in late-life depression, in Clinical Geriatric Psychopharmacology, 3rd Edition. Edited by Salzman C. Baltimore, MD, Williams & Wilkins, 1998, pp 262–309

Sackeim HA, Rush AJ: Melancholia and response to ECT. Am J Psychiatry 152:1242–1243, 1995

Sackeim HA, Prudic J, Devanand DP, et al: The impact of medication resistance and continuation pharmacotherapy on relapse following response to electroconvulsive therapy in major depression. J Clin Psychopharmacol 10:96–104, 1990

Sackeim HA, Prudic J, Devanand DP, et al: Effects of stimulus intensity and electrode placement on the efficacy and cognitive effects of electroconvulsive therapy. N Engl J Med 328:839–846, 1993

Sackeim HA, Haskett RF, Mulsant BH, et al: Continuation pharmacotherapy in the prevention of relapse following electroconvulsive therapy: a randomized controlled trial. JAMA 285:1299–1307, 2001

Sackeim HA, Prudic J, Fuller R, et al: The cognitive effects of electroconvulsive therapy in community settings. Neuropsychopharmacology 32:244–254, 2007

Saito S: Anesthesia management for electroconvulsive therapy: Hemodynamic and respiratory management. J Anesth 19:142–149, 2005

Sajatovic M, Meltzer HY: The effect of short-term electroconvulsive treatment plus neuroleptics in treatment-resistant schizophrenia and schizoaffective disorder. Convuls Ther 9:167–173, 1993

Shorter E, Healy D: Shock Therapy: A History of Electroconvulsive Treatment in Mental Illness. New Brunswick, NJ, Rutgers University Press, 2007

Small JG, Klapper MH, Kellams JJ, et al: Electroconvulsive treatment compared with lithium in the management of manic states. Arch Gen Psychiatry 45:727–732, 1988

Sobin C, Prudic J, Devanand DP, et al: Who responds to electroconvulsive therapy? A comparison of effective and ineffective forms of treatment. Br J Psychiatry 169:322–328, 1996

Stern L, Hirschmann S, Grunhaus L: ECT in patients with major depressive disorder and low cardiac output. Convuls Ther 13:68–73, 1997

Stoppe A, Louza M, Rosa M, et al: Fixed high-dose electroconvulsive therapy in the elderly with depression: a double-blind, randomized comparison of efficacy and tolerability between unilateral and bilateral electrode placement. J ECT 22:92–99, 2006

Takada JY, Solimene MC, da Luz PL, et al: Assessment of the cardiovascular effects of electroconvulsive therapy in individuals older than 50 years. Braz J Med Biol Res 38:1349–1357, 2005

Tew JD Jr, Mulsant BH, Haskett RF, et al: Acute efficacy of ECT in the treatment of major depression in the old-old. Am J Psychiatry 156:1865–1870, 1999

Thompson JW, Weiner RD, Myers CP: Use of ECT in the United States in 1975, 1980, 1986. Am J Psychiatry 151:1657–1661, 1994

Tomac TA, Rummans TA, Pileggi TS, et al: Safety and efficacy of electroconvulsive therapy in patients over age 85. Am J Geriatr Psychiatry 5:126–130, 1997

UK ECT Review Group: Efficacy and safety of electroconvulsive therapy in depressive disorders: a systematic review and meta-analysis. Lancet 361:799–808, 2003

van der Wurff FB, Stek ML, Hoogendijk WJ, et al: The efficacy and safety of ECT in depressed older adults: a literature review. Int J Geriatr Psychiatry 18:894–904, 2003

Weiner RD, Coffey CE: Indications for use of electroconvulsive therapy, in Review of Psychiatry, Vol 7. Edited by Frances AJ, Hales RE. Washington, DC, American Psychiatric Press, 1988, pp 458–481

Weiner RD, Krystal AD: Electroconvulsive therapy, in Treatments of Psychiatric Disorders, 3rd Edition. Edited by Gabbard GO, Rush AJ. Washington, DC, American Psychiatric Press, 2001, pp 1267–1293

Weiner RD, Rogers HJ, Davidson JR, et al: Effects of stimulus parameters on cognitive side effects. Ann N Y Acad Sci 462:315–325, 1986

Weiner RD, Coffey CE, Krystal AD: The monitoring and management of electrically induced seizures. Psychiatr Clin North Am 14:845–869, 1991

Weiner RD, Coffey CE, Krystal AD: Electroconvulsive therapy in the medical and neurologic patient, in Psychiatric Care of the Medical Patient, 2nd Edition. Edited by Stoudemire A, Fogel BS, Greenberg D. New York, Oxford University Press, 2000, pp 419–428

Wesson ML, Wilkinson AM, Anderson DN, et al: Does age predict the long-term outcome of depression treated with ECT? (A prospective study of the long-term outcome of ECT-treated depression with respect to age.) Int J Geriatr Psychiatry 12:45–51, 1997

Wyche MC, O'Reardon J, Carpenter LL: Neurostimulation therapies for depression: acute and long-term outcomes. Depression: Mind and Body 3:106–114, 2007

Zielinski RJ, Roose SP, Devanand DP, et al: Cardiovascular complications of ECT in depressed patients with cardiac disease. Am J Psychiatry 150:904–909, 1993

Suggested Readings

Abrams R: Electroconvulsive Therapy, 4th Edition. New York, Oxford University Press, 2002

American Psychiatric Association: The Practice of ECT: Recommendations for Treatment, Training, and Privileging. Washington, DC, American Psychiatric Press, 2001

Beyer J, Weiner RD, Glenn MD: Practical Aspects of ECT: A Programmed Text, 2nd Edition. Washington, DC, American Psychiatric Press, 1998

Dukakis K, Tye L: Shock: The Healing Power of Electroconvulsive Therapy. New York, Avery, 2006

Endler NS: Holiday of Darkness, Revised. Toronto, ON, Wall and Davis, 1990

Fink M: Electroshock: Restoring the Mind. New York, Oxford University Press, 1999

CHAPTER 28

Nutrition and Physical Activity

Connie Watkins Bales, Ph.D., R.D.
Martha Elizabeth Payne, Ph.D., R.D., M.P.H.

Health Promotion in the Elderly

The attainment of 65 years or more of living carries with it all the positive attributes (such as apparent resistance to early mortality) and negative consequences (including the effects of a lifetime of environmental exposures and health insults) of being an older adult. However, the quality and quantity of life from age 65 years onward remains very responsive to the impact of lifestyle factors, particularly the type of dietary and physical activity patterns maintained. In fact, with the onslaught of age-related decrements in physiological function and the concomitant onset of the chronic diseases of aging, it could be argued that this period in the life cycle offers one of the most important opportunities for lifestyle interventions to make a difference in health-related quality of life (Wellman 2007). This chapter provides a detailed discussion of the complex interactions of diet and physical activity with mental health and treatments for mental health disorders. In addition, the last section of this chapter provides a thorough discussion of assessment techniques and clinical guidelines for both nutrition and physical activity in the elderly.

As during all stages of the life cycle, good nutrition and healthy patterns of physical activity are basic requirements for optimal health in later life. Essential nutrients are required to support the structural and metabolic functions of the body, the components of which are constantly being turned over and replenished, even in mature individuals. For example, essential amino acids are the required building blocks for protein synthesis (for both structural and functional proteins), whereas vitamins and minerals are required as cofactors for a host of essential enzymes in metabolic pathways. Of particular relevance to mental health and cognitive function are select nutrients (see next section) that are essential for nervous system function because of their roles in membrane health, myelin production, and neurotransmitter synthesis, as well as their participation in key enzymatic reactions. The commonly quoted caveat to "use it or lose it" aptly applies to physical activity; maintaining an active lifestyle preserves muscle mass and muscle strength, as well as bone mineral density, and has been linked with improved mood, sleep patterns, and quality of life.

In addition to maintaining essential life-sustaining functions, judiciously applied diet and exercise regimens can help prevent or at least delay the onset of many age-related chronic diseases and thus play a critical health-preserving role for high-risk individuals. Many of the leading causes of illness and death in the second half of life, including cardiovascular disease, stroke, diabetes mellitus, osteoporosis, certain cancers, anxiety, and depression, are amenable to modification with diet and/or physical activity intervention strategies. Beyond these disease prevention effects, healthy diet and activity patterns also contribute to functional status and overall well-being. For example, reducing the risk of falls and associated injuries is a key benefit of physical activity. Although healthy diet patterns and physical activity play important roles in promoting optimal mental health, it is also true that mental/cognitive parameters can have considerable impact on nutritional status and physical

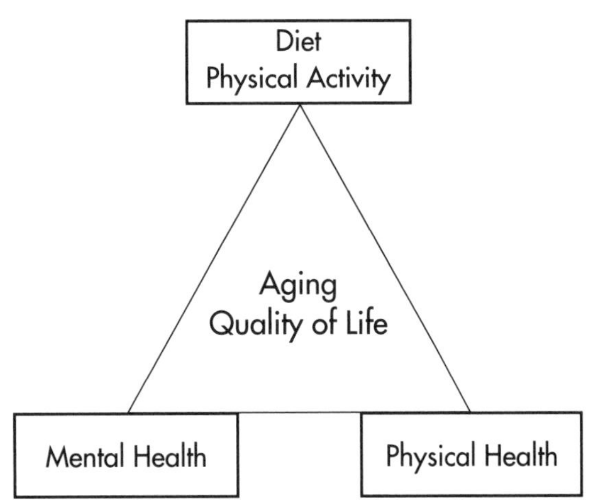

FIGURE 28–1. Determinants of quality of life in the elderly.

Lifestyle factors including diet and physical activity are critical determinants of not only physical health but also mental health of older adults. Together, these components determine quality of life and the success of aging.

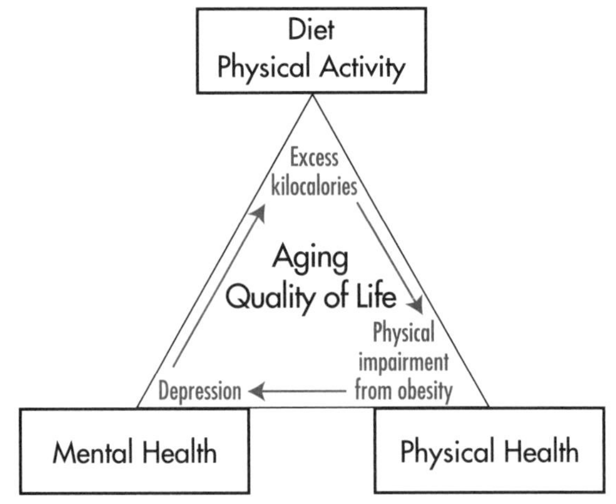

FIGURE 28–2. Example of a cascading problem.

Excess food intake can lead to overweight and obesity that in turn can lead to physical impairment (e.g., mobility problems). Physical impairment may then promote psychiatric symptoms and even depression. To exacerbate the cycle, depression itself may lead to detrimental changes in dietary intake and physical fitness.

activity patterns (Vreeland 2007). As illustrated in Figure 28–1, determinants of the quality of life during aging include physical and mental health, along with both diet and physical activity. These interactions are explored in more detail in the following sections.

Mental Health, Nutritional Status, and Physical Activity: A Complex Interplay

Effect of Diet and Physical Activity on Mental Health and Cognitive Well-Being

Although the specific etiological mechanisms have not been fully delineated, it is well recognized that mental function can be adversely affected by poor dietary choices. As shown in Figure 28–1, the interrelationships among diet and physical activity, mental health, and physical health are critical determinants of health and quality of life among older adults. A problem in any one component can lead to deterioration in other components and in overall health. For example, as shown in Figure 28–2, excess kilocalorie intake may lead to obesity and related physical impairments that may in turn promote depression.

The role of nutrition in the structure and function of the central nervous system is well substantiated, and this effect is manifested throughout the life course. Many of the studies examining nutritional interventions to preserve cognitive function focus on the important roles of inflammation and oxidative stress in normal aging of the brain. Thus, one line of research targets antioxidants that, when consumed from dietary sources, could help slow typical age-related changes in the brain. It is proposed that dietary components such as the polyphenolic compounds found in foods (e.g., blueberries) have favorable effects on signal transduction and neural communications (Lau et al. 2007). Studies of supplementation with these and other compounds are actively underway. Although discussion of preventive nutrition to benefit brain function is beyond the scope of this chapter, the clinical practitioner should be aware of the popularity of this topic with patients and the possibility that patients may be "self-medicating" with foods or supplements that claim to enhance cognitive function.

When a patient presents with mental difficulties for the first time, there is a diverse laundry list of possible nutritional concerns that needs to be considered. Although the effects of nutritional deficits might be transitory, the symptoms can be disabling and are likely to obscure any other underlying mechanisms of impairment. Chronic inadequate food intake is a concern and can lead to weakness, fatigue, and other vague symptoms because of negative energy balance. Certain vitamin deficiencies can have cognitive components; these are addressed more comprehensively in the following section. Dehydration is an important contributor to delirium and confusion in the elderly, who are known to have a diminished thirst response compared with younger adults (Luckey and Parsa 2003). Lack of compliance with therapeutic diet restrictions and instructions can also contribute to poor mental status. For example, when diabetic control is poor, the cognitive effects of both hyperglycemia and hypoglycemia can be marked. The elderly are especially susceptible to hyperglycemia as well as dehydration (Gaglia et al. 2004). Poor glycemic control can also contribute to poor cognitive outcomes in the long term. Gregg et al. (2000) utilized repeated clinical neuropsychological testing to evaluate the relationship of diabetes and disease duration to cognitive function in a large population-based study of older women and found an increased risk of cognitive decline in individuals with diabetes mellitus.

Role of Nutrition in the Etiology of Dementia

The possibility that the lifelong intake of key nutrients or sustained dietary patterns might fundamentally modify the development of major dementias such as Alzheimer's disease is the subject of intense study. If altering a modifiable factor such as diet could preclude the onset of devastating conditions such as dementia and depression, this would, of course, be of incredible public health significance. Nutrients and diet constituents of interest in regard to this question have included consumption patterns for alcohol and fish, the intakes of various types of fats, and vitamins related to homocysteine metabolism. Although no definitive recommendations can be made based on current findings, some of the most recently available related evidence is presented in this section.

Alcohol

Although there are distinct disadvantages to advocating regular alcohol consumption for adults of any age, there is a considerable amount of evidence linking modest to moderate alcohol intake with preservation of cognitive function. A longitudinal study of 1,624 Japanese Americans over age 65 years assessed cognitive performance over time and associated moderate alcohol consumption with beneficial effects on cognitive performance (Bond et al. 2005). Ganguli et al. (2005) monitored a representative elderly cohort for 7 years and reported that a pattern of mild to moderate drinking, compared with nondrinking, was associated with a lower average rate of decline in cognitive domains. Modest intake of alcohol, particularly of wine, has also been linked with lower risk of developing Alzheimer's disease (Luchsinger et al. 2004). It remains to be determined whether alcohol has direct benefits to cognition or whether alcohol use is associated with other factors (e.g., physiological, cultural) that promote these benefits.

Type of Fat and Intake of Fish

Type of fat consumed may be an important determinant of cognitive health. Dietary fats are divided into four general categories: saturated, trans-unsaturated, mono-unsaturated, and poly-unsaturated, with the latter subdivided into omega-6 and omega-3 fats. Saturated and trans-unsaturated fats are likely detrimental to cognitive as well as overall health, whereas mono-unsaturated and poly-unsaturated (especially omega-3) fats are associated with a reduced risk of cognitive decline and dementia (Solfrizzi et al. 2006). Adherence to the Mediterranean diet, characterized by high intake of mono-unsaturated and omega-3 fats, moderate ethanol consumption, and low intake of saturated fats, has been associated with a reduced risk for cognitive decline (Scarmeas et al. 2006).

Because certain fish are the primary food sources of omega-3 fatty acids, several studies have evaluated associations between fish intake and cognitive health. A study of subjects of all ages (>15 yrs; N=4,644) in New Zealand linked good mental health with the consumption of fish (Silvers and Scott 2002). Morris et al. (2005) studied dietary intake of fish and omega-3 fatty acids in relation to cognitive decline in a prospective cohort study of adults age 65 years or older. Although fish consumption was linked with slower rates of cognitive decline in this study, the relationship seemed to be associated with fats (saturated, poly-unsaturated, and trans-unsaturated) other than the omega-3 fatty acid component of the diet.

Vitamins

Epidemiological studies, including longitudinal observations, have been conducted to examine the relationships between vitamin intake and incident dementia. The most commonly studied are folate and vitamin B_{12}, the deficiencies of which have been linked with symptoms of dementia in the elderly (Clarke 2007). A recently reported longitudinal study of adults older than age 65 years who were dementia free at baseline looked at predictors of incident Alzheimer's disease over 6.1±1.3 person-years. Intakes of folate at baseline (assessed by food frequency questionnaire) were associated with a decreased risk of Alzheimer's disease, independent of other risk factors as well as intakes of vitamin B_6 and B_{12} (Luchsinger et al. 2007b). However, Cochrane reviews for folate (M. Malouf et al. 2003) and for vitamins B_{12} (R. Malouf and Areosa Sastre 2003) and B_6 (R. Malouf and Grimley Evans 2003) have not supported a cognitive benefit for these nutrients (Luchsinger et al. 2007a), and there are other such findings in the recent literature (Eussen et al. 2006; Paulionis et al. 2005).

A role of vitamin D in cognitive function has also been suggested (Przybelski and Binkley 2007). Other studies have linked low plasma antioxidant levels with cognitive impairment (*N*=589 elderly subjects) (Akbaraly et al. 2007) and brain white matter hyperintense lesions (*N*=355 subjects ages 45–75 years) (Schmidt et al. 1996). It is likely that other nutrients will also emerge as candidates for promoting optimal cognitive status. Already, some investigators have tried interventions using nutritional supplements to enhance cognitive function in the elderly, with limited success (Wouters-Wesseling et al. 2005). Despite mechanistic theories and encouraging preliminary findings, however, there is no clear consensus on the use of dietary modifications to affect the development of dementia. The available scientific evidence does not support a recommendation of specific nutrients, foods, or diet patterns for the prevention of Alzheimer's disease (Luchsinger et al. 2007a).

Nutrition and Late-Life Depression

Another important concern relating diet with mental health is its potential role in the etiology of depression. Diet may exert its influence on depression risk by promoting physical illnesses that lead to depression, by causing brain changes or other intermediate conditions that are favorable to the development of depression, or potentially by directly promoting depression (see Figure 28–3).

Depression in the elderly is inextricably linked to vascular diseases, including heart disease, diabetes, and stroke. Vascular disease and depression promote one another. Key nutrients are known to be critical factors in determining vascular disease risk and may thus lead indirectly to late-life depression, as shown in Figure 28–3. Vascular promoters include saturated fat, trans-unsaturated fat, cholesterol, high-fat dairy products,

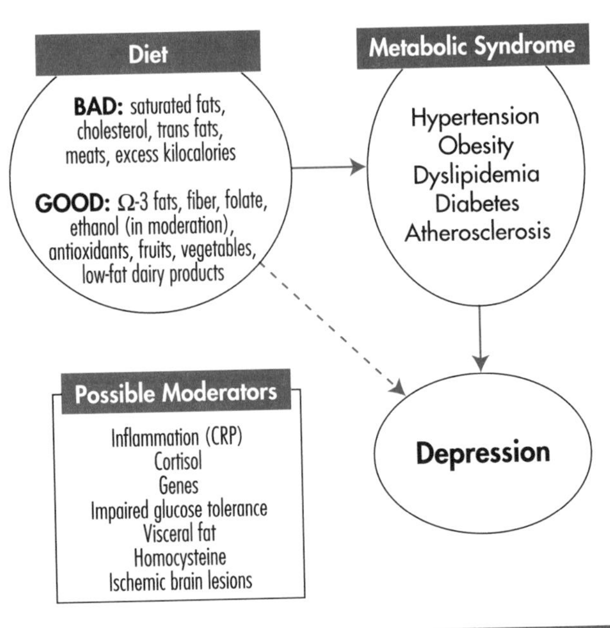

FIGURE 28–3. A dietary mechanism for late-life depression.

Diet may promote (or prevent) depression by influencing one's risk of vascular diseases, including atherosclerosis and diabetes. These vascular diseases are known to promote late-life depression. In addition, diet may directly promote (or prevent) depression by altering neuronal health or neurotransmitter levels. Potential moderators of both pathways include ischemic brain lesions and inflammation.

meats, and excess total energy (kcals) intake. Preventive dietary factors for vascular diseases include monounsaturated and poly-unsaturated fats (including omega-3 fatty acids), fiber, folate, ethanol (in moderation), phytochemicals, fruits, and vegetables. In addition, obesity has been shown to increase risk of depression in the elderly (Roberts et al. 2003).

A number of nutrients, including the B vitamins and omega-3 fatty acids, have been specifically linked to depression. Of the B vitamins, pyridoxine (B_6), cobalamin (B_{12}), and folate (B_9) are essential for serotonin production and myelin formation and have been implicated in depression. Pyridoxine deficiency is common in the elderly, and low levels of pyridoxine have been correlated with depression (Bell et al. 1991; Stewart et al. 1984; Tolonen et al. 1988). However, studies of these factors have not demonstrated that low pyridoxine levels or pyridoxine deficiency cause depression.

Cobalamin deficiency, also common in the elderly, is mostly attributable to an insufficiency of intrinsic factor, necessary for gastrointestinal absorption of B_{12} (Andres et al. 2004). Although prolonged B_{12} deficiency has been shown to cause irreversible neurological damage, its relationship to depression is less clear. Although cross-sectional population studies have associated depression with low B_{12} (Penninx et al. 2000; Tiemeier et al. 2002), longitudinal studies have failed to find an association between depression and B_{12} (Eussen et al. 2002; Sachdev et al. 2005). Folate has been studied extensively in relationship to depression, and its importance may relate to neuronal (serotonin or myelin production) or vascular (including homocysteine metabolism) functions. Clinical studies have found folate levels to be inversely associated with both depression and depression severity (Abou-Saleh and Coppen 1986; Bell et al. 1990; Botez et al. 1982; Bottiglieri et al. 1990; Ghadirian et al. 1980; Hunter et al. 1967; Levitt and Joffe 1989). However, many of these studies failed to control for comorbid disease and other risk factors for depression. In addition, the majority of population and community studies have found no association between folate status and depression (Bjelland et al. 2003; Eussen et al. 2002; Lindeman et al. 2000a; Penninx et al. 2000). The effect of folate status may vary according to genetic profile and may be related to treatment response (see treatment section of this chapter).

There is evidence that omega-3 fatty acid metabolism is altered with depression, but dietary studies have been conflicting (Adams et al. 1996; Maes et al. 1999). Population studies have shown that fish consumption may be protective for depression, associating a higher fish consumption with a decreased risk of depression (Hibbeln 1998; Tanskanen et al. 2001). However, a fish and fish oil supplementation trial conducted in the United Kingdom did not confirm a beneficial effect on depression (Ness et al. 2003). Likewise, a large epidemiological study (*N*=29,133 men ages 50–69 years) did not confirm any beneficial effects of dietary omega-3 fatty acids on mood. In fact, in this study, *higher* intakes of omega-3 fatty acids were reported by subjects with anxiety or depressed mood (Hakkarainen et al. 2004a, 2004b). It may be that some component of fish other than omega-3 fatty acids is responsible for epidemiological studies that link fish intake with beneficial effects on mental health.

Physical Activity as a Determinant of Cognitive Status

Physical activity has been associated with numerous cognitive benefits, including delayed onset of dementia (Larson et al. 2006), higher Mini-Mental State Examination scores (Almeida et al. 2006), and increased brain volumes (Colcombe et al. 2006). Also encouraging are recent reports linking greater aerobic fitness with white matter integrity in certain regions of the brain (Marks et al. 2007). Reported mental well-being is higher in older adults with good mobility status (Lampinen et al. 2006). Acree et al. (2006) measured Health Related Quality of Life (HRQL) in older (mean age=70± 8 years) adults and categorized them by physical activity level. They concluded that older adults who were regular participants in physical activity of at least moderate intensity for more than 1 hour per week had higher HRQL than those who were less active. In contrast, older men living in neighborhoods in which "walkability" was lower were more likely to be depressed than those in environments more supportive of physical activity (Berke et al. 2007).

Even when cognitive deficits are already present, as in depression or dementia patients, a carefully tailored program of physical activity can be beneficial. In a randomized, controlled trial in 134 patients with mild to severe Alzheimer's disease, a simple exercise intervention resulted in a slower decline in the ability to perform activities of daily living (Rolland et al. 2007).

Indirect Effects of Lifestyle Factors on Mental Health

When diet and physical activity behaviors promote medical illnesses, there also may be deterioration in mental health (see Figure 28–1) and in factors that are known to affect brain health. For example, heart disease is known to promote late-life depression. Physical inactivity and numerous nutrients are known to promote heart disease, which may in turn promote late-life depression. Preventive factors for heart disease may thus similarly prevent late-life depression.

In summary, although the effects of lifestyle factors on mental health have been given considerable study, many questions about the specific interplay of nutrition and physical activity remain unanswered.

Impact of Mental Health Status on Diet and Physical Fitness

Mental disorders and other causes of cognitive decline can have profound direct effects on nutritional status and physical activity level. This may be especially important in the elderly, who are likely to be accruing age-related decrements in both the mental and physical domains over time. As shown in Figure 28–1, the interrelationships between diet and physical activity, mental health, and physical health are critical determinants of health and quality of life among older adults. A problem in any one component can lead to deterioration in other components and in overall health.

Mood Disorders

Mood disorders, including major depression and bipolar illness, and situational conditions, such as bereavement and living alone, can significantly affect health behaviors, including diet and physical activity. Depression among the elderly is often characterized by reduced appetite and weight loss (Kolasa et al. 1995; Morley 1996; Pirlich and Lochs 2001; Reife 1995). In fact, many geriatricians consider depression to be the most common cause of poor food intake and nutritional frailty in the elderly (Morley 2001). The loneliness and loss experienced by many elderly individuals affect both mood and dietary status, contributing to the anorexia and malnutrition of aging (Ferry et al. 2005). Locher et al. (2005) conducted in-depth interviews with isolated elderly individuals and reported that when eating alone, they consumed on average 114 fewer calories per meal than when someone joined them at mealtime. In a French survey of 150 adults ages 80 years and older who were living alone, Ferry et al. (2005) documented high rates of undernutrition. In these situations, inadequate nutrient intakes may lead to muscle loss, an increased risk of bone fractures, and nursing home admission (Christensen and Somers 1994).

Although depression can interfere with food intake by affecting general interest in daily activities, there are also possible physiological mechanisms whereby depression could lead to decreased appetite and weight loss. One potential explanation points to corticotrophin-releasing factor, a potent anorectic agent known to be elevated in depressed individuals (Morley 1996). Some have blamed antidepressants for the weight loss associated with depression; however, this relationship was observed long before the advent of psychotropic medications. In addition, only a subset of antidepressants is known to cause weight loss.

Patients who suffer from atypical depression may experience weight gain as a result of increased appetite and inactivity. Obesity may develop or be exacerbated in this situation. In addition to changes in quantity of food consumed in those with depression, food quality may decline. Carbohydrate-rich foods that are lacking in micronutrients (i.e., "junk foods") may be preferred by depressed individuals (Wurtman and Wurtman 1996). Elderly individuals with depression have higher intakes of saturated fat and cholesterol when compared with those without depression (Payne et al. 2006). In addition, lack of energy may curtail healthy eating in depressed people. For example, individuals may eat fast food rather than preparing healthier meals at home.

With regard to physical activity, the loss of energy that may accompany depression naturally makes efforts to exercise extremely difficult. At the other end of the spectrum, some people with depression, bipolar disorder, or other mood disorders experience agitation, an increase in energy, or excessive activity.

Brain Changes and Cognitive Dysfunction

Neurological and psychiatric conditions lead directly and indirectly to cognitive and behavioral difficulties that can greatly impair one's ability to consume a healthy diet and to be physically active. The most obvious of these is stroke, the aftereffects of which can hinder cognitive processes as well as motor skills and other functions. Stroke patients may experience problems chewing or swallowing food as well as cognitive changes that impair their ability to plan meals, shop for food, prepare meals, and make healthy food choices. Malnutrition at the time of hospital admission for stroke is common and contributes to poor outcomes, including increased length of stay, incidence and complications of dysphagia, and likelihood of subsequent need for enteral feeding (Martineau et al. 2005). Depending on its extent and location, paralysis may limit mobility and can cause physical difficulties with food preparation or consumption. Although eventual recovery of some body functions and activities following stroke is common, nutritional status can deteriorate in the 4–10 weeks this recovery can require (Kwakkel et al. 2006). In addition, some stroke patients do not fully recover their ability to eat but remain at high nutritional risk for months (Carlsson et al. 2004). In a study of patients admitted to a geriatric rehabilitation unit following an ischemic stroke, 35% were malnourished at 1 week poststroke, and 22% remained malnourished at 6 months (Brynningsen et al. 2007). Evidence-based guidelines for nutrition support in acute stroke have been developed and linked with improvements in some patient outcomes (Perry and McLaren 2003).

A variety of dementias, characterized by numerous cognitive deficits, may also lead to changes in dietary behavior. Along with vascular dementia, Alzheimer's disease is a leading cause of dementia in the elderly, affecting 4.9 million Americans ages 65 and older, with the following age group breakdowns:

- Ages 65–74: 2%, or 300,000 people
- Ages 75–84: 19%, or 2,400,000 people
- Ages 85+: 42%, or 2,200,000 people

Thus, the nutritional risks posed by this disease constitute a major geriatric concern. Patients with Alzheimer's disease tend to lose weight early in the disease process (White et al. 1996), which can lead to serious consequences, including increased mortality (White et al. 1998). Early weight loss may be caused by inadequate access to food and the inability to prepare food. Appetite alterations (caused by taste and/or smell alterations) and anorexia (caused by the effect of inflammatory mediators such as the cytokines) may also play a role. Some patients deteriorate to the point of being unable to consume sufficient oral intake to sustain life, and tube feedings may be initiated. Unfortunately, the survival rates are poor and are not improved by the tube feeding in most cases (Mitchell et al. 2003).

In addition to stroke and dementia, ischemic and other forms of damage may occur in the brain, particularly in elderly individuals. As with stroke, the brain regions affected are likely to determine the symptoms, which can include changes in appetite, psychomotor changes, and cognitive impairment. Cognitive impairment may also occur with depression, bipolar disorder, schizophrenia, delirium, and a variety of other disorders. As with stroke, cognitive impairment can lead to weight loss or malnutrition by hindering meal planning, food choices, and food purchasing and preparation. In severe cases individuals may forget to eat or how to eat.

Stroke, dementia, and other cognitive problems are likely to affect physical activity in addition to nutritional status. Although many individuals impaired by these conditions have the ability to be active at some level, for safety reasons they need to be carefully supervised, and it may be difficult for them to follow instructions about proper performance and safety aspects of the exercise.

Alcoholism

Alcoholism is a condition with considerable impact on both mental and physical health because it occurs at the intersection of nutritional imbalance and mental disorders. People with alcoholism often consume inadequate amounts of vitamins and minerals and may have an insufficient intake of protein. Not only does ethanol displace healthier dietary components, but behavioral manifestations of alcoholism may hinder consumption of a nutritionally adequate diet. In addition, alcoholic individuals may develop deficiencies of certain nutrients (e.g., folate, other B vitamins) because of malabsorption (Halsted et al. 2002). Chronic alcohol misuse can lead to severe vitamin depletion and the development of Wernicke-Korsakoff syndrome in susceptible individuals (Thomson 2000).

Interaction of Treatments With Nutrition and Physical Activity

Nutritional status can affect and be affected by mental health treatments, particularly pharmacological ones. The most obvious concern is for nutrient-drug interactions. Other issues are weight changes caused by drug treatment and side effects that affect dietary habits. Diet and physical activity have also been used as treatments for mental illness. Finally, nutritional status can influence treatment outcomes.

Nutrient-Drug Interactions

Use of medications, including polypharmacy, is higher among the elderly than among younger adults. This situation, combined with the physiological changes of aging, contributes to drug-related problems including nutrient-drug interactions (Knight-Klimas and Boullata 2004). The poor nutritional state that is common in elderly individuals can exacerbate nutrient-drug interactions. A serious example of a nutrient-drug interaction is a hypertensive crisis resulting from consumption of tyramine-containing foods during monoamine oxidase inhibitor (MAOI) therapy (McCabe 1986). Although addressing the list of possible nutrient-drug interactions with psychotropic medications is beyond the scope of this chapter, a general approach is recommended. Clinicians should 1) consider the patient's nutritional status (including malnutrition, nutrient deficiencies, and body weight) and current diet (including intake of vitamin, mineral, and herbal dietary supplements), 2) evaluate the potential for known nutrient-drug interactions for the medication being considered (which can be obtained from a nutrient-drug interaction reference book or a pharmacist), and 3) discontinue the offending agent and/or institute appropriate dietary modifications, if indicated.

Other Treatment Concerns

In addition to nutrient-drug interactions, side effects from medications can lead to changes in diet and nutritional status. For example, tricyclic antidepressants and conventional antipsychotics often lead to weight gain, whereas some selective serotonin reuptake inhibitors (SSRIs) cause weight loss. Side effects such as dry mouth or nausea may affect the quality or quantity of food intake. The potential nutritional consequences of psychotropic medications should be considered before and throughout treatment.

Diet and Physical Activity as Psychiatric Treatment

Dietary manipulation and physical activity regimens have been used to treat mental disorders. For example, aerobic exercise has been shown to be as effective as antidepressants in treating major depression in the elderly (Blumenthal and Babyak 1999). Omega-3 fatty acids have been used successfully in bipolar disorder (Osher et al. 2005) and schizophrenia (Peet 2003). Nutritional status may also affect treatment outcomes of these disorders. For example, baseline folate status has been positively associated with response to SSRIs in elderly depressed patients (Alpert et al. 2003). Finally, it should be noted that some individuals who have mental health problems take dietary supplements, including vitamins, minerals, and herbal supplements, as a means of treating their condition. For example, St. John's wort (*Hypericum perforatum*) shows some antidepressant properties (Kasper et al. 2006) but has not been studied sufficiently in elderly populations. In addition to safety concerns about a minority of herbal supplements, dietary supplement users are at risk for consuming specific nutrients in amounts far exceeding those which would be attainable through diet, with possible detriment to health.

Achieving Optimal Nutrition and Physical Fitness in Later Life

Nutritional Issues and Wellness Barriers for Older Adults

Elderly individuals are at increased nutritional risk caused by the normal changes of aging (e.g., loss of lean muscle and bone mass, decline in immune function and oral health) (Morley 2001) as well as the difficulties associated with chronic and acute medical conditions (Chernoff 2005). Age-related changes lead to a variety of problems with eating, including difficulties with chewing, swallowing, digestion, and absorption of nutrients. For example, atrophic gastritis occurs in 10%–30% of adults over age 50 years, reducing the absorption of vitamin B_{12} and mineral nutrients that require an acid environment for optimal absorption (Ho et al. 1999).

Age-associated decrements in energy requirements (discussed later in this chapter) lead to reduced food intake and thus a decrease in nutrient consumption. As appetites diminish, overall diet quality may also suffer as foods that are less well liked (e.g., vegetables) may be the first to be eliminated and comfort foods that are high in fat and low in micronutrients may tend to predominate in the diet (Chernoff 2005). Chronic medical conditions lead to impaired nutritional and functional status and are linked with overall decline (Black and Rush 2002; Fried and Guralnik 1997). The complications of chronic illness and the side effects of medications and other medical interventions for chronic conditions (e.g., special diets, surgery, chemotherapy) decrease the likelihood of achieving nutritional adequacy on a regular basis. The introduction of therapeutic diets for these conditions also increases the likelihood of poor nutritional status (Niedert 2005). In addition, environmental, social, financial, and functional barriers can compound nutritional risk.

To promote ideal health behaviors through lifestyle changes, it is first necessary to recognize the potential barriers to behavior change that inevitably present themselves. Environmental and social factors strongly influence dietary intake and ultimate nutritional adequacy (Locher et al. 2005). Limited social contact (e.g., eating meals alone) affects dietary intake, as does inadequate assistance with shopping and preparing food. Institutionalization (hospital, assisted living, nursing home) is almost always linked with increased nutritional risk. Fixed-income limitations put some elders in the position of choosing between other essential expenses such as prescription medications and money to be spent on nutritious foods.

Primer on Nutritional Assessment

The major elements of nutritional assessment are its dietary, biochemical, and clinical components. A thorough nutritional assessment should combine elements of all three domains. Conventionally accepted methods of dietary assessment include diet histories, 24-hour recall interviews, food records, and abbreviated food frequency questionnaires. These tools often are difficult to implement because of time and effort burdens, cognitive and/or memory limitations of the patient, or the lack of a proxy source in the cases where the patient is not able to give a firsthand account of foods eaten. Assessment approaches that rely solely on memory (e.g., 24-hour recall) may be less accurate than information enriched by an ongoing record or checklist that can be completed as soon as a meal is eaten (van Staveren et al. 1994).

The most commonly used biochemical assessment is for one or more markers of protein status. Albumin is one of the most abundant and commonly measured serum proteins. However, it has a relatively long half-life (18 days) and is also known to decrease with age. Because chronic or acute inflammation, advanced liver disease, heart failure, nephrotic syndrome, and protein-losing enteropathy can all result in hypoalbuminemia, serum albumin is not recommended as a sole marker of nutritional status (Sullivan et al. 2002). Other serum proteins that have been studied as protein status markers are prealbumin (or transthyretin) and insulin-like growth factor (IGF-1). Prealbumin is a transport protein for thyroxine with a half-life of 2 days. Prealbumin levels usually show daily improvements with good nutritional repletion. IGF-1 is a peptide produced by the liver for which levels drop rapidly during starvation and increase during nutritional repletion. IGF-1 has a very short half-life of 2–4 hours and a relatively small body pool, making it very sensitive to nutritional changes. In hospitalized older adults, low IGF-1 levels are associated with higher morbidity and life-threatening complications (Sullivan and Carter 1994). Blood tests for levels of individual micronutrients are rarely done because they are expensive, difficult to obtain (not routinely performed in most clinical laboratories), and not always indicative of actual nutrient status.

Clinical indications of poor nutritional status include fatigue, weakness, changes in ability to taste or smell, gastrointestinal complaints (poor appetite, oral problems, nausea, vomiting, diarrhea, constipation), and changes in mental or emotional status (Fabiny and Kiel 1997). For the detection of underweight status and risk of frailty, serial measurement of body weight offers the simplest and most helpful indicator. A decrease in weight exceeding 2% of baseline body weight in 1 month, 5% in 3 months, or 10% in 6 months is considered clinically significant. Even a stable weight may not ensure that all is well. Age-related loss of muscle mass, or sarcopenia, is very common and is strongly associated with disability, independent of morbidity (Baumgartner 1998). Anthropometrically, arm muscle area can be calculated by using a triceps skin fold (TSF) and the mean arm circumference (MAC), although the measurement requires relatively complex equations (Heymsfield 1982), as shown here:

Men:
$$\text{Arm muscle area} = [(\text{MAC} - \pi \times \text{TSF})^2 / 4\pi] - 10$$

Women:
$$\text{Arm muscle area} = [(\text{MAC} - \pi \times \text{TSF})^2 / 4\pi] - 6.5$$

It should also be noted that overnutrition (and, in particular, increased fat mass with decreased muscle mass, or "sarcopenic obesity") may be masked by normal to slightly above normal body weight.

Another approach to nutritional assessment makes use of indices such as the Mini Nutritional Assessment (MNA) or the Subjective Global Assessment (SGA). The MNA (http://www.mna-elderly.com) is a validated tool (predictive value for detecting undernutrition of 97%) that incorporates several domains, including functional status, lifestyle, diet, self-perception of health, and anthropometric indices (Donini 2003). The SGA uses a history and physical examination and is used to derive a clinical grade of nutritional status (Detsky et al. 1994; Sacks et al. 2000). However, neither of these indices addresses the potential that overweight could be masking the existence of micronutrient deficiencies.

General Nutrition Recommendations

Dietary Reference Intakes

Although calorie needs decline with age (see next section), the requirements for most other nutrients do not, making dietary nutrient density important at a time when the added complications of chronic illness and the side effects of medications and other medical interventions for chronic conditions (e.g., special diets, surgery, chemotherapy) decrease the likelihood of achieving it. Dietary requirements are expressed as Dietary Reference Intakes (DRIs), including Recommended Daily Allowances (RDAs) or Adequate Intakes (AIs) as appropriate, for all recognized essential nutrients, including macronutrients, vitamins, and minerals (Institute of

Medicine 1997, 1998, 2000, 2005). In previously released versions of these recommendations, the oldest age category was 51 years and older, so it is important to note that the most recently released recommendations include recommendations for those older than 70 years of age. Tables 28–1 and 28–2 show the DRIs (consisting of RDAs, or AIs when RDAs are not available) for the older adult age categories. These recommendations are most helpful in terms of guiding nutritional assessment and supplementation with regard to the micronutrients (vitamins and minerals). More specific guidelines are needed to individualize recommendations for energy and macronutrient intakes.

Energy-Yielding Nutrients and Alcohol

The DRI recommendations for macronutrients are given in Table 28–1. The Institute of Medicine has also published formulas for calculation of total daily energy expenditures (TDEE) based on height, weight, age, activity level, and gender (Institute of Medicine 2005). These equations (replacing the previously used Harris Benedict equations) were developed for use in normal and overweight individuals age 19 years or older, and are as follows:

Men:

$$\text{TDEE} = 864 - (9.72 \times \text{age [y]}) + \text{PA} \times (14.2 \times \text{weight [kg]} + 503 \times \text{height [m]})$$

Women:

$$\text{TDEE} = 387 - (7.31 \times \text{age [y]}) + \text{PA} \times (10.9 \times \text{weight [kg]} + 660.7 \times \text{height [m]})$$

where PA=1.00 assumes that physical activity level is sedentary.

Energy requirements decline with age because of reductions in metabolic rate, loss of lean body mass, and a diminution of energy expenditure for physical activity. A progressive reduction in TDEE occurs with age, assumed to be about 7 kcal and 10 kcal per year for adult women and men, respectively. Although food intake and calorie (energy) intakes also decrease with age, before age 60 years there is rarely a detrimental effect, the reduced energy intake being more than offset by the aforementioned decrements in requirements. In fact, overweight and excess adiposity pose serious health risks in middle and early old age and persist as a late-life concern for some individuals (Villareal et al. 2005). However, energy deficits and poor nutrient intakes are the most likely nutritional concerns in late life. From the decades of the 20s through 80s, mean energy intakes were reduced by up to 1,200 kcal in men and up to 800 kcal in women, according to the Third National Health and Nutrition Examination Survey (NHANES-III; Wakimoto and Block 2001). It is well recognized that inadequate energy intakes and low body mass indices (BMIs) are linked with frailty in the elderly (Markson 1997). Poor food intake also jeopardizes the adequacy of micronutrients; food choices may be poor when appetites falter.

The current RDA for protein (4 kcal/g) is 0.80 g/kg/day and is the same for adults of all ages. Protein intakes decrease with age; however, because typical protein intakes generously exceed the recommended levels, the amount of protein intake usually remains sufficient to meet the needs of healthy elderly populations. However, as is the case with energy, protein insufficiency is a concern in some high-risk individuals, especially during the stress of medical illness and commonly when institutionalization occurs.

Fat is another macronutrient that provides energy and is, in fact, the major fuel source for the body (providing 9 kcal/g). In addition, it is needed for the absorption of fat-soluble vitamins and other dietary components. As was stated previously, dietary fats are divided into four general categories: saturated, trans-unsaturated, mono-unsaturated, and poly-unsaturated, with the latter subdivided into omega-6 and omega-3 fats. Only certain fatty acids must be consumed from the diet (essential fatty acids)—namely, two of the long-chain poly-unsaturated fatty acids: linolenic (an omega-3) and linoleic (an omega-6). Saturated fatty acids, mono-unsaturated fatty acids, and cholesterol can be synthesized by the body. Trans fats are not needed by the body and are, in fact, detrimental to health. The dietary intake of fat, as well as cholesterol, declines with age. The percentage of calories coming from fat in the diet also declines and reaches its lowest value in the oldest age groups (Wakimoto and Block 2001).

Carbohydrates are divided into starches and sugars (monosaccharides and disaccharides) and are also an important energy source for the body (providing 4 kcal/gram). A minimum amount of carbohydrate (130 grams for adults) must be consumed daily in order to meet needs that cannot be met by another fuel source (e.g., fat). Glucose is the only fuel source used by erythrocytes and is the preferred energy source for the brain, which accounts for 20% of the body's resting metabolic rate (Siegel 1999). In the absence of sufficient dietary

TABLE 28–1. Dietary Reference Intakes for adults ages 51 years and older

				Fat[c] (g)	
Age (years)	Protein[a] (g)	Carbohydrate (g)	Fiber (total)[b] (g)	Linoleic acid[b]	α-Linolenic acid[b]
Men					
51–70	56	130	30	14	1.6
>70	56	130	30	14	1.6
Women					
51–70	46	130	21	11	1.1
>70	46	130	21	11	1.1

[a]0.80 g/kg/day
[b]Adequate Intakes (AIs) represent the recommended average daily intake level based on observed or experimentally determined approximations. AIs are used when there is insufficient information to determine a Recommended Dietary Allowance.
[c]There is no Dietary Reference Intake for total fat because of insufficient data. AIs are given in this table for essential fatty acids.

Source. Institute of Medicine 2005.

carbohydrate, liver glycogen and skeletal muscle are broken down to generate glucose.

In recent years, the popularity of low-carbohydrate diets for weight loss (Yancy et al. 2004) and findings regarding the benefits of protein for satiety have renewed interest in manipulations of macronutrient proportions in the diet. In fact, a number of different distributions of macronutrients (e.g., Mediterranean diet pattern, vegetarian diet) other than the more traditional low-fat diet can be used to achieve a healthy dietary pattern (Malik and Hu 2007).

Although alcohol does yield calories (7 kcal/g), recommendations about alcohol for older adults are difficult to reconcile based on the available scientific evidence. The intake of moderate amounts of alcohol by older adults is linked with decreased risk of cardiovascular disease (thought to be caused by decreased inflammation and increased high-density lipoproteins) (Mukamal et al. 2006), risk of ischemic stroke (except in *APOE*E4*-positive individuals) (Mukamal et al. 2005), bone density of the hip (Mukamal et al. 2007), and even dementia (Mukamal et al. 2003). Yet the issue of alcohol misuse and abuse among the elderly is a concern, and particularly so when any cognitive impairment is present. Therefore it is difficult to apply these research findings given the inadvisability of promoting ethanol consumption in the elderly because of concerns about falls and alcohol abuse (see section on alcoholism earlier in this chapter). However, if a patient already consumes light to moderate amounts of alcohol on a regular basis and is not having problems, it may be acceptable for this level of consumption to continue, and it may be beneficial to suggest consumption of red wine, which is the alcoholic beverage that contains the highest levels of beneficial phytochemical compounds.

Fiber and Water

Recommended fiber intakes (20–30 grams per day) are almost never met. Improving the intakes of dietary fiber may help prevent age-related chronic diseases such as diabetes (Meyer et al. 2000) and cancer (Dreosti 1998). The importance of hydration is well recognized in geriatric individuals, and most typically the concern is about dehydration, because the thirst response is diminished in the elderly (Kayser-Jones 2006). But there are also potential negative effects of excessive water consumption, including dilutional hyponatremia (water intoxication) and increased nocturia (Morley 2000). It is recommended that healthy older adults consume approximately six glasses of fluid a day (Lindeman et al. 2000b), except during stressful situations when more is needed because of fluid loss (e.g., severely hot weather, heavy exertion).

Use of Nutritional Supplements

Elderly individuals are more likely to use vitamin and other nutrient supplements than younger adults, with the rate of their use among older Americans estimated at 31%–56%, based on data from NHANES-III (Ervin et al. 1999). Trends are for greater use of vitamins and supplements by women than by men and in white individuals compared with black individuals (Houston 1997; Subar and Block 1990). As is commonly found for all adults, the choice to take a nutritional supple-

TABLE 28–2. Dietary Reference Intakes for adults ages 51 years and older

Gender Age (years)	Vitamin A (μg retinol activity equivalents)	Vitamin D[a] (μg)	Vitamin E (mg)	Vitamin K[a] (μg)	Vitamin C (mg)	Thiamin (mg)	Riboflavin (mg)	Niacin (mg)	Folacin (μg)
Men									
51–70	900	10	15	120	90	1.2	1.3	16	400
>70	900	15	15	120	90	1.2	1.3	16	400
Women									
51–70	700	10	15	90	75	1.1	1.1	14	400
>70	700	15	15	90	75	1.1	1.1	14	400
	Vitamin B_6 (mg)	**Vitamin B_{12} (μg)**	**Calcium[a] (mg)**	**Magnesium (mg)**	**Iron (mg)**	**Zinc (mg)**	**Copper (μg)**	**Chromium[a] (μg)**	**Selenium (μg)**
Men									
51–70	1.7	2.4	1,200	420	8	11	900	30	55
>70	1.7	2.4	1,200	420	8	11	900	30	55
Women									
51–70	1.5	2.4	1,200	320	8	11	900	20	55
>70	1.5	2.4	1,200	320	8	11	900	20	55

[a]Adequate Intakes (AIs) represent the recommended average daily intake level based on observed or experimentally determined approximations. AIs are used when there is insufficient information to determine a Recommended Dietary Allowance.

Source. Institute of Medicine 1997, 1998, 2000.

ment does not seem linked to severity of health problems but rather is more likely to occur in those with strong health-seeking behaviors (Payette and Gray-Donald 1991). Thus, the health benefits of nutritional supplements may be subtle and related more to health promotion than to the prevention of overt deficiency. However, these benefits can still be important and include reduced plasma homocysteine levels (McKay et al. 2000), improved antioxidant status (Girodon et al. 1999), and enhanced immune function (Bogden et al. 1994; Chandra 1992).

Although most experts support the recommendation that all older adults take a multivitamin/mineral supplement, it is important to carefully consider the types and amounts of supplements being chosen. Potential risks from excessive intakes of specific nutrients include the possibility of increased risk of hip fractures with vitamin A (Feskanich et al. 2002; Melhus et al. 1998) and the aggravation of iron overload by mineral supplements containing iron. Supplemental iron, unless given to remedy an anemic condition, may be unwise for those who are homozygous or heterozygous for mutations of the hemochromatosis-associated gene, because even relatively modest amounts of supplemental iron could increase the likelihood of diabetes and cardiovascular disease in these individuals (Garry et al. 1982). A meta-analysis linked use of high-dose vitamin E supplements with an increase in all-cause mortality (Miller et al. 2005). Long-term zinc supplementation, especially at higher doses, can interfere with copper status and impair immune function (Bogden 2004; McClain et al. 2002). Of particular concern in regard to nutrition and mental health is the possibility that large intakes of folate (or folic acid) could mask symptoms of a vitamin B_{12} deficiency. The interaction of folate and vitamin B_{12} with metabolism makes it essential to ensure that intake and status of these two nutrients are in balance. A recent study of serum levels of folate and vitamin B_{12} in the elderly (N=1,459) found that in seniors with low vitamin B_{12} levels, high serum folate was linked with cognitive impairment. However, in subjects with normal B_{12} levels, high serum folate was protective against cognitive impairment (Morris et al. 2007). Deficiencies of vitamin B_{12} are more likely than folate deficiencies in this age group, particularly since the institution of wide-scale folic acid fortification of U.S. grain foods in the late 1990s for the purpose of reducing birth defects. With the 85%–100% higher bioavailability of the synthetic form of folate (folic acid) found in supplements and fortified foods (including breakfast cereals, which are frequently consumed by the elderly), all adults, including the elderly, now have higher intakes of this nutrient. Individuals who consume both a folate supplement and fortified cereals may be at risk for excess folate intake (Mulligan et al. 2007). In this case, and whenever folic acid supplements are given, it is important that a supplement of vitamin B_{12} should also be included.

When a nutritional supplement is needed, it is generally best to rely on a multivitamin/mineral-type supplement that meets approximately 100% of the DRI recommendations. However, it should be noted that the amount of calcium contained in a multitype supplement is too low (generally less than 200 mg) to be physiologically important. If supplemental calcium is needed, it should be provided as a single nutrient supplement or as part of a fortified food such as calcium-fortified orange juice. Vitamin D should also be taken to ensure adequate calcium uptake and may have other beneficial properties as well. Vitamin D can be administered as part of a calcium supplement or separately.

General Physical Activity Recommendations

Benefits of Exercise

Physical activity is essential for optimal health throughout the life cycle, providing protection against a diverse array of diseases and disorders linked with aging, including cardiovascular disease, thromboembolic stroke, diabetes mellitus, osteoporosis, certain cancers, anxiety, and depression (Nelson et al. 2007). Prevention of the risk of falls and associated injuries is another key benefit. Physical activity preserves muscle mass and strength as well as bone mineral density and has been linked with improved mood and sleep patterns.

Initiating a fitness program to increase activity levels in a sedentary person requires an exercise assessment and subsequent individualization of the exercise prescription to avoid injuries to the musculoskeletal or cardiovascular system. Physical limitations must be identified, specific exercises selected, and exertion ranges established. The American College of Sports Medicine (2005) provides detailed guidance for fitness assessments and exercise prescriptions. Ongoing reassessment will allow upgrades of the program in response to progress by the participant. It should be stressed that some level of physical activity is almost always beneficial, even in individuals with physical limitations or chronic health conditions.

Recommendations for Physical Activity and Exercise in Older Adults

A panel composed of public health, behavioral science, epidemiology, exercise science, medicine, and gerontology experts has released recommendations on physical activity for older adults based on prior recommendations from the American College of Sports Medicine and the American Heart Association as well as relevant evidence from primary research and existing consensus statements (Nelson et al. 2007). These new recommendations advise on the types and amount of physical activity that will benefit the health of older adults and include the following:

- *Aerobic activities.* Moderate-intensity activity beyond routine activities of daily living and lasting greater than 10 minutes in duration is necessary to benefit the health of older adults. Moderate-intensity aerobic activity is best described as producing noticeable increases in heart rate and breathing and ranking on a level of 5 or 6 on a 10-point scale, in which sitting is 0 and maximal effort is 10. To promote and maintain health, older adults should participate in such aerobic activity for at least 30 minutes, 5 days each week.
- *Muscle-strengthening activities.* Older adults will also benefit from resistance weight training that will maintain or enhance muscular strength. Exercises should be repeated 10–15 times at a moderate to high level of effort. The benefits of prescribed and supervised resistance training include the enhancement of muscular strength and endurance, functional capacity, independence, and quality of life; these and other attributes of resistance exercise were recently summarized in a scientific statement from the American Heart Association (Williams et al. 2007). The American Geriatrics Society published specific guidelines for resistance training in the elderly in 2001 (American Geriatrics Society Panel on Exercise and Osteoarthritis 2001) as follows:

Low:	40% 1RM; 10–15 reps
Moderate:	40–60% 1RM; 8–10 reps
High:	>60% 1RM; 6–8 reps

  where RM=range of motion and reps=repetitions.
- *Activities to increase flexibility.* Flexibility is important in everyday physical activity, and therefore older adults should spend at least 10 minutes, 2 days each week, on exercises that will maintain or increase flexibility.
- *Exercises to improve balance.* Many older adults are at risk of falls, and in order to reduce the ensuing risk of injury, they should participate in activity that focuses on maintaining or improving balance.
- *Development and implementation of an activity plan.* Older adults seeking to reach the recommended levels of physical activity should implement a plan of gradual increase in exercise over time. It is acceptable to spend time with activity that is lower than the recommended amount as long as there is a stepwise increase toward sufficiency. Each recommended type of activity, as well as how, when, and where such exercise should occur, must be addressed in the plan, and older adults should self-monitor and reevaluate their individual activity plans as their physical ability and health status vary.

Special Caveats for Older Adults

Older adults are capable of reaching high levels of physical activity, although it may be difficult for some to do. Physical activity should therefore be promoted in particular ways so as to encourage older adults in reaching their potential. Although achieving the recommended level of exercise is ideal, those who participate in lower levels of activity still benefit in terms of health, and this should be emphasized to those who cannot reach the recommended goal. Similarly, engaging in moderate activity at recommended levels is more important than working toward vigorous activity, because the latter increases the risk of injury and reduces adherence to the exercise plan (Franklin et al. 2000). Vigorous activity may be difficult to reach because of age-related loss of fitness, chronic diseases, or functional limitations and should not be emphasized in promoting physical activity of the elderly. In reaching a level of moderate activity, older adults should take care to increase exercise over time so as to reduce risk of injury from overuse and allow for attainment of intermediate goals. Experience, fitness, and self-confidence are all necessary in reaching the optimal level of physical activity and may be acquired through spending a period of time at one step. Part of such exercise should focus on muscle-strengthening activity, because this plays a strong role in preventing loss of muscle mass (Tseng et al. 1995) and bone (Nelson et al. 2004). Given that only 12% of older adults currently partake in such activities, the importance of muscle-strengthening activities should be promoted in recommending type of exercise.

Minimizing Risk During Exercise

Almost all older adults can and should be physically active on a regular basis. Although there are always concerns about safety, the majority of older persons experience few problems if they receive appropriate guidance in planning their activity program. However, heart disease, osteoporosis, and musculoskeletal injuries may increase the risk of adverse events and should be managed appropriately (Hootman et al. 2002). Cardiac arrest is a rare event, and exercise incorporated in leisure-time activity has been shown to reduce the risk of sudden death (Albert et al. 2000; Lemaitre et al. 1999). The risk of musculoskeletal injuries can be kept to a minimum by providing appropriate supervision and guidance for the use of warm-up routines and suitable equipment. Alternatives such as t'ai chi and pool exercises with motion against water resistance often can be safely employed (Hartman et al. 2000). In individuals with osteoporosis, fractures caused by falls or unsafe movements are a concern. Fractures are exceedingly painful and necessitate cessation of exercise until healing is complete. Specialized instructions for exercise programs in patients with osteoporosis have been developed (Bonner et al. 2003).

Conclusion

Diet and physical activity are important determinants of both overall health and mental health. Although the specific mechanisms by which these lifestyle parameters affect mental function are not fully understood, there is no question that healthy dietary intakes and a physically active lifestyle promote and help sustain optimal cognitive function. The guidelines presented here can benefit all patients and should be a part of the regular care plan. In order to assist patients in setting and achieving realistic behavioral goals, the physician should partner with other professionals, consulting with dietitians, speech language pathologists, dentists, and pharmacists regarding dietary needs and involving physical and occupational therapy as well as other specialists to individualize the physical activity program.

Key Points

- Nutrition and physical activity are important determinants of overall health and also play an important role in key elements of mental health and cognitive status.
- Although a number of lifestyle factors have been implicated in the etiology of mental disorders, the available scientific evidence does not support a recommendation of specific nutrients, foods, or diet patterns for the prevention of dementia.
- Because late-life depression is known to interact with vascular disease, depressed individuals should be encouraged to adhere to a diet that will reduce their vascular risk.
- Regular physical activity appears to benefit cognitive health and is therapeutic for depression and dementia in terms of function and quality of life.
- Mental disorders that can negatively affect nutritional and physical fitness status include depression and dementia. Treatments for these conditions also may affect nutrition and activity patterns.
- Older adults should consume a varied diet that provides the recommended amounts of all essential nutrients and meets, but does not exceed, energy requirements.

References

Abou-Saleh MT, Coppen A: The biology of folate in depression: implications for nutritional hypotheses of the psychoses. J Psychiatr Res 20:91–101, 1986

Acree LS, Longfors J, Fjeldstad AS, et al: Physical activity is related to quality of life in older adults. Health Qual Life Outcomes 4:37, 2006

Adams PB, Lawson S, Sanigorski A, et al: Arachidonic acid to eicosapentaenoic acid ratio in blood correlates positively with clinical symptoms of depression. Lipids 31(suppl):S157–S161, 1996

Akbaraly NT, Faure H, Gourlet V, et al: Plasma carotenoid levels and cognitive performance in an elderly population: results of the EVA Study. J Gerontol A Biol Sci Med Sci 62:308–316, 2007

Albert CM, Mittleman MA, Chae CU, et al: Triggering of sudden death from cardiac causes by vigorous exertion. N Engl J Med 343:1355–1361, 2000

Almeida OP, Norman P, Hankey G, et al: Successful mental health aging: results from a longitudinal study of older Australian men. Am J Geriatr Psychiatry 14:27–35, 2006

Alpert M, Silva RR, Pouget ER: Prediction of treatment response in geriatric depression from baseline folate level: interaction with an SSRI or a tricyclic antidepressant. J Clin Psychopharmacol 23:309–313, 2003

American College of Sports Medicine: ACSM's Guidelines for Exercise Testing and Prescription, 7th Edition. Philadelphia, PA, Lippincott Williams & Wilkins, 2005

American Geriatrics Society Panel on Exercise and Osteoarthritis: Exercise prescriptions for older adults with osteoarthritis pain: consensus practice recommendations: a supplement to the AGS Clinical Practice Guidelines on the management of chronic pain in older adults. J Am Geriatr Soc 49:808–823, 2001

Andres E, Loukili NH, Noel E, et al: Vitamin B12 (cobalamin) deficiency in elderly patients. CMAJ 171:251–259, 2004

Baumgartner RN, Koehler KM, Gallagher D, et al: Epidemiology of sarcopenia among the elderly in New Mexico. Am J Epidemiol 147:755–763, 1998

Bell IR, Edman JS, Marby DW, et al: Vitamin B12 and folate status in acute geropsychiatric inpatients: affective and cognitive characteristics of a vitamin nondeficient population. Biol Psychiatry 27:125–137, 1990

Bell IR, Edman JS, Morrow FD, et al: B complex vitamin patterns in geriatric and young adult inpatients with major depression. J Am Geriatr Soc 39:252–257, 1991

Berke EM, Gottlieb LM, Moudon AV, et al: Protective association between neighborhood walkability and depression in older men. J Am Geriatr Soc 55:526–533, 2007

Bjelland I, Tell GS, Vollset SE, et al: Folate, vitamin B12, homocysteine, and the MTHFR 677C→T polymorphism in anxiety and depression: the Hordaland Homocysteine Study. Arch Gen Psychiatry 60:618–626, 2003

Black SA, Rush RD: Cognitive and functional decline in adults aged 75 and older. J Am Geriatr Soc 50:1978–1986, 2002

Blumenthal JA, Babyak MA, Moore KA, et al: Effects of exercise training on older patients with major depression. Arch Intern Med 159:2349–2356, 1999

Bogden JD: Influence of zinc on immunity in the elderly. J Nutr Health Aging 8:48–54, 2004

Bogden JD, Bendich A, Kemp FW, et al: Daily micronutrient supplements enhance delayed-hypersensitivity skin test responses in older people. Am J Clin Nutr 60:437–447, 1994

Bond GE, Burr RL, McCurry SM, et al: Alcohol and cognitive performance: a longitudinal study of older Japanese Americans. The Kame Project. Int Psychogeriatr 17:653–668, 2005

Bonner FJ Jr, Sinaki M, Grabois M, et al: Health professional's guide to rehabilitation of the patient with osteoporosis. Osteoporos Int 14 (suppl 2):S1–S22, 2003

Botez MI, Young SN, Bachevalier J, et al: Effect of folic acid and vitamin B12 deficiencies on 5-hydroxyindoleacetic acid in human cerebrospinal fluid. Ann Neurol 12:479–484, 1982

Bottiglieri T, Hyland K, Laundy M, et al: Enhancement of recovery from psychiatric illness by methylfolate. Lancet 336:1579–1580, 1990

Brynningsen PK, Damsgaard EM, Husted SE: Improved nutritional status in elderly patients 6 months after stroke. J Nutr Health Aging 11:75–79, 2007

Carlsson E, Ehrenberg A, Ehnfors M: Stroke and eating difficulties: long-term experiences. J Clin Nurs 13:825–834, 2004

Chandra R: Effect of vitamin and trace-element supplementation on immune responses and infection in elderly subjects. Lancet 340:1124–1127, 1992

Chernoff R: Micronutrient requirements in older women. Am J Clin Nutr 81:1240S–1245S, 2005

Christensen L, Somers S: Adequacy of the dietary intake of depressed individuals. J Am Coll Nutr 13:597–600, 1994

Clarke R: Homocysteine, B vitamins, and the risk of dementia. Am J Clin Nutr 85:329–330, 2007

Colcombe SJ, Erickson KI, Scalf PE, et al: Aerobic exercise training increases brain volume in aging humans. J Gerontol A Biol Sci Med Sci 61:1166–1170, 2006

Detsky AS, Smalley PS, Chang J: The rational clinical examination. Is this patient malnourished? JAMA 271:54–58, 1994

Donini LM, Savina C, Rosano A, et al: MNA predictive value in the follow-up of geriatric patients. J Nutr Health Aging 7:282–293, 2003

Dreosti IE: Nutrition, cancer, and aging. Ann N Y Acad Sci 854:371–377, 1998

Ervin R, Wright J, Kennedy-Stephenson J: Use of dietary supplements in the United States, 1988–94. Vital Health Stat 11:1–14, 1999

Eussen SJ, Ferry M, Hininger I, et al: Five year changes in mental health and associations with vitamin B12/folate status of elderly Europeans. J Nutr Health Aging 6:43–50, 2002

Eussen SJ, de Groot LC, Joosten LW, et al: Effect of oral vitamin B-12 with or without folic acid on cognitive function in older people with mild vitamin B-12 deficiency: a randomized, placebo-controlled trial. Am J Clin Nutr 84:361–370, 2006

Fabiny AR, Kiel DP: Assessing and treating weight loss in nursing home patients. Clin Geriatr Med 13:737–751, 1997

Ferry M, Sidobre B, Lambertin A, et al: The SOLINUT study: analysis of the interaction between nutrition and loneliness in persons aged over 70 years. J Nutr Health Aging 9:261–268, 2005

Feskanich D, Singh V, Willett WC, et al: Vitamin A intake and hip fractures among postmenopausal women. JAMA 287:47–54, 2002

Franklin B, Whaley M, Howley E (eds): ACSM's Guidelines for Exercise Testing and Prescription, 6th Edition. Philadelphia, PA, Lippincott Williams & Wilkins, 2000, pp 137–164

Fried LP, Guralnik JM: Disability in older adults: evidence regarding significance, etiology, and risk. J Am Geriatr Soc 45:92–100, 1997

Gaglia JL, Wyckoff J, Abrahamson MJ: Acute hyperglycemic crisis in the elderly. Med Clin North Am 88:1063–1084, 2004

Ganguli M, Vander Bilt J, Saxton JA, et al: Alcohol consumption and cognitive function in late life: a longitudinal community study. Neurology 65:1210–1217, 2005

Garry PJ, Goodwin JS, Hunt WC, et al: Nutritional status in a healthy elderly population: dietary and supplemental intakes. Am J Clin Nutr 36:319–331, 1982

Ghadirian AM, Ananth J, Engelsmann F: Folic acid deficiency and depression. Psychosomatics 21:926–929, 1980

Girodon F, Galan P, Monget AL, et al: Impact of trace elements and vitamin supplementation on immunity and infections in institutionalized elderly patients: a randomized controlled trial. MIN. VIT. AOX. geriatric network. Arch Intern Med 159:748–754, 1999

Gregg EW, Yaffe K, Cauley JA, et al: Is diabetes associated with cognitive impairment and cognitive decline among older women? Study of Osteoporotic Fractures Research Group. Arch Intern Med 160:174–180, 2000

Hakkarainen R, Partonen T, Haukka J, et al: Food and nutrient intake in relation to mental wellbeing. Nutr J 3:14, 2004a

Hakkarainen R, Partonen T, Haukka J, et al: Is low dietary intake of omega-3 fatty acids associated with depression? Am J Psychiatry 161:567–569, 2004b

Halsted CH, Villanueva JA, Devlin AM, et al: Metabolic interactions of alcohol and folate. J Nutr 132:2367S–2372S, 2002

Hartman CA, Manos TM, Winter C, et al: Effects of t'ai chi training on function and quality of life indicators in older adults with osteoarthritis. J Am Geriatr Soc 48:1553–1559, 2000

Heymsfield SB, McManus C, Smith J, et al: Anthropometric measurement of muscle mass: revised equations for calculating bone-free arm muscle area. Am J Clin Nutr 36:680–690, 1982

Hibbeln JR: Fish consumption and major depression. Lancet 351:1213, 1998

Ho C, Kauwell GP, Bailey LB: Practitioners' guide to meeting the vitamin B-12 recommended dietary allowance for people aged 51 years and older. J Am Diet Assoc 99:725–727, 1999

Hootman JM, Macera CA, Ainsworth BE, et al: Epidemiology of musculoskeletal injuries among sedentary and physically active adults. Med Sci Sports Exerc 34:838–844, 2002

Houston DK Johnson MA, Daniel TD, et al: Health and dietary characteristics of supplement users in an elderly population. Int J Vitam Nutr Res 67, 183–191, 1997

Hunter R, Jones M, Jones TG, et al: Serum B12 and folate concentrations in mental patients. Br J Psychiatry 113:1291–1295, 1967

Institute of Medicine: Dietary Reference Intakes for Calcium, Phosphorus, Magnesium, Vitamin D, and Fluoride. Washington, DC, National Academy Press, 1997

Institute of Medicine: Dietary Reference Intakes for Thiamin, Riboflavin, Niacin, Vitamin B6, Folate, Vitamin B12, Pantothenic Acid, Biotin, and Choline. Washington, DC, National Academy Press, 1998

Institute of Medicine: Dietary Reference Intakes for Vitamin C, E, Selenium, and Carotenoids. Washington, DC, National Academy Press, 2000

Institute of Medicine: Dietary Reference Intakes for Energy, Carbohydrate, Fiber, Fat, Fatty Acids, Cholesterol, Protein, and Amino Acids. Washington, DC, National Academies Press, 2005

Kasper S, Anghelescu IG, Szegedi A, et al: Superior efficacy of St John's wort extract WS 5570 compared to placebo in patients with major depression: a randomized, double-blind, placebo-controlled, multi-center trial [ISRCTN77277298]. BMC Med 4:14, 2006

Kayser-Jones J: Preventable causes of dehydration: nursing home residents are especially vulnerable. Am J Nurs 106:45, 2006

Knight-Klimas TC, Boullata JI: Drug-nutrient interactions in the elderly, in Handbook of Drug-Nutrient Interactions. Edited by Boullata JI, Armenti VT. Totowa, NJ, Humana Press, 2004, pp 363–410

Kolasa KM, Mitchell JP, Jobe AC: Food behaviors of southern rural community-living elderly. Arch Fam Med 4:844–848, 1995

Kwakkel G, Kollen B, Twisk J: Impact of time on improvement of outcome after stroke. Stroke 37:2348–2353, 2006

Lampinen P, Heikkinen RL, Kauppinen M, et al: Activity as a predictor of mental well-being among older adults. Aging Ment Health 10:454–466, 2006

Larson EB, Wang L, Bowen JD, et al: Exercise is associated with reduced risk for incident dementia among persons 65 years of age and older. Ann Intern Med 144:73–81, 2006

Lau FC, Shukitt-Hale B, Joseph JA: Nutritional intervention in brain aging: reducing the effects of inflammation and oxidative stress. Subcell Biochem 42:299–318, 2007

Lemaitre RN, Siscovick DS, Raghunathan TE, et al: Leisure-time physical activity and the risk of primary cardiac arrest. Arch Intern Med 159:686–690, 1999

Levitt AJ, Joffe RT: Folate, B12, and life course of depressive illness. Biol Psychiatry 25:867–872, 1989

Lindeman RD, Romero LJ, Koehler KM, et al: Serum vitamin B12, C and folate concentrations in the New Mexico elder health survey: correlations with cognitive and affective functions. J Am Coll Nutr 19:68–76, 2000a

Lindeman RD, Romero LJ, Liang HC, et al: Do elderly persons need to be encouraged to drink more fluids? J Gerontol A Biol Sci Med Sci 55:M361–M365, 2000b

Locher JL, Robinson CO, Roth DL, et al: The effect of the presence of others on caloric intake in homebound older adults. J Gerontol A Biol Sci Med Sci 60:1475–1478, 2005

Luchsinger JA, Tang MX, Siddiqui M, et al: Alcohol intake and risk of dementia. J Am Geriatr Soc 52:540–546, 2004

Luchsinger JA, Noble JM, Scarmeas N: Diet and Alzheimer's Disease. Curr Neurol Neurosci Rep 7:366–372, 2007a

Luchsinger JA, Tang MX, Miller J, et al: Relation of higher folate intake to lower risk of Alzheimer disease in the elderly. Arch Neurol 64:86–92, 2007b

Luckey AE, Parsa CJ: Fluid and electrolytes in the aged. Arch Surg 138:1055–1060, 2003

Maes M, Christophe A, Delanghe J, et al: Lowered omega3 polyunsaturated fatty acids in serum phospholipids and cholesteryl esters of depressed patients. Psychiatry Res 85:275–291, 1999

Malik VS, Hu FB: Popular weight-loss diets: from evidence to practice. Nat Clin Pract Cardiovasc Med 4:34–41, 2007

Malouf M, Grimley EJ, Areosa SA: Folic acid with or without vitamin B12 for cognition and dementia. Cochrane Database Syst Rev 4:CD004514, 2003

Malouf R, Areosa Sastre A: Vitamin B12 for cognition. Cochrane Database Syst Rev 3:CD004326, 2003

Malouf R, Grimley Evans J: The effect of vitamin B6 on cognition. Cochrane Database Syst Rev 4:CD004393, 2003

Marks BL, Madden DJ, Bucur B, et al: Role of aerobic fitness and aging on cerebral white matter integrity. Ann N Y Acad Sci 1097:171–174, 2007

Markson EW: Functional, social, and psychological disability as causes of loss of weight and independence in older community-living people. Clin Geriatr Med 13:639–652, 1997

Martineau J, Bauer JD, Isenring E, et al: Malnutrition determined by the patient-generated subjective global assessment is associated with poor outcomes in acute stroke patients. Clin Nutr 24:1073–1077, 2005

McCabe BJ: Dietary tyramine and other pressor amines in MAOI regimens: a review. J Am Diet Assoc 86:1059–1064, 1986

McClain CJ, McClain M, Barve S, et al: Trace metals and the elderly. Clin Geriatr Med 18:801–818, 2002

McKay DL Perrone G, Rasmussen H, et al: Multivitamin/mineral supplementation improves plasma B-vitamin status and homocysteine concentration in healthy older adults consuming a folate-fortified diet. J Nutr 130:3090–3096, 2000

Melhus H, Michaelsson K, Kindmark A, et al: Excessive dietary intake of vitamin A is associated with reduced bone mineral density and increased risk for hip fracture. Ann Intern Med 129:770–778, 1998

Meyer KA, Kushi LH, Jacobs DR Jr, et al: Carbohydrates, dietary fiber, and incident type 2 diabetes in older women. Am J Clin Nutr 71:921–930, 2000

Miller ER 3rd, Pastor-Barriuso R, Dalal D, et al: Meta-analysis: high-dosage vitamin E supplementation may increase all-cause mortality. Ann Intern Med 142:37–46, 2005

Mitchell SL, Teno JM, Roy J, et al: Clinical and organizational factors associated with feeding tube use among nursing home residents with advanced cognitive impairment. JAMA 290:73–80, 2003

Morley J: Water, water everywhere and not a drop to drink. J Gerontol A Biol Sci Med Sci 55:M359–M360, 2000

Morley J: Decreased food intake with aging. J Gerontol Med Sci 56:81–88, 2001

Morley JE: Anorexia in older persons: epidemiology and optimal treatment. Drugs Aging 8:134–155, 1996

Morris MC, Evans DA, Tangney CC, et al: Fish consumption and cognitive decline with age in a large community study. Arch Neurol 62:1849–1853, 2005

Morris MS, Jacques PF, Rosenberg IH, et al: Folate and vitamin B-12 status in relation to anemia, macrocytosis, and cognitive impairment in older Americans in the age of folic acid fortification. Am J Clin Nutr 85:193–200, 2007

Mukamal KJ, Kuller LH, Fitzpatrick AL, et al: Prospective study of alcohol consumption and risk of dementia in older adults. JAMA 289:1405–1413, 2003

Mukamal KJ, Chung H, Jenny NS, et al: Alcohol use and risk of ischemic stroke among older adults: the cardiovascular health study. Stroke 36:1830–1834, 2005

Mukamal KJ, Chung H, Jenny NS, et al: Alcohol consumption and risk of coronary heart disease in older adults: the Cardiovascular Health Study. J Am Geriatr Soc 54:30–37, 2006

Mukamal KJ, Robbins JA, Cauley JA, et al: Alcohol consumption, bone density, and hip fracture among older adults: the cardiovascular health study. Osteoporos Int 18:593–602, 2007

Mulligan JE, Greene GW, Caldwell M: Sources of folate and serum folate levels in older adults. J Am Diet Assoc 107:495–499, 2007

Nelson ME, Layne JE, Bernstein MJ, et al: The effects of multidimensional home-based exercise on functional performance in elderly people. J Gerontol A Biol Sci Med Sci 59:154–160, 2004

Nelson ME, Rejeski WJ, Blair SN, et al: Physical activity and public health in older adults: recommendation from the American College of Sports Medicine and the American Heart Association. Med Sci Sports Exerc 39:1435–1445, 2007

Ness AR, Gallacher JE, Bennett PD, et al: Advice to eat fish and mood: a randomised controlled trial in men with angina. Nutr Neurosci 6:63–65, 2003

Niedert KC: Position of the American Dietetic Association: Liberalization of the diet prescription improves quality of life for older adults in long-term care. J Am Diet Assoc 105:1955–1965, 2005

Osher Y, Bersudsky Y, Belmaker RH: Omega-3 eicosapentaenoic acid in bipolar depression: report of a small open-label study. J Clin Psychiatry 66:726–729, 2005

Paulionis L, Kane SL, Meckling KA: Vitamin status and cognitive function in a long-term care population. BMC Geriatr 5:16, 2005

Payette H, Gray-Donald K: Dietary intake and biochemical indices of nutritional status in an elderly population, with estimates of the precision of the 7-d food record. J Clin Nutr 54:478–488, 1991

Payne ME, Hybels CF, Bales CW, et al: Vascular nutritional correlates of late-life depression. Am J Geriatr Psychiatry 14:787–795, 2006

Peet M: Eicosapentaenoic acid in the treatment of schizophrenia and depression: rationale and preliminary double-blind clinical trial results. Prostaglandins Leukot Essent Fatty Acids 69:477–485, 2003

Penninx BW, Guralnik JM, Ferrucci L, et al: Vitamin B(12) deficiency and depression in physically disabled older women: epidemiologic evidence from the Women's Health and Aging Study. Am J Psychiatry 157:715–721, 2000

Perry L, McLaren S: Nutritional support in acute stroke: the impact of evidence-based guidelines. Clin Nutr 22:283–293, 2003

Pirlich M, Lochs H: Nutrition in the elderly. Best Pract Res Clin Gastroenterol 15:869–884, 2001

Przybelski RJ, Binkley NC: Is vitamin D important for preserving cognition? A positive correlation of serum 25-hydroxyvitamin D concentration with cognitive function. Arch Biochem Biophys 460:202–205, 2007

Reife CM: Involuntary weight loss. Med Clin North Am 79:299–313, 1995

Roberts RE, Deleger S, Strawbridge WJ, et al: Prospective association between obesity and depression: evidence from the Alameda County Study. Int J Obes Relat Metab Disord 27:514–521, 2003

Rolland Y, Pillard F, Klapouszczak A, et al: Exercise program for nursing home residents with Alzheimer's disease: a 1-year randomized, controlled trial. J Am Geriatr Soc 55:158–165, 2007

Sachdev PS, Parslow RA, Lux O, et al: Relationship of homocysteine, folic acid and vitamin B12 with depression in a middle-aged community sample. Psychol Med 35:529–538, 2005

Sacks GS, Dearman K, Replogle WH, et al: Use of Subjective Global Assessment to identify nutrition-associated complications and death in geriatric long-term care facility residents. J Am Coll Nutr 19:570–577, 2000

Scarmeas N, Stern Y, Tang MX, et al: Mediterranean diet and risk for Alzheimer's disease. Ann Neurol 59:912–921, 2006

Schmidt R, Hayn M, Fazekas F, et al: Magnetic resonance imaging white matter hyperintensities in clinically normal elderly individuals: correlations with plasma concentrations of naturally occurring antioxidants. Stroke 27:2043–2047, 1996

Siegel GJ: Basic Neurochemistry: Molecular, Cellular, and Medical Aspects, 6th Edition. Philadelphia, PA, Lippincott-Raven, 1999

Silvers KM, Scott KM: Fish consumption and self-reported physical and mental health status. Public Health Nutr 5:427–431, 2002

Solfrizzi V, Colacicco AM, D'Introno A, et al: Dietary intake of unsaturated fatty acids and age-related cognitive decline: a 8.5-year follow-up of the Italian Longitudinal Study on Aging. Neurobiol Aging 27:1694–1704, 2006

Stewart JW, Harrison W, Quitkin F, et al: Low B6 levels in depressed outpatients. Biol Psychiatry 19:613–616, 1984

Subar AF, Block G: Use of vitamin and mineral supplements: demographics and amounts of nutrients consumed. The 1987 Health Interview Survey. Am J Epidemiol 132:1091, 1990

Sullivan DH, Carter WJ: Insulin-like growth factor I as an indicator of protein-energy undernutrition among metabolically stable hospitalized elderly. J Am Coll Nutr 13:184–191, 1994

Sullivan DH, Bopp MM, Roberson PK: Protein-energy undernutrition and life-threatening complications among the hospitalized elderly. J Gen Intern Med 17:923–932, 2002

Tanskanen A, Hibbeln JR, Hintikka J, et al: Fish consumption, depression, and suicidality in a general population. Arch Gen Psychiatry 58:512–513, 2001

Thomson AD: Mechanisms of vitamin deficiency in chronic alcohol misusers and the development of the Wernicke-Korsakoff syndrome. Alcohol Alcohol Suppl 35:2–7, 2000

Tiemeier H, van Tuijl HR, Hofman A, et al: Vitamin B12, folate, and homocysteine in depression: the Rotterdam Study. Am J Psychiatry 159:2099–2101, 2002

Tolonen M, Schrijver J, Westermarck T, et al: Vitamin B6 status of Finnish elderly. Comparison with Dutch younger adults and elderly. The effect of supplementation. Int J Vitam Nutr Res 58:73–77, 1988

Tseng BS, Marsh DR, Hamilton MT, et al: Strength and aerobic training attenuate muscle wasting and improve resistance to the development of disability with aging. J Gerontol A Biol Sci Med Sci 50:113–119, 1995

van Staveren WA, de Groot LC, Blauw YH, et al: Assessing diets of elderly people: problems and approaches. Am J Clin Nutr 59:221S–223S, 1994

Villareal DT, Apovian CM, Kushner RF, et al: Obesity in older adults: technical review and position statement of the American Society for Nutrition and NAASO, The Obesity Society. Am J Clin Nutr 82:923–934, 2005

Vreeland B: Bridging the gap between mental and physical health: a multidisciplinary approach. J Clin Psychiatry 68 (suppl 4):26–33, 2007

Wakimoto P, Block G: Dietary intake, dietary patterns, and changes with age: an epidemiological perspective. J Gerontol A Biol Sci Med Sci 56:65–80, 2001

Wellman NS: Prevention, prevention, prevention: nutrition for successful aging. J Am Diet Assoc 107:741–743, 2007

White H, Pieper C, Schmader K, et al: Weight change in Alzheimer's disease. J Am Geriatr Soc 44:265–272, 1996

White H, Pieper C, Schmader K: The association of weight change in Alzheimer's disease with severity of disease and mortality: a longitudinal analysis. J Am Geriatr Soc 46:1223–1227, 1998

Williams MA, Haskell WL, Ades PA, et al: Resistance exercise in individuals with and without cardiovascular disease: 2007 update: a scientific statement from the American Heart Association Council on Clinical Cardiology and Council on Nutrition, Physical Activity, and Metabolism. Circulation 116:572–584, 2007

Wouters-Wesseling W, Wagenaar LW, Rozendaal M, et al: Effect of an enriched drink on cognitive function in frail elderly persons. J Gerontol A Biol Sci Med Sci 60:265–270, 2005

Wurtman RJ, Wurtman JJ: Brain Serotonin, Carbohydrate-craving, obesity and depression. Adv Exp Med Biol 398:35–41, 1996

Yancy WS Jr, Olsen MK, Guyton JR, et al: A low-carbohydrate, ketogenic diet versus a low-fat diet to treat obesity and hyperlipidemia: a randomized, controlled trial. Ann Intern Med 140:769–77, 2004

Suggested Readings

American Geriatrics Society Panel on Exercise and Osteoarthritis: Exercise prescriptions for older adults with osteoarthritis pain: consensus practice recommendations: a supplement to the AGS Clinical Practice Guidelines on the management of chronic pain in older adults. J Am Geriatr Soc 49:808–823, 2001

Bonner FJ Jr, Sinaki M, Grabois M, et al: Health professional's guide to rehabilitation of the patient with osteoporosis. Osteoporos Int 14 (suppl 2):S1–S22, 2003

Malouf M, Grimley EJ, Areosa SA: Folic acid with or without vitamin B12 for cognition and dementia. Cochrane Database Syst Rev 4:CD004514, 2003

Malouf R, Areosa Sastre A: Vitamin B12 for cognition. Cochrane Database Syst Rev 3:CD004326, 2003

Malouf R, Grimley Evans J: The effect of vitamin B6 on cognition. Cochrane Database Syst Rev 4:CD004393, 2003

Morley J: Decreased food intake with aging. J Gerontol Med Sci 56:81–88, 2001

Nelson ME, Rejeski WJ, Blair SN, et al: Physical activity and public health in older adults: recommendation from the American College of Sports Medicine and the American Heart Association. Med Sci Sports Exerc 39:1435–1445, 2007

Payne ME, Hybels CF, Bales CW, et al: Vascular nutritional correlates of late-life depression. Am J Geriatr Psychiatry 14:787–795, 2006

Perry L, McLaren S: Nutritional support in acute stroke: the impact of evidence-based guidelines. Clin Nutr 22:283–293, 2003

Williams MA, Haskell WL, Ades PA, et al: Resistance exercise in individuals with and without cardiovascular disease: 2007 update: a scientific statement from the American Heart Association Council on Clinical Cardiology and Council on Nutrition, Physical Activity, and Metabolism. Circulation 116:572–584, 2007

CHAPTER 29

Individual and Group Psychotherapy

Thomas R. Lynch, Ph.D.
Moria J. Smoski, Ph.D.

Psychotherapy has been shown to be an effective treatment for a number of mental disorders seen in older adults. As a treatment modality it can be particularly useful for older adult psychiatric patients who cannot or will not tolerate medication or who are dealing with stressful conditions, interpersonal difficulties, limited levels of social support, or recurrent episodes of the disorder. However, it has been estimated that only 10% of older adults in need of psychiatric services actually receive professional care, and there has been minimal utilization of mental health services in this age group (Lebowitz et al. 1997; Weissman et al. 1981). Older adults report a longer delay in initiation of mental health treatment than do younger cohort groups (Wang et al. 2005). A review by Unützer et al. (2000) reports a slight improvement in treatment rates over earlier estimates, but a large proportion of older adults with mental disorders remain untreated.

Many practitioners assume that older adults have negative attitudes toward psychotherapy. Although research on attitudes toward treatment in elderly samples is not conclusive, contrary to clinical lore, growing descriptive research suggests that older adults may prefer counseling over medication treatment. In a large-scale study of depression treatment, a greater proportion of older adults preferred counseling (57%) over medication (43%) (Gum et al. 2006). Older adults have also been shown to report a greater number of positive attitudes toward mental health professionals and to be less concerned than younger adults about stigma attached to seeking treatment for depression (Rokke and Scogin 1995). However, when perceived stigma is present, it is predictive of treatment dropout (Sirey et al. 2001). A further preference for mental health treatment to be provided in a primary care context rather than through specialty clinics has been observed in older adults (Bartels et al. 2004; Chen et al. 2006). Whenever possible, patient preferences or biases regarding treatment should be considered before referral for psychotherapy.

In this chapter we review the theoretical and empirical evidence for psychotherapy in older adults. The material is organized by type of disorder and, for each disorder, by type of therapy. We begin with a brief set of considerations in modifying treatments originally developed for younger adults to treat older adults. When possible, we evaluate the evidence with respect to quality of data, generalizability, and long-term effects of treatment.

Adaptation of Existing Therapies to Older Adult Populations

As discussed in more detail in the sections on specific disorders, older adults will respond to many of the therapeutic interventions used with younger populations. For example, highly effective treatments originally developed in younger adult populations, such as cognitive-behavioral therapy (CBT) for mood and anxiety disorders and dialectical behavior therapy (DBT) for personality disorder, have been successfully modified for older adult populations. Certain age-specific considerations are useful when modifying treatments, however.

Given the higher incidence of confounding factors in older adult populations (e.g., declines in sensory functions and speed of processing), certain modifications to standard therapy procedures are advisable. The pace of therapy should be slower, and fonts for written material should be larger. In addition, providing memory aids such as handouts and session summaries can be very helpful. For example, in our work we audiotape each session and ask the patient to review the session during the week before the next meeting. Thorough pretreatment assessment and modifications specific to the individual's strengths and deficits can help to circumvent age-related pitfalls in psychological treatment. Additional areas to consider are listed in Table 29–1.

Depression

Cognitive-Behavioral Therapy

Cognitive-behavioral techniques currently in use generally combine earlier work that used either solely cognitive or solely behavioral therapies and now encompass a wide variety of treatment protocols. There has been ongoing debate in the literature as to whether strictly behavioral or strictly cognitive strategies have greater treatment utility. However, regardless of mechanistic explanations of change, cognitive-behavioral interventions have been the most frequently studied therapies and have repeatedly been found useful in treating depression in older adults (Koder et al. 1996; Scogin and McElreath 1994; Thompson and Gallagher 1984; Thompson et al. 1987).

Cognitive therapies focus on problematic thoughts that may perpetuate depression. The goal is to change and adapt cognitive patterns away from negative thoughts that have become automatic. By changing the thoughts, therapists hope to change underlying dysfunctional attitudes that are hypothesized to result in relapse (Floyd and Scogin 1998). However, research supporting the process by which cognitive therapy reduces depressive relapse has not been well articulated (Barber and DeRubeis 1989; Teasdale et al. 2002). Recent component analysis research suggests that behavioral activation and automatic thought modification have equal effectiveness and that both components together are no more effective in preventing relapse than when used alone (Dimidjian et al. 2006; Gortner et al. 1998; Jacobson et al. 1996). In addition, an increasing amount of data suggests that the salient mechanism of change in cognitive therapy is the development of metacognition (i.e., responding to negative thoughts as transitory events rather than as an inherent aspect of self or as necessarily true) rather than change in the dysfunctional attitude per se (Teasdale et al. 2002).

More purely behavioral interventions are derived from classic learning theory in which problem behaviors are viewed as the result of specific antecedent stimuli and consequential events that reinforce, punish, or maintain behavioral responses (e.g., Dougher and Hackbert 1994). Genetics and biology are considered to play important roles in the development of psychopathology; however, theorists believe that biological predispositions can be mediated by skill acquisition and learning that occur throughout the life span. This therapeutic approach views depression as a state in which there is a relative shift toward an increase in dysphoric or hopeless affective reactions and a concomitant reduction in the frequency of reinforcing overt activities. Problem behaviors are analyzed functionally. For example, dysphoric responses (e.g., sad facial expressions, self-denigration) may function to reduce hostility or increase sympathy by caregivers, yet over time the lack of recovery or recurrent depression may be seen as aversive to caregivers (Biglan 1991; Coyne 1976; Dougher and Hackbert 1994). Behavioral techniques include monitoring behavior and affect patterns; assigning pleasant events; controlling or avoiding depression-eliciting stimuli; and limiting worry and depressive ruminations with time limits, behavioral exposure, and skills training (relaxation, problem solving, interpersonal skills).

Using a form of behavioral activation, Blumenthal et al. (1999) studied the effects of exercise on depression in older adults. Supervised exercise therapy, medication (sertraline) alone, and combined exercise and medication therapy all produced significant improvements in depressive symptoms. There were no significant differences between treatment groups, which suggests that exercise training might be comparable to the use of medication in older adults. Interestingly, follow-up assessment at 10 months showed lower rates of depression in the exercise training group than in the medication or combined treatment groups (Babyak et al. 2000). A smaller-scale study of supervised and unsupervised exercise therapy versus a psychoeducation control group in an older sample (mean age of 71 years, versus 57 years in the Blumenthal study) also showed a greater reduction in depressive symptoms in the ex-

TABLE 29–1. Considerations in the adaptation of psychotherapy to older adult populations

Medical illness. Illness or problematic medicines can exacerbate symptoms of a mental disorder. During assessment, it is important to obtain a medical history and a medication list.

Sterotypes. The clinician should actively work against stereotypes (held by the patient, the clinician, and/or society) of elderly persons as being withdrawn, rigid, lonely, dependent, or unable to learn.

Memory problems. Older adults may have difficulty remembering troublesome events. The clinician should consider consulting family members or longtime friends.

Avoidance of feedback. Some patients may avoid feedback about their problems as a way to reduce anxiety. In addition, therapists may be reinforced in avoiding critical topics if patients become distressed or hostile when such topics are introduced or if patients seem to feel relieved when the topic is changed. From the outset of treatment, patients should be advised that therapeutic progress will likely involve some discomfort as they learn to cope differently (e.g., being assertive if normally avoidant), and the therapist should model and reinforce willingness to remain engaged in therapy despite occasional discomfort.

Cognitive deficits. Cognitive impairments can impede learning speed and memory. Therapists may need to slow the pace when teaching skills to patients and may need to ask patients to summarize the issues covered.

ercise treatment group, both at posttreatment and at a 26-month follow-up assessment. In addition, 33% of the exercise treatment group was still exercising at follow-up assessment (Singh et al. 2001).

In a study comparing cognitive, behavioral, and brief psychodynamic therapy to waiting-list control subjects, Thompson et al. (1987) found that all of the treatment modalities led to comparable and clinically significant reductions of depression. Overall, 52% of the sample attained complete remission after treatment, and 18% showed significant improvement, with some enduring depressive symptoms. These rates are comparable with treatment outcomes in younger adult populations and with response to pharmacotherapy (O'Rourke and Hadjistavropoulos 1997; Thompson et al. 1987). Follow-up research indicated that at 12 months after treatment, 58% of the sample was depression free and that at 24 months, 70% of the sample was not depressed. As in acute treatment, no differences were found between treatment modalities at follow-up (Gallagher-Thompson et al. 1990), although in previous research with a smaller sample size, depressed geriatric patients in cognitive and behavioral therapies maintained the gains longer than those treated with brief psychodynamic therapy (Gallagher and Thompson 1982).

In the first known randomized trial examining CBT as a medication augmentation strategy, Thompson et al. (2001) assessed 102 depressed older adults. Patients were assigned to one of three treatment conditions: 1) CBT alone, 2) medication alone, or 3) combined CBT and medication. Although all three groups showed improvements in depressive symptoms over 16–20 weeks of treatment, the combined-therapy group had the greatest improvements. A significant difference was found between the combined-therapy and the medication-only groups. The CBT-alone group showed similar improvements as the combined-therapy group, but the superiority of CBT alone over medication alone did not reach a significant level. This study supports conclusions by Reynolds et al. (1999) that a combined medication plus psychotherapy approach may be optimal for the treatment of depression in older adults.

Dialectical behavior therapy is another treatment approach that combines cognitive and behavioral strategies in managing affective symptoms. DBT groups teach specific skills to increase mindfulness, interpersonal effectiveness, emotion regulation, and distress tolerance. Originally designed to treat chronically suicidal younger adult women, DBT has been modified to treat a number of difficult-to-treat conditions, including chronic depression in older adults. The modification for older adults includes many of the standard features of DBT but also targets cognitive/behavioral rigidity and emotional constriction. In a randomized clinical trial, antidepressant medication plus clinical management alone was compared with the same therapy with the addition of DBT skills training and scheduled telephone coaching sessions (Lynch et al. 2003). At follow-up after 6 months, 73% of medication-plus-DBT patients were in remission, compared with only 38% of medication-only patients, a significant difference. Only patients receiving DBT showed significant improvements from pretreatment to posttreatment on scores of dependency and adaptive coping, which are theorized to create vulnerability to depression (Lynch et al. 2003). In a recent study of comorbid depression and personality disorder in older adults, DBT plus medication showed a faster reduction in depressive symptoms when compared with medication alone (Lynch et al. 2007). DBT shows great promise in alleviating depressive symptoms in individuals whose chronic symptoms and comorbid conditions place them at strong risk of treatment failure.

Another related therapy for depression in the elderly that utilizes elements associated with both cognitive and behavioral interventions described above examines problems associated with social problem solving. Social problem-solving therapy (PST) is based on a model in which ineffective coping under stress is hypothesized to lead to a breakdown of problem-solving abilities and subsequent depression (Nezu 1987; Thompson and Gallagher 1984). Patients are taught a structured format for solving problems that considers problem details, present goals, multiple solutions, specific solution advantages, and assessment of the final solution in context. PST ideally refines and augments patients' present strategies to improve their ability to handle day-to-day problems. As with interpersonal psychotherapy (IPT), PST bolsters an area of weakness in individuals with depression. PST attempts to increase coping and buffer factors that maintain and aggravate depression (Hegel et al. 2002). PST has been found to be more effective than reminiscence therapy or waiting-list control subjects both in initial treatment of depression and at a 3-month follow-up (Areán et al. 1993).

One of the attractions of PST is that it can be delivered in a limited space of time. Because many older adults do not seek treatment for depression beyond their primary care health providers, this is an ideal place to deliver psychotherapies for depression in older adults. Several studies have evaluated the adaptation of PST in primary care (PST-PC) (Hegel et al. 2002; Mynors-Wallis 2001; Unützer et al. 2001; Williams et al. 2000). In one study, primary care treatment options were compared in a population of older adults with depression or dysthymia (Williams et al. 2000). Subjects were randomly assigned to treatment with an antidepressant, treatment with a placebo, or PST-PC. Subjects who received PST-PC did not show significant improvements over subjects who received placebos. The antidepressant treatment group did show significant improvements over placebo. These findings suggest that the ideal use of PST-PC for older adults might include augmentation with medication. PST-PC was a component of the large-scale Improving Mood-Promoting Access to Collaborative Treatment (IMPACT) study, which tested collaborative care management (including the potential for medication, PST-PC, or a combination of both treatments implemented in a primary care environment) versus treatment as usual in 1,801 adults age 60 or older. Participants in the collaborative care condition showed greater improvements in depressive symptoms than control participants at posttreatment as well as in follow-up assessments up to 12 months posttreatment (Unützer et al. 2002).

Interpersonal Psychotherapy

IPT is a manualized treatment that focuses on four components that are hypothesized to lead to or maintain depression. Whatever its etiology, depression is seen to persist in a social context. The four components of treatment focus are 1) grief (e.g., death of spouse), 2) interpersonal disputes (e.g., conflict with adult children), 3) role transitions (e.g., retirement), and 4) interpersonal deficits (e.g., lack of assertiveness skills). Techniques utilized in treatment include role playing, communication analysis, clarification of the patient's wants and needs, and links between affect and environmental events (Hinrichsen 1997). Frank et al. (1993) developed separate treatment manuals for interpersonal therapy in late life and interpersonal maintenance therapy for older patients. These manuals include adaptations specific for use in elderly patients, including flexibility in length of sessions, long-standing role disputes, and the need to help the patient with practical problems.

Controlled trials in populations of depressed adults have demonstrated the efficacy of IPT for the treatment of acute depression (Frank and Spanier 1995; Hinrichsen 1997). IPT has also been found to be as effective as nortriptyline in the acute treatment of major depressive disorder in elderly patients (Sloane et al. 1985). Of additional importance are findings that elderly patients in IPT treatment were less likely to drop out of treatment than were those taking nortriptyline because of the medication's side effects.

IPT in combination with nortriptyline has been shown to be an effective treatment for depression in geriatric samples (Reynolds et al. 1992, 1994). In an attempt to understand more about the treatment of elderly patients with recurrent depression, Reynolds et al. (1992) selected patients only if they reported at least one prior episode of depression. Seventy-eight percent

(116 of 148) remitted during the acute phase of treatment (8–14 weeks). During the continuation phase, 15% (18 of 116) experienced relapse of major depression; therefore, a total of 66% of patients recovered fully (Reynolds et al. 1992, 1994). The authors concluded that older patients with recurrent major depression can be successfully treated with a combination of antidepressant medication and IPT and that older patients respond as well, albeit more slowly, as middle-aged patients (Reynolds et al. 1997). Importantly, a combination of IPT and medication was found to be the optimal maintenance treatment strategy in preventing recurrence of depression, with 20% of IPT-plus-medication patients relapsing in the 3 years after depression remittance, compared with 43% in the medication-only group, 64% in IPT plus placebo, and 90% in the placebo-alone group (Reynolds et al. 1999).

The large-scale Prevention of Suicide in Primary Care Elderly: Collaborative Trial (PROSPECT) tested the effectiveness of a collaborative case management intervention in reducing suicide risk factors (including depression) in an older adult sample (Bruce et al. 2004). Participants in the active condition received selective serotonin reuptake inhibitor (SSRI) medication, IPT, a combination of medication and therapy, or no treatment, depending on physician assessment and patient preference. Although it is difficult to determine the relative contributions of medication and IPT to treatment outcome, participants in the managed-intervention group showed a significant reduction in both suicidal ideation and depression treatments when compared with a treatment-as-usual group (Bruce et al. 2004). As with PST, IPT administered in primary care settings in conjunction with antidepressant medication has strong empirical support in the reduction of depressive symptoms.

Psychodynamic Psychotherapy

Psychodynamic psychotherapy is based on psychoanalytic theory, which views current interpersonal and emotional experience as having been influenced by early childhood experience (Bibring 1952). Revised conceptualizations have emphasized how relationships are internalized and transformed into a sense of self (e.g., Kohut and Wolf 1978; Mahler 1952). Psychopathology is theorized as being related to arrestments in the development of the self, and depression is viewed as a symptom state resulting from unresolved intrapsychic conflict that may be activated by life events such as loss. During therapy, patients are encouraged to develop insight into past experiences and how these experiences influence their current relationships.

Although short-term psychodynamic therapy has been less studied for older adults than other treatments (e.g., CBT, IPT), there have been several indications that short-term psychodynamic therapy, particularly as conducted by Thompson, Gallagher-Thompson, and colleagues, is an effective means to treat depression in samples of older adults. In studies with random assignment to a waiting-list control condition, short-term psychodynamic therapy, or CBT, no significant differences were found between the types of psychotherapy at the end of treatment or at 12- and 24-month follow-ups (Gallagher-Thompson et al. 1990; Thompson et al. 1987). Additional research on depressed caregivers demonstrated an interaction between the mode of therapy and length of caregiving, such that those who had been providing care for less than 44 months appeared to achieve greater improvement with dynamic therapy, whereas longer-term caregivers seemed to obtain greater benefit from CBT (Gallagher-Thompson and Steffen 1994). The authors suggested that the long-term caregivers needed the skills learned in CBT to care for family members with more pronounced deficits who required more complicated care. These interesting results call for additional controlled trials comparing different treatment modalities, continued component analysis research, and continued research that examines which type of treatment works best with which type of patient.

Life Review and Reminiscence Psychotherapy

Life review and reminiscence psychotherapy are both based on the patient reexperiencing personal memories and significant life experiences. In life review, individuals are encouraged to acknowledge past conflicts and to consider their meaning in their life as a whole. Reminiscence psychotherapy focuses more on positive memories in group settings to improve self-esteem and social cohesiveness.

Empirical support for life review and reminiscence psychotherapy as a treatment for depression is sparse. Much of the research in this area focuses on case studies, qualitative reports, and general functioning. Early work by Fry (1983) specifically assessed the use of reminiscence therapy in older adults with depression and addressed the degree of structure required to define clinically helpful reminiscence therapy. Study participants in structured or unstructured reminiscence therapy reported improvement in depression symptoms over a no-treatment control group. Those who participated in the structured reminiscence therapy also showed significantly greater improvement in depression symptoms than those who participated in the unstructured reminiscence therapy. More recently, small-scale studies have reported modest effects on improving self-esteem (Chao et al. 2006) but nonsignificant improvements in depression scores (Chao et al. 2006; Stinson and Kirk 2006).

As reported previously (see "Cognitive-Behavioral Therapy" in this chapter), Areán et al. (1993) conducted a randomized trial comparing reminiscence psychotherapy, social PST, and a waiting-list control condition in older adults with major depression. The reminiscence psychotherapy protocol in this study emphasized acceptance of past events and development of personal goals. Social PST was associated with significantly greater improvements in depressive symptoms compared with reminiscence therapy. Therefore, although reminiscence psychotherapy at first blush appeared to have theoretical and practical treatment utility for older adults, to date empirical results fail to support its use over more empirically validated approaches.

Group Psychotherapy

Our review of the literature found several published reports on controlled studies of group treatments for cognitively unimpaired elderly persons with depression. Perrotta and Meacham (1982) reported that group reminiscence therapy was no more effective than a waiting-list control condition. In contrast, self-management therapy and education groups were both equally effective and were superior to a waiting-list control condition (Rokke et al. 1999). In comparisons with medications, one nonrandomized, controlled study found that cognitive-behavioral and psychodynamic group therapies were both more effective than placebo pill but less effective than tricyclic antidepressants (Jarvik et al. 1982) and that although the cognitive-behavioral and psychodynamic groups were equivalent on most measures of depression and anxiety, the CBT group had lower posttreatment scores on one depression measure (Steuer 1984). A randomized, controlled study found that cognitive therapy with or without alprazolam (an anxiolytic) was more effective than alprazolam alone (Beutler et al. 1987). Also, the addition of behavioral group therapy to standard hospital care (which presumably included medication) led to higher remission rates among inpatients than standard care alone (Brand and Clingempeel 1992). In a study of a group treatment for low-income women that combined behavioral activation, psychoeducation, cognitive therapy, reminiscence, and social skills, treatment was found to be more effective in reducing depression scores than a treatment-as-usual control for white women but not black women (Husaini et al. 2004).

In summary, certain group therapy interventions, particularly cognitive-behavioral groups, appear promising for use with depressed older adults. Group therapy may also offer advantages for many elders; it is generally less expensive than individual treatment, and the social network provided by group therapy may provide significant therapeutic benefits to elders experiencing a loss of interpersonal relationships through the death of friends and spouses.

Bibliotherapy

Bibliotherapy, or book therapy, emphasizes a skills acquisition approach via selected readings from books. For example, Scogin and his associates (Floyd et al. 2004; Jamison and Scogin 1995; Scogin et al. 1989, 1990) have done a series of randomized, controlled studies to test the efficacy of bibliotherapy for mild to moderate depression in older adults. Individuals with depression read books such as *Feeling Good* (Burns 1980) to enhance behavioral skills that combat depression or to modify dysfunctional thoughts. Cognitive bibliotherapy was superior to psychoeducation and waiting-list control conditions in reducing depression symptoms in mildly to moderately depressed individuals age 60 or older (Scogin et al. 1989). At 2-year follow-up, those who had completed the cognitive bibliotherapy showed no significant changes in depressive symptoms from the initial posttreatment gains (Scogin et al. 1990). In a subsequent study, cognitive bibliotherapy was compared with individual CBT for depression. Although the individual CBT group showed greater reductions in depression scores than the bibliotherapy group at the end of treatment, the bibliotherapy group continued to improve after treatment, and differences at a 3-month follow-up were nonsignificant (Floyd et al. 2004).

Bibliotherapy has advantages for older adults. Because the intervention is delivered in a book format, adults with late-life depression are able to read and process material at their own pace. In addition, bibliotherapy can be privately self-administered, and consequently fears about stigmatization can be avoided. Also, for older adults who have limited mobility, these interventions do not require as many visits to a clinical site, and clinicians can monitor their progress intermittently through telephone calls. The optimal use of bibliotherapy appears to be as an adjunct to pharmacotherapy or individual therapy, and even bibliotherapy alone should be conducted under the care of a trained clinician. In addition, bibliotherapy obviously would not be appropriate for older adults who cannot read or who have poor eyesight or cognitive deficits that prevented them from attending to the book.

Anxiety Disorders

Anxiety Symptoms

Anxiety disorders are among the most prominent mental disorders of late life. The prevalence of anxiety disorders among younger adults was estimated at 7.3% of the population; a slightly lower rate of 5.5% was reported among older adults (Regier et al. 1988). Review of these reports, however, suggests that the rate of anxiety disorders in older adults may be underestimated because of older adults' reluctance to report symptoms, confusion of anxiety symptoms with symptoms of physical illness, and a lack of measurement instruments validated for geriatric populations. Across community surveys, prevalence rates for anxiety disorders in older adults ranged from 0.7% to 18.6% (Flint 1994; Klap et al. 2003). Another possible explanation for the range in reported prevalence rates is that the symptomatic makeup of anxiety disorders in older adults differs from that seen in younger adults. Older adults tend to report anxiety symptoms that do not necessarily fit a specific disorder. A naturalistic survey of primary care patients found that in older adults diagnosed with anxiety disorders, the most prevalent diagnosis was anxiety disorder not otherwise specified (Stanley et al. 2001). A portion of the empirical work on the psychotherapeutic treatment of anxiety in older adults focuses on symptoms rather than specific diagnostic categories.

The most frequently used and the most well substantiated treatments for anxiety in older adults are based on behavioral therapies. Specifically, a variety of relaxation training techniques have been pilot-tested as a treatment strategy for older adults. Work by DeBerry et al. (1982a, 1982b, 1989) showed that progressive muscle relaxation and meditation relaxation techniques reduced anxiety symptoms more effectively than treatment control conditions in older adults. Scogin et al. (1992) assessed the use of progressive muscle relaxation and imaginal relaxation, with mixed results. Both relaxation training groups showed improvements in state anxiety and general psychiatric symptoms after training, but there was no significant improvement in trait anxiety. General symptom improvements were maintained at a 1-month follow-up. In a 1-year follow-up assessment (Rickard et al. 1984) of older adults who had responded to relaxation training with a significant decrease in anxiety symptoms, the improvements from the pretraining assessment to the 1-year follow-up in state anxiety, trait anxiety, psychological symptoms, and relaxation level were all significant. Study participants also showed a nonsignificant trend of continuing treatment gains from posttreatment to 1-year follow-up. Given the small sample size of 26 study participants, these results indicate the possibility of promise in using relaxation strategies to treat distinct anxiety symptoms.

Relaxation training has some advantages for treating mild anxiety in older adults. The strategies can be taught in brief individual or group sessions. Theoretically, the strategies can be delivered during a regular visit to a primary care physician. As with many behavioral strategies, relaxation training has the advantage of masquerading as skills training for patients who might avoid traditional psychotherapy. Also, patients with cognitive deficits, who may have difficulty with more cognitively based strategies, may benefit from purely behavioral strategies.

CBT is a potentially useful treatment for anxiety symptoms. There is support for the use of CBT in the management of mixed anxious symptoms. Barrowclough et al. (2001) compared CBT and supportive counseling delivered in patients' homes for the treatment of anxiety symptoms in older adults (over age 55 years) who met criteria for a range of anxiety disorders. Participants who received CBT showed significantly greater decreases in self-reported anxiety symptoms after treatment than did participants who received supportive counseling. The CBT participants also showed a stronger decreasing trend in clinician-rated anxiety symptoms from posttreatment to 12-month follow-up; however, the differences between the two treatment groups on this measure did not reach statistical significance ($P < 0.08$), although the number of participants in the CBT group who attained criteria for treatment response was significantly higher than in the supportive counseling group. In a study targeting older adults (ages 60 years and older) with significant anxiety symptoms who wished to reduce their medication usage, individual CBT plus medication management was more effective than medication management alone in the reduction of anxiety symptoms, although both were equally effective in reducing medication usage (Gorenstein et al. 2005). A subset of anxiety symptom scores continued to show improvement at a 6-month follow-up. A challenging aspect of treatment outcome research on late-life anxiety is patient recruitment and maintenance. Both the Barrowclough et al. and Gorenstein et al. studies reported difficulty with identifying eligible patients. Despite strong efforts in the recruitment phases of these studies, a relatively small proportion of recruited participants qualified for the studies (55 qualifiers of 179 recruited in Barrowclough et al.; 42 of 147 in Gorenstein et al.). Further attrition due to dropouts or changes in health status among study participants reduced the final samples by an additional 22% and 33%, respectively. Recruitment challenges highlight the difficulty of treatment outcome research and also reflect the difficulties experienced by practitioners in preventing treatment dropouts. Despite these weaknesses, the results did support the efficacy of CBT for anxiety in older adults.

Generalized Anxiety Disorder

Among older adults, generalized anxiety disorder (GAD) is the most commonly diagnosed anxiety disorder. On the basis of data in Epidemiologic Catchment Area surveys, it is estimated that up to 1.9% of older adults currently experience GAD (Blazer et al. 1991). Although researchers tend to agree that rates of GAD are lower in older adults than in younger populations, several researchers have suggested that GAD is still underdiagnosed in this population (Palmer et al. 1997; Stanley and Novy 2000). Diagnostic criteria for GAD in younger adults may fail to take into account different ways that older adults experience anxiety. Older adults may focus on different targets of worry and on somatic symptoms that can be confused with medical illness (Sable and Jeste 2001). Evidence also suggests that GAD often appears in conjunction with depressive symptoms, which confuses both diagnostic criteria and the focal point for treatment strategies. One study reported that 91% of older adults with GAD diagnoses also met criteria for depression (Lindesay et al. 1989). The problems of variant symptom presentations, overemphasis on somatic symptoms, and depressive comorbidity create confusion in both diagnoses and treatment choices.

Given the issue of comorbidity with depression, the previously reported success of CBT in the treatment of depression in older adults makes it a logical area of treatment research for GAD in this population. Because of the nature of CBT, this treatment theoretically will also expose a variety of cognitive patterns of worry regardless of content and the cognitive and behavioral antecedents that link anxiety to somatic symptoms. CBT appears to be the best-equipped form of psychotherapy to manage the diagnostic and treatment issues that exist in older populations with GAD. Treatment research on GAD in late life is limited. Not surprisingly, though, the bulk of this literature focuses on the efficacy of CBT in this population (Stanley and Novy 2000; Stanley et al. 1996, 2004; Wetherell et al. 2003).

In one example of a randomized trial of GAD treatment, Stanley et al. (2003a) compared the efficacy of CBT with that of a minimal contact condition. The researchers' treatment protocol included education training, relaxation training, cognitive restructuring, and exposure to anxiety-provoking stimuli. CBT participants reported a significant within-group improvement in the severity of GAD symptoms from the point of their assessment immediately after the completion of the treatment protocol to an assessment 12 months after treatment completion. These findings suggest that CBT not only may provide effective immediate therapy but also may promote long-term gains in the management of GAD. Several other randomized trials have also supported the use of CBT for the treatment of GAD (Mohlman et al. 2003; Stanley et al. 1996, 2003b; Wetherell et al. 2003).

Because of the tendency for older adults to seek treatment for mental disorders in primary care facilities, current research is exploring an adaptation of CBT protocols that can be delivered in primary care. A pilot study by Stanley et al. (2004) presents a shortened CBT protocol for use in a primary care setting. This therapy was administered in eight sessions, either within the medical clinic or in the patients' homes. The treatment focused on six issues: education, relaxation training, cognitive therapy, problem-solving strategies, gradual exposure treatment, and sleep management. Further details may be found in the treatment manual (Stanley et al. 2004). Compared with a usual-care control condition, CBT was associated with significant decreases in GAD severity, anxiety symptoms, and depression symptoms. Although the sample size was very small (*N*=12), the positive results provide preliminary utility for the use of CBT in primary care settings. Adapting CBT to use in primary care facilities is a logical step that one hopes will prove efficacious. Primary care treatment will provide treatment where older adults are most likely to look for it, and it facilitates collaboration between CBT therapists and prescription providers. This integration may also be a cost-effective treatment option, as has been the case in primary care psychotherapy for depression.

Although CBT has strong promise for treating GAD in older adults, further empirical research must be conducted to verify its efficacy in this population and to determine mediators and moderators of treatment response. For example, it appears that CBT is not effective in older adults who have consistently low executive function abilities but is effective in individuals whose executive functioning improves along with their psychological symptoms (Mohlman and Gorman 2004). Likewise, Wetherell et al. (2005) pooled data from several studies of group-administered CBT for GAD to test predictors of treatment response. They found that the most consistent predictor of symptom change was completion of therapy homework assignments. In addition, and in contrast to younger adult populations, older individuals with more severe anxiety at baseline as well as psychiatric comorbidities showed the greatest benefit from treatment (Wetherell et al. 2005). A greater understanding of the mechanisms and predictors of treatment response will help further refine CBT as an effective treatment for late-life anxiety disorders.

Substance Use Disorders

Limited research is available on the prevalence of substance use disorders in older people, and much less is available on their treatment. With the exception of alcohol use, most substance use in late life is thought to be an extension of substance use from earlier periods of life into late life (Oslin et al. 2000). Although medical comorbidity becomes an increasing factor in older adults, most substance use in late life is presumed to differ from younger populations' use, more because of cohort differences than developmental differences. Treatment research on substance use in this population is nearly absent but is greatly needed.

The only substance whose use has been studied comprehensively in older adults is alcohol. Alcohol dependence is estimated to be lower in older adults than in younger cohorts. According to Epidemiologic Catchment Area surveys, current alcohol dependence and abuse prevalence rates ranged from 1.4% in North Carolina to 3.7% in Maryland in adults over 65 years of age compared with a prevalence rate of 8.6% in all adult Americans (Adams et al. 1993). Regular alcohol use that falls below diagnostic criteria can still be problematic in older adults. Given the possibility of interactions with prescription medications and increased risk of physical illness, even relatively low levels of alcohol can be potentially dangerous for older adults (Fingerhood 2000; Moore et al. 1999).

Research on effective therapy for alcohol-related disorders in older adults is sparse. In the review literature, standard treatment for older adults is to mainstream them into therapeutic groups for adults of any age, such as Alcoholics Anonymous. This treatment choice has not been empirically validated for older adults, and in fact some researchers suggest that older adults will demonstrate better treatment gains in peer support groups and age-specific treatment protocols (Dupree et al. 1984; Schonfeld et al. 2000).

Schonfeld et al. (2000) compared the success of veterans age 60 years or older who completed a cognitive-behavioral treatment for substance abuse with veterans who dropped out of the treatment program. Although the dropouts do not constitute an unbiased treatment control comparison group, the dropouts do allow some level of comparison between those who received full treatment and those who did not. Of the 110 veterans who enrolled in the program, 61 dropped out. The treatment program consisted of 22 weekly group sessions, including components of health education, cognitive-behavioral, and self-management strategies. The cognitive-behavioral and self-management strategies focused especially on identifying and managing situations that were risky for substance abuse, coping with depression and anxiety without substance abuse, and reestablishing goals after a relapse. Analysis found that the veterans who completed treatment were significantly more likely to have remained abstinent even after a brief relapse than were those who had dropped out of treatment. Veterans who dropped out of treatment were more likely to have died, to have evaded location, or to have returned to substance abuse. This study has several limitations, including a lack of division between alcohol abuse and other substance abuse and a biased control comparison group. However, given the positive preliminary findings, especially in a difficult-to-treat population in which 34.2% were homeless, this study shows a clear incentive to investigate the use of age-specific cognitive-behavioral treatments for substance abuse in older adults.

As in other Axis I disorders, such as depression and GAD, brief interventions in primary care have received increasing attention for the treatment of alcohol use in older adults. Because primary care physicians are most likely to identify overuse of alcohol in their patients, this is a natural area in which to develop treatment protocols. In a recent study, adults ages 65 years and older received either a brief cognitive-behavioral intervention from their physician or just a general health booklet (Fleming et al. 1999). The intervention consisted of two 10- to 15-minute counseling sessions in which the physician discussed consequences of alcohol consumption and personal cues for alcohol consumption. The physician also instructed the patient to keep a diary card of his or her drinking behavior and made a drinking agreement with each patient to control the patient's alcohol consumption. The investigators found that at 3-month and 12-month follow-ups, the patients who had received the intervention drank significantly less than those who received only a health booklet. Patients who participated in the intervention also had significantly less binge drinking and excessive drinking than those who did not receive the intervention.

The empirical studies described above provide groundwork for further research in this area. Age-specific CBT techniques show promise for the treatment of alcohol abuse in older adults. One avenue of research might examine group interventions to take advantage of peer support, whereas a second avenue of research might investigate primary care interventions to take advantage of older adults' relationships with their physicians. However, despite growing awareness that addictive disorders are common among older populations, it remains unclear whether treatments that have shown success in younger age groups (with the exception of brief alcohol interventions) can be applied with equal success among older adults (Oslin 2005). It is clear that more research is needed in this area.

Personality Disorders

According to DSM-IV and DSM-IV-TR (American Psychiatric Association 1994, 2000), a personality disorder is an enduring pattern of inner experience (e.g., cognition, affect, impulse control) and behavior (e.g., interpersonal difficulties) that has an onset in adolescence or early adulthood, is stable over time, deviates considerably from normal cultural expectations, and causes distress or impairment in functioning. Meta-analyses have concluded that the prevalence rate of personality disorder is between 10% and 20% of the older adult community (Abrams 1996; Abrams and Horowitz 1999), essentially analogous to the 13% prevalence rate among younger age groups (Torgersen et al. 2001). Overall, the emotionally constricted/risk-averse disorders in clusters A (paranoid and schizoid personality disorders) and C (obsessive-compulsive, avoidant, and dependent personality disorders) are the most commonly diagnosed in late life (Abrams 1996; Abrams and Horowitz 1999; Kenan et al. 2000; Morse and Lynch 2004), and there are also high rates of the Not Otherwise Specified category compared with other individual personality disorder diagnoses (Abrams 1996; Abrams and Horowitz 1999; Kenan et al. 2000). In addition, personality disorder rates are even higher (approximately 30%) among depressed older adult samples (Abrams 1996; Thompson et al. 1988).

Personality psychopathology has generally been associated with poorer response to treatment among older adults, whether treated with antidepressants or psychotherapy (Abrams et al. 1994; Lynch et al. 2007; Thompson et al. 1988; also see Gradman et al. 1999 for a review), and depressed older adult patients with comorbid personality disorder are four times more likely to experience maintenance or reemergence of depressive symptoms compared with those without personality disorder diagnoses (Morse and Lynch 2004). Despite this, with the exception of case studies, only one published outcome study has specifically focused on treating late-life personality disorders (Lynch et al. 2007; reviewed later in this chapter).

Although it was not the specific focus of the study, a well-controlled study by Thompson et al. (1988) examined the effect of personality disorder diagnosis obtained via structured interviews on depression treatment outcome. Seventy-five older adults who met diagnostic criteria for major depression were randomly assigned to receive either short-term cognitive, behavioral, or psychodynamic therapy. Results indicated that the likelihood of treatment failure was approximately four times greater for patients diagnosed with personality disorders (37%) than for those without (9.5%).

Individuals who had passive-aggressive or obsessive-compulsive personality disorders were more likely to experience treatment failure, whereas those with dependent or avoidant personality disorders were more likely to have their treatment succeed. A 2-year follow-up of this study concluded that patients with avoidant and mixed personality disorders were at a higher risk of relapse (Rose et al. 1991).

As observed in the Thompson et al. (1988) study cited previously, specific personality disorders may have different recovery trajectories and require different treatment approaches. Gradman et al. (1999) concluded that disorders such as dependent and avoidant personality disorders may respond better to treatment because patients with these disorders are more likely to comply with suggestions by the therapist and to work in a collaborative way. Alternatively, treatment response may be influenced by the degree to which the patient considers the personality dysfunction to be compatible with his or her character or sense of self and the extent to which the patient desires to change his or her personality style (Lynch and Cheavens 2008). For example, not only has it been shown that individuals with certain personality disorders do not seek treatment (e.g., paranoid personality disorder) (Tyrer et al. 2003), but with the exception of borderline personality disorder, individuals with personality disorder in general do not consider their personality dysfunction problematic (Bailey 1998; Beck et al. 2004; Hirschfeld 1993; Tyrer et al. 2003).

The only published randomized clinical trial specifically targeting personality disorders in older adults was conducted by Lynch et al. (2007) at Duke University Medical Center. The study focused on providing standard DBT (both group and individual sessions following Linehan's [1993] book), with depressed older adults presenting with at least one comorbid personality disorder. There were two phases of treatment. The *first phase* consisted of a standard 8-week medication trial of a physician's choice of SSRI (paroxetine, paroxetine controlled release, sertraline, or fluoxetine) plus clinical management. Results after 8 weeks of medication treatment showed that only 14% of the sample had at least a 50% reduction in Hamilton Rating Scale for Depression (Ham-D) scores, and only 12% were in remission (defined as a Ham-D score of 10 or less), suggesting that an 8-week course of antidepressant medication alone is not adequate to treat depressed personality-disordered older adults.

The *second phase* of this study included only those participants who had not fully responded to the standard medication trial. For this phase, participants were randomly assigned to 24 weeks, plus a taper of individual sessions, of either medication management alone plus clinical management (MED) or medication management plus standard DBT (DBT+MED). Examination of remission and time to remission findings suggested that the DBT+MED group reached the level of remission more quickly than the MED group. By use of the Inventory of Interpersonal Problems–Personality Disorders (IIP-PD) (Pilkonis et al. 1996), significant differences were found for interpersonal sensitivity and interpersonal aggression between the MED and DBT+MED groups at posttreatment and follow-up, suggesting that the DBT+MED condition significantly improved personality functioning compared with the MED condition. Interpersonal sensitivity and interpersonal aggression are two constructs that are theorized to be related to interpersonal difficulties often observed in individuals diagnosed with personality disorder.

Adaptations to standard DBT focusing on the most common older adult personality disorders (e.g., paranoid personality disorder, obsessive-compulsive personality disorder) are in development, with treatment targets that include reducing rigidity, cognitive inflexibility, emotional constriction, and risk aversion (Lynch and Cheavens 2008). The new DBT adaptation for emotionally constricted/risk-averse disorders emphasizes skills designed to maximize openness and flexibility to new experience and to reduce rigid thinking/behaving, as opposed to standard DBT, which is primarily focused on modulating extreme emotional experience/expression and reducing highly impulsive behavior. New skills include new states of mindfulness designed to help the patient find balance in the rigidity-to-openness continuum and a radical openness module that includes lovingkindness/forgiveness training. In addition, specific informal exposure techniques have been developed that are designed to help the patient successfully learn new responses to criticism or unwanted interpersonal feedback, including techniques to induce positive mood states prior to in vivo behavioral exposure (Lynch and Cheavens 2008).

Despite the promising nature of these findings, the empirical evidence suggests that the presence of a personality disorder in an older adult seriously compromises treatment. In addition, rates of personality disorders among older adults may be only slightly lower than in younger age groups, and subsyndromal personality disorders may be more prevalent in older populations relative to younger ones (Abrams and Bromberg 2006). It appears that psychotherapy interventions likely will be enhanced when they target the unique behavioral, cognitive, and interpersonal dynamics associated with older-adult personality disorders.

Dementia

The development of psychosocial interventions for dementia is a complicated area of research. Unlike some of the other disorders discussed in this chapter, dementia is unlikely to remit as a result of psychotherapy. Researchers in this area have struggled to find distinct goals and outcomes on which to focus. Because the dementia as a whole is not expected to abate, researchers have chosen specific variables to focus on in older adults with dementia, such as global quality of life, affective states, disruptive behavioral symptoms, functional impairment, and prevention of self-harm.

Another concern is whom to target in psychosocial interventions. Dementia is a disease with social consequences. The families of older adults with dementia gradually lose their loved ones to the disease and learn to cope with the demands of caring for an individual with dementia. In addition, individuals with dementia are likely to be institutionalized at some point in the disease process (Severson et al. 1994). Consensus is lacking on what is the best program of psychosocial care in an inpatient facility. For example, patients with dementia may cause social distress in patients without dementia but may also benefit from social contact with other patients (Lawton 1996). Because of the social impact of dementia, interventions for it may be delivered directly to treat the individual patient, alter his or her environment, or help the caregiver.

Because of the cognitive deterioration experienced by dementia patients, most empirical research on interventions for dementia is based on behavioral strategies. Studies of psychosocial interventions can be categorized by the treatment outcome goals and by the intervention targets. Typical targets include cognitive functioning, affect, and problematic behaviors, with interventions often attempting to address multiple targets. Reviews of empirically supported interventions by Teri et al. (2005b) and Livingston et al. (2005) provide overviews of current treatment approaches. Treatments that specifically target the physical or sensory environment (such as managing ambient lighting levels or obscuring windows and doors to reduce cues for wandering) may also be effective in managing problem behaviors but are beyond the scope of this chapter.

Cognitive symptoms such as disorientation and confusion can cause distress and injury in patients and increased stress in caregivers. One proposed psychotherapeutic technique to cope with the cognitive symptoms of dementia is cognitive stimulation therapy. Derived from reality-orientation therapy, which aims to continuously reorient patients' attention to the present situation and surroundings by repeating who they are and where they are, cognitive stimulation therapy focuses on improving information processing abilities. Treatment can take place in formal groups and/or through training of professional or lay caregivers to administer intervention activities during the course of day-to-day activities. Several recent randomized, controlled studies have found improved performance in patients receiving cognitive stimulation therapy, whether as a standalone intervention (Quayhagen et al. 1995; Spector et al. 2001, 2003) or as an augmentation of cholinesterase inhibitor medication (Onder et al. 2005). Cognitive abilities were generally preserved and/or improved in the treatment groups relative to control subjects (Onder et al. 2005; Spector et al. 2003). Relative improvements in mood (Spector et al. 2001) and behavior (Quayhagen et al. 1995) were observed, but not all studies showed improvements in these areas (e.g., Onder et al. 2005; Quayhagen et al. 2000; Spector et al. 2003). Overall, cognitive stimulation therapy appears to be a promising approach to preserving cognitive function in older adults with dementia, but further study is necessary to determine its influence on mood and/or problem behaviors.

Individuals with dementia are often at risk for anxiety, depression, or other negative affective states. Successful treatments of noncognitive affective symptoms in dementia can be thought to have one of two goals: to increase positive affect or to decrease negative affect. Many of the treatments that have been proposed to promote positive experience in individuals with dementia, such as art therapy, music therapy, religious participation, or social participation, lack empirical validation (Lawton 1996). Treatment research on decreasing negative affective states, such as depression, has a stronger empirical base.

Several behavioral therapies involving a combination of caregiver training in problem solving and communication, as well as structured behavioral activation for patients, have been found to be effective in reducing depressive symptoms (Beck et al. 2004; McCallion et al. 1999; Proctor et al. 1999; Teri et al. 1997, 2003). For example, Teri et al. (1997) assessed two protocols: behavior therapy with pleasant events and behavior therapy with problem solving. In both therapies, the therapists helped the caregiver develop behavioral strategies in response to the patient's behavior. Participants in the pleasant-events group were also encouraged to increase pleasant activities. Participants in the problem-solving group were taught systematic problem-solving strategies along with the behavior therapy. Control participants included both a waiting-list group and a treatment-as-usual group. At posttreatment, both problem-solving groups showed significant improvement in depression scores compared with the two control groups. Gains in depression status were maintained at 6 months posttreatment. The two active treatments did not differ in effectiveness, nor did the two control conditions. Both the use of problem solving for problem behaviors and the introduction of more pleasant events into patients' experience appear to function as successful behavioral management strategies for depressive moods in patients with dementia.

Behavioral therapy also has a strong history of controlling patients' problem behaviors, such as aggression, withdrawal, or resistance. These therapies generally train those who care for individuals with dementia—whether in the community or in inpatient facilities—to manage patient behavior using principles of operant conditioning. The behavioral interventions found effective in reducing depressive symptoms have also been found to be helpful in reducing problem behaviors (Bourgeois et al. 2002; Proctor et al. 1999; Teri et al. 1997, 2003, 2005a). Another set of treatments with growing empirical support are based on the progressively lowered stress threshold (PLST) theory (Hall and Buckwalter 1987). From this perspective, the disease processes underlying dementia progressively lower the patient's ability to cope with stressors such as fatigue, change in routine, or physical illness. Treatment consists of educating and training caregivers in managing the patient's environment to minimize such stressors. Gerdner et al. (2002) found that their PLST-based caregiver training maintained the frequency of problem behaviors among dementia patients cared for by a nonspouse, whereas the frequency of such behaviors increased significantly over time in the control group. The effect for patients cared for by a spouse was not significant. Caregiver distress over patient behavior problems decreased in both spouse and nonspouse caregivers. Huang et al. (2003) also found a reduction in problem behaviors among patients whose caregivers received PLST-based training when compared with a group receiving education and social support. This effect was present at both 3 weeks and 3 months posttreatment. Although further research is necessary to match the empirical validation of behavioral therapies for problem behaviors in dementia, the PLST approach shows great promise.

Several treatments for mood and behavior problems in dementia are frequently used in nursing homes and assisted living facilities but unfortunately lack solid empirical support. One example is validation therapy. The premise of validation therapy is that patients who experience dementia use their remaining cognitive abilities to communicate with others. When communication efforts are validated through simple speech, empathetic voice tone, and attempts to reflect speech and behavior, the hypothesized result is a reduction in negative behavior and affect. The largest controlled study of validation therapy with a group of nursing home residents with dementia revealed only mildly positive effects (Toseland et al. 1997). After participation in a validation therapy group, nurses reported significant decreases in verbal and physical aggression. They also reported significantly greater confidence in their ability to manage problem behaviors. Similar results were obtained at 3- and 12-month follow-up. According to ratings by trained observers, though, there was not a significant decrease in agitation or a significant increase in positive behavior. The researchers also compared validation therapy with a social contact control. Treatment gains from validation therapy were not significantly different from those found in the social contact condition. There is no strong support for validation therapy having greater efficacy than other interventions such as social support. However, validation therapy remains a popular therapeutic intervention in practical care. Likewise, reminiscence therapy, which uses memory cues and structured group activities to facilitate memories and to encourage the sharing of past experiences, has not been consistently shown to improve mood, behaviors, or functioning in elders with dementia (see Livingston et al. 2005 for a review).

Several well-supported, broad-based psychosocial interventions are available to manage cognitive, affective, and behavioral challenges in elders with dementia. Although none of these interventions offers a cure, they are important tools for symptom management that have the potential to benefit both patients and their caregivers.

Conclusion

It is evident that psychotherapy offers significant promise for the treatment of psychopathology in elderly persons and at times may be the treatment of choice in terms of both efficacy and patient preference. We encourage practitioners to select treatments that have been tested with randomized clinical trials rather than basing their choices on theoretical preference or ease of application. The use of treatments without this type of empirical support can slow or reduce recovery. For example, reminiscence, life review, and validation therapy have readily apparent face validity. Yet research to date has failed to support the use of these therapies in isolation for certain disorders.

Future research should continue to examine the beneficial effects of strategies combining medication and psychotherapy. The large-scale PROSPECT and IMPACT studies of depression treatment in primary care provide excellent models for treatment outcome research and for clinical practice. In addition, research examining the mechanisms of change and issues associated with treatment response by disorder and type of therapy remain to be more fully developed. Finally, continued research is needed to focus on populations with treatment-resistant illnesses such as personality disorders and comorbid disorders.

Key Points

- Psychotherapy is a good option for treating mental disorders in older adults who have trouble tolerating medications, who prefer psychotherapy over medication treatment, or who have conditions for which psychotherapy is the most effective treatment.
- Modifications of traditional therapies may be necessary to compensate for age-related problems with vision, hearing, mobility, and memory.
- Effective treatments for depression include several different individual and group cognitive-behavioral therapies, interpersonal psychotherapy, and short-term psychodynamic therapy.
- The most common anxiety disorders among older adults are generalized anxiety disorder and anxiety disorder not otherwise specified. Behavioral treatments such as relaxation training and cognitive-behavioral therapy are the most effective treatments for these disorders.
- Personality pathology is associated with poorer treatment response to other comorbid conditions such as depression and anxiety. Few treatments targeting personality disorder in older adults have been tested. One promising and empirically validated treatment is a modification of dialectical behavior therapy for older adults.
- Dementia is unlikely to abate as a result of psychotherapy, but treatments targeting patients and their caregivers are effective in improving global quality of life, affective states, disruptive behavioral symptoms, and functional impairment.

References

Abrams RC: Personality disorders in the elderly. Int J Geriatr Psychiatry 11:759–763, 1996

Abrams RC, Bromberg CE: Personality disorders in the elderly: a flagging field of inquiry. Int J Geriatr Psychiatry 21:1013–1017, 2006

Abrams RC, Horowitz SV: Personality disorders after age 50: a meta-analytic review of the literature, in Personality Disorders in Older Adults: Emerging Issues in Diagnosis and Treatment. Edited by Rosowsky E, Abrams RC. Mahwah, NJ, Erlbaum, 1999, pp 55–68

Abrams RC, Rosendahl E, Card C, et al: Personality disorder correlates of late and early onset depression. J Am Geriatr Soc 42:727–731, 1994

Adams WL, Yuan Z, Barboriak JJ, et al: Alcohol-related hospitalizations of elderly people: prevalence and geographic variation in the United States. JAMA 270:1222–1225, 1993

American Psychiatric Association: Diagnostic and Statistical Manual of Mental Disorders, 4th Edition. Washington, DC, American Psychiatric Association, 1994

American Psychiatric Association: Diagnostic and Statistical Manual of Mental Disorders, 4th Edition, Text Revision. Washington, DC, American Psychiatric Association, 2000

Areán PA, Perri MG, Nezu AM, et al: Comparative effectiveness of social problem-solving therapy and reminiscence therapy as treatments for depression in older adults. J Consult Clin Psychol 61:1003–1010, 1993

Babyak M, Blumenthal JA, Herman S, et al: Exercise treatment for major depression: maintenance of therapeutic benefit at 10 months. Psychosom Med 62:633–638, 2000

Bailey GR Jr: Cognitive-behavioral treatment of obsessive-compulsive personality disorder. Journal of Psychological Practice 4:51–59, 1998

Barber JP, DeRubeis RJ: On second thought: where the action is in cognitive therapy for depression. Cognit Ther Res 13:441–457, 1989

Barrowclough C, King P, Colville J, et al: A randomized trial of the effectiveness of cognitive-behavioral therapy and supportive counseling for anxiety symptoms in older adults. J Consult Clin Psychol 69:756–762, 2001

Bartels SJ, Coakley EH, Zubritsky C, et al: Improving access to geriatric mental health services: a randomized trial comparing treatment engagement with integrated versus enhanced referral care for depression, anxiety, and at-risk alcohol use. Am J Psychiatry 161:1455–1462, 2004

Beck AT, Freeman A, Davis DD: Cognitive Therapy of Personality Disorders, 2nd Edition. New York, Guilford, 2004

Beutler LE, Scogin F, Kirkish P, et al: Group cognitive therapy and alprazolam in the treatment of depression in older adults. J Consult Clin Psychol 55:550–556, 1987

Bibring E: [The problem of depression.] Psyche 6:81–101, 1952

Biglan A: Distressed behavior and its context. Behav Anal 14:157–169, 1991

Blazer D, George LK, Hughes D: The epidemiology of anxiety disorders: an age comparison, in Anxiety in the Elderly: Treatment and Research. Edited by Salzman C, Lebowitz BD. New York, Springer, 1991, pp 17–30

Blumenthal JAP, Babyak MAP, Moore KAP, et al: Effects of exercise training on older patients with major depression. Arch Intern Med 159:2349–2356, 1999

Bourgeois MS, Schulz R, Burgio LD, et al: Skills training for spouses of patients with Alzheimer's disease: outcomes of an intervention study. Journal of Clinical Geropsychology 8:53–73, 2002

Brand E, Clingempeel WG: Group behavioral therapy with depressed geriatric inpatients: an assessment of incremental efficacy. Behav Ther 23:475–482, 1992

Bruce ML, Ten Have TR, Reynolds CF, et al: Reducing suicidal ideation and depressive symptoms in depressed older primary care patients. JAMA 291:1081–1091, 2004

Burns D: Feeling Good. New York, New American Library, 1980

Chao SY, Liu HY, Wu CY, et al: The effects of group reminiscence therapy on depression, self-esteem, and life satisfaction of elderly nursing home residents. J Nurs Res 14:36–45, 2006

Chen H, Coakley EH, Cheal K, et al: Satisfaction with mental health services in older primary care patients. Am J Geriatr Psychiatry 14:371–379, 2006

Coyne JC: Depression and the response of others. J Abnorm Psychol 85:186–193, 1976

DeBerry S: The effects of meditation-relaxation on anxiety and depression in a geriatric population. Psychotherapy: Theory, Research and Practice 19:512–521, 1982a

DeBerry S: An evaluation of progressive muscle relaxation on stress related symptoms in a geriatric population. Int J Aging Hum Dev 14:255–269, 1982b

DeBerry S, Davis S, Reinhard KE: A comparison of meditation-relaxation and cognitive behavioral techniques for reducing anxiety and depression in a geriatric population. J Geriatr Psychiatr 22:231–247, 1989

Dimidjian S, Hollon SD, Dobson KS, et al: Randomized trial of behavioral activation, cognitive therapy, and antidepressant medication in the acute treatment of adults with major depression. J Consult Clin Psychol 74:658–670, 2006

Dougher MJ, Hackbert L: A behavior-analytic account of depression and a case report using acceptance-based procedures. Behav Anal 17:321–334, 1994

Dupree LW, Broskowski H, Schonfeld LI: The Gerontology Alcohol Project: a behavioral treatment program for elderly alcohol abusers. Gerontologist 24:510–516, 1984

Fingerhood M: Substance abuse in older people. J Am Geriatr Soc 48:985–995, 2000

Fleming MFM, Manwell LB, Barry KLP, et al: Brief physician advice for alcohol problems in older adults: a randomized community-based trial. J Fam Pract 48:378–384, 1999

Flint AJ: Epidemiology and comorbidity of anxiety disorders in the elderly. Am J Psychiatry 15:640–649, 1994

Floyd M, Scogin F: Cognitive-behavior therapy for older adults: how does it work? Psychotherapy 35:459–463, 1998

Floyd M, Scogin F, Mc-Kendree-Smith NL, et al: Cognitive therapy for depression: a comparison of individual psychotherapy and bibliotherapy for depressed older adults. Behav Modif 28:297–318, 2004

Frank E, Spanier C: Interpersonal psychotherapy for depression: overview, clinical efficacy, and future directions. Clinical Psychology Science and Practice 2:349–369, 1995

Frank E, Frank N, Cornes C, et al: Interpersonal psychotherapy in the treatment of late-life depression, in New Applications of Interpersonal Psychotherapy. Edited by Klerman GL, Weissman MM. Washington, DC, American Psychiatric Press, 1993, pp 167–198

Fry PS: Structured and unstructured reminiscence training and depression among the elderly. Clin Gerontol 1:15–37, 1983

Gallagher DE, Thompson LW: Treatment of major depressive disorder in older adult outpatients with brief psychotherapies. Psychotherapy: Theory, Research and Practice 19:482–490, 1982

Gallagher-Thompson D, Steffen AM: Comparative effects of cognitive-behavioral and brief psychodynamic psychotherapies for depressed family caregivers. J Consult Clin Psychol 62:543–549, 1994

Gallagher-Thompson D, Hanley-Peterson P, Thompson LW: Maintenance of gains versus relapse following brief psychotherapy for depression. J Consult Clin Psychol 58:371–374, 1990

Gerdner LA, Buckwalter KC, Reed D: Impact of a psychoeducational intervention on caregiver response to behavioral problems. Nurs Res 51:363–374, 2002

Gorenstein EE, Kleber MS, Moblman J, et al: Cognitive-behavioral therapy for management of anxiety and medication taper in older adults. Am J Geriatr Psychiatr 13:901–909, 2005

Gortner ET, Gollan JK, Dobson KS, et al: Cognitive-behavioral treatment for depression: relapse prevention. J Consult Clin Psychol 66:377–384, 1998

Gradman TJ, Thompson LW, Gallagher-Thompson D: Personality disorders and treatment outcome, in Personality Disorders in Older Adults: Emerging Issues in Diagnosis and Treatment. Edited by Rosowsky E, Abrams RC. Mahwah, NJ, Erlbaum, 1999, pp 69–94

Gum AM, Areán PA, Hunkeler E, et al: Depression treatment preferences in older primary care patients. Gerontologist 46:14–22, 2006

Hall GR, Buckwalter KC: Progressively lowered stress threshold: a conceptual model for care of adults with Alzheimer's disease. Arch Psychiatr Nurs 1:399–406, 1987

Hegel MTP, Barrett JE, Cornell JE, et al: Predictors of response to problem solving treatment of depression in primary care. Behav Ther 33:511–527, 2002

Hinrichsen GA: Interpersonal psychotherapy for depressed older adults. J Geriatr Psychiatry 30:239–257, 1997

Hirschfeld RM: Personality disorders: definition and diagnosis. J Personal Disord 7:9–17, 1993

Huang HL, Shyu YIL, Chen MC, et al: A pilot study on a home-based caregiver training program for improving caregiver self-efficacy and decreasing the behavioral problems of elders with dementia in Taiwan. Int J Geriatr Psychiatry 18:337-345, 2003

Husaini BA, Cummings S, Kilbourne B, et al: Group therapy for depressed elderly women. Int J Group Psychother 54:295–319, 2004

Jacobson NS, Dobson KS, Truax PA, et al: A component analysis of cognitive-behavioral treatment for depression. J Consult Clin Psychol 64:295–304, 1996

Jamison C, Scogin F: The outcome of cognitive bibliotherapy with depressed adults. J Consult Clin Psychol 63:644–650, 1995

Jarvik LF, Mintz J, Steuer JL, et al: Treating geriatric depression: a 26-week interim analysis. J Am Geriatr Soc 30:713–717, 1982

Koder DA, Brodaty H, Anstey KJ: Cognitive therapy for depression in the elderly. Int J Geriatr Psychiatry 11:97–107, 1996

Kohut H, Wolf ES: The disorders of the self and their treatment: an outline. Int J Psychoanal 59:413–425, 1978

Kenan MM, Kendjelic EM, Molinari VA, et al: Age-related differences in the frequency of personality disorders among inpatient veterans. Int J Geriatr Psychiatry 15:831–837, 2000

Klap R, Unroe KT, Unützer J: Caring for mental illness in the United States: a focus on older adults. Am J Geriatr Psychiatry 11:517–524, 2003

Lawton MP: Behavioral problems and interventions in Alzheimer's disease: research needs. Int Psychogeriatr 8:95–98, 1996

Lebowitz BD, Pearson JL, Schneider LS, et al: Diagnosis and treatment of depression in late life: consensus statement update. JAMA 278:1186–1190, 1997

Lindesay J, Briggs K, Murphy E: The Guy's/Age Concern Survey: prevalence rates of cognitive impairment, depression and anxiety in an urban elderly community. Br J Psychiatry 155:317–329, 1989

Linehan MM: Cognitive-Behavioral Treatment of Borderline Personality Disorder. New York, Guilford, 1993

Livingston G, Johnston K, Katona C, et al: Systematic review of psychological approaches to the management of neuropsychiatric symptoms of dementia. Am J Psychiatry 162:1996–2021, 2005

Lynch TR, Cheavens JS: Dialectical behavior therapy for co-morbid personality disorders. J Clin Psychol 64:154–167, 2008

Lynch TR, Morse JQ, Mendelson T, et al: Dialectical behavior therapy for depressed older adults: a randomized pilot study. Am J Geriatr Psychiatry 11:33–45, 2003

Lynch TR, Cheavens JS, Cukrowicz KC, et al: Treatment of older adults with co-morbid personality disorder and depression: a dialectical behavior therapy approach. Int J Geriatr Psychiatry 22:131–143, 2007

Mahler MS: On child psychosis and schizophrenia: autistic and symbiotic infantile psychoses. Psychoanal Study Child 7:286–305, 1952

McCallion P, Toseland RW, Freeman K: An evaluation of a family visit education program. J Am Geriatr Soc 47:203-214, 1999

Mohlman J, Gorman JM: The role of executive functioning in CBT: a pilot study with anxious older adults. Behav Res Ther 43:447–465, 2004

Mohlman J, Gorenstein EE, Kleber M, et al: Standard and enhanced cognitive-behavior therapy for late-life generalized anxiety disorder: two pilot investigations. Am J Geriatric Psychiatry 11:24-32, 2003

Moore AA, Morton SC, Beck JC, et al: A new paradigm for alcohol use in older persons. Med Care 37:165–179, 1999

Morse JQ, Lynch TR: Personality disorders in late-life. Curr Psychiatry Rep 2:24–31, 2000

Morse JQ, Lynch TR: A preliminary investigation of self-reported personality disorders in late life: prevalence, predictors of depressive severity, and clinical correlates. Aging Ment Health 8:307-315, 2004

Mynors-Wallis LM: Pharmacotherapy is more effective than psychotherapy for elderly people with minor depression or dysthymia. Evidence-Based Healthcare 5:61, 2001

Nezu AM: A problem-solving formulation of depression: a literature review and proposal of a pluralistic model. Clin Psychol Rev 7:121–144, 1987

Onder G, Zanetti O, Giocobini E, et al: Reality orientation therapy combined with cholinesterase inhibitors in Alzheimer's disease: randomised controlled trial. Br J Psychiatry 187:450–455, 2005

O'Rourke N, Hadjistavropoulos T: The relative efficacy of psychotherapy in the treatment of geriatric depression. Aging Ment Health 1:305–310, 1997

Oslin DW: Evidence-based treatment of geriatric substance abuse. Psychiatr Clin North Am 28:897–911, 2005

Oslin DW, Katz IR, Edell WS, et al: Effects of alcohol consumption on the treatment of depression among elderly patients. Am J Geriatr Psychiatry 8:215–220, 2000

Palmer BW, Jeste DV, Sheikh JI: Anxiety disorders in the elderly: DSM-IV and other barriers to diagnosis and treatment. J Affect Disord 46:183–190, 1997

Perrotta P, Meacham JA: Can a reminiscing intervention alter depression and self-esteem? Int J Aging Hum Dev 14:23–30, 1982

Pilkonis PA, Kim Y, Proietti JM, et al: Scales for personality disorders developed from the Inventory of Interpersonal Problems. J Personal Disord 10: 355–369, 1996

Proctor R, Burns A, Powell HS, et al: Behavioural management in nursing and residential homes: a randomised controlled trial. Lancet 354:26–29, 1999

Quayhagen MP, Quayhagen M, Corbeil RR, et al: A dyadic remediation program for care recipients with dementia. Nurs Res 44:153–159, 1995

Quayhagen MP, Quayhagen M, Corbeil RR, et al: Coping with dementia: evaluation of four nonpharmacologic interventions. Int Psychogeriatr 12:249–265, 2000

Regier DA, Boyd JH, Burke JD, et al: One-month prevalence of mental disorders in the United States: based on five epidemiologic catchment area sites. Arch Gen Psychiatry 45:977–986, 1988

Reynolds CF 3rd, Frank E, Perel JM, et al: Combined pharmacotherapy and psychotherapy in the acute and continuation treatment of elderly patients with recurrent major depression: a preliminary report. Am J Psychiatry 149:1687–1692, 1992

Reynolds CF 3rd, Frank E, Perel JM, et al: Treatment of consecutive episodes of major depression in the elderly. Am J Psychiatry 151:1740–1743, 1994

Reynolds CF 3rd, Frank E, Houck PR, et al: Which elderly patients with remitted depression remain well with continued interpersonal psychotherapy after discontinuation of antidepressant medication? Am J Psychiatry 154:958–962, 1997

Reynolds CF 3rd, Frank E, Perel JM, et al: Nortriptyline and interpersonal psychotherapy as maintenance therapies for recurrent major depression: a randomized controlled trial in patients older than 59 years. JAMA 281:39–45, 1999

Rickard HC, Scogin F, Keith S: A one-year follow-up of relaxation training for elders with subjective anxiety. Gerontologist 34:121–122, 1984

Rokke PD, Scogin F: Depression treatment preferences in younger and older adults. Journal of Clinical Geropsychology 1:243–257, 1995

Rokke PD, Tomhave JA, Jocic Z: The role of client choice and target selection in self-management therapy for depression in older adults. Psychol Aging 14:155–169, 1999

Rose J, Schwarz M, Steffen AM, et al: Personality disorder and outcome in the treatment of depressed elders: two year follow-up. Poster presented at the 44th Annual Conference of the Gerontological Society of America, San Francisco, CA, November 22–26, 1991

Sable JA, Jeste DV: Anxiety disorders in older adults. Curr Psychiatr Rep 3:302–307, 2001

Schonfeld L, Dupree LW, Dickson-Fuhrmann E, et al: Cognitive-behavioral treatment of older veterans with substance abuse problems. J Geriatr Psychiatry Neurol 13:124–129, 2000

Scogin F, McElreath L: Efficacy of psychosocial treatments for geriatric depression: a quantitative review. J Consult Clin Psychol 62:69–73, 1994

Scogin F, Jamison C, Gochneaur K: Comparative efficacy of cognitive and behavioral bibliotherapy for mildly and moderately depressed older adults. J Consult Clin Psychol 57:403–407, 1989

Scogin F, Jamison C, Davis N: Two-year follow-up of bibliotherapy for depression in older adults. J Consult Clin Psychol 58:665–667, 1990

Scogin F, Rickard HC, Keith S, et al: Progressive and imaginal relaxation training for elderly persons with subjective anxiety. Psychol Aging 7:419–424, 1992

Severson MA, Smith GE, Tangalos EG, et al: Patterns and predictors of institutionalization in community-based dementia patients. J Am Geriatr Soc 42:181–185, 1994

Singh NA, Clements KM, Fiatarone Singh MA: The efficacy of exercise as a long-term antidepressant in elderly subjects: a randomized, controlled trial. J Gerontol A Biol Sci Med Sci 56:M497–M504, 2001

Sirey JA, Bruce ML, Alexopoulos GS, et al: Perceived stigma as a predictor of treatment discontinuation in young and older outpatients with depression. Am J Psychiatry 158:479–481, 2001

Sloane RB, Staples FR, Schneider LSM: Interpersonal therapy versus nortriptyline for depression in the elderly: case reports and discussion, in Clinical and Pharmacological Studies of Psychiatric Disorders. Edited by Burrows G, Norman TR, Dennerstein L. London, John Libbey, 1985, pp 344–346

Spector A, Orrell M, Davies S, et al: Can reality orientation be rehabilitated? Development and piloting of an evidence-based programme of cognition-based therapies for people with dementia. Neuropsychol Rehabil 11:377–379, 2001

Spector A, Thorgrimsen L, Woods B, et al: Efficacy of an evidence-based cognitive stimulation therapy programme for people with dementia: randomised controlled trial. Br J Psychiatry 183:248–254, 2003

Stanley MA, Novy DM: Cognitive-behavior therapy for generalized anxiety in late life: an evaluative overview. J Anxiety Disord 14:191–207, 2000

Stanley MA, Beck JG, Glassco JD: Treatment of generalized anxiety in older adults: a preliminary comparison of cognitive-behavioral and supportive approaches. Behav Ther 27:565–581, 1996

Stanley MA, Roberts RE, Bourland SL, et al: Anxiety disorders among older primary care patients. Journal of Clinical Geropsychology 7:105–116, 2001

Stanley MA, Beck JG, Novy DM, et al: Cognitive behavioral treatment of late-life generalized anxiety disorder. J Consult Clin Psychol 71:309–319, 2003a

Stanley MA, Hopko DR, Diefenbach GJ, et al: Cognitive-behavioral therapy for older adults with late-life anxiety disorder in primary care: preliminary findings. Am J Geriatr Psychiatry 11:92–96, 2003b

Stanley MA, Diefenbach GJ, Hopko DR: Cognitive behavioral treatment for older adults with generalized anxiety disorder: a therapist manual for primary care settings. Behav Mod 28:73–117, 2004

Steuer JL: Cognitive-behavioral and psychodynamic group psychotherapy in treatment of geriatric depression. J Consult Clin Psychol 52:180–189, 1984

Stinson CK, Kirk E: Structured reminiscence: an intervention to decrease depression and increase self-transcendence in older women. J Clin Nursing 15:208–218, 2006

Teasdale JD, Moore RG, Hayhurst H, et al: Metacognitive awareness and prevention of relapse in depression: empirical evidence. J Consult Clin Psychol 70:275–287, 2002

Teri L, Logsdon RG, Uomoto J, et al: Behavioral treatment of depression in dementia patients: a controlled clinical trial. J Gerontol B Psychol Sci Soc Sci 52:P159–P166, 1997

Teri L, Gibbons LE, McCurry SM, et al: Exercise plus behavioral management in patients with Alzheimer disease: a randomized controlled trial. JAMA 290:2015-2022, 2003

Teri L, McCurry SM, Logsdon RG, et al: Training community consultants to help family members improve dementia care: a randomized controlled trial. Gerontologist 45:802–811, 2005a

Teri L, McKenzie G, LaFazia D: Psychosocial treatment of depression in older adults with dementia. Clinical Psychology: Science and Practice 12:303–316, 2005b

Thompson LW, Gallagher D: Efficacy of psychotherapy in the treatment of late-life depression. Advances in Behaviour Research and Therapy 6:127–139, 1984

Thompson LW, Gallagher D, Breckenridge JS: Comparative effectiveness of psychotherapies for depressed elders. J Consult Clin Psychol 55:385–390, 1987

Thompson LW, Gallagher D, Czirr R: Personality disorder and outcome in the treatment of late-life depression. J Geriatr Psychiatry 21:133–146, 1988

Thompson LW, Coon DW, Gallagher-Thompson D, et al: Comparison of desipramine and cognitive/behavioral therapy in the treatment of elderly outpatients with mild-to-moderate depression. Am J Geriatr Psychiatry 9:225–240, 2001

Torgersen S, Kringlen E, Cramer V: The prevalence of personality disorders in a community sample. Arch Gen Psychiatry 58: 590–596, 2001

Toseland RW, Diehl M, Freeman K, et al: The impact of validation group therapy on nursing home residents with dementia. J Appl Gerontol 16:31–50, 1997

Tyrer P, Seivewright H, Johnson T: The core elements of neurosis: mixed anxiety–depression (cothymia) and personality disorder. J Personal Disord 17:129–138, 2003

Unützer J, Simon G, Belin TR, et al: Care for depression in HMO patients aged 65 and older. J Am Geriatr Soc 48:871–878, 2000

Unützer JM, Katon WM, Williams JWJ, et al: Improving primary care for depression in late life: the design of a multicenter randomized trial. Med Care 39:785–799, 2001

Unützer JM, Katon W, Callahan CM, et al: Collaborative care management of late-life depression in the primary care setting: a randomized controlled trial. JAMA 228:2836–2845, 2002

Wang PS, Berglund P, Olfson M, et al: Failure and delay in initial treatment contact after first onset of mental disorders in the national comorbidity survey replication. Arch Gen Psychiatry 62:629–640, 2005

Weissman MM, Myers JK, Thompson WD: Depression and its treatment in a U.S. urban community—1975–1976. Arch Gen Psychiatry 38:417–421, 1981

Wetherell JL, Gatz M, Craske MG: Treatment of generalized anxiety disorder in older adults. J Consult Clin Psychol 71:31–40, 2003

Wetherell JL, Hopko DR, Diefenbach GJ, et al: Cognitive-behavioral therapy for late-life generalized anxiety disorder: who gets better? Behav Ther 36:147-156, 2005

Williams JW Jr, Barrett J, Oxman T, et al: Treatment of dysthymia and minor depression in primary care: a randomized controlled trial in older adults. JAMA 284:1519–1526, 2000

Suggested Readings

Barrowclough C, King P, Colville J, et al: A randomized trial of the effectiveness of cognitive-behavioral therapy and supportive counseling for anxiety symptoms in older adults. J Consult Clin Psychol 69:756–762, 2001

Bartels SJ, Coakley EH, Zubritsky C, et al: Improving access to geriatric mental health services: a randomized trial comparing treatment engagement with integrated versus enhanced referral care for depression, anxiety, and at-risk alcohol use. Am J Psychiatry 161:1455–1462, 2004

Bruce ML, Ten Have TR, Reynolds CF, et al: Reducing suicidal ideation and depressive symptoms in depressed older primary care patients. JAMA 291:1081–1091, 2004

Lebowitz BD, Pearson JL, Schneider LS, et al: Diagnosis and treatment of depression in late life: consensus statement update. JAMA 278:1186–1190, 1997

Livingston G, Johnston K, Katona C, et al: Systematic review of psychological approaches to the management of neuropsychiatric symptoms of dementia. Am J Psychiatry 162:1996–2021, 2005

Lynch TR, Cheavens JS, Cukrowicz KC, et al: Treatment of older adults with co-morbid personality disorder and depression: a dialectical behavior therapy approach. Int J Geriatr Psychiatry 22:131–143, 2007

Mohlman J, Gorman JM: The role of executive functioning in CBT: a pilot study with anxious older adults. Behav Res Ther 43:447–465, 2004

Oslin DW: Evidence-based treatment of geriatric substance abuse. Psychiatr Clin North Am 28:897–911, 2005

Thompson LW, Coon DW, Gallagher-Thompson D, et al: Comparison of desipramine and cognitive/behavioral therapy in the treatment of elderly outpatients with mild-to-moderate depression. Am J Geriatr Psychiatry 9:225–240, 2001

Unützer JM, Katon W, Callahan CM, et al: Collaborative care management of late-life depression in the primary care setting: a randomized controlled trial. JAMA 228:2836–2845, 2002

CHAPTER 30

Working With Families of Older Adults

Lisa P. Gwyther, M.S.W.
Diane E. Meglin, M.S.W.

No single model exists for working with families of older adults. Clinicians need to provide both patients and families with individualized family assessment and treatment, taking into account issues of diversity and heterogeneity. Despite the need for family-specific treatment, there are patterns of family issues that consistently emerge, based on trajectories of psychiatric illness. Perhaps the most specific guidance in the literature comes from meta-analyses of clinical research on families of older adults with progressive degenerative dementias (Gallagher-Thompson and Coon 2007; Pinquart and Sorenson 2006b; Sorensen et al. 2002).

Over the course of an older adult's degenerative dementia, families will confront depression, delusions, agitation, behavioral changes, and other psychiatric symptoms in their cognitively impaired relative (Lyketsos et al. 2000; Olin et al. 2002; Tractenberg et al. 2002). The burden on the family can be great, information can be insufficient, and doubt can be overwhelming (Gwyther 2000). Families caring for older members with dementia need reminders from psychiatrists to focus on maintaining family quality of life as well as quality of care within the constraints imposed by psychiatric, functional, and behavioral changes (Hughes et al. 1999).

In this chapter, we take a chronological approach to working with families over the course of the dementia of an older adult. Dementias are the focus because of ample evidence that dementia is more disruptive of family life and more likely to result in negative mental health outcomes for family caregivers (especially females) (Pinquart and Sorensen 2006a). Compared with family caregivers of older adults with normal cognition, family caregivers of older adults with Alzheimer's disease spend more hours per week providing care, with measurable negative impacts on caregivers' mental health, personal and family time (Langa et al. 2001), and family relationships (Gwyther 2005). Psychiatrists working with families of persons with dementia should expect to treat vulnerable primary family caregivers as well as families in conflict (Rabins et al. 2006). Alzheimer's has forced long-term care services, policy, and treatment to move from a narrow focus on aging to a more dynamic family focus that is still inclusive of the person with dementia (Gwyther 2005).

Family Care for Older Adults With Dementia

Half of family caregivers live with the older adult over a disease course of 3–20 years. Despite the high rates of

Lisa P. Gwyther gratefully acknowledges support for preparing this manuscript from grant P30-AG028377 from the National Institute on Aging to the Joseph and Kathleen Bryan Alzheimer's Disease Research Center at Duke University Medical Center.

shared residence, increasing evidence suggests that 30% of older adults with moderate to severe dementia live alone, often with extensive supervision and assistance from local and long-distance family caregivers (Tierney 2004). Certain trends have emerged from studies of family care in dementia. A shift is occurring away from the direct provision of care by families toward more long-distance care or family care coordination. Dementia care may precipitate moves by retired adult children or a move by the older person to be closer to adult children. More female family caregivers are employed full or part time, and employment appears to have unanticipated benefits as well as commonly assumed burdens associated with role overload. Dementia care frequently precipitates the family's first experience with seeking help from agencies and other family members. Increasing evidence shows that the lack of an available and affordable long-term care system is pushing the limits of family capacity and solidarity.[1]

Family care is universally preferred, based in strong family values that cross cultural and ethnic lines. Yet exclusive reliance on family care has well-documented personal and social costs. Family caregivers may become overwhelmed, exhausted, depressed, or anxious. Many family caregivers report loss of pleasure, motivation, friends, activities, privacy, intimacy, or identity. Gradual and sometimes sudden loss of the person "as he once was" can precipitate significant grief in family members.

Research even documents that premature death is associated with spousal caregiver strain in the care of persons with Alzheimer's disease, suggesting an urgent public health preventive or protective focus for work with spouses of older adults with dementia (Schulz and Beach 1999).

Despite this apparent investment of families in care for older adults, some families never comprehend minimal safety risks associated with dementia care. Elder mistreatment—whether abuse or passive or active neglect—may be associated with exceeding these family limits (Fulmer et al. 2005). Families may feel powerless and overwhelmed when they cannot predictably control the symptoms and course of dementia. The role of the psychiatrist with the family becomes one of assessment of tolerance limits, education, treatment of psychiatric consequences of caregiver burden, and management of family expectations of the disease course and of themselves.

Despite a research focus on primary family caregivers, often a change in primary caregiver occurs when a spouse dies or when siblings pass a cognitively impaired parent among themselves in a futile attempt to equalize responsibility.

Increasing dependency, loss, and grief are realities of family care in Alzheimer's disease, but not all family outcomes are negative or burdensome. Although depression is the most frequently reported psychiatric symptom among caregivers of Alzheimer's disease patients, some families express pride in their care as a legacy of their commitment to family values.

The following clinical reminders about family care may prove useful in working with families of older adults:

1. Family care is an adaptive challenge: the family is not necessarily the problem, nor is the family necessarily the obstacle to effective care. Few incentives (financial, religious, or counseling) will make an unwilling family assume care. The reverse is equally true. Few disincentives will keep a determined spouse or child from honoring his or her commitment.
2. The family rarely has one voice. Different perceptions and expectations of close and distant family members frequently precipitate family conflict. There is no perfectly fair and equal division of family care responsibility. Families can expect a permanent imbalance in the normal give and take of family relationships while working toward a more equitable sharing of responsibility.

---

[1] In November 2007, Evercare, a health care coordination program, in collaboration with the National Alliance for Caregiving (NAC), released their findings from a comprehensive survey on the personal financial costs of family caregiving. Although not limited to families caring for a person with dementia, the data revealed that costs (including food, household goods, clothing, travel, transportation, medical copayments, and medications) for as many as 17 million people in the United States averaged more than 10% of caregivers' own household incomes. The financial burden of family care is clearly a significant factor, and its implications need to be addressed by practitioners as well as policy makers (http://www.evercare-healthplans.com/pdf/CareGiversStudy.pdf).

3. Few families have the luxury of one person needing care at a time. Manipulation by dependent elders is much less common than are real unmet dependency needs. There is more underutilization of services and underreporting of burden than the reverse.
4. There is no one right way or ideal place to offer family care. Many families are forced to choose between equally unacceptable options. Successful family caregivers gather information, take direct action when possible, and often reframe things that they cannot change in more positive terms ("It could be worse—at least she is still with me").
5. Successful family caregivers are flexible in adjusting expectations of themselves, the older adult, and other family members as they work to fit the needs and capacities of all. Coping with family care is facilitated by a sense of humor, a strong faith or value system, creativity, practical problem-solving skills, and emotional support from other family members or friends.
6. Families caring for older adults with dementia must define and negotiate complex situations, perform physically intimate tasks, manage emotions and communication, modify expectations, and capitalize on the older adult's preserved capacities.
7. A family caregiver's awareness of an available service, need for the service, or knowledge of how to access the service does not necessarily lead to their appropriate or timely use of that service.
8. There is no perfect control in a family care situation. Families are better off if they work on their reactions to stress or lack of control.
9. Denial is a common defense of family caregivers. Some people need to deny the inevitable outcome (loss of a beloved spouse or eventual placement of a parent in a nursing home) to provide hopeful, consistent daily care.
10. A primary caregiver at home is efficient and preferred. Primary caregivers, however, need breaks, respite, backup people, and services to supplement their personalized care. Even in ideal situations, contingency plans are necessary (Derence 2005).

Goals in Working With Families of Older Adults

Clinical goals with families of older adults will vary with presenting problems and family resources. Common goals, however, are to normalize variability, address safety issues, mobilize secondary family support, facilitate appropriate decision making at care transitions, and help family members to accept help or let go of direct care as necessary. In essence, the family is forced to adapt to a new state of "normal" in their family life, often with resistance from the member with dementia. Well-timed psychiatric help in interpreting the family's and the elder's reluctance to accept new realities can promote appropriate decision making and help smooth care transitions.

Other goals in working with family caregivers include treatment of their own mood, substance abuse, or anxiety disorders. Additionally, goals include providing individual and family treatment around issues of grief, loss, or conflict in family relationships that limit the effectiveness of care. In general, family work should enhance the effectiveness of family care and coping, the self-efficacy of caregivers (Fortinsky 2002a), and the family's satisfaction with their preferred levels of involvement.

Psychiatrists working with family caregivers over time will monitor the quality of family care, the mental health, capacity, and vulnerability of caregivers, and the impact of the demands of care on family relationships (Yates et al. 1999). Psychiatrists should be especially alert to escalating anxiety, self-neglect, suicidal ideation, depression, or anger in caregivers, as well as abuse or neglect of the patient. These indications should prompt immediate recommendations for treatment, respite, or relinquishment of primary care responsibility. Exigent negative caregiver outcomes on which to focus therapy include decrements in mental health, social participation, personal or family time, and loss of privacy.

Interdisciplinary Partnerships

Focused work with families of older adults holds great potential for positive outcomes, particularly in the context of an interdisciplinary partnership or team (Fortinsky et al. 2002b). Research suggests that social workers' individual and family counseling with spouse caregivers can mobilize and sustain community and secondary family support, reduce and prevent further primary caregiver depression, preserve caregiver self-reported health, change negative appraisals of behavioral symptoms, and even delay nursing home placement by over a year compared with a control group (Mittelman et al. 1996, 2004, 2007).

Psychiatrists may work collaboratively with social workers or nurses. These mental health professionals can provide timely or sustained assistance during the particularly vulnerable times of care transitions (Gwyther 2005). The psychiatrist's role is to assess and treat a family caregiver's psychiatric illness and to treat the cognitively impaired patient's psychiatric symptoms. Over time, the social worker or nurse may provide case management and monitor family capacity and tolerance while educating the family about common symptoms and care transitions (Callahan et al. 2006).

Some families will initially resist referrals to a social worker but may become more amenable if the social worker is described as an expert consumer guide or family consultant. At care transition times, a family consultant can provide assessment, intervention, and information. The family consultant can help families learn how to be their own case managers and actually increase their level of independence in handling the requisite tasks. The consultant may serve as a teacher, coach, advocate, counselor, cheerleader, or support person who can provide energy and a fresh perspective to promote family resilience.

Referrals to well-developed and validated psychoeducational group treatment programs have demonstrated equally positive results (Hepburn et al. 2007; Ostwald et al. 1999). Participation in peer counseling or support groups can have positive outcomes for active caregiver participants (Pillemer and Suitor 1996). One particularly helpful resource is the Rosalynn Carter Institute for Caregiving (www.rosalynncarter.org), which offers an Evidence-Based Caregiver Intervention Resource Center and detailed information on interventions that have been found to positively affect caregiver outcomes.

Another way to monitor goals in the psychiatric treatment of families of older adults is to base treatment on known precipitants of the breakdown of family care. Major precipitants of placement include both patient and caregiver factors (Yaffe et al. 2002). One of the patient factors that strongly predicts placement is disruptive psychiatric and behavioral symptoms. Changes in behavior and personality are also major causes of caregiver burden and depression. To the extent that psychiatric consultation is available to the older adult for treatment of psychiatric symptoms, and to the extent the family can be taught nonpharmacological approaches (see Chapter 25 in this book, "Agitation and Suspiciousness"), the health of the family and caregivers and effective home care for the older adult can be preserved.

Other predictors of family care breakdown are unresolved family conflicts or mood disorders, substance abuse, or anxiety disorders of the primary caregiver. Treating depression in a family caregiver generally has a positive impact on the mood, function, and behavior of the cognitively impaired older adult (Brodaty and Luscombe 1998; Teri et al. 1997), and the reverse is equally true.

The Family as Information Seeker

Families are more likely than older adults with dementia to initiate and seek psychiatric care throughout the course of the illness. The stigma of psychiatric illness often delays psychiatric diagnosis, and ethnic and cultural beliefs that equate cognitive decline with normal aging can produce the same result. Psychiatrists must remind families that a specific diagnosis suggests treatment options. Stigma is best addressed by correcting misconceptions or lack of information. An unconvinced family can be told that Alzheimer's disease is a brain disorder that can and does happen to anyone. The brain becomes the vulnerable organ in dementia, and psychiatric symptoms are brain symptoms just as angina is a symptom of a heart disorder. When damaged, both organs require special diagnosis and care.

Many family caregivers do not seek a diagnosis until psychiatric symptoms (e.g., suspiciousness) emerge or personality changes (e.g., uncharacteristic irritability) disrupt family life. Unfortunately, the patient is most likely to resist an evaluation once these symptoms have emerged. Psychiatrists typically are reluctant to speak with family members without the consent of the patient. An evaluation can be facilitated if the psychiatrist agrees to see the patient about a less threatening symptom such as headaches, loss of interest, or low energy.

Diagnostic Office Visits

Although the patient is entitled to time alone with the psychiatrist initially, later time alone with family informants is invaluable to the psychiatrist as he or she assesses the effects of functional loss and other family stressors. Most family caregivers prefer to talk privately with the psychiatrist to avoid confronting the older adult about his or her symptoms and declining condition. It may be helpful to have two family members accompany the patient for an evaluation. One family member can distract or sit with the older adult while another speaks privately with the psychiatrist.

Initial Communication With Older Adults and Their Families

Initially, communication with patients and their family members will likely be in response to the common emotional reactions to learning that there is a diagnosis of degenerative dementia. Elders and family members may express doubt about the diagnosis. Rather than confront their doubt or denial, it may be helpful to suggest to them that they behave as if the diagnosis of Alzheimer's disease had been confirmed while awaiting confirmation based on symptoms or progression of the disease. Asking directly about common early changes, such as difficulty handling money or increased irritability, may highlight expectable mental status changes while offering them a preview of psychiatric expertise. Sometimes, explaining the symptoms of apathy and loss of executive function can help families understand why their efforts to get the elder to try harder at tasks are likely to prove frustrating and futile.

Initial family sessions often elicit fear from family caregivers about their interdependent future or risks of heritability. Frustration is another common theme that emerges in early family treatment. Family caregivers frequently express frustration with the elder's obsessive need for repetition and reassurance. Clinicians can help families cope by offering information to clear up misconceptions about the presumed intentionality of the elder's resistance. Additionally, the elder's confabulations are typical and predictable attempts to fill in gaps for a failing memory. Encouraging the family to get angry at the disease rather than at professionals, the services, or each other can be extremely helpful. Families should be reminded that conflict among their members will only limit needed help (Coon et al. 2003). It is important for the family to understand that the elder's realistic dependency does not imply weakness of character or lack of will.

Fatigue and exhaustion are also common issues. Encouraging rest, exercise, and energy economies can be helpful for family members. Another common theme in family work is the guilt that family members feel about losing patience. They appreciate reminders from clinicians that everyone experiences regret based on unique but certain limits.

After the psychiatric evaluation, key themes, tailored to the family's capacity to understand or utilize them, should be highlighted and repeated in writing for distant or absent family members. Older couples in first marriages are generally more comfortable facing threatening health information together. Spouses of older adults with Alzheimer's disease often are put off by attempts to separate them from their impaired spouse. Providing the same information to both spouses at the same time helps older couples preserve their couple identity and accept the psychiatric recommendations as a mutual and shared adaptive challenge.

Family Expectations of Psychiatrists

Vulnerable family caregivers may seek a private place and time, undivided professional attention, and the comfort of initial familiar, polite small talk. Families want psychiatrists to listen without rushing to implied understanding or suggestions. Families of older adults expect to be asked what they have tried in coping with their relative's impairment. Even more, these families appreciate the psychiatrist's asking about what else is going on in their lives.

Wandering is a common problem that emerges for these families. Older spouse caregivers may expect expert advice and immediate cures for the dementia patient's most disruptive symptoms, such as wandering from home. Caregivers often seek explanations about why antipsychotic medications do not "treat" wandering as well as environmental and activity strategies do. They need specific referrals to the Alzheimer's Association's Safe Return identification system (see http://www.alz.org/we_can_help_medicalert_safereturn.asp). They also need help in coping with the toll taken by the prolonged hypervigilance required to protect a wandering spouse.

Families of older adults want psychiatrists to tailor information and education relevant to their immediate, pressing concerns. For example, a family concerned about the combative behavior of an older adult may be helped by a psychiatrist who responds, "First, let's get the guns out of the house" (Spangenberg et al. 1999).

When depleted primary caregivers are confronting the range of behavioral symptoms of an older adult with Alzheimer's disease, they may look to the psychiatrist to lend energy, a proactive attitude and perspective, and objectivity. They want acknowledgment of their contributions to the older adult's quality of life or absolution and forgiveness for what they were unable to achieve despite their best intentions. The psychiatrist must be careful with well-intentioned attempts to commend families for doing "a great job." Some family caregivers are quick to point out, "I am not her caregiver—I am her husband, and I promised to take care of her in sickness and in health."

Families also appreciate preventive self-care reminders from psychiatrists, but vague suggestions that caregivers need to take care of themselves often frustrate overwhelmed families that have few resources (Burton et al. 1997). Family members need help translating principles of respite in ways that are congruent with their personal values and cultural expectations. Specific examples may help. For example, some husbands respond to statements such as "Family care without respite is like expecting your car to run on empty. It doesn't." Respite options can be presented as opportunities to "recharge your battery" (Gitlin et al. 2006).

Also, increasing evidence shows that encouraging physical activity (King and Brassington 1997; Teri et al. 2003) and actively assessing and treating sleep disorders in older adults and their family caregivers are associated with positive care and family outcomes (McCurry et al. 2005a).

Families look to psychiatrists for support in making certain decisions and may ask for help in mobilizing other family members. Expertise in family communication and family systems theory is particularly helpful and relevant at these junctures (Eisdorfer et al. 2003). Family caregivers expect psychiatrists to let them express feelings even when these feelings are judged to be unacceptable. They may want help managing anger toward the older adult, other family members, service providers, or God. These families appreciate psychiatrists who create new choices by reframing the problem or situation. For example, a family caregiver may seek permission from the psychiatrist to be less than perfect or a "good-enough-for-now" family caregiver. At such times, a psychiatrist's use of humor and compassion can produce dramatic relief.

Assessing the Family of an Older Adult

A targeted assessment of the family of an older adult may result in referrals to Alzheimer's Association services, private or public geriatric care management, family or peer counseling, home help, day programs, assisted living, or nursing home care. Cultural values, expectations, and health beliefs will influence how and when families decide to pursue referrals, as well as their receptivity to family treatment by psychiatrists. Pinquart and Sorensen (2005) investigated the ethnic differences in stressors, resources, and psychological outcomes of family caregiving. They suggested that more specific theories are needed to explain some of the differential effects of ethnic minority groups of caregivers.

One of the most useful ways to elicit a picture of family functioning is to ask the family to describe a typical day. Clues about how much time the patient is left alone and about potential safety risks come from such open-ended questions. The psychiatrist should probe further if the caregiver hints about increased use of alcohol or psychoactive medications in response to stress. Older husband caregivers are particularly at risk of increased alcohol use in response to care demands.

The psychiatrist should encourage or support positive activities such as regular exercise, social stimulation, and secondary family support. A husband caring for his wife may be frustrated by her loss of interest in cooking. A suggestion to try regular restaurant meals at a familiar diner may conserve his energy and better meet the couple's nutritional and social needs.

Questions about a typical day often elicit family anger at the patient's apathy and withdrawal or a family's lack of awareness of safety issues. The family may complain that the cognitively impaired older adult is becoming more irritable and jealous of grandchildren. Probing may reveal that the impaired grandparent is still providing childcare despite significant declines in judgment or function.

It is wise to assess the home and neighborhood environment. People with dementia are easy targets for exploitation by telephone and mail fraud and people who come to the door. High-crime neighborhoods pose additional risks. An older adult who spends his or her time at the corner store buying alcohol and cigarettes may be especially vulnerable.

The psychiatrist should ask specifically about the primary caregiver's health. The psychiatrist should be alert to offhand comments such as "I'm fine as long as he can drive me to chemotherapy." The caregiver should be asked about his or her sleep and how it is affected by the older adult's sleep pattern. Many family caregivers will report being frustrated, overwhelmed, edgy, or exhausted but will deny having depression, anxiety, or psychiatric symptoms. Although psychiatrists are well advised to respond promptly to poorly controlled rage or suicidal or violent threats, skillful probing may be required to elicit frank symptoms.

A brief review of family relationships may further elicit new or resurfacing family conflict that can complicate care. For example, a distant, estranged sister may insist that her local sister is exaggerating their mother's dependency needs in an attempt to take control. The psychiatrist's written explanation of the mother's need for constant supervision may mobilize support from the distant daughter or at least may reassure the local daughter that her supervision is in fact what her mother needs. The psychiatrist must be alert to reports by family caregivers of exacerbated somatic symptoms or chronic illnesses of their own that they may not attribute to caregiver burden.

Another key to effective family assessment is to ask about other family commitments. For example, a daughter backing up her mother's care of her father may be distracted by anxiety about her own husband's failing business or a child's drug addiction. Cultural expectations must be carefully assessed along with each family member's subjective perceptions of financial resources. When paid or formal services are needed, family decision making is often related to subjective perceptions of future financial adequacy rather than the objective cost or affordability of services. Some family members may be saving for a rainy day, whereas others may value preserving their inheritance above meeting the elder's current care needs.

It is wise to assess family strengths, skills, and goals. For example, some families may cope well with providing care for incontinence, or end-of-life care, but were unable to tolerate the disruptive behaviors or sleep patterns of moderate dementia. Families who have coped with chronic mental illness or substance abuse in other family members may have well-developed coping strategies or support systems (such as Alcoholics Anonymous) that help them adapt to care for an impaired elder.

Finally, assessment should include some review of the family's experience with previous and current help from family members or paid services. Some key issues include the adequacy, quality, cost, and dependability of the help. For example, if a previous home care worker stole from them or failed to show up, the family would be less likely to accept another home health referral. Previous family conflict over elder care is likely to limit the family's willingness to ask for help. If a family believes the help they give each other is adequate, dependable, or sufficient, they often are unwilling to consider formal services.

Selecting Interventions for Families of Older Adults

Families of persons with dementia need a continuing source of reliable information. Referrals to the Alzheimer's Association (800-272-3900; http://www.alz.org) and the Alzheimer's Disease Education and Referral Center of the National Institute on Aging (800-438-4380; http://www.nia.nih.gov/alzheimers) meet this need.

Multidimensional interventions have been shown to enhance positive caregiver outcomes (Belle et al. 2006). The most effective multidimensional interventions for family caregivers emphasize psychological and/or skill-building strategies for behavior change over purely educational approaches. Effective multidimensional approaches are flexible and tailored to individual risk factors, are timed to key transition points or stressors in care trajectories, and are offered in sufficient dosages or amounts of assistance over time to ensure sustained or long-term outcomes. Combining individual and family counseling, family education, support group participation, and sustained availability of a care manager is associated with decreased caregiver burden and depression; decreases in the elder's disruptive symptoms; and increased caregiver satisfaction, subjective well-being, and self-efficacy (Sorensen et al. 2002). Psychoeducational and psychotherapeutic interventions produce the most consistent short-term effects on all outcome measures (Burgio et al. 2003). Although interventions with dementia caregivers appear effective in meta-analyses, effects are small and domain-specific rather than global (McCurry et al. 2005b). For example, a reasonable multimodal approach to treating an elder's disruptive agitation could include treatment of depression in the elder or in the family caregiver with pharmacological and nonpharmacological strategies; participation by the family caregiver in psychoeducational, skills training, or caregiver support groups; and participation by the elder and the family caregiver in structured exercise programs.

Nonpharmacological approaches to the treatment of depression in eldercare family dyads could be based on increasing the frequency of individually selected pleasant events (Teri et al. 1997). Once the elder and caregiver have identified which activities are the most enjoyable, the goal becomes one of increasing the frequency and duration of these activities relative to less enjoyable daily activities. Another recent dyadic intervention study showed that individuals with early-stage dementia and their family caregivers were able to participate in and benefit from a structured intervention that focused on care planning for future needs (Whitlatch et al. 2006).

Referrals to support groups should be balanced, and participation not oversold. Research on participation in support groups documents specific benefits from experiential similarity, consumer information, coping and survivor models, expressive or advocacy outlets, and (for some participants) the creation of substitute family or social outlets. Indeed, early studies of support group participation showed that participants knew more about Alzheimer's disease and services (although participants did not necessarily use that information) and that participants felt less isolated and misunderstood than nonparticipants. There are, however, realistic limits to the benefits of support group participation.

One support group does not fit all. Black individuals frequently do not feel the need to talk about family business among strangers. In an open mutual help group with revolving membership, not all participants will be dealing with the same care issues. The exclusive focus on Alzheimer's disease as just one aspect of family life may not meet certain families' needs. Some families cannot get to meetings regularly, and some groups are not consistently available. These factors limit the benefits of such a minimalist intervention. The benefits of participation can be enhanced by encouraging families to shop around for a group that best meets their needs and reminding them that they may be able to obtain comparable social support from groups to which they already belong, such as a church, synagogue, or retiree organization.

Internet information can be quite useful for seeking resources at care transition points as well. For example, if placement becomes an issue, statewide lists for nursing homes and assisted living facilities are available online. There are online guides to choosing a nursing home (e.g., http://www.medicare.gov/Publications/Pubs/pdf/nursinghome.pdf; http://www.medicare.gov/Publications/Pubs/pdf/02174.pdf). State ombudsman offices also offer online information about local facilities. Online discussion boards and Alzheimer's disease–focused discussion groups can be helpful as well.

Educational Strategies With Families of Older Adults

Many families are too overwhelmed at a first psychiatric consultation to absorb information or instructions. Teachable moments with families come at crisis points with specific psychiatric symptoms, such as when there are accusations of family theft or spousal infidelity or when the older adult asks his or her spouse to find his "real" wife or husband.

A medicine metaphor is appropriate. The timing and "dosing" of information may enhance effective use of that information in adapting care over time. Some families have read or heard inaccurate or partially correct information about symptoms that can be easily corrected, such as myths about all older men with dementia becoming sexual predators. Just like medication management in geriatrics, the maxim "start low and go slow" applies equally well to family education about dementia. Overwhelming families with too many treatment suggestions or referrals is just as likely to lead to poor compliance as is changing multiple medication regimens all at once. Finally, information should be presented in hopeful terms, such as "Treating your depression should have positive effects on your husband's mood as well" or "Many families surprise themselves with their resilience."

The presentation of information in a timed and dosed manner also offers opportunities for repetition of key themes. The key messages for family caregivers listed in Table 30–1 can be presented at intervals and in "doses" that are based on the frequency of contact with the family, the family's need to know, and the family's capacity to understand.

Responding to Families Over the Course of Progressive Impairment

Over the course of a dementia, family caregivers become not only information seekers but also care managers, consumer advocates, surrogate decision makers, and health care providers. It is difficult enough to negotiate these complex roles, and it is even more difficult if the family caregiver is burdened by role overload. Assessing caregiver vulnerability can be facilitated by asking family members to self-assess their pressure points or signs of increasing caregiver overload (Kaufer et al. 1998).

TABLE 30–1. Key messages for family caregivers

1. Be willing to listen to the older adult, but understand that you cannot fix or do everything he or she may want or need. Know that it will not necessarily get easier, but things will change, and the experience will change you forever.
2. You are living with a situation you did not create, and your choices are limited by circumstances beyond your control. Seek options that are good enough for now.
3. You can only do what seems best at the time. Identify what you can and will tolerate, then set limits and call in reinforcements. Doubts are inevitable.
4. Find someone with whom you can be brutally honest, express those doubts and negative feelings, and move on.
5. Solving problems is much easier than living with the solutions. It is tempting for distant relatives to second-guess or criticize. Hope for the best but plan for the worst.
6. It is not always possible to compare how one person handles things with how another relative would handle them if the positions were reversed.
7. The older adult is not unhappy or upset because of what you have done. He or she is living with unwanted dependency. Sick people often take out their frustration on close family members.
8. Considering what is best for your family involves compromise among competing needs, loyalties, and commitments. Everyone may get some of what he or she needs. Think twice before giving up that job, club, or church group. Make realistic commitments, and avoid making promises that include the words *always, never,* or *forever.*
9. Find ways to let your older relative give to or help you. He or she needs to feel purposeful, appreciated, and loved.
10. Take time to celebrate small victories when things go well.

Clinical red flags may signal imminent danger resulting from the caregiver's precarious health. Unsubtle hints may be a caregiver's comments such as "after my last stroke," "before he totaled the car," or "sometimes I feel like just letting him wander away." Pursuing these threads with standard clinical protocols is certainly warranted.

Other issues surface when working with families of moderately impaired older adults. Isolation of the caregiver and elder is common as friends drop off in response to disruptive behavioral symptoms or the need for constant supervision of the older adult. Families need to be reminded that being vulnerable does not make older people grateful or lovable and that cabin fever among cohabitating elders and family caregivers is a real threat to mental health and safety. Families are especially sensitive to elders who confuse or mistake family identities or suggest that family members are impostors. Making suggestions that family caregivers say something like "I'll try to do it like your mother would" may help them understand and respond to accusations of this type.

Family members need to be warned not to give up cherished activities—social engagement has positive mental health effects at any age, and maintenance of a strong religious faith or community has been shown to have positive effects on elders and family caregivers. Expressive outlets such as sports, the arts, or advocacy can help families cope with frustration and anger. Prayer, meditation, exercise, massage, and yoga, in combination with active treatment of depression or anxiety, are all worthy treatment recommendations. An elder's participation at an adult day center can be presented to the family as a source of social stimulation for the elder and a stress-reduction strategy for the family caregiver (Zarit et al. 1998).

Helping Families Assess Capacity of Older Adults

Many families turn to psychiatrists to assess the judgment and decision-making capacity of older adults, whether it is related to handling money, making health decisions, living alone, or driving.

Money-handling and health care decisions should be addressed soon after diagnosis to ensure time for patients to select a surrogate. Often families seek psychiatric consultation when family conflict surfaces over the patient's selection of a surrogate or the surrogate's handling of the older adult's funds. Questions about whether the patient had sufficient capacity at the time he or she wrote a will or assigned power of attorney can become adversarial and unrelated to family treatment.

Effective work with families regarding capacity is done early with a preventive focus. It is wise for one family member to make sure bills are paid. This can be done with different levels of involvement of the patient, from making decisions about which bills to pay to signing checks.

Assessment of and Limitations on Driving

Families can be encouraged to assess driving capacity based on observations of current driving, with reminders that dementia affects judgment, reaction time, and problem solving. Psychiatric assessment of the patient along with current observations from the family will provide direction on when driving should be limited. Unfortunately, by the time there is evidence of a decline in driving abilities, many patients cannot adequately report or judge their safety on the road. Anonymous reports to the Department of Motor Vehicles may lead to required testing or removal of the patient's license, but the absence of a license rarely stops a determined older adult with dementia.

Driving is one area in which the family must be encouraged and prepared to assess capacity over time. The signs listed in Table 30–2 may guide family observations and reports to the psychiatrist.

Psychiatrists may suggest a range of successful ways to limit driving, such as the following:

- A prescription reminder to stop driving can be tempered with a qualifier such as "until the end of your treatment." The patient's forgetfulness can be put to work for the psychiatrist. However, patients have been known to keep driving, making comments such as "That doctor doesn't know anything."
- Shaving the patient's keys, substituting another key, removing a distributor cap, or otherwise disabling a car can sometimes reduce the need to confront the patient with lost skills. However, patients have been known to fix the car, replace the keys, or even buy a new car while the old one was "in the shop."
- The car could be sold, moved to an undisclosed location, or put up on blocks. One family of a taxi driver put the taxi on blocks in the backyard to help the patient remember that it was broken.
- The family can also work on solutions that limit the need for driving—delivery services, senior vans, or offers of regular rides to church or for visits. Some families find that a taxi charge account works best.

TABLE 30–2. Signs of decline in driving skills
Incorrect signaling
Trouble navigating turns
Moving into the wrong lane
Getting confused about exits
Parking in inappropriate places
Driving at inappropriate speeds
Delayed responses to unexpected situations
Failure to anticipate dangerous situations
Scrapes or dents on car, garage, or mailbox
Becoming lost in familiar places
Arriving unusually late from a short-distance drive
Receiving moving violations or warnings about near misses
Confusing the brake and the accelerator
Stopping in traffic for no apparent reason

Addressing Questions of Capacity to Live Alone

Families may go to extremes to keep an older adult with dementia in a familiar environment, allowing values of autonomy and choice to temporarily trump safety. In addition to peforming a psychiatric assessment of the patient's cognition, judgment, functional impairment, and decision-making capacity, the psychiatrist can suggest that the family consider the following questions:

- Can the person with dementia use the telephone to call for help from a family member or to call 911? Will he or she respond inappropriately to telemarketers? Have mysterious packages or bills for unusual items begun appearing? Does he or she make repetitive calls every few minutes to the police or the same family member at work or at home?
- Can the family member with dementia get to the store or to his or her regular activities? Does he or she overbuy or underbuy certain items?
- Can the individual handle money and pay bills, or if not, is he or she willing to let others do this for him or her?
- Can he or she take medicine appropriately, on time, and in correct doses? Does he or she self-medicate or risk overdoses of unnecessary medications?
- Is he or she bathing, changing clothes, and dressing appropriately for the weather?

- Is he or she leaving the house after dark or traveling in dangerous areas alone? Does he or she let strangers in or buy from or contribute to questionable causes based on visits to his or her home?
- Is he having problems positioning his body to use a toilet, or is he urinating in wastebaskets or outdoors?
- Is he or she falling or getting lost by wandering outside a safe area?
- Are there significant changes in his or her appetite, weight, sleep, appearance, or eating habits?
- Is discreet surveillance by neighbors, friends, or family readily available?

The question of discreet surveillance is paramount. Persons with moderate dementia may live alone successfully if they have regular contact with, surveillance by, or checking from neighbors or family members. Environmental demand varies considerably and must be assessed along with patient variables.

Families and Institutionalization of the Older Adult

Not only does family stress not stop at the door of the nursing home, but ample evidence shows that families experience the greatest burden, disruption, and conflict in the time immediately before and after nursing home placement. Family members may seek psychiatric services to deal with guilt, grief, and often anger toward the nursing facility, reimbursement system, and each other. Many families are disappointed by the lack of medical or psychiatric treatment available to residents of nursing homes. Families should be encouraged to work with the facility and the nursing home ombudsman while dealing with their affective, anxiety, and grief symptoms.

Conclusion

Work with families of older adults is about adaptation to change and loss. Much of psychiatric treatment of families helps them modify expectations for new dependency while learning to forgive themselves and others for inevitable doubts and mistakes. Interdisciplinary partnerships and teamwork with the Alzheimer's Association or with nurses or social workers offer the most effective and efficient models for psychiatric services to families of older adults. There is often as much need for "timed and dosed" patient and family education as there is need for treatment of specific psychiatric symptoms or syndromes of the elder or family members. Families will expect psychiatrists to provide active treatment and monitoring of psychiatric symptoms, reassurance, interpretation of information, and referrals. In addition, it is always helpful to acknowledge losses and contributions to care by individual family members, to encourage caregiver self-care, to offer authoritative absolution for inevitable mistakes, and to offer decisional support, especially with transitions in care or with end-of-life care.

Key Points

- Psychiatric treatment of families helps them modify expectations about the newly dependent family member and learn to forgive themselves and others for inevitable doubts and mistakes.
- Interdisciplinary partnerships and teamwork with the Alzheimer's Association or with social workers or nurses offer the most effective and efficient models for psychiatric services to families of older adults.
- Psychiatrists should provide active treatment and monitoring of family caregivers' psychiatric symptoms, outline reasonable expectations, and offer families information about outcomes of treatment.
- It is helpful to acknowledge family caregivers' losses and their contributions to care. It is also important to encourage their own self-care and to offer them expert decisional support during transitions in care.

References

Belle SH, Burgio L, Burns R, et al: Enhancing the quality of life of dementia caregivers from different ethnic or racial groups: a randomized, controlled trial. Ann Intern Med 145:727–738, 2006

Brodaty H, Luscombe G: Psychological morbidity in caregivers is associated with depression in patients with dementia. Alzheimer Dis Assoc Disord 1:62–70, 1998

Burgio L, Stevens A, Guy D, et al: Impact of two psychosocial interventions on white and African-American family caregivers of individuals with dementia. Gerontologist 43:568–579, 2003

Burton LC, Newsom JT, Schulz R, et al: Preventive health behaviors among spousal caregivers. Prev Med 26:162–169, 1997

Callahan CM, Boustani MA, Unverzagt FW, et al: Effectiveness of collaborative care for older adults with Alzheimer disease in primary care: a randomized controlled trial. JAMA 295:2148–2157, 2006

Coon DW, Thompson L, Steffen A, et al: Anger and depression management: psychoeducational skill training intervention for women caregivers of a relative with dementia. Gerontologist 43:678–689, 2003

Derence K: Dementia-specific respite: the key to effective caregiver support. N C Med J 66:48–51, 2005

Eisdorfer C, Czaja SJ, Loewenstein DA, et al: The effect of a family therapy and technology-based intervention on caregiver depression. Gerontologist 43:521–531, 2003

Fortinsky RH, Kercher K, Burant CJ: Measurement and correlates of family caregiver self-efficacy for managing dementia. Aging Ment Health 6:153–160, 2002a

Fortinsky RH, Unson CG, Garcia RI: Helping family caregivers by linking primary care physicians with community-based dementia care services. Dementia 1:227–240, 2002b

Fulmer T, Paveza G, Van de Weerd C, et al: Dyadic vulnerability and risk profiling for elder neglect. Gerontologist 45:525–534, 2005

Gallagher-Thompson D, Coon DW: Evidence-based psychological treatments for distress in family caregivers of older adults. Psychol Aging 22:37–51, 2007

Gitlin LN, Reever K, Dennis MP, et al: Enhancing quality of life of families who use adult day services: short-and long-term effects of the Adult Day Services Plus Program. Gerontologist 46:630–639, 2006

Gwyther LP: Family issues in dementia: finding a new normal. Neurol Clin 18:993–1010, 2000

Gwyther LP: Family care and Alzheimer's disease: What do we know? What can we do? N C Med J 66:39–44, 2005

Hepburn K, Lewis M, Tornatore J, et al: The Savvy Caregiver program: the demonstrated effectiveness of a transportable dementia caregiver psychoeducation program. J Gerontol Nurs 33:30–36, 2007

Hughes SL, Giobie-Hurder A, Weaver FM, et al: Relationships between caregiver burden and health-related quality of life. Gerontologist 39:534–545, 1999

Kaufer DI, Cummings JL, Christine D, et al: Assessing the impact of neuropsychiatric symptoms in Alzheimer's disease: the Neuropsychiatric Inventory Caregiver Distress Scale. J Am Geriatr Soc 46:210–215, 1998

King AC, Brassington G: Enhancing physical and psychological functioning in older family caregivers: the role of regular physical activity. Ann Behav Med 19:91–100, 1997

Langa KM, Chernew ME, Kabeto MU, et al: National estimates of the quantity and cost of informal caregiving for the elderly with dementia. J Gen Intern Med 16:770–776, 2001

Lyketsos CG, Steinberg M, Tschanz JT, et al: Mental and behavioral disturbances in dementia: findings from the Cache County Study on Memory in Aging. Am J Psychiatry 157:708–714, 2000

McCurry SM, Gibbons LE, Logsdon RG, et al: Nighttime insomnia treatment and education for Alzheimer's disease: a randomized controlled trial. J Am Geriatr Soc 53:793–802, 2005a

McCurry SM, Logsdon R, Gibbons LE: Training community consultants to help family members improve dementia care: a randomized controlled trial. Gerontologist 45:802–811, 2005b

Mittelman MS, Ferris SH, Shulman E, et al: A family intervention to delay nursing home placement of patients with Alzheimer disease: a randomized controlled trial. JAMA 276:1725–1731, 1996

Mittelman MS, Roth DL, Haley WE, et al: Effects of a caregiver intervention on negative caregiver appraisals of behavior problems in patients with Alzheimer's disease: results of a randomized trial. J Gerontol B Psychol Sci Soc Sci 59:P27–P34, 2004

Mittelman MS, Roth DL, Clay OJ, et al: Preserving health of Alzheimer caregivers: impact of a spouse caregiver intervention. Am J Geriatr Psychiatry 15:780–789, 2007

Olin JT, Schneider LS, Katz IR, et al: Provisional diagnostic criteria for depression of Alzheimer's disease. Am J Geriatr Psychiatry 10:125–128, 2002

Ostwald SK, Hepburn KW, Caron W, et al: Reducing caregiver burden: a randomized psychoeducational intervention for caregivers of persons with dementia. Gerontologist 39:299–309, 1999

Pillemer K, Suitor JJ: "It takes one to help one": effects of similar others on the well-being of caregivers. J Gerontol B Psychol Sci Soc Sci 51:S250–S257, 1996

Pinquart M, Sorensen S: Ethnic differences in stressors, resources, and psychological outcomes of family caregiving: a meta-analysis. Gerontologist 45:90–106, 2005

Pinquart M, Sorensen S: Gender differences in caregiver stressors, social resources, and health: an updated meta-analysis. J Gerontol B Psychol Sci Soc Sci 61:P33–P45, 2006a

Pinquart M, Sorensen S: Helping caregivers of persons with dementia: which interventions work and how large are the effects? Int Psychogeriatr 18:577–595, 2006b

Rabins PV, Lyketsos C, Steele C: Practical Dementia Care. Oxford, UK, Oxford University Press, 2006

Schulz R, Beach SR: Caregiving as a risk factor for mortality: the Caregiver Health Effects Study. JAMA 282:2215–2219, 1999

Sorensen S, Pinquart M, Duberstein P, et al: How effective are interventions with caregivers? An updated meta-analysis. Gerontologist 42:356–372, 2002

Spangenberg KB, Wagner MT, Hendrix S, et al: Firearm presence in households of patients with Alzheimer's disease and other dementias. J Am Geriatr Soc 47:1183–1186, 1999

Teri L, Logsdon RG, Uomoto J, et al: Behavioral treatment of depression in dementia patients: a controlled clinical trial. J Gerontol B Psychol Sci Soc Sci 52:P159–P166, 1997

Teri L, Gibbons LE, McCurry SM, et al: Exercise plus behavioral management in patients with Alzheimer's disease: a randomized controlled trial. JAMA 290:2015–2022, 2003

Tierney MC, Charles J, Naglie G, et al: Risk factors for harm in cognitively impaired seniors who live alone: a prospective study. J Am Geriatr Soc 52:1435–1441, 2004

Tractenberg RE, Weiner MF, Thal LJ: Estimating the prevalence of agitation in community-dwelling persons with Alzheimer's disease. J Neuropsychiatry Clin Neurosci 14:11–18, 2002

Whitlatch CJ, Judge K, Zarit SH, et al: Dyadic intervention for family caregivers and care receivers in early stage dementia. Gerontologist 46:688–694, 2006

Yaffe K, Fox P, Newcomer R, et al: Patient and caregiver characteristics and nursing home placement in patients with dementia. JAMA 287:2090–2097, 2002

Yates ME, Tennstedt S, Chang BH: Contributors to and mediators of psychological well-being for informal caregivers. J Gerontol B Psychol Sci Soc Sci 54:P12–P22, 1999

Zarit SH, Stephens MA, Townsend A, et al: Stress reduction for family caregivers: effects of adult day care use. J Gerontol B Psychol Sci Soc Sci 53:S267–S277, 1998

Suggested Readings

Belle SH, Burgio L, Burns R, et al: Enhancing the quality of life of dementia caregivers from different ethnic or racial groups: a randomized, controlled trial. Ann Intern Med 145:727–738, 2006

Gallagher-Thompson D, Coon DW: Evidence-based psychological treatments for distress in family caregivers of older adults. Psychol Aging 22:37–51, 2007

Mittelman MS, Roth DL, Clay OJ, et al: Preserving health of Alzheimer caregivers: impact of a spouse caregiver intervention. Am J Geriatr Psychiatry 15:780–789, 2007

Pinquart M, Sorensen S: Helping caregivers of persons with dementia: which interventions work and how large are the effects? Int Psychogeriatr 18:577–595, 2006

Rabins PV, Lyketsos C, Steele C: Practical Dementia Care. Oxford, UK, Oxford University Press, 2006

CHAPTER 31

Clinical Psychiatry in the Nursing Home

Joel E. Streim, M.D.
Ira R. Katz, M.D., Ph.D.

Nursing homes provide long-term care for elderly patients with chronic illness and disability as well as rehabilitation and convalescent care for those recovering from acute illness. As documented in previous reviews (Katz et al. 2000; Streim et al. 2004), clinical studies have consistently provided evidence that the diagnosis, management, and treatment of mental disorders are important components of nursing home care. The delivery of mental health services in nursing homes continues to be shaped by several factors, including growing scientific knowledge, availability of new treatments, evolving federal regulations, public dissemination of survey data, and changes in the medical marketplace. In this chapter we review current information on the psychiatric problems that are common in the nursing home, discuss current trends affecting clinical care, and present a conceptual model for the organization of mental health services.

Nursing Home Populations

Although the number of nursing homes in the United States has decreased by 16% since 1985, the total number of beds remains relatively constant (National Center for Health Statistics 2004). According to the 2004 National Nursing Home Survey, 4% of Americans age 65 years or older—1.5 million people—resided in 16,100 long-term care facilities. Compared with 1995 survey data from the National Center for Health Statistics (Dey 1997), this percentage actually represents a 0.11% decline in the proportion of adults over age 65 residing in nursing homes, although the proportion of residents in the oldest age groups has been continuously increasing. Between 1977 and 1999, the proportion of nursing home residents 65–84 years of age decreased from 52.2% to 43.8%, whereas the proportion of residents 85 years of age and older increased from 34.8% to 46.5% (Decker 2005). Not surprisingly, with the increasing age of residents in nursing homes, there has been a decline in the proportion of residents who are independent in the performance of basic activities of daily living (ADLs). For example, in 1977, 30% of residents could dress without assistance, compared with only 13% in 1999. In that same period, the proportion of residents who were completely independent in bathing declined from 13% to 5.6% (Decker 2005). These trends suggest that despite the increased availability of long-term care services at home and in assisted living facilities, nursing homes continue to be utilized to care for the oldest and most frail elderly.

Persons living in nursing homes in recent years have tended to be very disabled: 96% of residents required assistance with bathing, 86% with dressing, 57% with toileting, and 45% with feeding. Thirty percent had ambulatory dysfunction, and 24% required assistance getting in and out of bed. The proportion needing help with three or more ADLs was 83.3%, and only 8% were independent in all ADLs (Krauss and Altman 1998;

Rhoades and Krauss 1999). Among residents 65 years of age and older, 27% had visual impairment and 23% had hearing impairment. Approximately half of nursing home residents had some incontinence of both bladder and bowel. These statistics show that nursing home residents are characterized by extreme old age and high levels of disability. The prediction that future nursing home populations will be composed of increasingly older, sicker, and more functionally dependent residents (Evans et al. 1995) has been realized, and this trend appears to be continuing (National Center for Health Statistics 2004).

Prevalence of Psychiatric Disorders

Epidemiological studies conducted between 1986 and 1993 uniformly reported high prevalence rates for psychiatric disorders among nursing home residents. Rovner et al. (1990a) reported the prevalence of psychiatric disorders among persons newly admitted to a proprietary chain of nursing homes to be 80.2%. Parmelee et al. (1989) found psychiatric disorders diagnosed according to DSM-III-R (American Psychiatric Association 1987) criteria in 91% of the residents of a large urban geriatric center. On the basis of psychiatric interviews of subjects in randomly selected samples, other investigators found prevalence rates of DSM-III (American Psychiatric Association 1980) or DSM-III-R disorders to be as high as 94% (Chandler and Chandler 1988; Rovner et al. 1986; Tariot et al. 1993). Although some studies reported lower rates, those investigations used less rigorous methods for sampling or diagnosis (Burns et al. 1988; Custer et al. 1984; German et al. 1986; National Center for Health Statistics 1987; Teeter et al. 1976). In one study, case ascertainment by review of selected medical records revealed a 68% prevalence of psychiatric diagnosis (Linkins et al. 2006), suggesting that chart documentation of mental disorders by nursing home clinicians may underestimate the actual rates of mental disorders. An interview-based study of the distribution of various psychiatric disorders among nursing home residents found that 67.4% of residents had dementia, 10.4% had depressive disorders, and 2.4% had schizophrenia or other psychotic disorders (Rovner et al. 1990a). Although there have been no interview-based epidemiological studies in nursing homes published since 1993, subsequent prevalence data from the Medical Expenditures Panel Survey (MEPS) revealed that 70%–80% of residents had cognitive impairment and 20% had a diagnosis of a depressive disorder (Krauss and Altman 1998). Although the MEPS data were not derived from clinical interviews, they indicate prevalence rates of dementia and depression that are greater than the prevalence rates found in nursing home studies a decade earlier. These prevalence data also suggest that nursing homes are de facto neuropsychiatric institutions, although they were not originally intended for this purpose. The challenge of providing long-term care services in nursing homes is therefore complicated by the extensive psychiatric comorbidity found in this setting.

Cognitive Disorders and Behavioral Disturbances

In all studies, the most common psychiatric disorder was dementia, with prevalence rates of 50% – 75% (Chandler and Chandler 1988; Katz et al. 1989; Parmelee et al. 1989; Rovner et al. 1986, 1990a; Tariot et al. 1993; Teeter et al. 1976). Alzheimer's disease (DSM-III-R primary degenerative dementia) accounted for about 50%–60% of cases of dementia, and vascular dementia accounted for about 25%–30% (Barnes and Raskind 1980; Rovner et al. 1986, 1990a). Other causes of dementia were reported with lower prevalence and greater variability between sites. The prevalence of Lewy body dementia has not been ascertained in nursing home populations.

Delirium is common in nursing homes and occurs primarily in patients made more vulnerable by a dementing illness. Available studies indicated that approximately 6%–7% of residents were delirious at the time of evaluation (Barnes and Raskind 1980; Rovner et al. 1986, 1990a). However, this figure probably underestimates the number of patients who have cognitive impairment associated with reversible toxic or metabolic factors. In one study, investigators found that nearly 25% of impaired residents had potentially reversible conditions (Sabin et al. 1982); in another study it was found that 6%–12% of residential care patients with dementia actually improved in cognitive performance over the course of 1 year (Katz et al. 1991). A large study of residents with severe cognitive impairment found improvement at 6-month follow-up in 14% of the sample, associated with the following baseline findings: higher function, antidepressant medication use, and falls (Buttar et al. 2003). In the nursing home, as in other settings, a common reversible cause of cognitive impairment may be cognitive toxicity from drugs used to treat medical or psychiatric disorders. However, there is evidence that long-acting opioids, previously thought to have adverse effects on cognitive function, may actually lead to improvements in functional status and social engagement without decrements in cognitive status or increases in the rate of delirium among nursing home residents who are treated for nonmalignant chronic pain (Won et al. 2006). For residents admitted to the nursing home for post–acute care rehabilitation, unresolved delirium is associated with poor functional recovery (Kiely et al. 2007).

The clinical features of dementing disorders include treatable behavioral and psychological symptoms of dementia—such as hallucinations, delusions, depression, anxiety, and agitation—that can contribute to disability. Combined 1-year prevalence of psychosis, agitation, and depression has been estimated between 76% and 82% (Ballard et al. 2001). In nursing home populations, psychotic symptoms have been reported in approximately 25%–50% of residents with a primary dementing illness (Berrios and Brook 1985; Chandler and Chandler 1988; Rovner et al. 1986, 1990a; Teeter et al. 1976). Clinically significant depression is seen in approximately 25% of patients with dementia; one-third of such patients exhibit symptoms of secondary major depression (Parmelee et al. 1989; Rovner et al. 1986, 1990a). Dementia complicated by mixed agitation and depression accounts for more than one-third of complicated dementia in nursing home populations and is associated with multiple psychiatric and medical needs, psychotropic drug use, and hospital admissions (Bartels et al. 2003).

MEPS data revealed that 30% of residents exhibit behavioral problems, including 11.8% with verbal abuse, 9.1% with physical abuse, 14.5% with socially inappropriate behavior, 12.5% with resistance to care, and 9.4% with wandering (Krauss and Altman 1998). In earlier studies, behavioral disturbances were found in up to 75% of residents, and multiple behavior problems were found in at least half (Chandler and Chandler 1988; Cohen-Mansfield 1986; National Center for Health Statistics 1979; Rovner et al. 1986, 1990a; Tariot et al. 1993; Zimmer et al. 1984). It is likely that the lower rates reported in MEPS reflect a different method of case ascertainment rather than improvement in behavioral management leading to a subsequent decrease in prevalence. In addition to impaired ability to perform ADLs, disturbances of behavior have been identified as the most common reasons that patients with dementia are admitted to nursing homes (Steele et al. 1990), and disruptive behaviors frequently complicate care after admission (Cohen-Mansfield et al. 1989; Teeter et al. 1976; Zimmer et al. 1984). The majority of psychiatric consultations in long-term care settings are for the evaluation and treatment of behavioral disturbances such as pacing and wandering, verbal abusiveness, disruptive shouting, physical aggression, destructive acts, and resistance to necessary care (Fenton et al. 2004; Loebel et al. 1991). Behavioral disturbances most frequently occur in patients with dementia, often in those with psychotic symptoms—an association that remains even after controlling for level of cognitive impairment (Rovner et al. 1990b). Agitation and hyperactivity can also be caused by agitated depression (Heeren et al. 2003) as well as delirium, sensory deprivation or overload, occult physical illness, pain, constipation, urinary retention, and adverse drug effects (including akathisia due to neuroleptics) (Cohen-Mansfield and Billig 1986). Depressive symptoms are associated with disruptive vocalizations in nursing home residents, even after controlling for gender, age, and cognitive status (Dwyer and Byrne 2000). In a subsequent study comparing verbal and physical nonaggressive agitation, verbal agitation was correlated with female gender, depressed affect, poor performance of ADLs, and impaired social functioning (Cohen-Mansfield and Libin 2005).

In addition to agitation, symptoms such as apathy, inactivity, and withdrawal occur among nursing home residents with and without a diagnosis of depression. Although these symptoms are less disturbing to staff and less frequently lead to psychiatric consultation (Fenton et al. 2004), they can be disabling and may be associated with decreases in socialization and self-care.

Depression

Among community-dwelling elders in the United States and Europe, depression increases the risk of nursing home admission (Ahmed et al. 2007; Harris and Cooper 2006; Onder et al. 2007), and this association remains after controlling for age, physical illness, and functional status (Harris 2007). Among those who reside in nursing homes, depressive disorders represent the second most common psychiatric diagnosis. Most studies in U.S. nursing homes show depression prevalence rates of 15%–50%, depending on the population studied and the instruments used, whether major depression or depressive symptoms are being reported, and whether primary depression and depression occurring secondary to dementia are considered together or separately (Baker and Miller 1991; Chandler and Chandler 1988; Hyer and Blazer 1982; Katz et al. 1989; Kaup et al. 2007; Lesher 1986; Levin et al. 2007; Parmelee et al. 1989; Rovner et al. 1986, 1990a, 1991; Tariot et al. 1993; Teeter et al. 1976). Studies from other countries have shown similar rates (Ames 1990, 1991; Ames et al. 1988; Chahine et al. 2007; Harrison et al. 1990; Horiguchi and Inami 1991; Jongenelis et al. 2004; Mann et al. 1984; Snowdon 1986; Snowdon and Donnelly 1986; Spagnoli et al. 1986; Trichard et al. 1982). Thus, the high rates of depression in the United States cannot be attributed solely to problems in this country's approach to long-term care for elderly persons. Approximately 6%–10% of all nursing home residents, and 20%–25% of those who are cognitively intact, meet DSM-III or DSM-III-R criteria for major depression; the latter figure is an order of magnitude greater than rates among community-dwelling elderly persons (Blazer and Williams 1980; Kramer et al. 1985).

The prevalence of less severe but clinically significant (e.g., minor or subsyndromal) depression is even higher. In one study, Parmelee et al. (1992a) reported that the 1-year incidence of major depression was 9.4% and that patients with preexisting minor depression were at increased risk; the incidence of minor depression among those who were euthymic at baseline was 7.4%. Other smaller-scale studies have shown comparable rates (Foster et al. 1991; Katz et al. 1989). These data show that minor depression in nursing home residents appears to be a risk factor for major depression and might represent an opportunity for preventive treatment in this population.

Depression among nursing home residents tends to be persistent. Although there may be moderate decreases in self-rated depression in the initial 2 weeks to 6 months after nursing home admission (Engle and Graney 1993; Smalbrugge et al. 2006), Ames et al. (1988) found that only 17% of patients with diagnosable depressive disorders had recovered after an average 3.6 years of follow-up. Smallbrugge et al. (2006) found persistence of symptoms in two-thirds of residents at 6-month follow-up, although rates were significantly higher in those with more severe symptoms at baseline. Evidence for morbidity associated with depression comes from studies that showed an increase in pain complaints among residents with depression (Parmelee et al. 1991) and an association between depression and biochemical markers of subnutrition (Katz et al. 1993). Depression in nursing home residents, both with and without dementia, is associated with disability (Kaup et al. 2007). Among individuals admitted to nursing homes for post–acute care rehabilitation, those with depression have poorer functional outcomes (Webber et al. 2005). In addition to its association with morbidity and disability, depression has been found to be associated with an increase in mortality rate, with effect sizes ranging from 1.6 to 3 (Ashby et al. 1991; Katz et al. 1989; Parmelee et al. 1992b; Rovner et al. 1991; Sutcliffe et al. 2007). There is, however, controversy about the mechanism involved. Whereas Rovner et al. (1991) reported that the increased mortality rate remained apparent after controlling for the patients' medical diagnoses and level of disability, Parmelee et al. (1992a) found that the effect could be attributed to the interrelationships among depression, disability, and physical illness. Resolution of this issue still requires further study.

The literature on depression as it presents in patients with significant medical illness is marked by recurring questions about the extent to which diagnostic criteria developed in younger and healthier adults remain valid among patients with significant psychiatric and medical comorbidity. It might seem logical to expect that the somatic and vegetative symptoms that characterize major depression in other populations lose their diagnostic value among long-term care residents and that long-term care patients who have symptoms consistent with a diagnosis of major depressive disorder may instead be experiencing a combination of medical symptoms and an existential reaction to disease, disability, and residential care placement. However, it has been demonstrated that DSM diagnostic criteria remain valid as predictors of treatment response and that the symptoms of major depression in frail elderly patients characterize a disease similar to that which occurs among younger adult psychiatric patients (Katz et al. 1990), even though most nursing home patients have concurrent medical illnesses and disabilities that complicate diagnosis and treatment.

In addition to the high level of complexity that characterizes major depression among nursing home residents, there is evidence for heterogeneity in these patients that may reflect the existence of clinically relevant subtypes of depression. The treatment study by Katz et al. (1990) demonstrated that measures of self-care deficits and serum levels of albumin were highly intercorrelated and that both predicted a lack of response to treatment with nortriptyline. Therefore, although this study demonstrated that major depression is a specific, treatable disorder—even in long-term care patients with medical comorbidity—there is also evidence in this setting for a treatment-relevant subtype of depression characterized by high levels of disability and low levels of serum albumin. This latter condition may be related to failure to thrive in infants, as discussed by Braun et al. (1988) and by Katz et al. (1993).

Progress in Treatment of Psychiatric Disorders in the Nursing Home

As described earlier, the high levels of psychiatric morbidity in nursing home residents did not diminish over the last 15 years of the twentieth century. However, during the 1990s and beyond, there was significant progress in the development and evaluation of treatments for psychiatric disorders in nursing homes. An appreciation of the unique characteristics of nursing home populations—particularly the extremes of old age and the high prevalences of cognitive impairment, psychiatric and medical comorbidity, and disability, all in the context of residential long-term care institutions—has led to increased recognition that results of efficacy studies conducted in general adult outpatient populations may not be readily generalizable to nursing home residents. This recognition points to the need for treatment studies conducted specifically with nursing home patients. Although the number of randomized, controlled studies is limited, there is a growing body of literature on treatment outcomes in the nursing home.

Nonpharmacological Management of Behavioral Disturbances

Since 1990, numerous studies have been published describing nonpharmacological interventions for behavioral disturbances associated with dementia in the nursing home setting. Few of these are randomized, controlled trials. The reader is referred to comprehensive reviews of these studies by Cohen-Mansfield (2001), Snowden et al. (2003), and Livingston et al. (2005). Several nonpharmacological interventions have been shown to be effective, although only behavior management therapies, specific types of caregiver and residential care staff education, and possibly cognitive stimulation appear to have lasting effectiveness (Livingston et al. 2005). One promising approach combined enhanced activities, guidelines for the use of psychotropic medication, and educational rounds for nursing home staff (Rovner et al. 1996). In a randomized clinical trial, this approach was shown to reduce the prevalence of problem behaviors and the use of antipsychotic drugs and physical restraints. Activities matched to skills and interests of residents with dementia have also been shown to reduce agitation and negative affect (Kolanowski et al. 2005). Individualized consultation for staff nurses about the management of patients with dementia was also shown to diminish the use of physical restraints (Evans et al. 1997). Reductions in agitation were observed in a study of a daytime physical activity intervention combined with a nighttime program to decrease noise and sleep-disruptive nursing care practices (Alessi 1999). Bright light therapy has been shown to increase observed nocturnal sleep time but not to improve agitated behavior in nursing home residents with dementia (Lyketsos et al. 1999). Although some studies have claimed that aromatherapy with lavender oil is effective in reducing agitated behaviors, results have not been consistently replicated when controlling for nonolfactory aspects of treatment in residents with severe dementia (Snow et al. 2004). Other programs decrease behavioral difficulties through individualized modifications in the physical environment (van Weert et al. 2005). Research on individualized behavioral interventions for patients with behavioral disturbances of dementia has been limited to case series and small-scale controlled trials that are often difficult to replicate, although some of the results are promising (Allen-Burge et al. 1999).

Psychotherapy

The evidence for the efficacy of psychotherapy in other settings suggests that it may be of value for treating mental disorders of aging in patients whose cognitive abilities allow them to participate. However, a search of the PsycINFO, PubMed, and Cochrane databases for the terms *psychotherapy* and *nursing homes* from 1987 to the time of writing this chapter identified only a small number of controlled studies of the effectiveness of specific psychotherapeutic modalities, individual or group, for nursing home residents (Table 31–1). Bharucha et al. (2006) identified and reviewed 18 controlled "talk" psychotherapy studies conducted in nursing home populations and found that a majority showed at least short-term benefits on measures of mood, hopeless-

TABLE 31–1. Randomized, controlled studies of the outcomes of psychotherapeutic interventions in elderly nursing home residents

Study	Type of intervention	Sample	Outcome measures	Results and comments
Moran and Gatz 1987	Task-oriented group vs. insight-oriented group vs. waiting-room control group	*N*=59; mean age, 76.3 years; conversant, mobile	Self-reported psychosocial competence in a) sense of control, b) trust, c) active coping, d) striving for social approval; life satisfaction	Task group improved on all measures except trust. Task group had significant increase in life satisfaction compared with insight and control groups. Insight group improved on sense of control and trust.
Baines et al. 1987	Reality orientation vs. reminiscence therapy vs. no-therapy control group (crossover design)	*N*=15; mean age, 81.5 years; moderately to severely cognitively impaired	Cognitive function; life satisfaction; communication; behavior; staff knowledge of residents	Only the group that received reality orientation first, followed by reminiscence therapy, showed sustained improvement in communication and behavior and nonsustained improvement in function (information/orientation). No improvement was found in other groups. Intervention was associated with improved staff knowledge of residents.
Goldwasser et al. 1987	Reminiscence group therapy vs. supportive group therapy vs. no-treatment control group	*N*=27; dementia (MMSE range, 1–22; mean, 10.4)	Depression; cognitive function; behavioral/ADL function	Reminiscence group showed nonsustained improvement in self-reported depression on BDI. Neither intervention showed significant effects on cognitive or behavioral function.
Orten et al. 1989	Reminiscence group vs. control group	*N*=56; mean age, 82.6 years; moderately confused	Social behavior; ADL function; agitation; somatic complaining; attitude	Significant improvement for one of three experimental groups; no improvement when all groups were analyzed together. Investigators suggest that therapist skills are an important variable.
Rattenbury and Stones 1989	Reminiscence group vs. current topics discussion group vs. no group	*N*=24; mean ages of groups, 83–87 years; judged by nursing home staff not to be cognitively impaired	Psychological well-being (happiness-depression scale); activity level; functional level; mood	Both intervention groups improved on happiness-depression scale. No improvement on other measures, including mood scale. Positive correlation between happiness scores and increased verbal activity level between first and fourth weeks.
Youssef 1990	Group reminiscence counseling for young-old subjects vs. group reminiscence counseling for old-old subjects vs. control group	*N*=60, all women; young-old, 65–74 years; old-old, ≥75 years	Depression	Young-old group had significant improvement in depression scores on BDI. Old-old group showed improvement only on social withdrawal and somatic preoccupation items but not on total BDI scores. Control condition was not described.

TABLE 31–1. Randomized, controlled studies of the outcomes of psychotherapeutic interventions in elderly nursing home residents *(continued)*

Study	Type of intervention	Sample	Outcome measures	Results and comments
Ames 1990	Psychogeriatric team recommendations vs. routine clinical care	*N*=93; mean age, 82.3 years	Depression; ADL performance	No difference between intervention and control groups. Only 27 of 81 recommended interventions were actually implemented (e.g., medication changes, referral for mental health services). Role of psychogeriatric services in management of the facilities and medical care of the residents was not clearly defined.
Zerhusen et al. 1991	Group cognitive therapy vs. music group (control) vs. routine clinical care (control)	*N*=60; mean age, 77 years	Depression; performance ratings of group leaders	Cognitive therapy group had 30% improvement in self-rated depression scores on BDI; no significant improvement in control subjects. Group gains did not vary with group leader ratings.
Williams-Barnard and Lindell 1992	Group therapy with high nurse prizing vs. group therapy with low nurse prizing vs. control group (control had 3 meetings vs. 16 meetings for experimental groups)	*N*=73; age ≥65 years	Self-concept	Self-concept improved in 68.4% of residents in high-prizing group, 29.4% of residents in low-prizing groups, and 10.8% of residents in control group. Self-concept declined in 40% of low-prizing group and 5.3% of high-prizing group.
Bensink et al. 1992	PR group vs. activity group (control)	*N*=28; age ≥65 years; mean age, 77 years; MMSE score ≥20	Locus of control; self-esteem	Only PR group showed increase in perceived internal locus of control. Both PR and activity groups showed improvement in self-esteem, with greater effect in PR group.
Abraham et al. 1992	CB group therapy vs. FVI group therapy vs. control groups (control had 3 meetings vs. 16 meetings for experimental groups)	*N*=76; mean age, 84 years; depressed and mildly to moderately cognitively impaired	Cognitive function; depression; hopelessness; life satisfaction	No effects of group therapy on geriatric depression, hopelessness, or life satisfaction. Both CB and FVI groups showed improved cognitive function on modified MMSE, with greater gains in FVI participants. No significant cognitive change in ED control groups.
McMurdo and Rennie 1993	Exercise sessions vs. reminiscence groups	*N*=49; mean age, 81 years	Physical function; ADL performance; depression; life satisfaction; cognitive function	Physical function improved in exercise group, declined in reminiscence group. Self-reported depression (BDI scores) declined in both groups; exercise group showed significantly greater improvement than reminiscence group.
Abraham et al. 1997	CB group therapy vs. FVI group therapy vs. control groups	*N*=76; mean age, 84 years; depressed with mild to moderate cognitive impairment	Depression factors; cognitive factors	Secondary analyses. Both CB and FVI reduced depressive symptoms over 24 weeks.

TABLE 31–1. Randomized, controlled studies of the outcomes of psychotherapeutic interventions in elderly nursing home residents *(continued)*

Study	Type of intervention	Sample	Outcome measures	Results and comments
Toseland et al. 1997	VT group vs. social contact group (control) vs. usual care group (control)	*N*=88; mean age, 87 years; dementia	Behavioral disturbances; depression; use of physical restraints; use of psychotropic medication	VT group had less physical and verbal aggression and less depression than social contact or usual care group. VT not effective in reducing physical restraints or psychotropic drug use. Social contact and usual care groups had great reductions in nonaggressive behavioral problems.
C.K. Beck et al. 2002	ADL group vs. psychosocial activity intervention vs. both vs. placebo vs. no intervention	*N*=127; mean age, 83 years; mean MMSE score=10; with disruptive behaviors	Positive and negative affect; frequency of disruptive behaviors	Significantly more positive affect in treatment groups; no decrease in negative affect and no change in disruptive behaviors.
Politis et al. 2004	Reminiscence-based activity intervention vs. "time and attention" one-on-one meetings with activities therapist (control)	*N*=37; dementia diagnosis	Apathy; quality of life; activity level	Significant reduction in NPI apathy scores in both groups, but no difference between groups; greater within-group improvement on quality-of-life measure for control group only.
Chao et al. 2006	Reminiscence group therapy vs. usual care (matched controls)	*N*=24	Depression; self-esteem; life satisfaction	Significant improvement on self-esteem measure; no significant effects on depression or life satisfaction.

Note. ADL=activities of daily living; BDI=Beck Depression Inventory (A.T. Beck et al. 1961); CB=cognitive-behavioral; ED=education-discussion; FVI=focused visual imagery; MMSE=Mini-Mental State Exam (Folstein et al. 1975); NPI=Neuropsychiatric Inventory (Wood et al. 2000); PR=progressive relaxation; VT=validation therapy.

ness, perceived control, self-esteem, or other psychological variables. However, the authors noted that interpretation of findings of many of these studies was limited by small sample sizes, variable study entry criteria, short duration of trials, heterogeneous outcome assessment methods, and lack of detail on intervention methods. Controlled research on psychotherapeutic interventions has included studies of task-oriented versus insight-oriented therapy (Moran and Gatz 1987); reality orientation (Baines et al. 1987); reminiscence groups (Baines et al. 1987; Chao et al. 2006; Goldwasser et al. 1987; McMurdo and Rennie 1993; Orten et al. 1989; Politis et al. 2004; Rattenbury and Stones 1989; Youssef 1990); exercise, activity, and progressive relaxation groups (Bensink et al. 1992; McMurdo and Rennie 1993); supportive group psychotherapy (Goldwasser et al. 1987; Williams-Barnard and Lindell 1992); validation therapy (Tondi et al. 2007; Toseland et al. 1997); cognitive or cognitive-behavioral group therapies (Abraham et al. 1992; Zerhusen et al. 1991); focused visual imagery therapy (Abraham et al. 1997); and a psychosocial activity intervention (Beck et al. 2002). With the exception of the investigations by Abraham and colleagues, patients in most of these studies were not selected on the basis of specific psychiatric symptoms or syndromes but rather on the basis of age, cognitive status, or mobility.

Some of these studies reported improvements on measures of communication, behavior, cognitive performance, mood, social withdrawal, physical function, somatic preoccupation, self-esteem, perceived locus of control, quality of life, and life satisfaction. Case reports and demonstration projects by experienced clinicians also documented the value of psychotherapy for treating depressed nursing home residents (Leszcz et al. 1985; Ollech 2006; Sadavoy 1991). Overall, there is a paucity of research on the outcomes of well-described psychotherapies among nursing home residents who have well-characterized psychiatric disorders. Nevertheless, the available evidence from nursing home research, considered together with outcomes of psychotherapy for older adults in other clinical settings, suggests that psychotherapy should be regarded as an important component of mental health treatment for the more cognitively intact nursing home residents with depression.

Pharmacotherapy

Pharmacological treatments are commonly used in nursing homes for dementia and its associated psychological and behavioral symptoms, and for depression. For a more comprehensive review of the evidence for pharmacological treatment of neuropsychiatric symptoms of dementia, the reader is referred to the article by Sink et al. (2005).

Before 1985 there were few randomized, placebo-controlled clinical trials of psychotropic drugs that were conducted specifically in nursing home populations; those that have been published since that time are summarized in Table 31–2. Some of the earlier studies provided evidence for the efficacy of antipsychotic drugs in managing agitation and related symptoms in nursing home residents with dementia, but the effect sizes were often modest, and high placebo response rates were common (Barnes et al. 1982; Schneider et al. 1990; Sunderland and Silver 1988). Subsequently, several multicenter, randomized, double-blind, placebo-controlled clinical trials demonstrated efficacy of some of the atypical antipsychotic agents for the treatment of psychotic symptoms and agitated behavior in nursing home residents with dementia. These include published studies of risperidone (Brodaty et al. 2003; Katz et al. 1999), olanzapine (Meehan et al. 2002; Street et al. 2000), quetiapine (Zhong et al. 2007), and aripiprazole (Mintzer et al. 2007). Secondary analyses of data from the nursing home trials of risperidone showed that it had antipsychotic effects and also had independent effects on aggression or agitation. Other studies of atypical antipsychotic drugs in nursing home residents with dementia failed to show statistically significant benefits on the *a priori* designated primary outcome measures related to psychosis or behavioral disturbances (DeDeyn et al. 1999, 2004; Mintzer et al. 2006; Streim et al., in press), although some of these studies found possible benefits on secondary behavioral measures. Widespread interest in studying atypical antipsychotics for treatment of elderly nursing home residents was partly attributable to the expectation that these agents would be better tolerated than conventional antipsychotics in this population. For example, early follow-up studies had suggested that risperidone may cause less tardive dyskinesia than do typical antipsychotic agents (Jeste et al. 2000).

These controlled clinical trials have examined only the acute effects of treatment, typically for 6–12 weeks of treatment, and little is known about the effectiveness of treatment for longer periods. However, there is evidence to suggest that the need for and benefit from antipsychotic drug treatment changes over the course of

TABLE 31–2. Randomized, placebo-controlled studies of the efficacy of psychotropic medications in elderly nursing home residents

Study	Medication and dosage (mg/day)	Sample	Efficacy measures	Results and comments
Beber 1965	Oxazepam (10–80) vs. placebo	*N*=100; mean age, 79 years; nonpsychotic with chronic brain syndrome (*n*=28), mixed anxiety/depression (*n*=26), anxiety (*n*=43), or depression (*n*=3)	Anxiety and tension; depression, lethargy, and autonomic reactions; irritability, insomnia, agitation, phobic reactions	Improvement in all parameters was significantly greater in oxazepam-treated group than in placebo-treated group; 44 subjects received concomitant treatment with other drugs, including neuroleptics, antidepressants, hypnotics, antiparkinsonian agents, and analgesics.
Barnes et al. 1982	Thioridazine (mean, 62.5) vs. loxapine (mean, 10.5) vs. placebo	*N*=53; mean age, 83 years; dementia and three or more behavioral symptoms	BPRS; SCAG; NOSIE; CGI	Total scores and global ratings showed modest efficacy with thioridazine and loxapine, but not statistically better than placebo; high placebo response rate; significant improvement in anxiety, excitement, emotional lability, and uncooperativeness in active treatment groups, but no significant differences in overall efficacy between thioridazine and loxapine; significant improvement on BPRS and SCAG only in subjects with high-severity baseline scores.
Stotsky 1984	Thioridazine (10–200) vs. diazepam (20–40) vs. placebo	*N*=237 nursing home patients; mean age, 80 years; all nonpsychotic with cognitive impairment, emotional lability, ADL dysfunction and agitation, anxiety, depressed mood, or sleep disturbance (also studied were 273 patients on geriatric wards of state hospitals)	Modified Ham-A; modified NOSIE; global evaluations	Thioridazine was well tolerated, with few side effects. Thioridazine-treated group improved significantly more than placebo group on all Ham-A items (74% vs. 42%) and global evaluations. Thioridazine-treated group improved significantly more than diazepam group on NOSIE and global ratings. Insomnia responded better to diazepam, but there was more overall improvement on Ham-A rating with thioridazine.
Dehlin et al. 1985	Alaproclate (400) (serotonin reuptake inhibitor) vs. placebo	N=40; mean age, 82 years; primary degenerative, multi-infarct, or mixed dementia; not selected on the basis of affective or behavioral symptoms	Intellectual function; motor function (ADL); emotional function (including depressive symptoms); clinical global evaluation	No difference in efficacy between alaproclate and placebo. Severity of dementia ranged from mild to severe. Behavioral problems not described.

TABLE 31–2. Randomized, placebo-controlled studies of the efficacy of psychotropic medications in elderly nursing home residents *(continued)*

Study	Medication and dosage (mg/day)	Sample	Efficacy measures	Results and comments
Katz et al. 1990	Nortriptyline (mean, 65.25) vs. placebo	*N*=30 residents of nursing home or congregate housing; mean age=84 years; major depression (Ham-D scores ≥18)	Ham-D*; Geriatric Depression Scale; CGI	Significant improvement in patients treated with nortriptyline compared with placebo on Ham-D and CGI but not on Geriatric Depression Scale. Location (in nursing home vs. congregate housing) not significantly related to response. Trend toward decreased nortriptyline response in nursing home related to higher levels of disability and lower serum albumin in nursing home patients.
Nyth and Gottfries 1990	Citalopram (10–30; mean, 25) vs. placebo	*N*=98; mean age, 77.6 years; primary degenerative (Alzheimer's disease) or multi-infarct dementia (vascular dementia)	GBS; CGI; MADRS	Compared with control subjects, Alzheimer's disease patients in citalopram group had significant reduction in irritability and depressed mood on GBS. From baseline to week 4, Alzheimer's disease patients in citalopram group improved significantly on MADRS and on GBS emotional blunting, confusion, irritability, anxiety, fear-panic, depressed mood, and restlessness. No treatment benefits found in vascular dementia patients. Placebo group worsened on CGI. Few adverse effects, with no drug–placebo differences.
Finkel et al. 1995	Thiothixene (0.25–18; mean, 4.6) vs. placebo	*N*=33; mean age, 85 years; dementia with agitated or aggressive behavior	CMAI; MMSE; GDS; ADLs	Thiothixene-treated group had significantly greater reduction in agitation than placebo group after 11 weeks of treatment and 6 weeks after crossover from placebo; no between-group differences on MMSE, GDS, ADLs.
Tariot et al. 1998	Carbamazepine (modal dose, 300; mean serum level, 5.3 μg/mL) vs. placebo	*N*=51; dementia with agitation	BPRS; CGI; agitation; aggression; cognition; functional status; staff time	Carbamazepine-treated group had significantly greater improvement on BPRS compared with placebo group at 6 weeks. Global improvement in 77% of patients taking carbamazepine and in 22% of those taking placebo. Secondary analyses showed that improvement was attributable to decreased agitation and aggression. Nurses reported perception of decreased time required to manage agitation in carbamazepine group. Significantly more adverse events with carbamazepine (59%) than with placebo (29%).

TABLE 31–2. Randomized, placebo-controlled studies of the efficacy of psychotropic medications in elderly nursing home residents *(continued)*

Study	Medication and dosage (mg/day)	Sample	Efficacy measures	Results and comments
DeDeyn et al. 1999	Risperidone (0.5–4; mean, 1.1) vs. haloperidol (0.5–4; mean, 1.2) vs. placebo; 12 weeks	*N*=344; Alzheimer's, vascular, and mixed dementia (mean MMSE score=8.7)	BEHAVE-AD*; CMAI; CGI; MMSE Response defined as ≥30% reduction in BEHAVE-AD scores	No significant difference in response rates on BEHAVE-AD between risperidone and placebo, but reduction in BEHAVE-AD total and aggression subscale and CMAI aggression item scores, and CGI was significantly greater with risperidone than with placebo; post hoc analysis showed significantly greater reduction in BEHAVE-AD aggression scores with risperidone compared with haloperidol. Somnolence greater with risperidone (12.2%) than placebo (4.4%). Extrapyramidal symptoms were significantly greater with haloperidol (22%) than with risperidone (15%) or placebo (11%). Slight but significant decline in MMSE scores in haloperidol group.
Katz et al. 1999	Risperidone (0.5–2) vs. placebo; 12 weeks	*N*=625; mean age, 82.7 years; psychotic and behavioral symptoms and Alzheimer's disease, vascular dementia, or mixed Alzheimer's disease and vascular dementia (mean MMSE score=6.6)	BEHAVE-AD*; CMAI; CGI; MMSE; FAST; PSMS Response defined as ≥50% reduction in BEHAVE-AD score	Significantly greater reductions in BEHAVE-AD total scores and in Aggressiveness and Psychosis subscale scores with risperidone 1 mg and 2 mg compared with placebo. Response rates significantly greater with risperidone 1 mg (45%) and 2 mg (50%) than placebo (33%). More extrapyramidal symptoms and somnolence with 2 mg than 1 mg of risperidone; 1 mg appears to be optimal dosage for nursing home patients with severe dementia.
Street et al. 2000	Olanzapine (5, 10, 15) vs. placebo; 6 weeks	*N*=206; mean age, 83.8 years; Alzheimer's disease with psychotic and/or behavioral symptoms (mean MMSE score=6.9)	NPI-NH core* and total (including Occupational Disruptiveness scores); BPRS; MMSE	Olanzapine 5 mg and 10 mg produced significant improvement in summary measures of agitation, aggression, and psychosis. Olanzapine 5 mg significantly reduced disruptive effects on caregivers compared with placebo. Olanzapine was associated with somnolence and gait disturbance but not with increased extrapyramidal symptoms, central anticholinergic effects, or cognitive impairment compared with placebo; 18% of placebo group and 44% of olanzapine group dropouts were due to adverse events.
Magai et al. 2000	Sertraline vs. placebo	*N*=31; all women with late-stage Alzheimer's disease and depression	Depression; facial affect	Both groups were improved at 8 weeks; sertraline had no significant benefits over placebo. "Knit-brow" facial response approached significance for treatment × time effect.
Olin et al. 2001	Carbamazepine (mean, 388) vs. placebo; 6 weeks	*N*=21; Alzheimer's dementia (mean MMSE score=6.0)	BPRS*; CGI-C; Ham-D	Both groups improved on CGI-C (56% on carbamazepine, 58% on placebo), but no significant differences on BPRS, CGI, Ham-D. Adverse events mild, similar in drug and placebo.

TABLE 31–2. Randomized, placebo-controlled studies of the efficacy of psychotropic medications in elderly nursing home residents *(continued)*

Study	Medication and dosage (mg/day)	Sample	Efficacy measures	Results and comments
Porsteinsson et al. 2001	Divalproex (mean, 826; mean serum level, 45.4 μg/mL) vs. placebo; 6 weeks	*N*=56; mean age, 85.0 years; probable or possible Alzheimer's disease, vascular dementia, or mixed dementia with agitation (mean MMSE score=6.8)	BPRS*; OAS; BRSD; CMAI; CGI-C;	Divalproex group showed significant improvement on BPRS at 6 weeks compared with placebo only in a secondary analysis after adjustment for several covariates; 68% of divalproex group and 52% of placebo group had reduced agitation on CGI (NS). Significantly more side effects in divalproex vs. placebo group (68% vs. 33%), generally mild, but sedation 39% with divalproex vs. 11% with placebo.
Tariot et al. 2001a	Donepezil (5–10) vs. placebo	*N*=208; mean age, 85.7 years; probable or possible Alzheimer's disease or Alzheimer's disease with cerebrovascular disease (mean MMSE score=14.4)	NPI-NH; CDR-SB; MMSE; PSMS	Both groups improved on NPI-NH, with no significant difference between donepezil and placebo. Significantly greater improvement with donepezil than with placebo on CDR-SB at week 24 and on MMSE at weeks 8, 16, 20, but not on PSMS. Improvement not influenced by advanced age. No difference in adverse events between drug and placebo.
Tariot et al. 2001b	Divalproex (mean, 1,000) vs. placebo; 6 weeks	*N*=172; Alzheimer's disease, vascular or mixed dementia with symptoms of mania (mean MMSE score=7.4)	BRMS*; BPRS; CMAI; CGI-C	Study discontinued early due to significantly greater rate of adverse events with divalproex, especially somnolence.
Meehan et al. 2002	Olanzapine (2.5–5 IM single dose) vs. lorazepam vs. placebo; 24 hours	*N*=204; recruited from nursing home *and* hospital sites; Alzheimer's, vascular, and mixed Alzheimer's/vascular dementia (mean MMSE score=11.8)	PANSS-EC*, ACES	Significantly greater mean reduction in PANSS-EC scores 2 hours post-dose for olanzapine 2.5 and 5 mg vs. placebo; no difference between olanzapine and lorazepam; adverse events not significantly different across groups.
Brodaty et al. 2003	Risperidone (0.5–2; mean, 0.95) vs. placebo; 12 weeks	*N*=345; mean age, 83 years; Alzheimer's, vascular, or mixed dementia, with aggressive behavior (mean MMSE score=5.5)	CMAI aggression*; CMAI non-aggression subscales; BEHAVE-AD; CGI-S; CGI-C	Compared with placebo group, risperidone group had significant improvement on CMAI total aggression and nonaggressive agitation scores, on BEHAVE-AD total scores and psychosis subscale, and on CGI severity and change scores. More somnolence, falls, urinary tract infections, and cerebrovascular adverse events in risperidone group but no drug–placebo difference in extrapyramidal side effects.

TABLE 31–2. Randomized, placebo-controlled studies of the efficacy of psychotropic medications in elderly nursing home residents *(continued)*

Study	Medication and dosage (mg/day)	Sample	Efficacy measures	Results and comments
DeDeyn et al. 2004	Olanzapine (1, 2.5, 5, or 7.5) vs. placebo; 10 weeks	*N*=652; Alzheimer's dementia, with psychosis (mean MMSE score=13.7)	NPI-NH psychosis subscale*; CGI-C*; NPI total, individual item, and occupational disruptiveness scores	No significant difference between any dose of olanzapine and placebo on primary outcomes. More weight gain with olanzapine, but no difference in anticholinergic or extrapyramidal adverse effects or dropout rates due to adverse effects.
Tariot et al. 2005	Divalproex (800) vs. placebo; 6 weeks	*N*=153; probable or possible Alzheimer's disease with agitation	BPRS agitation factor*; BPRS total, CGI-C, CMAI.	72% of enrolled subjects completed the trial. No significant drug-placebo differences on primary or secondary outcome measures.
Winblad et al. 2006	Donepezil (10) vs. placebo; 26 weeks	*N*=248; severe Alzheimer's disease (MMSE score=1–10)	SIB*; ADCS-ADL severe*; MMSE; NPI; CGI-I	Significant improvement in SIB scores and less decline in ADL function on donepezil at 6 months. CGI-I only significant for donepezil in completer analysis. No significant behavioral benefits. Rate of adverse events comparable in drug and placebo groups, but more patients discontinued treatment because of adverse events in donepezil group.
Mintzer et al. 2006	Risperidone (1 or 1.5; mean 1.03) vs. placebo; 8 weeks	*N*=473; Alzheimer's dementia with psychosis (mean MMSE score=12.4)	BEHAVE-AD psychosis subscale*; CGI-C*	Both groups improved, with no significant differences on primary outcome measures. Subgroup analysis showed patients with MMSE<10 had significantly greater improvement on CGI-C with risperidone. No difference in discontinuation rates between risperidone and placebo groups, but risperidone group had higher rates of somnolence (16.2% vs 4.6%) and death (3.8% and 2.5%).
Zhong et al. 2007	Quetiapine (100 or 200) vs. placebo; 10 weeks	*N*=333; Alzheimer's and mixed dementia	PANSS-EC*; CGI-C; response rate (defined as ≥40% reduction in PANSS-EC, or "much" or "very much" improved on CGI-C); NPI-NH; CMAI	No significant differences between quetiapine and placebo by LOCF analysis of PANSS-EC, NPI-NH, or CMAI scores at endpoint. However, quetiapine 200 mg/day (but not 100 mg/day) was significantly better than placebo on CGI-C scores and CGI-C response rates using both LOCF and OC (observed case) analyses and on PANSS-EC using OC analysis. No differences in incidence of postural hypotension, falls, cerebrovascular adverse events. There were more deaths with quetiapine, although rates were not statistically different from placebo.

TABLE 31–2. Randomized, placebo-controlled studies of the efficacy of psychotropic medications in elderly nursing home residents *(continued)*

Study	Medication and dosage (mg/day)	Sample	Efficacy measures	Results and comments
Mintzer et al. 2007	Aripiprazole (2, 5, or 10 fixed dose) vs. placebo; 10 weeks	*N*=487; mean age 82.5 years; Alzheimer's dementia with psychosis (mean MMSE score=12.4)	NPI-NH psychosis subscale*; NPI-NH total; CGI-S; CGI-I (improvement); BPRS psychosis, core, and total scores; CMAI; response defined as ≥50% decrease in NPI scores	Aripiprazole 10 mg/day group had significantly greater improvement than placebo on NPI psychosis scores and response rates, BPRS core and total, and CMAI scores. Aripiprazole 5 mg/day showed significantly greater improvement only on BPRS and CMAI. Aripiprazole 2 mg/day was not efficacious. There was a dose-dependent occurrence of cerebrovascular adverse events in the aripiprazole groups. Death rates in the placebo, 2, 5, and 10 mg groups were 3%, 3%, 2%, and 7%, respectively, although the differences were not statistically significant.
Streim et al. 2008	Aripiprazole (2, 5, 10, 15 flexible dose titration) vs. placebo; 10 weeks	*N*=256; mean age 83 years; Alzheimer's dementia with psychosis (mean MMSE score=13.6)	NPI-NH psychosis subscale*; CGI-S*; NPI-NH total; BPRS psychosis, core, and total scores; CMAI; Cornell Scale for Depression; NPI caregiver distress; ADCS ADL scores; CGI-I (improvement); response defined as ≥50% decrease in NPI scores	No significant difference between aripiprazole and placebo on NPI psychosis or CGI severity at endpoint. However, significantly greater improvement in the aripiprazole group on secondary outcomes: NPI and BPRS total scores, CMAI, CGI-I, Cornell Depression Scale. More somnolence with aripiprazole (14%) than placebo (4%); other adverse effects were similar for aripiprazole and placebo, with low rate of extrapyramidal side effects in both groups.

Note. *Primary outcome measure.

ACES=Agitation-Calmness Evaluation Scale; ADCS=Alzheimer's Disease Cooperative Study; ADL=activities of daily living; BEHAVE-AD=Behavioral Pathology in Alzheimer's Disease (Reisberg et al. 1996); BPRS=Brief Psychiatric Rating Scale (Overall and Gorham 1962); BRMS=Bech-Rafaelsen Mania Scale (Bech et al. 1979); BRSD=Behavior Rating Scale for Dementia (by the Consortium to Establish a Registry for Dementia); CDR-SB=Clinical Dementia Rating (Nursing Home Version)–Sum of the Boxes (Hughes et al. 1982); CGI=Clinical Global Impression Scale (Guy 1976); CGI-C=Clinical Global Impression of Change; CGI-I=Clinical Global Impression of Improvement; CGI-S=Clinical Global Impression of Severity; CMAI=Cohen-Mansfield Agitation Inventory (Cohen-Mansfield et al. 1989); FAST=Functional Assessment Staging (Reisberg 1988); GBS=Gottfries-Brane-Steen Geriatric Rating Scale (Gottfries et al. 1982); GDS=Global Deterioration Scale (Reisberg et al. 1988); Ham-A=Hamilton Anxiety Scale (Hamilton 1959); Ham-D=Hamilton Rating Scale for Depression (Hamilton 1960); LOCF=last observation carried forward; MADRS=Montgomery-Åsberg Depression Rating Scale (Montgomery and Åsberg 1979); MMSE=Mini-Mental State Examination (Folstein et al. 1975); NOSIE=Nurses' Observation Scale for Inpatient Evaluation (Honigfeld et al. 1966); NPI-NH=Neuropsychiatric Inventory–Nursing Home Version (Wood et al. 2000); OAS=Overt Aggression Scale; PANSS-EC=Positive and Negative Symptom Scale-Excited Component; PSMS=Physical Self-Maintenance Scale (Lawton and Brody 1969); SCAG=Sandoz Clinical Assessment–Geriatric (Shader et al. 1974); SIB=self-injurious behavior.

months in nursing home patients with dementia. Several double-blind, placebo-controlled studies of antipsychotic drug discontinuation demonstrated that the majority of patients who had been receiving longer-term treatment could be withdrawn from these agents without reemergence of psychosis or agitated behaviors (Bridges-Parlet et al. 1997; Cohen-Mansfield et al. 1999; Ruths et al. 2004). This is consistent with findings from older discontinuation studies (Barton and Hurst 1966; Risse et al. 1987). Therefore, it is important to periodically reevaluate the need for continuing antipsychotic drug treatment.

Since 2003, analyses of safety data from randomized, controlled studies of atypical antipsychotic drugs in elderly patients with dementia, including the aforementioned nursing home studies, have revealed significantly increased risks of cerebrovascular adverse events and mortality in this population. Although elevated risks were not found in every study, pooled analyses showed that the rate of cerebrovascular adverse events (including stroke and transient ischemic attacks) is greater than placebo by 2.3% in elderly patients treated with risperidone, 0.9% in patients treated with olanzapine, and 0.7% in those treated with aripiprazole. Most of the affected individuals had known cerebrovascular risk factors prior to starting drug treatment. These findings led to regulatory warnings in the United States, Canada, and the United Kingdom regarding the safety of these drugs in elderly patients with dementia.

The U.S. Food and Drug Administration (FDA) also warned that elderly patients with dementia-related psychosis who are treated with atypical antipsychotics have a risk of death between 1.6 and 1.7 times greater than those treated with placebo (4.5% vs. 2.6%), with a reminder that atypical antipsychotics are not FDA-approved for the treatment of patients with dementia-related psychosis. Consistent with this FDA warning, a meta-analysis by Schneider et al. (2005), examining results of 15 randomized, controlled trials, many of which were conducted in nursing home patients, found that the risk of mortality was 3.5% in elderly patients treated with atypical antipsychotics versus 2.3% of patients treated with placebo. Although no placebo-controlled trials of ziprasidone or clozapine are known to have been conducted in elderly patients with dementia, it is reasonable to view the increased mortality as a class effect. Although the FDA mortality warning applies to all atypicals but not to conventional antipsychotic drugs, a study by Wang et al. (2005) found a significantly higher adjusted risk of death in elderly patients taking conventional antipsychotics compared with those taking atypical antipsychotic medications, whether or not the patients had dementia or resided in a nursing home. The authors suggested that conventional antipsychotic medications are at least as likely as atypical agents to increase the risk of death in older adults and that conventional drugs should not be used to replace atypical agents discontinued in response to the FDA warning.

In light of the concerns about risks of antipsychotic drugs in elderly nursing home residents with dementia, experts in the field have suggested that nonpharmacological approaches should be considered first when treating noncognitive behavioral symptoms. However, for those nursing home patients whose behavioral symptoms do not respond to nonpharmacological interventions, the decision to use an atypical antipsychotic should be based on a careful assessment of individual risk-benefit profile.

Five randomized clinical trials evaluated the efficacy of mood-stabilizing anticonvulsant drugs for the treatment of agitation and aggression in nursing home residents. The first was a study of carbamazepine that showed it to be effective for agitation and aggression but not for psychotic symptoms such as delusions and hallucinations (Tariot et al. 1998). In this study, nursing reports indicated that less staff time was required for patient care in the group treated with carbamazepine. Another trial of carbamazepine found high rates of improvements in drug- and placebo-treated patients, with nonsignificant between-group differences (Olin et al. 2001). Several placebo-controlled studies evaluated divalproex with few encouraging results, including one trial that was discontinued before completion because of adverse effects in the drug treatment group; overall, these studies failed to provide evidence for efficacy in reducing agitated behavior (Porsteinsson et al. 2001; Tariot et al. 2001b, 2005). It is of note that the tolerability of divalproex was limited by somnolence, weakness, and diminished oral intake in this population of elderly nursing home subjects with dementia.

Acetylcholinesterase inhibitors have been shown to delay the decline in cognitive function in patients with mild to severe Alzheimer's disease, although few studies have been conducted specifically in nursing home samples. One randomized clinical trial of donepezil in nursing home residents showed effects on cognitive performance that were comparable with those observed in less impaired outpatients (Tariot et al. 2001a). A subsequent study demonstrated that donepezil improves cognition and preserves function in Alzheimer's disease patients with severe dementia residing in nursing homes (Winblad et al. 2006). These studies also examined the effects of donepezil on behavioral disturbances, as a secondary outcome measure, and did not find significant benefits. A more recent study of patients with severe dementia failed to show improvement on secondary behavioral measures, but this study excluded nursing home residents (Black et al. 2007). Clinical trials of memantine, conducted in outpatient populations, have included secondary measures of behavior, with conflicting findings. One study by Tariot et al. (2004) reported significant improvement on Neuropsychiatric Inventory scores with memantine, but it is not yet known whether this generalized to the nursing home setting. Prospective trials are still needed to evaluate effects of these drugs on behavioral disturbances, specifically in nursing home populations.

There have been only four randomized clinical trials evaluating the effects of antidepressants in nursing home residents. The first study, which was placebo controlled, showed a positive response to nortriptyline for treatment of major depression in a long-term care population with high levels of medical comorbidity (Katz et al. 1990). In the second study, patients were randomized to receive regular or low-dosage nortriptyline, and significant plasma level–response relationships were demonstrated in cognitively intact patients (Streim et al. 2000). These findings again confirmed the validity of the diagnosis of depression in nursing home residents in the context of significant medical comorbidity and disability. However, in patients with dementia, the plasma level–response relationship was significantly different, suggesting that the depression occurring in dementia might be a treatment-relevant subtype of depression or a distinct disorder. A controlled antidepressant trial in nursing home residents with late-stage Alzheimer's disease showed no significant benefits of sertraline over placebo (Magai et al. 2000). Available open-label studies of the efficacy of selective serotonin reuptake inhibitors (SSRIs) in nursing home residents with depression have had mixed results, some consistent with the findings of Magai et al. (2000), suggesting that SSRIs may be less effective for depression in patients with dementia than in those who are cognitively intact (Oslin et al. 2000; Rosen et al. 2000; Trappler and Cohen 1996, 1998).

Although the SSRIs might be expected to be well tolerated by frail elderly nursing home patients because of their side-effect profile, there is evidence that these drugs can cause serious adverse events in this population. Thapa et al. (1998) demonstrated that the use of SSRIs was associated with a nearly twofold increase in the risk of falls in nursing home residents, comparable with the risk found with tricyclic antidepressant drugs. Investigators in the United Kingdom reported that antidepressant use was associated with better physical functioning but also with greater frequency of falls in residential care patients (Arthur et al. 2002). A randomized, double-blind comparison trial found that venlafaxine was less well tolerated compared with sertraline in frail nursing home patients without conferring more treatment benefits, as might be expected from an agent with mixed serotonergic and noradrenergic effects (Oslin et al. 2003).

History of Deficient Mental Health Care as an Impetus for Nursing Home Reform

Although psychiatric disorders are extraordinarily common among nursing home residents, and efficacious treatments exist, psychiatric services are often not adequate. Historically, nursing home design, staffing, programs, services, and funding have not evolved to meet the needs of patients with mental disorders (Streim and Katz 1994). In the 1980s, it was estimated that as many as two-thirds of nursing home residents with psychiatric disorders were misdiagnosed (German et al. 1986; Sabin et al. 1982) and that as little as 5% of nursing home residents' needs for mental health services were being met (Burns and Taube 1990). This mismatch of psychiatric needs and available treatment led not only to neglect but also to inappropriate treatment; psychiatric problems were often mismanaged by using physical or chemical restraints.

Physical Restraints

A 1977 survey of American nursing home residents showed that 25% of 1.3 million people were restrained by geriatric chairs, cuffs, belts, or similar devices, primarily in an attempt to control behavioral symptoms (National Center for Health Statistics 1979). Other early surveys demonstrated rates of restraint as high as 85%. Patient factors predicting the use of restraints, in addition to agitation and behavior problems, include age, cognitive impairment, risk of injuries to self (e.g., from falls) or others (e.g., from combative behavior), physical frailty, the presence of monitoring or treatment devices, and the need to promote body alignment. Institutional and systemic factors associated with restraint use include pressure to avoid litigation, staff attitudes, insufficient staffing, and the availability of restraint devices. Potential adverse effects include an increased risk of falls and other injuries (Capezuti et al. 1996) as well as functional decline, skin breakdown, physiological effects of immobilization stress, disorganized behavior, and demoralization. Although mechanical restraints have frequently been used in attempts to control agitation, they do not in fact decrease behavioral disturbances (Werner et al. 1989), and cross-national studies indicated that it is possible to manage nursing home residents without such measures (Cape 1983; Evans and Strumpf 1989; Innes and Turman 1983).

Misuse of Psychotropic Drugs

Concerns about inadequate and inappropriate care have also focused on the overuse of psychotropic drugs in nursing home residents, especially the misuse of these drugs as "chemical restraints" to control patient behaviors. Studies in the 1970s and 1980s reported that approximately 50% of residents had orders for psychotropic medications, with 20%–40% being given antipsychotic drugs, 10%–40% given anxiolytics or hypnotics, and 5%–10% given antidepressants (Avorn et al. 1989; Beers et al. 1988; Buck 1988; Burns et al. 1988; Cohen-Mansfield 1986; Custer et al. 1984; DeLeo et al. 1989; Ray et al. 1980; Teeter et al. 1976; Zimmer et al. 1984). Psychotropic drugs were frequently prescribed without adequate regard for the residents' psychiatric diagnosis or medical status. In one study, Zimmer et al. (1984) reported that only 15% of residents being given psychotropic drugs had received a psychiatric consultation. Other studies reported that 21% of patients without a psychiatric diagnosis were receiving psychotropic medication (Burns et al. 1988), that physicians'—as opposed to patients'—characteristics predicted drug dosages (Ray et al. 1980), and that psychotropic drugs were often prescribed in the absence of any documentation of the patient's mental status in the clinical record (Avorn et al. 1989).

The greatest concerns about inappropriate overprescribing of medications have related to the misuse of neuroleptics as chemical restraints to control resident behaviors. Despite evidence for the efficacy of antipsychotic drugs in managing psychosis and agitation in nursing home residents with dementia, patients with nonpsychotic behavioral problems may be appropriately managed with other medications, behavioral treatments, interpersonal approaches, or environmental interventions. Moreover, it is important to note that whereas all the evidence for the efficacy of antipsychotic medications comes from short-term studies, these medications are frequently prescribed for long-term treatment. In this context, concerns about overuse of antipsychotic drugs were supported by findings from drug discontinuation studies (cited earlier). One classic double-blind study of neuroleptic withdrawal showed that only 16% of patients who had been receiving medications on a chronic basis exhibited significant deterioration when the drugs were withdrawn (Barton and Hurst 1966). A subsequent small-scale withdrawal study in patients who had been receiving neuroleptics for several months showed that 22% experienced increased agitation on withdrawal, indicating a need for continued treatment, but that 22% were unchanged and 55% actually showed improvement (Risse et al. 1987).

Inadequate Treatment of Depression

Although the focus of public concern and regulatory scrutiny in the 1970s and 1980s was on overprescription of antipsychotic medications in patients with dementia, undertreatment of other psychiatric conditions in the nursing home has also been a serious problem. The Institute of Medicine Committee on Nursing Home Regulation (1986) report "Improving the Quality of Care in Nursing Homes," which did much to stimulate nursing home reform, highlighted problems both in the overuse of antipsychotic drugs and in the underuse of antidepressants for treatment of affective disorders. Similarly, in reviewing epidemiological studies on the use of psychotropics in nursing homes, Murphy (1989) noted that antidepressants were the one class of drugs that appeared to be underused and that, as a result, major depression in this setting often remained untreated.

Federal Regulations and Psychiatric Care in the Nursing Home

The misuse of physical and chemical restraints was a rallying point for advocacy groups that urged the federal government to institute a process of nursing home reform. In addition, the U.S. General Accounting Office was concerned that states were admitting patients with chronic and severe psychiatric problems to Medicaid-certified nursing homes not because patients needed this type of care but because admission would shift a substantial portion of the costs of patients' care from the state to the federal government. Apparently in response to both sets of concerns, Congress enacted the Nursing Home Reform Act as part of the Omnibus Budget Reconciliation Act of 1987 (OBRA '87). This legislation provided for government regulation of the operation of nursing facilities and of the care that they provide (Elon and Pawlson 1992). This legislation directed the Health Care Financing Administration (HCFA)—reorganized and renamed in 2001 as the Centers for Medicare and Medicaid Services (CMS)—to issue regulations (Health Care Financing Administration 1991) that operationalize the laws and to develop guidelines (Centers for Medicare and Medicaid Services 2007) that assist federal and state surveyors in interpreting the regulations. Mental health screening, assessment, care planning, and treatment are addressed under sections of the regulations that pertain to resident assessment, resident rights and facility practices, and quality of care (Health Care Financing Administration 1991, 1992a, 1992b).

The regulations include provisions for preadmission screening and annual resident review that require assessment of each resident before admission to any nursing facility that receives federal funds (Health Care Financing Administration 1992a). When an initial first-stage screening reveals that a serious mental disorder (other than dementia) might be present, a second-stage assessment that includes a psychiatric evaluation must be made in order to ascertain whether the patient has a mental disorder, to make a specific psychiatric diagnosis, and to determine whether there is a need for acute psychiatric care that precludes adequate or appropriate treatment in a nursing home. Patients found to have dementia on the initial screen are exempt from the preadmission psychiatric evaluation. Thus, preadmission screening is intended 1) to prevent inappropriate admission to nursing homes of patients who do not have dementia but who have severe psychiatric disorders and 2) to help ensure that patients with disabilities due in large part to treatable psychiatric disorders (such as depression) are not placed in long-term care facilities before they receive the benefits of adequate psychiatric treatment. For eligible patients who are admitted to a nursing home, an annual reassessment must be made in order to determine whether nursing home care remains appropriate. Regulations requiring comprehensive assessment for all residents (Health Care Financing Administration 1991) have led to development of a uniform Resident Assessment Instrument, which includes the Minimum Data Set (MDS) (Morris et al. 1990). This instrument must be administered on a regular basis by members of an interdisciplinary health care team, usually a nurse or sometimes a social worker, and ultimately the nursing home administrator is responsible for its completion (Health Care Financing Administration 1992c). Areas of assessment relevant to mental illness and behavior include mood, cognition, communication, functional status, medications, and other treatments.

Responses on the MDS suggesting that there may be a need to reevaluate a patient's clinical status and treatment plan serve as triggers for completing Resident Assessment Protocols (RAPs). These protocols 1) define medical conditions, psychiatric disorders, adverse treatment effects, functional impairments, and disabilities that are common among nursing home residents, 2) note differential diagnoses and potential causal and aggravating factors, 3) outline procedures for evaluation, and 4) list key elements of management or treatment (Health Care Financing Administration 1992c). The MDS and RAPs together are designed as a two-stage assessment system, with a screening survey followed by a focused clinical evaluation. RAP problem areas related to mental disorders and behavior include delirium, cognitive loss and dementia, psychosocial well-being, mood state, behavior problems, psychotropic drug use, and physical restraints. The individual RAPs are designed to 1) help nursing home staff recognize common signs and symptom clusters that are indicators of clinically significant problems, 2) conduct evaluations using standardized algorithms, and 3) determine whether it is necessary to alter the treatment plan. The regulations hold facilities responsible for ensuring that RAPs are followed appropriately. Although physicians have no mandated role in this process, physician involvement is clearly necessary for proper diagnosis and treatment of conditions covered by the RAPs (Elon and Pawlson 1992). Psychiatric consultation may be needed when RAPs indicate a need for the evaluation of problems related to mental health.

Regulations related to resident rights and facility practices restrict the use of physical restraints and antipsychotic drugs when they are "administered for purposes of discipline or convenience and not required to treat the resident's medical symptoms" (Health Care Financing Administration 1991, p. 48,875). Regulations related to quality of care further require that residents not receive "unnecessary drugs" and specify that antipsychotic medications may not be given "unless these are necessary to treat a specific condition as diagnosed and documented in the clinical record" (p. 48,910). An *unnecessary drug* is defined as any drug used 1) in excessive dose (including duplicate therapy), 2) for excessive duration, 3) without adequate monitoring, 4) without adequate indications for its use, 5) in the presence of adverse consequences that indicate that it should be reduced or discontinued, or 6) for any combination of the first five reasons (Health Care Financing Administration 1991). The guidelines based on these regulations further limit the use of antipsychotic medications, antianxiety agents, sedative-hypnotics, and related medications (Centers for Medicare and Medicaid Services 2007). For each of these classes, the guidelines specify a list of acceptable indications, upper limits for daily dosages, requirements for monitoring treatment and adverse effects, and time frames for attempting dosage reductions and discontinuation. These guidelines were updated in 2006 to reflect new clinical knowledge and the availability of new drugs approved by the FDA (Centers for Medicare and Medicaid 2007).

To minimize concerns about federal interference with medical practice, the current guidelines include qualifying statements that recognize cases in which strict adherence to prescribing limits or gradual dosage reduction or discontinuation is "clinically contraindicated." Although the focus is on limiting the use of psychotropic drugs, the guidelines acknowledge that appropriate medical treatment can entail continuing treatment with psychotropic medications. The guidelines instruct surveyors monitoring nursing facilities to allow the facilities the opportunity to present a rationale for the use of medications prescribed outside the guidelines and to explain why such use is in the best interest of the resident before finding that the facility is not in compliance with regulations. Thus, the physician's options for treating nursing home residents need not be unduly restricted by the regulations if the clinical rationale—explaining that the benefits of treatment (in terms of symptom relief, improved health status, or improved functioning) outweigh the risks—is clearly documented in the medical record. Although the facility, not the physician, is accountable for compliance with the regulations, the physician's clinical reasoning and judgment play a critical role in the process of ensuring quality care.

In addition to addressing the use of psychotropic drugs, the interpretive guidelines also outline conditions for the use of physical restraints. According to the guidelines, restraints may not be used unless there is documentation that 1) efforts were made to identify and correct preventable or treatable factors that cause or contribute to the problem, 2) prior attempts to use less restrictive measures failed, and 3) use of restraints enables the resident to achieve or maintain the highest practicable level of function. Physical or occupational therapists must be consulted if restraints are deemed necessary to enhance body positioning or improve mobility.

Although much of the emphasis of the federal regulations is on eliminating inappropriate treatment, there are also requirements for the provision of necessary and appropriate care for residents with mental health problems. Under the provisions designed to ensure quality of care, federal regulations define a need for geriatric psychiatry services in nursing homes, requiring that "the facility must ensure that a resident who displays mental or psychosocial adjustment difficulties receives appropriate services to correct the assessed problem" (Health Care Financing Administration 1991, p. 48,896). More recently, within the scope of its responsibility as a payer, CMS developed a system for assessing the quality of care provided in U.S. nursing homes. To enable surveyors to compare individual facilities within the same state, HCFA introduced quality indicators derived from MDS data (Nursing Home Quality Indicators Development Group 1999). There are 24 quality indicators in 11 different domains, including behavior and emotional problems, cognitive patterns, and psychotropic drug use.

The domain of behavioral and emotional patterns covers the prevalence of behavioral symptoms affecting others (e.g., verbally or physically abusive, socially inappropriate, or disruptive behavior), prevalence of symptoms of depression, and prevalence of depression without antidepressant therapy. The cognitive pattern domain examines the incidence of cognitive impairment when consecutive MDS assessments reveal new onset of impairments in short-term memory or decision-making capacity. The psychotropic drug use domain includes the prevalence of antipsychotic use for patients without psychotic conditions, the prevalence of anxiolytic and hypnotic use, and the prevalence of hypnotic use more than twice in a 7-day period. Quality indicators that are indirectly related to mental disorders and their treatment include the use of nine or more different medications and the prevalence of falls, weight loss, daily application of physical restraints, and little or no activity.

Whenever a review in any of these areas results in a citation of deficiency, a plan of correction must be developed and submitted for approval. This system is a first step in monitoring quality of care, although the face validity of some of the quality indicators has been questioned and the results of quality surveys may be difficult to interpret. Nevertheless, the results from every nursing home surveyed are available for public inspection, and consumers of nursing home services (and their families) can access the quality indicators reports online.

Changing Patterns of Psychiatric Care

Since the implementation of the Nursing Home Reform Act in 1990, there have been significant changes in nursing home care, including mental health care. Some of these changes may be attributed to the process of conducting surveys and enforcing federal regulations; however, several other factors appear to have contributed, including the dissemination of information about regulatory requirements, availability and marketing of new medications, advances in scientific knowledge from nursing home research, and cumulative effects of professional education regarding good clinical practice. Increasing consumer awareness is also likely to have played a role.

Shifts in Antipsychotic Medication Use

Studies of the effect of federal regulations in the early years after implementation showed a substantial decline in the use of antipsychotic drugs (Shorr et al. 1994) and physical restraints (Hawes et al. 1997) and increases in antidepressant use (Lantz et al. 1996). Between 1991 and 1997 there was a 52.2% decrease in the use of antipsychotic medications, from 33.7% to 16.1% (Health Care Financing Administration 1998). One study reported that greater reductions in antipsychotic use during this period were found in nursing facilities with an emphasis on psychosocial care, a less severe case mix, and a higher nurse-to-resident ratio (Svarstad et al. 2001). Soon after the regulations were introduced, several investigators developed educational programs for physicians, nurses, and aides to teach practice principles consistent with federal guidelines. Studies evaluating these educational interventions demonstrated reductions of 23%–72% in the use of antipsychotic drugs (Avorn et al. 1992; Meador et al. 1997; Ray et al. 1993; Rovner et al. 1992; Schnelle et al. 1992). Studies of the appropriateness of antipsychotic use examining documentation of OBRA '87–approved diagnostic indications and appropriate target symptoms, and dosing within the recommended limits in the HCFA guidelines, suggested relatively high rates of compliance with the OBRA '87 regulations (Llorente et al. 1998; Siegler et al. 1997).

Although the changes found by the studies were generally interpreted as an indication of improvement in care, the studies did not examine health care outcomes or effects on residents' quality of life (Snowden and Roy-Byrne 1998) and did not address concerns that reductions in medication use might have an adverse effect on patients who required antipsychotic treatment. A retrospective study in a single nursing facility, which described attempts to discontinue or lower the dosage of antipsychotic drugs in 75% of subjects studied, found that residents with appropriate indications for antipsychotic use according to the federal regulations were significantly less likely to have their antipsychotic agents stopped (Semla et al. 1994). Nevertheless, for 20% of residents whose antipsychotic was discontinued or reduced in dosage, the agent was subsequently resumed or its dosage was increased. This result, which is consistent with reports from earlier discontinuation studies, suggests that the finding of a reduction in overall rates of antipsychotic use may reflect a beneficial trend for a majority of patients, but this result cannot be interpreted as an indication of across-the-board improvement in the quality of residents' care (Lantz et al. 1996).

In contrast to the declining rates of antipsychotic use in the early 1990s, Online Survey Certification and Reporting (OSCAR) data showed a reversal in this trend from 1995 to 1999, with the national rate for antipsychotic drug use in nursing homes increasing from 16% to 19.4% during that period (American Society of Consultant Pharmacists 2000). Despite this increase, a survey conducted by the Office of the Inspector General of the Department of Health and Human Services, based on data from the year 2000, found that psychotropic drugs were appropriately prescribed in 85% of 485 cases reviewed (Office of Inspector General 2001c).

However, the findings of the Office of the Inspector General are contradicted by a large retrospective analysis of Medicare databases merged to MDS assessments from the same time period (Briesacher et al. 2005). In this analysis, 27.6% of all Medicare beneficiaries in nursing homes received antipsychotic medications between 2000 and 2001; of the treated patients, only 41.8% received antipsychotic therapy within federal prescribing guidelines. There are still no prospective studies that have examined the effect of compliance with the federal guidelines or of the changing rates of psychotropic medication use on resident outcomes such as symptom control, functional status, and quality of life.

The increased rates of antipsychotic medication use, coupled with the safety concerns related to the risk of cerebrovascular adverse events and mortality, have prompted a closer look at alternatives to antipsychotic drug treatment of behavioral disturbances in nursing home residents with dementia. A study by Fossey et al. (2006), conducted in the wake of the safety findings described earlier in this chapter, examined 12-month outcomes of an intervention that provided training and support to nursing home staff in psychosocial approaches for managing agitated behavior associated with dementia. The rate of antipsychotic medication use was 19.1% lower in the intervention homes, with no significant differences in the level of agitated or disruptive behavior between intervention and control facilities. Thus it appears that a significant proportion of residents may be managed with less risk without a concomitant increase in behavioral problems. Nevertheless, changes in the prevalence of antipsychotic medication use specifically in response to safety concerns have not yet been documented in nursing home populations.

Increase in Antidepressant Drug Use

Despite the decline in use of antipsychotic drugs in the early 1990s, it has been estimated that the overall use of psychotherapeutic medications in U.S. nursing homes actually increased, from 21.7% in 1991 to 46.1% in 1997 (Health Care Financing Administration 1998). This increase was partly attributable to a rise in the use of antidepressants from 12.6% to 24.9% (a 97.6% increase) during that period. Since the mid-1990s, there has been emerging evidence of further increases in the prevalence of antidepressant use. A retrospective chart review of psychiatric referrals in seven Massachusetts nursing homes during 1995–1996 found that 61% of patients were being given antidepressants and 53% were being given SRIs (Lasser and Sunderland 1998). Rates of antidepressant use also increased in the United Kingdom, from 11% in 1990 to 18.9% in 1997 (Arthur et al. 2002). According to OSCAR data (American Society of Consultant Pharmacists 2000), 35.5% of U.S. nursing home patients had prescriptions for antidepressant medication in 2001, ranging from 27.9% in Hawaii to 62.7% in Utah. A study of 12 Pennsylvania nursing homes similarly found that 47.6% of residents were taking antidepressants (Datto et al. 2002). Before 1990, fewer than 15% of residents with a known diagnosis of depression were receiving antidepressant medication (Heston et al. 1992).

Considered together, these data represent an extraordinary change in the pattern of drug use in a population that has traditionally received inadequate pharmacotherapy for depression. The dramatic increase in antidepressant prescriptions is probably due in part to the wide availability of newer antidepressants that are thought to be well tolerated by elderly nursing home residents with medical and psychiatric comorbidity. Aggressive marketing to primary care physicians may also play a role. With current antidepressant drug use rates that appear comparable with or greater than the estimated prevalence of depression in nursing homes, it is possible that a significant proportion of antidepressant prescriptions are intended for indications other than depression, such as sleep, pain, anxiety, or agitation. Research is needed to determine whether the reported changes in prescribing have had a positive effect on the mental health of nursing home residents with depression.

Decline in Physical Restraint Use

Although questions remain about the interpretation of trends in psychotropic drug use (Lantz et al. 1996), the effect of the federal regulations on restraints appears to be positive, with several studies showing significant reductions in the use of physical restraints (Castle et al. 1997). One study found restraint use rates of 37.4% in 1990 (before OBRA '87 implementation in October 1990) and 28.1% in 1993 (after introduction of the standardized Resident Assessment Instrument required by OBRA '87) (Hawes et al. 1997). Siegler et al. (1997) found that restraint use could be significantly reduced without a resultant increase in antipsychotic or benzodiazepine use. There is no published evidence of an increase in fall-related injuries associated with lower rates of physical restraint use.

Special Care Units

Encouraged by consumer demand to better meet the needs of nursing home residents with dementia, 10% of U.S. nursing homes had established special care units (SCUs) by 1991. A decade later, it was estimated that 22% of nursing homes had designated SCUs for patients with dementia. Research on the effectiveness of SCUs is difficult to interpret and generalize because of the heterogeneity of these facilities (Office of Technology Assessment 1992; Ohta and Ohta 1988). In an effort to characterize the population served by these units, Holmes et al. (1990) reported that SCU patients had more severe cognitive, behavioral, and functional deficits than non-SCU patients with dementia who lived in the same nursing home. More than 90% of residents in SCUs have behavior problems (Wagner et al. 1995).

Some studies indicate that the facilities, services, and programs offered by SCUs may not be significantly better than those available on conventional nursing home units. A study of Minnesota nursing homes described unit and facility characteristics, noting that the designation of SCU was not associated with more services or more individualized dementia care than were units without the designation; however, the study found that some dementia-specific features were less likely to be found in regular units of nursing homes that had designated SCUs (Grant et al. 1995). In the 2004 National Nursing Home Survey, 23.8% of facilities reported having special programs for the management of behavior problems, although not all of these were provided exclusively on a dedicated SCU (National Center for Health Statistics 2004).

A case-control study of 625 patients in 31 SCUs and 32 traditional units found that residence in an SCU was associated with reduced use of physical restraints but not with less use of "pharmacological restraints" (Sloane et al. 1991). A subsequent study that included data on more than 1,100 residents in 48 SCUs reported that the use of physical restraints was not different, and the likelihood of psychotropic medication use was actually greater, for patients on SCUs than for their counterparts on traditional units (Phillips et al. 2000). Although evidence suggests that mobility may be maintained for longer periods of time among residents of SCUs (Saxton et al. 1998), others have found that the rate of decline in ADL function is not significantly slower for SCU residents (Phillips et al. 1997). Studies showing benefits of SCUs for behavioral disturbances are limited, although one randomized clinical trial reported a reduced frequency of catastrophic reactions (Swanson et al. 1993)—sudden agitated behavior in response to overwhelming external stimuli—as a positive outcome for residence on a dementia SCU. Some studies have demonstrated psychological benefits not only for patients (Lawton et al. 1998) but also for caregivers (Kutner et al. 1999; Wells and Jorm 1987), with evidence of increased family involvement (Hansen et al. 1988; Sloane et al. 1998).

Studies have also examined the extent to which agitation is associated with aspects of the treatment environment in SCUs. Independent correlates of low agitation levels in these units included low rates of physical restraint use, a high proportion of residents in bed during the day, small unit size, fewer comorbid conditions, low levels of functional dependency, and favorable scores on measures of physical environment and unit activities. Despite the efforts of these investigators, there is still insufficient knowledge about the essential elements of treatment in SCUs, and evidence for the effectiveness of these units has not been adequately demonstrated.

Subacute Care in Nursing Homes

Since 1983, when the Medicare Prospective Payment System established reimbursement for acute-care hospitals on the basis of diagnosis-related groups rather than number of inpatient days, hospitals have had a strong incentive to limit lengths of stay by discharging patients earlier. Over the past 20 years, therefore, many patients have been discharged to nursing homes that serve as step-down facilities, providing subacute medical treatment, convalescent care, and rehabilitation services. Subsequently, the trend toward decreasing lengths of stay in hospitals and the transfer of subacute-care patients to nursing homes has been reinforced by additional efforts on the part of insurers and managed care organizations to contain hospital costs. In response both to heavy demand and to nursing home reimbursement rates that were substantially higher for short-stay patients with rehabilitation needs (compared with the per diem rates for long-term care patients), the availability of nursing home beds designated for subacute care increased dramatically in the mid-1990s. It was estimated that subacute-care patients constituted about one-third of nursing home admissions during that period. Medicare reimbursement rates for the first 100 days of nursing home care, computed according to the Resource Utilization Groups system, combined with increased use of the facilities, resulted in significant increases in Medicare spending on subacute care patients in the nursing home setting. Alarm about the increase in spending occurring in the late 1990s prompted changes in Medicare reimbursement that resulted in dramatic reductions in payments to nursing homes from the late 1990s onward.

In general, short-stay residents—patients who, after relatively brief stays in nursing homes, are discharged to the community or die—differ from long-term care patients in that they are younger; more likely to be admitted directly from an acute-care hospital; less likely to have irreversible cognitive impairment, incontinence, or ambulatory dysfunction; and more likely to have a primary diagnosis of hip fracture, stroke, or cancer. The objectives of mental health care for short-stay patients are related not so much to managing behavior problems associated with dementia as to helping patients cope with disease and disability, to searching for delirium and reversible causes of cognitive impairment, and to treating disorders such as depression and anxiety that can be impediments to rehabilitation and recovery. In short, the objectives of mental health care for these patients are similar to goals of traditional consultation-liaison psychiatry in the general hospital. As the opportunities for psychiatric intervention follow these patients from the acute-care hospital into the nursing homes, the services required may need to be more frequent or intensive than those usually available to long-term care residents. For subacute care patients in nursing homes, an investment in psychiatric care can lead to improved participation in rehabilitation efforts, with more efficient recovery and return to independent functioning and more rapid discharge to the community. It is hoped that the benefits of mental health care, in terms of both cost offsets and improved quality of life, will provide a strong incentive for insurers, public and private, to establish reimbursement policies that facilitate such treatment.

Adequacy of Care

The high prevalence of psychiatric problems and the federal mandate to ensure quality of care define a need for geriatric mental health services in nursing homes (Smith et al. 1990). Although the OBRA '87 regulations are having the intended impact (Snowden and Roy-Byrne 1998) and have resulted in measurable improvements in patient care, it has not been shown that the federal requirements for assessment and treatment of mental disorders have led to improved case identification, access to mental health care, receipt of appropriate care, or improved health care outcomes. Medicare claims data in 1992, 2 years after implementation of the Nursing Home Reform Act of 1987, indicated that only 26% of all nursing home residents and 36% of residents with a mental illness received psychiatric services (Smyer et al. 1994), and evidence shows continued low levels of mental health treatment in nursing homes (Shea et al. 2000). Although Medicare payments for psychiatric services in nursing facilities increased in the mid-1990s, expenditures declined from $221 million in 1996 to $194 million in 1999 (Office of Inspector General 2001a).

Borson et al. (1997) found that the required preadmission assessment is inadequate for identifying nursing home applicants who require mental health services. This inadequate assessment occurs, in part, because patients with dementia are exempt from initial psychiatric evaluation; therefore, a large number of patients with psychiatric disturbances secondary to dementia are not identified. Although 88% of patients in the sample in this study were appropriately placed on the basis of their personal and nursing care needs, 55% had unmet mental health needs. There are also concerns that required periodic assessments using the MDS *after* admission do not provide adequate detection of depression (Brown et al. 2002; McCurren 2002; Office of Inspector General 2001b; Schnelle et al. 2001; Snowden 2004). McCurren (2002) found poor correlation between the MDS mood disturbance items and the Geriatric Depression Scale, a well-validated screening instrument for depression in older adults. Ruckdeschel et al. (2004) have shown evidence to support the use of a self-report approach to detection of depression by the MDS. In examining the data from 1,492 nursing homes across five states, Brown et al. (2002) found that 11% of residents were identified on the MDS as depressed, half the rate that was expected on the basis of epidemiological studies that used direct clinical assessments. Of the 11% detected, only 55% received antidepressant therapy. Thus, even when mental disorders are identified, detection does not routinely result in treatment.

Limited access to care appears to be at least part of the problem. In a survey of nursing homes across six states, conducted by Reichman et al. (1998), 47.6% of 899 respondents indicated that the frequency of on-site psychiatric consultation was inadequate. The 2004 National Nursing Home Survey similarly reported that only 40.4% of nursing homes had mental health services available at the facility, and only 48.5% had formal contracts for psychology or psychiatry services (National Center for Health Statistics 2004). Directors of nursing judged 38% of nursing home residents as needing a psychiatric evaluation, but more than one-fourth of rural facilities and more than one-fifth of small facilities reported that no psychiatric consultant was available to them. Meeting the demand for mental health treatment may also be more difficult for nursing facilities that are part of a chain or contain Medicaid beds (Castle and Shea 1997). Thus, there is evidence that the federal requirement that patients receive services to "attain or maintain the highest practicable physical, mental, and psychosocial well-being" has not remedied the problem of access to mental health services in U.S. nursing homes (Colenda et al. 1999). Despite this evidence for the continuing lack of available services, the Office of Inspector General reported in 2001 that 27% of mental health services provided in nursing homes and paid for by Medicare were "medically unnecessary" (Office of Inspector General 2001a). However, it is important to recognize that many of the services identified as resulting in "inappropriate" payments were specifically for excessive psychological testing and group psychotherapy for patients with severe cognitive impairment who were determined by reviewers to be incapable of benefiting from these specific procedures. This survey by the Office of Inspector General did not examine the adequacy of appropriate, medically necessary psychiatric care.

Even among patients whose mental disorders are recognized and for whom treatment is initiated, there is evidence that treatment is often inadequate. A report by Brown et al. (2002) indicated that, of nursing home residents known to be depressed and receiving antidepressants, 32% were taking dosages less than the manufacturers' recommended minimum effective dosage for treating depression. In a survey of 12 nursing homes, Datto et al. (2002) found 47% of patients were taking antidepressants, but nearly half of these patients were still depressed. Although a small proportion of these residents may have been in the early stages of treatment, before a treatment response could reasonably be expected, it appears likely that many residents did not receive proper follow-up care with required dosage adjustments or changes in therapy for those who were not responsive to initial treatment. This finding points to a need for nursing home providers to improve adherence to practice guidelines for the follow-up care of depression.

A federal quality indicator introduced in 1999 focuses on persistence of depression (Nursing Home Quality Indicators Development Group 1999). Prescription of an antidepressant suggests that depression has been recognized and diagnosed and that the first step has been taken to manage it. However, persistence of depression in a patient who is receiving an antidepressant drug suggests that the treatment may not be adequate. Thus, if the proportion of depressed patients receiving antidepressants is high, it may indicate that the facility is doing a good job of recognizing depression and initiating treatment, but it may also suggest it is not doing an adequate job of monitoring patients' response to treatment and modifying treatments as needed to produce optimal outcomes. Clearly, there is a need to improve care processes and to further refine the federal quality indicators for depression care in the nursing home. For a more comprehensive treatment of this subject, the reader is referred to consensus recommendations for improving the quality of mental health care in nursing homes (American Geriatrics Society and American Association for Geriatric Psychiatry 2003).

Mental Health Care in Nursing Homes: A Model for Service Delivery

The high prevalence of psychiatric disorders in nursing homes argues for the importance of establishing systems that incorporate mental health into the basic services provided (Borson et al. 1987). In addition, several factors argue for the importance of the professional components of care: 1) the complex nature of the psychiatric disorders exhibited by nursing home residents, 2) the need to evaluate medical as well as social and environmental factors as causes of mental health problems, 3) the potential benefits of specific treatments, and 4) the need for careful monitoring to assess treatment responses and prevent serious adverse effects of medications. Thus, clinical needs demand that mental health services in nursing homes have two distinct but interacting systems: one that is intrinsic to the facility and is contextual, and another that is professional and is concerned primarily with the delivery of specific treatments.

It has been suggested that mental health training should be provided to facility staff to develop basic skills in assessment and clinical management that can help staff handle problems that occur when specific professional services are lacking. However, it is important to recognize that the intrinsic and the professional systems cannot readily replace each other and that adequate care requires both. Although there is a real need for staff training, a realistic goal is to develop staff skills that complement rather than replace the activities of mental health professionals. This two-system model has obvious implications with respect to the financing of mental health services in nursing homes: it demonstrates the need to fund mental health care both as a necessary part of the per diem costs of nursing home care and as a reimbursable professional service.

Although the intrinsic and the professional systems for mental health services are distinct, they must interact: geriatric psychiatrists and psychologists and geropsychiatric nurse practitioners can play important intrinsic roles as administrative and staff consultants, in-service educators, moderators of case conferences, participants in interdisciplinary team meetings, and contributors in other activities familiar to the consultation-liaison psychiatrist. Facility staff must be effective in recognizing problems, facilitating referral, supporting treatment, and monitoring outcome to enable the professional system to function optimally.

Intrinsic System

The intrinsic system of mental health care in nursing homes can be conceptualized as including a wide range of components: design of the environment; implementation of psychosocial programs; formulation of institutional policies and procedures for assessment, care delivery, monitoring, and quality improvement; and optimization of the ways in which staff and residents interact. The importance of the intrinsic system is recognized in nursing home regulations that require training of nursing aides; in the nursing staff assessments required for completion of the MDS and RAPs; and in OBRA '87 requirements that nursing homes provide assessments, treatment planning, and services to attain or maintain the highest practicable level of mental and physical well-being for each resident. Because psychiatric disorders are common in nursing homes, nurses and aides should be knowledgeable about the nature of the cognitive and functional deficits associated with dementia and the manifestations of delirium and depression. Staff members should understand how to modify their approach to working with residents when cognitive impairment or communication deficits interfere with care. Staff should also know how to apply basic principles of behavioral psychology to identify the causes of agitation and related behavioral symptoms in patients with dementia as well as how to plan environmental and behavioral interventions.

A number of approaches to providing such staff training have been developed. Evaluation studies have demonstrated that improved mental health care through staff training is an attainable goal and have identified barriers that must be overcome (Smyer et al. 1992). As mental health care is incorporated into the basic fabric of the nursing home, it must include provisions for patients with variable degrees of cognitive impairment and depression in both the extent of residents' autonomy and the design of activities.

The concept that several key components of mental health services are intrinsic to the nursing home is perhaps best developed in the design of SCUs for patients with dementing illnesses. Nonetheless, the need for these services applies to all patients, not only to those with dementia. Moreover, the potential benefits of such services are not limited to their effects on residents with diagnosed disorders; there is also the potential for prevention. For example, evidence indicates that contextual interventions designed to encourage a sense of empowerment in residents can have positive effects on both mental and physical health.

Knowledge of the benefits of encouraging autonomy is derived from the classic study by Langer and Rodin (1976), who evaluated a controlled intervention designed to increase nursing home residents' sense of control over day-to-day events. Residents were randomized to either 1) a treatment group in which staff gave the message that residents were expected to be responsible for making decisions for themselves or 2) a control condition in which the message conveyed was that the staff was responsible for residents' care. Both immediately after the intervention and at 18-month follow-up, the treatment groups exhibited benefits in mood, alertness, and active participation. The effects of control-enhancing interventions have been confirmed in a number of other studies (e.g., Banziger and Roush

1983; Schulz 1976; Thomasma et al. 1990) and have been discussed in terms of "learned helplessness" models (Avorn and Langer 1982).

Benefits of interventions designed to enhance the predictability of the environment have also been confirmed (Krantz and Schulz 1980). In summary, these studies demonstrate that the social environment within which care is provided can have a significant effect on nursing home residents; environmental design should be viewed as a component of mental health care.

Professional System

The intrinsic system for mental health services as just described is necessary but not sufficient to meet the needs of nursing home residents. In addition, the services of mental health professionals are important in evaluating the interactions between medical and mental health problems, in establishing psychiatric diagnoses, and in planning and administering specific treatments for mental disorders. This component of the professional system must encompass medically oriented psychiatric care, including psychopharmacological treatment. A position statement by the major provider groups in this field (American Association for Geriatric Psychiatry et al. 1992) acknowledged the history of misuse of psychotropic drugs in nursing homes, but the statement emphasized that psychopharmacological treatment of diagnosed mental disorders is an important part of the medical and mental health care of nursing home residents. The evidence base for the appropriate use of psychotropic medications in the nursing home setting is described earlier in the chapter, in the section titled "Pharmacotherapy." The complexity of psychopharmacological treatment in frail nursing home residents with medical comorbidity requires that the skills of psychiatrists knowledgeable in geriatrics be an integral part of the professional system.

The professional system should include care with a psychosocial as well as a biomedical focus. For example, psychiatrists, psychologists, and psychiatric nurse practitioners and advanced practice nurses with specific expertise in behavioral treatment may be successful in evaluating the antecedents and causes of agitation and related symptoms among patients with dementia and in developing environmental and behavioral interventions, even when efforts by the facility's nursing staff have proven ineffective. As described earlier in this chapter, psychotherapy may be of value for residents whose cognitive abilities allow them to participate. Further research is needed in order to determine how existing treatments should be modified and how they can be administered to optimize their effectiveness in the nursing home. However, despite the need for more research, psychotherapy for the more cognitively intact nursing home residents with depression should be considered an important treatment among the professional mental health services made available to nursing home residents.

Integration of the professional and intrinsic components of mental health care in the nursing home is required because of the inherent interdependence of these systems. To conduct valid assessments and make diagnoses, mental health professionals must rely on nursing home staff to report their shift-by-shift observations of residents' behavior and other clinical signs. Mental health professionals must also depend on nursing home staff to implement and monitor the treatments they prescribe. Conversely, to succeed in providing appropriate mental health care to nursing home residents, staff members in the intrinsic system must have access to ongoing consultation from, and must receive direct support from, mental health professionals who are knowledgeable in geriatrics.

Key Points

- According to the 2004 National Nursing Home Survey, 4% of Americans age 65 years or older—1.5 million people—resided in 16,100 long-term care facilities.
- Epidemiological studies have consistently shown that 80%–94% of nursing home residents have diagnosable psychiatric disorders. These prevalence data suggest that nursing homes are de facto neuropsychiatric institutions, although they were not originally intended for this purpose.
- Since the implementation of federal nursing home regulations in 1991, the rate of antipsychotic medication use has declined, and the use of antidepressants has increased. However, approximately half of nursing home residents who are receiving antidepressant medications continue to have symptoms of depression.
- Since 2003, analyses of safety data from randomized, controlled studies of atypical antipsychotic drugs in elderly patients with dementia, including nursing home studies, have revealed significantly increased

risks of cerebrovascular adverse events and mortality in this population.

- Although mechanical restraints have frequently been used in attempts to control agitation, they do not decrease behavioral disturbances, and cross-national studies have indicated that it is possible to manage nursing home residents without such measures.
- The social environment within which care is provided can have a significant effect on nursing home residents; environmental design should be viewed as a component of mental health care.

References

Abraham IL, Neundorfer MM, Currie LJ: Effects of group interventions on cognition and depression in nursing home residents. Nurs Res 41:196–202, 1992

Abraham IL, Onega LL, Reel SJ, et al: Effects of cognitive group interventions on depressed frail nursing home residents, in Depression in Long Term and Residential Care: Advances in Research and Treatment. Edited by Rubinstein RL, Lawton MP. New York, Springer, 1997, pp 154–168

Ahmed A, Lefante CM, Alam N: Depression and nursing home admission among hospitalized older adults with coronary artery disease: a propensity score analysis. Am J Geriatr Cardiol 16:76–83, 2007

Alessi CA: A randomized trial of a combined physical activity and environmental intervention in nursing home residents: do sleep and agitation improve? J Am Geriatr Soc 47:784–791, 1999

Allen-Burge R, Stevens AB, Burgio LD: Effective behavioral interventions for decreasing dementia-related challenging behavior in nursing homes. Int J Geriatr Psychiatry 14:213–228, 1999

American Association for Geriatric Psychiatry, American Geriatrics Society, American Psychiatric Association: Psychotherapeutic medications in the nursing home. J Am Geriatr Soc 40:946–949, 1992

American Geriatrics Society, American Association for Geriatric Psychiatry: The American Geriatrics Society and American Association for Geriatric Psychiatry recommendations for policies in support of quality mental health care in U.S. nursing homes. J Am Geriatr Soc 51:1299–1304, 2003

American Psychiatric Association: Diagnostic and Statistical Manual of Mental Disorders, 3rd Edition. Washington, DC, American Psychiatric Association, 1980

American Psychiatric Association: Diagnostic and Statistical Manual of Mental Disorders, 3rd Edition, Revised. Washington, DC, American Psychiatric Association, 1987

American Society of Consultant Pharmacists: Fact Sheet. Alexandria, VA, American Society of Consultant Pharmacists, September 2000

Ames D: Depression among elderly residents of local-authority residential homes: its nature and the efficacy of intervention. Br J Psychiatry 156:667–675, 1990

Ames D: Epidemiological studies of depression among the elderly in residential and nursing homes. Int J Geriatr Psychiatry 6:347–354, 1991

Ames D, Ashby D, Mann AH, et al: Psychiatric illness in elderly residents of part III homes in one London borough: prognosis and review. Age Ageing 17:249–256, 1988

Arthur A, Matthews R, Jagger C, et al: Factors associated with antidepressant treatment in residential care: changes between 1990 and 1997. Int J Geriatr Psychiatry 17:54–60, 2002

Ashby D, Ames D, West CR, et al: Psychiatric morbidity as prediction of mortality for residents of local authority homes for the elderly. Int J Geriatr Psychiatry 6:567–575, 1991

Avorn J, Langer E: Induced disability in nursing home patients: a controlled trial. J Am Geriatr Soc 30:397–400, 1982

Avorn J, Dreyer P, Connelly K, et al: Use of psychoactive medication and the quality of care in rest homes: findings and policy implications of a statewide study. N Engl J Med 320:227–232, 1989

Avorn J, Soumerai SD, Everitt DE, et al: A randomized trial of a program to reduce the use of psychoactive drugs in nursing homes. N Engl J Med 327:168–173, 1992

Baines S, Saxby P, Ehlert K: Reality orientation and reminiscence therapy. Br J Psychiatry 151:222–231, 1987

Baker FM, Miller CL: Screening a skilled nursing home population for depression. J Geriatr Psychiatry Neurol 4:218–221, 1991

Ballard CG, Margallo-Lana M, Fossey J, et al: A 1-year follow-up study of behavioral and psychological symptoms in dementia among people in care environments. J Clin Psychiatry 62:631–636, 2001

Banziger G, Roush S: Nursing homes for the birds: a control-relevant intervention with bird feeders. Gerontologist 23:527–531, 1983

Barnes R, Raskind MA: DSM-III criteria and the clinical diagnosis of dementia: a nursing home study. J Gerontol 36:20–27, 1980

Barnes R, Veith R, Okimoto J, et al: Efficacy of antipsychotic medications in behaviorally disturbed dementia patients. Am J Psychiatry 139:1170–1174, 1982

Bartels SJ, Horn SD, Smout RJ, et al: Agitation and depression in frail nursing home elderly patients with dementia: treatment characteristics and service use. Am J Geriatr Psychiatry 11:231–238, 2003

Barton R, Hurst L: Unnecessary use of tranquilizers in elderly patients. Br J Psychiatry 112:989–990, 1966

Beber CR: Management of behavior in the institutionalized aged. Dis Nerv Syst 26:591–596, 1965

Bech P, Bolwig TG, Kramp P, et al: The Bech-Rafaelsen Mania Scale and the Hamilton Depression Scale. Acta Psychiatr Scand 59:420–430, 1979

Beck AT, Ward CH, Mendelson M, et al: An inventory for measuring depression. Arch Gen Psychiatry 4:561–571, 1961

Beck CK, Vogelpohl TS, Rasin JH, et al: Effects of behavioral interventions on disruptive behavior and affect in demented nursing home residents. Nurs Res 51:219–228, 2002

Beers M, Avon J, Soumerai SB, et al: Psychoactive medication use in intermediate-care facility residents. JAMA 260:3016–3020, 1988

Bensink GW, Godbey KL, Marshall MJ, et al: Institutionalized elderly: relaxation, locus of control, self-esteem. J Gerontol Nurs 18:30–36, 1992

Berrios GE, Brook P: Delusions and psychopathology of the elderly with dementia. Acta Psychiatr Scand 75:296–301, 1985

Bharucha AJ, Dew MA, Miller MD, et al: Psychotherapy in long-term care: a review. J Am Med Dir Assoc 7:568–580, 2006

Black SE, Doody R, Li H, et al: Donepezil preserves cognition and global function in patients with severe Alzheimer disease. Neurology 69:459–469, 2007

Blazer DG, Williams CD: Epidemiology of dysphoria and depression in an elderly population. Am J Psychiatry 137:439–444, 1980

Borson S, Liptzin B, Nininger J, et al: Psychiatry and the nursing home. Am J Psychiatry 144:1412–1418, 1987

Borson S, Loebel JP, Kitchell M, et al: Psychiatric assessments of nursing home residents under OBRA-87: should PASARR be reformed? Pre-Admission Screening and Annual Review. J Am Geriatr Soc 45:1173–1181, 1997

Braun JV, Wykle MH, Cowling WR: Failure to thrive in older persons: a concept derived. Gerontologist 28:809–812, 1988

Bridges-Parlet S, Knopman D, Steffes S: Withdrawal of neuroleptic medications from institutionalized dementia patients: results of a double-blind, baseline-treatment-controlled pilot study. J Geriatr Psychiatry Neurol 10:119–126, 1997

Briesacher BA, Limcangco R, Simoni-Wastila L, et al: The quality of antipsychotic drug prescribing in nursing homes. Arch Intern Med 165:1280–1285, 2005

Brodaty H, Ames D, Snowdon J, et al: A randomized placebo-controlled trial of risperidone for the treatment of aggression, agitation, and psychosis of dementia. J Clin Psychiatry 64:134–143, 2003

Brown MN, Lapane KL, Luisi AF: The management of depression in older nursing home residents. J Am Geriatr Soc 50:69–76, 2002

Buck JA: Psychotropic drug practice in nursing homes. J Am Geriatr Soc 36:409–418, 1988

Burns BJ, Taube CA: Mental health services in general medical care and in nursing homes, in Mental Health Policy for Older Americans: Protecting Minds at Risk. Edited by Fogel BS, Furino A, Gottlieb GL. Washington, DC, American Psychiatric Press, 1990, pp 63–84

Burns BJ, Larson DB, Goldstrom ID, et al: Mental disorder among nursing home patients: preliminary findings from the National Nursing Home Survey Pretest. Int J Geriatr Psychiatry 3:27–35, 1988

Buttar AB, Mhyre J, Fries BE, et al: Six-month cognitive improvement in nursing home residents with severe cognitive impairment. J Geriatr Psychiatry Neurol 16:100–108, 2003

Cape RD: Freedom from restraint. Gerontologist 23:217, 1983

Capezuti E, Evans L, Strumpf N, et al: Physical restraint use and falls in nursing home residents. J Am Geriatr Soc 44:627–633, 1996

Castle NG, Shea D: Institutional factors of nursing homes that predict the provision of mental health services. J Ment Health Adm 24:44–54, 1997

Castle NG, Fogel B, Mor V: Risk factors for physical restraint use in nursing homes: pre- and post-implementation of the Nursing Home Reform Act. Gerontologist 37:737–747, 1997

Centers for Medicare and Medicaid: State Operations Manual, Appendix PP: Guidance to Surveyors for Long Term Care Facilities. Baltimore, MD, Centers for Medicare and Medicaid. 2007. Available at http://www.cms.hhs.gov/manuals/Downloads/som107ap_pp_guidelines_ltcf.pdf. Accessed August 6, 2008.

Chahine LM, Bijlsma A, Hospers AP, et al: Dementia and depression among nursing home residents in Lebanon: a pilot study. Int J Geriatr Psychiatry 22:283–285, 2007

Chandler JD, Chandler JE: The prevalence of neuropsychiatric disorders in a nursing home population. J Geriatr Psychiatry Neurol 1:71–76, 1988

Chao SY, Liu HY, Wu CY, et al: The effects of group reminiscence therapy on depression, self esteem, and life satisfaction of elderly nursing home residents. J Nurs Res 14:36–45, 2006

Cohen-Mansfield J: Agitated behaviors in the elderly: preliminary results in the cognitively deteriorated. J Am Geriatr Soc 34:722–727, 1986

Cohen-Mansfield J: Nonpharmacologic interventions for inappropriate behaviors in dementia: a review, summary, and critique. Am J Geriatr Psychiatry 9:361–381, 2001

Cohen-Mansfield J, Billig N: Agitated behaviors in the elderly: a conceptual review. J Am Geriatr Soc 34:711–721, 1986

Cohen-Mansfield J, Libin A: Verbal and physical non-aggressive agitated behaviors in elderly persons with dementia: robustness of syndromes. J Psychiatr Res 39:325–332, 2005

Cohen-Mansfield J, Marx MS, Rosenthal AS: A description of agitation in a nursing home. J Gerontol 44:M77–M84, 1989

Cohen-Mansfield J, Lipson S, Werner P, et al: Withdrawal of haloperidol, thioridazine, and lorazepam in the nursing home: a controlled, double-blind study. Arch Intern Med 159:1733–1740, 1999

Colenda CC, Streim JE, Greene JA, et al: The impact of the Omnibus Budget Reconciliation Act of 1987 (OBRA '87) on psychiatric services in nursing homes. Am J Geriatr Psychiatry 7:12–17, 1999

Custer RL, Davis JE, Gee SC: Psychiatric drug usage in VA nursing home care units. Psychiatr Ann 14:285–292, 1984

Datto C, Oslin D, Streim J, et al: Pharmacological treatment of depression in nursing home residents: a mental health services perspective. J Geriatr Psychiatry Neurol 15:141–146, 2002

Decker FH: Nursing Home, 1977–1999: What Has Changed, What Has Not? Hyattsville, MD, National Center for Health Statistics, 2005

DeDeyn PP, Rabheru K, Rasmussen A, et al: A randomized trial of risperidone, placebo, and haloperidol for behavioral symptoms of dementia. Neurology 53:946–955, 1999

De Deyn PP, Katz IR, Brodaty H, et al: Management of agitation, aggression, and psychosis associated with dementia: a pooled analysis including three randomized, placebo-controlled double-blind trials in nursing home residents treated with risperidone. Clin Neurol Neurosurg 107:497–508, 2005

Dehlin O, Hedenrud B, Jansson P, et al: A double-blind comparison of alaproclate and placebo in the treatment of patients with senile dementia. Acta Psychiatr Scand 71:190–196, 1985

DeLeo D, Stella AG, Spagnoli A: Prescription of psychotropic drugs in geriatric institutions. Int J Geriatr Psychiatry 4:11–16, 1989

Dey AN: Characteristics of elderly nursing home residents: data from the 1995 National Nursing Home Survey. Adv Data 289:1–8, 1997

Dwyer M, Byrne GJ: Disruptive vocalization and depression in older nursing home residents. Int Psychogeriatr 12:463–471, 2000

Elon R, Pawlson LG: The impact of OBRA on medical practice within nursing facilities. J Am Geriatr Soc 40:958–963, 1992

Engle VF, Graney MJ: Stability and improvement of health after nursing home admission. J Gerontol 48:S17–S23, 1993

Evans JM, Chutka DS, Fleming KC, et al: Medical care of nursing home residents. Mayo Clin Proc 70:694–702, 1995

Evans LK, Strumpf NE: Tying down the elderly: a review of the literature on physical restraint. J Am Geriatr Soc 37:65–74, 1989

Evans LK, Strumpf NE, Allen-Taylor SL, et al: A clinical trial to reduce restraints in nursing homes. J Am Geriatr Soc 45:675–681, 1997

Fenton J, Raskin A, Gruber-Baldini AL, et al: Some predictors of psychiatric consultation in nursing home residents. Am J Geriatr Psychiatry 12:297–304, 2004

Finkel SI, Lyons JS, Anderson RL, et al: A randomized, placebo-controlled trial of thiothixene in agitated, demented nursing home patients. Int J Geriatr Psychiatry 10:129–136, 1995

Folstein MF, Folstein SE, McHugh PR: "Mini-Mental State": a practical method for grading the cognitive state of patients for the clinician. J Psychiatr Res 12:189–198, 1975

Fossey J, Ballard C, Juszczak E, et al: Effect of enhanced psychosocial care on antipsychotic use in nursing home residents with severe dementia: cluster randomized trial. Br Med J 332:756–761, 2006

Foster JR, Cataldo JK, Boksay IJE: Incidence of depression in a medical long-term care facility: findings from a restricted sample of new admissions. Int J Geriatr Psychiatry 6:13–20, 1991

German PS, Shapiro S, Kramer M: Nursing home study of eastern Baltimore epidemiologic catchment area, in Mental Illness in Nursing Homes: Agenda for Research. Edited by Harper MS, Lebowitz BD. Rockville, MD, National Institute of Mental Health, 1986, pp 21–40

Goldwasser AN, Auerbach SM, Harkins SW: Cognitive, affective, and behavioral effects of reminiscence group therapy of demented elderly. Int J Aging Hum Dev 25:209–222, 1987

Gottfries CG, Brane G, Gullberg B, et al: A new rating scale for dementia syndromes. Arch Gerontol Geriatr 1:311–330, 1982

Grant LA, Kane RA, Stark AJ: Beyond labels: nursing home care for Alzheimer's disease in and out of special care units. J Am Geriatr Soc 43:569–576, 1995

Guy W (ed): ECDEU Assessment Manual for Psychopharmacology, Revised (DHEW Publ No ADM-76-388). Rockville, MD, U.S. Department of Health, Education and Welfare, 1976

Hamilton M: The assessment of anxiety states by rating. Br J Med Psychol 32:50–55, 1959

Hamilton M: A rating scale for depression. J Neurol Neurosurg Psychiatry 23:56–62, 1960

Hansen SS, Patterson MA, Wilson RW: Family involvement on a dementia unit: the Resident Enrichment and Activity Program. Gerontologist 28:508–510, 1988

Harris Y: Depression as a risk factor for nursing home admission among older individuals. J Am Med Dir Assoc 8:14–20, 2007

Harris Y, Cooper JK: Depressive symptoms in older people predict nursing home admission. J Am Geriatr Soc 54:593–597, 2006

Harrison R, Savla N, Kafetz K: Dementia, depression, and physical disability in a London borough: a survey of elderly people in and out of residential care and implications for future developments. Age Ageing 19:97–103, 1990

Hawes C, Mor V, Phillips CD, et al: The OBRA-87 nursing home regulations and implementation of the Resident Assessment Instrument: effects on process quality. J Am Geriatr Soc 45:977–985, 1997

Health Care Financing Administration: Medicare and Medicaid: Requirements for Long Term Care Facilities, Final Regulations. Fed Regist 56:48865–48921, 1991

Health Care Financing Administration: Medicare and Medicaid Programs: Preadmission Screening and Annual Resident Review. Fed Regist 57:56450–56504, 1992a

Health Care Financing Administration: Medicare and Medicaid: Resident Assessment in Long Term Care Facilities. Fed Regist 57:61614–61733, 1992b

Health Care Financing Administration: State Operations Manual: Provider Certification (Transmittal No 250). Washington, DC, Health Care Financing Administration, 1992c

Health Care Financing Administration: Report to Congress: Study of Private Accreditation (Deeming) of Nursing Homes, Regulatory Incentives and Non-Regulatory Incentives, and Effectiveness of the Survey and Certification System. Washington, DC, Health Care Financing Administration, 1998. Available at http://cms.hhs.gov/medicaid/reports/default.asp. Accessed July 17, 2003.

Heeren O, Borin L, Raskin A, et al: Association of depression with agitation in elderly nursing home residents. J Geriatr Psychiatry Neurol 16:4–7, 2003

Heston LL, Garrard J, Makris L, et al: Inadequate treatment of depressed nursing home elderly. J Am Geriatr Soc 40:1117–1122, 1992

Holmes D, Teresi J, Weiner A, et al: Impact associated with special care units in long-term care facilities. Gerontologist 30:178–181, 1990

Honigfeld G, Roderic D, Klett JC: NOSIE-30: a treatment-sensitive ward behavior scale. Psychol Rep 19:180–182, 1966

Horiguchi J, Inami Y: A survey of the living conditions and psychological states of elderly people admitted to nursing homes in Japan. Acta Psychiatr Scand 83:338–341, 1991

Hughes CD, Berg L, Danziger L, et al: A new clinical scale for the staging of dementia. Br J Psychiatry 140:566–572, 1982

Hyer L, Blazer DG: Depressive symptoms: impact and problems in long term care facilities. International Journal of Behavioral Gerontology 1:33–44, 1982

Innes EM, Turman WG: Evolution of patient falls. Q Rev Biol 9:30–35, 1983

Institute of Medicine Committee on Nursing Home Regulation: Improving the Quality of Care in Nursing Homes. Washington, DC, National Academy Press, 1986

Jeste DV, Okamoto A, Napolitano J, et al: Low incidence of persistent tardive dyskinesia in elderly patients with dementia treated with risperidone. Am J Psychiatry 157:1150–1155, 2000

Jongenelis K, Pot AM, Eisses AM, et al: Prevalence and risk indicators of depression in elderly nursing home patients: the AGED study. J Affect Disord 83:135–142, 2004

Katz IR, Lesher E, Kleban M, et al: Clinical features of depression in the nursing home. Int Psychogeriatr 1:5–15, 1989

Katz IR, Simpson GM, Curlik SM, et al: Pharmacological treatment of major depression for elderly patients in residential care settings. J Clin Psychiatry 51(suppl):41–48, 1990

Katz IR, Parmelee P, Brubaker K: Toxic and metabolic encephalopathies in long-term care patients. Int Psychogeriatr 3:337–347, 1991

Katz IR, Beaston-Wimmer P, Parmelee PA, et al: Failure to thrive in the elderly: exploration of the concept and delineation of psychiatric components. J Geriatr Psychiatry Neurol 6:161–169, 1993

Katz IR, Jeste DV, Mintzer JE, et al: Comparison of risperidone and placebo for psychosis and behavioral disturbances associated with dementia: a randomized, double-blind trial. J Clin Psychiatry 60:107–115, 1999

Katz IR, Streim JE, Smith BD: Psychiatric aspects of long-term care, in Kaplan and Sadock's Comprehensive Textbook of Psychiatry, 7th Edition, Vol 2. Edited by Sadock BJ, Sadock VA. Philadelphia, PA, Lippincott Williams & Wilkins, 2000, pp 3145–3150

Kaup BA, Loreck D, Gruber-Baldini AL, et al: Depression and its relationship to function and medical status, by dementia status, in nursing home admissions. Am J Geriatr Psychiatry 15:438–442, 2007

Kiely DK, Jones RN, Bergmann MA, et al: Association between delirium resolution and functional recovery among newly admitted postacute facility patients. J Gerontol A Biol Sci Med Sci 62:107–108, 2007

Kolanowski AM, Litaker M, Buettner L: Efficacy of theory-based activities for behavioral symptoms of dementia. Nurs Res 54:219–228, 2005

Kramer M, German PS, Anthony JC, et al: Patterns of mental disorders among the elderly residents of eastern Baltimore. J Am Geriatr Soc 33:236–245, 1985

Krantz DS, Schulz PR: Personal control and health: some applications to crises of middle and old age. Advances in Environmental Psychology 2:23–57, 1980

Krauss NA, Altman BM: Characteristics of Nursing Home Residents, 1996. MEPS Research Findings No 5 (AHCPR Publ No 99-0006). Rockville, MD, Agency for Health Care Policy and Research, 1998

Kutner N, Mistretta E, Barnhart H, et al: Family members' perceptions of quality of life change in dementia SCU residents. J Appl Gerontol 18:423–439, 1999

Langer E, Rodin J: The effects of choice and enhanced personal responsibility for the aged: a field experiment in an institutional setting. J Pers Soc Psychol 34:191–198, 1976

Lantz MS, Giambanco V, Buchalter EN: A ten-year review of the effect of OBRA-87 on psychotropic prescribing practices in an academic nursing home. Psychiatr Serv 47:951–955, 1996

Lasser RA, Sunderland T: Newer psychotropic medication use in nursing home residents. J Am Geriatr Soc 46:202–207, 1998

Lawton MP, Brody EM: Assessment of older people: self-maintaining and instrumental activities of daily living. Gerontologist 9:179–186, 1969

Lawton MP, Van Haitsma K, Klapper J, et al: A stimulation-retreat special care unit for elders with dementing illness. Int Psychogeriatr 10:379–395, 1998

Lesher E: Validation of the Geriatric Depression Scale among nursing home residents. Clinics in Gerontology 4:21–28, 1986

Leszcz M, Sadavoy J, Feigenbaum E, et al: A men's group psychotherapy of elderly men. Int J Group Psychother 33:177–196, 1985

Levin CA, Wei W, Akincigil A, et al: Prevalence and treatment of diagnosed depression among elderly nursing home residents in Ohio. J Am Med Dir Assoc 8:585–594, 2007

Linkins KW, Lucca AM, Housman M, et al: Use of PASRR programs to assess serious mental illness and service access in nursing homes. Psychiatr Serv 57:325–332, 2006

Livingston G, Johnston K, Katona C, et al: Systematic review of psychological approaches to the management of neuropsychiatric symptoms of dementia. Am J Psychiatry 162:1996–2021, 2005

Llorente MD, Olsen EJ, Leyva O, et al: Use of antipsychotic drugs in nursing homes: current compliance with OBRA regulations. J Am Geriatr Soc 46:198–201, 1998

Loebel JP, Borson S, Hyde T, et al: Relationships between requests for psychiatric consultations and psychiatric diagnoses in long-term care facilities. Am J Psychiatry 148:898–903, 1991

Lyketsos CG, Lindell Veiel L, Baker A, et al: A randomized, controlled trial of bright light therapy for agitated behaviors in dementia patients residing in long-term care. Int J Geriatr Psychiatry 14:520–525, 1999

Magai C, Kennedy G, Cohen CI, et al: A controlled clinical trial of sertraline in the treatment of depression in nursing home patients with late-stage Alzheimer's disease. Am J Geriatr Psychiatry 8:66–74, 2000

Mann AH, Graham N, Ashby D: Psychiatric illness in residential homes for the elderly: a survey in one London borough. Age Ageing 13:257–265, 1984

McCurren C: Assessment for depression among nursing home elders: evaluation of the MDS mood assessment. Geriatr Nurs 23:103–108, 2002

McMurdo MET, Rennie L: A controlled trial of exercise by residents of old people's homes. Age Ageing 22:11–15, 1993

Meador KG, Taylor JA, Thapa PB, et al: Predictors of antipsychotic withdrawal or dose reduction in a randomized controlled trial of provider education. J Am Geriatr Soc 45:207–210, 1997

Meehan KM, Wang H, David SR, et al: Comparison of rapidly acting intramuscular olanzapine, lorazepam, and placebo: a double-blind, randomized study in acutely agitated patients with dementia. Neuropsychopharmacology 26:494–504, 2002

Mintzer J, Greenspan A, Caers I, et al: Risperidone in the treatment of psychosis of Alzheimer disease: results from a prospective clinical trial. Am J Geriatr Psychiatry 14:280–291, 2006

Mintzer JE, Tune LE, Breder CD, et al: Aripiprazole for the treatment of psychoses in institutionalized patients with Alzheimer dementia: a multicenter, randomized, double-blind, placebo-controlled assessment of three fixed doses. Am J Geriatr Psychiatry 15:918–931, 2007

Montgomery SA, Åsberg M: A new depression scale designed to be sensitive to change. Br J Psychiatry 134:381–382, 1979

Moran JA, Gatz M: Group therapies for nursing home adults: an evaluation of two treatment approaches. Gerontologist 27:588–591, 1987

Morris JN, Hawes C, Fries BE, et al: Designing the national Resident Assessment Instrument for nursing homes. Gerontologist 30:293–307, 1990

Murphy E: The use of psychotropic drugs in long-term care (editorial). Int J Geriatr Psychiatry 4:1–2, 1989

National Center for Health Statistics: The National Nursing Home Survey (DHEW Publ No PHS-79-1794). Hyattsville, MD, National Center for Health Statistics, 1979

National Center for Health Statistics: Use of Nursing Homes by the Elderly: Preliminary Data From the 1985 National Nursing Home Survey (DHHS Publ No PHS-87-1250). Hyattsville, MD, National Center for Health Statistics, 1987

National Center for Health Statistics: The National Nursing Home Survey. Hyattsville MD, National Center for Health Statistics. 2004. Available at http://cdc.gov/nchs/nnhs.htm. Accessed December 26, 2007.

Nursing Home Quality Indicators Development Group: Facility Guide for the Nursing Home Quality Indicators. National Data System. September 28, 1999. Available at http://www.cms.hhs.gov/MinimumDataSets20/Downloads/CHSRA%20QI%20Fact%20Sheet.pdf. Accessed August 6, 2008.

Nyth AL, Gottfries CG: The clinical efficacy of citalopram in treatment of emotional disturbances in dementia disorders: a Nordic multicentre study. Br J Psychiatry 157:894–901, 1990

Office of Inspector General: Medicare Payments for Psychiatric Services in Nursing Homes: A Follow-Up (Publ No OEI-02-99-00140). Washington, DC, U.S. Department of Health and Human Services. 2001a. Available at http://oig.hhs.gov/oei/reports/oei-02-99-00140.pdf. Accessed July 17, 2003.

Office of Inspector General: Nursing Home Resident Assessment, Quality of Care (Publ No OEI-02-99-00040). Washington, DC, U.S. Department of Health and Human Services. 2001b. Available at http://oig.hhs.gov/oei/reports/oei-02-99-00040.pdf. Accessed July 17, 2003.

Office of Inspector General: Psychotropic Drug Use in Nursing Homes (Publ No OEI-02-00-00490). Washington, DC, U.S. Department of Health and Human Services. 2001c. Available at http://oig.hhs.gov/oei/reports/oei-02-00-00490.pdf. Accessed July 17, 2003.

Office of Technology Assessment: Special Care Units for People With Alzheimer's and Other Dementias: Consumer Education, Research, Regulatory, and Reimbursement Issues (OTA-H-543). Washington, DC, U.S. Government Printing Office, August 1992

Ohta RJ, Ohta BM: Special units for Alzheimer's disease patients: a critical look. Gerontologist 28:803–808, 1988

Olin JT, Fox LS, Pawluczyk S, et al: A pilot randomized trial of carbamazepine for behavioral symptoms in treatment-resistant outpatients with Alzheimer disease. Am J Geriatr Psychiatry 9:400–405, 2001

Ollech D: An analyst's experience working in a skilled nursing facility: a case study. Am J Psychoanal 66:381–390, 2006

Omnibus Budget Reconciliation Act of 1987, Pub L No 100-203. Subtitle C: Nursing home reform.

Onder G, Liperoti R, Soldato M, et al: Depression and risk of nursing home admission among older adults in home care in Europe: results from the Aged in Home Care (AdHOC) study. J Clin Psychiatry 68:1392–1398, 2007

Orten JD, Allen M, Cook J: Reminiscence groups with confused nursing center residents: an experimental study. Soc Work Health Care 14:73–86, 1989

Oslin DW, Streim JE, Katz IR, et al: Heuristic comparison of sertraline with nortriptyline for the treatment of depression in frail elderly patients. Am J Geriatr Psychiatry 8:141–149, 2000

Oslin DW, Ten Have TR, Streim JE, et al: Probing the safety of medications in the frail elderly: evidence from a randomized clinical trial of sertraline and venlafaxine in depressed nursing home residents. J Clin Psychiatry 64:875–882, 2003

Overall JE, Gorham DR: The Brief Psychiatric Rating Scale. Psychol Rep 10:799–812, 1962

Parmelee PA, Katz IR, Lawton MP: Depression among institutionalized aged: assessment and prevalence estimation. J Gerontol 44:M22–M29, 1989

Parmelee PA, Katz IR, Lawton MP: The relation of pain to depression among institutionalized aged. J Gerontol 46:P15–P21, 1991

Parmelee PA, Katz IR, Lawton MP: Depression and mortality among institutionalized aged. J Gerontol 47:P3–P10, 1992a

Parmelee PA, Katz IR, Lawton MP: Incidence of depression in long-term care settings. J Gerontol 47:M189–M196, 1992b

Phillips CD, Sloane PD, Hawes C, et al: Effects of residence in Alzheimer's disease special care units on functional outcomes. JAMA 278:1340–1344, 1997

Phillips CD, Spry KM, Sloane PD, et al: Use of physical restraints and psychotropic medications in Alzheimer special care units in nursing homes. Am J Public Health 90:92–96, 2000

Politis AM, Vozzella S, Mayer LS, et al: A randomized, controlled, clinical trial of activity therapy for apathy in patients with dementia residing in long-term care. Int J Geriatr Psychiatry 19:1087–1094, 2004

Porsteinsson AP, Tariot PN, Erb R, et al: Placebo-controlled study of divalproex sodium for agitation in dementia. Am J Geriatr Psychiatry 9:58–66, 2001

Rattenbury C, Stones MJ: A controlled evaluation of reminiscence and current topics discussion groups in a nursing home context. Gerontologist 29:768–771, 1989

Ray WA, Federspiel CF, Schaffner W: A study of antipsychotic drug use in nursing homes: epidemiologic evidence suggesting misuse. Am J Public Health 70:485–491, 1980

Ray WA, Taylor JA, Meador KG, et al: Reducing antipsychotic drug use in nursing homes: a controlled trial of provider education. Arch Intern Med 153:713–721, 1993

Reichman WE, Coyne AC, Borson S, et al: Psychiatric consultation in the nursing home: a survey of six states. Am J Geriatr Psychiatry 6:320–327, 1998

Reisberg B: Functional Assessment Staging (FAST). Psychopharmacol Bull 24:653–659, 1988

Reisberg B, Ferris SH, deLeon MJ, et al: Global Deterioration Scale (GDS). Psychopharmacol Bull 24:661–663, 1988

Reisberg B, Auer SR, Monteiro IM: Behavioral Pathology in Alzheimer's Disease (BEHAVE-AD) rating scale. Int Psychogeriatr 8(suppl):301–308, 1996

Rhoades J, Krauss N: Nursing Home Trends, 1987 and 1996. MEPS Chartbook No 3 (AHCPR Publ No 99-0032). Rockville, MD, Agency for Health Care Policy and Research, 1999

Risse SC, Cubberley L, Lampe TH, et al: Acute effects of neuroleptic withdrawal in elderly dementia patients. Journal of Geriatric Drug Therapy 2:65–77, 1987

Rosen J, Mulsant BH, Pollock BG: Sertraline in the treatment of minor depression in nursing home residents: a pilot study. Int J Geriatr Psychiatry 15:177–180, 2000

Rovner BW, Kafonek S, Filipp L, et al: Prevalence of mental illness in a community nursing home. Am J Psychiatry 143:1446–1449, 1986

Rovner BW, German PS, Broadhead J, et al: The prevalence and management of dementia and other psychiatric disorders in nursing homes. Int Psychogeriatr 2:13–24, 1990a

Rovner BW, Lucas-Blaustein J, Folstein MF, et al: Stability over one year in patients admitted to a nursing home dementia unit. Int J Geriatr Psychiatry 5:77–82, 1990b

Rovner BW, German PS, Brant LJ, et al: Depression and mortality in nursing homes. JAMA 265:993–996, 1991

Rovner BW, Edelman BA, Cox MP, et al: The impact of antipsychotic drug regulations (OBRA 1987) on psychotropic prescribing practices in nursing homes. Am J Psychiatry 149:1390–1392, 1992

Rovner BW, Steele CD, Shmuely Y, et al: A randomized trial of dementia care in nursing homes. J Am Geriatr Soc 44:7–13, 1996

Ruckdeschel K, Thompson R, Datto CJ, et al: Using the Minimum Data Set 2.0 mood disturbance items as a self-report screening instrument for depression in nursing home residents. Am J Geriatr Psychiatry 12:43–49, 2004

Ruths S, Straand J, Nygaard HA, et al: Effect of antipsychotic withdrawal on behavior and sleep/wake activity in nursing home residents with dementia: a randomized, placebo-controlled, double-blinded study. The Bergen District Nursing Home Study. J Am Geriatr Soc 52:1737–1743, 2004

Sabin TD, Vitug AJ, Mark VH: Are nursing home diagnosis and treatment inadequate? JAMA 248:321–322, 1982

Sadavoy J: Psychotherapy for the institutionalized elderly, in Practical Psychiatry in the Nursing Home: A Handbook for Staff. Edited by Conn DK, Herrman N, Kaye A, et al. Toronto, ON, Canada, Hogrefe and Huber, 1991, pp 217–236

Saxton J, Silverman M, Ricci E, et al: Maintenance of mobility in residents of an Alzheimer's special care facility. Int Psychogeriatr 10:213–224, 1998

Schneider LS, Pollock VE, Lyness SA: A meta-analysis of controlled trials of neuroleptic treatment in dementia. J Am Geriatr Soc 38:553–563, 1990

Schneider LS, Dagerman KS, Insel P: Risk of death with atypical antipsychotic drug treatment for dementia: meta-analysis of randomized placebo-controlled trials. JAMA 294:1934–1943, 2005

Schnelle JF, Newman DR, White M, et al: Reducing and managing restraints in long-term-care facilities. J Am Geriatr Soc 40:381–385, 1992

Schnelle JF, Wood S, Schnelle ER, et al: Measurement sensitivity and the Minimum Data Set depression quality indicator. Gerontologist 41:401–405, 2001

Schulz PR: Effect of control and predictability on the psychological well-being of the institutionalized aged. J Pers Soc Psychol 33:563–573, 1976

Semla TP, Palla K, Poddig B, et al: Effect of the Omnibus Reconciliation Act 1987 on antipsychotic prescribing in nursing home residents. J Am Geriatr Soc 42:648–652, 1994

Shader RI, Harmatz JS, Salzman C: A new scale for clinical assessment in geriatric populations: Sandoz Clinical Assessment—Geriatric (SCAG). J Am Geriatr Soc 22:107–113, 1974

Shea DG, Russo PA, Smyer MA: Use of mental health services by persons with a mental illness in nursing facilities: initial impacts of OBRA 87. J Aging Health 12:560–578, 2000

Shorr RI, Fought RL, Ray WA: Changes in antipsychotic drug use in nursing homes during implementation of the OBRA-87 regulations. JAMA 271:358–362, 1994

Siegler EL, Capezuti E, Maislin G, et al: Effects of a restraint reduction intervention and OBRA '87 regulations on psychoactive drug use in nursing homes. J Am Geriatr Soc 45:791–796, 1997

Sink KM, Holden KF, Yaffe K: Pharmacological treatment of neuropsychiatric symptoms of dementia: a review of the evidence. JAMA 293:596–608, 2005

Sloane PD, Mathew LS, Scarborough M, et al: Physical and pharmacologic restraint of nursing home patients with dementia: impact of specialized units. JAMA 265:1278–1282, 1991

Sloane PD, Mitchell CM, Preisser JS, et al: Environmental correlates of resident agitation in Alzheimer's disease special care units. J Am Geriatr Soc 46:862–869, 1998

Smalbrugge M, Jongenelis L, Pot AM, et al: Incidence and outcome of depressive symptoms in nursing home patients in the Netherlands. Am J Geriatr Psychiatry 14:1069–1076, 2006

Smith M, Buckwalter KC, Albanese M: Geropsychiatric education programs: providing skills and understanding. J Psychosoc Nurs Ment Health Serv 28:8–12, 1990

Smyer M, Brannon D, Cohn M: Improving nursing home care through training and job redesign. Gerontologist 32:327–333, 1992

Smyer MA, Shea DG, Streit A: The provision and use of mental health services in nursing homes: results from the National Medical Expenditure Survey. Am J Public Health 84:284–287, 1994

Snow LA, Hovanec L, Brandt J: A controlled trial of aromatherapy for agitation in nursing home patients with dementia. J Altern Complement Med 10:431–437, 2004

Snowden M: The Minimum Data Set depression rating scale (MDSDRS) lacks reliability for identifying depression among older adults living in nursing homes. Evid Based Ment Health 7:7, 2004

Snowden M, Roy-Byrne P: Mental illness and nursing home reform: OBRA-87 ten years later. Omnibus Budget Reconciliation Act. Psychiatr Serv 49:229–233, 1998

Snowden M, Sato K, Roy-Byrne P: Assessment and treatment of nursing home residents with depression or behavioral symptoms associated with dementia: a review of the literature. J Am Geriatr Soc 51:1305–1317, 2003

Snowdon J: Dementia, depression, and life satisfaction in nursing homes. Int J Geriatr Psychiatry 1:85–91, 1986

Snowdon J, Donnelly N: A study of depression in nursing homes. J Psychiatr Res 20:327–333, 1986

Spagnoli A, Foresti G, Macdonald A, et al: Dementia and depression in Italian geriatric institutions. Int J Geriatr Psychiatry 1:15–23, 1986

Steele C, Rovner BW, Chase GA, et al: Psychiatric symptoms and nursing home placement in Alzheimer's disease. Am J Psychiatry 147:1049–1051, 1990

Stotsky B: Multicenter study comparing thioridazine with diazepam and placebo in elderly, nonpsychotic patients with emotional behavioral disorders. Clin Ther 6:546–559, 1984

Street JS, Clark WS, Gannon KS, et al: Olanzapine treatment of psychotic and behavioral symptoms in patients with Alzheimer disease in nursing care facilities, a double-blind, randomized, placebo-controlled trial. Arch Gen Psychiatry 57:968–976, 2000

Streim JE, Katz IR: Federal regulations and the care of patients with dementia in the nursing home. Med Clin North Am 78:895–909, 1994

Streim JE, Oslin DW, Katz IR, et al: Drug treatment of depression in frail elderly nursing home residents. Am J Geriatr Psychiatry 8:150–159, 2000

Streim JE, Rovner BW, Katz IR: Psychiatric aspects of long-term care, in Comprehensive Textbook of Geriatric Psychiatry, 3rd Edition. Edited by Sadavoy J, Jarvik LF, Grossberg GT, et al. New York, WW Norton, 2004, pp 1071–1102

Streim JE, Porsteinsson AP, Breder CD, et al: A randomized, double-blind, placebo-controlled study of aripiprazole for the treatment of psychosis in nursing home patients with Alzheimer's disease. Am J Geriatr Psychiatry 16:537–550, 2008

Sunderland T, Silver MA: Neuroleptics in the treatment of dementia. Int J Geriatr Psychiatry 3:79–88, 1988

Sutcliffe C, Burns A, Challis D, et al: Depressed mood, cognitive impairment, and survival in older people admitted to care homes in England. Am J Geriatr Psychiatry 15:708–715, 2007

Svarstad BL, Mount JK, Bigelow W: Variations in the treatment culture of nursing homes and responses to regulations to reduce drug use. Psychiatr Serv 52:666–672, 2001

Swanson E, Maas M, Buckwalter K: Catastrophic reactions and other behaviors of Alzheimer's residents: special unit compared with traditional units. Arch Psychiatr Nurs 7:292–299, 1993

Tariot PN, Podgorski CA, Blazina L, et al: Mental disorders in the nursing home: another perspective. Am J Psychiatry 150:1063–1069, 1993

Tariot PN, Erb R, Podgorski CA, et al: Efficacy and tolerability of carbamazepine for agitation and aggression in dementia. Am J Psychiatry 155:54–61, 1998

Tariot PN, Cummings JL, Katz IR, et al: A randomized, double-blind, placebo-controlled study of the efficacy and safety of donepezil in patients with Alzheimer's disease in the nursing home setting. J Am Geriatr Soc 49:1590–1599, 2001a

Tariot PN, Schneider LS, Mintzer J, et al: Safety and tolerability of divalproex sodium in the treatment of signs and symptoms of mania in elderly patients with dementia: results of a double-blind, placebo-controlled trial. Curr Ther Res Clin Exp 62:51–67, 2001b

Tariot PN, Farlow MR, Grossberg GT, et al: Memantine treatment in patients with moderate to severe Alzheimer disease already receiving donepezil: a randomized controlled trial. JAMA 291:317–324, 2004

Tariot PN, Raman R, Jakimovich L, et al: Divalproex sodium in nursing home residents with possible or probable Alzheimer disease complicated by agitation: a randomized, controlled trial. Am J Geriatr Psychiatry 13:942–949, 2005

Teeter RB, Garetz FK, Miller WR, et al: Psychiatric disturbances of aged patients in skilled nursing homes. Am J Psychiatry 133:1430–1434, 1976

Thapa PB, Gideon P, Cost TW, et al: Antidepressants and the risk of falls among nursing home residents. N Engl J Med 339:875–882, 1998

Thomasma M, Yeaworth R, McCabe B: Moving day: relocation and anxiety in institutionalized elderly. J Gerontol Nurs 16:18–24, 1990

Tondi L, Ribani L, Bottazzi M, et al: Validation therapy (VT) in nursing home: a case-control study. Arch Gerontol Geriatr 44(suppl):407–411, 2007

Toseland RW, Diehl M, Freeman K, et al: The impact of validation group therapy on nursing home residents with dementia. J Appl Gerontol 61:31–50, 1997

Trappler B, Cohen CI: Using fluoxetine in "very old" depressed nursing home residents. Am J Geriatr Psychiatry 4:258–262, 1996

Trappler B, Cohen CI: Use of SSRIs in "very old" depressed nursing home residents. Am J Geriatr Psychiatry 6:83–89, 1998

Trichard L, Zabow A, Gillis LS: Elderly persons in old age homes: a medical, psychiatric and social investigation. S Afr Med J 61:624–627, 1982

van Weert JC, van Dulmen AM, Spreeuwenberg PM, et al: Behavioral and mood effects of snoezelen integrated into 24-hour dementia care. J Am Geriatr Soc 53:24–33, 2005

Wagner AW, Teri L, Orr-Rainey N: Behavior problems of residents with dementia in special care units. Alzheimer Dis Assoc Disord 9:121–127, 1995

Wang PS, Schneeweiss S, Avorn J, et al: Risk of death in elderly users of conventional vs. atypical antipsychotic medications. N Engl J Med 353:2335–2321, 2005

Webber AP, Martin JL, Harker JO, et al: Depression in older patients admitted for postacute nursing home rehabilitation. J Am Geriatr Soc 53:1017–1022, 2005

Wells Y, Jorm FA: Evaluation of a special nursing home unit for dementia suffers: a randomized controlled comparison with community care. Aust N Z J Psychiatry 21:524–531, 1987

Werner P, Cohen-Mansfield J, Braun J, et al: Physical restraint and agitation in nursing home residents. J Am Geriatr Soc 37:1122–1126, 1989

Williams-Barnard CL, Lindell AR: Therapeutic use of "prizing" and its effect on self-concept of elderly clients in nursing homes and group homes. Issues Ment Health Nurs 13:1–17, 1992

Winblad B, Kilander L, Eriksson S, et al: Donepezil in patients with severe Alzheimer's disease: double-blind, parallel-group, placebo-controlled study. Lancet 367:1057–1065, 2006

Won A, Lapane KL, Vallow S, et al: Long-term effects of analgesics in a population of elderly nursing home residents with persistent nonmalignant pain. J Gerontol A Biol Sci Med Sci 61:165–169, 2006

Wood S, Cummings JL, Hsu MA, et al: The use of the Neuropsychiatric Inventory in nursing home residents: characterization and measurement. Am J Geriatr Psychiatry 8:75–83, 2000

Youssef FA: The impact of group reminiscence counseling on a depressed elderly population. Nurse Pract 15:32–38, 1990

Zerhusen JD, Boyle K, Wilson W: Out of the darkness: group cognitive therapy for depressed elderly. J Psychosoc Nurs Ment Health Serv 29:16–21, 1991

Zhong KX, Tariot PN, Mintzer J, et al: Quetiapine to treat agitation in dementia: a randomized, double-blind, placebo-controlled study. Curr Alzheimer Res 4:81–93, 2007

Zimmer JG, Watson N, Treat A: Behavioral problems among patients in skilled nursing facilities. Am J Public Health 74:1118–1121, 1984

Suggested Readings

American Geriatrics Society, American Association for Geriatric Psychiatry: The American Geriatrics Society and American Association for Geriatric Psychiatry recommendations for policies in support of quality mental health care in U.S. nursing homes. J Am Geriatr Soc. 51:1299–1304, 2003

Bharucha AJ, Dew MA, Miller MD, et al: Psychotherapy in long-term care: a review. J Am Med Dir Assoc 7:568–580, 2006

Centers for Medicare and Medicaid: State Operations Manual, Appendix PP: Guidance to Surveyors for Long Term Care Facilities. Baltimore, MD, Centers for Medicare and Medicaid. 2007. Available at http://www.cms.hhs.gov/manuals/Downloads/som107ap_pp_guidelines_ltcf.pdf. Accessed December 31, 2007.

Sink KM, Holden KF, Yaffe K: Pharmacological treatment of neuropsychiatric symptoms of dementia: a review of the evidence. JAMA 293:596–608, 2005

Snowden M, Sato K, Roy-Byrne P: Assessment and treatment of nursing home residents with depression or behavioral symptoms associated with dementia: a review of the literature. J Am Geriatr Soc 51:1305–1317, 2003

Streim JE, Katz IR: Federal regulations and the care of patients with dementia in the nursing home. Med Clin North Am 78:895–909, 1994

CHAPTER 32

The Continuum of Caring in the Long Term

Movement Toward the Community

George L. Maddox, Ph.D.
Elise J. Bolda, M.S.P.H., Ph.D.

Among health care policy analysts, care providers, and consumers in the United States, the conversation about the role of communities in chronic care over the long term has changed significantly over the past two decades. A primary stimulus for this change has been increased awareness of how badly the currently dominant medical model of hospital care is mismatched with the increasingly obvious needs for more effective care of chronic conditions in nonhospital settings. This mismatch has been illustrated dramatically by a report of the Institute of Medicine of the National Academy of Sciences, *Crossing the Quality Chasm: A Health System for the 21st Century* (Institute of Medicine 2001), which emphasizes the importance of multidisciplinary care in community settings and the necessary involvement of patients in that type of care. Involving the community in caregiving becomes increasingly necessary as well as desirable as populations age. In recent decades, federal policies guiding the provision of long-term care have devolved to give states and communities increasing responsibility for how that care is provided. How this devolution of long-term care policy, which began as a requirement, has become an opportunity for innovation is the issue of interest here.

As long ago as 1980, James Fries anticipated the importance of multidisciplinary community care when he argued persuasively that the demographics of the aging population in the United States were changing. Although the population was demonstrably aging, evidence indicated that the onset of disabling chronic illness was apparently being delayed, in part, by a variety of successful social, psychological, and biomedical interventions. He anticipated correctly that implications of these epidemiological changes would be need for and use of noninstitutional forms of care for chronic conditions and greater use of preventive care in the community. Whereas three decades ago these conclusions were only informed guesses, evidence increasingly has confirmed them (Fries 2001). (For an illustration online of the practical implications of Fries' argument for health care in an aging population, see http://healthproject.stanford.edu.)

Confirming evidence also indicates that disability in the U.S. population resulting in institutional care has been declining at the rate of about 1% a year over the past several decades (Cutler 2001). And in the past decade the occupancy rate of available nursing home beds has continued to decline as alternative forms of supportive care in the community have increased (Smith 2003).

The anticipated long-term care needs of an aging population have changed the conversation among policy analysts and care providers regarding care in the community. As is often the case in guiding public policy regarding the provision of social services, court decisions have specified community alternatives to institutional care. Advocates of disabled persons of all ages jointly achieved the passage of the Americans With Disabilities Act in 1990 that facilities easier access to public places and services (Vachon 2001), and the Supreme Court in the *Olmstead* decision (1999) declared that publicly funded services must be supplied in the least restrictive environment (Fox-Grage et al. 2008). These legal decisions came at the end of more than three decades of interest and renewed debate about federal dominance in social welfare policy and the appropriate role of states. Across those decades, a process of devolution of decision making had occurred, particularly regarding social welfare policies, that proposed to give states more responsibility for funding as well as for regulating health and welfare services (Caro and Morris 2002). The full implications of the devolution of health and welfare policy toward more state responsibility, and of the Americans With Disabilities Act and the *Olmstead* decision, remain to be seen. At a minimum, many states are taking great care to certify that they intend to be in compliance. There are also indications that for some states, necessity to take responsibility for the redesign and implementation of care in the long term has become an opportunity for innovation. Some illustrations of such innovations in community care are the focus here.

Emerging Long-Term Care Policy in the United States: Muddling Through

Historians have documented the difficulties of achieving and adapting effective health care policies in democratic societies. Public preferences for care and who provides it, where it is provided, and at what cost vary and change. Political circumstances change. There is no compelling evidence that there is a single effective way to design an effective, affordable health care system. This pessimistic observation leads some health policy analysts to suggest, despite the risk of fragmenting the policy process, that policy pragmatism, sometimes called "muddling through," may be the strategy of choice in rapidly changing circumstances of democratic societies with complex, sometimes conflicting, values. Although "muddling" might suggest a lack of thoughtfulness, quite the opposite is the case (Lindblom 1959). Organizational theorists know there is no single correct way to organize sustainable, effective organizations; successful policy design and implementation depend substantially on an understanding of changing societal contexts and on leadership that realistically aligns public policies with the changing needs, values, and resources observed (Mitchell and Shortell 2000; von Bertalanffy 1968). Grand theories of what policies should work to provide desired public outcomes tend to give way to "grounded research" (Glaser 1998) that focuses not only on how public policy is formulated but also on whether in fact it is implementable (Pressman and Wildavsky 1984). For example, in 1948 Great Britain created a relatively low-cost but effective National Health Service (NHS) that remained relatively stable until the 1990s when a conservative government proposed greater emphasis on primary care and increased privatization of the system. A succeeding Labour government that had vowed to oppose such changes in fact failed to do so (Maddox 1971, 1999). Long-term care policy in the NHS initially designated some hospitals beds as "long stay" and developed domiciliary beds in the community supported by general practitioners and visiting nurses. In recent years Britain, in contrast to other countries in the European Union, has increasingly permitted the development of nursing homes in the private sector (Maddox 1992). The long-term care policy in the United States, in contrast, was embodied in Medicare/Medicaid legislation in 1965 that authorized limited posthospital care under Medicare but financed care in nursing homes for the poor under Medicaid. In fact, Medicaid encouraged and financed the development of a substantial nursing home industry in the private sector. In recent decades the federal policy of devolution that gives additional authority to states and communities in allocating funds for long-term care has encouraged development and allocation of nonfederal funds for community- and home-based care and alternative sources of assisted-living housing in the private sector (Maddox 2001; Smith 2003). Although these were positive developments, nursing homes, and the incorrect assumption that their use would be covered by Medicare, remained the dominant image of long-term care in the United States. That image is now changing.

As Theodore Marmor (2000) argued in his original and subsequent account of the creation of Medicare and Medicaid in 1965, the enabling legislation was a marvelously complex political creation. Proponents of community-based health care services underwritten by public dollars faced not only opposing medical and hospital interests but also, and perhaps more daunting, deeply held public values favoring personal health care in the private sector and personal responsibility for that care (Maddox 1992). The initial outcome of this complex political contest was the decision to make public dollars available to private sector entrepreneurs to create, literally, what is now observed as a hospital-like system of nursing homes whose facilities are described in terms of numbers of beds to be occupied by patients and serviced by medical directors and nurses and their various aides. The private sector nursing home industry is estimated currently to provide over 1.7 million beds that have an occupancy rate of 83% at a cost of $115 billion annually. Fifty-eight percent of the annual cost is paid with federal dollars, primarily by Medicaid (44%) (National Center for Health Statistics 2006). Although nursing homes continue to be the principal providers of institutional long-term care, alternative sources of care have consistently increased as interest in the reinvention of long-term care, particularly various forms of nonmedical residential care, such as assisted-living housing and community- and home-based care, has increased (Maddox 2001; Smith 2003).

Medicare's provision of services was initially intended to serve predominantly older adults as indicated by the near universal association of age 65 years as the age of eligibility. There was, however, no intention to provide long-term care underwritten by Medicare beyond limited posthospital care in nursing homes. Medicaid was authorized to pay for nursing home care, and as the "new federalism," emphasizing federal/state cooperation, has matured, it has increased resources for community and home care. In 1970, Medicaid allocated minimal dollars to home and community care. By 2004 the home- and community-care dollars approached half the dollars allocated to institutional long-term care.

Federal policy on long-term care has been slow to change. Beginning with federal devolution of responsibility for long-term care to states in the mid-1980s, federal interest focused on cost containment. Perhaps the most notable example of federal policy innovation in long-term care is the modification of Medicaid under the Reagan administration's home- and community-based care (HCBS) waivers. This provision enabled states to seek waivers creating home- and community-based options for older and disabled beneficiaries who otherwise would require nursing home care. Federal approval of such waivers required states to document that Medicaid expenditures would be less than the expenses incurred if care were provided in nursing homes. With the impetus of HCBS waivers and growing state expenditures, the 1990s were years of growth in innovation of state long-term care policy as many states chose not to wait for further federal innovation (Goldsmith and Eggers 2002). Articulation of the critical role of states and communities in long-term care policy began to evolve more systematically after 2000, as evidenced by the long-term care agenda announced in October 2004 by the Chairman of the National Governors Association promoting "A Lifetime of Health and Dignity: Confronting Long-Term Care Challenges in America" (National Governors Association 2003).

Care in the Community: A New Dynamic

Concentrating solely, and pessimistically, on notable gaps in availability and access to long-term care services produced by decades of fragmentation of federal long-term care and financing policy emphasizing cost containment, however, is giving way to a new dynamic focused on reinventing long-term care. Innovative alternatives to the dominant initial focus of Medicare and Medicaid on medicine, hospitals, and nursing homes are increasingly evident (Smith 2003). The new focus is on coordinating health and welfare resources and services in the community.

The devolution of policy and the "new federalism" that encouraged greater state and community responsibility for health and welfare resources and services has turned out to be both permission and encouragement to explore alternative ways to reinvent long-term care. The new dynamic encourages communities to explore new ways to reinvent caring in the long term that is affordable, accessible, and effective for older adults. The new conversation focuses on creating in communities a sustainable sense of social efficacy in making it possible for older adults to age in place.

Interest in the reinvention of community-based care in the long term comes with convergence of new thinking from many perspectives. For example, a growing sense of empowerment and self-efficacy has been noted among consumers of health and social services, and an increased sense of collective efficacy in solving problems has tended to accompany these changes (Bandura 1997; Kiwachi and Berkman 2000; Maddox

2001; Schulz et al. 1998). Communities have become increasingly interested in local initiatives to make their communities more livable for older adults.

The devolution of responsibility for the allocation of health and social resources and services toward the community, however, is not without risk. Policy analysts have noted, for example, that devolution risks the uneven distribution of resources among political districts and populations and the shifting of risk from society to individuals (Hacker 2007). These caveats should be kept in mind in reading the following illustrations of devolution of long-term care for older adults toward the community, which stress the positive aspects of increased community involvement in innovative provision of accessible and sustainable caring for older adults in the long term.

In the six initiatives illustrating notable innovations in community-based long-term care discussed in this chapter—hospice, chronic-care management, consumer-directed care, assisted-living housing, community mental health initiatives, and collaborative partnerships for older adults—the importance of a sense of collective efficacy and the current interest in initiating and sustaining innovative caring in the long term will be apparent. All of the innovations are works in progress that illustrate innovative care of older adults in communities. The brief description of each innovation includes key references to relevant sources that will facilitate further inquiry.

Six Illustrative Innovations in Community-Based Long-Term Care

Hospice

Hospice is an ancient provision of community care for dying persons and their families that reemerged in the modern era with establishment of St. Christopher's Hospice outside London in 1967. The idea migrated to the United States in the 1970s but with a difference (Mor and Allen 2001). Whereas the English hospice was a community of caring for the dying within institutional walls, the American version has emphasized home care, or "hospice without walls." Hospice facilities did not receive federal financial support until the 1980s. The inadequacy of care at the end of life has been widely documented, particularly in hospital and nursing home settings (Field and Cassel 1997; Meier and Morrison 1999). The Institute of Medicine review reported by Field and Cassel documents widespread neglect of dying patients and their families in hospital wards, in nursing homes, and in medical education. The perceived inadequacy of care at the end of life in hospital settings, disenchantment with the unfulfilled promise of curative medicine, and a new sensitivity to the possibility of better care at the end of life have combined to promote the implementation in hospice of a new philosophy about care at the end of life in the community. This philosophy emphasizes the importance of developing and maintaining a homelike environment for terminal care, pain control, absence of high-technology medical and surgical interventions characteristic of hospitals, and emotional support for the dying patients and their families.

Hospice care is designed to maximize a sense of self-efficacy of individuals and a sense of collective efficacy for families in managing as much as possible a terminal patient's final transition in a minimally medical environment and with the promise of a collective assurance that social and emotional support reliably will remain available. The life-prolonging high-technology interventions characteristic of hospitals are simply not available by design, and this, economists have conjectured, is one likely explanation of why the cost of hospice remains relatively low when compared with hospitalization.

Hospice is an innovation in long-term care that has been extensively evaluated. This strategy of terminal care that has, since the mid-1980s, been covered by Medicare does tend to reduce cost of care at the end of life. And, overall, the quality of medical care provided within the low-tech environment of hospice care compares favorably with the care that hospitals provide for comparable patients. Consequently, terminal care provided by hospice has become increasingly popular as a service and widely supported in communities. By the late 1990s more than 1,000 hospices were serving over 350,000 patients in the United States. In 2004 there were more than 2,600 hospice facilities. Hospice, in sum, has become a major community alternative for terminal care, particularly for patients with cancer and more recently for those with AIDS. Current information on hospice and how it has stimulated interest in palliative care in medicine is available online at http://www.hospicefoundation.org.

Chronic-Care Management

Curative medicine has produced the paradox of facilitating the survival of an increasing number of individuals who in an earlier era would have died young but who now face the challenge of decades of managing chronic illness. Critics increasingly note that the dominant medical-hospital complex in the United States is not providing effective care for a population with increasing rates of chronic conditions and illness. The current health system, they conclude, in fact cannot do the job.

The Institute of Medicine, National Academy of Sciences, has become a principal advocate of designing a new, more adequate health care system (Institute of Medicine 2001) that emphasizes care in the community. An executive summary and the full text of Institute of Medicine conclusions and their proposal for corrective action are available for free online (Institute of Medicine 2001). In 2004, the first annual Crossing the Quality Chasm Summit specified the role of communities in developing care that focuses on prevention and coalition building in the development of community-based care services (Institute of Medicine 2004). Key recommendations emphasize the importance of involving patients in decisions about their care, understanding that health is a broader concept than medicine, and that the integration of the skills of multiple caregivers is necessary in providing adequate care in the long term. In brief, in the achievement and maintenance of health, communities are involved.

An initiative of the Robert Wood Johnson Foundation, chronic-care management also provides a related evaluated illustration of how a new way of thinking about caring for patients with chronic conditions can be implemented in health care organizations of various sizes (Wagner et al. 2001). An overview of the idea of chronic-care management and its current implementation is available online at http://www.improvingchroniccare.org. Chronic-care management applies the principles of chronic-care management identified as essential by the Institute of Medicine, such as the importance of continuous relationships among members of a care team, the primacy of anticipating as well as recognizing patient needs, and accessible information available to patients about care options. The intention is not to make decisions for an uninformed patient but to provide decision support for an informed patient.

The principles of chronic-care management are not new. Emphasis on the benefits of their implementation in managing chronic conditions in the community is new.

Consumer-Directed Care

Self-care is a typical "first response" when symptoms of acute illness appear. Self-care when chronic conditions occur is more likely to involve consideration of health-promoting activities such as diet, exercise, rest, and stress control (DeFriese 2001). In either case, emphasis is on self-management. When activities of daily living (ADLs) are compromised, assistance by others is likely to be required. Recent interest in consumer-directed care, particularly since the enactment of the Americans With Disabilities Act of 1990, focuses rather on whether and how the management of community medical alliance/ Medicaid resources, including personal assistance services, might be appropriately maintained by the consumer. Consumer-directed care as a strategy to empower individuals to remain involved in the design and implementation of their care has increased the prospects of many older adults to age in the community. Two major reviews of consumer-directed home and community service programs that have reviewed such programs in the United States and abroad have endorsed their usefulness (Cuellar et al. 2000; National Council on Disability 2004).

Disabled Americans of all ages frequently require the assistance of some other person to function adequately in their daily lives. Additionally, about 80% of persons needing personal supportive care, a majority of whom are elderly, reside in the community, mostly at home and frequently living alone. One survey (Benjamin 2001) reports that about one-third of more than 12 million Americans of all ages need some kind of personal service. For the past two decades most personal care services have been provided and supervised by designated agencies and social services organizations. The past decade has produced, however, new programs in more than half the states that offer to chronically disabled persons services they can employ and direct.

Programs of consumer-directed care vary widely across countries and across states in the United States. An overview article that displays with clarity the observed variety and issues is offered online by the Urban Institute (Tilly et al. 2000). Prominent issues when older consumers are involved include the competence of the consumer to make decisions and manage finances, the consumer's or other person's control of cash and cash payments, the availability of consumer training for care direction, the availability of family members to be employed, or of appropriate care providers to be hired, and the provision of quality assurance. Consumer-directed care has been slower to develop among older adults because of concerns about whether older persons are capable of directing their services and about how the quality of care can be ensured without agency oversight and accountability. Although definitive answers are not yet available for such questions, consumer-directed personal assistance services continue to flourish internationally and have achieved the endorsement of the National Council on Disability in the United States.

Consumer-directed care, as with chronic-care management, is consistent with current interest in the empowerment of health care consumers and with the enhancement of both self-efficacy and collective efficacy in communities (Meiners et al. 2002). The relatively passive and grateful patients of an earlier day are now encouraged to be involved and informed consumers, and sometimes directors, of their health care.

In addition to the potential benefit of expanding the workforce, public officials might be expected to be interested in quality consumer-directed care if it is cost-effective, which early evidence indicates it probably is. Early evidence also indicates that the risk of poor care is not higher for consumers who direct the use of their resources and how their needs are met than for those using established service organizations. Evaluation research accompanying the Robert Wood Johnson Foundation's cash and counseling initiative promises to provide policy makers with more definite answers for such key questions (see also Mahoney et al. 2001 and Polivka 2000).

Consumer-directed personal services care does appear to enhance the competence of chronically disabled individuals to care for themselves, increase these individuals' sense of self-efficacy in achieving a satisfactory quality of life, and encourage communities to develop a sense of collective efficacy in providing reliably available support for chronically disabled persons.

Assisted-Living Housing

A home locates families socially in a community and is the locale for reliably available social support when it is needed. For a minority, there is neither home nor family. Particularly in the case of elderly chronically disabled persons, even if housing is available, they live alone or in settings they cannot negotiate safely. In earlier decades, frail chronically disabled adults were housed in homes for the poor and elderly. In more recent decades such vulnerable individuals became patients in nursing homes or residents in adult care homes or similar nonmedical residential care settings. None of the typically available housing arrangements for frail and chronically disabled elderly was designed to maintain or enhance a sense of self-efficacy in patients/residents; nor have usually available housing arrangements promised reliably available compensatory care for frail, disabled residents.

Fortunately, recent studies of housing and living arrangements in the United States indicate that, overall, older persons are among the best-housed adults in a well-housed nation. Only a minority of older adults, though a significant minority, live alone. Periodic reviews of housing in the United States have documented the quality of housing available but only recently have questioned the appropriateness of that housing and various housing alternatives for frail, disabled adults. The medicalized environment of nursing homes provides reliably available nursing care for their patients, but for a minority, too much care is provided, increasing the risk of creating dependency. Nonmedical residential care homes for older adults have not typically provided reliably available care designed to meet the measured needs of residents. (For an overview of current Census of Housing information about housing and living arrangements in the United States, behavioral and social scientific theory and research about the significance of housing over the life course, and new housing options for frail disabled adults, see Maddox 2001.) An introduction to assisted-living housing from an industry perspective is online at http://www.alfa.org.

In response to the clear mismatch between housing needs and availability of supportive services for chronically disabled older adults, a distinctive new type of housing has appeared: assisted-living housing. The four basic concepts of the distinctive philosophy of assisted-living housing in its ideal form are 1) offering a private, self-contained space of one's own, 2) matching reliably available services with measured individual need, 3) sharing responsibility for care among residents, family, and staff, and 4) enhancing in residents the availability of information for informed choice and control of their lives. These concepts clearly resonate with the philosophy of the community care innovations discussed previously (enhancement of self-efficacy and collective-efficacy in responsive communities such as hospice, chronic-care management, and consumer-directed services).

Currently there are over 28,000 assisted-living housing facilities in the United States serving over 600,000 residents. The number of these facilities and their residents continues to increase rapidly. Assisted-living housing clearly has appealed to economically secure older adults who value its philosophy. Affordability, however, is clearly a problem. The average annual income of current assisted-living housing residents is $31,000. Despite a few innovative state efforts and the Robert Wood Johnson Foundation's *Coming Home* initiative, there is not in prospect a national commitment to subsidize such housing routinely for frail disabled adults. More information on affordable assisted-living housing is available online at http://www.elderweb.com/home/node/2112.

Nevertheless, assisted-living housing has attracted attention because its philosophy is so consistent with current values that emphasize self-efficacy, autonomy, and the reliable availability of needed compensatory services in the community. Of particular interest in current theories of adult development is Paul and Margret Baltes' (1990) theory of selective optimization with compensation. In brief, they argue that as energy and personal resources wane in late adulthood, autonomous individuals select how they will concentrate their resources and search for environments in which compensatory services are reliably available when needed. These are precisely the conditions that the philosophy of assisted-living housing offers (see Maddox 2001 for a review of the history of assisted-living housing and of relevant research assessing its philosophy and its outcomes in practice). The initial evidence suggests that assisted-living housing delivers the promised outcomes when its philosophy, emphasizing autonomy, self-direction, social involvement, and reliable availability of care when needed, is implemented.

Community Mental Health Care: From Deinstitutionalization to Empowerment

Mental health care has remained at the margins of the dominant medical care system in the United States. In the twentieth century, when chronic mood disorders ranked as the second most common disability among adults, mental health problems tended to be considered the problems of individuals and families until the problems became severe. The response then tended to be hospitalization.

Movement toward reform of mental health services was evident in the 1950s and 1960s, beginning with federal policy to deinstitutionalize persons in mental hospitals. (For the history of reforming mental health care in the United States that promoted community care, see Morrissey et al. 1980.) In the 1950s, for example, the risk of placement in a mental institution fell from 339/100,000 to 29/100,000 adults. Although research indicates that, overall, mental health outreach services were associated with improved or maintained psychiatric status (Van Citters 2004), an unfortunate outcome of returning behaviorally challenged individuals to the community turned out to be, for many, placement in nursing homes or adult care homes, and, for some, homelessness (see Kahana 2001). Mental health services in the community were enhanced in the mid-1970s by federal mandates to create community health centers and a Supreme Court mandate in the *Olmstead* decision to provide services in the least restrictive environment. Additionally, mental health services were broadened to include special populations such as the mental retardation, developmental disability, or substance abuse problems. Mental health services for older adults, however, were rarely featured in community programs, and information regarding the availability and effectiveness of community-based mental health services for older adults is quite limited.

In health services research on mental health in the United States, the issue of cost tends to be raised early and often. Discussion of mental health care in one of the most prestigious journals has focused on economic issues such as 1) concern of employers underwriting health care for employees that demand for mental health services might be limitless, 2) concern of consumers and consumer advocates that insurance for mental health care might be arbitrarily limited, and 3) concern of ethicists that mental health services, already marginalized and undercapitalized in the dominant medicalized care system, may, in the interest of cost control, be even more inequitably treated. One symptom of the current interest in cost control of mental health services is the practice of "carving out" of such services from managed care insurance. This practice refers to contracting with "behavioral health" companies specifically to manage mental health services. This practice has demonstrably reduced cost by limiting the number of services provided and by limiting days in the hospital (see Health Affairs 1999).

Current literature summarizing the consequences of moving mental health services from institutions toward the community and relating this movement to theory and research, although relatively spare, identifies some positive developments. The Robert Wood Johnson Foundation, for example, funded and evaluated in the 1990s a demonstration in nine communities in the United States of the effects of having a central mental health authority coordinate community-based services (Goldman et al. 1994). The focus on community coordination was an explicit response of the new federalism that increased opportunities as well as responsibilities of communities to integrate a broad range of uncoordinated federally funded services. The evaluation of this intervention documented that although "there was no one best way to coordinate mental health services in the nine communities studied," because each responded appropriately to the specific contextual issues of their communities and no community produced a sustainable, comprehensive system of mental health care, several important outcomes were documented. A key factor in improving mental health care in the community was ensuring the availability of adequate housing, and although the program produced minimal client-level effects, family burdens in caring for the mentally ill were reduced and coordination of services was improved. The most important outcome of this program was said to be the building of social capital in the community that reinforced the belief that communities can enhance community-based mental health services that produce positive results.

A monograph providing an adequately comprehensive review of research and theory underlying the movement of mental health toward the community in Canada is also available. *Shifting the Paradigm in Community Mental Health: Towards Empowerment and the Community* (Nelson et al. 2001) provides a particularly readable account of how mental health services in a middle-sized Canadian city were transformed to implement three primary values:

1. Enhanced personal empowerment of individual consumers of mental health care
2. Effective integration of mental health organizations and programs through collaboration and partnering
3. More equitable distribution of community resources and services to mental health

Beyond a clear statement of the history of movement of mental health services toward the community, theories of personal empowerment, of organizational collaboration, and of equitable distribution of social capital are discussed and related to the research involving interventions to enhance such values in Waterloo, Ontario. Qualitative research was used to demonstrate how mental health services were effectively shifted toward the community. Secondary benefits of this achievement were a sense of personal empowerment and a more equitable distribution of community resources, achieved through effective organizational partnering.

The continuing need for similar community-based mental health initiatives for the elderly in the United States is noted in the Surgeon General's Report on Mental Health (1999) and the Administration on Aging's report *Older Adults and Mental Health: Issues and Opportunities* (2001). These and other mental health and aging services information are available through the Elders and Families link on the Administration on Aging's Web site (http://www.aoa.gov/eldfam/healthy_lifestyles/mental_health/mental_health.asp). The American Society on Aging's Mental Health and Aging Network and the National Coalition on Mental Health and Aging have promoted state and community coalitions to improve the integration into the care system of mental health care for the aging (see http://www.empowermentzone.com/coalesce.txt). A new advocacy network also seeks to increase the voice of older mental health consumers and advocates in public policies regarding home and community-based mental health services (see Our Own Voice online at http://www.bazelon.org/issues/elders/index.htm).

Collaborative Partnerships of Community Care for Older Adults

The preceding five illustrations of movement toward the community in the design and delivery of services for older adults have focused on *discrete* initiatives to enhance community-based long-term care for older adults—hospice, health care needs of the chronically ill, self-directed care, assisted-living housing, and mental health care. Policy and funding addressing specific needs for various specific services at the community level have given less attention to coordinating and facilitating access to essential services. The sixth and last illustration of innovations in improving community-based care for older adults is distinctive in focusing on improving the coordination of and communication about access to health and social services that facilitate aging in the community.

Arizona responded early to the opportunity for innovation provided by devolution with an integrated suite of community-based programs for older adults (see http://www.ahcccs.state.az.us/Services/Programs/ALTCS.asp). California, Minnesota, Texas, Wisconsin, and Vermont provide additional illustrations of moving long-term care options toward the community. A useful summary of information about long-term care policy, practice, and funding in various states in the era of devolution is available from the Aging and Disability Resource Center (http://www.adrc-tae.org/tiki-index.php?page=p_FedPolicy; select CMS TA Tool for Assessing Long Term Care Systems"). In anticipation of an increased need for long-term care for baby boomers, civic leaders have been encouraged by foundations as well as federal and state agencies to create more elder-friendly communities (see http://www.aarp.org/community/search.bt?query=livable+communities&x=128&y=13 and http://www.smartgrowth.org/library/articles.asp?art=2100). The Robert Wood Johnson Foundation has continued to fund programs that explore ways to improve accessible, affordable community-based services (e.g., through personal long-term care insurance and exploration of how collaborative community partnerships might improve the coordination of care in the community). The Robert Wood Johnson Foundation also joined other foundations in underwriting an assessment of whether and how collaborative community health partnerships improve community accountability of providers, focus community interest on health, provide access to a continuum of services, and promote economic efficiency in provision of services. The design, implementation, and outcomes of this ambitious project have been well documented in published accounts by Hasnaim-Wynia (2003) and Shortell and colleagues (Mitchell and Shortell 2000; Shortell et al. 2002). This work has led to the identification and conceptualization of key issues in forecasting the sustainability and effectiveness of partnerships that stress the importance of partnership governance in aligning the composition of partnerships and their programs with priority community needs, resources, and values. Further, this work posits that effective governance must ensure that community *centrality* is achieved (i.e., fulfillment of program promises are appropriately monitored, achieved, and publicly recognized). Evidence of the achievement of centrality forecasts sustainability of community partnerships.

Between 1994 and 1999, the Kate B. Reynolds Charitable Trust in North Carolina funded a program that identified team building as another important dimension of developing effective partnerships that coordinate community services for older adults. The Aging at Home Program at the Duke University Center for Aging (Bell and Leak 1999) created successful community partnerships in caring in 39 counties across the state using Senge's (1990) theory of learning organizations. Learning organizations stress leadership development and a philosophy of teaching and learning in which every teacher is a learner and every learner a teacher. Although timely technical assistance is useful in the development of collaborative partnering, a primary source of empowerment of participants is the discovery that they share a sense of the importance of what they are doing and share a sense of leadership in which each teacher is a learner, each learner a teacher.

The Community Partnerships for Older Adults (CPFOA) program was created to promote local efforts to improve long-term care and supportive services systems to meet the needs of current and future older adults. Sixteen communities were selected through a national competitive process to

- Mobilize and strengthen community resources to meet the growing needs for long-term care and supportive services.
- Increase communication and coordination among providers and between providers and consumers.
- Promote a better quality of life for vulnerable older adults and their caregivers.

(The CPFOA program objectives, selection process, and communities selected are described in Bolda et al. (2005, 2006; see also http://www.CPFOA.org.) Central tenets of the program were

- Inclusion of older adults and hard-to-reach community groups and the broader community in identifying priorities for improvement and community solutions.
- Understanding that in creating collaborative partnerships, no one size fits all because of their unique constellation of populations, preferences and assets.
- Technical assistance for partnerships would come substantially from the implementation of a philosophy of teaching and learning among participants. Technical assistance to implement this philosophy during the development phase of the program was provided by the Duke Long-Term Care Resources Program, building on experience with creating teaching and learning communities in North Carolina.

Although the CPFOA collaborative partnerships are mid-course, early evidence of program performance suggests significant accomplishments. The first of two funding cohorts is now completing its work under Robert Wood Johnson Foundation funding, and the second cohort is in the midst of its 4-year implementation grant. It is this first cohort of eight communities that provides the basis for observations about the effectiveness of collaborative community partnerships in achieving sustainable improvement in community capacity to make available needed long-term care options for older adults.

Evidence of progress toward achieving centrality among the first cohort of eight CPFOA partnerships has been noted in the assessment of the achievement of objectives proposed in logic models and in the evolving strategic plans of partnerships, as well as in partnerships' achievement of specific pilot initiatives and interventions, the receipt of financial support from community private sectors, and indications that the advice of partnerships has been sought locally, regionally, and nationally. Foundations have requested information about the priority of needs for use in setting their own priorities for allocating resources. Of particular significance are plans for continuing the functions of the partnerships after termination of support from the Robert Wood Johnson Foundation.

The achievements of CPFOA partnerships have been noted far beyond their own communities. Three of the communities have received national recognition as "livable communities" by the U.S. Administration on Aging. Also at the national level, CPFOA partnerships were featured during the opening session of the 2006 National Leadership Summit "Working Together to Build a Better Future of Long-Term Care." Congressional committees have requested testimony about what partnerships have learned about innovative ways to improve coordination of community resources and systems that assist older adults to age in place.

Over the next several years, evidence will provide additional insight into how community partnerships can play an important role in the development and coordination of community-based long-term care resources for older adults. In the meantime, the experience of CPFOA in developing community partnerships suggests several useful lessons about the role of communities in long-term care development and the creation of effective, sustainable partnerships.

Partnership Design

In designing community partnerships, no one model will fit all communities. Diversity in the composition of effective partnerships is virtually assured by the process of aligning their design and programs with the perceived needs, values, and resources of communities they intend to serve through improving coordination of existing resources or, as needed, developing new resources and options to meet the needs of older adults in the long term.

Communication and Facilitation

Although any community may lack one or another service of importance for older adults, the common problem for even service-rich communities is lack of information about and convenient access to existing services. The experience of CPFOA partnerships documents that providing information about and access to services is universal and tends to take precedence over creation of new services.

Understanding Why Community Partnerships Succeed

Organizational theory stresses the importance of governance of partnerships in aligning partnerships with community interests and values to increase the prospects of effectiveness and sustainability of partnership objectives. Successful CPFOA partnerships have developed neutral forums where decision-making procedures developed by community leaders can address community priorities that are beyond the scope of individual partners and community organizations. As a result, they are responding to community needs and developing new relationships through strategies of empowerment and leadership characteristic of learning organizations

Successful Partnering

The eventual success of an individual CPFOA partnership cannot be adequately assessed and understood at this point. Survival of a CPFOA partnership as a separate organization with its own financing will, however, be only one outcome that might be considered successful. Experience suggests at least two other types of successful outcomes: 1) the embedding of a partnership's collaborative approach to addressing the broader interests of the community within an existing organization or coalition of organizations, with the partnership playing a distinctive role as a research and planning unit, or

2) the intentional discontinuation of the original partnership after successful demonstration of the benefits of the original partnering and devolving the partnership functions to those neighborhoods and newly organized groups in which new social capital and resources for long-term care have been created.

Conclusion

The preceding six illustrations of movement toward the community in developing resources and services to improve access to community-based care in the long term for older adults illustrate that older adults are increasingly recognized as a national resource as well as a challenge. Options for where and how older adults will find needed supportive services will continue to evolve. Movement toward the community in meeting the long-term needs of today's older adults will continue to benefit the collaborative, cross-disciplinary communication of professionals, older adults, and community leadership.

Key Points

- Aging at home in the community remains the preference for most older adults.
- Redesign of community services for older adults to increase access and to coordinate options for receiving health services outside traditional medical and hospital settings has enhanced options for aging at home.
- Improving information about and coordination of access to long-term care services remains a priority for most communities.
- Collaborative partnerships are a strategy of choice in facilitating the coordination of and access to community-based long-term care services.
- Effective community partnership in caring takes many forms. With leadership, different ways of aligning long-term care services with the needs, preferences, and resources of communities can be equally effective.

References

Baltes P, Baltes M: Psychological perspectives on successful aging: the model of selective optimization with compensation, in Successful Aging. Edited by Baltes P, Baltes M. New York, Cambridge University Press, 1990, pp 1–34

Bandura A: Self-Efficacy: The Exercise of Control. New York, WH Freeman, 1997

Bell JP, Leak SC: The aging at home project: a successful partnership in caring. Duke LTC Policy Paper Series, No 8. July 1999. Available at www.ltc.duke.edu/occasional_8.htm. Accessed March 3, 2008.

Benjamin AE: Consumer-directed services at home. Health Aff (Millwood) 20:80–95, 2001

Bolda E, Lowe JI, Maddox GL, et al: Community Partnerships for Older Adults: a case study. Fam Soc 86:411–418, 2005

Bolda E, Saucier P, Maddox GL, et al: Governance and management structures for community partnerships: experiences from the Robert Wood Johnson Foundation's Community Partnerships for Older Adults Program. Gerontologist 46:398–403, 2006

Caro F, Morris R: Devolution and Aging Policy. New York, Haywood Press, 2002

Cuellar E, Tilly J, Wiener J: Consumer directed home and community service programs in five countries: policy issues for people and government. October 1, 2000. Available at http://www.urban.org/publication1410330.html. Accessed March 2, 2008.

Cutler DM: Declining disability among the elderly. Health Aff (Millwood) 20:1–27, 2001

DeFriese G: Self-care activities, in Encyclopedia of Aging, 3rd Edition. Edited by Maddox G. New York, Springer, 2001, pp 900–902

Field M, Cassel C: Approaching Death: Improving Care at the End of Life. Washington, DC, National Academy Press, 1997

Fox-Grage W, Folkemer D, Lewis J: The States' Response to the Olmstead Decision: How Are States Complying? 2008. Available at http://www.ncsl.org/programs/health/forum/olmsreport.htm. Accessed March 4, 2008.

Fries J: Aging, natural death, and the compression of morbidity. N Engl J Med 303:130–135, 1980

Fries J: Compression of morbidity, in Encyclopedia of Aging, 3rd Edition. Edited by Maddox G. New York, Springer, 2001, pp 234–236

Glaser B: Doing Grounded Theory: Issues and Discussions. Mill Valley, CA, Sociology Press, 1998

Goldman HH, Morrissey JP, Ridgely MS: Evaluating the Robert Wood Johnson Foundation program on chronic mental illness. Milbank Q 72:37–47, 1994

Goldsmith S, Eggers W: Governing by Network: The New Shape of the Public Sector. Washington, DC, Harvard University and the Brookings Institution, 2002

Hacker J: "The Great Risk Shift": Issues for Aging and Public Policy. Public Policy and Aging Report 17:2, 2007

Hasnain-Wynia R: Overview of the community care network demonstration program and its evaluation. Med Care Res Review 60:5S–16S, 2003

Health Affairs: New Mental Health Care Market 18(5):1–255, 1999

Health Affairs: Chronic Care in America 20(6):1–286, 2001

Institute of Medicine: Crossing the Quality Chasm. Washington, DC, National Academies Press. 2001. Available at http://books.nap.edu/openbook.php?record_id=10027&page=R1. Accessed March 4, 2008.

Institute of Medicine: First Annual Quality Chasm Summit: Focus on Communities. Washington, DC, National Academies Press. 2004. Available at http://books.nap.edu/openbook.php?record_id=11085&page=R1. Accessed March 4, 2008.

Kahana E: "De-institutionalization," in Encyclopedia of Aging, 3rd Edition. Edited by Maddox G. New York, Springer, 2001, pp 273–276

Kiwachi I, Berkman L: Social cohesion, social capital, and health, in Social Epidemiology. Edited by Berkman L, Kawachi I. New York, Oxford University Press, 2000, pp 174–190

Lindblom C: The science of "muddling through." Public Adm Rev 19:79–88, 1959

Maddox G: Muddling through: planning health services in England. Med Care 9:439–448, 1971

Maddox G: Long-term care in comparative perspective. Ageing Soc 12:335–368, 1992

Maddox G: General practice fundholding in the British National Health Service: accounts of the dynamics of change. J Health Polit Policy Law 24:815–834, 1999

Maddox G: Housing and living arrangements, in Handbook of Aging and the Social Sciences, 5th Edition. Edited by Binstock R, George L. San Diego, CA, Academic Press, 2001, pp 426–443

Mahoney K, Simon-Rasinowitz L, Mares L: Cash payments for care, in Encyclopedia of Aging, 3rd Edition. Edited by Maddox G. New York, Springer, 2001, pp 167–70

Marmor T: The Politics of Medicare. New York, Aldine de Gruyter, 2000

Meier D, Morrison R (eds): Care at the End of Life: Restoring a Balance. Generations 23, 1999

Meiners M, Mahoney K, Shoop D, et al: Consumer direction in managed long-term care: an exploratory survey of practices and perceptions. Gerontologist 42:32–38, 2002

Mitchell S, Shortell S: The governance and management of effective community health partnerships: a typology of research, policy and practice. Milbank Q 78:241–289, 2000

Mor V, Allen S: Hospice, in Encyclopedia of Aging, 3rd Edition. Edited by Maddox G. New York, Springer, 2001, pp 507–509

Morrissey JP, Goldman HH, Klerman LV: The Enduring Asylum. New York, Grune & Stratton, 1980

National Center for Health Statistics: Health, United States 2006, With Chartbook on Trends in the Health of Americans (DHHS Publ No 2006-1232). Hyattsville, MD, U.S. Department of Health and Human Services, 2006

National Council on Disability: Consumer-directed health care: how well does it work? October 26, 2004. Available at http://www.ncd.gov/newsroom/publications/2004/consumerdirected.htm. Accessed March 5, 2008.

National Governors Association: A Lifetime of Health and Dignity: Confronting Long-Term Care Challenges in America. February 1, 2003. Available at http://www.nga.org/portal/site/nga/menuitem.5cd31a89efe1f1e122d81fa6501010a0/?vgnextoid=295c4c33c7732010VgnVCM1000001a01010aRCRD&vgnextchanel=4b18f074f0d9ff00VgnVCM1000001a 01010aRCRD. Accessed March 4, 2008.

Nelson G, Lord J, Ochoocka J: Shifting the Paradigm in Community Mental Health: Towards Empowerment and the Community. Toronto, Canada, University of Toronto Press, 2001

Olmstead v L.C (98-536) 527 US 581 138 F3d 893 (1999), affirmed in part, vacated in part, and remanded.

Polivka L: The ethical and empirical basis for consumer-directed care for frail elderly. Contemp Gerontol 7:50–52, 2000

Pressman J, Wildavsky A: Implementation. San Francisco, University of California Press, 1984

Schulz R, Maddox G, Lawton P (eds): Interventions Research With Older Adults. Annu Rev Gerontol Geriatr 18, 1998

Senge P: The Fifth Discipline: The Art and Practice of Learning Organization. New York, Doubleday/Currency, 1990

Shortell SM, Zukoski AP, Alexander JA, et al: Evaluating partnerships for community health improvement: tracking the footprints. J Health Polit Policy Law 27:49–91, 2002

Smith D: Reinventing Care: Assisted Living in New York City. Nashville, TN, Vanderbilt University Press, 2003

Tilly J, Wiener J, Cueller A: Consumer-directed home and community care in five countries: policy issues for older adults and government. October 2000. Available at http://www.urban.org/publications/410330.html. Accessed March 3, 2008.

Vachon A: Americans With Disabilities Act, in Encyclopedia of Aging, 3rd Edition. Edited by Maddox G. New York, Springer, 2001, pp 91–83

Van Citters AD, Bartus S: A systematic review of the effectiveness of community-based outreach mental health services for older adults. Psychiatr Serv 55:1237–1249, 2004

von Bertalanffy B: General Systems Theory. New York, George Braziller, 1968

Wagner EH, Austin BT, Davis C, et al: Improving chronic illness care: translating evidence into action. Health Aff (Millwood) 20:64–78, 2001

Suggested Readings

Adams A, Grenier AC, Corrigan JM (eds): First Annual Crossing the Quality Chasm Summit: Focus on Communities. Washington, DC, National Academies Press, 2004

Cassel C: Medicare Matters: What Geriatric Medicine Can Teach American Health Care. Berkeley, University of California Press, 2005

Nelson G, Ochoocka J: Shifting the Paradigm in Community Mental Health: Toward Empowerment and the Community. Toronto, ON, Canada, University of Toronto Press, 2006

Rodwin V, Gusmano G (eds): Growing Older in World Cities: New York, London, Paris and Tokyo. Nashville, TN, Vanderbilt University Press, 2006

Schulz J, Binstock R: Aging Nation: The Economics and Politics of Growing Old in America. Westport, CT, Praeger, 2006

Smith D: Reinventing Care: Assisted Living in New York City. Nashville, TN, Vanderbilt University Press, 2003

Web Resources

Federal and State Resources Providing Information About Care for Older People

An overview of federal initiatives supporting home- and community-based services is provided by the Administration on Aging, which implements the Older Americans Act (http://www.aoa.gov). The Association of Area Agencies on Aging (http://www.n4a.org) provides information about state and local services for older adults. For example, an elder care locator provides information about long-term care services.

Hospice

Comprehensive information is available online from http://www.hospicefoundation.org.

Chronic Pain Management

To view proposed changes in the U.S. health care system recommended by the Institute of Medicine, visit the National Academies Press Web site:

Crossing the Quality Chasm: http://books.nap.edu/openbook.php?record_id=10027&page=R1

First Annual Quality Chasm Summit: Focus on Communities: http://books.nap.edu/openbook.php?record_id=11085&page=R1

Consumer-Directed Care

The National Council on Disability delivered a report to the U.S. Congress that provides the history of consumer-directed care and an evaluation of its effects and effectiveness (see http://www.ncd.gov/newsroom/publications/2004/consumerdirected.htm). For an overview of consumer-directed home and community services for older adults in five countries, see the Urban Institute Web site (http://www.urban.org/publications/410330.html).

Assisted-Living Housing

An introduction and overview of assisted-living housing for older adults from a trade association perspective is available from the Assisted-Living Housing Association of America at http://www.alfa.org.

Mental Health Care

Documents on mental health and aging services and on collaborative partnerships to develop state- and community-coordinated programs are described by the Administration on Aging (http://www.aoa.gov/press/publications/Older-Adults-and-Mental-Health-2001.pdf). For a description of a mental health advocacy network, Our Own Voice, see http://www.bazelon.org/issues/elders/index.htm.

Livable Communities

A national initiative to characterize and build livable communities for older adults is summarized on the National Area Agency on Aging Web site (http://www.n4a.org); search for *Livable Communities.*

PART V

Special Topics

CHAPTER 33

Legal, Ethical, and Policy Issues

William E. Reichman, M.D.
Joel E. Streim, M.D.
Jason H.T. Karlawish, M.D.
J. Pierre Loebel, M.D.

With the explosive growth anticipated in the ranks of the elderly over the coming decades, clinicians, educators, researchers, patient advocates, and policy makers have become increasingly focused on society's ability to meet the anticipated health care needs of older adults. This focus has involved ongoing reexamination of the financing structure and workforce dedicated to supporting the health care of the nation's elderly population. In addition, increasingly open dialogues have occurred regarding other important and related social themes, including the ethical issues that must be confronted and managed in caring for patients at the end of life (Institute for Health and Aging 1996). Reform and redesign of health care services directed to the care of an aging and increasingly infirm population is a dynamic and highly politicized process. The same holds true for the social and ethical dimensions of geriatric health care. In the midst of this evolving and complex process, one conclusion has been widely embraced by all especially interested stakeholders: the current U.S. mental health care system serves older patients with mental disorders poorly and is largely unprepared to meet what has been described as an upcoming crisis (Jeste et al. 1999).

In 2000, the U.S. Surgeon General's Report on Mental Health highlighted in depth the challenges confronting all of those committed to ensuring the optimal provision of health care to elderly persons suffering from psychiatric illness (U.S. Department of Health and Human Services 1999a). That seminal report concluded that "there are barriers to access in the organization and financing of health care services for aging citizens. There are specific problems with Medicare, Medicaid, nursing homes, and managed care." Since the issuance of that report, the United States and many other developed nations have continued to lack the ability to make substantial gains in senior mental health policy and service implementation. In this chapter, we review the dominant themes that have emerged in the present debate on how best to meet the growing mental health care needs of an aging population. These themes touch on legal, ethical, and policy concerns. We focus particular attention on the financing of mental health care for older patients, the clear imperative to train a larger workforce to meet the needs of this population, and the cardinal ethical issues that must be confronted when caring for older patients toward the end of life.

Geriatric Mental Health Policy

Financing of Mental Health Care for Older Adults

Policies on paying for mental health care for older adults in the United States have been shaped by the federal government since the inception of Medicare and Medicaid in the mid-1960s. These policies, which have been mirrored by private health insurance carriers, have consistently restricted coverage for mental health services more stringently than coverage for general medical care (Frank 2000).

After several years of failed attempts to undo enduring inequities in mental health and substance dependence insurance coverage, the Congress finally successfully addressed the issue. On October 3, 2008, the United States House of Representatives voted to approve, by a vote of 263 to 171, the Emergency Economic Stabilization Act (H.R. 1424). This initiative included mental health and substance use disorder parity legislation, the Paul Wellstone and Pete Domenici Mental Health Parity and Addiction Equity Act of 2008 <http://www.govtrack.us/congress/bill.xpd?bill=h110-6983> (introduced as H.R. 6983). The same package cleared the Senate on October 1 by a vote of 74 to 25. Subsequently signed into law by the President, this legislation requires health insurance companies that provide mental health and substance use benefits to ensure the same level of coverage as they would for any other medical condition.

Medicare

Between 1966 and 1988, Medicare Part B covered outpatient psychiatric services up to a maximum of $500, subject to a 50% copayment; thus, Medicare paid only $250 per year. The Omnibus Budget Reconciliation Act of 1987 (OBRA-87) raised the $500 cap for psychotherapy reimbursement to $2,200 per year but retained the 50% copayment, thereby limiting actual Medicare payments for psychotherapy to $1,100 per year. However, medical management of psychotropic medications was exempted from this limit, and the copayment for these services was reduced to 20% under OBRA-87. Although the Omnibus Budget Reconciliation Act of 1989 eliminated the cap on outpatient mental health services, the 50% copayment was retained for psychotherapy services, and that disparity with coverage for general medical care (which requires only a 20% copayment) remained as a matter of dispute in Congress until very recently. Consumer and professional groups had lobbied to change this discriminatory policy. Over several years bills, were introduced in Congress that would have provided mental health care coverage on a par with coverage for other medical and surgical care. None of these bills had enough support to pass.

On July 15, 2008, the House and Senate overrode the President's veto of H.R. 6331, the Medicare Improvements for Patients and Providers Act of 2008. The bill reversed the 10.6% reduction in Medicare reimbursements for physicians that were slated to take effect on July 1, 2008. Critically, it also provided Medicare mental health equity by phasing in, over 6 years, a reduction in the 50% mental health copayment requirement to the 20% required for all other outpatient services. Specifically, the bill provided for cost sharing for outpatient mental health services to be phased down from 50% to 20% by 2014. Cost sharing will be 45% in 2010 and 2011, 40% in 2012, 35% in 2013, and 20% in 2014 and thereafter. In addition, there is a provision allowing an adjustment for Medicare mental health services such that for the period of July 1, 2008, through December 31, 2009, Medicare psychotherapy codes will be increased by 5%. This will effectively reverse some of the payment reductions that occurred as a result of the budget-neutral implementation of the most recent 5-year review of relative values (American Association of Geriatric Psychiatry 2008).

In 1990, the Medicare Part B psychiatric benefit was expanded to allow licensed clinical psychologists and certified social workers to bill Medicare for mental health services. This led to a substantial increase in Medicare payments for mental health services, especially in nursing homes, during the early and mid-1990s, although it is not known whether the increased spending was associated with better access to care or provision of more appropriate mental health services.

Despite increasing incentives to use outpatient rather than inpatient services in the private sector, Medicare payment policies for mental health care continue to encourage the use of acute inpatient services (Bartels and Colenda 1998). Traditional fee-for-service Medicare Part A coverage for inpatient psychiatric hospital care sets a 190-day lifetime limit for care rendered in freestanding psychiatric hospitals but no time limit on care rendered on psychiatric units in general hospitals. In 2000, Medicare paid for inpatient care up to 90 days during a benefit period, paying all but a 1-day deductible of $768 for the first 60 days and all but $192 for days 61–90 (Health Care Financing Administration 2000).

In the context of these reimbursement policies, outpatient service utilization remains low. Despite the 14%–17% prevalence of clinically significant mental disorders among older adults residing in community settings, it is estimated that only 6%–8% of older adults actually receive outpatient mental health services. Overall, Medicare expenditures for mental health care

are similarly disproportionate to the need. In 1996, only 4.9% of total Medicare expenditures were directed to mental health and substance abuse disorders (Witkin et al. 1998). Most of these expenditures were for hospital-based services.

The Balanced Budget Act of 1997 established Medicare Part C (Medicare Plus Choice), a managed care program offered through private insurance companies. Before 1997, Medicare's managed care products included Medicare Risk Contracting (MRC) plans, point-of-service options, social health maintenance organizations (Kane et al. 1997), and programs of all-inclusive care for the elderly (Eng et al. 1997). The latter two were demonstration projects that combined Medicare and Medicaid funding to provide a continuum of health services that included inpatient, outpatient, and long-term care settings (Colenda et al. 1999). Medicare Plus Choice expanded managed care options to include medical savings accounts, point-of-service options that permit patients to select from a broader panel of practitioners outside the health maintenance organization network, religious fraternal benefit plans, and other coordinated care plans.

MRC plans typically "carve out" mental health care as a separate provider plan, which helps vendors manage costs and services. However, these programs may not contract with mental health providers who are geographically accessible for older adults, and communication between providers of general medical care and mental health care is more cumbersome, hampering the coordination of services. Some experts advocate a "carve-in" model for mental health services that better integrates behavioral and medical care, reduces stigma, improves access, increases coordination of care, and produces cost offsets in general health expenditures for elderly patients with medical-psychiatric comorbidity (Bartels et al. 1999; Mechanic 1997).

Participation in Medicare Plus Choice plans declined in the late 1990s. In 2000, 16.4% of all Medicare beneficiaries were enrolled in these plans. Many managed care companies have withdrawn since 1999 because of low payment rates and heavy regulatory burdens (Medicare Payment Advisory Commission 1999). Despite predictions that a large proportion of Medicare beneficiaries would elect managed Medicare options because of enticements such as prescription drug coverage, preventive care, and optical benefits (Hogan et al. 2000; Langwell et al. 1999), the future of managed Medicare is uncertain.

Medicare Part D (Centers for Medicare and Medicaid Services 2008), a federal program to provide support for the costs of prescription drugs for Medicare beneficiaries, was enacted as part of the Medicare Prescription Drug Improvement and Modernization Act of 2003 (MMA). It went into effect January 1, 2006, and is administered by private insurance sponsors or plans. These plans are reimbursed by the Centers for Medicare and Medicaid Services (CMS).

Beneficiaries can obtain the Medicare drug benefit through two types of private plans: they can either use a Prescription Drug Plan (PDP) for drug coverage only or join a Medicare Advantage (MA) plan, a component of Medicare Part C that covers both prescription drugs and medical services (MA-PD).

The MMA established a standard drug benefit that Part D plans may offer. The standard benefit is defined in terms of the benefit structure and not in terms of the drugs that must be covered. In 2008, this defined standard benefit required the beneficiary to make a deductible payment of $275. The beneficiary would then pay 25% of the cost of a covered Part D prescription drug up to an initial coverage limit of $2,510. The defined standard benefit is not the most common benefit offered by Part D plans. Only 10% of plans for 2008 offered the defined standard benefit. Most sponsors eliminated the deductible and introduced tiered drug copayments.

Once the initial coverage limit is reached, the beneficiary is subject to an added deductible, designated the Coverage Gap. This is commonly noted as the "doughnut hole," within which the insured pays the entire cost of medication. When total out-of-pocket expenses on formulary covered medications for the year, including the deductible and initial coinsurance, reach $4,050, the beneficiary then attains catastrophic coverage, in which he or she pays $2.25 for a generic or preferred drug and $5.65 for other drugs, or 5% coinsurance, whichever is the greater amount. Most low-income beneficiaries are exempt from the total amount or a portion of the expense gap and the deductible.

It should be noted that the thresholds above refer only to the standard defined benefit structure. Specific health sponsors typically offer enhanced benefit plans, consisting of their own variations on the standard benefit. Some of these plans completely remove the deductible or extend the limits of the initial coverage, thus reducing the size of the coverage gap. Typically, the beneficiary pays a higher annual premium for these enriched plans.

Beneficiary premiums for Part D plans vary considerably, but overall, they increased from 2006 to 2008. Importantly, Part D plans are not required to pay for all covered Part D drugs, being free to develop their own tiered formularies.

Medicaid

Medicaid is the joint federal-state program that pays for long-term care in nursing homes and for acute care services for poor patients. It is not possible to determine the proportion of Medicaid dollars spent on mental health care for patients ages 65 years and older (Witkin et al. 1998), and the effect of managed Medicaid enrollment on mental health service use by elders has not been evaluated (Colenda et al. 2002). However, approximately 75% of Medicaid expenditures for older adults are spent on long-term care services. Approximately 40% of nursing home costs are paid "out of pocket" by patients. Although some individuals have purchased long-term care insurance policies in addition to their medical insurance, only a small proportion of nursing home costs are covered by private insurance. Many older adults spend down their life savings to pay for nursing home care, and they then become eligible for Medicaid benefits, usually at a lower per diem rate. Overall, the Medicaid program covers about 68% of nursing home residents and more than 59% of nursing home costs (Streim et al. 2002).

Reimbursement of Nursing Homes

Although Medicare pays for psychiatric services rendered in the nursing home by consulting physicians, psychologists, and nurse practitioners, the nursing facility is responsible for ensuring the psychosocial well-being of residents and the provision of other mental health care by nursing home staff. Federal financial support for these nursing home–based mental health services decreased for many facilities after the Balanced Budget Act of 1997 repealed federal standards for reimbursing nursing homes, giving states the freedom to set payment rates. In 1999, payment policy was changed again, requiring that social work services be furnished as one of many services bundled together under payments made directly to nursing facilities, rather than on a fee-for-service basis under Medicare. Nursing homes must therefore rely on per diem reimbursement, with Medicaid rates that vary substantially across states, to cover these nursing home–based mental health care costs.

Department of Veterans Affairs

Another major provider of geriatric mental health care for older Americans is the Department of Veterans Affairs (VA) health care system. More than 9 million veterans are older than age 65, and 510,000 are age 85 or older. The VA supports an extensive system of care for older adults with mental disorders, including acute inpatient psychiatric hospitalization, outpatient mental health and substance abuse clinics, a network of more than 120 long-term care facilities, and domiciliary care. Between 1990 and 2000, the number of veterans ages 45–54 who received mental health services from the VA more than tripled. These were mostly Vietnam-era veterans, the baby boomers who are now beginning to, and will continue to, swell the ranks of those who require geriatric care. However, the most rapid growth in demand during the same period was among the oldest of older veterans. From 1990 to 2000, the number of veterans ages 75–84 who received VA mental health services increased fourfold. It is projected that from 2000 to 2015, the number of veterans over age 75 will continue to increase, with a tripling of those age 85 or older (U.S. Department of Veterans Affairs 2007). To promote mental health care for veterans, Congress has authorized funding for 10 Mental Illness Research, Education, and Clinical Centers to conduct research, disseminate findings, and translate new knowledge into practice, as well as several Geriatric Research, Education, and Clinical Centers and several Parkinson Disease Research, Education, and Clinical Centers that address, among other problems, cognitive disorders in older adults.

Federal Regulation of Mental Health Care in Nursing Homes

The substantial role of the federal government in paying for health care has given Congress and the Centers for Medicare and Medicaid Services (CMS; formerly the Health Care Financing Administration, or HCFA) the license to impose stringent regulations on the delivery of mental health care to elderly patients who reside in long-term care facilities. Regulatory focus on nursing homes was prompted in the 1980s by a combination of factors: 1) concerns about the inappropriate use of physical and chemical restraints, 2) concerns about inadequate treatment of depression (Institute of Medicine 1986), and 3) cautions from the federal Office of Management and Budget that older adults with chronic mental illness were being discharged from state mental hospitals and admitted to nursing homes, thereby shifting the cost of their care from the states to the federal government. Congress responded by passing the Nursing Home Reform Act as part of OBRA-87. Mental health aspects of federally mandated nursing home reform are detailed in Chapter 31 of this volume.

When it enacted OBRA-87, Congress directed HCFA to take steps to ensure that unmet mental health needs of nursing home residents were addressed. The resultant HCFA regulations require preadmission assessment to identify nursing home applicants with mental illness who require acute psychiatric care and to ensure that applicants are appropriately placed in residential or treatment settings (Health Care Financing Administration 1992). For individuals admitted to a nursing home, the regulations require the facility to conduct periodic assessments of mental health and to "ensure that a resident who displays mental or psychosocial adjustment difficulties receives appropriate services to correct the assessed problem" (Health Care Financing Administration 1991, p. 48,896 [tag F272]), including treatment not otherwise provided for by the state (U.S. Department of Health and Human Services 2001). Together, these regulations provide a clear federal mandate for detection and treatment of mental illness in nursing home residents.

Quality of care is addressed in regulations that are intended to limit the inappropriate use of psychotropic medications. Although after implementation of nursing home reforms the use of antipsychotic drugs and physical restraints declined (Health Care Financing Administration 1998; Rovner et al. 1992; Shorr et al. 1994) and the use of antidepressant drugs increased (Datto et al. 2002; Lantz et al. 1996; Lasser and Sunderland 1998), the effect of the federal regulations on symptom control, functional status, quality of life, and other important outcome measures has not been studied (Llorente et al. 1998; Streim et al. 2002).

According to Reichman et al. (1998), despite the federal mandate for assessment and treatment, 48% of nursing home administrators reported that the frequency of on-site psychiatric consultation was inadequate, leaving nursing home staff to provide mental health care without sufficient expert support. More than one-fourth of rural nursing homes and more than one-fifth of small nursing homes reported that no psychiatric consultant was available to them, despite high rates of psychiatric problems among residents. Studies in the 1990s found that many nursing home patients had undetected psychiatric symptoms (Snowden and Roy-Byrne 1998) and that 55% of residents had unmet mental health services needs (Borson et al. 1997). Thus, the HCFA requirement that patients receive needed mental health care did not remedy the lack of access to mental health services in U.S. nursing homes (Colenda et al. 1999). More recently, the 2004 National Nursing Home Survey found that only 40% of nursing homes had mental health services available at the facility (National Center for Health Statistics 2004).

Federal Quality Improvement Initiatives

Nursing homes have also been the setting for government efforts to use the regulatory and payment systems to encourage improvement in the quality of care for older adults. Assessment, survey, and payment data can be used to analyze the quality of care and, in turn, feedback can inform refinements in care (Nyman 1988). In 1999, HCFA introduced 24 quality indicators, derived from the standardized assessment data that all nursing homes are required to report, to enable facilities and surveyors to compare individual facility performance within the same state. Results are used to identify and address potential quality problems (Clark 1999) and to inform consumers about the quality of individual nursing home performance. Quality indicators that pertain to geriatric mental health encompass behavioral and emotional problems, cognitive patterns, and psychotropic drug use. Whenever a review in any of these areas results in a citation of a deficiency, a plan of correction must be developed and submitted to the state's department of health for approval. This system is a first step in monitoring quality of care, although the face validity of some of the quality indicators has been questioned, and the results of quality surveys may be difficult to interpret. Nevertheless, quality monitoring is a potent mechanism by which the assessment data required by the payment system can drive quality improvement efforts (Institute of Medicine 2001).

Systems of Care for Older Adults With Serious Mental Illness

At least 1% of individuals over age 55 have a serious mental illness, such as schizophrenia, schizoaffective disorder, and bipolar disorder, and this population of older adults is expected to double by the year 2030 (U.S. Department of Health and Human Services 1999a). In the 1970s and 1980s, with the widespread downsizing and closure of state mental hospitals and other facilities with long-term psychiatric inpatient units, many older patients were transferred to nursing home beds instead of being discharged to community-based care as were their younger counterparts. Despite the provisions of OBRA-87 that limit the use of nursing homes for people with severe mental illness who do not require skilled nursing facility care, inappropriate nursing home placement continues (Office of the Inspector General 2001). To counter this trend, there has been increasing attention over the past decade to providing home- and community-based alternatives to long-term institutional care for older adults (Kane 1998; Meeks et al. 1990). These efforts were bolstered by the 1999 *Olmstead v. L.C.* decision, which requires that states develop plans to end unnecessary institutionalization through creation of opportunities for community living (Williams 2000).

The challenge of caring for older adults with severe mental illness in community settings is substantial. Although patients with serious mental illness account for only 22% of older adults receiving services in community mental health centers, these patients account for 60% of mental health services costs. Among patients with schizophrenia, the greatest per capita expenditures for mental health care are for the youngest and the oldest patients (Cuffel et al. 1996). Nevertheless, Medicare recipients over age 65 with a diagnosis of schizophrenia are half as likely overall to receive ambulatory care services (Dixon et al. 2001), and this is likely to be associated with a lack of general medical care.

Of particular concern is the high prevalence of medical comorbidity in this population of elderly patients (Dixon et al. 1999; Goldman 1999; Sheline 1990; Vieweg et al. 1995; Zubenko et al. 1997). However, there is disagreement about the ideal model for providing integrated medical and psychiatric care for these patients. Policies that encourage the provision of psychiatric services that are "carved into" general medical care may be more likely to result in coordinated care, but such policies have been criticized for failing to meet the specialized care needs of older adults with serious mental illness (Bartels and Colenda 1998; Mechanic 1997). On the other hand, policies that promote "carved-out" mental health services may result in higher-quality specialized services but also run the risk of fragmenting medical and psychiatric services. Regardless of the arrangement, Medicare and Medicaid pay for most of the health care for older adults with serious mental illness, and the cost of their health care is projected to grow exponentially over the next 10 years (Heffler et al. 2002). Alternatives to traditional financing of mental health care, such as Medicaid's long-term care waiver programs and Medicare's programs of all-inclusive care for the elderly and social health maintenance organizations, have begun to increase the availability and use of home- and community-based services for the sickest elderly patients.

Workforce and Training Issues

According to the American Association for Geriatric Psychiatry, there are currently about 1,500 board certified geriatric psychiatrists in the United States, and fewer than 80 psychiatrists graduate from fellowship training programs in geriatrics each year. Clearly, the number of psychiatrists with subspecialty training and certification is insufficient to meet the growing need for geriatric psychiatric care in the United States. Most of the clinical training in geriatric psychiatry in the United States is funded by Medicare graduate medical education (GME) payments, plus support of some training positions from the VA and the U.S. Department of Health and Human Services Health Research and Services Administration. Under current law, hospitals receive 100% GME reimbursement for initial residency training up to 5 years, depending on specialty board requirements. After that, programs receive only 50% of GME funding for subspecialty fellowship training. However, the law now includes a geriatric exception, under which programs training fellows in geriatric medicine or psychiatry are eligible to receive full funding for an additional 2 years beyond the initial residency. Legislation has also been introduced that provides up to $35,000 per year in educational loan forgiveness for trainees who choose to pursue research fellowships in geriatrics. Even with this legislation, recruitment to the field of geriatric psychiatry continues to lag behind the projected workforce needs and is expected to fall far short of the mark for at least the next decade.

Ethical Issues and End-of-Life Care

Advances in medical technologies, such as mechanical ventilation and enteral nutrition and hydration, present ethical challenges for patients, families, and physicians. These technologies can extend the course of a patient's chronic and progressive disease to an advanced stage, leading the patient or persons who care for that patient to question the value of the treatment. In short, medicine has increasing control over how and when a patient dies.

Numerous reviews and professional organizations' position statements have set forth guidelines for what constitutes good care at the end of life (American Geriatrics Society 2007; Institute of Medicine 1997; Rabow et al. 2000; Sachs 2000). Despite considerable progress in recognizing the importance of quality of care for the dying, there is uncertainty and poor agreement about the characteristics of "the good death"; wide variation exists in attitudes among patients, physicians, other professional care providers, and family members concerning the specific attributes of this concept (Steinhauser et al. 2000). Nevertheless, some common fundamentals have emerged (see Table 33–1).

Acceptable interventions should allow dying patients to fulfill goals that are highly personal.

> The healthy and the mildly chronically ill want prevention and cure. Those with disabling, progressive, eventually fatal chronic illness have much broader priorities. For example, when patients are very sick, they want to be comfortable, retain control and dignity, leave a legacy, live longer, and bring closure to their lives. (Lynn 2001, p. 930)

Underlying all efforts must be the primary objective of enabling the individual "to live well on their own terms right up to the time of death" (Lynn 1997, p. 1635).

Medical organizations such as the American Geriatrics Society, the American Medical Association, and the American Psychiatric Association have attempted to define the characteristics of good care at the end of life. Using these characteristics, the Joint Commission on Accreditation of Healthcare Organizations has developed a list of core principles for care at the end of life (Cassell and Foley 1999):

1. Respect the dignity of both patient and caregivers.
2. Be sensitive to and respectful of the patient's and family's wishes.
3. Use the most appropriate measures that are consistent with the patient's choices.
4. Encompass alleviation of pain and other physical symptoms.
5. Assess and manage psychological, social, and spiritual/religious problems.
6. Offer continuity (the patient should be able to continue to be cared for, if so desired, by his or her primary care and specialist providers).
7. Provide access to any therapy that may realistically be expected to improve the patient's quality of life, including alternative or nontraditional treatments.
8. Provide access to palliative care and hospice care.
9. Respect the right to refuse treatment.
10. Respect the physician's professional responsibility to discontinue some treatments when appropriate, with consideration for both patient and family preferences.
11. Promote clinical and evidence-based research on providing care at the end of life.

TABLE 33–1. Fundamental concerns in providing end-of-life care

Advance planning and preparation for death
Attention to quality of life, maximizing as many features as possible:
—Respect and dignity
—Autonomy
—Continuity of care, nonabandonment
—Alleviation of suffering of physical and mental symptoms
—Pain management
—Spirituality
Support of family and caregivers before and after death of patient
Removal of regulatory barriers to facilitate access to care
Education and training of both professional and informal caregivers

Collaborative Care

Quality end-of-life care relies on collaboration among the patient, all treating professionals, and the patient's family. Organizations have developed programs to educate physicians and others about the numerous services that are available to assist them (home care, hospice programs, nursing homes, palliative care units). It is important to take cultural and religious variants into account when designing and offering these services (Kagawa-Singer and Blackhall 2001; Lo et al. 2002).

Role of the Psychiatrist

Psychiatrists can have a key role in the care of older adults who are chronically ill. Psychiatric sensitivity to the interplay of multifactorial influences and the biopsychosocial paradigm, as well as to developmental stages and their dynamics, is valuable in enabling psychiatrists to make in-depth individualized assessment and to give attention to the special requirements of the dying person and his or her family. These skills are especially helpful when there are disagreements among family members or among family, patient, and the health care team over what is the right plan of care for a seriously ill patient. Table 33–2 lists some areas for consideration by the psychiatrist.

The American Association for Geriatric Psychiatry (2001) has developed its own Position Statement on care at the end of life. Two of the principles are of special interest to care of the seriously ill. Principle 1 calls for psychiatrists to respect the dignity of both the patient and the caregiver, paying special attention to the changes in mental state and in psychodynamic and social functioning and behavior that are an integral part of the aging process and that are not to be considered psychopathological per se. The rationale for this principle is that a person's mental state is affected not only by the terminal condition(s) but also by the aging process. The elderly patient's own perspective on this time of closure is an issue that must be assessed and knowledgably managed. Other issues include support of psychodynamic defenses, life review, countering fears of helplessness and abandonment, and assistance with active conflicts (e.g., within the family).

Principle 4 involves giving high priority to the alleviation of pain and distress in psychological and social domains in addition to the physical arena. The rationale for this principle is that alleviating pain and distress includes sensitively working with elderly patients' feelings of hopelessness (not only those that arise in the context of depression), the absence of self-worth that patients feel when they are not productive, their weariness with life, and their desire not to be a burden to others.

A variety of techniques are available to psychiatrists to improve the quality of communication between patients, families, and health care professionals. These techniques draw from the skills used for psychotherapy, with particular attention to permitting people to tell their stories. Such stories are the foundation for achieving common understandings of key issues such as the patient's prognosis, his or her quality of life, and the goals of care. Table 33–3 lists useful questions to efficiently and effectively structure the end-of-life discussion with a patient (Karlawish 1999).

TABLE 33–2. Areas in end-of-life care for consideration by the psychiatrist

Quality of life
Pain and suffering
Diagnostic foci
—Decision-making capacity
—Axis I
—Axis II
Family conflict
Patient–physician relationship
Withholding or withdrawal of treatment
Assistance in dying
Treatment

Source. Data from American Psychiatric Association 1994; Larson and Tobin 2000; Quill 2000; Von Gunten et al. 2000.

Hospice Care

One particular service of value in the care of persons with late-stage dementia is the Medicare hospice benefit (Volicer and Hurley 1998). Hospice care is not limited to institutional sites and may also be delivered at home. A wide array of interventions are offered, including medication, oxygen, companions and aides, spiritual counseling, advance planning, and family support (Health Care Financing Administration 2000; National Task Force on End-of-Life Care in Managed Care 1999).

Unfortunately, significant barriers exist for patient access to hospice programs (Hanrahan and Luchins 1995; Luchins 1995). One of the chief barriers is the requirement that there be a prognosis of 6 months or less to live. This requirement is problematic in view of the uncertain nature of the course and rate of decline of various diseases (e.g., Alzheimer's disease). To determine whether a patient should be deemed terminal, one can consider this question: "Would I be surprised if I had learned today that the patient had died last night?" A "no" answer to this question suggests that the balance of data and overall clinical picture describe a patient who is seriously ill and potentially at the terminal stage.

TABLE 33–3. Questions to structure the end-of-life discussion with the patient

Identify the patient's present concerns, with attention to both the patient and the family.
What concerns you most about your illness?
How is treatment going for you? What about for your family?
What has been most difficult about this illness for you? What about for your family?

Learn the patient's understanding about potential outcomes. Correct any misunderstandings of pertinent facts.
When you think about your illness, what's the best that could happen?
When you think about your illness, what's the worst that could happen?

Identify the patient's concerns about the future.
What are your fears for the future?
As you think about the future, what matters most to you?

Identify how the patient conceives of quality of life.
If you were dying, where would you want to receive medical care? At home? In a hospital? In a hospice?
What makes life worth living?

Clarify vague terms.
What do you mean by "being a vegetable"?

Identify a proxy decision maker.
If you were to become ill and could not speak for yourself like you are talking with me now, who would you want to speak on your behalf? Who do you trust?

Source. Adapted from Karlawish et al. 1999.

Legal Issues

Advance Directives for Health Care, Living Wills, and Powers of Attorney

The Patient Self-Determination Act of 1991 (PSDA) requires hospitals, nursing homes, and organizations receiving Medicare and Medicaid funds from the federal government to notify patients of their right to express their wishes concerning life-sustaining care and of the laws of the relevant state with respect to advance directives. The law does not require patients to sign such a document.

Advance directives for health care should include the following:

- *A living will.* In some states, witnesses to the signing are required.
- *A power of attorney for health care.* In some states, this document requires notarization. Power of attorney differs from guardianship in that the power of attorney is given by a competent individual, whereas the guardianship is imposed on a person who is deemed incompetent. A durable power of attorney takes effect when the person is unable to make the decisions the document addresses.

In many states, the living will relates only to 1) a terminal condition (incurable and irreversible) and 2) a permanently unconscious condition (persistent vegetative state). Hence, the living will is generally made in association with a durable power of attorney for health care, which confers wider scope for the decision-making right.

In spite of a long series of informational and legislative initiatives (Emanuel et al. 1991; Luptak and Boult 1994; Spears et al. 1993), only 10%–30% of older adults, and a somewhat higher percentage of the nursing home population, have stated their preferences for life-sustaining treatment (Molloy et al. 2000; Sachs et al. 1992; SUPPORT Principal Investigators 1995; Teno 2000; Teno et al. 1997). Even if people do create such documents, however, these documents may not be as valuable in practice as in theory. Individuals' preferences may change in concert with the patient's changing mood, experience of illness, and degree of hope (Menon et al. 2000). Therefore, directives that set forth general principles to guide care and designate a person who can serve as a proxy are perhaps the most valuable kinds of advance planning documents.

When patients are unable to explicitly state their preferences, the process of *substituted judgment* should become operative. This means that another person makes a decision for a patient on the basis of what the patient's wishes would be if the patient were capable of making the decision. Several studies that have assessed the accuracy of substituted judgment have found what could be considered a disturbing result: poor congruence between patients' preferences and their spouses' and physicians' predictions of those preferences (see, e.g., Miles et al. 1996; Uhlmann 1988). However, these data are not on the whole as disturbing as they may seem. Sehgal et al. (1992) found that many patients, although capable of stating their advance directive for treatment, are willing to allow their trusted proxy to exercise leeway, or freedom, to overrule this directive and do the opposite.

When a patient who lacks the capacity to make his or her own decisions lacks an advance directive or a legally appointed proxy, certain individuals, by virtue of their relationship with the patient, are authorized to make decisions. The laws of the state where the patient resides dictate the specific order of the hierarchy of relatives (e.g., spouse; if spouse is not available, then adult child; if adult child is not available, then sibling; etc.). Decisions by surrogates need to be informed by an understanding of the benefits, risks, and burdens of the course chosen, the criterion being the attainment of the "best interests" of the patient. This criterion, the broadest standard used in the United States and in the United Kingdom (Brahams 1989), is not without difficulties (Wikler 1988). Assessment of best interests should include consideration of relief of suffering, preservation or restoration of function, and quality and extent of sustained life.

The motivation for advance directives, especially living wills, arises principally from considerations of the right of a mentally incapacitated patient to refuse or to withdraw from life-sustaining treatment (e.g., artificial nutrition and hydration). Although the right of mentally incapacitated persons and their properly appointed proxies to refuse or discontinue artificial nutrition and hydration has been affirmed by the U.S. Supreme Court (*Cruzan v. Director* 1990; *Washington v. Glucksberg* 1997), the legal standards applied by states vary widely. For example, some states require "clear and convincing evidence" that the patient would have wanted treatment discontinued.

In the United States, Catholic and Jewish religious groups have adopted the position that the right to refuse or discontinue life-sustaining treatment does apply to events in which such refusal could lead to death or to cases in which the patient is not terminally ill (National Conference of Catholic Bishops 1995; Rosin and Sonnenblick 1998). Courts have also legitimized the withdrawal of life-sustaining treatment, basing the decisions in part on the rejection of the distinction between withholding and withdrawing treatments, with artificial feeding included in the category of treatment (*Barber v. Superior Court* 1983; *Brophy v. New England Sinai Hospital* 1986). It has been concluded that the right to refuse medical treatments, including artificial nutrition and hydration, outweighed states' interest in the preservation of life, the prevention of suicide, and the ethical integrity of the medical profession. The discontinuation of feeding has not been found to be suicide or active euthanasia; rather, it has been viewed as allowing the underlying disease to take its natural course. The American Medical Association (1999) has concurred with this interpretation.

Competency and Decision-Making Capacity

A core ethic of medicine is informed consent. The term *informed consent* describes the voluntary choice of a competent patient following a physician's disclosure of the relevant facts (Appelbaum 2007). Informed consent has four elements: disclosure, voluntariness, competency, and choice. Of these elements, competency is the one that most often affects psychiatrists' work. Common psychiatric illnesses such as dementia, delirium, and psychosis can impair cognition to the degree that a person is no longer capable, or competent, to make a decision (Appelbaum 2007), and psychiatrists are often consulted to assess whether such a patient is capable of making a decision. For example, the Oregon criteria for providing assisted suicide to a terminally ill patient require the determination by a qualified professional that the patient is capable of consenting to assisted suicide

Competency in this context refers to the judgment that a person has adequate capacity to make a decision (Grisso and Appelbaum 1998a). Critical to this definition is that competency requires a judgment. Society entrusts this judgment to judges and, in the day-to-day conduct of clinical care and research, to clinicians and clinical investigators. The consensus in both law and ethics is that two criteria should inform this judgment: the person's decision-making capacity and the risks and benefits of the various options.

Decision-making capacity describes a dimensional construct akin to weight, blood pressure, and height.

Table 33–4 provides definitions of the four abilities—understanding, choice, appreciation, and reasoning—that constitute decision-making capacity. A clinician or judge assesses these abilities to measure a person's decision-making capacity. These findings, together with an assessment of the risks and benefits of the options available to the patient, support the judgment as to whether the person lacks the capacity to make the decision. This is called a risk-sensitive model of capacity assessment (Appelbaum 2007). For example, a patient with end-stage renal disease who refuses dialysis faces the likely outcome of death by renal failure within 30 days. This risk—death—is sufficiently significant that a reasonable clinician should assess that the person understands this outcome of his or her choice.

Assessments of capacity require professionals to balance two core ethical principles of medicine: respect for autonomy and beneficence. Clinicians should respect the choice of persons who have the capacity to make a decision (and all adults are presumed to have this capacity unless shown otherwise). However, clinicians also have a beneficence-based obligation to seek out other persons, commonly called proxies or surrogates, to make a decision for a person who lacks the ability or capacity to make a decision.

Over the last 20 years, considerable progress has been made in developing instruments to assist clinicians in assessing patients' decision-making abilities. The MacArthur Competency Assessment instruments, for example, include instruments to assess research and treatment capacity (Appelbaum and Grisso 2001; Grisso and Appelbaum 1998b). Studies have demonstrated that conditions such as depression and psychosis have some but not a substantial impact on a patient's performance on measures of decision-making ability. Specifically, impairment in mood or the severity of psychiatric symptoms explains little variance in performance on the decision-making abilities (Raymont et al. 2004). Instead, cognition explains much of the variance in patient performance. This does not mean that tests of cognition can substitute for an assessment of capacity. What it does mean is that as cognition worsens, the probability increases that a person has clinically significant loss in capacity.

The term *competency* has been reserved for a legal judgment that can be made only by judges. Determination of competency is particularly relevant in cases of guardianship. However, these judgments address the same question as the clinical judgment that a person lacks the capacity to provide informed consent, which physicians make on a daily basis in hospitals and clinics. In either case—competency or capacity—the outcome is the same: the person does or does not have the ability to make the decision at hand.

TABLE 33–4. Abilities required for decision-making capacity

Understanding: The ability to state the meaning of the information disclosed.

Example of assessing a person's ability to understand the indication for a procedure:

—"Can you tell me in your own words the reason why I am recommending hospice?"

Choice: The ability to state a decision. This is often linked to consistency, or the ability to state the same decision over the course of an assessment of decision-making abilities.

Example of assessing a person's ability to make a choice:

—"I just want to make sure. Do you still not want to enroll in hospice?"

Appreciation: The ability to recognize that the facts of a decision apply to the person (e.g., the ability to recognize that a procedure might benefit the patient). A useful example to demonstrate the difference between appreciation and understanding is the case of a person with psychosis who can say back what schizophrenia is but does not accept that he or she has delusions that are actually false.

Example of assessing a person's ability to appreciate benefit:

—"I know you said that you do not want to receive hospice services, but can you tell me how hospice might benefit you?"

Reasoning: There are two kinds of reasoning: *consequential* (inferring the potential results of a choice) and *comparative* (weighing the merits vs. the demerits of options).

Example of assessing a person's ability to reason consequentially:

—"How might enrolling in hospice affect your everyday activities?"

Example of assessing a person's ability to reason comparatively:

—"You say you are more likely not to choose to enroll in hospice. How is not having it better than enrolling in it?"

Conclusion

The number of older patients with mental disorders is expected to grow dramatically in coming decades. In response, a number of professional and consumer advocates, government agencies, policy analysts, policy planners, and university-based academics have opened a vigorous dialogue focused on how best to meet the mental health needs of older adults. Preliminary but important discussions have begun on how best to structure and finance mental health care for older persons, how to strengthen an inadequately sized and undertrained workforce to deal with these issues, and how to resolve the ethical and legal questions that arise toward the end of life. What will probably emerge is a mandate to implement a research and policy agenda for aging and mental health that focuses on prevention, early detection, evidence-based intervention, and training. Without such forethought and planning, those stakeholders who predict a crisis in geriatric mental health in coming decades may prove to be clairvoyant.

Key Points

- With regard to the mental disorders of late life, the current U.S. mental health care system serves older patients poorly and is largely unprepared to meet what has been described as an upcoming crisis as the numbers of older adults increase.
- Recruitment to the field of geriatric psychiatry continues to lag behind the projected workforce needs and is expected to fall far short of the mark for at least the next decade.
- Despite considerable progress in recognizing the importance of quality of care for the dying, there is uncertainty and poor agreement about the characteristics of "the good death."
- Assessments of capacity have a critical role in mediating the balance between two core ethical principles of medicine: respect for autonomy and beneficence.

References

American Association for Geriatric Psychiatry: End-of-Life Care: position statement of the American Association for Geriatric Psychiatry. Adopted by the AAGP Board of Directors. February 2001. Available at http://www.aagponline.org/prof/position_end.asp. Accessed April 13, 2008.

American Association for Geriatric Psychiatry: H.R. 6331, Medicare Improvements for Patients and Providers Act of 2008 as passed by the House and Senate: summary of provisions. 2008. Available at http://www.aagponline.org/Uploads/Web/HR6331summary.HPA.Jul08.pdf. Accessed July 20, 2008.

American Geriatrics Society Ethics Committee: The Care of Dying Patients. New York, American Geriatrics Society. 2007. Available at http://www.americangeriatrics.org/products/positionpapers/careofd.shtml. Accessed April 12, 2008.

American Medical Association: Medical futility in end-of-life care: report of the Council on Ethical and Judicial Affairs. JAMA 281:937–941, 1999

American Psychiatric Association: The role of the psychiatrist in end-of-life decisions: report of the Subcommittee on Psychiatric Aspects of Life-Sustaining Technology. Washington, DC, American Psychiatric Association, May 1994

Appelbaum PS, Grisso T: MacArthur Competence Assessment Tool for Clinical Research (MacCAT-CR). Sarasota, FL, Professional Resource Press, 2001

Appelbaum PS: Assessments of patients' competence to consent to treatment. N Engl J Med 357:1834–1840, 2007

Balanced Budget Act of 1997, Pub L No 105-33, 111 Stat. 251

Barber v Superior Court, 195 Cal Rptr 484, 147 Cal App 3d 1006 (1983)

Bartels SJ, Colenda CC: Mental health services for Alzheimer's disease: current trends in reimbursement and public policy, and the future under managed care. Am J Geriatr Psychiatry 6 (suppl 1):S85–S100, 1998

Bartels SJ, Levine KJ, Shea D: Community-based long-term care for older persons with severe and persistent mental illness in an era of managed care. Psychiatr Serv 50:1189–1197, 1999

Borson S, Loebel JP, Kitchell M, et al: Psychiatric assessments of nursing home residents under OBRA-87: should PASARR be reformed? Pre-Admission Screening and Annual Review. J Am Geriatr Soc 45:1173–1181, 1997

Brahams D: Sterilization of a mentally incapable woman. Lancet 1:1275–1276, 1989

Brophy v New England Sinai Hospital Inc, 497 NE2d 626 (Mass 1986)

Cassell CK, Foley KM: Principles for care of patients at the end of life: an emerging consensus among the specialties of medicine. New York, Milbank Memorial Fund. 1999. Available at http://www.milbank.org/reports/endoflife. Accessed April 13, 2008.

Centers for Medicare and Medicaid Services: Prescription drug coverage: general information. 2008. Available at http://www.cms.hhs.gov/PrescriptionDrugCovGenIn. Accessed July 20, 2008.

Clark TR (ed): Nursing Home Survey Procedures and Interpretive Guidelines: A Resource for the Consultant Pharmacist. Alexandria, VA, American Society of Consultant Pharmacists, 1999, pp 1–8

Colenda CC, Streim JE, Greene JA, et al: The impact of the Omnibus Budget Reconciliation Act of 1987 (OBRA'87) on psychiatric services in nursing homes. Am J Geriatr Psychiatry 7:12–17, 1999

Colenda CC, Bartels SC, Gottlieb GL: The North American system of care, in Principles and Practice of Geriatric Psychiatry, 2nd Edition. Edited by Copeland J, Abou-Saleh M, Blazer D. London, Wiley, 2002, pp 689–696

Cruzan v Director, Missouri Department of Health, 497 U.S. 261, 279 (1990)

Cuffel BJ, Jeste DV, Halpain M, et al: Treatment costs and use of community mental health services for schizophrenia by age cohorts. Am J Psychiatry 153:870–876, 1996

Datto C, Oslin D, Streim J, et al: Pharmacological treatment of depression in nursing home residents: a mental health services perspective. J Geriatr Psychiatry Neurol 15:141–146, 2002

Dixon L, Postrado L, Delahanty J, et al: The association of medical comorbidity in schizophrenia with poor physical and mental health. J Nerv Ment Dis 187:496–502, 1999

Dixon L, Lyles A, Smith C: Use and costs of ambulatory care services among Medicare enrollees with schizophrenia. Psychiatr Serv 52:786–792, 2001

Emanuel LL, Barry MJ, Stoeckle JD, et al: Advance directives for medical care: a case for greater use. N Engl J Med 324:889–895, 1991

Eng C, Pedulla J, Eleazer GP, et al: Program of all-inclusive care for the elderly (PACE): an innovative model of integrated geriatric care and financing. J Am Geriatr Soc 45:223–232, 1997

Frank RG: The creation of Medicare and Medicaid: the emergence of insurance and markets for mental health services. Psychiatr Serv 51:465–468, 2000

Goldman LS: Medical illness in patients with schizophrenia. J Clin Psychiatry 60 (suppl 21):10–15, 1999

Grisso T, Appelbaum PS: Assessing Competence to Consent to Treatment: A Guide for Physicians and Other Health Professionals. New York, Oxford University Press, 1998a

Grisso T, Appelbaum S: MacArthur Competence Assessment Tool for Treatment (MacCAT-T). Sarasota, FL, Professional Resource Press, 1998b

Hanrahan P, Luchins DJ: Access to hospice programs in end-stage dementia: a national survey of hospice programs. J Am Geriatr Soc 43:56–59, 1995

Health Care Financing Administration: Medicare and Medicaid: Requirements for Long-Term Care Facilities, Final Regulations. Fed Regist 56:48865–48921, September 26, 1991

Health Care Financing Administration: Medicare and Medicaid Programs: Preadmission Screening and Annual Resident Review. Fed Regist 57:56450–56504, November 30, 1992

Health Care Financing Administration: Report to Congress: Study of Private Accreditation (Deeming) of Nursing Homes, Regulatory Incentives and Non-Regulatory Incentives, and Effectiveness of the Survey and Certification System. Washington, DC, Health Care Financing Administration, 1998

Health Care Financing Administration: Medicare and Your Mental Health Benefits. Washington, DC, U.S. Government Printing Office, 2000

Heffler S, Smith S, Won G, et al: Health spending projections for 2001–2011: the latest outlook. Health Aff (Millwood) 21:207–218, 2002

Hogan C, Lynn J, Gabel J, et al: Medicare Beneficiaries' Costs and Use of Care in the Last Year of Life. Washington, DC, Medicare Payment Advisory Commission, 2000

Institute for Health and Aging: Chronic Care in America: A 21st Century Challenge. Princeton, NJ, Robert Wood Johnson Foundation, 1996

Institute of Medicine, Committee on Nursing Home Regulation: Improving the Quality of Care in Nursing Homes. Washington, DC, National Academy Press, 1986

Institute of Medicine, Committee on Care at the End of Life: Approaching Death: Improving Care at the End of Life. Edited by Field MJ, Cassel CK. Washington, DC, National Academy Press, 1997

Institute of Medicine, Committee on Improving Quality in Long-Term Care: Improving the Quality of Long-Term Care. Edited by Wunderlich GS, Kohler P. Washington, DC, National Academy Press, 2001, pp 235–247

Jeste DV, Alexopoulos GS, Bartels SJ, et al: Consensus statement on the upcoming crisis in geriatric mental health: research agenda for the next 2 decades. Arch Gen Psychiatry 56:848–853, 1999

Kagawa-Singer M, Blackhall L: Negotiating cross-cultural issues at the end of life: "you got to go where he lives." JAMA 286:2993–3001, 2001

Kane RL: Managed care as a vehicle for delivering more effective chronic care for older persons. J Am Geriatr Soc 46:1034–1039, 1998

Kane RL, Kane RA, Finch M, et al: S/HMOs, the second generation: building on the experience of the first social health maintenance organization demonstrations. J Am Geriatr Soc 45:101–107, 1997

Karlawish JH, Quill T, Meier DE: A consensus-based approach to providing palliative care to patients who lack decision-making capacity. Ann Intern Med 130:835–840, 1999

Langwell K, Topoleski C, Sherman D: Analysis of Benefits Offered by Medicare HMOs, 1999: Complexities and Implications. Menlo Park, CA, Henry J. Kaiser Foundation, 1999

Lantz MS, Giambanco V, Buchalter EN: A ten-year review of the effect of OBRA-87 on psychotropic prescribing practices in an academic nursing home. Psychiatr Serv 47:951–955, 1996

Larson DG, Tobin DR: End-of-life conversations. JAMA 284:1573–1578, 2000

Lasser RA, Sunderland T: Newer psychotropic medication use in nursing home residents. J Am Geriatr Soc 46:202–207, 1998

Llorente MD, Olsen EJ, Leyva O, et al: Use of antipsychotic drugs in nursing homes: current compliance with OBRA regulations. J Am Geriatr Soc 46:198–201, 1998

Lo B, Ruston D, Kates LW, et al: Discussing religious and spiritual issues at the end of life: a practical guide for physicians. JAMA 287:749–754, 2002

Luchins DJ: Access to hospice programs in end-stage dementia: a national survey of hospice programs. J Am Geriatr Soc 43:56–59, 1995

Luptak MK, Boult C: A method for increasing elders' use of advance directives. Gerontologist 34:409–412, 1994

Lynn J: Clinical crossroads: an 88-year-old woman facing the end of life. JAMA 277:1633–1640, 1997

Lynn J: Perspectives on care at the close of life: serving patients who may die soon and their families: the role of hospice and other services. JAMA 285:925–932, 2001

Mechanic D: Approaches for coordinating primary and specialty care for persons with mental illness. Gen Hosp Psychiatry 19:395–402, 1997

Medicare Payment Advisory Commission: Medicare Plus Choice: a program in transition, in Report to Congress: Medicare Payment Policy. Washington, DC, Medicare Payment Advisory Commission, 1999, pp 27–46

Meeks S, Carstensen LL, Stafford PB, et al: Mental health needs of the chronically mentally ill elderly. Psychol Aging 5:163–171, 1990

Menon AS, Campbell D, Ruskin P, et al: Depression, hopelessness, and the desire for life-saving treatments among elderly medically ill veterans. Am J Geriatr Psychiatry 8:333–342, 2000

Miles SH, Koepp R, Weber EP: Advance end-of-life treatment planning: a research review. Arch Intern Med 156:1062–1068, 1996

Molloy DW, Guyatt GH, Russo R, et al: Systematic implementation of an advance directive program in nursing homes: a randomized controlled trial. JAMA 283:1437–1443, 2000

National Center for Health Statistics: The National Nursing Home Survey. Hyattsville, MD, National Center for Health Statistics. 2004. Available at http://cdc.gov/nchs/nnhs.htm. Accessed April 13, 2008.

National Conference of Catholic Bishops: Ethical and Religious Directives for Catholic Health Care Services. Washington, DC, U.S. Catholic Conference, 1995

National Task Force on End-of-Life Care in Managed Care: Meeting the Challenge: Twelve Recommendations for Improving End-of-Life Care in Managed Care. Newton, MA, Education Development Center, 1999

Nyman JA: Improving the quality of nursing home outcomes: are adequacy- or incentive-oriented policies more effective? Med Care 26:1158–1171, 1988

Office of the Inspector General, Department of Health and Human Services: Medicare Payments for Psychiatric Services in Nursing Homes: A Follow-up. January 2001. Available at http://oig.hhs.gov/oei/reports/oei-02-99-00140.pdf. Accessed April 13, 2008.

Omnibus Budget Reconciliation Act of 1987, Pub L No 100-203

Omnibus Budget Reconciliation Act of 1989, Pub L No 101-239

Patient Self-Determination Act of 1991. Pub L No 101-508 §§ 4206, 4751 (codified in scattered sections of 42 U.S.C., especially §§ 1395cc, 1396a [West Supp. 1991]

Paul Wellstone and Pete Domenici Mental Health Parity and Addiction Equity Act of 2008. Text available at http://www.govtrack.us/congress/bill.xpd? bill=h110-6983. Accessed October 10, 2008.

Quill TE: Initiating end-of-life discussions with seriously ill patients. JAMA 284:2502–2507, 2000

Rabow MW, Hardie GE, Fair JM, et al: End-of-life care content in 50 textbooks from multiple specialties. JAMA 283:771–778, 2000

Raymont V, Bingley W, Buchanan A, et al: Prevalence of mental incapacity in medical inpatients and associated risk factors: cross-sectional study. Lancet 364:1421–1427, 2004

Reichman W, Coyne A, Borson S, et al: Psychiatric consultation in the nursing home: a survey of six states. Am J Geriatr Psychiatry 6:320–327, 1998

Robert Wood Johnson Foundation: Death and Dying in America: Too Much Technology, Too Little Care. Princeton, NJ, Robert Wood Johnson Foundation, May 1998

Rosin AJ, Sonnenblick M: Autonomy and paternalism in geriatric medicine: the Jewish ethical approach to issues of feeding terminally ill patients, and to cardiopulmonary resuscitation. J Med Ethics 24:44–48, 1998

Rovner BW, Edelman BA, Cox MP, et al: The impact of antipsychotic drug regulations (OBRA 1987) on psychotropic prescribing practices in nursing homes. Am J Psychiatry 149:1390–1392, 1992

Sachs GA: A piece of my mind: sometimes dying still stings. JAMA 284:2423, 2000

Sachs GA, Stocking CB, Miles SH: Empowerment of the older patient? A randomized, controlled trial to increase discussion and use of advance directives. J Am Geriatr Soc 40:269–273, 1992

Sehgal A, Galbraith A, Chesney M, et al: How strictly do dialysis patients want their advance directive followed? JAMA 267:59–63, 1992

Sheline YI: High prevalence of physical illness in a geriatric psychiatric inpatient population. Gen Hosp Psychiatry 12:396–400, 1990

Shorr RI, Fought RL, Ray WA: Changes in antipsychotic drug use in nursing homes during implementation of the OBRA-87 regulations. JAMA 271:358–362, 1994

Snowden M, Roy-Byrne P: Mental illness and nursing home reform: OBRA-87 ten years later. Psychiatr Serv 49:229–233, 1998

Spears R, Drinka PJ, Voeks SK: Obtaining a durable power of attorney for health care from nursing home residents. J Fam Pract 36:409–413, 1993

Steinhauser KE, Christakis NA, Clipp EC, et al: Factors considered important at the end of life by patients, family, physicians and other care providers. JAMA 284:2476–2482, 2000

Streim JE, Beckwith EW, Arapakos D, et al: Regulatory oversight, payment policy, and quality improvement in mental health care in nursing homes. Psychiatr Serv 53:1414–1418, 2002

SUPPORT Principal Investigators: A controlled trial to improve care for seriously ill hospitalized patients: the Study to Understand Prognoses and Preferences for Outcomes and Risks of Treatment (SUPPORT). JAMA 274:1591–1598, 1995

Teno JM: Advance directives for nursing home residents: achieving compassionate, competent, cost-effective care. JAMA 283:1481–1482, 2000

Teno JM, Lynn J, Wenger NS, et al: Advance directives for seriously ill hospitalized patients: effectiveness with the Patient Self-Determination Act and the SUPPORT intervention. J Am Geriatr Soc 45:500–507, 1997

Uhlmann RF, Pearlman RA, Cain KC: Physicians' and spouses' predictions of elderly patients' resuscitation preferences. J Gerontol 43:M115–M121, 1988

U.S. Department of Health and Human Services: Older adults and mental health, in Mental Health: A Report of the Surgeon General. Bethesda, MD, National Institute of Mental Health, 1999a, pp 335–401. Available at http://www.surgeongeneral.gov/library/mentalhealth/home.html. Accessed April 13, 2008.

U.S. Department of Health and Human Services: Organizing and financing mental health services, in Mental Health: A Report of the Surgeon General. Bethesda, MD, National Institute of Mental Health, 1999b, pp 405–433. Available at http://www.surgeongeneral.gov/library/mentalhealth/home.html. Accessed April 13, 2008.

U.S. Department of Health and Human Services, Office of the Inspector General: Medicare Payments for Psychiatric Services in Nursing Homes: A Follow-up (DHHS Publ No OEI-02-99-00140). New York, Office of Evaluation and Inspections. 2001. Available at http://oig.hhs.gov/oei/reports/oei-02-99-00140.pdf. Accessed April 13, 2008.

U.S. Department of Veterans Affairs: Facts about the Department of Veterans Affairs. December 2007. Available at http://www1.va.gov/opa/fact/docs/vafacts.doc. Accessed July 17, 2008.

Vieweg V, Levenson J, Pandurangi A, et al: Medical disorders in the schizophrenic patient. Int J Psychiatry Med 25:137–172, 1995

Volicer L, Hurley A: Hospice Care for Patients With Advanced Progressive Dementia. New York, Springer, 1998

Von Gunten CF, Ferris FD, Emanuel LL: Ensuring competency in end-of-life care. JAMA 284:3051–3057, 2000

Washington v Glucksberg, 117 S. Ct. 2258, 2270 (1997)

Wikler D: Patient interests: clinical implications of philosophical distinctions. J Am Geriatr Soc 36:951–958, 1988

Williams L: Long-term care after Olmstead v. L.C.: will the potential of the ADA's integration mandate be achieved? J Contemp Health Law Policy 17:205–239, 2000

Witkin MJ, Atay JE, Manderscheid RW, et al: Highlights of organized mental health services in 1994 and major national and state trends, in Mental Health, United States 1998 (HHS Pub No 99-3285). Rockville, MD, Substance Abuse and Mental Health Services Administration, 1998

Zubenko GS, Marino LJ, Sweet RA, et al: Medical comorbidity in elderly psychiatric inpatients. Biol Psychiatry 41:724–736, 1997

Suggested Readings

Appelbaum PS: Assessments of patients' competence to consent to treatment. N Engl J Med 357:1834–1840, 2007

Heffler S, Smith S, Won G, et al: Health spending projections for 2001–2011: the latest outlook. Health Aff (Millwood) 21:207–218, 2002

Jeste DV, Alexopoulos GS, Bartels SJ, et al: Consensus statement on the upcoming crisis in geriatric mental health: research agenda for the next 2 decades. Arch Gen Psychiatry 56:848–853, 1999

Raymont V, Bingley W, Buchanan A, et al: Prevalence of mental incapacity in medical inpatients and associated risk factors: cross-sectional study. Lancet 364:1421–1427, 2004

CHAPTER 34

The Past and Future of Geriatric Psychiatry

Dan G. Blazer, M.D., Ph.D.
David C. Steffens, M.D., M.H.S.

The Path of Geriatric Psychiatry in the United States

The relatively recent emergence of geriatric psychiatry in North America is based on two centuries of interest and work by both Americans and non-Americans. For example, Benjamin Franklin (1706–1790) maintained a strong belief that science would eventually discover the aging process, control it, and be able to rejuvenate people. He apparently was convinced that if the patriarchs of the antediluvian era, described in the Hebrew Scriptures (Old Testament), could achieve extended life spans, so could the human of the future. It appears that Franklin was a man who both talked the talk and tried to walk the walk. Many of his most lasting historical contributions came after his 70th year, most notably his service in Europe during the Revolutionary War and subsequent reconstruction of the United States, the negotiation of the peace treaty with Great Britain, and, upon his return from Europe, his role as a delegate to the Constitutional Convention. Two of his inventions have contributed to the well-being of elderly persons: the Franklin stove and bifocal eyeglasses (Gruman 1966).

Benjamin Rush (1745–1830), a famous American physician, "father of American psychiatry" according to the American Psychiatric Association (APA), and a signer of the Declaration of Independence, wrote extensively and lucidly on a variety of subjects, including old age. In 1805, he published *An Account of the State of the Body and Mind in Old Age: With Observations on Its Diseases and Remedies* (Butterfield 1976).

The 1930s was a time of increased interest in old age research. Walter R. Miles and his associates developed the Stanford Greater Maturity Project with the objective of investigating systematically the psychological aspects of aging. Medical research was enhanced by the publication of *Problems of Aging* by Edmund V. Cowdry (1938), which brought together discussions of physical and health-related problems in one volume. Cowdry played a major role in organizing the American Geriatrics Society, the Gerontological Society of America, and the International Association of Gerontology. Also in the late 1930s, two important sociologists, Leo Simmons and Ernest W. Burgess, independently published studies on social aspects of aging. In 1945, Simmons published a pioneer study of aging in 70 preliterate societies (Simmons 1945). Burgess and his associates at the University of Chicago developed instruments to measure personality adjustment in old age.

Ignatz Leo Nascher (1863–1944) is thought to have coined the term *geriatrics* with the publication of his text *Geriatrics: The Diseases of Old Age and Their Treatment* (Nascher 1914). He published numerous articles that helped shape the field of geriatrics and influenced a generation of geriatricians. In an article on the aging mind published just before his death in 1944, Nascher tabulated the characteristics of chronic brain syndrome and suggested that the condition was a primary change of senescence that must have a familial determinant (Nascher 1944).

In 1946, the American Psychological Association created the division of later maturity in old age. In the same year, the first issue of the *Journal of Gerontology* was published by the Gerontological Society of America. The first national conference of that society was held in 1950 and was followed by several White House Conferences on Aging, the last occurring in 2005. Also in 1950, the International Association of Gerontology was organized in Liege, Belgium. In 1955, psychiatrist Ewald W. Busse established the Duke University Center for Aging, the first research center of its kind in the nation.

In 1969, one of the first American books on aging and psychiatry was published. This text, *Behavior and Adaptation in Late Life,* edited by Ewald Busse and Eric Pfeiffer (1969), derived in large part from ongoing Duke University studies of the longitudinal aspects of normal aging. Another study of normal aging, the Baltimore Longitudinal Study on Aging, was sponsored by the National Institutes of Health. Before the appearance of Busse and Pfeiffer's book, among the best-known English-language texts about geriatric psychiatry were *The Clinical Psychiatry of Late Life* by Felix Post (1965) and *Normal Psychology of the Aging Process* by Zinberg and Kaufman (1963).

The Emergence of Geriatric Psychiatry in Professional Organizations

Authorized by the constitution of the American Psychiatric Association, the APA Council on Aging was established in 1979 to address six areas of activity: 1) evaluation and diagnosis, 2) training, 3) interface problems between psychiatry and other geriatric care disciplines, 4) design of services and third-party payment for psychiatric disorders of older adults, 5) decisions made by the government that influence the mental health of older adults, and 6) identification and implementation of research in the problems of geriatric psychiatry. The Council on Aging is responsible for developing and maintaining liaison with groups involved in the mental health care of aging Americans, including other APA components, appropriate non-APA organizations, and federal agencies.

Psychiatrists have played leading roles in the activities of two major U.S. societies concerned with aging: the Gerontological Society of America and the American Geriatrics Society. The Gerontological Society of America, founded in 1945, is a multidisciplinary organization with four distinct sections: biological sciences, medical sciences, social sciences, and psychological sciences. Four psychiatrists have served as presidents of this organization. The American Geriatrics Society, established in 1942, is composed largely of physicians and members of the health care professions. Psychiatrists also have led this medical society.

The American Association for Geriatric Psychiatry was founded in 1978. Its membership now exceeds 1,700, including about 100 affiliates. Of the active members, about 800 have reported that they have Certification in the Subspecialty of Geriatric Psychiatry from the American Board of Psychiatry and Neurology. About 1,100 persons attend the annual meeting. In 2000, the American Association for Geriatric Psychiatry established the Geriatric Mental Health Foundation to raise awareness of psychiatric and mental health disorders affecting older adults, eliminate the stigma of mental illness and treatment, promote healthy aging strategies, and increase access to quality mental health care for older adults.

The American Association for Geriatric Psychiatry played a significant role in the effort to obtain recognition for geriatric psychiatry as a subspecialty and to establish the certifying examination for this subspecialty by the American Board of Psychiatry and Neurology. The first examination was given in 1991; more than 800 persons sat for the examination, and more than 500 passed it. The original certification was for 10 years, and the first recertifying examination was given in 2001. Between 1991 and 2006, the American Board of Psychiatry and Neurology issued 2,823 certificates in geriatric psychiatry. The current examination is a 200-item multiple-choice test administered via computer over 4 hours. Recertifying examinations are also computer administered. The American Board of Psychiatry and Neurology is also planning to implement over the next several years a maintenance of certification program in which board-certified geriatric psychiatrists will need to provide documentation in four areas: 1) professional standing, 2) self-assessment and lifelong learning, 3) cognitive expertise, and 4) performance in practice.

The Center for the Study of Mental Health of the Aging was established at the National Institute of Mental Health (NIMH) in 1975, but it was later disbanded during reorganizational efforts by NIMH. In 1977, the center received funds to support and coordinate research, research training, and clinical training projects.

Its original efforts focused primarily on research and clinical training, with long-term support of fellowship stipends for approved geriatric psychiatry training programs, which greatly increased the number of psychiatrists with specialty training. Recently, efforts have been renewed at NIMH to reinvigorate the research agenda of the institute. These efforts resulted in the release of a report, "Mental Health for a Lifetime: Research for Mental Health Needs of Older Americans" (National Institute of Mental Health 2003). Currently, much of the clinical research supported by NIMH is managed through the Geriatrics Research Branch of the Division of Adult Translational Research and Treatment Development.

The National Institute on Aging (NIA) was established in May 1974 as part of the National Institutes of Health. The first director of NIA, Robert N. Butler, was a psychiatrist. Enabling legislation was passed designating NIA as the chief federal agency responsible for promoting, coordinating, and supporting basic research and training relevant to the aging process and to the diseases and problems of older adults. A unique aspect of NIA's mandate was that it was the first component of the National Institutes of Health to be formally charged by Congress with conducting research in the biological, biomedical, behavioral, and social sciences. This broad mandate has resulted in activities differing from those of other national research institutes. NIA has led the effort in Alzheimer's disease research, whereas research in other geriatric psychiatric disorders, especially major depression, has been led by NIMH.

For many years, medical and health care education related to geriatrics received little attention. The first training program in geriatric psychiatry supported by NIMH was established at Duke University Medical Center in 1965, and it was the only such program for almost a decade. Although an increasing number of geriatric psychiatry fellowship programs now exist, few currently receive NIMH support. These programs have been funded primarily through the Department of Veterans Affairs (VA), state support, and support from individual medical centers. The establishment of these training programs and lobbying by groups (including the American Association for Geriatric Psychiatry) convinced the American Board of Psychiatry and Neurology to establish an examination for Added Qualifications in Geriatric Psychiatry (now called Certification in the Subspecialty of Geriatric Psychiatry, which was previously mentioned).

Geriatric Psychiatry: Present and Future

Although general psychiatrists, generalist physicians, and geriatricians may provide mental health care to older adults, the geriatric psychiatrist has made a significant and unique contribution to clarifying the role of psychiatry in relation to other specialties in caring for older adults who are mentally ill. The current emphasis on primary care has challenged the viability of all medical specialties during recent years. Nevertheless, geriatric psychiatry has established itself solidly on a foundation of knowledge and skill in caring for older persons with psychiatric disorders, using the most advanced technologies and clinically proven therapies. In most settings, the geriatric psychiatrist has established a unique and meaningful role on interdisciplinary teams caring for older adults.

In many ways, geriatric psychiatrists assume the role of primary care physicians. They not only must maintain proficiency in general medicine but also must apply special knowledge of epidemiology, as well as of behavioral and social factors, to patient care. For example, geriatric psychiatrists have no alternative but to recognize that many of the disorders they treat, such as Alzheimer's disease, cannot currently be cured or prevented, but these clinicians know that the patients' suffering can be relieved and the disability reduced. Focusing on improving function encourages clinicians to make observations that can contribute to a better understanding of the course of chronic illness. These observations can also motivate investigations that may in the future lead to improved convalescence from, or even eradication of, such disorders when they are recognized earlier in the course of illness.

To achieve the goal of effective care of chronically ill older adults with psychiatric problems, geriatric psychiatrists must broaden their skills to include proficiency in geriatric medicine, neurology, and the neurosciences, as well as focus their skills on advances in geriatric psychiatry specifically and in neuropsychiatry more broadly. Proficient geriatricians and geriatric psychiatrists must be aware of aging-related changes that affect the human organism's capacity to respond to stress, disease, and trauma and that may eventually result in death (Busse and Blazer 1980). Specific procedures, such as the treatment of urinary tract infection, moderate hypertension, and peripheral edema, should not require that geriatric psychiatrists consult internists or geriatricians for appropriate management. The role of geriatric psychiatrists may indeed be such that specialty consultation is frequent and that combined management of the patient is conducted by a geriatrician and a geriatric psychiatrist (e.g., in a tertiary-care center). However, the skill of geriatric psychiatrists should be such that in the absence of a geriatrician, they can administer adequate medical care. As care moves increasingly from inpatient to ambulatory settings, the independent skills of geriatric psychiatrists will be required to a greater extent.

At the same time, significant advances will emerge in the epidemiology, pathophysiology, diagnosis, and treatment of the most frequently encountered late-life psychiatric disorders. These disorders span at least the range described in this volume, and even a short list must include dementias, mood disorders, anxiety disorders, schizophrenic disorders, light disorders, sleep disorders, and psychological and social factors affecting medical conditions. Advances in the neuroscience and clinical management of dementia of the Alzheimer's type alone illustrate the substantial knowledge base on which geriatric psychiatry is practiced. Previous trends have been such that when a biological etiology has been identified for a behavioral disorder, that disorder is passed from psychiatry to another specialty, usually neurology. Surely this cannot be tolerated in the future by geriatric psychiatrists. For example, geriatric psychiatrists must maintain a central role in the clinical management of patients with dementia, especially because patients' primary problems are usually behavioral. To maintain this role, psychiatrists must have skills of a level that prevents those skills from becoming overshadowed by those of neurologists and geriatricians. Psychiatrists must keep up with current advances in the genetics, neurochemistry, and molecular biology of dementia and other late-life neuropsychiatric disorders. Awareness of trends in research will continue to be important; for example, recent NIMH-sponsored conferences point to the need for research into depression, cognitive impairment, and cognitive decline (Steffens et al. 2006), as well as translational research in late-life mood disorders (Smith et al. 2007).

Geriatric psychiatry faces special problems in the future regarding referrals. Managed care systems discourage referrals (although managed care penetration of Medicare is still limited), and geriatric psychiatry must help identify for the primary care physician the cases in which the unique skills of the geriatric psychiatrist can contribute to cost-effective care of the older adult. Although geriatric psychiatry is a broad-based specialty, in practice it rarely receives primary referrals. Patients do not usually consider the psychiatrist as the coordinator or the provider of general medical care. The geriatric psychiatrist has special skills in the management of acute schizophrenia-like disorders, the more severe mood disorders, severe anxiety and panic disorders, behavioral disorders resulting from dementing illness, complex personality and behavioral disturbances that interfere with appropriate medical management, and severe problems with sleep. Appropriate referral by the primary care physician to the geriatric psychiatrist, especially if initial therapy by the primary care physician proves ineffective, can be cost-effective and provide relief of considerable suffering by the older adult with psychiatric impairment.

Therefore, geriatric psychiatrists in the twenty-first century find themselves in a paradoxical situation. On the one hand, they are better trained, and their training rests on a firmer knowledge base, than at any time in the past. Of more importance, advances in understanding of the diagnosis and treatment of psychiatric disorders in late life have led to significantly improved and cost-effective therapies for older adults with psychiatric disorders. On the other hand, specialty care, in particular psychiatric care, could lose badly in the struggle for scarce health care resources. Administrators of fellowship programs in geriatric medicine as well as psychiatry are finding that recruitment to these programs has been more difficult in recent years. Training has never been better, and the original hesitation of many young physicians to treat older persons because of prejudices about aging has been largely overcome. Yet the uncertain future of medical specialties and the difficulty of receiving reimbursement for the care of older persons render geriatric medicine and geriatric psychiatry less desirable financially than procedure-driven medical specialties and primary care.

Financing Psychiatric Care for Older Adults

The future of health care financing, much less the financing of psychiatric care, is uncertain. The federal government has shaped the financing of psychiatric care for older adults since the mid-1960s with the transfer of financial responsibility from state and private insurance to Medicare and Medicaid. Since that time, Medicare has tended to lead rather than follow health care financing reform in this country. For example, the capitation of payments for certain illnesses via diagnosis-related groups was instituted in 1983, although diagnosis-related groups have yet to be applied to inpatient psychiatric disorders.

The Omnibus Budget Reconciliation Act of 1987 increased coverage for outpatient psychiatric services from a total annual reimbursement of $500, with a 62.5% reimbursement of charges, to $2,200 annually for 1989. Services for the medical management of psychiatric disorders were exempted from this $2,200 limit. The Omnibus Budget Reconciliation Act of 1989 further improved outpatient psychiatric benefits: effective July 1, 1990, annual dollar limits for outpatient mental health services were eliminated. The higher copayment required for mental health services, however, continued to be the subject of considerable debate regarding parity for mental health services with other health services paid for by Medicare.

Then, in October 2008, a 50% copayment for Part B services, in place for many years, was eliminated by legislation. Now mental health benefits no longer are discriminated against by Medicare. Given present budgetary constraints, however, the burden for mental health payments that will fall on older adults remains to be determined.

Inpatient services have not been capitated in terms of reimbursement for individual hospitalizations, yet a 190-day lifetime psychiatric hospitalization limit remains in effect. This limit applies to freestanding psychiatric hospitals, not to psychiatric units in general hospitals. Medicare requires a one-time deductible of $768 for a hospital stay of up to 60 days and daily deductibles after 60 days until the 150th day of a hospitalization, and Medicare does not pay after day 150 of a single hospitalization. Recent legislation reduces average payments to all physicians by 5.4% below the 2001 level, which will undoubtedly jeopardize future care of older adults. Each year since 2001, Congress has passed emergency legislation to reinstate funds that cover (or come close to covering) inflationary costs. If the reductions in average payments remain in place for even a year, the impact on geriatric psychiatrists in private practice could be devastating.

Two additional providers of care directly affect the delivery of health services to older adults with psychiatric impairments. First, the VA provides care for many older adults, primarily, although not exclusively, for men. The VA currently supports the most comprehensive system of care for older adults with mental impairments; coverage is provided for acute inpatient hospitalization, outpatient clinics, long-term care facilities, and domiciliary care. Blurring of the boundaries between the VA and Medicare reimbursement for mental health services may occur, however, as length of stay decreases and outpatient care replaces inpatient care. In the future, the VA's extensive network of hospitals could be used for a broader constituency, with reimbursements from other health plans.

A second important sector of the health care delivery system for older adults with psychiatric impairments is long-term care. Support for long-term care in existing health plans is limited. Therefore, many older adults must use their life savings to support long-term care until only a small sum remains, at which time the older person becomes eligible for Medicaid support. Medicare supports long-term care only for rehabilitation and only for 120 days.

The Medicaid system reimburses about 42% of all nursing home care for older adults. The development of humane and effective treatment facilities for persons with chronic psychiatric disorders, especially persons with Alzheimer's disease and chronic schizophrenia, will depend in large part on the availability of funds to support long-term care. According to a 2008 report from the Centers for Medicare and Medicaid Services, 26% of nursing home expenditures in 2006 were out-of-pocket (Catlin et al. 2006). Although some older persons are purchasing long-term care insurance, the inability to actuate the needs of long-term care over the lifetimes of a cohort of older adults, coupled with the relatively short life of these insurance programs to date, does not ensure that long-term care will be adequately financed in the future.

Finally, any discussion of the financing of psychiatric care for older adults must recognize the dramatic and probably unsustainable burden of Medicare and Medicaid upon the federal budget if no changes are enacted. Neglect of the burgeoning cost of these programs, by merely providing year-to-year Band-Aids or gradually chipping away at services and fees, will not solve the problem. David Walker, comptroller general of the United States (Walker 2005), noted that the percentage of the federal budget that goes to Medicare and Medicaid jumped from 9% to 19% between 1984 and 2004. He predicted that with the retirement of the baby boom generation, a tsunami of demand upon the system will bankrupt the country if changes are not made. No person or group has developed a plan that easily or painlessly addresses these financial challenges. Nevertheless, geriatric psychiatrists must be constantly aware of the financial pressures against expanding even the woefully inadequate existing services.

Geriatric Psychiatrists and Public Health

The number of older persons in North America is ever increasing, and resources for the psychiatric care of these individuals are limited. Therefore, to be able to advocate for humane and cost-effective mental health care for these older adults, geriatric psychiatrists of the future must understand the prevalence and distribution of psychiatric disorders in the population and the delivery of psychiatric services to these older adults. Most older adults with psychiatric disorders do not receive any care for their conditions. For those who do receive care, most of it is provided by primary care physicians (German et al. 1985).

In planning for more effective and efficient delivery of psychiatric services to older adults, the geriatric psychiatrist must consider interventions at one of three points in the natural course of a disorder. These points—primary, secondary, and tertiary—correspond to the three classic types of prevention described by public health specialists (Last 1980). Primary prevention is prevention of the occurrence of disease or injury. Secondary prevention is early detection and intervention. Tertiary prevention minimizes the effects of disease and disability.

The geriatric psychiatrist can effect primary prevention for the older adult by identifying potential stressful events and elements in the environment, both social and physical, that contribute to the onset of a psychiatric disorder. For example, forced isolation and the absence of effective communication with other persons contribute to the onset of major depression and paranoid psychoses; in this case, intervention would encourage social interaction. The appropriate use of psychotropic medications may prevent the occurrence of acute organic brain syndromes in an older adult who is bereaved; the clinical intervention in this situation would focus on education. Early supportive intervention has also been demonstrated to prevent the onset of major depression in the bereaved. As evidence mounts for a possible link between development of geriatric neuropsychiatric disorders and deficiencies in folic acid, vitamin B_{12}, and other nutrients, the geriatric psychiatrist may also play a role in nutrition (Bhat et al. 2005).

Secondary prevention requires the geriatric psychiatrist to intervene early enough in the course of an illness to facilitate the prescription of effective treatment to prevent a complicated convalescence. It is at this level that the geriatric psychiatrist may achieve the greatest success, given the limited resources available. For example, early diagnosis of major depression permits the psychiatrist to attempt a rational course of outpatient antidepressant therapy before the complications of excess medication or neglect of physical health ensue during the course of a depressive illness.

Tertiary prevention is directed toward preventing the disability that may result from mental illness. Rehabilitation techniques are important in long-term care facilities, especially in the management of the patient with dementia. These techniques include reality orientation, adequate hygiene efforts, and maintenance of mobility. Although the activities themselves may not be the direct responsibility of geriatric psychiatrists, development of a comprehensive treatment and rehabilitation plan must involve these clinicians.

Geriatric Psychiatry and Successful Aging

Physicians have traditionally focused on illness, and the success of the practice of medicine, including psychiatry, has been determined by the removal of illness or disability. However, an interest in *successful aging*—an idea that has implicitly undergirded gerontological research since its inception—has assumed prime importance in gerontological circles since the 1980s. The construct arose primarily as a response to a perceived need to view aging as something other than loss, decline of functioning, and approaching death. In addition, physicians working with older adults have been faulted for not looking beyond the absence of disease as a marker for health (Baltes and Baltes 1990). Criteria that have been suggested as markers of successful aging include length of life, biological health, life satisfaction and morale, cognitive efficacy, social competence and productivity, personal control, and resiliency and adaptivity (Baltes and Baltes 1990; Nowlin 1977, 1985; Palmore 1979; Rowe and Kahn 1987). Rowe and Kahn (1987) emphasized the need to explore how greatly extrinsic factors can play positive as well as negative roles in the aging process. For example, they noted studies of social support demonstrating that the availability of perceived connectedness and membership in a network of family and friends decreases the likelihood of illness and mortality (Berkman and Syme 1979; Blazer 1982). Rodin (1986) emphasized the greater positive effects on health and well-being in older adults who were involved in and asserted more control over their environments compared with older adults who assumed a passive role.

Another theme that has traversed studies of successful aging is that of resiliency and adaptation. For example, Busse (1985) equated successful aging in part with the capacity to respond with resilience to challenges arising from changes within one's body, mind, and environment. A central task for older adults is to adopt effective strategies for dealing with losses and to be able to change goals and aspirations as either physical or psychosocial changes occur.

Baltes (1993) emphasized the importance of wisdom in successful aging, something that cannot be measured quantitatively. For example, he suggested that wisdom includes 1) factual knowledge (the data necessary to respond to a situation); 2) procedural knowledge (strategies of acquiring data, making decisions, and providing advice); 3) life-span contextualization (recognizing the inner relationships, tensions, and priorities of different life domains within the context of the life span); 4) value relativism (the ability to separate one's own values from those of others); and 5) acceptance of uncertainty (recognizing that no perfect solution exists and optimizing the resolution of a situation as well as possible). Baltes noted that wisdom falls generally within the domain of cognitive pragmatics, or cognitive functioning that is primarily culture based and therefore potentially stable over time in persons who reach old age without specific brain pathology. In contrast, cognitive mechanics is roughly comparable to fluid intelligence and is primarily determined by the neurophysiological functioning of the brain.

Depp and Jeste (2006) identified 28 studies in which the construct of successful aging was operationalized. Approximately one-third of elderly individuals were classified as aging successfully. The most frequent significant correlates of the various definitions of successful aging were age (young-old), nonsmoking, and absence of disability, arthritis, and diabetes. Moderate support was found for greater physical activity, more social contacts, better self-rated health, absence of depression and cognitive impairment, and fewer medical conditions. Gender, income, education, and marital status generally did not relate to successful aging.

Not all commentators have accepted the construct of successful aging. Cole (1991) noted that this change in perspective regarding late life may be secondary to the dramatic increase in the proportion of the adult population over age 65. Specifically, as more people have aged, it is less acceptable to view aging as a time of frailty, poor health, and death. Cole pointed out that questions about the quality of life of the oldest old (persons age 85 or older) remain at the center of the health care debate regarding ordinary versus extraordinary life-extending therapies and even health care monitoring. He suggested that our society does not apply the construct of success to other stages of the life cycle and that the natural consequence of the construct of successful aging is the assumption that growing old presents a problem that must be solved "successfully." Aging continues to present many problems, not the least of which are the finitude of life, preservation of personal integrity, and quality of life. Yet Cole believes our culture has distanced itself from these troubling issues, in part through its emphasis on successful aging.

Baltes and Baltes (1990) proposed the third and fourth ages of the life cycle—the third age corresponding to our conceptions of the young old (for whom the construct of successful aging is quite pertinent) and the fourth age (after the age span of 80–85) being a period when a different construct may be needed. These authors suggested that this new construct be selection, optimization, and compensation. This model is based on recognition of the realities of aging, including the recognition that 1) late-life development is a specialized and age-graded adaptation, 2) elderly persons experience a reduction in general reserve capacity, and 3) losses occur in specific functions. Such recognition leads to selection, optimization, and compensation, which in turn lead to a reduced and transformed life. In other words, self-efficacy results when the elderly person realistically accepts the limits of aging and at the same time compensates for these limits through recognition of other potentials for happiness and productivity. Selection, optimization, and compensation ensure the efficacious life.

It is far from clear, however, that conflict is inevitable between the idea of successful aging and the care of frail elderly persons. For example, emphasis on successful aging has decreased fatalism about health and health habits in late life. Through diet, exercise, and strengthening (especially of the lower extremities), older persons can improve their balance, decrease their risk of falling, and improve their quality of life. On the other hand, when illness does occur that is chronic and about which outcomes are better known, there is no reason that health care professionals cannot realistically and seriously address the proper and realistic, not to mention the humane, care of these persons.

Key Points

- Important figures in the emergence of geriatrics in the twentieth century include Ewald Busse, Edmund Cowdry, Walter Miles, Ignatz Nascher, and Felix Post.
- The American Association for Geriatric Psychiatry has been instrumental in obtaining recognition for geriatric psychiatry as a subspecialty by the American Board of Psychiatry and Neurology and in advocating for mental health care and research by establishing the Geriatric Mental Health Foundation.
- At the federal level, much of the research in geriatric psychiatry is supported through the Geriatric Research Branch at the National Institute of Mental Health and through the National Institute on Aging.
- Future research will seek to improve mental health outcomes of older adults by focusing not only on factors related to frailty and cognitive decline but also on successful aging.

References

Baltes PB: The aging mind: potential and limits. Gerontologist 33:580–594, 1993

Baltes PB, Baltes MM: Successful Aging: Perspectives From the Behavioral Sciences. New York, Cambridge University Press, 1990

Berkman LF, Syme SL: Social network, host resistance, and mortality: a 9-year follow-up study of Alameda County residents. Am J Epidemiol 109:186–204, 1979

Bhat HS, Chiu E, Jeste DV: Nutrition and geriatric psychiatry: a neglected field. Curr Opin Psychiatry 18:609–614, 2005

Blazer DG: Social support and mortality in an elderly community population. Am J Epidemiol 115:684–694, 1982

Busse EW: Mental health and mental illness, in Normal Aging, III. Edited by Palmore E, Busse EW, Maddox G, et al. Durham, NC, Duke University Press, 1985, pp 81–91

Busse EW, Blazer DG (eds): Handbook of Geriatric Psychiatry. New York, Van Nostrand Reinhold, 1980

Busse EW, Pfeiffer E (eds): Behavior and Adaptation in Late Life. Boston, MA, Little, Brown, 1969

Butterfield LH: Benjamin Rush, the American Revolution and the American millennium. Harv Med Alumni Bull 50:16–22, 1976

Catlin A, Cowan C, Hartman M, et al: National health spending in 2006: a year of change for prescription drugs. Health Aff (Millwood) 27:14–29, 2008

Cole TR: The Journey of Life: A Cultural History of Aging in America. New York, Cambridge University Press, 1991

Cowdry EV: Problems of Aging: Biological and Medical Aspects. Baltimore, MD, Williams & Wilkins, 1938

Depp CA, Jeste DV: Definitions and predictors of successful aging: a comprehensive review of larger quantitative studies. Am J Geriatr Psychiatry 14:6–20, 2006

German PS, Shapiro S, Skinner EA: Mental health of the elderly: use of health and mental health services. J Am Geriatr Soc 33:246–252, 1985

Gruman GJ: A history of ideas about the prolongation of life: the evolution of prolongevity hypotheses to 1800 (Transactions of the American Philosophical Society, Vol 56, Part 9). Philadelphia, PA, American Philosophical Society, 1966

Last JM (ed): Public Health and Preventive Medicine, 11th Edition. New York, Appleton-Century-Crofts, 1980

Nascher IL: Geriatrics: The Diseases of Old Age and Their Treatment. Philadelphia, PA, P Blakiston's Sons, 1914

Nascher IL: The aging mind. Medical Record 157:669, 1944

National Institute of Mental Health: Mental Health for a Lifetime: Research for Mental Health Needs of Older Americans. Rockville, MD, National Institute of Mental Health, October 22, 2003

Nowlin JB: Successful aging. Black Aging 2:4–6, 1977

Nowlin JB: Successful aging, in Normal Aging, III. Edited by Palmore E, Busse EW, Maddox G, et al. Durham, NC, Duke University Press, 1985, pp 34–46

Omnibus Budget Reconciliation Act of 1987, Pub L No 100-203

Omnibus Budget Reconciliation Act of 1989, Pub L No 101-239

Palmore E: Predictors of successful aging. Gerontologist 19:427–431, 1979

Post F: The Clinical Psychiatry of Late Life. Oxford, UK, Pergamon, 1965

Rodin J: Aging and health: effects of the sense of control. Science 233:1271–1276, 1986

Rowe JW, Kahn RL: Human aging: usual and successful. Science 237:143–149, 1987

Simmons LW: The Role of the Aged in Primitive Societies. New Haven, CT, Yale University Press, 1945

Smith GS, Gunning-Dixon FM, Lotrich FE, et al: Translational research in late-life mood disorders: implications for future intervention and prevention research. Neuropsychopharmacology 32:1857–1875, 2007

Steffens DC, Otey E, Alexopoulos GS, et al: Perspectives on depression, mild cognitive impairment, and cognitive decline. Arch Gen Psychiatry 63:130–138, 2006

Walker DM: Social Security and America's Long Term Fiscal Challenge. Washington, DC, Government Accounting Office, 2005

Zinberg NE, Kaufman I: Normal Psychology of the Aging Process. New York, International Universities Press, 1963

Suggested Readings

Colenda CC, Mickus MA, Marcus SC, et al: Comparison of adult and geriatric psychiatric practice patterns: findings from the American Psychiatric Association's Practice Research Network. Am J Geriatr Psychiatry 10:609–617, 2002

Colenda CC, Wilk JE, West JC: The geriatric psychiatry workforce in 2002: analysis from the 2002 National Survey of Psychiatric Practice. Am J Geriatr Psychiatry 13:756–765, 2005

Cutler DM: Disability and the future of Medicare. N Engl J Med 349:1084–1085, 2003

Jeste DV: Geriatric psychiatry may be the mainstream psychiatry of the future. Am J Psychiatry 157:1912–1914, 2000

Lieff SJ, Kirwin P, Colenda CC: Proposed geriatric psychiatry core competencies for subspecialty training. Am J Geriatr Psychiatry 13:815–821, 2005

INDEX

Page numbers printed in **boldface** type refer to tables or figures.